Nutrition: An Applied Approach

Janice Thompson, Ph.D., FACSM
University of New Mexico

Melinda Manore, Ph.D., RD, FACSM
Oregon State University

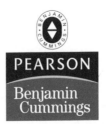

PEARSON

Benjamin Cummings

San Francisco   Boston   New York
Cape Town   Hong Kong   London   Madrid   Mexico City
Montreal   Munich   Paris   Singapore   Sydney   Tokyo   Toronto

Publisher: Daryl Fox
Senior Acquisitions Editor: Deirdre Espinoza
Development Manager: Claire Alexander
Development Editor: Laura Bonazzoli
Art Development Editor: Laura Southworth
Project Editor: Marie Beaugureau, Ellen Keohane
Editorial Assistant: Alison Rodal
Production Supervisor: Steven Anderson
Project Coordination: Elm Street Publishing Services, Inc.
Manufacturing Buyer: Stacey Weinberger
Senior Marketing Manager: Sandra Lindelof
Market Development Manager: Cheryl Cechvala
Text and Cover Designer: Kathleen Cunningham
Art Coordinator: Laura Murray, Kelly Murphy
Photo Researcher: Brian Donnelly, Cypress Integrated Systems
Copyeditor: Carla Breidenbach
Compositor: Carlisle Communications

Cover Photo: Mark Tomalty/Masterfile.

Credits can be found on page CR-1.

ISBN 0-8053-5532-4

Library of Congress Cataloging-in-Publication Data
Thompson, Janice,
    Nutrition : an applied approach / Janice Thompson, Melinda Manore.
       p. ; cm.
    Includes bibliographical references and index.
    ISBN 0-8053-5532-4 (pbk.)
I. Nutrition.
    [DNLM: I. Nutrition. QU 145 T473n 2005] I. Manore, Melinda, 1951–. II.
Title.
    QP141.T467 2005
    613.2—dc22
          2004012643

2 3 4 5 — CRK — 07 06 05

www.aw-bc.com

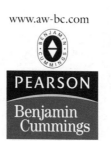

PEARSON

Benjamin
Cummings

Tolerable Upper Intake Levels (UL[a])

Vitamins

Life Stage Group	Vitamin A (μg/d)[b]	Vitamin C (mg/d)	Vitamin D (μg/d)	Vitamin E (mg/d)[c,d]	Niacin (mg/d)[d]	Vitamin B6 (mg/d)	Folate (μg/d)[d]	Choline (g/d)
Infants								
0–6 mo	600	ND[e]	25	ND	ND	ND	ND	ND
7–12 mo	600	ND	25	ND	ND	ND	ND	ND
Children								
1–3 y	600	400	50	200	10	30	300	1.0
4–8 y	900	650	50	300	15	40	400	1.0
Males, Females								
9–13 y	1,700	1,200	50	600	20	60	600	2.0
14–18 y	2,800	1,800	50	800	30	80	800	3.0
19–70 y	3,000	2,000	50	1,000	35	100	1,000	3.5
> 70 y	3,000	2,000	50	1,000	35	100	1,000	3.5
Pregnancy								
≤18 y	2,800	1,800	50	800	30	80	800	3.0
19–50 y	3,000	2,000	50	1,000	35	100	1,000	3.5
Lactation								
≤18 y	2,800	1,800	50	800	30	80	800	3.0
19–50 y	3,000	2,000	50	1,000	35	100	1,000	3.5

Elements

Life Stage Group	Boron (mg/d)	Calcium (g/d)	Copper (μg/d)	Fluoride (mg/d)	Iodine (μg/d)	Iron (mg/d)	Magnesium (mg/d)[f]	Manganese (mg/d)	Molybdenum (μg/d)	Nickel (mg/d)	Phosphorus (g/d)	Selenium (μg/d)	Vanadium (mg/d)[g]	Zinc (mg/d)
Infants														
0–6 mo	ND	ND	ND	0.7	ND	40	ND	ND	ND	ND	ND	45	ND	4
7–12 mo	ND	ND	ND	0.9	ND	40	ND	ND	ND	ND	ND	60	ND	5
Children														
1–3 y	3	2.5	1,000	1.3	200	40	65	2	300	0.2	3	90	ND	7
4–8 y	6	2.5	3,000	2.2	300	40	110	3	600	0.3	3	150	ND	12
Males, Females														
9–13 y	11	2.5	5,000	10	600	40	350	6	1,100	0.6	4	280	ND	23
14–18 y	17	2.5	8,000	10	900	45	350	9	1,700	1.0	4	400	ND	34
19–70 y	20	2.5	10,000	10	1,100	45	350	11	2,000	1.0	4	400	1.8	40
> 70 y	20	2.5	10,000	10	1,100	45	350	11	2,000	1.0	3	400	1.8	40
Pregnancy														
≤18 y	17	2.5	8,000	10	900	45	350	9	1,700	1.0	3.5	400	ND	34
19–50 y	20	2.5	10,000	10	1,100	45	350	11	2,000	1.0	3.5	400	ND	40
Lactation														
≤18 y	17	2.5	8,000	10	900	45	350	9	1,700	1.0	4	400	ND	34
19–50 y	20	2.5	10,000	10	1,100	45	350	11	2,000	1.0	4	400	ND	40

Source: Adapted from the Dietary Reference Intakes series, National Academies Press. Copyright 1997, 1998, 2000, 2001, by the National Academy of Sciences. These reports may be accessed via www.nap.edu. Courtesy of the National Academies Press, Washington D.C.

[a] UL = The maximum level of daily nutrient intake that is likely to pose no risk of adverse effects. Unless otherwise specified, the UL represents total intake from food, water, and supplements. Due to lack of suitable data, ULs could not be established for vitamin K, thiamin, riboflavin, vitamin B12, pantothenic acid, biotin, or carotenoids. In the absence of ULs, extra caution may be warranted in consuming levels above recommended intakes.

[b] As preformed vitamin A only.

[c] As α-tocopherol; applies to any form of supplemental α-tocopherol.

[d] The ULs for vitamin E, niacin, and folate apply to synthetic forms obtained from supplements, fortified foods, or a combination of the two.

[e] ND = Not determinable due to lack of data of adverse effects in this age group and concern with regard to lack of ability to handle excess amounts. Source of intake should be from food only to prevent high levels of intake.

[f] The ULs for magnesium represent intake from a pharmacological agent only and do not include intake from food and water.

[g] Although vanadium in food has not been shown to cause adverse effects in humans, there is no justification for adding vanadium to food, and vanadium supplements should be used with caution. The UL is based on adverse effects in laboratory animals, and this data could be used to set a UL for adults but not children and adolescents.

To our Moms—your consistent love and support are the keys to our happiness and success. You have been incredible role models.

To our Dads—you raised us to be independent, intelligent, and resourceful. We miss you and wish you were here to be proud of, and to brag about, our accomplishments.

Welcome to *Nutrition: An Applied Approach!*

Why We Wrote the Book

Nutrition gets a lot of press. Pick up a magazine and you'll read the latest debate over high-protein/low-carbohydrate diets; turn on the TV and you'll hear a Hollywood star describe how she lost 50 pounds without exercising; scan the newspaper and you'll discover the politics surrounding the creation of the new food guide pyramid. How can you evaluate these sources of nutrition information and find out whether the advice they provide is reliable? How do you navigate through the endless recommendations and come up with a way of eating that's right for you—one that supports your physical activity, allows you to maintain a healthful weight, and helps you avoid chronic disease?

We Wrote this Book to Help You Answer These Questions

Nutrition: An Applied Approach began with the conviction that both students and instructors would benefit from an accurate and clear textbook that links nutrients to their functional benefit. As authors and instructors, we know that students have a natural interest in their bodies, their health, their weight, and their success in sports and other activities. By demonstrating how nutrition relates to these interests, *Nutrition: An Applied Approach* empowers students to reach their personal, health, and fitness goals. We used several strategies to capture students' interest, from our functional organization to the variety of features and activities described below. In addition, throughout the chapters, material is presented in lively narrative that continually links the facts to students' situations, lifestyles, and goals. Information on current events and research keep the inquisitive spark alive, illustrating that nutrition is not a "dead" science, but rather the source of considerable debate. The content of *Nutrition: An Applied Approach* is appropriate for non-nutrition majors, but it also includes information to challenge students who have a more advanced understanding of chemistry and math. We present the "science side" in an easy-to-read, friendly narrative, with engaging features that reduce students' fears and encourage them to apply the material to their lives. Also, because this book is not a derivative of a majors text, the writing and the figures are cohesive and always level-appropriate. The organization and flow of the information and the art come together to provide a learning experience that is enjoyable for both instructors and students.

As teachers, we are familiar with the myriad challenges of presenting nutrition information in the classroom, and we have included ancillary package tools to assist instructors in successfully meeting these challenges. Through broad instructor and student support with print and media supplements, we hope to contribute to the excitement of teaching and learning about nutrition: a subject that affects every one of us, a subject so important and relevant that correct and timely information can make the difference between health and disease.

Content Is Applied to Life

Because students are most interested in how nutrition applies to their own lives, we have developed several learning tools throughout the book to illustrate real-life implications of nutrition. For instance, to teach students the effect of vitamins and minerals in the body, we organized the micronutrients chapters according to their function. We also developed case studies, math activities, and nutrition label activities that encourage students to put the information they've just learned into practice.

Functional Organization

Students have traditionally learned about micronutrients by memorizing each one along with their deficiency symptoms and toxicity syndromes. We have found with this traditional approach that they quickly forget the information they have learned, and they never really understand why micronutrients are important. To respond to this problem, we decided to illustrate the immediate health issues and physiological functions of vitamins and minerals by discussing them within the context of fluid and electrolyte balance, antioxidant function, bone health, and energy metabolism and blood formation. We've found through our own experience teaching, and through extensive class testing, that this functional approach helps students to think about these micronutrients on a conceptual level, enabling them to answer the questions "Why are vitamins and minerals important?" and "What do they do?" This approach also promotes better retention of the material and application to real life.

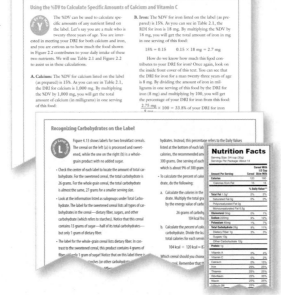

Nutri-Cases

In Chapter 1, we introduce five characters of various ages, ethnic backgrounds, and nutritional needs. In the **Nutri-Cases** throughout the rest of the book, we discuss the implications of nutrition on these characters. By prompting students to help characters think about a variety of nutrition-related issues, these Nutri-Cases help students apply the material they have just learned to real life.

You Do the Math

You Do the Math boxes show students how to perform nutritional calculations, such as determining their own Body Mass Index (BMI), step by step. Knowledge of these calculations helps students determine their own nutritional needs.

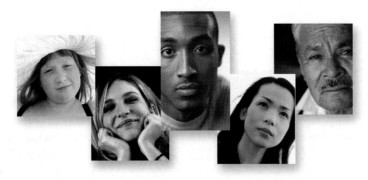

Nutrition Label Activities

Nutrition Label Activities teach students how to read and evaluate labels from real food products so they can make educated choices about the foods they eat. Students can use the skills they learn when they do their food shopping.

Teaching How to Evaluate Nutrition Information

One of our goals with *Nutrition: An Applied Approach* is to teach students how to evaluate the nutrition information they encounter every day. Each chapter discusses how to find and evaluate reliable sources for nutrition facts, and provides references students can trust for answers to common nutrition questions. In addition, the following features help to debunk some commonly held myths about nutrition.

Test Yourself Questions

A brief **Test Yourself** quiz at the beginning of each chapter piques students' interest in the topics to be covered by raising and dispelling common myths about nutrition. The answers to these questions can be found at the end of each chapter.

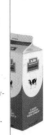

Test Yourself True or False?

1. Sometimes you may have an appetite even though you are not hungry. T or F

2. Your stomach is the primary organ responsible for telling you when you are hungry. T or F

3. The entire process of digestion and absorption of one meal takes about twenty-four hours. T or F

4. Most ulcers result from a type of infection. T or F

5. Irritable bowel syndrome is a rare disease that mostly affects older people. T or F

Test Yourself answers can be found at the end of the chapter.

Bottled Water is No Safer to Drink than Tap Water

Bottled water has become increasingly popular over the past 20 years. It is estimated that Americans drink almost 3 billion gallons of bottled water each year (Bottled Water Web‰ 2002). Many people prefer the taste of bottled water to that of tap water. They also feel that bottled water is safer than tap water. Is this true?

The water we drink in the U.S. generally comes from two sources: surface water and ground water. Surface water comes from lakes, rivers, and reservoirs. Common contaminants of surface water include runoff from highways, pesticides, animal wastes, and industrial wastes. Many of the cities across the U.S. obtain their water from surface water sources. Ground water comes from underground rock formations called aquifers. People who live in rural areas generally pump ground water from a well as their water source. Hazardous substances leaking from waste sites, dumps, landfills, and oil and gas pipelines can contaminate ground water.

The most common chemical used to treat and purify our water is chlorine. Chlorine is effective in killing many contaminants in our water supply. Water treatment plants also routinely check our water supp... chemicals, minerals, and other contami... the U.S. has on...

Although bottled water may taste better than tap water, there is no evidence that it is always safer to drink. Look closely at the label of your favorite bottled water. It may come directly from the tap! Some types of bottled water may contain more minerals than tap water, but there are no other additional nutritional benefits of drinking bottled water. Most bottling plants use an ozone treatment to disinfect water instead of chlorine, and many people feel this process leaves the water tasting better than water treated with chlorine.

Should you spend money on bottled water? The answer depends on personal preference and your source of drinking water. For instance, many supermarkets have a water filtration machine in front of the store where you can purchase and fill your own bottles of water. These machines may not be cleaned and the filters not changed on a regular basis, making this water less safe than tap water. Some people may not have access to safe drinking water where they live, making bottled water the safest alternative water source. If you choose to drink bottled water, look for brands that carry the trademark of the International Bottled Water Association. This association follows the regulations... water cooler, ...

Nutrition Myth or Fact

Nutrition Myth or Fact boxes provide the facts behind the hype on many current nutrition and dietary issues. They dispel common misconceptions and teach students how to critically evaluate information on the Internet, in the mass media, and from their peers.

Nutrition Debates

Nutrition Debates contain in-depth coverage of current events and hot topics, such as vitamin and mineral supplementation. By presenting both sides of the argument, these debates encourage students to think critically about controversial issues and become more informed and discriminating consumers of nutrition and health information.

Nutrition Debate:

Can Reducing Sugar Intake Be the Answer to Obesity?

Almost every day in the news we see headlines about obesity: "More Americans Overweight!", "The Fattening of America," "Obesity is a National Epidemic!" These headlines accurately reflect the state of weight in the United States. Over the past thirty years, obesity rates have increased dramatically for both adults and children. Obesity has become public health enemy number one, as many chronic diseases such as type 2 diabetes, heart disease, high blood pressure, and arthritis go hand-in-hand with obesity.

Of particular concern are the rising obesity rates in children. It is estimated that the rate of overweight in children has increased 100% since the mid-1970s, while the rate of obesity has increased 50% over this same time period (Troiano et al. 1995). Why should we concern ourselves with fighting obesity in children? First, it is well established that the treatment of existing obesity is extremely challenging, and our greatest hope of combating ... se is through prevention. Most agree ... start with children at ... 0% of chil...

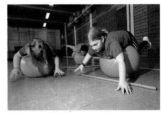

It is estimated that the rate of overweight in children has increased 100% since the mid 1970s.

One factor that has recently come to the forefront f nutrition research and policy making ... ntribu- ded sugars to overwei... ed earli...

Captivating Student Interest

In order to capture students' interest and motivate them to read on, we have created chapter-opening scenarios and Highlight boxes that stimulate students' curiosity, and we have included appealing and informative illustrations and photos that draw students into the text and create an engaging learning environment.

Chapter-Opening Scenarios

Each chapter opens with a real-life story that teaches students about the sometimes life-altering effects of diet and exercise. These scenarios grab students' attention and motivate them to delve deeper into the chapter material.

Highlight Boxes

Highlight boxes provide further insight into topics that students will recognize from the mass media and popular culture, such as mad cow disease or sports beverages. These boxes discuss the nutritional facts and theories behind these often complex issues.

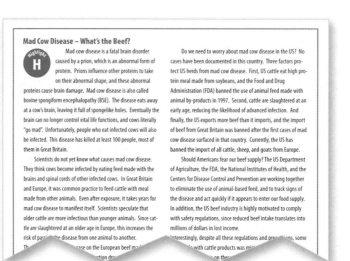

Mad Cow Disease – What's the Beef?

Mad cow disease is a fatal brain disorder caused by a prion, which is an abnormal form of protein. Prions influence other proteins to take on their abnormal shape, and these abnormal proteins cause brain damage. Mad cow disease is also called bovine spongiform encephalopathy (BSE). The disease eats away at a cow's brain, leaving it full of spongelike holes. Eventually the brain can no longer control vital life functions, and cows literally "go mad." Unfortunately, people who eat infected cows will also be infected. This disease has killed at least 100 people, most of them in Great Britain.

Scientists do not yet know what causes mad cow disease. They think cows become infected by eating feed made with the brains and spinal cords of other infected cows. In Great Britain and Europe, it was common practice to feed cattle with meal made from other animals. Even after exposure, it takes years for mad cow disease to manifest itself. Scientists speculate that older cattle are more infectious than younger animals. Since cattle are slaughtered at an older age in Europe, this increases the risk of passing the disease from one animal to another.

Do we need to worry about mad cow disease in the US? No cases have been documented in this country. Three factors protect US herds from mad cow disease. First, US cattle eat high protein meal made from soybeans, and the Food and Drug Administration (FDA) banned the use of animal feed made with animal by-products in 1997. Second, cattle are slaughtered at an early age, reducing the likelihood of advanced infection. And finally, the US exports more beef than it imports, and the import of beef from Great Britain was banned after the first cases of mad cow disease surfaced in that country. Currently, the US has banned the import of all cattle, sheep, and goats from Europe.

Should Americans fear our beef supply? The US Department of Agriculture, the FDA, the National Institutes of Health, and the Centers for Disease Control and Prevention are working together to eliminate the use of animal-based feed, and to track signs of the disease and act quickly if it appears to enter our food supply. In addition, the US beef industry is highly motivated to comply with safety regulations, since reduced beef intake translates into millions of dollars in lost income.

Interestingly, despite all these regulations and precautions, some

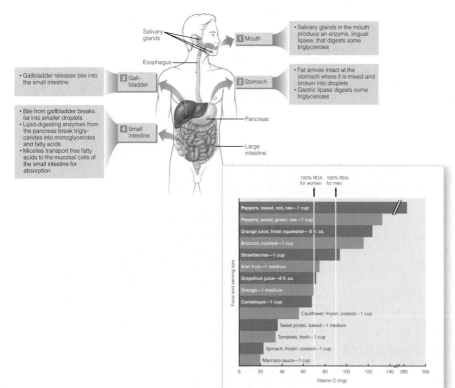

Art, Photos, and Tables

The art program was specially designed to walk students through the body's processing of nutrients. Insets on digestion diagrams illustrate context, so students understand where in the body a given process is located. The photos were chosen to provide illustration for conditions created by nutrient deficiencies, as well as to show students foods that they may not immediately think of as good sources for specific nutrients. Tables integrate nutrition information, and special figures act as "shopper's guides," indicating foods that are good sources of Dietary Reference Intakes of specific vitamins and minerals.

Support for the Student

In writing *Nutrition: An Applied Approach*, we worked to develop pedagogical features that would benefit students by helping them learn and remember all the information in the chapter. These features help students review the material they just learned, find more information, check their understanding of the materials, and stay focused on the most important points.

Recaps

We have placed **Recap** paragraphs consistently throughout each chapter of the text. The Recaps rephrase what students just learned in the preceding sections, providing a quick summary and using new wording to help students remember the concept (not just the words) before moving on to the next topic.

> **Recap:** All complex carbohydrates are polysaccharides. They include starch, glycogen, and fiber. Starch is the storage form of glucose in plants, while glycogen is the storage form of glucose in animals. Fiber forms the support structures of plants; our bodies cannot digest fiber.

Test Yourself Answers

Answers to each chapter's **Test Yourself** questions are located after the review questions at the end of the chapter. Using the Test Yourself answers, students can evaluate their responses to these basic, but sometimes deceiving, questions about nutrition.

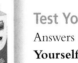

Test Yourself Answers

1. **True.** Sometimes you may have an appetite even though you are not hungry. These feelings are referred to as "cravings" and are associated with physical or emotional cues.

2. **False.** Your brain, not your stomach, is the primary organ responsible for telling you when you are hungry.

3. **True.** Although there are individual variations in how we respond to food, the entire process of digestion and absorption of one meal usually takes about twenty-four hours.

4. **True.** Most ulcers result from an infection of the bacterium *Helicobacter pylori* (*H. pylori*). Contrary to popular belief, ulcers are not caused by stress or food.

Chapter Objectives

Chapter objectives help students stay focused by listing the most important concepts in the chapter. After reading the chapter, students can go back and review the objectives to make sure that they understand each point.

Chapter Summaries

Our chapter summaries provide quick reviews of the major points and topics covered in each chapter. By going through the chapter summaries, students can determine whether they have understood information about the chapter's main concepts.

Review Questions

Review questions at the end of each chapter allow students to assess their retention and understanding of the material they have covered in the chapter. Answers to review questions appear at the end of the book.

Web Links and References

The references and web links sections provide students with all of the references used in the chapter, as well as related web links for further information and study.

Media Reinforces and Applies Concepts

A comprehensive media package is offered with *Nutrition: An Applied Approach*, including diet analysis software, a website, videos, the Classroom Response System, and MyNutritionLab. Our media reinforces and applies concepts presented in the book and promotes interactive learning with animations and exercises.

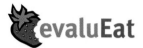

EvaluEat Diet Analysis Software

Our **EvaluEat diet analysis software** is accurate, user-friendly, and comprehensive, and contains an extensive food database. Students can use the software to perform a single or multi-day diet analysis, create a variety of reports (for example, the balance between fats, carbohydrates, and proteins in their diets), calculate how many calories they are consuming versus how many they are expending in exercise, and determine whether they are meeting the DRIs for various vitamins and minerals. A copy of the EvaluEat software is included with each new copy of the text.

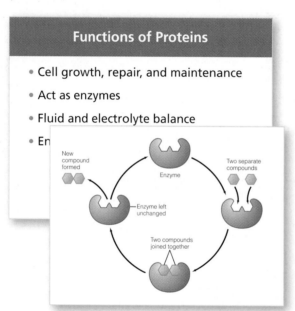

Functions of Proteins

- Cell growth, repair, and maintenance
- Act as enzymes
- Fluid and electrolyte balance
- En

Instructor's Resource CD-ROM

The **Instructor's Resource CD-ROM** provides instructors with PowerPoint® lecture outlines as well as PowerPoint® and JPEG files of all the art, tables, and selected photos from the text. The PowerPoint® slides can be fully customized.

Companion Website
www.aw-bc.com/thompson

The *Nutrition: An Applied Approach* **open-access website** offers interactive exercises and study tools for students. The site includes immediate feedback for chapter-specific as well as cumulative self-quizzes, web links, critical thinking activities, flashcards, a glossary, and current articles from the *New York Times* selected specifically for use with our book. The website also provides further discussion and exercises related to the Nutri-Cases and Nutrition Debates that appear in the text. In addition, the website provides instructors with password-protected resources, such as an instructor's manual, PowerPoint® slides, and the Computerized Test Bank. The companion website can be found at www.aw-bc.com/thompson.

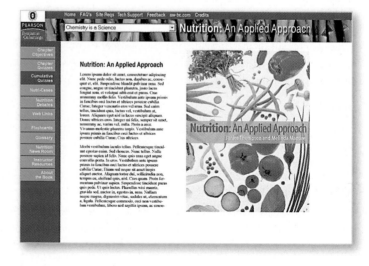

Nutrition Video Series

Our nutrition and fitness video series from **Films for the Humanities** includes programs on topics such as supplements, diet and cancer, the Food Guide Pyramid, and life in the fast food lane. Instructors can use these videos to introduce topics or spark debate. Available through your Benjamin Cummings sales representative.

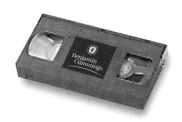

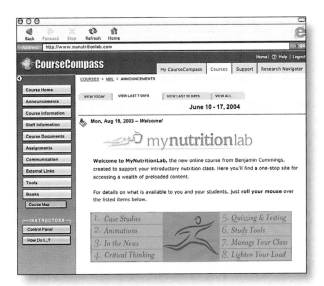

MyNutritionLab

This online standard course management system is loaded with teaching and learning resources that make giving assignments and tracking student progress easy. **MyNutritionLab**, powered by CourseCompass™, features a wealth of pre-loaded content for instructors including PowerPoint® slides, Test Bank questions, Instructor's Manual material, and more. Features for students include interactive label activities, animations, and drag-and-drop activities. Research Navigator™, which provides three databases of credible and reliable source materials, is also included.

Classroom Response System

The **Classroom Response System** can be offered with *Nutrition: An Applied Approach*, using either EduCue or H-ITT software. The wireless polling system lets instructors take attendance, pose questions, and assess students' progress instantly. Each student uses a wireless transmitter to communicate their answers to in-class questions; a receiver immediately tabulates answers and displays them graphically. Ask your sales representative for more information on the Benjamin Cummings rebate coupon that can be packaged with *Nutrition: An Applied Approach*.

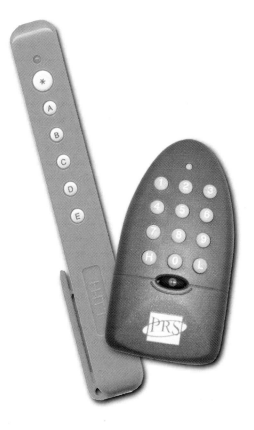

Ancillaries Help Students and Instructors

Instructors and students have access to a wide variety of ancillary material to facilitate teaching, help learning and retention, and contribute to the classroom experience.

Instructor Supplements

Instructor's Manual (0-8053-7953-3)
The Instructor's Manual contains chapter summaries; objectives; lecture outlines; and activity ideas, including an EvaluEat activity and a Nutrition Debate activity, for each chapter. The Instructor's Manual will help instructors create engaging lectures and additional activities to develop effective student learning.

Printed Test Bank (0-8053-7956-8)
The Test Bank contains more than 80 questions for each chapter, including multiple-choice, true/false, short answer, matching, and essay questions.

Computerized Test Bank (0-8053-7957-6)
Created in TestGen, the Computerized Test Bank contains all the questions from the printed Test Bank in a user-friendly, cross-platform CD-ROM. The Computerized Test Bank lets instructors create and customize quizzes and tests, using pre-written questions or inserting questions of their own.

Transparency Acetates (0-8053-7955-X)
The transparency acetates include all of the art and tables from the text. There are more than 200 full-color transparencies in this package.

Instructor's Resource CD-ROM (0-8053-7954-1)
The Instructor's Resource CD-ROM allows instructors to seamlessly integrate the text into their lecture presentations by providing PowerPoint® and JPEG files of all the art, tables, and selected photos from the text, as well as providing a full set of PowerPoint® lecture slides that correspond directly to each chapter of the book.

Great Ideas in Teaching Nutrition
This newsletter compiles your colleagues' best teaching ideas from the classroom. It offers instructors access to innovative ideas suitable for teaching to a large lecture hall or a small group.

MyNutritionLab Instructor Access Kit (0-8053-7905-3)
Provides full instructor access to MyNutritionLab.

Course Management Technologies
In addition to MyNutritionLab, WebCT (0-8053-7959-2) and Blackboard (0-8053-7958-4) are also available. Contact your Benjamin Cummings sales representative for details.

Nutrition Video Series
Nutrition and fitness videos by Films for the Humanities include videos on supplements, diet and cancer, the Food Guide Pyramid, and life in the fast food lane. Contact your Benjamin Cummings sales representative for details.

Student Supplements

Student Study Guide (0-8053-7962-2)
The Study Guide will help students get the best grade possible with terminology questions, text outlines, study questions, completion exercises, and critical thinking sections for each chapter.

Companion Website
www.aw-bc.com/thompson
The *Nutrition: An Applied Approach* website offers students chapter and cumulative quizzes with immediate feedback, web links, flashcards, a glossary, the Nutrition News Room containing current articles from the *New York Times*, as well as further discussion and exercises related to the Nutri-Cases and Nutrition Debates.

MyNutritionLab Student Access Kit (0-8053-7906-1)
Provides full student access to MyNutritionLab including the entire companion website plus interactive exercises, animations, self-assessments, news, and study tools.

EvaluEat Dietary Analysis Software
EvaluEat is included with every new copy of the textbook. Students can use this software to do a single or multi-day diet analysis, create a variety of reports, and determine whether they are meeting the RDAs for various vitamins and minerals. *The EvaluEat software is also available for purchase separately from the textbook* (ISBN 0-8053-7949-5).

Acknowledgments

It is eye opening to author a textbook and to realize that the work of so many people contributes to the final product. There are numerous people to thank and we'd like to begin by extending our gratitude to our contributors, Cindy Beck of Evergreen State College and Kendra Golden of Whitman College. Cindy and Kendra wrote Chapters 14 and 15, respectively, and their efforts are greatly appreciated. In addition we offer our sincere thanks to Judy Sheeshka, of the University of Guelph, who created the Canadian Recommendations and Guidelines appendix for this book, and Patricia Brown, of Cuesta College, for her consultation on the Nutrient Values of Common Foods table that also appears as an appendix.

We would like to thank the fabulous staff at Benjamin Cummings for their incredible support and dedication to this book. Our Acquisitions Editor, Deirdre Espinoza, encouraged us to be authors, and she has provided unwavering support and guidance throughout the entire process of writing and publishing this book. Publisher Daryl Fox has committed extensive resources to ensuring the quality of this text, and his support and enthusiasm has helped us maintain the momentum we needed to complete this project. We could never have written this text without the exceptional editing skills of Laura Bonazzoli, our Developmental Editor. In addition to her content guidance, she wrote the chapter-opening stories and the Nutri-Cases. Laura's energy, enthusiasm, and creativity significantly enhanced the quality of this textbook. We are also deeply indebted to Art Development Editor Laura Southworth. She developed a spectacular art program and guided two non-artists through the arduous process of creating informative and attractive textbook illustrations. Three individuals guided our efforts as Project Editors: Erin Joyce, who got us started and moving in the right direction; Ellen Keohane, who worked diligently to keep us on course; and Marie Beaugureau, who joined us during the most hectic phase of publishing, and kept us sane with her sense of humor and excellent organizational skills. Michelle Cadden, Assistant Editor, and Alison Rodal, Editorial Assistant, provided us with editorial and administrative support that we would have been lost without.

Multiple talented players helped build this book in the production and design process as well. Steven Anderson, Production Supervisor, and Brandi Nelson and the whole group at Elm Street Publishing Services, kept manuscripts moving through the entire process, and they never lost track of the minute details. And speaking of minute details, Carla Breidenbach, Copyeditor, never let the smallest thing slip. Laura Murray and Kelly Murphy, Art and Photo Coordinators, supervised the art and photo programs. Kathleen Cunningham created a beautiful text and cover design. Brian and Eloise Donnelly, of Cypress Integrated Inc., performed research for hundreds and hundreds of photos.

We can't go without thanking the marketing and sales teams, especially Cheryl Cechvala, Market Development Manager, and Sandra Lindelof, Senior Marketing Manager, who coordinated class testing, nutrition forums, and extensive market research to ensure that we directed our writing efforts to meet the needs of students and instructors, and who have been working incredibly hard to get this book out to those who will benefit most from it.

Our goal of meeting instructor and student needs could not have been realized without the team of educators and editorial staff who worked on the substantial supplements package for *Nutrition*. Dr. Kim Aaronson of Truman College wrote the inventive and useful Student Study Guide; Ruth Reilly and Jesse Morell, both of the University of New Hampshire, created a comprehensive Test Bank; and Linda Flemming of Middlesex Community College, authored the wonderful Instructor's Manual; all of which were managed by editor Ziki Dekel. Ryan Shaw, Assistant Editor, and Dr. Amy Marion of New Mexico State University worked on the Instructor's Resource CD-ROM and PowerPoint lecture slides. Alex Levering, Media Producer, headed up the coordination and development of the companion website to the text, working with content contributors Marie Dunford; Judy

Kaufman of Monroe Community College; Colleen Kvaska of Mt. San Antonio College; Kristy Long; Wendy Cunningham of California State University of Sacramento; Andria Pescatello of University of California, Irvine; Priya Venkatesan of Pasadena City College; Sandra Weatherilt of Mt. San Antonio College; and Jennifer Weddig of Metropolitan State College of Denver.

We would also like to thank the many colleagues, friends, and family members who helped us along the way. Janice would specifically like to thank the hard-working staff at the University of New Mexico Office of Native American Diabetes Programs. Venita Wolfe, Novaline Wilson, Carla Herman, Ayn Whyte, Peggy Allen, Georgia Perez, and Kim Giang were incredibly supportive and were willing to cover our incredibly busy workload so that I could take time off to write and edit this book. My family and friends have been so incredibly wonderful throughout my career. Mom, Dianne, Pam, Steve, Susie, Karen, and Amanda are always there for me to offer a sympathetic ear, a shoulder to cry on, and endless encouragement. You are incredible people who keep me sane and healthy and help me to remember the most important things in life. Melinda would specifically like to thank her husband, Steve Carroll, for the patience and understanding he has shown through this process—once again. He has learned that there is always another chapter due! Melinda would also like to thank her family, friends, and professional colleagues for their support and listening ear through this whole process. You have all helped make life a little easier during this incredibly busy time.

Reviewers

Helen Alexanderson-Lee
California State University, Long Beach

Janet Anderson
Utah State University

Laura Avila
Glendale Community College

James Bailey
University of Tennessee, Knoxville

Bobby Baldridge
Asbury College

Beverly Benes
University of Nebraska, Lincoln

Ethan Bergman
Central Washington University

Nancy Berkoff
Los Angeles Trade Technical College

Jaqueline Berning
University of Colorado, Colorado Springs

Carlton Bessinger
Winthrop University

Gregory Blake Biren
Rowan University

M. Ann Bock
New Mexico State University

Nancy Bradley
Central Florida Community College, Ocala

Ellen Brennan
San Antonio College

K. Shane Broughton
University of Wyoming

Ardith Brunt
North Dakota State University

Joanne Burke
Boston College

John Capeheart
University of Houston, Downtown

Denise Cazes
University of Houston, Clearlake

Dorothy Chen-Maynard
California State University, San Bernardino

Debbie Cohen
Southeast Missouri State University

Priscilla Connors
University of North Texas

Margaret Craig-Schmidt
Auburn University

Wendy Cunningham
California State University, Sacramento

Diane Dembicki
Dutchess County Community College

Richard Dowdy
University of Missouri, Columbia

Virginia Englert
Colorado State University

Bruce Evans
Huntington College

Sally Feltner
Western Carolina University

Gary Fosmire
Pennsylvania State University

Bernard Frye
University of Texas, Arlington

Peggy Gorbach
Evergreen Valley College

Cynthia Gossage
Prince George's Community College

Sandra Gross
Westchester University

Nancy Harris
East Carolina University

William Helferich
University of Illinois, Urbana–Champaign

Beckee Hobson
College of the Sequoias

Carolyn Holcroft
Foothill College

Claire Hollenbeck
San Jose State University

Peter Horvath
State University of New York, Buffalo

Cara Hoyt
California State University, Hayward

Jasminka Ilich
University of Connecticut

Rao Ivaturi
Indiana State University

Thunder Jalili
University of Utah

Catherine Jen
Wayne State University

Jay Kandiah
Ball State University

Judy Kaufman
Monroe Community College

Margaret Kessel
Ohio State University

Laura Kruskall
University of Nevada, Las Vegas

Melody Kyzer
University of North Carolina, Wilmington

Larry Lanciotti
Morton College

Deirdre Larkin
California State University, Northridge

Barbara Lohse
Kansas State University

Bernadene Magnuson
University of Maryland, College Park

Teresa Marcus
Chattanooga State Technical Community College

Rose Martin
Pennsylvania State University

Karen Mason
Western Kentucky University

Marlene McCall
Community College of Allegheny County

Jaqueline McClelland
North Carolina State University

Shelley McGuire
Washington State University

Glen McNeil
Fort Hays State University

Renee Melton
State University of New York, Buffalo

Sharon Michael
Tacoma Community College

Gina Marie Morris
Frank Phillips College

Donna Mueller
Drexel University

Mary Murimi
Louisiana Tech University

Michelle Neyman
California State University, Chico

Anne O'Donnell
Santa Rosa Junior College

Millie Owens
College of the Sequoias

Erwina Peterson
Yakima Valley Community College

Linda Rankin
Idaho State University

Ruth Reed
Juniata College

Amy Reeder
University of Utah

Larry Reichard
Maple Woods Community College

Ruth Reilly
University of New Hampshire

Raylene Reimer
University of Calgary

Tonia Reinhard
Wayne State College

Bob Reynolds
University of Illinois, Chicago

Nuha Rice
University of Phoenix

Jennifer Ricketts
University of Arizona

Leah Robinson
Bucks County Community College

Judith Rodriguez
University of North Florida

Lisa Sasson
New York University

Susan Saylor
University of Alabama

Monique Schaefer
El Camino College

Donal Scheidel
University of South Dakota

Connie Vinton Schoepske
Iowa Central Community College

Jiri Seltzer
Valdosta State University

Terry Shaw
Austin Community College

Tina Shepard
Arizona State University East

Sarah Short
Syracuse University

Kathryn Silliman
California State University, Chico

Clifford Singh
California State University, San Bernardino

Neeta Singh
University of the Incarnate Word

Elizabeth Skendzic
University of Wisconsin, Parkside

Carole Sloan
Henry Ford Community College

Mollie Smith
California State University, Fresno

Anastasia Snelling
American University

Diana Marie Spillman
Miami University

Stasinos Stavrianeas
Williamette University

Tammy Stephenson
University of Kentucky

Lianne Summerfield
Marymount University

Steven Swoap
Williams College

Robin Sytsma
Solano Community College

Elsie Takeguchi
Sacramento City College

Norman Temple
Athabasca University

Ann Thompson
South Plains College

Linda Vaughn
Arizona State University

Priya Venkatesan
Pasadena City College

Daryle Wane
Pasco-Hernando Community College

Beverly Webber
University of Utah

Jennifer Weddig
Metropolitan State College of Denver

Sally Weerts
University of North Florida

Stacie Wing
University of Utah

Cynthia Wright
Southern Utah University

Gloria Young
Virginia State University

Maureen Zimmerman
Mesa Community College

Donna Zoss
Purdue University

Nutrition Forum and Focus Group Participants

Amy Allen-Chabot
Anne Arundel Community College

Janet Anderson
Utah State University

James Bailey
University of Tennessee, Knoxville

Beverly Benes
University of Nebraska, Lincoln

Patricia Brown
Cuesta College

Alison Campbell
Brigham Young University

Paula Cochrane
TVI Community College

Priscilla Connors
University of North Texas

Robert Cullen
Illinois State University

Earlene Davis
Bakersfield College

Linda Davis
Virginia Polytechnic Institute and State University

Gail Frank
California State University, Long Beach

Bernard Frye
University of Texas, Arlington

Art Gilbert
University of California, Santa Barbara

Cynthia Gossage
Prince Georges Community College

Lisa Gurule
TVI Community College

Beckee Hobson
College of the Sequoias

Clarie Hollenbeck
San Jose State University

Thunder Jalili
University of Utah

Mary Kelso
Antelope Valley College

Laura Kruskall
University of Nevada, Las Vegas

Renee Melton
SUNY Buffalo

Debra Pearce
Northern Kentucky University

Ruth Reilly
University of New Hampshire

Nidia Romer
Miami Dade College

Margaret Craig Schmidt
Auburn University

Roseann Schnoll
Brooklyn College

Sarah Short
Syracuse University

Priya Venkatesan
Pasadena City College

Jennifer Weddig
Metropolitan College of Denver

Sally Weerts
University of North Florida

Jurist Willis-Morris
Miami Dade College

Cynthia Wright
Southern Utah University

Research Consultants

The authors wish to thank the following individuals who provided research materials for their consultation. Their contributions helped ensure the exceptional currency and accuracy of the textbook.

Janet Anderson
Utah State University

Beverly Benes
University of Nebraska, Lincoln

Ethan Bergman
Central Washington University

Priscilla Connors
University of North Texas

Stacy Gehrig
Illinois Central College

Silvia Giraudo
University of Georgia

David Holben
Ohio University

Clarie Hollenbeck
San Jose State University

Peter Horvath
SUNY Buffalo

Thunder Jalili
University of Utah

Laura Kruskall
University of Nevada, Las Vegas

Janet Sundberg
Southern Illinois University

Alan Titchenal
University of Hawaii, Manoa

Cynthia Wright
Southern Utah University

Class Testers

Kim Aaronson
Truman College

Kwaku Addo
University of Kentucky

Amy Allen-Chabot
Anne Arundel Community College

Julianne Arient
Triton College

Jennifer Asher
Southeast Missouri State University

Garry Auld
Colorado State University

James Bailey
University of Tennessee, Knoxville

Susan Balinsky
College of Charleston

Sharon Barron
Brevard Community College

Cynthia Beck
Evergreen State College

Nancy Berkoff
LA Trade Technical College

Jean Boone
Palm Beach Community College

Ardith Brunt
North Dakota State University

Alison Campbell
Brigham Young University

Nancy Canolty
University of Georgia

Catherine Christie
University of North Florida

Elizabeth Chu
San Diego Mesa College

Debbie Cohen
Southeast Missouri State University

Fabio Comona
San Diego State University

Rhena Cooper
North Idaho College

Wendy Cunningham
California State University, Sacramento

Noemi Custodia-Lora
Northern Essex Community College

Earlene Davis
Bakersfield College

Cindy Dostal
Hawkeye Community College

Sally Feltner
Western Carolina University

Brian Findley
Palm Beach Community College

Anthony Giusti
American River College

Cynthia Gonzalez
Santa Monica College

Peggy Gorbach
Evergreen Valley College

Meledath Govindan
Fitchburg State College

Carolyn Holcroft
Foothill College

Julie Hood
Central Oregon Community College

Debra Hook
California State University, San Bernardino

Brian Hug
Olivet College

Linda Ibarra–Gonzalez
Palo Alto College

Thunder Jalili
University of Utah

James Kahora
Middlesex Community College

Judy Kaufman
Monroe Community College

Susan Kazen
Palo Alto College

Mary Kelso
Antelope Valley College

Linda Kollett
Massasoit Community College

Dorothy Koteski
Community College of Philadelphia

Laura Kruskall
University of Nevada, Las Vegas

Alison Leahy
Shoreline Community College

Jeannie Luther
Albuquerque Technical Vocational Institute

Susan Meyers
Miami Dade College

Lauren Morgan
Gloucester County College

Gina Marie Morris
Frank Phillips College

Rose Ann Neff
Lock Haven University of Pennsylvania

Terry O'Toole
Lynchburg College

Anna Page
Johnson County Community College

Stephanie Perry
University of North Florida

Roseann Poole
Tallahassee Community College

Ralph Price
University of Arizona

Peggy Ramsey
University of California, Irvine

Linda Rankin
Idaho State University

Ruth Reilly
University of New Hampshire

Carol Reynolds
Fullerton College

Tom Richard
Keene State College

Christian Roberts
University of California, Los Angeles

Leah Robinson
Bucks County Community College

Nidia Romer
Miami Dade College

Donal Scheidel
University of South Dakota

Connie Schneider
California State University, Fresno

Roseanne Schnoll
Brooklyn College

A.I. Clifford Singh
California State University, San Bernardino

Neeta Singh
University of the Incarnate Word

Lorraine Siniscaro
Herkimer County Community College

Eleanor Skelley
Palo Alto College

Mollie Smith
California State University, Fresno

Debra St. George
Massasoit Community College

Ann Thompson
South Plains College

Joan Thompson
Weber State University

Alan Titchenal
University of Hawaii, Manoa

Simin Vaghefi
University of North Florida

Linda Vaughan
Arizona State University

Marva Volk
Tulsa Community College

Sandra Weatherilt
Mt. San Antonio College

Jennifer Weddig
Metropolitan College of Denver

Sally Weerts
University of North Florida

Kathy White
St. Philips College

Jurist Willis–Morris
Miami Dade College

Jean York
Mt. San Antonio College

Wendy Zins
Anoka Ramsey Community College

Brief Contents

Contents

Chapter 14
Food Safety and Technology: Impact on Consumers 495

Chapter 15
Nutrition Through the Lifecycle: Pregnancy and the First Year of Life 535

Chapter 16
Nutrition Through the Lifecycle: Childhood to Late Adulthood   575

Appendices

Nutrition: An Applied Approach

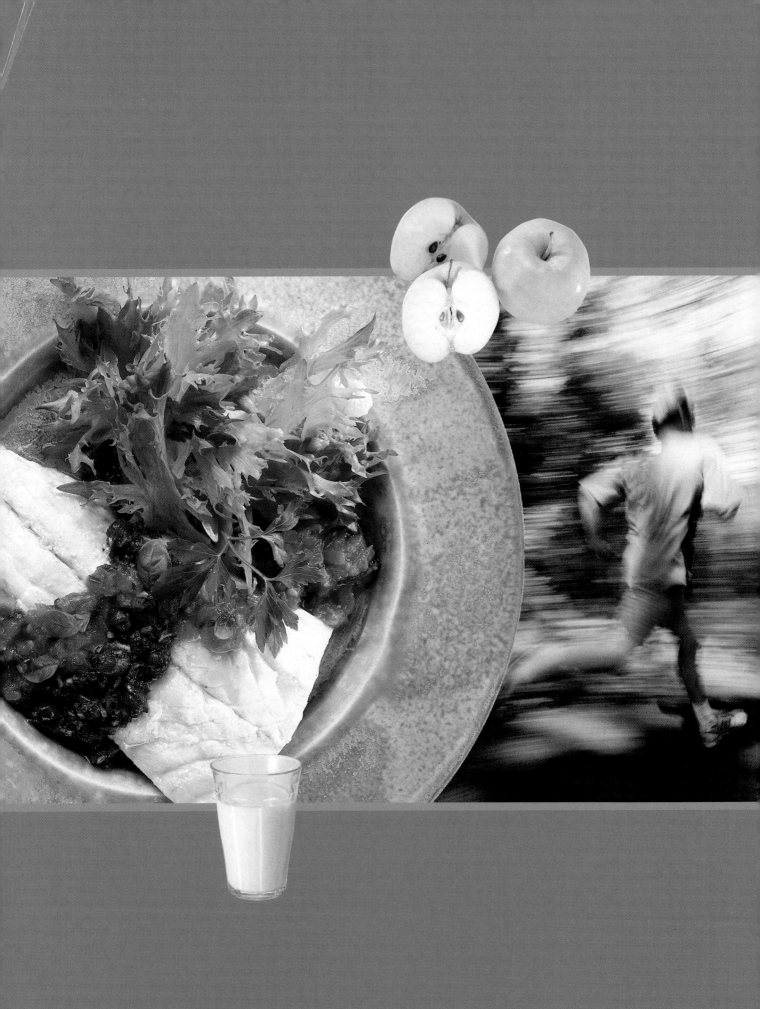

Chapter 1
The Role of Nutrition in Our Health

Chapter Objectives

After reading this chapter you will be able to:

1. Define the term *nutrition*, p. 4.

2. Discuss why nutrition is important to health, pp. 5–8.

3. List three *Healthy People 2010* nutrition-related goals or objectives, pp. 8–9.

4. Identify the six classes of nutrients essential for health, pp. 10–11.

5. Discuss the three energy nutrients, pp. 11–13.

6. Describe how vitamins and minerals differ from each other, pp. 14–17.

7. Identify the Dietary Reference Intakes for nutrients, pp. 18–21.

8. List at least four sources of reliable and accurate nutrition information, pp. 21–25.

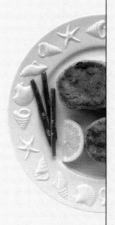

Test Yourself True or false?

1. Nutrition is the science that studies food and how food nourishes our body and influences health. T or F

2. Proteins are a primary energy source for our bodies. T or F

3. All vitamins must be consumed daily to support optimal health. T or F

4. The Recommended Dietary Allowance is the maximum amount of nutrient that people should consume to support normal body functions. T or F

5. Federal agencies in the United States are typically poor sources of reliable nutrition information. T or F

Test Yourself answers can be found at the end of the chapter.

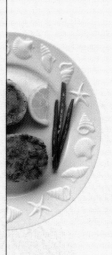

Miguel hadn't expected that college life would make him feel so tired. After classes, he just wanted to go back to his dorm and sleep. Plus he had been having difficulty concentrating and was worried that his first-semester grades would be far below those he'd achieved in high school. Scott, his roommate, had little sympathy. "It's all that junk food you eat!" he insisted. "Let's go down to the organic market for some real food." Miguel dragged himself to the market with Scott but rested at the juice counter while his roommate went shopping. A middle-aged woman wearing a white lab coat approached him and introduced herself as the market's staff nutritionist. "You're looking a little pale," she said. "Anything wrong?" Miguel explained that he had been feeling tired lately. "I don't doubt it," the woman answered. "I can see from your skin tone that you're anemic. You need to start taking an iron supplement." She took a bottle of pills from a shelf and handed it to him. "This one is the easiest for you to absorb, and it's on special this week. Take it three times a day, and you should start feeling better in a day or two." Miguel purchased the supplement and began taking it that night with the meal his roommate prepared. He took it the next day as well, three times as the nutritionist had recommended, but didn't feel any better. After two more days, he visited the university health clinic, where a nurse drew some blood for testing. When the results of the blood tests came in, the physician told him that his thyroid gland wasn't making enough of the hormone that he needed to keep his body functioning properly. She prescribed a medication and congratulated Miguel for catching the problem early. "If you had waited," she said, "it would only have gotten worse, and you could have become seriously ill." Miguel asked if he should continue taking his iron supplements. The physician looked puzzled. "Where did you get the idea that you needed iron supplements?"

Like Miguel, you've probably been offered nutrition-related advice from well-meaning friends and self-professed "experts." Perhaps you found the advice helpful, or maybe, as in Miguel's case, it turned out to be all wrong. Where can you go for reliable advice about nutrition? What exactly *is* nutrition anyway, and why does what we eat have such an influence on our health? In this chapter, we'll begin to answer these questions, and you'll gain a deeper understanding as you work through the rest of this book. Our goal is that, by the time you finish this course, you'll be the expert on your own nutritional needs!

What Is Nutrition?

If you think that the word *nutrition* means pretty much the same thing as *food*, you're right—partially. But the word has a broader meaning that will gradually become clear as you make your way in this course. Specifically, **nutrition** is the science that studies food and how food nourishes our bodies and influences our health. It encompasses how we consume, digest, metabolize, and store nutrients and how these nutrients affect our bodies. Nutrition also involves studying the factors that influence our eating patterns, making recommendations about the amount we should eat of each type of food, attempting to maintain food safety, and addressing issues related to the global food supply. You can think of nutrition, then, as the discipline that encompasses everything about food.

Nutrition is a relatively new scientific discipline. Although food has always played a major role in the lives of humans since the beginning of time, the importance of nutrition to our health has only been formally recognized and studied over the past one hundred years or so. Early research in nutrition focused on making the link between nutrient deficiencies and illness. For instance, the cause of scurvy, which is a vitamin C deficiency, was discovered in the mid-1700s. At that time, however, vitamin C had not been identified—what was known was that some ingredient found in citrus fruits could prevent scurvy. Another example of early discoveries in nutrition is presented in the accompanying Highlight box on the Mystery of Pellagra. As is the case with scurvy and vitamin C, this early research was able to pinpoint a deficiency disease and foods that could prevent it; it would only be later in the twentieth century that the exact nutrient responsible for the deficiency symptoms would be discovered. Thus, unlike sciences such as physics and mathematics, the majority of discoveries in the field of nutrition are relatively recent, and we still have much to learn.

nutrition   The science that studies food and how food nourishes our bodies and influences our health.

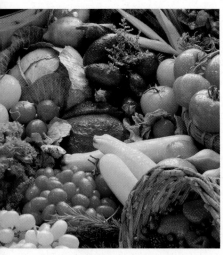

The study of nutrition encompasses everything about food.

Solving the Mystery of Pellagra

In the first few years of the twentieth century, Dr. Joseph Goldberger successfully controlled outbreaks of several fatal infectious diseases, from yellow fever in Louisiana to typhus in Mexico. So it wasn't surprising that, in 1914, the Surgeon General of the United States chose him to tackle another disease thought to be infectious that was raging throughout the South. Called pellagra, the disease was characterized by a skin rash, diarrhea, and mental impairment. At the time, it afflicted more than 50,000 people each year, and in about 10% of cases, it resulted in death.

Goldberger began studying the disease by carefully observing its occurrence in groups of people. He asked, if it is infectious, then why would it occur in prison inmates, yet leave their guards unaffected? Why, in fact, did it overwhelmingly affect impoverished Southerners, while leaving their affluent (and well-fed) neighbors healthy? Could a dietary deficiency cause pellagra? Before he could confirm his hunch, he first had to prove that pellagra was not spread by germs. To do so, he and his colleagues deliberately injected or ingested patients' scabs or bodily fluids. When he and his team remained healthy, he conducted a series of experiments in which he fed his patients different nutrient-rich foods.

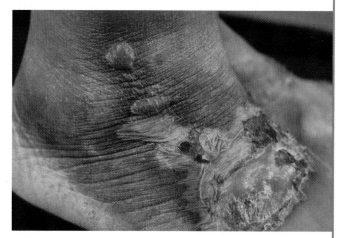

Pellagra is often characterized by a scaly skin rash.

Finally he found an inexpensive and widely available substance—brewer's yeast—that cured the disease.

Shortly after Goldberger's death in 1937, scientists identified the precise nutrient that was deficient in the diet of pellagra patients: niacin, one of the B vitamins, which is plentiful in brewer's yeast.

Source: Based on Howard Markel, "The New Yorker Who Changed the Diet of the South," *New York Times,* 12 August 2003, p. D5. ●

Why Is Nutrition Important?

Thousands of years ago, people in some cultures believed that the proper diet could cure criminal behavior, cast out devils, and bring us into alignment with the divine. Although modern science has failed to find evidence to support these claims, we do know that proper nutrition can help us improve our health, prevent certain diseases, achieve and maintain a desirable weight, and maintain our energy and vitality. As you'll learn in Chapter 3, you are what you eat: the substances you take into your body are broken down and reassembled into your brain cells, bones, muscles—all of your tissues and organs. Think about it: if you eat three meals a day, then by this time next year, you'll have had more than a thousand chances to influence your body's make-up! Let's take a closer look at how nutrition supports health and wellness.

Nutrition Is One of Several Factors Contributing to Wellness

Wellness can be defined in many ways. Traditionally, wellness was defined simply as the absence of disease. However, as we have learned more about our health and what it means to live a healthful lifestyle, our definition of wellness has expanded. Wellness is now considered to be a multidimensional process, one that includes physical, emotional, and spiritual health (Figure 1.1). Wellness is not an endpoint in our lives, but is an active process we work on every day.

In this book, we focus on two critical aspects of wellness: nutrition and physical activity. The two are so closely related that you can think of them as two sides of the same coin: our overall state of nutrition is influenced by how much energy we expend

wellness A multidimensional, lifelong process that includes physical, emotional, and spiritual health.

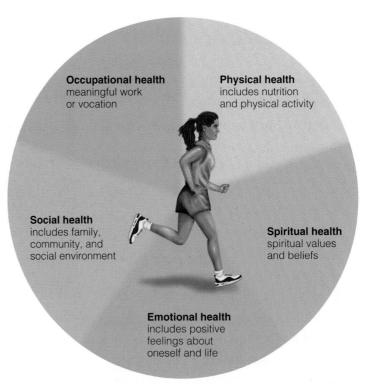

Figure 1.1   Many factors contribute to an individual's wellness. Primary among these are a nutritious diet and regular physical activity.

doing daily activities, and our level of physical activity has a major impact on how we use the nutrients in our food. We can perform more strenuous activities for longer periods of time when we eat a nutritious diet, whereas an inadequate or excessive food intake can make us lethargic. A poor diet, inadequate or excessive physical activity, or a combination of these also can lead to serious health problems. Finally, several studies have suggested that healthful nutrition and regular physical activity can increase feelings of well-being and reduce feelings of anxiety and depression. In other words, wholesome food and physical activity just plain feel good!

A Healthful Diet Can Prevent Some Diseases and Reduce Your Risk for Others

Early work in the area of nutrition focused on nutrient deficiencies and how we can prevent them. As you read in the Highlight box on pellagra, nutrient deficiencies can cause serious, even life-threatening illnesses; diseases such as scurvy, goiter, and rickets are other examples. The discoveries of the causes of nutrient deficiencies have aided nutrition experts in developing guidelines for healthful diets that can prevent deficiency diseases. An ample food supply and fortifying foods with nutrients have ensured that the majority of nutrient deficiency diseases are no longer of concern in developed countries. However, these diseases are still major problems in many developing nations. Some of the nutritional issues impacting developing nations will be discussed throughout this book in Highlight boxes on Global Nutrition.

In addition to preventing nutrient-related diseases, a healthful diet can reduce your risk for chronic diseases. In the United States and many developed nations, the prevalence of obesity (Figure 1.2) and such chronic diseases as heart disease, stroke, type 2 diabetes, and cancer has dramatically increased over the past sixteen years. We know that obesity and its accompanying diseases are significantly affected by nutrition and activity: regularly consuming foods that are high in total energy (or calories),

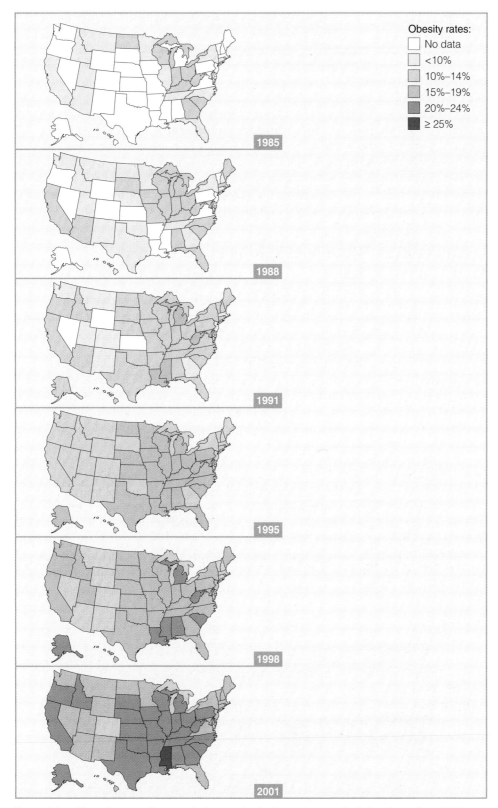

Figure 1.2 These diagrams illustrate the increase in obesity rates across the United States from 1985 to 2001 as documented in the Behavioral Risk Factor Surveillance Survey. Obesity is defined as a body mass index greater than or equal to 30, or approximately 30 pounds overweight for a 5'4" woman. (Data from A. H. Mokdad et al. *JAMA* 1999; 282:16, 2001; 286:10. Graphics from Centers for Disease Control and Prevention, U.S. Obesity Trends 1985 to 2001 [CDC Nutrition and Physical Activity Web page, 2003], www.cdc.gov/nccdphp/dnpa/obesity/trend/index.htm)

total fat, and saturated fat, and low in fiber, fruits, vegetables, and whole grains is associated with an increased risk for obesity, heart disease, type 2 diabetes, and some forms of cancer. The imbalance of consuming too much food and exercising too little also greatly increases our risk for these diseases. Throughout this text, we will discuss in more detail how nutrition and physical activity affect the development of obesity and other chronic diseases.

Nutrition appears to play a role in many diseases. Its role can vary from mild influence, to a strong association, to directly causing a disease (Figure 1.3). For instance, poor nutrition is known to cause deficiency diseases such as anemia and scurvy. Poor nutrition has a strong impact on certain diseases such as type 2 diabetes and heart disease, and it appears to play some role in diseases such as osteoporosis and some forms of cancer. The strength of the association between nutrition and various diseases will continue to be modified as nutrition research continues.

Healthy People 2010 Includes Nutrition-Related Goals for the United States

Healthy People 2010 An agenda that emphasizes health promotion and disease prevention across the United States by identifying goals and objectives that we hope to reach as a nation by the year 2010.

Because of its importance to the wellness of all Americans, nutrition has been included in the national health promotion and disease prevention plan of the United States. *Healthy People 2010* is an agenda that promotes optimal health and disease prevention across the United States by identifying a set of goals and objectives that we hope to reach as a nation by the year 2010 (U.S. Department of Health and Human Services 2000). This agenda was developed by a team of experts from a variety of federal agencies under the direction of the Department of Health and Human Services. Input was gathered from a large number of individuals and organizations, including hundreds of national and state health organizations, and the general public was asked to share their ideas.

The two overarching goals of *Healthy People 2010* are: 1) to increase quality and years of healthy life; and 2) to eliminate health disparities. These goals are supported by hundreds of more specific goals and objectives. The importance of nutrition is underscored by the number of nutrition-related objectives in the agenda. Other objectives address physical activity and the problem with overweight and obesity, both of which are of course influenced by nutrition.

Table 1.1 identifies some of the specific *Healthy People 2010* goals and objectives related to nutrition and physical activity. This textbook includes a wealth of information and activities that can assist you in achieving these health objectives.

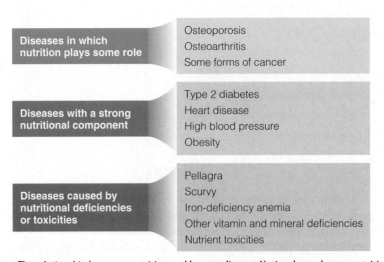

Figure 1.3 The relationship between nutrition and human disease. Notice that, whereas nutritional factors are only marginally implicated in the diseases on the top, they are strongly linked to the development of the diseases in the middle column, and truly causative of those on the bottom.

Table 1.1 Nutrition and Fitness Goals and Objectives from *Healthy People 2010*

Focus Area	Goal	Objective Number and Description
Nutrition and overweight	Promote health and reduce chronic disease associated with diet and weight.	19–1. Increase the proportion of adults who are at a healthy weight from 42% to 60%.
		19–2. Reduce the proportion of adults who are obese from 23% to 15%.
		19–5. Increase the proportion of persons aged 2 years and older who consume at least two daily servings of fruit from 28% to 75%.
		19–6. Increase the proportion of persons aged 2 years and older who consume at least three daily servings of vegetables, with at least one-third being dark green or orange vegetables from 3% to 50%.
		19–9. Increase the proportion of persons aged 2 years and older who consume no more than 30% of calories from total fat from 33% to 75%.
Physical activity and fitness	Improve health, fitness, and quality of life through daily physical activity.	22–1. Reduce the proportion of adults who engage in no leisure-time physical activity from 40% to 20%.
		22–2. Increase the proportion of adults who engage regularly, preferably daily, in moderate physical activity for at least 30 minutes per day from 15% to 30%.
		22–4. Increase the proportion of adults who perform physical activities that enhance and maintain muscular strength and endurance from 18% to 30%.
		22–5. Increase the proportion of adults who perform physical activities that enhance and maintain flexibility from 30% to 43%.

Source: U.S. Department of Health and Human Services. *Healthy People 2010: Understanding and Improving Health*, 2d ed. (Washington, DC: U.S. Governmental Printing Office, November 2000. Available at www.health.gov/healthypeople [accessed June 2003]).

Recap: Nutrition is the science that studies food and how food impacts our body and our health. Nutrition is an important component of wellness and is strongly associated with physical activity. One goal of a healthful diet is to prevent nutrient deficiency diseases such as scurvy and pellagra; a second goal is to lower the risk for chronic diseases such as type 2 diabetes and heart disease. *Healthy People 2010* is a health promotion and disease prevention plan for the United States.

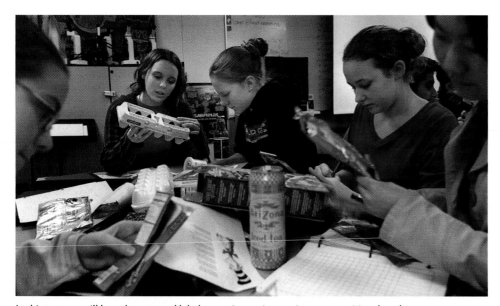

In this text you will learn how to read labels to assist you in meeting your nutritional goals.

What Are Nutrients?

A glass of milk or a spoonful of peanut butter may seem as if it is all one substance, but in reality most foods are made up of many different chemicals. Some of these chemicals are not useful to the body, whereas others are critical to human growth and function. These latter chemicals are referred to as **nutrients.** The six groups of nutrients found in the foods we eat are (Figure 1.4):

nutrients Chemicals found in foods that are critical to human growth and function.

- carbohydrates
- fats and oils (two types of lipids)
- proteins
- vitamins
- minerals
- water

As you may know, the term *organic* is commonly used to describe foods that are grown without the use of non-natural fertilizers or chemicals. But when scientists

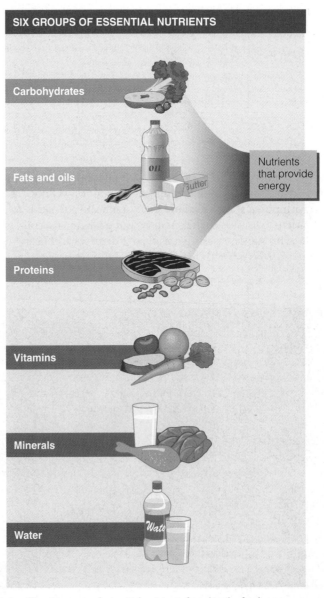

Figure 1.4   The six groups of essential nutrients found in the foods we consume.

What Is a Kilocalorie?

Have you ever wondered what the difference is between the terms *energy*, *kilocalories,* and *calories*? Should these terms be used interchangeably, and what do they really mean? The brief review provided in this highlight should broaden your understanding. First, some precise definitions:

- *Energy* is defined as the capacity to do work. We derive energy from the energy-containing nutrients in the foods we eat; namely, carbohydrates, fats, and proteins.

- A *kilocalorie* (kcal) is the amount of heat required to raise the temperature of one kilogram of water by one degree Celsius. It is a unit of measurement we use to quantify the amount of energy in food that can be supplied to the body. For instance, we can say that the energy found in one gram of carbohydrate is equal to 4 kcal.

- A *calorie* (cal) is also a unit of measurement: technically, one kilocalorie is equal to 1000 calories. *Kilo-* is a prefix used in the metric system to indicate one thousand (think of *kilometer* or *kilobytes*). In science, the term Calorie, with a capital "C", is also equal to kilocalorie. It is the capital "C" Calories that are always listed on food labels. However, the term calorie, with a lower case "c", is sometimes used on food labels and elsewhere to represent the unit of kilocalorie. So remember that when you see the term calorie, it may really be referring to kilocalories, especially if it is on a food label.

It is most appropriate to use the term *energy* when you are referring to the general concept of energy intake or energy expenditure. If you are discussing the specific *units* related to energy, use either kilocalories or calories. In this textbook, we use the term kilocalories as a unit of energy; we will only use the term calories when reviewing information about food labels. ●

---

describe individual nutrients as **organic,** they mean that these nutrients contain an element called carbon that is an essential component of all living organisms. Minerals and water are **inorganic** because they do not contain carbon. Both organic and inorganic nutrients are equally important for sustaining life but differ in their structures, functions, and basic chemistry.

Carbohydrates, Fats, and Proteins Are Nutrients That Provide Energy

Carbohydrates, fats, and proteins are the only nutrients in foods that provide energy. By this we mean that these nutrients break down and reassemble into a fuel that our body uses to support physical activity and basic functioning. Although taking a multivitamin and a glass of water might be beneficial in other ways, it will not provide you with the energy you need to do your twenty minutes on the stair-climber! The energy nutrients are also referred to as **macronutrients.** *Macro* means "large," and our bodies need relatively large amounts of these nutrients to support normal function and health.

Alcohol is a chemical found in food, and it provides energy—but it is not considered a nutrient essential for good health. This is because it does not support the regulation of body functions or the building or repairing of tissues. In fact, alcohol is considered to be both a drug and a toxin.

We express energy in units of *kilocalories* (kcal). Refer to the Highlight box, "What Is a Kilocalorie?" for an explanation of energy and kilocalories. Both carbohydrates and proteins provide 4 kcal per gram, alcohol provides 7 kcal per gram, while fats provide 9 kcal per gram. Thus, for every gram of fat we consume, we obtain more than twice the energy as compared to a gram of carbohydrate or protein. Refer to the You Do the Math box to learn how to calculate the energy contribution of carbohydrate, fat, and protein in a given food.

organic A substance or nutrient that contains the element carbon.

inorganic A substance or nutrient that does not contain carbon.

macronutrients Nutrients that our bodies need in relatively large amounts to support normal function and health. Carbohydrates, fats, and proteins are macronutrients.

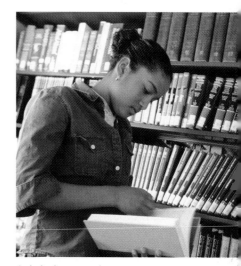

Carbohydrates are the primary source of fuel for our bodies, particularly for our brain.

Calculating Energy Contribution of Carbohydrate, Fat, and Protein

Have you ever wondered how you can determine the percentage of the total energy you eat that comes from carbohydrates, fats, or protein? There is a simple equation you can use to calculate these values. To begin, you need to know how much energy you consume and how many grams of carbohydrates, fats, and protein you eat. You also need to know the kilocalorie (kcal) value of each of these nutrients. Remember that the energy value for carbohydrate and protein is 4 kcal per gram, the energy value for alcohol is 7 kcal per gram, and the energy value for fat is 9 kcal per gram. Working along with the following example will help you perform the calculations for yourself:

1. Let's say you have completed a personal diet analysis, and you consume 2,500 kcal per day. From your diet analysis you also find that you consume 300 grams of carbohydrates, 90 grams of fat, and 123 grams of protein.
2. To calculate your percentage of total energy that comes from carbohydrate, you must do two things:
   a. Take your total grams of carbohydrate, and multiply by the energy value for carbohydrate to give you how many kcal of carbohydrate you have consumed.

$$300 \text{ grams of carbohydrate} \times 4 \text{ kcal/gram} = 1200 \text{ kcal of carbohydrate}$$

   b. Take the kcal of carbohydrate you have consumed, divide this number by the total number of kcal you consumed, and multiply by 100. This will give you the percentage of the total energy you consume that comes from carbohydrate.

$$(1200 \text{ kcal}/2500 \text{ kcal}) \times 100 = 48\%$$
of total energy comes from carbohydrate

3. To calculate your percentage of total energy that comes from fat, you follow the same steps but incorporate the energy value for fat:
   a. Take your total grams of fat and multiply by the energy value for fat to find the kcal of fat consumed.

$$90 \text{ grams of fat} \times 9 \text{ kcal/gram} = 810 \text{ kcal of fat}$$

   b. Take the kcal of fat you have consumed, divide this number by the total number of kcal you consumed, and multiply by 100 to get the percentage of total energy you consume that comes from fat.

$$(810 \text{ kcal}/2500 \text{ kcal}) \times 100 = 32.4\%$$
of total energy comes from fat

Now try these steps to calculate the percentage of the total energy you consume that comes from protein. These calculations will be very useful throughout this course as you learn more about how to design a healthful diet and how to read labels to assist you in meeting your nutritional goals. Later in this book, in Chapter 11, you will learn how to estimate your unique energy needs and determine the ideal amount of energy you need from carbohydrates, fat, and protein. ●

Carbohydrates Are a Primary Fuel Source

carbohydrates The primary fuel source for our bodies, particularly for our brain and for physical exercise.

Carbohydrates are the primary source of fuel for our bodies, particularly for our brain and during physical exercise (Figure 1.5). A close look at the word "carbohydrate" reveals the chemical structure of this nutrient. *Carbo-* refers to carbon, and *-hydrate* refers to water. You may remember that water is made up of hydrogen and oxygen. Thus, carbohydrates are composed of chains of carbon, hydrogen, and oxygen.

Carbohydrates encompass a wide variety of foods; rice, wheat, and other grains, as well as vegetables are carbohydrates, and fruits contain natural sugars that are carbohydrates. Carbohydrates are also found in legumes (including lentils, dry beans, and peas), milk and other dairy products, seeds, and nuts. Carbohydrates and their role in health are the subject of Chapter 4.

Fats Provide Energy and Other Essential Nutrients

fats An important energy source for our bodies at rest and during low intensity exercise.

Fats, a type of *lipids,* are another important source of energy for our bodies (Figure 1.6). Lipids are a diverse group of organic substances that are insoluble in water. Lipids include triglycerides (more commonly known as fats), phospholipids, and sterols. Like

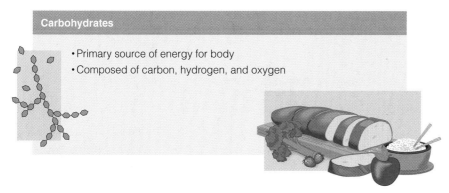

Figure 1.5 Carbohydrates are a primary source of energy for our bodies and are found in a wide variety of foods.

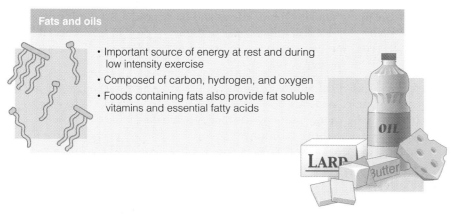

Figure 1.6 Fats are an important energy source during rest and low intensity exercise. Foods containing fat also provide other important nutrients.

carbohydrates, fats are comprised of carbon, hydrogen, and oxygen; however, they contain proportionally much less oxygen and water than carbohydrates do. This quality allows them to pack together tightly, which explains why they yield more energy per gram than either carbohydrates or proteins.

Fat is an important energy source for our bodies at rest and during low intensity exercise. Our body is capable of storing large amounts of fat as adipose tissue. These fat stores can be broken down for energy during periods of fasting, for example, while we are asleep. Foods that contain fats are also important in providing fat-soluble vitamins and essential fatty acids.

Dietary fats come in a variety of forms. Solid fats include such things as butter, lard, and margarine. Liquid fats are referred to as oils and include vegetable oils such as canola and olive oils. Cholesterol is a form of lipid that is synthesized in our bodies, and it can also be consumed in the diet. Chapter 5 provides a thorough review of lipids.

Proteins Support Tissue Growth, Repair, and Maintenance

Proteins also contain carbon, hydrogen, and oxygen, but they are different from carbohydrates and fats in that they contain the element *nitrogen* (Figure 1.7). Within proteins, these four elements assemble into small building blocks known as amino acids. We break down dietary proteins into amino acids and reassemble them to build our own body proteins—for instance, the proteins in our muscles and blood.

Although proteins can provide energy, they are not a primary source of energy for our bodies. Proteins play a major role in building new cells and tissues, maintaining the structure and strength of bone, repairing damaged structures, and assisting in regulating metabolism and fluid balance.

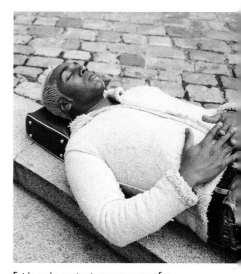

Fat is an important energy source for our bodies at rest and can be broken down for energy during periods of fasting, for example, while we are asleep.

proteins The only macronutrient that contains nitrogen; the basic building blocks of proteins are amino acids.

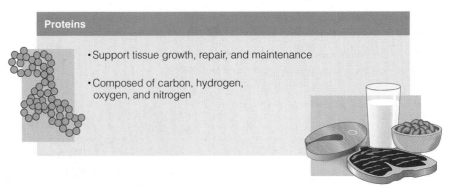

Figure 1.7   Proteins contain nitrogen in addition to carbon, hydrogen, and oxygen. Proteins support the growth, repair, and maintenance of body tissues.

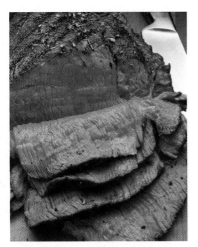

Meats are one of our primary sources of proteins.

vitamins Organic compounds that assist us in regulating our bodies' processes.

micronutrients Nutrients needed in relatively small amounts to support normal health and body functions. Vitamins and minerals are micronutrients.

fat-soluble vitamins Vitamins that are not soluble in water, but soluble in fat. These include vitamins A, D, E, and K.

Proteins are found in many foods. Meats and dairy products are our primary sources of proteins, but we also obtain small amounts of protein from vegetables and whole grains. Seeds, nuts, and legumes are good sources of protein. Proteins are reviewed in detail in Chapter 6.

Recap: The six essential nutrient groups found in foods are carbohydrates, fats, proteins, vitamins, minerals, and water. Carbohydrates, fats, and proteins are referred to as the energy nutrients, as they provide our bodies with the energy necessary to thrive. Carbohydrates are the primary energy source for our bodies; fats provide fat-soluble vitamins and essential fatty acids and act as energy storage molecules; and proteins support tissue growth, repair, and maintenance.

Vitamins Assist in the Regulation of Biological Processes

Vitamins are organic compounds that assist us in regulating our bodies' processes. Vitamins are critical in building and maintaining healthy bone and muscle tissue, supporting our immune system so we can fight illness and disease, and ensuring healthy vision. They also assist in maintaining the health of our blood. Contrary to popular belief, vitamins do not contain energy (or calories); however, vitamins do play an important role in assisting our bodies with releasing and utilizing the energy found in carbohydrates, fats, and proteins. Because we need relatively small amounts of these nutrients to support normal health and body functions, the vitamins (in addition to minerals) are referred to as **micronutrients.**

Vitamins are classified as two types: fat-soluble and water-soluble (Table 1.2). This classification is based upon their solubility in water, which affects how vitamins are absorbed, transported, and stored in our bodies. As our bodies cannot synthesize most vitamins, we must consume them in our diets. Both types of vitamins are essential for our health and are found in a variety of foods. Let's now review the different properties of fat-soluble and water-soluble vitamins.

Fat-Soluble Vitamins Are Stored in the Body

Vitamins A, D, E, and K are **fat-soluble vitamins.** As you will learn in more detail in Chapter 3, fat-soluble vitamins are absorbed in our intestines along with dietary fat. They are then transported to the liver or other organs, where they are either utilized or stored for later use.

Our ability to store fat-soluble vitamins sets them apart from the water-soluble vitamins. Because we are capable of storing these vitamins, we do not have to consume the recommended intakes of these nutrients on a daily or weekly basis. As long as our diet contains the average amounts recommended over a given time period, intakes of these vitamins will be sufficient to support healthy function.

Table 1.2   Overview of Vitamins

Type	Names	Distinguishing Features
1) Fat Soluble	A, D, E, and K	Soluble in fat Stored in the human body Toxicity can occur from consuming excess amounts, which accumulate in the body
2) Water Soluble	C, B vitamins (thiamin, riboflavin, niacin, vitamin B_6, vitamin B_{12}, pantothenic acid, biotin, and folate)	Soluble in water Not stored to any extent in the human body Excess excreted in urine Toxicity generally only occurs as a result of vitamin supplementation

Storing fat-soluble vitamins can have its disadvantages. Consuming large amounts of these vitamins, particularly from supplements, can cause an excessive build-up and lead to dangerously toxic levels. Toxicity can occur relatively quickly for some of these vitamins. Toxicity symptoms include damage to our hair, skin, bone, eyes, and nervous system.

Even though we can store fat-soluble vitamins, deficiencies can and do occur, although they are relatively uncommon. Eating too little fat in our diet or excreting these vitamins from our digestive tract along with undigested fat can lead to deficiencies. Using mineral oil as a laxative can result in a significant loss of fat-soluble vitamins in our feces. Diets that are extremely low in fat, as well as diseases that prevent the normal absorption of fat can also result in fat-soluble vitamin deficiencies. Deficiencies of fat-soluble vitamins can lead to serious health problems such as night blindness and osteoporosis and even death in the most severe cases.

Fat-soluble vitamins are found in a variety of fat-containing foods. Meats, dairy products, vegetable oils, avocados, nuts, and seeds are all potentially good sources. You will learn more about the specific functions, toxicity and deficiency symptoms, and food sources of these vitamins in Chapters 7 through 10.

Water-Soluble Vitamins Should Be Consumed Daily or Weekly

In contrast to the fat-soluble vitamins, **water-soluble vitamins** dissolve in water. Vitamin C and the B vitamins (thiamin, riboflavin, niacin, vitamin B_6, vitamin B_{12}, pantothenic acid, biotin, and folate) are absorbed through the intestinal wall directly into the bloodstream. These vitamins then travel to the cells of the body where they are needed.

Precisely because these vitamins dissolve in water, we cannot store large amounts of them. Our kidneys filter out any excess water-soluble vitamins we consume, and we then excrete this excess in our urine. Because we cannot store large amounts of these vitamins, toxicity rarely occurs when we consume excess amounts in our diet. We *can* consume toxic levels of these nutrients through supplementation, however, if we consume higher amounts than our bodies can eliminate.

Another consequence of our inability to store large amounts of water-soluble vitamins is that we need to consume adequate amounts of these nutrients on a daily or weekly basis. If we do not regularly consume these nutrients in our diets, deficiency symptoms and even disease can result fairly quickly. However, this does not mean that we must take vitamin supplements to obtain adequate amounts of these nutrients. The water-soluble vitamins are abundant in many foods, including whole grains, fruits, vegetables, meat, and dairy products. The toxicity symptoms, deficiency diseases, and food sources of these vitamins are described in detail in Chapters 7 through 10 in relation to their specific functions.

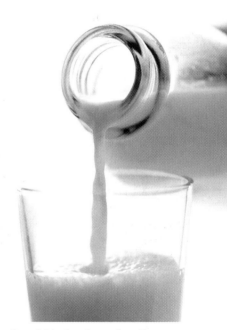

Fat-soluble vitamins are found in a variety of fat-containing foods, including dairy products.

water-soluble vitamins Vitamins that are soluble in water. These include vitamin C and the B vitamins.

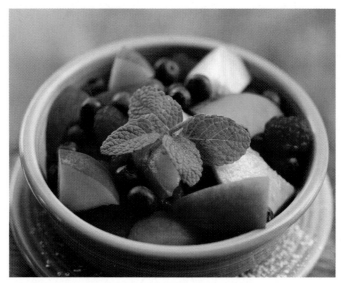

Fruits are an abundant source of water-soluble vitamins.

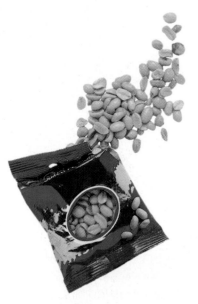

Peanuts are a good source of magnesium and phosphorus, which play an important role in formation and maintenance of our skeleton.

minerals Inorganic substances that are not broken down during digestion and absorption and are not destroyed by heat or light. Minerals assist in the regulation of many body processes and are classified as major minerals or trace minerals.

major minerals Minerals we need to consume in amounts of at least 100 milligrams per day and of which the total amount in our bodies is at least 5 grams.

Recap: Vitamins are organic compounds that assist with regulating a multitude of body processes. Fat-soluble vitamins are soluble in fat and include vitamins A, D, E, and K. We can store fat-soluble vitamins in our liver, adipose, and other fatty tissues. Water-soluble vitamins are soluble in water and include vitamin C and the B vitamins (thiamin, riboflavin, niacin, vitamin B_6, vitamin B_{12}, pantothenic acid, biotin, and folate). Our bodies excrete excess amounts of water-soluble vitamins in our urine.

Minerals Assist in the Regulation of Many Body Functions

Minerals are inorganic substances, meaning that they do not contain carbon. Some important dietary minerals include sodium, potassium, calcium, magnesium, and iron. Minerals are different from the macronutrients and vitamins in that they are not broken down during digestion or when our bodies use them to promote normal function; they are also not destroyed by heat or light. Thus, all minerals maintain their structure no matter what environment they are in. This means that the calcium in our bones is the same as the calcium in the milk we drink, and the sodium in our cells is the same as the sodium in our table salt.

Minerals have many important functions in our bodies. They assist in fluid regulation and energy production, are essential to the health of our bones and blood, and help rid our body of harmful by-products of metabolism. Chapters 7 through 10 discuss the various minerals and the roles they play in maintaining human health and function.

Minerals are classified according to the amounts we need in our diet and according to how much of the mineral is found in our bodies. The two categories of minerals in our diets and bodies are the major minerals and the trace minerals (Table 1.3).

Major Minerals Are Required in Amounts Greater than 100 Milligrams per Day

Major minerals earned their name from the fact that we need to consume at least 100 milligrams (mg) per day of these minerals in our diets and because the total amount found in our bodies is at least 5 grams (or 5000 mg). The major minerals calcium, phosphorus, and magnesium play an important role in formation and maintenance of our skeletons. Sodium, potassium, and chloride play critical roles in fluid balance, while sulfur is primarily recognized as a component of specific vitamins and amino acids. Food sources of major minerals are varied and include meats, dairy products, fresh fruits and vegetables, and nuts.

Table 1.3   Overview of Minerals

Type	Names	Distinguishing Features
1) Major Minerals	Calcium, phosphorus, sodium, potassium, chloride, magnesium, sulfur	Needed in amounts greater than 100 mg/day in our diets Amount present in the human body is greater than 5 grams (or 5000 mg)
2) Trace Minerals	Iron, zinc, copper, manganese, fluoride, chromium, molybdenum, selenium, iodine	Needed in amounts less than 100 mg/day in our diets Amount present in the human body is less than 5 grams (or 5000 mg)

Trace Minerals Are Required in Amounts Less than 100 Milligrams per Day

Trace minerals are those we need to consume in amounts less than 100 mg per day, and the total amount in our bodies is less than 5 grams (or 5000 mg) of these minerals. The primary trace minerals discussed in this textbook are iron, zinc, copper, manganese, selenium, iodine, fluoride, and chromium. Iron is recognized as important in maintaining the health of our blood and supporting oxygen transport to all parts of our bodies. Zinc has numerous functions, including ensuring reproductive health and appropriate cell growth and development. Copper, manganese, and selenium play roles in antioxidant function, while iodine is critical for the adequate production of hormones that control body temperature regulation, metabolic rate, and growth. Fluoride helps reduce tooth decay and strengthens our bones and teeth. Chromium is necessary for the proper metabolism of carbohydrates and fats. Food sources of the trace minerals are the same as those for major minerals.

trace minerals   Minerals we need to consume in amounts less than 100 milligrams per day and of which the total amount in our bodies is less than 5 grams.

Water Supports All Body Functions

Water is an inorganic nutrient that is vital for our survival. We consume water in its pure form, in juices, soups, and other liquids, and in solid foods such as fruits and vegetables. Adequate water intake ensures the proper balance of fluid both inside and outside of our cells, and also assists in the regulation of nerve impulses, muscle contractions, nutrient transport, and excretion of waste products. Because of the key role that water plays in our health, Chapter 7 focuses on water and its function in our bodies.

Recap: Minerals are inorganic elements that maintain their structure throughout the processes of digestion, absorption, and metabolism. Major minerals are needed in amounts greater than 100 milligrams per day, and the total amount found in our bodies is at least 5 grams (or 5000 mg). Trace minerals are needed in amounts less than 100 milligrams per day, and the total amount found in our bodies is less than 5 grams (or 5000 mg). Minerals play critical roles in virtually all aspects of human health and function. Water is critical for our survival and is important for regulating nervous impulses, muscle contractions, nutrient transport, and excretion of waste products.

How Can I Figure Out My Nutrient Needs?

Now that you know what the six classes of nutrients are, you are probably wondering how much of each you need each day. But before you can learn more about specific nutrients and how to plan your own healthful diet, you need to become familiar with current dietary standards and how these standards shape nutrition recommendations.

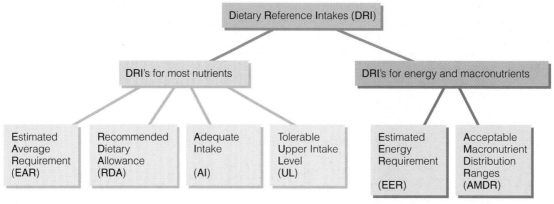

Figure 1.8   The Dietary Reference Intakes (DRIs) for all nutrients. Note that the Estimated Energy Requirement (EER) only applies to energy, and the Acceptable Macronutrient Distribution Ranges (AMDR) only apply to the macronutrients and alcohol.

Use the Dietary Reference Intakes to Check Your Nutrient Intake

In the past, the dietary standards in the United States were referred to as the *Recommended Dietary Allowances (RDAs)*, and the standards in Canada were termed the *Recommended Nutrient Intakes (RNIs)*. These standards define recommended intake values for various nutrients and can be used to plan diets for both individuals and groups. They were developed from the perspective of preventing nutrient-deficiency diseases; however, in developed countries like the United States, these diseases are now extremely rare. Thus, much of our current work in nutrition is focused on the associations between nutrition and wellness. We want to learn more about the role of nutrition in preventing and reducing the risks for chronic diseases such as diabetes, heart disease, and cancer and to design diets that promote optimal health. In response to these changes in focus, a new set of reference values have been developed to replace and expand upon the RDA and RNI values. These new reference values in both the United States and Canada are termed the **Dietary Reference Intakes (DRIs)** (Figure 1.8). These standards were developed to include and expand upon the former RDA values and to set new recommendation standards for nutrients that do not have RDA values.

Dietary Reference Intakes (DRIs)   A set of nutritional reference values for the United States and Canada that apply to healthy people.

The DRIs are dietary standards for healthy people only; they do not apply to people with diseases or those who are suffering from nutrient deficiencies. Like the RDAs and RNIs, they identify the amount of a nutrient needed to prevent deficiency diseases in healthy individuals, but they also consider how much of this nutrient may reduce the risk for chronic diseases in healthy people. The DRIs establish an upper level of safety for nutrients and represent one set of values for both the United States and Canada.

The DRIs for most nutrients consist of four values:

- Estimated Average Requirement (EAR)
- Recommended Dietary Allowances (RDA)
- Adequate Intake (AI)
- Tolerable Upper Intake Level (UL)

In the case of energy and the macronutrients, different standards are used. The standards for energy and the macronutrients include the Estimated Energy Requirement (EER) and the Acceptable Macronutrient Distribution Ranges (AMDR). Let's now define each of these DRI values.

Estimated Average Requirement (EAR)   The average daily nutrient intake level estimated to meet the requirement of half of the healthy individuals in a particular life stage or gender group.

The Estimated Average Requirement Guides the Recommended Dietary Allowance

The **Estimated Average Requirement (EAR)** represents the average daily nutrient intake level estimated to meet the requirement of half of the healthy individuals in a particular life stage or gender group (Institute of Medicine 2003). Figure 1.9 pro-

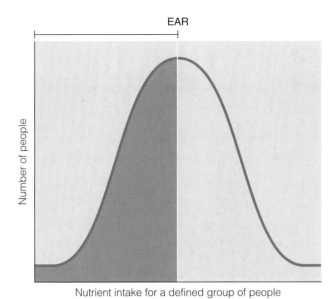

Figure 1.9 The Estimated Average Requirement (EAR) represents the average daily nutrient intake level that meets the requirements of half of the healthy individuals in a given group.

vides a graph representing this value. As an example, the EAR for phosphorus for women between the ages of nineteen and thirty years represents the average daily intake of phosphorus that meets the requirement of half of the women in this age group. The EAR is used by scientists to define the Recommended Dietary Allowance (RDA) for a given nutrient. Obviously, if the EAR meets the needs of only half the people in a group, then the recommended intake will be higher.

The Recommended Dietary Allowance Meets the Needs of Nearly All Healthy People

As previously introduced, the **Recommended Dietary Allowance (RDA)** was the term previously used to refer to all nutrient recommendations in the United States. The RDA is now considered one of many reference standards within the larger umbrella of the DRIs. The RDA represents the average daily nutrient intake level that meets the nutrient requirements of 97 to 98% of healthy individuals in a particular life stage and gender group (Figure 1.10) (Institute of Medicine 2003). For example, the RDA for phosphorus is 700 mg per day for women between the ages of nineteen and thirty years. This amount of phosphorus will meet the nutrient requirements of almost all women in this age category.

Again, scientists use the EAR to establish the RDA. In fact, if an EAR cannot be determined for a nutrient, then this nutrient cannot have an RDA. When this occurs, an Adequate Intake value is determined for a nutrient.

Recommended Dietary Allowance (RDA) The average daily nutrient intake level that meets the nutrient requirements of 97 to 98% of healthy individuals in a particular life stage and gender group.

The Adequate Intake is Based on Estimates of Nutrient Intakes

The **Adequate Intake (AI)** value is a recommended average daily nutrient intake level based on observed or experimentally determined estimates of nutrient intake by a group of healthy people (Institute of Medicine 2003). These estimates are assumed to be adequate and are used when an RDA cannot be determined. There are numerous nutrients that have an AI value, including calcium, vitamin D, vitamin K, and fluoride. More research needs to be done on human requirements for the nutrients assigned an AI value so that an EAR, and subsequently an RDA, can be established.

In addition to establishing RDA and AI values for nutrients, an upper level of safety for nutrients, or Tolerable Upper Intake Level, has also been defined.

Adequate Intake (AI) A recommended average daily nutrient intake level based on observed or experimentally determined estimates of nutrient intake by a group of healthy people.

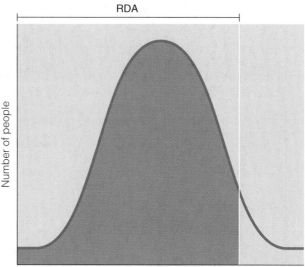

Figure 1.10   The Recommended Dietary Allowance (RDA). The RDA represents the average daily nutrient intake level that meets the requirements of almost all (97 to 98%) healthy individuals in a given life stage or gender group.

The Tolerable Upper Intake Level Is the Highest Level That Poses No Health Risk

Tolerable Upper Intake Level (UL) The highest average daily nutrient intake level likely to pose no risk of adverse health effects to almost all individuals in a particular life stage and gender group.

The **Tolerable Upper Intake Level (UL)** is the highest average daily nutrient intake level likely to pose no risk of adverse health effects to almost all individuals in a particular life stage and gender group (Institute of Medicine 2003). This does not mean that we should consume this intake level or that we will receive more benefits from a nutrient by meeting or exceeding the UL. In fact, as our intake of a nutrient increases in amounts above the UL, the potential for toxic effects and health risks increase. The UL value is a helpful guide to assist you in determining the highest average intake level that is deemed safe for a given nutrient.

> **Recap:** The Dietary Reference Intakes (DRIs) are dietary standards for nutrients established for healthy people in a particular life stage or gender group. The Estimated Average Requirement (EAR) represents the nutrient intake level that meets the requirement of half of the healthy individuals in a group. The Recommended Dietary Allowances (RDA) represent the nutrient intake level that meets the requirements of 97 to 98% of healthy individuals in a group. The Adequate Intake (AI) is a recommended nutrient intake level based on estimates of nutrient intake by a group of healthy people when there is not enough information to set an RDA. The Tolerable Upper Intake Level (UL) is the highest daily nutrient intake level that likely poses no risk of adverse health effects to almost all individuals in a group.

The Estimated Energy Requirement Is the Intake Predicted to Maintain a Healthy Weight

Estimated Energy Requirement (EER) The average dietary energy intake that is predicted to maintain energy balance in a healthy adult.

The **Estimated Energy Requirement (EER)** is defined as the average dietary energy intake that is predicted to maintain energy balance in a healthy adult. This dietary intake is defined by a person's age, gender, weight, height, and level of physical activity that is consistent with good health (Institute of Medicine 2002). It is recommended that an individual maintain an active lifestyle to maintain health and decrease risk for chronic diseases; thus, the EER for an active person is higher than the EER for an inactive person even if all other factors (age, gender, etc.) are the same.

Table 1.4 Acceptable Macronutrient Distribution Ranges (AMDR) for Healthful Diets

Nutrient	AMDR*
Carbohydrate	45–65%
Fat	20–35%
Protein	10–35%

* AMDR values expressed as percent of total energy or as percent of total calories.

Source: Institute of Medicine, Food and Nutrition Board, *Dietary Reference Intakes for Energy, Carbohydrates, Fiber, Fat, Protein and Amino Acids (Macronutrients)* (Washington, DC: National Academies Press, 2002).

The Acceptable Macronutrient Distribution Ranges Are Associated with Reduced Risk for Chronic Diseases

The **Acceptable Macronutrient Distribution Ranges (AMDR)** are a range of intakes for a particular energy source that is associated with reduced risk of chronic disease while providing adequate intakes of essential nutrients (Institute of Medicine 2002). The AMDR is expressed as a percentage of total energy or as a percentage of total calories. The AMDR also has a lower and upper boundary; if we consume nutrients above or below this range, there is a potential for increasing our risk for chronic diseases and for increasing our risk of consuming inadequate levels of nutrients essential for health. The AMDR for carbohydrate, fat, and protein are listed in Table 1.4.

Calculating Your Unique Nutrient Needs

The primary goal of dietary planning is to develop a diet or eating plan that is nutritionally adequate, meaning that the chances of consuming too little or too much of any nutrient are very low. By eating foods that give you nutrient intakes that meet the RDA or AI values, you help your body to maintain a healthy weight, support your daily physical activity, and prevent nutrient deficiencies and toxicities.

The DRI values are listed in a table on the inside cover of this book; they are also reviewed with each nutrient as it is introduced throughout this text. Find your life stage group and gender in the left-hand column, then simply look across to see each nutrient's value for you. Using the DRI values in conjunction with diet planning tools such as the Food Guide Pyramid or Dietary Guidelines for Americans will ensure a healthful and adequate diet. Chapter 2 provides details on how you can use these tools to develop a healthful diet.

> **Recap:** The Estimated Energy Requirement (EER) is the average daily energy intake that is predicted to maintain energy balance in a healthy adult. The EER is defined by a person's age, gender, weight, height, and physical activity level. The Acceptable Macronutrient Distribution Ranges (AMDR) are ranges of intakes for a particular energy source that are associated with reduced risk of chronic disease while also providing adequate intakes of essential nutrients. The DRI values can be used to plan diets that are nutritionally adequate and healthful.

Nutrition Advice: Who Can You Trust?

After reading this chapter, you can see that one of the major nutritional concerns in the United States is our high risk for many chronic diseases. One result of this concern has been the publication of an almost overwhelming quantity of nutritional information on television shows, on Web sites, in newspapers, magazines, newsletters, journals, and many other forums. In addition to this information overload, we continually discover

Acceptable Macronutrient Distribution Ranges (AMDR) A range of intakes for a particular energy source that is associated with reduced risk of chronic disease while providing adequate intakes of essential nutrients.

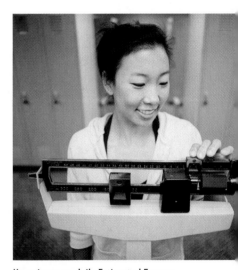

Knowing your daily Estimated Energy Requirement (EER) is a helpful way to maintain a healthy body weight. Your EER is defined by your age, gender, weight, height, and physical activity level.

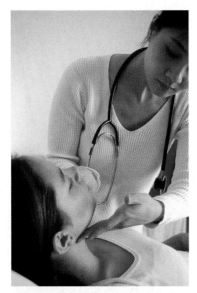

Your medical doctor may have limited experience and training in the area of nutrition, but they can refer you to a Registered Dietitian (RD) or licensed nutritionist to assist you in meeting your dietary needs.

that the nutritional messages from these supposedly "expert" sources are confusing, dissimilar, or even contradictory. On certain issues, even nutrition scientists and physicians cannot seem to agree! If you are wondering how to sort nutritional fact from fiction, the following discussion should help.

Trustworthy Experts Are Educated and Credentialed

There are a considerable number of health professionals who can assist us with reliable and accurate nutrition information. It is not possible to list all individuals who can provide information in this chapter. The following is a list of a few groups that provide reputable nutrition information:

- Registered Dietitian (or RD) — A registered dietitian is an individual who possesses at least a baccalaureate (bachelor's) degree and has completed a defined content of course work and experience in nutrition and dietetics. This individual has also successfully completed the Registration Exam for Dietitians. For a list of individuals who are registered dietitians in your community, you can look in the yellow pages of your phone book or contact the American Dietetic Association at www.eatright.org.

- Licensed Nutritionist — A licensed nutritionist is an individual who is educated, trained, and holds a professional license in nutrition. This individual may also be a registered dietitian, but a person can be a licensed nutritionist independent of being an RD. Each state in the United States has its own laws regulating dietitians or nutritionists. These laws specify which types of licensure or registration a nutrition professional must obtain in order to provide nutrition services or advice to individuals. Individuals who practice nutrition and dietetics without the required license or registration can be prosecuted for breaking the law.

- Nutritionist — this term generally has no definition or laws regulating it. This term may refer to anyone who thinks he or she is knowledgeable about nutrition.

- Professional with an advanced degree (a master's degree [MA or MS] or doctoral degree [PhD]) in nutrition — there are many individuals who are educated and experienced in nutrition and hold an advanced degree. Some of these individuals teach at community colleges and universities or work in fitness and health settings. Not all of these individuals are licensed nutritionists or registered dietitians. Such individuals who do not have a license or RD designation are very knowledgeable about nutrition and health, but they are not certified to provide clinical dietary counseling or treatment for individuals with diseases or illnesses.

- Medical doctor — A medical doctor, also called a physician or MD, is educated, trained, and licensed to practice medicine in the United States. This individual typically has limited experience and training in the area of nutrition. However, if you become ill, the medical doctor is usually one of the first health professionals to see for an accurate medical diagnosis. If you require a dietary plan to treat an illness or disease, most medical doctors will refer you to an RD or licensed nutritionist to assist you in meeting your dietary needs.

Remember that, as an educated consumer, it is important to seek out individuals who can provide you with reliable nutrition information. Even highly educated and credentialed people have limits on their knowledge and can make mistakes. Seeking a second opinion about nutrition information that impacts your health is strongly advised.

Government Sources of Information Are Usually Trustworthy

Many government health agencies have come together in the last twenty years to address the growing problem of nutrition-related disease in the United States. These organizations are funded with taxpayer dollars, and many of these agencies provide financial support for research in the areas of nutrition and health. Thus, these agencies have the resources to organize and disseminate the most recent and reliable information related to nutrition and other areas of health and wellness. A few of the most recognized and respected of these government agencies are discussed here.

The Centers for Disease Control and Prevention Protects the Health and Safety of Americans

The **Centers for Disease Control and Prevention (CDC)** is considered to be the leading federal agency in the United States that protects the health and safety of people. The CDC is located in Atlanta, Georgia, and works in the areas of health promotion, disease prevention and control, and environmental health. The CDC's mission is to promote health and quality of life by preventing and controlling disease, injury, and disability. Among its many activities, the CDC supports two large national surveys that provide us with important nutrition and health information. These surveys are discussed below. To learn more about the CDC, go to www.cdc.gov.

Centers for Disease Control and Prevention (CDC) The leading federal agency in the United States that protects the health and safety of people. It's mission is to promote health and quality of life by preventing and controlling disease, injury, and disability.

The National Health and Nutrition Examination Survey
The **National Health and Nutrition Examination Survey (NHANES)** is a survey conducted by the National Center for Health Statistics and the CDC. NHANES tracks the nutrient consumption of Americans and includes carbohydrates, fats, protein, vitamins, minerals, fiber, and other food components. Nutrition and other health information are gathered during an interview conducted in a person's household and during an examination in a mobile unit. The nutritional data is gathered using a tool called the **24-hour recall** interview, which is a data collection tool that assesses everything a person has consumed over the past 24 hours. The database for the NHANES survey is extremely large, and an abundance of research papers have been generated from it. To learn more about the NHANES and other national health surveys, go to the Web site for the National Center for Health Statistics at www.cdc.gov/nchs/express.htm.

National Health and Nutrition Examination Survey (NHANES) A survey conducted by the National Center for Health Statistics and the CDC; this survey tracks the nutrient and food consumption of Americans.

24-hour recall A data collection tool that assesses everything a person has consumed over the past 24 hours.

The Behavioral Risk Factor Surveillance System
The **Behavioral Risk Factor Surveillance System (BRFSS)** was established by the CDC. The BRFSS is the world's largest telephone survey, and it tracks lifestyle behaviors that increase our risk for chronic disease. Prior to the development of the BRFSS, such data were only available for the nation as a whole, and they were not gathered regularly. The BRFSS was developed to regularly gather this data at the state level. Many states have expanded on these efforts and developed methods to assess health behavior risks at regional levels within their state.

The BRFSS includes questions related to injuries, infectious diseases, and chronic diseases. This survey places a particularly strong focus on the health behaviors that increase our risk for the nation's leading killers: heart disease, stroke, cancer, and diabetes. These health behaviors include (U.S. Department of Health and Human Services 2002):

Behavioral Risk Factor Surveillance System (BRFSS) The world's largest telephone survey that tracks lifestyle behaviors that increase our risks for chronic diseases.

- Lack of adequate physical activity
- Consuming a diet that is low in fiber and high in fat
- Using tobacco and alcohol
- Not getting medical care that is known to save lives; includes regular Pap smears, mammograms, flu shots, and screening for cancer of the colon and rectum

These behaviors have garnered significant interest because it is estimated that four out of ten deaths (or 40%) in the United States can be attributed to smoking, alcohol misuse, lack of physical activity, and eating an unhealthful diet (U.S. Department of Health and Human Services 2002).

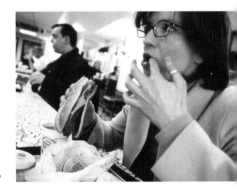

Lifestyle behaviors, such as eating an unhealthful diet, can increase your risk for chronic disease.

The National Institutes of Health Is The Leading Medical Research Agency in the World

The **National Institutes of Health (NIH)** is the world's leading medical research center, and it is the focal point for medical research in the United States. The NIH is one of the agencies of the Public Health Services, which is part of the U.S.

National Institutes of Health (NIH) The world's leading medical research center and the focal point for medical research in the United States.

Department of Health and Human Services. The mission of the NIH is to uncover new knowledge that leads to better health for everyone. This mission is accomplished by support of medical research throughout the world and by fostering communication of medical information. The NIH has many institutes and centers that focus on a broad array of nutrition-related health issues. Some of these institutes include:

- National Cancer Institute (NCI)
- National Eye Institute (NEI)
- National Heart, Lung, and Blood Institute (NHLBI)
- National Institute of Diabetes and Digestive and Kidney Diseases (NIDDK)
- National Center for Complementary and Alternative Medicine (NCCAM)

NIH headquarters are located in Bethesda, Maryland. To find out more about the NIH, go to www.nih.gov.

Professional Organizations Provide Reliable Nutrition Information

There are a number of professional organizations whose members are qualified nutrition professionals, scientists, and educators. These organizations publish cutting-edge nutrition research studies and educational information in journals that are accessible in most university and medical libraries. Some of these organizations include:

- The American Dietetic Association (ADA) — This is the largest organization of food and nutrition professionals in the United States. The mission of this organization is to promote nutrition, health, and well-being. The ADA publishes a professional journal called the *Journal of the American Dietetic Association;* information about ADA can be found at www.eatright.org.
- The American Society for Clinical Nutrition (ASCN) — The ASCN is the clinical division of the American Society for Nutritional Sciences. Its goal is to improve the quality of life through the science of nutrition. The ASCN publishes a professional journal called the *American Journal of Clinical Nutrition,* which focuses on basic and clinical studies in the area of human nutrition. More information about the ASCN can be found at www.faseb.org/ascn.
- The Society for Nutrition Education (SNE)—The SNE is dedicated to promoting healthy, sustainable food choices in communities through nutrition research and education. The primary goals of SNE are to educate individuals, communities, and professionals about nutrition education and to influence policy makers about nutrition, food, and health. The professional journal of SNE is the *Journal of Nutrition Education and Behavior.* Information about SNE can be found at www.sne.org.
- The American College of Sports Medicine (ACSM) — The ACSM is the leading sports medicine and exercise science organization in the world. The mission of the ACSM is to advance and integrate scientific research to provide educational and practical applications of exercise science and sports medicine. Many members are nutrition professionals who combine their nutrition and exercise expertise to promote health and athletic performance. *Medicine and Science in Sports and Exercise* is the professional journal of the ACSM. You can learn more about the ACSM at www.acsm.org.

If you aren't sure whether or not the source of your information is reliable, or can't tell whether the results of a particular study apply to you, how do you find out? What if two studies seem sound, but their findings contradict each other? The Nutrition Debate at the end of this chapter (page 30) explains how you can become a more informed and critical consumer of nutrition-related research.

Recap: The Centers for Disease Control and Prevention is the leading federal agency in the United States that protects the health and safety of people. The CDC supports two large national surveys that provide important nutrition and health information. These two surveys are the National Health and Nutrition Examination Survey (NHANES) and the Behavioral Risk Factor Surveillance System (BRFSS). The National Institutes of Health is the leading medical research agency in the world. The American Dietetic Association, the American Society for Clinical Nutrition, the Society for Nutrition Education, and the American College of Sports Medicine are examples of professional organizations that provide reliable nutrition information.

Nutri-Case: You Play the Expert!

A multitude of features throughout this book challenge you to think about how the various recommendations of the so-called "experts" apply to your unique health issues, metabolism, activity level, energy requirements, food preferences, and lifestyle. For example, the Nutrition Myth or Fact boxes explore the science supporting or challenging common beliefs about foods, and the Highlight boxes describe research on specific nutritional issues. In providing these features, we hope that, by the time you finish this book, you'll have become the expert on your own nutritional needs.

We'll also give you lots of chances to play the expert by offering nutritional advice to five individuals who are seeking advice from a variety of sources —some reliable and others questionable. As you do this, keep in mind that these case scenarios are offered to assist you in gaining a more complete understanding of the nutrition information presented. In the real world, only properly trained and licensed health professionals are qualified to offer nutritional advice to people. The people presented in these scenarios represent a wide range of personal backgrounds and nutritional challenges. You will learn more about each of these people in subsequent chapters, and they briefly introduce themselves here.

- I'm Hannah and I'm nine years old and I go to Valley Elementary School. I get really good grades in school, especially in science. It's my favorite class. Last week, my science teacher taught us about what we're supposed to eat, and then the school nurse weighed us. She said I weigh more than a kid my age should, and I need to play outside more and eat less. I told my mom and dad about it, but they said that's just the way I'm built and we don't have lots of money to eat fancy stuff anyway. I wish I knew what to do, because I feel kind of bad when we go swimming at the YMCA and I see kids staring at me. I always think they're thinking how fat I am.

- Hi, I'm Theo. Let's see, I'm nineteen, and my parents moved to the Midwest from Nigeria eleven years ago. The first time I ever played basketball, in junior high, I was hooked. I won lots of awards in high school and then got a full scholarship to the state university, where I'm a sophomore studying political science. I decided to take a nutrition course because, in my freshman year, I had a hard time making it through the playing season, plus keeping up with my classes and homework. I want to have more energy, and when I get stressed out, I can get really constipated, so I thought maybe I'm not eating right. Anyway, I want to figure out this food thing before basketball season starts again.

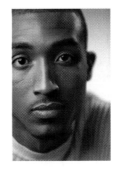

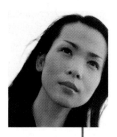

- I'm Liz, I'm twenty, and I'm a dance major at the School for Performing Arts. Last year, two other dancers from my class and I won a state championship and got to dance in the New Year's Eve celebration at the Governor's mansion. This spring, I'm going to audition for the City Ballet, so I have to be in top condition. I wish I had time to take a nutrition course, but I'm too busy with dance classes and rehearsals and teaching a class for kids. But it's okay, because I get lots of tips from other dancers and from the Internet. Like last week, I found a Web site especially for dancers that explained how to get rid of bloating before an audition. I'm going to try it for my audition with the City Ballet!

- My name is Nadia. I'm twenty-eight years old, and I'm a buyer for a chain of discount clothing stores. But the real news is that, after trying for three years, I am finally pregnant! My husband and I were ecstatic for weeks after we found out, until they tested my blood sugar and told me that I have what's called gestational diabetes. I have my first appointment with the clinic's registered dietitian next week, and I'm afraid she's going to tell me that I'll have to give myself insulin shots 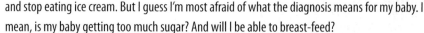 and stop eating ice cream. But I guess I'm most afraid of what the diagnosis means for my baby. I mean, is my baby getting too much sugar? And will I be able to breast-feed?

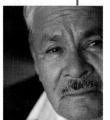

- Hello. My name is Gustavo. Almost sixty years ago, when I was thirteen, I came to the U.S. from Mexico with my father and mother and three sisters to pick crops in California, and now I manage a vineyard. They ask me when I'm going to retire, but I can still work as hard as a man half my age. Health problems? None. Well, maybe my doctor tells me my blood pressure is high, but that's normal for my age! I guess what keeps me going is thinking about how my father died six months after he retired, of colon cancer, and he never knew he had it until it was too late. Anyway, I watch the nightly news and read the papers, so I keep up on what's good for me, eating less fat and salt and all that. I'm doing fine.

Throughout this text you will interact with these five characters as they are dealing with nutrition-related challenges in their lives. As you do, you might find that they remind you of people you may know in your life, and you may also discover you have something in common with one or more of them. Think about how much you differ from each one in regard to your age, developmental stage, family and personal history, food issues, physical activity level, and nutrition and health goals. Our hope is that these characters and their challenges will assist you in applying the nutrition knowledge you acquire in this course not only to their situation, but also to your own life.

Chapter Summary

- Nutrition is the science of food and how food nourishes the body and impacts health.
- Nutrition is an important component of wellness, and healthful nutrition plays a critical role in eliminating nutritional deficiency disease and can help reduce our risks for various chronic diseases.
- *Healthy People 2010* is a national health agenda that focuses on health promotion and disease prevention; its two primary goals are to increase quality and years of life and to eliminate health disparities in the U.S. population.
- *Healthy People 2010* includes numerous objectives categorized into twenty-eight focus areas that target factors including physical activity, overweight and obesity, tobacco use, and access to health care.
- Nutrients are chemicals found in food that are critical to human growth and function.
- The six essential nutrients found in the foods we eat are carbohydrates, fats, proteins, vitamins, minerals, and water.

- The nutrients that provide energy for our bodies are the macronutrients: carbohydrates, fats, and proteins.

- Carbohydrates are composed of carbon, hydrogen, and oxygen. Carbohydrates are the primary energy source for our bodies, particularly our brains.

- Fats provide us with fat-soluble vitamins and essential fatty acids in addition to storing large quantities of energy.

- Proteins can provide energy if needed, but they are not a primary fuel source. Proteins support tissue growth, repair, and maintenance.

- Vitamins assist with the regulation of body processes.

- Fat-soluble vitamins are soluble in fat and can be stored in our tissues; these include vitamins A, D, E, and K.

- Water-soluble vitamins are soluble in water, and we excrete excess amounts in our urine. These include vitamin C and the B vitamins (thiamin, riboflavin, niacin, vitamin B_6, vitamin B_{12}, pantothenic acid, biotin, and folate).

- Minerals are inorganic substances that are not changed by digestion or other metabolic processes.

- Major minerals are found in our bodies in amounts greater than 5 grams (or 5000 mg), and we need to consume at least 100 mg of these minerals each day.

- Trace minerals are found in our bodies in amounts less than 5 grams (or 5000 mg), and we need to consume less than 100 mg of these minerals each day.

- Water is critical to support numerous body functions, including fluid balance, conduction of nervous impulses, and muscle contraction.

- The Dietary Reference Intakes (DRIs) are reference standards for nutrient intakes for healthy people in the United States and Canada.

- The DRIs should be used for dietary planning for individuals and groups.

- The DRIs include the Estimated Average Requirement, the Recommended Dietary Allowance, the Adequate Intake, and the Tolerable Upper Intake Level.

- Potentially good sources of reliable nutrition information include individuals who are registered dietitians, licensed nutritionists, or hold an advanced degree in nutrition.

- The Centers for Disease Control and Prevention (CDC) is the leading federal agency that protects the health and safety of people.

- The National Health and Nutrition Examination Survey (NHANES) is a survey conducted by the CDC and the National Center for Health Statistics that tracks the nutritional status of people in the United States.

- The Behavioral Risk Factor Surveillance System (BRFSS) was established by the CDC and is the world's largest telephone survey; the BRFSS tracks the health behaviors and risks of Americans.

- The National Institutes of Health (NIH) is the leading medical research agency in the world. The mission of NIH is to uncover new knowledge that leads to better health for everyone.

Review Questions

1. Vitamins A and C, thiamin, calcium, and magnesium are considered
   a. water-soluble vitamins.
   b. fat-soluble vitamins.
   c. energy nutrients.
   d. micronutrients.

2. *Healthy People 2010* is
   a. a set of health-related goals and objectives for the United States.
   b. a set of recommendations for intake levels of nutrients and alcohol.
   c. a survey developed by the CDC to track the health behaviors and risks of Americans.
   d. a collection of data on nutrient consumption in the United States.

3. Ten grams of fat
   a. contain 40 kilocalories of energy.
   b. constitute the Dietary Reference Intake for an average adult male.
   c. contain 90 kilocalories of energy.
   d. constitute the Tolerable Upper Intake Level for an average adult male.

4. Which of the following statements about hypotheses is true?
   a. Hypotheses can be proven by clinical trials.
   b. "Many inactive people have high blood pressure" is an example of a hypothesis.
   c. If the results of multiple experiments consistently support a hypothesis, it is confirmed as fact.
   d. "A high-protein diet increases the risk for porous bones" is an example of a hypothesis.

5. Which of the following foods contains all six nutrient groups?
   a. strawberry ice cream
   b. an egg-salad sandwich
   c. creamy tomato soup
   d. all of the above

6. **True or false?** Fat-soluble vitamins provide energy.

7. **True or false?** The Recommended Dietary Allowance represents the average daily intake level that meets the requirements of almost all healthy individuals in a given life stage or gender group.

8. **True or false?** Nutrition significantly affects a person's risk for heart disease.

9. **True or false?** Nutrition-related reports in the *American Journal of Clinical Nutrition* are usually trustworthy.

10. **True or false?** Carbohydrates, fats, and proteins all contain carbon, hydrogen, and oxygen.

11. Explain the difference between a trace mineral and a major mineral.

12. Compare the Estimated Average Requirement to the Recommended Dietary Allowance.

13. Your uncle has learned that you are taking a nutrition course and says, "How can I find reliable nutrition information?" How would you answer?

14. Your mother, who is a self-described "chocolate addict," phones you. She has read in the newspaper a summary of a research study suggesting that the consumption of a moderate amount of bittersweet chocolate reduces the risk of heart disease in older women. You ask her who funded the research. She says she doesn't know and asks you why it would matter. Explain why such information is important.

15. Intrigued by the idea of a research study on chocolate, you obtain a copy of the full report. In it, you learn that:
    • twelve women participated in the study;
    • the women's ages ranged from 65 to 78;
    • the women had all been diagnosed with high blood pressure;
    • they all described themselves as sedentary; and
    • six of the twelve smoked at least half a pack of cigarettes a day, but the others did not smoke.
    Your mother is fifty-one years old, walks daily, and takes a weekly swim class. Her blood pressure is on the upper end of the normal range. She does not smoke. Identify at least three aspects of the study that would cause you to doubt its relevance to your mother.

 Test Yourself Answers

1. **True.** Nutrition is the science that studies food and how food nourishes our body and influences health.

2. **False.** Carbohydrates and fats are the primary energy sources for our bodies.

3. **False.** Most water-soluble vitamins need to be consumed daily. However, we can consume foods that contain fat-soluble vitamins less frequently because our bodies can store these vitamins.

4. **False.** The Recommended Dietary Allowance is the average daily nutrient intake level that meets the nutrient requirements of 97 to 98% of healthy individuals in a particular life stage and gender group.

5. **False.** Other good sources are professional organizations in the field of nutrition research and education and individuals who are licensed or registered as nutrition professionals.

Web Links

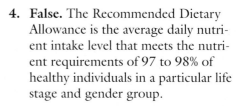

www.healthypeople.gov
Healthy People 2010
Search this site for a list of the 467 *Healthy People 2010* objectives that have been designed to identify the most significant preventable threats to health in the United States and to establish national goals to reduce these threats.

www.eatright.org
American Dietetic Association (ADA)
Obtain a list of registered dietitian in your community from the largest organization of food and nutrition professionals in the United States.

www.cdc.gov
Centers for Disease Control and Prevention (CDC)
Visit this site for additional information about the leading federal agency in the United States that protects the health and safety of people.

www.cdc.gov/nchs/express.htm
National Center for Health Statistics
Go to this site to learn more about the National Health and Nutrition Examination Survey (also referred to as NHANES) and other national health surveys.

www.nih.gov
National Institutes of Health (NIH)
Find out more about the National Institutes of Health, an agency under the U.S. Department of Health and Human Services.

www.faseb.org/ascn
The American Society for Clinical Nutrition (ASCN)
Learn more about the American Society for Clinical Nutrition, the clinical division of the American Society for Nutritional Sciences, and its goal to improve the quality of life through the science of nutrition.

www.sne.org
Society for Nutrition Education (SNE)
Go to this site for further information about the Society for Nutritional Education and its goals to educate individuals, communities, and professionals about nutrition education and influence policy makers about nutrition, food, and health.

www.acsm.org
American College of Sports Medicine (ACSM)
Obtain information about the leading sports medicine and exercise science organization in the world.

References

Institute of Medicine, Food and Nutrition Board. 2003. *Dietary Reference Intakes: Applications in Dietary Planning.* Washington, DC: National Academies Press.

Institute of Medicine, Food and Nutrition Board. 2002. *Dietary Reference Intakes for Energy, Carbohydrates, Fiber, Fat, Protein and Amino Acids (Macronutrients).* Washington, DC: National Academy Press.

U.S. Department of Health and Human Services. 2000, November. *Healthy People 2010: Understanding and Improving Health.* 2d ed. Washington, DC: U.S. Governmental Printing Office. (Available at www.health.gov/healthypeople accessed June 2003.)

U.S. Department of Health and Human Services. Accessed June 2003. Centers for Disease Control and Prevention. CDC at a Glance. Health Risks in America: Behavioral Risk Factor Surveillance System 2002. www.cdc.gov/nccdphp/aag/aag_brfss.htm. Accessed June 2003.

Nutrition Debate:

Research Study Results: Who Can We Believe?

"Reduce your fat intake! Make sure at least 60% of your diet comes from carbohydrates!"

"Eat more protein and fat! Carbohydrates cause obesity!"

Do you ever feel overwhelmed by the abundant and often conflicting advice in media reports related to nutrition? If so, you are not alone. In addition to the "high-carb, low-carb" controversy, we've been told that calcium supplements are essential to prevent bone loss and that calcium supplements have no effect on bone loss; that high fluid intake prevents constipation and that high fluid intake has no effect on constipation. For years, we were told that coffee and tea could be bad for our health; now, it appears that coffee is not unhealthful and tea may actually contain nutrients that are beneficial! When even nutrition researchers cannot agree, who can we believe?

Recall that we acknowledged at the beginning of this chapter that nutrition is a relatively young science. New experiments are being designed every day to determine how nutrition affects our health, and new discoveries are being made. So just as Dr. Goldberger's experiments toppled the theory that pellagra was caused by germs, the results of current experiments will topple the theories we hold today. Viewing conflicting evidence as essential to the advancement of our understanding may help you to feel more comfortable with the contradictions. In fact, controversy is what stimulates researchers to explore unknown areas and attempt to solve the mysteries of nutrition and health.

It is important to recognize that media reports rarely include a thorough review of the research findings on a given topic. Typically, they focus only on the most recent study. Thus, one article in a newspaper or magazine should never be taken as absolute fact on any topic.

To become a more educated consumer and informed critic of nutrition reports in the media, you need to understand the research process and how the results of different types of studies should be interpreted. Let's now learn more about research.

Research Involves Applying the Scientific Method

The *scientific method* is a multistep process that involves observation, experimentation, and development of a theory. This method was developed as a way to apply standardized procedures to minimize the influence of personal prejudices and biases on our understanding of natural phenomena. Thus, this method is used to perform quality research studies in any discipline, including nutrition.

Observation of a Phenomenon Initiates the Research Process

The first step in the scientific method is the observation and description of a phenomenon. As an example, let's say you are working in a healthcare office that caters to mostly elderly clients. You have observed that many of the elderly have high blood pressure, but there are some who have normal blood pressure. After talking with a large number of elderly clients, you notice a pattern developing in that the clients who report being more physically active are also those having lower blood pressure readings. This observation leads you to question the relationship that might exist between physical activity and blood pressure. Your next step is to develop a *hypothesis,* or possible explanation for your observation.

A Hypothesis Is a Possible Explanation for an Observation

A hypothesis is also sometimes referred to as a research question. In this example, your hypothesis would be something like, "Regular physical activity lowers blood pressure in elderly people." You must generate a hypothesis before you can conduct experiments to determine what factors may explain your observation.

Experiments Are Conducted to Test Research Hypotheses

An *experiment* is a scientific study that is conducted to test a research question or hypothesis. In the case of your hypothesis, we could design a variety of research studies to determine the impact of regular physical activity on blood pressure in elderly people. Later in this debate, we will review the different types of research that can be done to assist us in answering your question.

A well-designed experiment attempts to control for factors that may coincidentally influence the results. In the case of your research study, it is well known that weight loss can reduce blood pressure in people with high blood pressure. Thus, in performing your experiment on the effects of exercise on blood pressure, you would want to control for weight loss. You could do this by making sure people eat enough food so that they do not lose weight during your study.

It is important to emphasize that one research study does not prove or disprove a hypothesis. Ideally, multiple experiments are conducted over many years to thoroughly examine a hypothesis. Science exists to allow us to continue to challenge existing hypotheses and expand what we currently know.

A Theory May be Developed Following Extensive Research

If multiple experiments do not support a hypothesis, then the hypothesis is rejected or modified. On the other hand, if the results of multiple experiments consistently support a hypothesis, then it is possible to develop a theory. A *theory* represents a hypothesis or group of related hypotheses that have been confirmed through repeated scientific experiments. Theories are strongly accepted principles, but they can be challenged and changed as a result of applying the scientific method. Remember that centuries ago, it was theorized that the Earth was flat. People were so convinced of this that they refused to sail beyond known boundaries because they believed they would fall off the edge. Only after multiple explorers challenged this theory was it discovered that the Earth is round. We continue to apply the scientific method today to test hypotheses and challenge theories.

Various Types of Research Studies Tell Us Different Stories

You have just learned how the scientific method is applied to test an hypothesis. Establishing nutrition guidelines and understanding the role of nutrition in health involves constant experimentation. Depending upon how the research study is designed, we can gather information that tells us different stories. Let's now learn more about the different types of research conducted and what they tell us.

Epidemiological Studies Inform Us of Existing Relationships

Epidemiological studies are also referred to as observational studies. These types of studies involve assessing nutritional habits, disease trends, or other health phenomenon of large populations and determining the factors that may influence these phenomena. The NHANES survey introduced earlier in this chapter is an example of an epidemiological study. Epidemiological studies are very important in helping us study populations and health trends in large groups. However, these studies can only indicate relationships between factors, and the results do not indicate a cause-and-effect relationship.

Using your hypothesis as an example, we can gain a better understanding of what epidemiological studies can tell us. Let's say you are working with a researcher who has access to the NHANES database. Based on your original hypothesis, your experiment includes gathering blood pressure and physical activity information from all of the elderly study participants in the NHANES survey. After studying the data, you find that the blood pressure values of physically active elderly people are lower than those of inactive elderly people. These results do not indicate that regular physical activity reduces blood pressure or that inactivity causes high

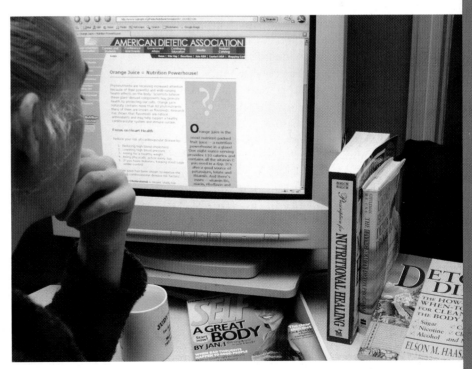

To become a more educated consumer and informed critic of nutrition reports in the media, you need to understand the research process and how the results of different types of studies should be interpreted.

blood pressure. All these results can tell us is that there is a relationship between higher physical activity and lower blood pressure in elderly people.

Laboratory Studies

Laboratory studies generally involve experiments with animals. In many cases, animal studies provide preliminary information that can assist us in designing and implementing human studies. Animal studies also are used to conduct research that cannot be done with humans. For instance, it is possible to study nutritional deficiencies in animals by causing a deficiency and studying its adverse health effects over the lifespan of the animal; this type of experiment is not acceptable to do in humans. One drawback of animal studies is that the results may not apply directly to humans. However, these studies can guide us in determining how we need to proceed to design experiments with humans.

Human Studies

The two primary types of studies conducted with humans include case control studies and clinical trials. *Case control studies* are epidemiological studies done on a smaller scale. Case control studies involve comparing a group of individuals with a particular condition (for instance, elderly with high blood pressure), to a similar group without this condition (for instance, elderly with low blood pressure). This comparison allows the researcher to identify factors other than the defined condition that differ between the two groups. By identifying these factors, researchers can gain a better understanding of things that may cause and help prevent disease. In the case of your experiment, you may find that elderly with low blood pressure are not only more physically active, but they eat more fruits and vegetables and eat less sodium. These findings indicate that other factors in addition to physical activity may play a role in affecting the blood pressure levels of elderly people.

Clinical trials are tightly controlled experiments in which an intervention is given to determine its effect on a given disease or health condition. Interventions may include medications, nutritional supplements, controlled diets, or exercise programs. Clinical trials include the experimental group, who are given the intervention, and the control group, who are not given the intervention. The responses of the intervention group are compared to those of the control group. In the case of your experiment, you could assign one group of elderly people with high blood pressure to an exercise program and assign a second group of elderly people with high blood

pressure to a program where no exercise is done. After the exercise program is completed, you can measure the blood pressure of the elderly people who exercised to those who did not exercise. If the blood pressure of the intervention group decreased and was statistically lower than the blood pressure of the control group, you can feel confident that the exercise program caused a decrease in blood pressure.

There are other important things to consider when conducting a quality clinical trial. Ideally, it is best to randomly assign research participants to intervention and control groups. Randomizing participants is like flipping a coin or drawing names from a hat; doing this reduces prejudice or bias within each group. If possible, it is also important to "blind" both researchers and participants to the treatment being given. A double-blind experiment is one in which neither researchers nor participants know which group is really getting the treatment. Blinding helps prevent the researcher from seeing only the results he or she wants to see, even if these results do not actually occur. In the case of testing medications or nutrition supplements, the blinding process can be assisted by giving the control group a placebo. A *placebo* is an imitation treatment that has no effect on participants; for instance, a sugar pill may be given in place of a vitamin supplement.

Use Your Knowledge of Research to Help You Evaluate Media Reports

How can all of this research information assist you in becoming a better consumer and critic of media reports? By having a better understanding of the research process and types of research conducted, you are more capable of discerning the truth or fallacy within media reports. Keep the following points in mind when examining any media report:

- Who is reporting the information? Is it an article in a newspaper, magazine, or on the Internet? If the report is made by a person or group who may financially benefit from you buying their products, you should be skeptical of the reported results. Also, many people who write for popular magazines and newspapers are not trained in science and are capable of misinterpreting research results.

- Is the report based on reputable research studies? Did the research follow the scientific method, and were the results reported in a reputable scientific journal? Ideally, the journal is peer-reviewed; that is, the articles are critiqued by other specialists working in the same scientific field. A reputable report should include the reference, or source of the information, and should identify researchers by name. This allows the reader to investigate the original study and determine its merit. Reputable journals include the *American Journal of Clinical Nutrition, Journal of Nutrition, Journal of the American Dietetic Association,* the *New England Journal of Medicine,* and the *Journal of the American Medical Association* (*JAMA*).

- Is the report based on testimonials about personal experiences? Are sweeping conclusions made from only one study? Be aware of personal testimonials, as they are fraught with bias. In addition, one study cannot answer all of our questions or prove any hypothesis, and the findings from individual studies should be placed in their proper perspective.

- Are the claims in the report too good to be true? Are claims made about curing disease or treating a multitude of conditions? If something sounds too good to be true, it probably is. Claims about curing diseases or treating many conditions with one product should be a signal to question the validity of the report.

Throughout this text we provide you with information to assist you in becoming a more educated consumer regarding nutrition. You will learn about labeling guidelines, the proper use of supplements, and whether various nutrition topics are myths or facts. Armed with this knowledge, you will become more confident when trying to determine who you can believe when it comes to nutrition claims in the media.

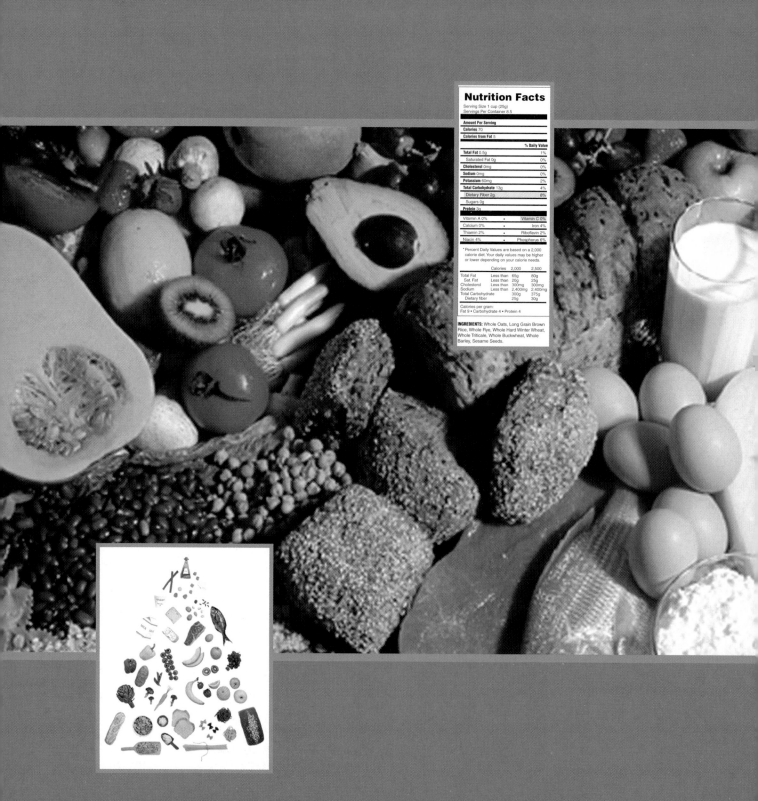

Nutrition Facts

Serving Size 1 cup (25g)
Servings Per Container 8.5

Amount Per Serving

Calories 70

Calories from Fat 5

	% Daily Value
Total Fat 0.5g	1%
Saturated Fat 0g	0%
Cholesterol 0mg	0%
Sodium 0mg	0%
Potassium 60mg	2%
Total Carbohydrate 13g	4%
Dietary Fiber 2g	8%
Sugars 0g	
Protein 3g	

Vitamin A 0%	•	Vitamin C 0%
Calcium 0%	•	Iron 4%
Thiamin 2%	•	Riboflavin 2%
Niacin 4%	•	Phosphorus 6%

* Percent Daily Values are based on a 2,000 calorie diet. Your daily values may be higher or lower depending on your calorie needs.

	Calories	2,000	2,500
Total Fat	Less than	65g	80g
Sat. Fat	Less than	20g	25g
Cholesterol	Less than	300mg	300mg
Sodium	Less than	2,400mg	2,400mg
Total Carbohydrate		300g	375g
Dietary fiber		25g	30g

Calories per gram:
Fat 9 • Carbohydrate 4 • Protein 4

INGREDIENTS: Whole Oats, Long Grain Brown Rice, Whole Rye, Whole Hard Winter Wheat, Whole Triticale, Whole Buckwheat, Whole Barley, Sesame Seeds.

Chapter 2
Designing a Healthful Diet

Chapter Objectives

After reading this chapter you will be able to:

1. Define the components of a healthful diet, pp. 36–38.

2. Read a food label and use the Nutrition Facts Panel to determine the nutritional adequacy of a given food, pp. 38–45.

3. Describe the Dietary Guidelines for Americans, and discuss how these guidelines can be used to design a healthful diet, pp. 45–50.

4. Identify the food groups, number of servings, and serving sizes included in the USDA Food Guide Pyramid, pp. 50–57.

5. Describe how the Food Guide Pyramid can be used to design a healthful diet, pp. 58–63.

6. Discuss the characteristics of the 5-A-Day for Better Health Program and the DASH diet plan, pp. 64–67.

7. Describe the components of the Exchange System, pp. 67–69.

8. List at least four ways to practice moderation, and apply healthful dietary guidelines when eating out, pp. 69–71.

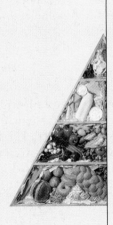

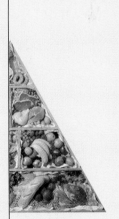

Test Yourself True or False?

1. A healthful diet should always include vitamin supplements. T or F

2. Food labels are designed to assist us in planning a healthful diet. T or F

3. The USDA Food Guide Pyramid is limited in scope and cannot be used by most Americans to design a healthful diet. T or F

4. The 5-A-Day for Better Health Program encourages us to eat 5 servings of fruit and 5 servings of vegetables each day. T or F

5. It is impossible to eat a healthful diet when eating out. T or F

Test Yourself answers can be found at the end of the chapter.

Guess how many school-age children in the United States consume a diet that meets national recommendations for the basic food groups? According to a 2001 report to Congress (Hueter 2002), the answer is just 2%! So how are American adults doing? A 1998 study indicates that as a nation we eat less than one-quarter of the recommended daily servings of dark-green leafy vegetables and less than half the recommended servings of fruits, but we consume plenty of saturated fats (Kantor 1998). Maybe that's one reason why so many Americans are overweight: according to the Centers for Disease Control and Prevention (CDC 2003), 13% of U.S. children and adolescents and an alarming 61% of adults are now overweight.

What are the recommended daily servings of fruits and vegetables anyway? Why are they important? Does your diet meet them? What factors do you think contribute to our poor diets? If you had a friend who had asked your advice about trying to lose weight, and you noticed her skipping lunch in the cafeteria in favor of a diet soda from the vending machine, what might you say to her?

Many factors contribute to the confusion surrounding healthful eating. First, nutrition is a relatively young science. In contrast to physics, chemistry, and astronomy, which have been studied for thousands of years, the science of nutrition emerged around 1900, with the first vitamin being discovered in 1897. The initial RDA values for the United States were published in 1941. Because nutritional research is in its infancy, new findings on the benefits of foods and nutrients are discovered almost daily. These new findings contribute to regular changes in how we define a healthful diet. Second, as stated in Chapter 1, the popular media typically report the results of only selected studies, usually the most recent. This practice does not give a complete picture of all the research conducted in any given area. Indeed, the results of a single study are often misleading. Third, there is no one right way to eat what is healthful and acceptable for everyone. We are individuals with unique needs, food preferences, and cultural influences. For example, a person with diabetes may benefit from eating lower amounts of added sugars and higher amounts of protein or monounsaturated fats than a person without diabetes. People following certain religious practices may limit or avoid foods like specific meats and dairy products. Thus there are literally millions of different ways to design a healthful diet to fit individual needs.

Given all this potential confusion, it's a good thing there are nutritional tools to guide us in designing a healthful diet. In this chapter, we introduce these tools, including the Dietary Guidelines for Americans, the USDA Food Guide Pyramid, and others. Before we explore the question of how to design a healthful diet, however, we should first make sure we understand what a healthful diet *is*.

What Is a Healthful Diet?

healthful diet   A diet that provides the proper combination of energy and nutrients and is adequate, moderate, balanced, and varied.

A **healthful diet** provides the proper combination of energy and nutrients. It has four characteristics: it is adequate, moderate, balanced, and varied. No matter if you are young or old, overweight or underweight, healthy, or coping with illness, if you keep in mind these characteristics of a healthful diet, you will be able to consciously select foods that provide you with the optimal combination of nutrients and energy each day.

A Healthful Diet Is Adequate

adequate diet   A diet that provides enough of the energy, nutrients, and fiber to maintain a person's health.

An **adequate diet** provides enough of the energy, nutrients, and fiber to maintain a person's health. A diet may be inadequate in only one area. For example, many people in the United States do not eat enough vegetables. Their intake of breads, meats, fruits, and dairy products is sufficient. By failing to eat enough vegetables, these people are not consuming enough of many of the important nutrients found in vegetables, such as fiber, vitamin C, beta carotene, and potassium. However, their intake of

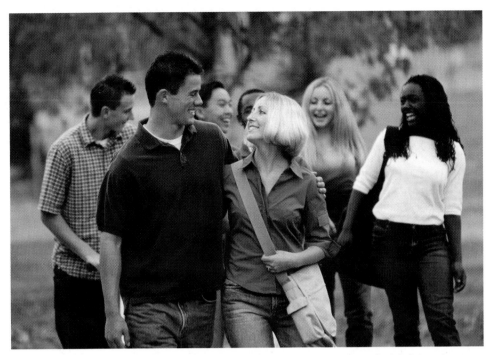

A diet that is adequate for one person may not be adequate for another. A woman who is lightly active may require less kilocalories of energy per day than a highly active male.

protein, fat, carbohydrate, and calcium may be adequate. In fact, many people who eat too few vegetables are overweight or obese, which means that they are eating a diet that exceeds their energy needs but may not be adequate in the nutrients found predominantly in vegetables.

On the other hand, a generalized state of undernutrition can occur if an individual's diet contains an inadequate level of several nutrients for a long period of time. This situation occurs when a person severely limits his or her intake of all foods to avoid gaining weight. For example, many teenage girls and college-aged women follow a very restrictive eating pattern to maintain a thin figure. These individuals may skip multiple meals each day, avoid foods that contain any fat, and limit their meals to only a few foods such as a bagel, a banana, a diet soda, or a small green salad. This type of restrictive eating pattern practiced over a prolonged period can cause low energy levels, loss of bone and hair, impair memory and cognitive function, and cause menstrual dysfunction in women.

A diet that is adequate for one person may not be adequate for another. For example, a small woman who is lightly active may require approximately 1,700 to 2,000 kilocalories of energy each day to support her body's functions. In contrast, a highly active male athlete may require more than 4,000 kilocalories of energy each day to support his body's demands. These two individuals differ greatly in their activity level and in their quantity of body fat and muscle mass, which means they require very different levels of fat, carbohydrate, protein, and other nutrients to support their daily needs.

A Healthful Diet Is Moderate

Moderation is the key to a healthful diet. **Moderation** refers to eating the right amounts of foods to maintain a healthy weight and to optimize our body's metabolic processes. If a person eats too much or too little of certain foods, healthful goals cannot be reached. For example, some people drink a lot of sugared soft drinks, as they enjoy the sweet taste and the energetic feelings produced by the caffeine found in

moderation Eating the right amounts of foods to maintain a healthy weight and to optimize our bodies' metabolic processes.

these drinks. It is not uncommon for many people to drink at least 60 fluid ounces (or three 20-ounce bottles) of soft drinks on some days. Drinking this much contributes an extra 765 kilocalories of energy to a person's diet. In order to maintain weight, a person would need to either reduce his or her food intake, exercise more, or both to make up for these extra kilocalories. This could lead to a person cutting healthful food choices from his or her diet. By consuming a more moderate amount of soft drinks, or switching to diet soft drinks or water, people can consume more healthful foods and maintain a healthy body weight.

A Healthful Diet Is Balanced

balanced diet A diet that contains the combinations of foods that provide the proper proportions of nutrients.

A **balanced diet** is one that contains the combinations of foods that provide the proper balance of nutrients. As you will learn in this course, our bodies need many types of foods in varying amounts to maintain health. For example, fruits and vegetables are excellent sources of fiber, vitamin C, beta carotene, potassium, and magnesium. In contrast, meats are not good sources of these nutrients. However, meats are excellent sources of protein, iron, zinc, and copper. By eating the proper balance of all healthful foods, including fruits, vegetables, and meats (or meat substitutes), we can be confident that we are consuming the proper balance of the nutrients we need to maintain health.

A Healthful Diet Is Varied

variety Eating a lot of different foods each day.

Variety refers to eating a lot of different foods each day. There are literally thousands of healthful foods we can choose from each day. Trying new foods on a regular basis can assist us in eating a more varied diet. Do not be afraid to eat a new green vegetable each week. Or, try putting spinach on your turkey sandwich in place of iceberg lettuce. By selecting a variety of foods, we optimize our chances of consuming the multitude of nutrients our bodies need. As an added benefit, eating a varied diet prevents boredom and avoids our getting into a "food rut." Later in this chapter we provide suggestions for eating a varied diet.

> **Recap:** A healthful diet provides adequate nutrients and energy, and it includes sweets, fats, and salty foods in moderate amounts only. A healthful diet includes an appropriate balance of foods and a wide variety of foods.

What Tools Can Help Me Design a Healthful Diet?

Many people feel it is impossible to eat a healthful diet. They may mistakenly believe that the foods they would need to eat are too expensive or not available to them, or they may feel too busy to do the necessary planning, shopping, and cooking. Some people rely on dietary supplements to get enough nutrients instead of focusing on eating a variety of foods. But is it really that difficult to eat a healthful diet?

Although designing and maintaining a healthful diet is not as simple as eating whatever you want, most of us can do it with a little practice and a little help. Let's look now at some tools for designing a healthful diet.

Reading Food Labels Can Be Easy and Fun

Learning to read food labels is an important skill to possess when planning and eating a healthful diet. It may surprise you to learn that prior to 1973, there were no federal regulations for including nutrition information on food labels! The U.S. Food and Drug Administration (FDA) first established regulations for nutrition information on food labels in 1973. These regulations were not as specific as they are today and were not required for many of the foods available to consumers. Throughout the 1970s and 1980s, consumer interest in food quality substantially grew, and many watchdog groups were formed to protect consumers from unclear labeling and false claims made by some manufacturers.

Public interest and concern about how food affects our health became so strong that in 1990, the U.S. Congress passed the Nutrition Labeling and Education Act. This act specifies which foods require a food label, provides detailed descriptions of the information that must be included on the food label, and describes the companies and food products that are exempt from publishing complete nutrition information on food labels. For example, detailed food labels are not required for meat or poultry, as these products are regulated by the U.S. Department of Agriculture, not the FDA. In addition, foods such as coffee and most spices are not required to follow the FDA labeling guidelines, as they contain insignificant amounts of all nutrients that must be listed in nutrition labeling.

Five Components Must be Included on Food Labels

There are five primary components of information that must be included on food labels (Figure 2.1):

1. **A statement of identity:** the common name of the product or an appropriate identification of the food product must be prominently displayed on the label. This information tells us very clearly what the product is.

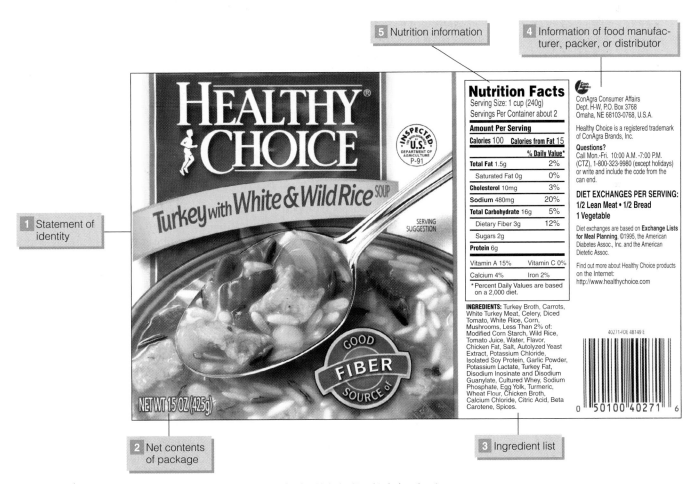

Figure 2.1 The five primary components that are required for food labels. (Food Label © Con Agra Brands, Inc. Used with permission.)

2. **The net contents of the package:** the quantity of the food product in the entire package must be accurately described. Information may be listed as weight (e.g., grams), volume (e.g., fluid ounces), or numerical count (e.g., 4 each).

3. **Ingredient list:** the ingredients must be listed by their common name, in descending order by weight. This means that the first product listed in the ingredient list is the predominant ingredient in that food. This information can be very useful in many situations, such as when you are looking for foods that are lower in fat or sugar, or when you are attempting to identify foods that contain whole grain flour instead of processed wheat flour.

4. **The name and address of the food manufacturer, packer, or distributor:** this information can be used if you want to find out more detailed information about a food product and to contact the company if there is something wrong with the product or you suspect that the food product caused an illness.

5. **Nutrition information:** the Nutrition Facts Panel contains the nutrition information required by the FDA. This panel is the primary tool to assist you in choosing more healthful foods. An explanation of the components of the Nutrition Facts Panel follows.

How to Read and Use the Nutrition Facts Panel on Foods

Figure 2.2 shows an example of a **Nutrition Facts Panel**. There is a variety of information on the label that is useful when designing a healthful diet. You can use this information to learn more about an individual food, and you can also use the Panel to compare one food to another. Let's start at the top of the Panel and work our way down to better understand how to use this information.

1. **Serving size and servings per container:** describes the serving size in a common household measure (e.g., cup), a metric measure (e.g., grams), and how many servings are contained in the package. The FDA has defined serving sizes based on the amounts people typically eat for each food. However, keep in mind that the serving size listed on the package may not be the same as the amount *you* eat. You must factor in how much of the food you eat when determining the amount of nutrients that this food contributes to your actual diet.

2. **Calories and calories from fat per serving:** describes the total number of calories and the total amount of calories that come from fat per one serving of that food. By looking at this section of the label, you can determine if this food is relatively high in fat. For example, one serving of the food on this label (as prepared) contains 320 total calories, with 90 of those calories coming from fat. This means that this food contains 28% of its total calories as fat (90 fat calories ÷ 320 total calories), making it relatively low in fat.

3. **List of nutrients:** describes various nutrients that are found in this food. Those nutrients listed toward the top, including total fat, saturated fat, cholesterol, and sodium, are generally nutrients that we strive to limit in a healthful diet. Some of the nutrients listed toward the bottom are those we try to consume more of, including fiber, vitamins A and C, calcium, and iron.

4. **Percent daily values (%DV):** tells you how much a serving of food contributes to your overall intake of nutrients listed on the label. Because we are all individuals with unique nutritional needs, it is impractical to include nutrition information that applies to each person consuming this food. That would require thousands of individual labels for each food! Thus, the FDA used standards based on a 2,000 calorie diet when they defined the %DV. You can use these percentages to determine whether a food is high or low in a given nutrient,

Nutrition Facts Panel The label on a food package that contains the nutrition information required by the FDA.

percent daily values (%DV) Information on a Nutrition Facts Panel that identifies how much a serving of food contributes to your overall intake of nutrients listed on the label; based on an energy intake of 2,000 calories per day.

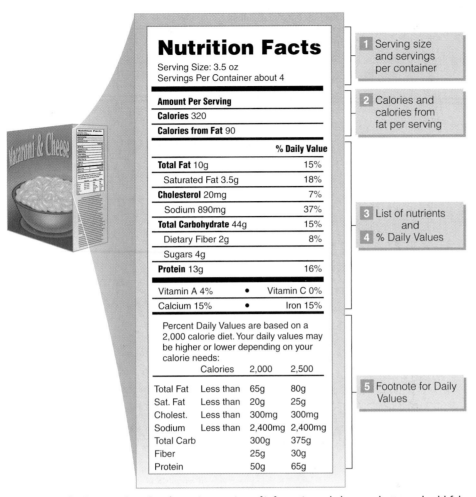

Nutrition Facts

Serving Size: 3.5 oz
Servings Per Container about 4

Amount Per Serving

Calories 320

Calories from Fat 90

	% Daily Value
Total Fat 10g	15%
Saturated Fat 3.5g	18%
Cholesterol 20mg	7%
Sodium 890mg	37%
Total Carbohydrate 44g	15%
Dietary Fiber 2g	8%
Sugars 4g	
Protein 13g	16%

Vitamin A 4%	•	Vitamin C 0%
Calcium 15%	•	Iron 15%

Percent Daily Values are based on a 2,000 calorie diet. Your daily values may be higher or lower depending on your calorie needs:

	Calories	2,000	2,500
Total Fat	Less than	65g	80g
Sat. Fat	Less than	20g	25g
Cholest.	Less than	300mg	300mg
Sodium	Less than	2,400mg	2,400mg
Total Carb		300g	375g
Fiber		25g	30g
Protein		50g	65g

1. Serving size and servings per container

2. Calories and calories from fat per serving

3. List of nutrients and
4. % Daily Values

5. Footnote for Daily Values

Figure 2.2   The Nutrition Facts Panel contains a variety of information to help you select more healthful food choices.

even if you do not consume a 2,000 calorie diet each day. For example, foods that contain less than 5% DV of a nutrient are considered low in that nutrient, while foods that contain more than 20% DV are considered high in that nutrient. If you are trying to consume more calcium in your diet, selecting foods that contain more than 20% DV for calcium are excellent choices. In contrast, if you are trying to consume lower fat foods, selecting foods that contain less than 5% or 10% fat will help you reach your goals. By comparing the %DV between foods for any nutrient, you can quickly decide which food is higher or lower in that nutrient without having to know anything about how many calories you need.

You may be asking yourself the question, "How do the %DV relate to the Recommended Dietary Allowance (RDA) and Dietary Reference Intakes (DRI) we discussed in Chapter 1?" Remember that the DRI is an umbrella term that applies to a group of nutrient standards, including the RDA, Estimated Average Requirement (EAR), Adequate Intake (AI) and Tolerable Upper Intake Level (UL). Many of these values are specific to life-stage and gender. In contrast, the %DV is used as a food labeling device, and its value is determined by using two additional standardized values, the **Reference Daily Intakes (RDI)** and the **Daily Reference Values (DRV)**. The *RDIs* provide standardized values for nutrients with RDAs, including protein and vitamins.

Reference Daily Intakes (RDI)
Standardized food label values for nutrients with RDAs, including protein and vitamins.

Daily Reference Values (DRV)
Standardized food label values for food components that do not have an RDA, such as fiber, cholesterol, and saturated fats.

Table 2.1 The Reference Daily Intakes (RDI) and Daily Reference Values (DRV) Used for Food Labeling

Food Component	RDI[1]	Food Component	RDI[1]	Food Component	DRV[2]
Protein	50 grams (g)	Pantothenic acid	10 mg	Protein	50 g
Vitamin A	1,000 Retinol Equivalents (RE)	Calcium	1,000 mg	Fat	65 g
Vitamin D	400 International Units (IU)	Phosphorus	1,000 mg	Saturated Fat	20 g
				Cholesterol	300 mg
				Total carbohydrate	300 g
Vitamin E	30 IU	Iodide	150 μg	Fiber	25 g
Vitamin K	80 micrograms (μg)	Iron	18 mg	Sodium	2,400 mg
Vitamin C	60 mg	Magnesium	400 mg	Potassium	3,500 mg
Folate	400 μg	Copper	2 mg		
Thiamin	1.5 mg	Zinc	15 mg		
Riboflavin	1.7 mg	Chloride	3,400 mg		
Niacin	20 mg	Manganese	2 mg		
Vitamin B$_6$	2 mg	Selenium	70 μg		
Vitamin B$_{12}$	6 μg	Chromium	120 μg		
Biotin	0.3 mg	Molybdenum	70 μg		

[1]RDI values are for people older than four years of age; these values were developed based on older Recommended Dietary Allowances and do not reflect the new Dietary Reference Intakes.
[2]DRV based on a 2,000 calorie intake.
U.S. Food and Drug Administration. Daily Reference Values and Reference Daily Intakes. www.fda.gov Accessed September 2002.

The *DRVs* are standards for food components that do not have an RDA, such as fiber, cholesterol, and saturated fats. Table 2.1 lists the RDIs and DRVs used for labeling purposes. Note that protein has both an RDI and DRV. Refer to the You Do the Math box (page 44) to learn how to use the %DV to calculate specific amounts of nutrients.

5. *Footnote* (or lower part of Panel): the lower part of the Nutrition Facts Panel includes a footnote that must be on all food labels. This footnote tells you that the %DV are based on a 2,000 calorie diet and that your needs may be higher or lower based on your caloric needs. The remainder of the footnote includes a table with values that illustrate the differences in recommendations between a 2,000 calorie and 2,500 calorie diet; for instance, someone eating 2,000 calories should strive to eat less than 65 grams of fat per day, while a person eating 2,500 calories should eat less than 80 grams of fat per day. The table may not be present on the package if the size of the food label is too small. The footnote and the table, when present, are always the same because the information refers to general dietary advice for all Americans rather than to a specific food.

By comparing labels from various foods, you can start designing a more healthful diet today. Try looking at the two labels in Figure 2.3 to decide which food is a more nutritious choice. First, you must decide which nutrients are more important for you. Let's assume you are trying to eat foods with more fiber and vitamin C. The food label on the left shows that cereal 1 contains 2 grams of dietary fiber and 0% DV vitamin C per serving. The food label on the right shows that cereal 2 contains 5 grams of dietary fiber and 15% DV for vitamin C per serving if served with skim milk. For these two nutrients, cereal 2 on the right would be a more nutritious choice.

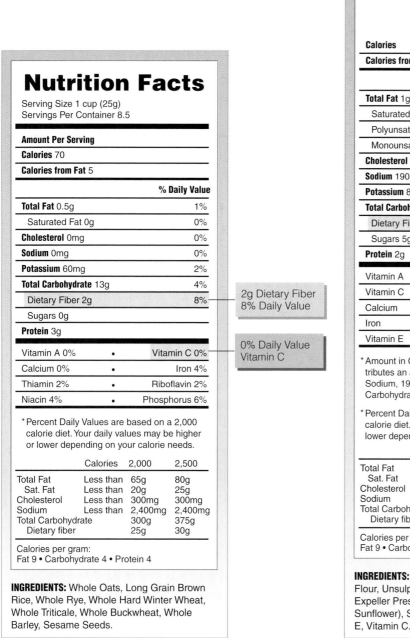

Nutrition Facts

Serving Size 1 cup (25g)
Servings Per Container 8.5

Amount Per Serving

Calories 70

Calories from Fat 5

	% Daily Value
Total Fat 0.5g	1%
Saturated Fat 0g	0%
Cholesterol 0mg	0%
Sodium 0mg	0%
Potassium 60mg	2%
Total Carbohydrate 13g	4%
Dietary Fiber 2g	8%
Sugars 0g	
Protein 3g	

Vitamin A 0%	•	Vitamin C 0%
Calcium 0%	•	Iron 4%
Thiamin 2%	•	Riboflavin 2%
Niacin 4%	•	Phosphorus 6%

* Percent Daily Values are based on a 2,000
calorie diet. Your daily values may be higher
or lower depending on your calorie needs.

	Calories	2,000	2,500
Total Fat	Less than	65g	80g
Sat. Fat	Less than	20g	25g
Cholesterol	Less than	300mg	300mg
Sodium	Less than	2,400mg	2,400mg
Total Carbohydrate		300g	375g
Dietary fiber		25g	30g

Calories per gram:
Fat 9 • Carbohydrate 4 • Protein 4

INGREDIENTS: Whole Oats, Long Grain Brown
Rice, Whole Rye, Whole Hard Winter Wheat,
Whole Triticale, Whole Buckwheat, Whole
Barley, Sesame Seeds.

2g Dietary Fiber
8% Daily Value

0% Daily Value
Vitamin C

(a)

Nutrition Facts

Serving Size 3/4 cup (27g)
Servings Per Container 13

Amount Per Serving

		With 1/2 Cup Vitamin A & D	
		Cereal alone	Fortified Skim Milk
Calories		90	130
Calories from Fat		10	10

		% Daily Value	
Total Fat 1g*		2%	2%
Saturated Fat 0g		0%	0%
Polyunsaturated Fat 0.5g			
Monounsaturated Fat 0.5g			
Cholesterol 0mg		0%	0%
Sodium 190mg		8%	11%
Potassium 85mg		2%	8%
Total Carbohydrate 23g		8%	10%
Dietary Fiber 5g		20%	20%
Sugars 5g			
Protein 2g			
Vitamin A		0%	4%
Vitamin C		10%	15%
Calcium		0%	15%
Iron		2%	2%
Vitamin E		2%	2%

* Amount in Cereal. One half cup skim milk con-
tributes an additional 40 calories, 65mg
Sodium, 190mg Potassium, 6g Total
Carbohydrate (6g sugars), and 4g Protein.

* Percent Daily Values are based on a 2000
calorie diet. Your daily values may be higher or
lower depending on your calorie needs:

	Calories	2,000	2,500
Total Fat	Less than	65g	80g
Sat. Fat	Less than	20g	25g
Cholesterol	Less than	300mg	300mg
Sodium	Less than	2,400mg	2,400mg
Total Carbohydrate		300g	375g
Dietary fiber		25g	30g

Calories per gram:
Fat 9 • Carbohydrate 4 • Protein 4

INGREDIENTS: Yellow Corn Flour, Corn Bran
Flour, Unsulphured Molasses, Oat Flour,
Expeller Pressed High Oleic Oil (Canola and/or
Sunflower), Salt, Baking Soda, Natural Vitamin
E, Vitamin C.

5g Dietary Fiber
20% Daily Value

15% Daily Value
Vitamin C (with
milk)

(b)

Figure 2.3   Labels from two breakfast cereals. Note that there is less fiber and vitamin C in **(a)** cereal 1 than in **(b)** cereal 2.

Using the %DV to Calculate Specific Amounts of Calcium and Vitamin C

The %DV can be used to calculate specific amounts of any nutrient listed on the label. Let's say you are a male who is twenty-three years of age. You are interested in meeting your DRI for both calcium and iron, and you are curious as to how much the food shown in Figure 2.2 contributes to your daily intake of these two nutrients. We will use Table 2.1 and Figure 2.2 to assist us in these calculations.

A. *Calcium:* The %DV for calcium listed on the label (as prepared) is 15%. As you can see in Table 2.1, the RDI for calcium is 1,000 mg. By multiplying the %DV by 1,000 mg, you will get the total amount of calcium (in milligrams) in one serving of this food:

$$15\% = 0.15 \qquad 0.15 \times 1,000 \text{ mg} = 150 \text{ mg}$$

How do we know how much this food contributes to your DRI for calcium? By looking at the inside back cover of this text, you can see that the DRI for calcium for a man twenty-three years of age is 1,000 mg calcium. This value happens to be the same as the DV for calcium used on the label, making this calculation very simple. Thus, this food contributes 15% of your total calcium needs (or DRI) for the day.

B. *Iron:* The %DV for iron listed on the label (as prepared) is 15%. As you can see in Table 2.1, the RDI for iron is 18 mg. By multiplying the %DV by 18 mg, you will get the total amount of iron in mg in one serving of this food:

$$15\% = 0.15 \qquad 0.15 \times 18 \text{ mg} = 2.7 \text{ mg}$$

How do we know how much this food contributes to your DRI for iron? Once again, look on the inside back cover of this text. You can see that the DRI for iron for a man twenty-three years of age is 8 mg. By dividing the amount of iron in milligrams in one serving of this food by the DRI for iron (8 mg) and multiplying by 100, you will get the percentage of your DRI for iron from this food:

$$\frac{2.7 \text{ mg}}{8 \text{ mg}} \times 100 = 33.8\% \text{ of your DRI for iron}$$

These calculations are very helpful when you need to determine how well a food meets your individual nutrient needs based on your gender and age. The %DV are a helpful guide in terms of determining whether a food is high or low in a given nutrient, and the calculations just shown can further assist you when you are someone who does not eat a 2,000 calorie diet or when you want to determine how well your diet is meeting the DRI standards. ●

Gustavo

Nutri-Case

"Until last night, I hadn't stepped inside of a grocery store for ten years, maybe more. But then my wife fell and broke her hip and had to go to the hospital. On my way home from visiting her, I remembered that we didn't have much food in the house, so I thought I'd do a little shopping. Was I ever in for a shock. I don't know how my wife does it, choosing between all the different brands, reading those long labels. She never went to school past sixth grade, and she doesn't speak English very well either! I bought a frozen chicken pie for my dinner, but it didn't taste right. So I got the package out of the trash and read all the labels, and that's when I realized there wasn't any chicken in it at all! It was made out of that soy stuff! This afternoon, my daughter is picking me up, and we're going to do our grocery shopping together!"

Given what you've learned about FDA food labels, what parts of a food package would you advise Gustavo to be sure to read before he makes a choice? What other advice might you give him to make his grocery shopping easier? Imagine that, like Gustavo's wife, you have only limited skills in mathematics and reading. In that case, what other strategies might you use when shopping for nutritious foods?

Recap: Reading food labels is a necessary skill when planning a healthful diet. Food labels must list the identity of the food, the net contents of the package, the contact information for the food manufacturer or distributor, the ingredients in the food, and a Nutrition Facts Panel. The Nutrition Facts Panel provides specific information about calories, macronutrients, and select vitamins and minerals.

Dietary Guidelines for Americans

The **Dietary Guidelines for Americans** (USDA and USDHHS 2000) are a set of principles developed by the U.S. Department of Agriculture and the U.S. Department of Health and Human Services to assist Americans in designing a healthful diet and lifestyle. They are updated every five years, and the current guidelines were published in 2000 (Table 2.2). The goal is to use these as general directives in assisting you with eating a healthful diet. These guidelines emphasize making changes in both food choices and physical activity habits to help reduce our risk for chronic diseases.

The United States is not the only country to develop dietary guidelines. Canada has its own specific nutrition recommendations (Table 2.3), and Canada's Food

Dietary Guidelines for Americans A set of principles developed by the U.S. Department of Agriculture and the U.S. Department of Health and Human Services to assist Americans in designing a healthful diet and lifestyle. These guidelines are updated every five years.

Table 2.2 The Dietary Guidelines for Americans, 2000

Aim for Fitness:	
Aim for a healthy weight.	Be physically active each day.
Build a Healthy Base:	
Let the Pyramid guide your food choices.	Choose a variety of grains daily; especially whole grains.
Choose a variety of fruits and vegetables daily.	Keep food safe to eat.
Choose Sensibly:	
Choose a diet that is low in saturated fat and cholesterol and moderate in total fat.	Choose beverages and foods to moderate your intake of sugars.
Choose and prepare foods with less salt.	If you drink alcoholic beverages, do so in moderation.

U.S. Department of Agriculture, and U.S. Department of Health and Human Services. 2000. Dietary Guidelines for Americans, 2000. 5th ed. Home and Garden Bulletin No. 232. (Available at www.health.gov/dietaryguidelines/dga2000/DIETGD.PDF)

Table 2.3 Nutrition Recommendations for Canadians

The Canadian diet should:
• Provide energy consistent with the maintenance of body weight within the recommended range.
• Include essential nutrients in amounts specified in the Recommended Nutrient Intakes.
• Include no more than 30% of energy as fat (33 grams/1000 calories or 39 grams/5000 kilojoules) and no more than 10% as saturated fat (11 grams/1000 calories or 13 grams/5000 kilojoules).
• Provide 55% of energy as carbohydrate (138 grams/1000 calories or 165 grams/5000 kilojoules) from a variety of sources.
• Be reduced in sodium content.
• Include no more than 5% of total energy as alcohol, or 2 drinks daily, whichever is less.
• Contain no more caffeine than the equivalent of 4 cups of regular coffee per day.
• Community water supplies containing less than 1 mg/liter should be fluoridated to that level.

Source: Health Canada. Office of Nutrition Policy and Promotion. Nutrition Recommendations for Canadians. July 16, 2003. Accessed December 2003. www.hc-sc.gc.ca/hpfb-dgpsa/onpp-bppn/nutrition-canadians-e.html

Guide to Healthy Eating, the corollary to the U.S. Food Guide Pyramid, is in the form of a rainbow (Figure 2.4) and emphasizes eating whole grains, vegetables, fruits, and dairy products each day.

Following is a brief description of each of the Dietary Guidelines for Americans. Refer to Table 2.4 for specific examples of how you might alter your current diet and physical activity habits to meet some of these guidelines.

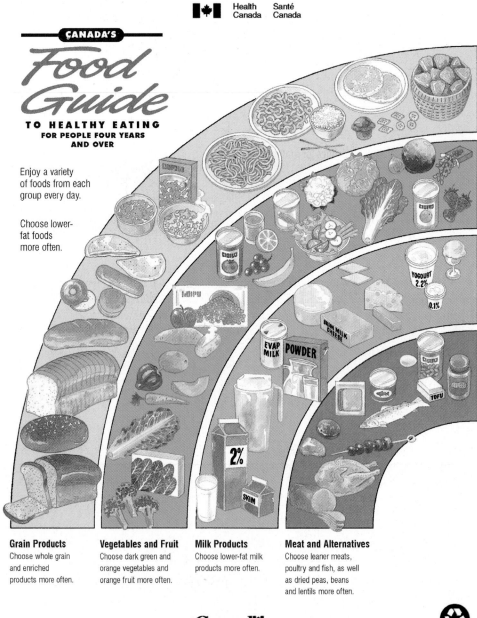

Figure 2.4   Canada's Food Guide to Healthy Eating. This guide emphasizes eating a variety of foods daily and eating lower-fat foods more often. Recommended daily servings for each group is: grain products — 5 to 12 servings per day; vegetables and fruits — 5 to 10 servings per day; milk products — 2 to 4 servings per day for adults; meat and alternatives — 2 to 3 servings per day. (Health Canada, Canada's Food Guide to Healthy Eating, Accessed August 2003, www.hc-sc.gc.ca/hppb/nutrition/pube/foodguid/)

Aim for a Healthy Weight

Being overweight or obese increases our risk for many chronic diseases, including heart disease, type 2 diabetes, stroke, and some forms of cancer. Evaluating your weight includes calculating your body mass index, which is a ratio of your weight to your height. We discuss how to calculate body mass index in Chapter 11. In addition, taking a measure of your waist can give you an indication of your level of overweight. A waist circumference greater than 35 inches for a woman or 40 inches for a man indicates excess abdominal fat, which increases your risk for chronic diseases.

Be Physically Active Each Day

By accumulating at least 30 minutes of moderate physical activity most, preferably all, days of the week can reduce your risk for chronic diseases. Moderate physical activity includes walking, riding a bike, mowing the lawn with a push mower, or performing heavy yard work or housework. Other activities that are beneficial include those that build strength, such as lifting weights, groceries, or other objects, carrying your golf clubs while you walk around the course, and participating in yoga or other flexibility activities. The 30-minute guideline is a minimum; if you are already doing more activity than this, then continue on your healthy path. If you are currently inactive, 30 minutes is a realistic and healthy goal.

Let the Pyramid Guide Your Food Choices

The Dietary Guidelines for Americans encourages using the Food Guide Pyramid when designing a healthful diet. Emphasis is placed on building the base of your diet to include plant foods such as whole grains, fruits, and vegetables and consuming only the recommended number of servings. We discuss how to use the Food Guide Pyramid in detail in the next section (page 50).

Table 2.4 Ways to Incorporate the Dietary Guidelines for Americans into Your Daily Life

If You Normally Do This:	Try Doing This Instead:
Watch television when you get home at night	Do 30 minutes of stretching or lifting of hand weights in front of the television
Drive to the store down the block	Walk to and from the store
Go out to lunch with friends	Take a 15 or 30 minute walk with your friends at lunchtime 3 days each week
Eat white bread with your sandwich	Eat whole wheat bread or some other bread made from whole grains
Eat white rice or fried rice with your meal	Eat brown rice or even try wild rice
Choose cookies or a candy bar for a snack	Choose a fresh nectarine, peach, apple, orange, or banana for a snack
Order French fries with your hamburger	Order a green salad with low-fat salad dressing on the side instead of French fries
Spread butter or margarine on your white toast each morning	Spread fresh fruit compote on whole grain toast
Order a bacon double cheeseburger at your favorite restaurant	Order a turkey burger or grilled chicken sandwich without the cheese and bacon, and add lettuce and tomato
Drink non-diet soft drinks to quench your thirst	Drink diet soft drinks, iced tea, or iced water with a slice of lemon
Eat salted potato chips and pickles with your favorite sandwich	Eat carrot slices and crowns of fresh broccoli and cauliflower dipped in low-fat or nonfat ranch dressing

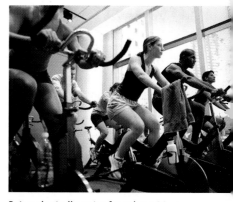

Being physically active for at least 30 minutes each day can reduce your risk for chronic diseases.

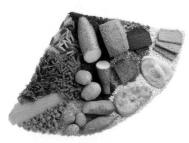

Eating a diet rich in whole grain foods like whole wheat bread and brown rice can enhance your overall health.

Choose a Variety of Grains Daily, Especially Whole Grains

Whole grains are more healthful food choices as they contain more vitamins, minerals, fiber, and other nutrients that enhance our health. Whole grain foods include brown rice, cracked wheat, oatmeal, whole wheat, whole rye, and popcorn.

Choose a Variety of Fruits and Vegetables Daily

Eating a variety of fruits and vegetables is important to ensure that we consume the various nutrients we need to enhance health. A few of the nutrients provided by fruits and vegetables include vitamin A, beta carotene, vitamin C, folate, and potassium. It is recommended that we eat at least 5 servings of fruits and vegetables every day, and healthy choices include fresh, canned, frozen and dried forms.

Keep Food Safe to Eat

A healthful diet is one that is safe from foodborne illnesses like those caused by bacteria, viruses, and other toxins. Food safety is discussed in more detail in Chapter 14. Important tips to remember include storing and cooking foods at the proper temperatures, avoiding unpasteurized juices and milk products and raw or undercooked meats and shellfish, and washing your hands and cooking surfaces before cooking and after handling raw meats, shellfish, and eggs.

Choose a Diet That is Low in Saturated Fat and Cholesterol and Moderate in Total Fat

Fat is an important part of a healthful diet, as it provides energy and important nutrients such as essential fatty acids and fat-soluble vitamins. However, eating a diet high in total fat can lead to overweight and obesity. Eating foods high in saturated fats and cholesterol causes an increase in our blood cholesterol levels, and high blood cholesterol levels increase our risk for heart disease. A healthful diet includes eating foods that provide low amounts of total fat, limiting our intake of solid fats like butter, lard, and margarine, and consuming healthier fat sources such as canola oil, olive oil, and other vegetable oils.

Choose Beverages and Foods to Moderate Your Intake of Sugars

It is important to moderate our intake of foods high in sugar and starch, as these foods promote tooth decay. Avoiding a lot of sugary snacks between meals and brushing our teeth after every meal and before bedtime reduces the risk for cavities. In addition, foods with a lot of added sugars, such as non-diet soft drinks, candies, cakes, and cookies, contribute excess calories to our diet and can cause overweight and obesity when eaten in excess. These foods should be eaten in small amounts only on occasion and should not predominate our regular diet.

Choose and Prepare Foods with Less Salt

Salt contains the mineral sodium, and eating a lot of sodium is linked to high blood pressure in some people. Eating high amounts of sodium also can cause us to lose calcium from our bones, which could increase our risk for bone loss and bone fractures. Much of the salt we consume in our diets comes from processed and prepared foods. Ways to decrease our salt intake include eating fresh, plain frozen, or canned vegetables without salt added, limiting our intake of processed meats such as cured ham, sausage, bacon, and most canned meats, and looking for foods with labels that say "low-sodium." In addition, adding little or no salt to foods at home and limiting our intake of salty condiments such as ketchup, mustard, pickles, soy sauce, and olives can help reduce our salt intake.

If You Drink Alcoholic Beverages, Do So in Moderation

Alcoholic beverages provide us with calories, but they do not contain any nutrients. Drinking alcoholic beverages in excess can lead to many health and social problems. Moderation is defined as no more than one drink per day for women and no more than two drinks per day for men. To learn more about whether or not alcohol can be part of a healthful diet, refer to the Nutrition Myth or Fact box on the next page.

When grocery shopping, try to select foods that are moderate in total fat, sugar, and salt.

Alcohol Can Be Part of a Healthful Diet

The effects of excessive alcohol consumption are well known. Alcohol is an addictive, toxic substance that can cause liver cirrhosis and brain damage, increase our risk for certain cancers and heart disease, and lead to numerous birth defects if consumed during pregnancy. Recent evidence has shown that even relatively small amounts of alcohol can cause birth defects and may possibly increase the risk for breast cancer. Although alcohol provides energy (7 kcal per gram) and is therefore considered a food, it is not considered a nutrient, as it is not essential to our bodies and performs no necessary functions.

Because alcohol is toxic and increases our risk for many diseases, the Dietary Guidelines for Americans recommend that, "If you drink alcoholic beverages, do so in moderation." *Drinking in moderation* is defined as no more than one drink per day for women and no more than two drinks per day for men. A drink is defined as:

- 12 ounces of regular beer (about 150 kcal)
- 5 ounces of wine (about 100 kcal)
- 1.5 ounces of 80-proof distilled spirits (hard liquor such as vodka or whiskey; about 100 kcal)

By the way, drinking 7 or 8 drinks in one night and abstaining for 6 nights does not average out to moderate drinking! This type of behavior, called *binge drinking,* is defined as the consumption of at least four drinks in a row for women and at least five drinks in a row for men. Binge drinking is common among college students and occurs more frequently in people with a past drinking history, a family history of alcohol abuse, and in members of athletic teams, fraternities, and sororities (Weschsler et al. 2000; Weschsler et al. 1995).

The negative health effects of binge drinking include liver damage, dehydration, loss of consciousness, and damage to the brain and heart—all due to the rapid accumulation of alcohol in the blood. In addition to the negative health effects of binge drinking, the behavioral consequences of binge drinking include damaged property, academic problems, having unprotected sex, getting injured, and drinking and driving. An interesting study done at Johns Hopkins University looked at the link between alcohol intake and bicycling accidents (Li et al. 2001). Of 124 accidents in Maryland involving bicyclists ages 15 years and older, 24% of those who died and 9% of those seriously injured had blood alcohol levels that would indicate impairment. Thus, just as with driving your car, riding your bike when you have been drinking significantly increases your chances of bodily injury or death. Many young people on college campuses have died as a result of binge drinking, highlighting the extreme dangers of this behavior.

People who should entirely avoid drinking alcoholic beverages include:

- Children and adolescents
- Individuals of any age who cannot restrict their drinking to moderate levels
- Women who may think they are or who are pregnant
- Individuals who plan to drive any sort of vehicle, operate machinery, or take part in other activities that require attention, skill, or coordination
- Individuals taking prescription or over-the-counter medications that can interact with alcohol

There are some studies showing that regular, moderate consumption of red wine reduces the risk for heart disease (Wollin and Jones 2001). The alcohol in wine may be partly responsible, as it can reduce the thickness of blood and has beneficial effects on our cholesterol levels. These are factors that are known to reduce heart disease risk. Although drinking red wine may have some health benefits, you can decrease your risk for heart disease much more effectively by adopting behaviors such as eating less total fat and saturated fat, reducing sodium intake, and exercising regularly. Interestingly, a recent study found that drinking only one drink per day significantly increased a woman's risk for breast cancer (Smith-Warner et al. 1998). More research is needed on this topic, however, before moderate alcohol intake can be defined as a risk factor for breast cancer. From this information you should be able to see that there is no strong justification to encourage people to drink alcoholic beverages on a regular basis. If you don't drink, don't start. If you do drink, do so in moderation. ●

Recap: The Dietary Guidelines for Americans emphasize healthful food choices and physical activity behaviors. The guidelines include achieving a healthy weight, being physically active each day, using the Food Guide Pyramid to select foods, eating whole grain foods, fruits and vegetables daily, keeping foods safe to eat, eating foods low in saturated fat and cholesterol and moderate in total fat, moderating sugar intake, eating less salt, and drinking alcohol in moderation, if at all.

The Food Guide Pyramid

Food Guide Pyramid   Illustration developed by the U.S. Department of Agriculture (USDA) to provide Americans with a conceptual framework for the types and amounts of foods we can eat in combination to achieve a healthful diet.

The U.S. Department of Agriculture (USDA) **Food Guide Pyramid** is another tool that can guide you in designing a healthful diet. It was created as a guide to provide a conceptual framework for the types and amounts of foods we can eat in combination to provide a healthful diet. It is important to remember that the Food Guide Pyramid is an evolving document, and it will continue to change as we learn more about the roles of specific nutrients and foods in promoting health and preventing disease.

As you can see in Figure 2.5, the pyramid is composed of sections that represent various categories of foods. Indicated beside each category is the recommended number of servings per day from each group. Notice that, as you look from the bottom to the top of the pyramid, the size of each group becomes smaller, indicating that a person should eat more of the foods at the base of the pyramid, and less of the foods at the top of the pyramid.

The base of the pyramid is the bread, cereal, rice, and pasta food group, and these foods should form the "base" of our daily dietary intake. The foods in this group are clustered together because they provide complex carbohydrates and fiber and are good sources of the nutrients riboflavin, thiamin, niacin, iron, folate, zinc, protein, and magnesium. Above this base sit the vegetable and the fruit groups. Fruits and vegetables are good sources of many of the same nutrients, including carbohydrate, fiber, vitamins A and C, folate, potassium, and magnesium. These two groups are separated in the pyramid as they do not contain all of the same nutrients and eating a variety of *both* fruits and vegetables is important in ensuring our consumption of many vital nutrients. Fruits and vegetables also contain differing amounts and types of naturally occurring chemicals that enhance our health, and these chemicals are referred to as phytochemicals. A detailed explanation of phytochemicals is presented in Chapter 8. You may be interested to learn that many nutrition experts are proposing that the government should switch the position of the bread, cereal, rice, and pasta group with that of the fruit and vegetable groups. This proposal is based on the fact that many individuals consume excess amounts of breads, pastas, and cereals made with refined flour, which has been speculated to lead to overweight and obesity. There is evidence to suggest that the base of a healthful diet may indeed revolve around eating ample servings of fruits and vegetables, supporting the reorganization of the current Food Guide Pyramid.

Perched above the fruits and vegetables are two groups of equivalent size: the milk, yogurt, and cheese group, and the meat, poultry, fish, dry beans, eggs, and nuts group. The milk, yogurt, and cheese group includes foods that are good sources of calcium, phosphorus, riboflavin, protein, vitamin B_{12}; many of these foods are also fortified with vitamins D and A. The meat, poultry, fish, dry beans, eggs, and nuts group is comprised of foods that are good sources of protein, phosphorus, vitamin B_6, vitamin B_{12}, zinc, magnesium, iron, zinc, niacin, riboflavin, and thiamin. Notice that legumes, which include dried beans, peas, and lentils, are included both in the meat group and in the vegetable group. This is because legumes are good sources of fiber and contain many of the vitamins found in vegetables and are also good sources of protein and of some of the minerals found in meat and poultry.

Food Guide Pyramid
A Guide to Daily Food Choices

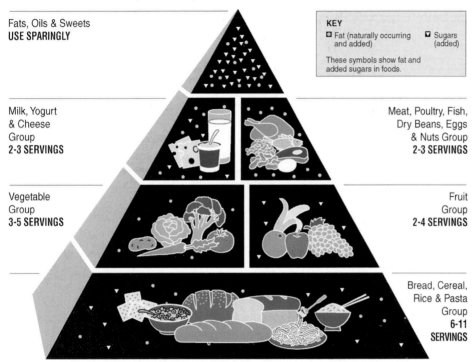

Source: U.S. Department of Agriculture/U.S. Department of Health and Human Services

Figure 2.5 The USDA Food Guide Pyramid. This Pyramid lists the various food groups and the recommended number of servings for each group. The number of servings you should eat is dependent upon your body size and activity level. In general, the lowest recommended number of servings is appropriate for inactive people, small females, and older individuals. The highest recommended number of servings is appropriate for very active, larger females and moderately active males. For more specific information on serving sizes and food groups, refer to the booklet at www.usda.gov/cnpp/pyrabklt.pdf.

At the top of the pyramid are fats, oils, and sweets. This is not really a food group, but a designation to draw attention to foods that we should eat sparingly. Foods included in this group are those high in fat such as butter, margarine, lard, salad dressings, oils, mayonnaise, sour cream, cream, and gravy. This group also includes high sugar foods such as candies, desserts, gelatin, soft drinks, and fruit drinks. Alcoholic beverages are also included in this group.

The Food Guide Pyramid also helps you decide *how much* of each food you should eat. Notice that, for each of the groups contained in the pyramid, there is a range of recommended servings. The lower number of suggested servings in each group applies to adults who are smaller in size or less active. The higher number of suggested servings in each group applies to adults who are larger in size or more active. Table 2.5 shows a sample diet at four different energy intake levels. As you can see in this table, highly active men may require over 3500 kcal per day. An individual with this high level of activity would need to eat more servings than suggested in the Food Guide Pyramid. Also notice that Table 2.5 identifies variations for infants, children, and pregnant and lactating women. Let's now discuss exactly what is meant by serving size when using the Food Guide Pyramid.

Table 2.5   Sample Diets from the Food Guide Pyramid at Four Different Energy Intakes

Energy Intake Food Group			
	Low (~1600 kcal/d[1])	Moderate (~2200 kcal/d[1])	High (~2800 kcal/d[1])	Very High (~3500 kcal/d[1])
Bread, cereal, rice, and pasta	6 servings	9 servings	11 servings	12 servings
Vegetables	3 servings	4 servings	5 servings	6 servings
Fruit	2 servings	3 servings	4 servings	10 servings
Milk, yogurt, and cheese	2–3 servings[2]	2–3 servings[2]	2–3 servings[2]	5 servings
Meat, poultry, fish, dry beans, eggs, and nuts	5 ounces	6 ounces	7 ounces	7 ounces
Total fat[3]	53 grams	73 grams	93 grams	~105 grams
Sugar[4]	6 teaspoons	12 teaspoons	18 teaspoons	~28 teaspoons

Note: Eat at least the lowest recommended number of servings for each food group in the Pyramid.
- About 1,600 kcal per day (kcal/d) is right for very sedentary women and some older adults.
- About 2,200 kcal/d is right for most children, teenage girls, moderately active women, and many sedentary men. Women who are pregnant or breastfeeding may need more.
- About 2,800 kcal/d is right for teenage boys, many active men, and some very active women.
- About 3,500 kcal/d is right for active teenage boys, active men, and some unusually active women.
- Very active men will need more than 3,500 kcal/d.

[1]These are the calorie levels if you choose low-fat, lean foods from the five major food groups and use foods from the fat, oils, and sweet group sparingly.
[2]Women who are pregnant or breastfeeding, teenagers, and young adults to age 24 need 3 servings per day.
[3]These are estimates based on the common fat content of foods (1 pat of butter or margarine = 4 grams of fat).
[4]These are estimates based on the common added sugar content of foods (1 tsp = 4 grams of sugar).

Source: Adapted from M. M. Manore and J. Thompson. 2000. Sport Nutrition for Health and Performance. Champaign, IL: Human Kinetics Publishers.

What Does Serving Size Mean in the Food Guide Pyramid?

What is considered a serving size for the foods listed in the Food Guide Pyramid? Figure 2.6 shows examples of serving sizes for foods in each group and includes a comparison to a familiar item that may make it easier to estimate serving size. A serving from the bread group is defined as one slice of bread, ½ of a regular hotdog or hamburger bun, or a 6-inch tortilla. A serving of vegetables is 1 cup of raw leafy vegetables such as spinach, or ½ cup of chopped raw or cooked vegetables such as broccoli. A serving of meat is 2 to 3 ounces, which is approximately the size of a deck of cards. Although it may seem unnatural and inconvenient to measure our food servings, understanding the size of a serving is critical to planning a nutritious diet.

It is important to understand that there is no standardized definition for a serving size for any food. A serving size as defined in the Food Guide Pyramid may not be equal to a serving size defined on a food label. For instance, the serving size for crackers in the Food Guide Pyramid is 3 to 4 small crackers, whereas a serving size for crackers on a food label can range from 5 to 18 crackers, depending upon the size and weight of the cracker. In addition, the defined weight of a "medium-sized" serving in the Food Guide Pyramid is typically much smaller than the foods we buy for consumption. Unfortunately, this lack of standardization in serving size leads to confusion among consumers. This confusion is illustrated by the results of a study conducted by Young and Nestle (1998) in which introductory nutrition students were asked to bring to class one sample of a "medium" bagel, baked potato, muffin, apple, or cookie. The weights of these foods were measured, and most of the foods the students brought to class well exceeded the definition of "medium" from the Food Guide Pyramid—in fact, many were twice as large as those defined in the Food Guide Pyramid. Thus, when using tools to assist you with designing a healthful diet, it is

Food group	Number of servings	Examples of serving sizes			
Milk, yogurt and cheese group	2-3	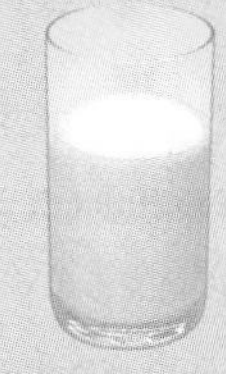 1 cup (8 fl. oz.) milk	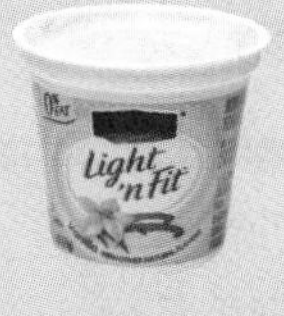 1 cup (8 fl. oz.) yogurt	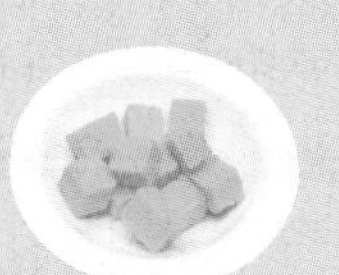 1.5 oz. hard cheese	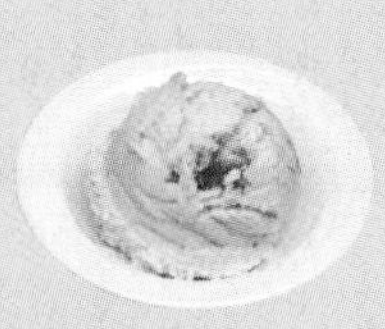 1 scoop of ice cream
Meat, Poultry, Fish, Dry Beans, Eggs and Nuts group	2-3	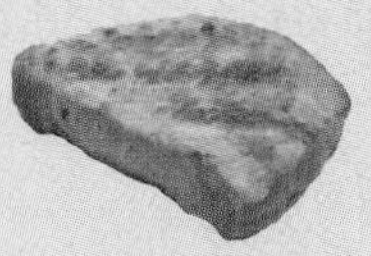 2-3 oz. pork loin chop	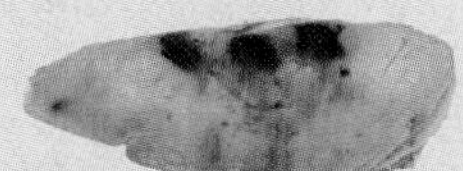 2-3 oz. chicken breast without skin	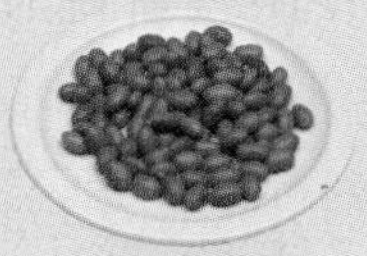 1/2 cup pinto beans	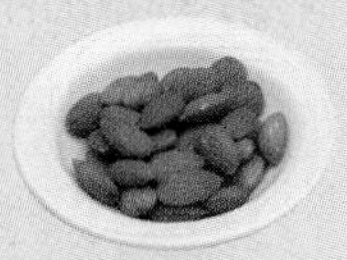 1/3 cup (~1 oz.) almonds
Vegetable group	3-5	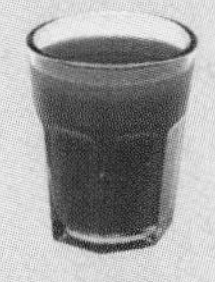 3/4 cup (6 fl. oz.) tomato juice	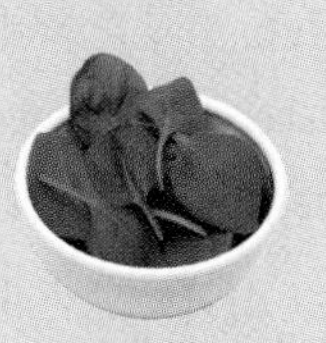 1 cup raw spinach	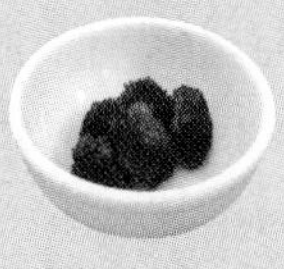 1/2 cup cooked broccoli	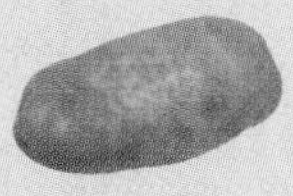 1 medium potato
Fruit group	2-4	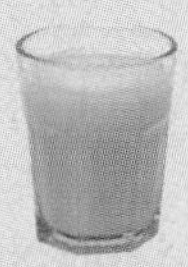 3/4 cup (6 fl. oz.) orange juice	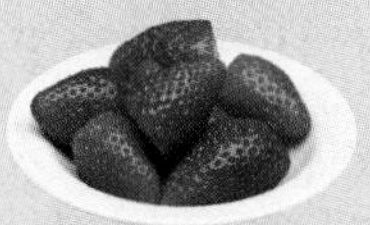 1/2 cup strawberries	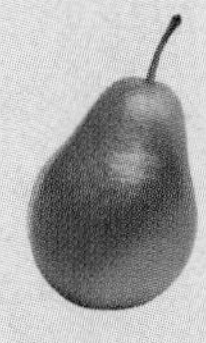 1 medium pear	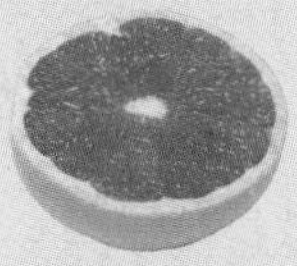 1/2 pink grapefruit
Bread, Cereal, Rice and Pasta group	6-11	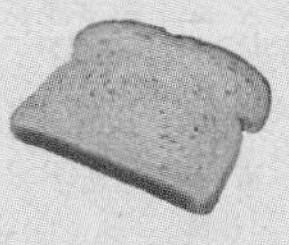 1 (1 oz.) slice of whole wheat bread	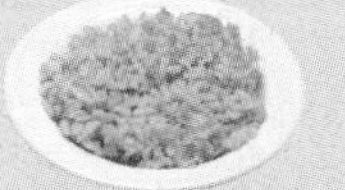 1/2 cup cooked brown rice	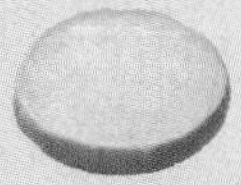 1/2 regular hamburger bun	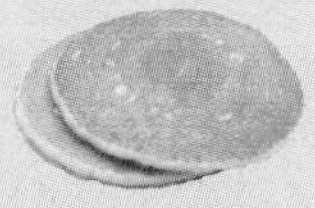 2 pancakes (4" diameter)

Figure 2.6   Examples of serving sizes for foods in each food group of the USDA Food Guide Pyramid. Here are some examples of household items that can help you estimate serving sizes: 1.5 ounce of hard cheese is equal to 4 stacked dice, 1 standard ice cream scoop is $1/2$ cup, 3 ounces of meat is equal in size to a deck of cards, a medium fruit is equal to a tennis ball, a medium potato is equal to a standard computer mouse, and $1/2$ of a regular hamburger bun is the size of a yo-yo.

How Realistic Are the Serving Sizes Listed on Food Labels?

Many people read food labels to determine the energy (i.e., caloric) value of foods, but it is less common to pay close attention to the actual serving size that corresponds to the listed caloric value. To test how closely your "naturally selected" serving size meets the actual serving size of certain foods, try these label activities:

- Choose a breakfast cereal that you commonly eat. Pour the amount of cereal that you would normally eat into a bowl. Before pouring any milk on your cereal, use a measuring cup to measure the actual amount of cereal you usually eat. Now read the label of the cereal to determine the serving size (for example, ½ cup or 1 cup) and the caloric value listed on the label. How do your "naturally selected" serving size and the label-defined serving size compare?

- At your local grocery store, locate various boxes of snack crackers. Look at the number of crackers and total calories per serving listed on the labels of crackers such as regular Triscuits, reduced fat Triscuits, Vegetable Thins, and Ritz crackers. How do the number of crackers and total calories per serving differ for the serving size listed on each box? How do the serving sizes listed in the nutrition facts label compare to how many crackers you would usually eat?

These activities are just two examples of ways to understand how nutrition labels can assist the consumer with making balanced and healthy food choices. As many people do not know what constitutes a serving size, they are inclined to consume too much of some foods (such as snack foods and meat) and too little of other foods (such as fruits and vegetables). ●

important to learn the definition of serving size for the tool you are using, and *then* measure your food intake to determine if you are meeting the guidelines.

When comparing a serving size from the Food Guide Pyramid with serving sizes listed on food labels, it is important to remember that food manufacturers identify the serving sizes of all canned and packaged foods on Nutrition Fact Labels. Unfortunately, relying on the labels of packaged foods to determine serving sizes can lead to higher food intakes than you may desire. The serving sizes defined in the Food Guide Pyramid are relatively small. Although in recent years food manufacturers have labeled serving sizes more realistically, in some cases they still do not match the sizes suggested in the Food Guide Pyramid. As a result, you must become an educated consumer and learn to read labels skeptically because the serving size you might typically eat can be very different from those defined by the Food Guide Pyramid or on food labels. Try the Nutrition Label Activity to determine whether the serving sizes listed on assorted food labels match the serving sizes that you normally consume.

> **Recap:** The USDA Food Guide Pyramid can be used to plan a healthful, balanced diet that includes 6 to 11 servings of whole grains, cereals and breads; 2 to 4 servings of fruit; 3 to 5 servings of vegetables; 2 to 3 servings of meat, poultry, fish, dried beans, eggs, and nuts; 2 to 3 servings of dairy foods; and few fats, oils, or sweets each day. The serving sizes of foods as defined in the Food Guide Pyramid typically are smaller than the amounts we normally eat or are served, so it is important to learn the definition of servings sizes when using the Food Guide Pyramid to design a healthful diet.

Variations of the Food Guide Pyramid

One of the most useful things about the Food Guide Pyramid is that it can be easily adapted to meet the dietary needs of a wide variety of people. For instance, Houtkooper (1994) modified the standard Food Guide Pyramid for athletes by including fluids as a new food category at the base of the pyramid, emphasizing the importance of daily fluid replacement for active people. There are also Pyramids for children and for adults over the age of 70 years (USDA 1999; Tufts University 1999).

The Mediterranean Diet and Pyramid

A Mediterranean-style diet has received significant attention in recent years, as the rates of cardiovascular disease in many Mediterranean countries are substantially lower than rates in the United States. There is actually not a single Mediterranean diet, as this region of the world includes Portugal, Spain, Italy, France, Greece, Turkey, and Israel. Each of these countries has different dietary patterns; however, there are similarities that have led nutrition researchers to speculate that this type of diet is more healthful than the typical U.S. diet:

- Meats, eggs, and sweets are eaten only a few times each week, making the diet low in saturated fats and refined sugars.

- The predominant fat used for cooking and flavor is olive oil, making the diet high in monounsaturated fats.

- Foods eaten daily include: grains such as bread, pasta, couscous, and bulgur; fruits; beans and other legumes; nuts; vegetables; and cheese and yogurt. These choices make this diet high in fiber and rich in vitamins and minerals.

As you can see in Figure 2.7b, the base of the Mediterranean Pyramid is similar to that of the U.S. Food Guide Pyramid, as it includes breads, cereals, and other grains. Another similarity is the daily intake of fruits and vegetables. The two Pyramids differ in several important aspects. The Mediterranean Pyramid includes beans, other legumes, and nuts daily; fish, poultry, and eggs are eaten a few times each week (not daily); and red meat is eaten only a few times each month. The Mediterranean Pyramid highlights cheese and yogurt as the primary dairy sources and recommends daily consumption of olive oil. Two unique features of the Mediterranean diet are the inclusion of wine and daily physical activity.

Interestingly, the Mediterranean diet is not lower in fat; in fact, about 40% of the total energy in this diet is derived from fat, which is much higher than the dietary fat recommendations made in the United States. This fact has led some nutritionists to criticize the Mediterranean diet. Supporters point out that the majority of fats in the Mediterranean diet are healthier fats than the animal fats found in the U.S. diet, which makes the Mediterranean diet more protective against cardiovascular disease. The potential benefits of the Mediterranean diet in reducing our cholesterol levels and reducing our risk for heart disease are discussed in Chapter 5.

Can following a Mediterranean-style diet really improve your health? In June of 1995, an entire supplement issue of the *American Journal of Clinical Nutrition* reviewed the most recent findings on the Mediterranean diet. Renaud et al. (1995) studied the effects of a Mediterranean diet on individuals living in Crete who were recovering from a heart attack. These researchers found that those who ate a Mediterranean diet had a much lower risk of recurrent heart attack and premature death than individuals who followed the heart healthy diet prescribed by their doctors. Tavani and La Vecchia (1995) reported that people from Italy who ate more fruits and vegetables as a part of a Mediterranean diet had significantly lower risks of some types of cancers, particularly cancers of the mouth, esophagus, stomach, lung, and intestines. These studies indicate that eating a Mediterranean-style diet that includes more fruits and vegetables, less meat, and few high-fat dairy products does reduce the risks for heart disease and some cancers. ●

There are also many ethnic and cultural variations of the Food Guide Pyramid. As you know, the population of the United States is culturally and ethnically diverse, and this diversity influences our food choices. Foods that we may typically consider a part of an Asian, Latin American, or Mediterranean diet can also fit into a healthful diet. Variations of the standard USDA Food Guide Pyramid that have been introduced include the Vegetarian Diet Pyramid, the Mediterranean Diet Pyramid, the Latin American Diet Pyramid, and the Asian Diet Pyramid (Figure 2.7). There are also variations for Arabic, Chinese, Cuban, Italian, Mexican, Portuguese, Russian, and Native American foods (Food and Nutrition Information Center 2002). These variations illustrate that anyone can design a healthful diet to accommodate their individual food preferences.

Of these variations, the Mediterranean Diet has enjoyed considerable popularity. Does it deserve its reputation as a healthful diet? Check out the Highlight box to learn more about the Mediterranean Diet.

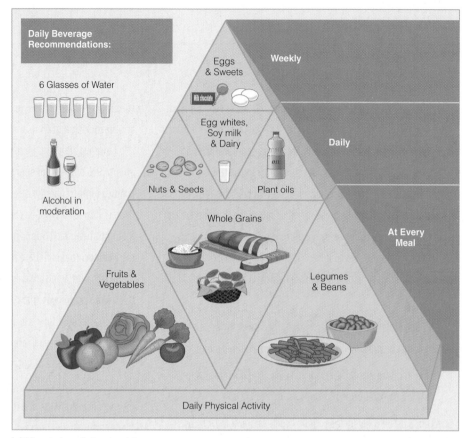

(a) Vegetarian diet pyramid

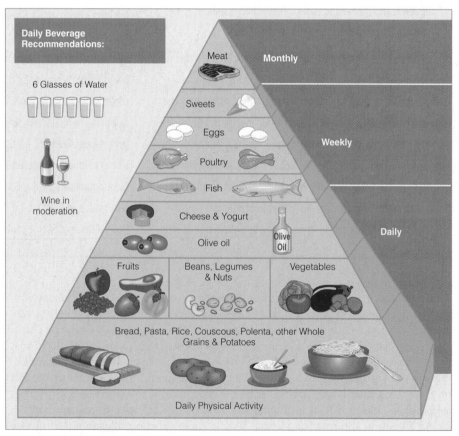

(b) Mediterranean diet pyramid

Figure 2.7 Ethnic and cultural variations of the USDA Food Guide Pyramid. **(a)** The Vegetarian Diet Pyramid. **(b)** The Mediterranean Diet Pyramid. (© 2000 Oldways Preservation and Exchange Trust. The Food Issues Think Tank. Healthy Eating Pyramids & Other Tools. www.oldwayspt.org. Accessed September 2002.)

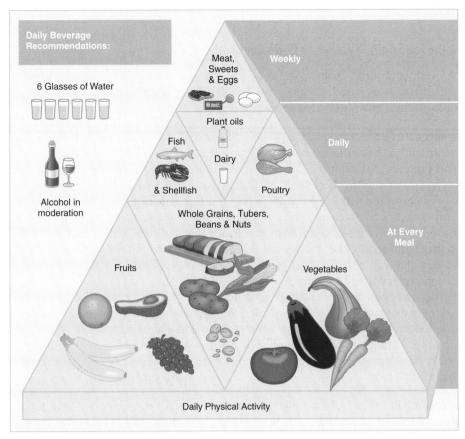

(c) Latin American diet pyramid

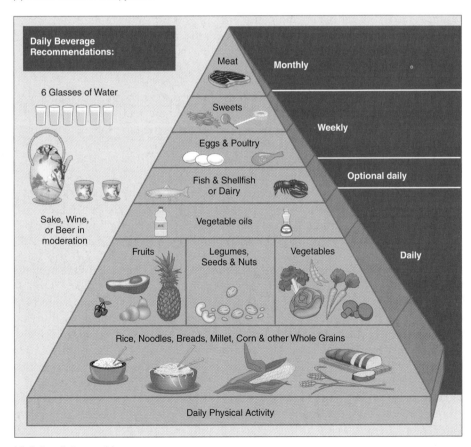

(d) Asian diet pyramid

Figure 2.7 *Continued.* **(c)** The Latin American Diet Pyramid. **(d)** The Asian Diet Pyramid. (© 2000 Oldways Preservation and Exchange Trust. The Food Issues Think Tank. Healthy Eating Pyramids & Other Tools. www.oldwayspt.org. Accessed September 2002.)

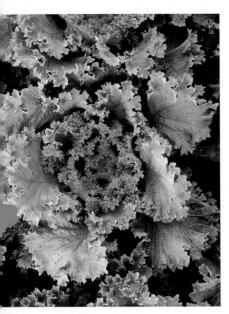

In addition to dairy products, kale is an excellent source of calcium.

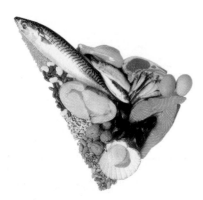

Seafood, meat, poultry, dry beans, eggs, and nuts are examples of foods that are high in protein.

Using The Food Guide Pyramid to Design a Healthful Diet

At the beginning of this chapter, we identified four key characteristics of a healthful diet: adequacy, moderation, balance, and variety. Let's look at how we can use the principles in the Food Guide Pyramid to design a diet with all four characteristics.

Eat an Adequate Diet   As we said earlier, an adequate diet provides enough of the energy, nutrients, and fiber to maintain a person's health. For example, the Food Guide Pyramid suggests that adults eat 2 to 3 servings of milk, yogurt, or cheese each day. However, you may avoid dairy products because they upset your digestive system, because of religious restrictions, or because you don't like the taste of them. As many dairy products are an excellent source of calcium, you will need to replace them with other foods that provide calcium, such as calcium-fortified orange juice and soy milk, turnip greens, broccoli, kale, black-eyed peas, or sardines. If you don't, your diet will be deficient in calcium, which puts you at risk for excessive bone loss and its related health consequences (see Chapter 9).

Eating an adequate diet means practicing optimal energy control. Failing to eat enough energy deprives your body of adequate nutrients. Eating too much energy will eventually result in weight gain, which will lead to obesity if left uncontrolled for too long. Eating an optimal number of servings as recommended in the Food Guide Pyramid helps you maintain the proper balance of energy in your diet. Refer to Chapter 11 (page 390) for a review on calculating your daily energy needs.

Eat in Moderation   You've heard the saying "Everything in moderation." This is an appropriate adage to keep in mind when planning your diet. The Food Guide Pyramid helps you eat moderately by recommending certain numbers of servings for you to consume each day. Eating too much of certain foods, such as those high in fat and added sugar, leads to weight gain and could prevent you from consuming adequate vitamins, minerals, and fiber. For this reason, foods at the top of the pyramid should be eaten only occasionally and in small amounts. Practicing moderation allows you to eat more nutritious foods without overeating.

Eat a Balanced Diet   The Food Guide Pyramid is designed to assist you with planning a diet that provides the proper balance of nutrients by eating the appropriate number of servings from each food group. If you are looking for foods high in protein, excellent sources are meat, poultry, fish, dry beans, eggs, nuts, milk, yogurt, and cheese. In general, meat, fish, and poultry are also high in iron and zinc, but dairy foods are low in these minerals. So if you use dairy products such as milk and yogurt as your primary protein sources, you could develop a deficiency of zinc and iron over time. Thus, designing a healthful diet is a balancing act, requiring you to eat enough (but not too much) of foods from each group. Each of the groups in the Pyramid plays a critical role in this balancing act, so no group should be completely substituted for another.

Eat a Variety of Foods   By following the Food Guide Pyramid, you will quite naturally be eating a variety of foods. Another way to see if you are varying your foods is to look at the colors on your plate. A healthy choice of foods generally is represented by many colors, including green, red, deep yellow or orange, brown, and white. But why should you strive to eat a wide variety of different foods each day? Well, even if all your food choices are healthful, you can limit the nutrients in your diet by always eating the same foods. Eating a wide variety of foods not only helps you to reach your nutrient goals, but also prevents you from feeling bored or deprived, as you could if your diet were extremely limited.

About ten years ago, the results of a national survey suggested that limiting your food choices might even be hazardous to your health! A study of the nutritional habits and health of people in the United States found that people who ate a limited variety of foods, or foods from two or fewer of the food groups in the Food Guide Pyramid, had a 1.5 times higher risk of premature death than people who ate foods from all five food groups (Kant et al. 1993). This was true across all age groups, at

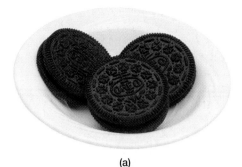
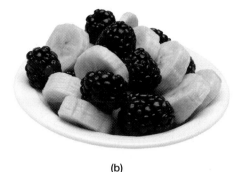

(a)   (b)

Figure 2.8   Examples of foods that are low and high in nutrient density. **(a)** Three chocolate sandwich cookies. **(b)** The combination of one medium banana and ½ cup fresh blackberries. Each bowl of food provides approximately 145 kcal. The cookies provide 56 kcal from fat (6.2 grams), 1 gram of fiber, and very few vitamins and minerals. The fruit combination provides almost 7 grams of fiber, 7.65 kcal from fat (0.85 grams), and a significant amount of other nutrients such as potassium (608 mg), vitamin A (21 RE), and vitamin C (26 mg). For our limited daily energy budget, the fruit is more nutrient dense and a more healthful choice. (Calculated using USDA Nutrient Database for Standard Reference, Release 15, September 2002.)

every level of education and income, for every race, and for both smokers and non-smokers. Unfortunately, the study did not attempt to explain the association between a limited diet and premature death; however, it is clear that limiting the variety of foods you eat can result in nutritional inadequacies.

Choose Foods High in Nutrient Density   As a general guideline, you should choose foods high in **nutrient density**. This means eating foods that give you the highest amount of nutrients for the least amount of energy (or calories). As an example, three Oreo cookies provide the same number of calories as a medium banana and ½ cup of fresh blackberries. Yet as you might guess, the density of nutrients in the fruit is far superior, giving you more true nourishment per calorie (Figure 2.8).

A helpful analogy for selecting nutrient-dense foods is shopping for clothes on a tight budget. If you had only $40 in your clothing budget, you would most likely buy two pairs of pants on sale for $20 each instead of one pair of pants for $40. Because you can only "afford" a certain number of calories each day to maintain a healthy weight, it makes sense to maximize the nutrients you can get for each calorie you consume. Table 2.6 provides a comparison of one day of meals that are high in nutrient density to meals that are low in nutrient density. This example can assist you in selecting the most nutrient-dense foods when planning your meals.

nutrient density The relative amount of nutrients per amount of energy (or number of calories).

Compare Your Diet to the Food Guide Pyramid   Considering these principles, how can you proceed with planning your diet? Try logging on to the Web site for the Interactive Healthy Eating Index (www.usda.gov/cnpp). This Web site is maintained by the USDA and contains an online dietary assessment tool that scores the overall quality of your diet based on the Food Guide Pyramid. You can analyze a diet for a single day or up to 20 days. The score for the highest quality diet is 100.

Nadia *Nutri-Case*

Before her pregnancy, Nadia used the USDA Web site to analyze one day of her diet. Figure 2.9 shows the results of this analysis. As you can see, Nadia's overall Healthy Eating Index (HEI) score was 66.4. Her diet for this day was too high in total fat, saturated fat, and sodium. Her personal pyramid did not match the recommended pyramid as she ate too few foods from the fruit, meat, dairy, and grains groups. What specific foods could Nadia eat to improve the quality of her diet?

Table 2.6   A Comparison of One Day's Meals that Contain Foods High in Nutrient Density
to Meals that Contain Foods Low in Nutrient Density

Meals with Foods High in Nutrient Density	Meals with Foods Low in Nutrient Density
Breakfast: 1 cup cooked oatmeal with ½ cup skim milk 1 slice whole-wheat toast with 1 tsp. butter 6 fl. oz. grapefruit juice	**Breakfast:** 1 cup puffed rice cereal with ½ cup whole milk 1 slice white toast with 1 tsp. butter 6 fl. oz. grape drink
Snack: 1 peeled orange 1 cup non-fat yogurt	**Snack:** 1 12-ounce can orange soft drink 1.5 ounces cheddar cheese

Lunch:
Turkey sandwich
    3 oz. turkey breast
    2 slices whole-grain bread
    2 tsp. Dijon mustard
    3 slices fresh tomato
    2 leaves red leaf lettuce
1 cup baby carrots with broccoli crowns
20 fl. oz. cola soft drink
	Lunch:
	Hamburger
	    3 oz. cooked regular ground beef
	    1 white hamburger bun
	    2 tsp. Dijon mustard
	    1 tbsp. tomato ketchup
	    2 leaves iceberg lettuce
	1 snack-sized bag potato chips
	20 fl. oz. (2.5 cups) water

Snack: ½ whole wheat bagel 1 tbsp. peanut butter 1 medium apple	**Snack:** 3 chocolate sandwich cookies 1 12-oz can diet soft drink 10 Gummi Bears candy

Dinner:
Spinach salad
    1 cup fresh spinach leaves
    ¼ cup diced tomatoes
    ¼ cup diced green pepper
    ½ cup kidney beans
    1 tbsp. fat-free Italian salad dressing
3 oz. broiled chicken breast
½ cup cooked brown rice
½ cup steamed broccoli
8 fl. oz. (1 cup) skim milk
	Dinner:
	Green salad
	    1 cup iceberg lettuce
	    ¼ cup diced tomatoes
	    1 tsp. green onions
	    ¼ cup bacon bits
	    1 tbsp. regular Ranch salad dressing
	3 oz. beef round steak, breaded and fried
	½ cup cooked white rice
	½ cup sweet corn
	8 fl. oz. (1 cup) iced tea

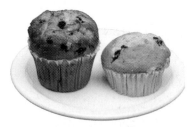

Although the serving size of a "medium" muffin in the Food Guide Pyramid is 1.5 ounces, many muffins sold today range in size from 2 to 8 ounces.

Limitations of the Food Guide Pyramid

Although the Food Guide Pyramid is a very useful tool you can use when designing a healthful diet, it does have its limitations. As discussed in the previous section, the serving sizes as defined in the Food Guide Pyramid are relatively small and do not always coincide with the standard amounts of food we buy, prepare, and serve. Some nutrition professionals believe these serving sizes are unrealistic, and it has been suggested that the serving sizes should be redefined to more closely match the amount of food people typically eat. For instance, the serving size of a "medium" muffin in the Food Guide Pyramid is 1.5 ounces, but many of the muffins sold today range in size from 2 to 8 ounces. This means that many people eat 2 to 4 servings as defined by the Food Guide Pyramid, even though they are eating only one muffin. It might be more realistic to define a serving size for a muffin as one-quarter or one-half of a "medium" muffin, as this would more closely match the size of muffins people choose and still meet the recommended weight of a muffin as defined by the Food Guide Pyramid. This type of alteration could reduce confusion for consumers.

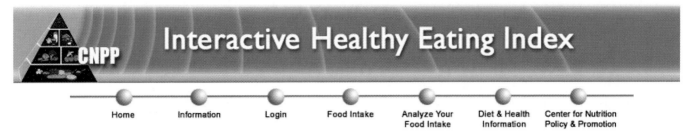

Here is the food displayed for Nadia on 10/1/2003

Select your serving sizes and specify how many servings you consumed for each. When you are done, click on Save & Analyze to save your food entry information and to analyze your food intake. If you want to make more than one day's food entry, click on Return to Login to save a day's food entry information and make another day's food entry. For a record of today's food entry, click Print Food Record prior to saving food entry. To return to initial values, click on the Reset Values. To add or remove food items, click on Enter Foods.

Foods Consumed	Select Serving Size	Number of Servings (Enter a number (e.g. 1.5))
BAGEL, W/ RAISINS	1 large (3-1/2" to 3-3/4" dia) ▼	1
CREAM CHEESE	1 tablespoon ▼	1
WATER	1 fl oz ▼	16
APPLE (APPLES), FRESH	1 medium (2-3/4 dia) (approx 3 per lb) ▼	1
HAM, FRESH, LEAN ONLY	1 thin slice (approx 4-1/2 x 2-1/2 x 1/8) ▼	6
BREAD, MARBLE RYE & PUMPERNICKEL	1 regular slice ▼	2
MUSTARD	1 teaspoon ▼	2
MAYONNAISE, REGULAR	1 tablespoon ▼	1
RED LEAF LETTUCE	1 small leaf ▼	2
POTATO CHIPS, BAKED	10 chips ▼	3
LETTUCE SALAD, W/ CHEESE, TOMATO/CARROTS, NO DRESSING	1 cup ▼	2
SALAD DRESSING, LOW CALORIE	1 tablespoon ▼	2
HERSHEY BAR	1 bar (1.45 oz) ▼	1
COFFEE, MADE FROM GROUND, REGULAR, FLAVORED	1 fl oz ▼	20
CHEDDAR OR COLBY, LOWFAT CHEESE	1 slice (1 oz) ▼	1

Save & Analyze	Enter Foods	Return to Login	Reset Values

Print Food Record

(a) Nadia's diet for one day

Figure 2.9 Analysis of one day of Nadia's diet using the Interactive Healthy Eating Index. **(a)** This is a list of all foods Nadia ate and recorded for one day.

Another drawback of the Food Guide Pyramid is that low-fat and low-calorie food choices are not clearly defined in each food category. For instance, 2 to 3 servings of meat, poultry, fish, dry beans, eggs, and nuts are suggested in the Pyramid, but these foods differ significantly in their fat content and in the type of fat they contain. Fish is well recognized for being low in fat and containing a healthier type of fat than that found in red meats. However, these two types of meat are treated equally in the Pyramid. This also holds true for the bread, cereal, rice, and pasta group. Whole grains are preferable choices, and breads, cereal, and pastas made with refined flour are not comparable in nutritional value to whole-grain foods. An attempt is made in the Pyramid to draw attention to the fact that fats and sugar are found in all food groups by sprinkling symbols for fat and sugar throughout these groups. However,

HEI Score For Nadia on 10/1/2003

Click directly on the 😊 😐 ☹️ emoticon (face) for more detailed dietary information.

HEI Component	Emoticon	Score (Out of 10)	Number of Pyramid Servings Eaten	Number of Pyramid Servings Recommended
Grain	😐	5.0	4.5	9
Vegetable	😊	10.0	4.5	4
Fruit	☹️	4.7	1.4	3
Milk	😐	6.5	1.3	2
Meat	😐	7.4	1.8	2.4

HEI Component	Emoticon	Score (Out of 10)	Amount Eaten	Recommendation or Goal
Total Fat	☹️	3.1	40.3% of total calories	no more than 30%
Saturated Fat	☹️	0.0	15.2% of total calories	less than 10%
Cholesterol	😊	10.0	193 mg	less than 300 mg
Sodium	😊	9.7	2472 mg	less than 2400 mg
Variety	😊	10.0	9	8

Total HEI Score: 66.4 out of a possible 100

More information about the Healthy Eating Index - **To view this document you need** Adobe Acrobat Reader

Back   Food Guide Pyramid   Nutrient Intakes   Compare to National Average   Calculate History

(b) Nadia's HEI score

Food Guide Pyramid For Nadia

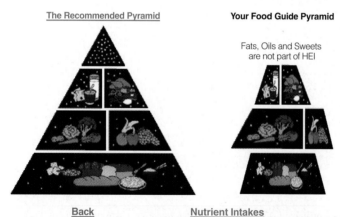

The Recommended Pyramid

Your Food Guide Pyramid

Fats, Oils and Sweets are not part of HEI

Your Food Guide Pyramid Stats

Pyramid Measure	Percent Recommendation
Fat	Fats, Oils and Sweets are not part of HEI
Milk	65%
Meat	75%
Vegetables	113%
Fruits	47%
Grains	50%

Back   Nutrient Intakes   HEI Score   Calculate History

(c) Nadia's food guide pyramid compared to the recommended food guide pyramid

Figure 2.9 *Continued.* **(b)** When Nadia entered her diet into the Interactive Healthy Eating Index program, she scored 66.4 points out of a possible 100 points. Her diet for this day was too low in fruit, grains, milk, and meat, and was too high in total and saturated fat. **(c)** As you can see, Nadia's personal food guide pyramid does not match the recommended USDA Food Guide Pyramid as she ate too few foods from the fruit, grains, milk, and meat groups.

the symbolism is not really helpful, as it does not clearly delineate high-fat and high-sugar foods from those lower in fat and sugar.

Similarly, you may eat the proper number of servings from all food groups in the Food Guide Pyramid, but this does not guarantee that you will be eating the proper balance of nutrients. This is because we may choose foods that are lower

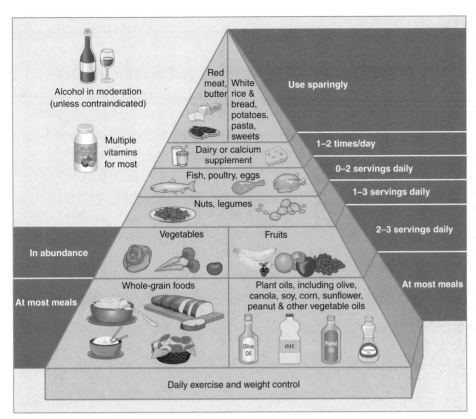

Figure 2.10 The Healthy Eating Pyramid. This is a pyramid suggested as a healthier alternative to the current USDA Food Guide Pyramid. (Walter C. Willett, Eat, Drink, and Be Healthy, in *Nutrition Source* Simon & Schuster, Harvard School of Public Health, Food Pyramids. 2001, www.hsph.harvard.edu/nutritionsource/pyramids.html [accessed September 2002].)

in nutrient density from each group, and these foods cannot provide us with the full complement of nutrients to maintain our health. For instance, many people prefer to eat potatoes as their vegetable for the day. If you eat 3 to 5 servings of vegetables each day, you meet the recommended number of servings for that food group, but potatoes do not contain all of the nutrients that other vegetables can provide.

In response to these limitations and others, researchers at the Harvard School of Public Health have revised the Food Guide Pyramid into the Healthy Eating Pyramid (Figure 2.10). The Healthy Eating Pyramid has been developed for informational purposes only and is not meant to endorse a particular product or to devalue the usefulness of the USDA Food Guide Pyramid. It is simply an illustration of how the current Food Guide Pyramid can be adapted to highlight more healthful food choices and to emphasize daily exercise and weight control.

Recap: There are many ethnic and cultural variations of the Food Guide Pyramid. The flexibility inherent in the Food Guide Pyramid allows anyone the ability to design a diet that meets the goals of adequacy, moderation, balance, variety, and nutrient density. Some of the limitations of the Food Guide Pyramid include relatively small serving sizes and the failure to distinguish between higher-fat and lower-fat food choices within food groups.

Hannah   *Nutri-Case*

"Today during class there was a lot of noise coming from the hallway. When the bell rang, and I went out to the hall to buy a snack and a soda from the vending machines, they were gone! I ran and told my teacher, and she said she knew all about it and was glad they'd taken the machines away. She said the stuff they sold was junk, but I say, as long as I eat my lunch every day, what's wrong with chips and soda? Why do adults always have to spoil everything?"

Vending machines are a source of extra income for many schools, whose contracts typically grant them an increased percentage of profits when sales volume increases (Hueter 2002). What ethical issues might arise from such a situation? What are the nutritional implications? If Hannah's vending-machine snacks do not replace her school lunch, then why shouldn't she be allowed to buy them? Using words that an elementary-school student would understand, explain to Hannah why adults might have made the decision to remove the machines from her school.

Diet Plans

As you already have learned, there is no single diet that is right for all individuals. By using the Food Guide Pyramid, each of us can design a healthful diet that fits our personal preferences and lifestyle. That said, there are a few diets that do seem to improve health for a majority of people. The 5-A-Day for Better Health Program and the DASH diet are two such diet plans, and we review them here. Try one on for a while, and see if the design works for you!

The 5-A-Day for Better Health Program

5-A-Day for Better Health Program A major public health initiative developed by the National Cancer Institute to promote nutrition and prevent cancer; recommends that Americans consume at least five servings of fruits and vegetables daily.

In 1991, the National Cancer Institute launched the **5-A-Day for Better Health Program**, a major public health initiative for nutrition and cancer prevention. Currently, a great deal of evidence links high fruit and vegetable consumption with cancer prevention (Heimendinger et al. 1996; Zhang et al. 1999; Greenwald, Clifford, and Milner 2001). Recent studies also suggest that eating more fruits and vegetables reduces the risk of heart disease in both men and women (Liu et al. 2001; Joshipura et al. 2001). These two diseases combined account for more than 60% of all deaths in the United States. Responding to research linking fruit and vegetable consumption to illness prevention, the message of the 5-A-Day Program is to eat a minimum of five fruits and vegetables each day.

Some consumers are confused by this advice, thinking it means to eat at least 5 fruits plus 5 vegetables each day. But in reality, the 5-A-Day message is consistent with the recommendations of the Food Guide Pyramid, which recommends 2 to 4 servings of fruit and 3 to 5 servings of vegetables each day. The lower end of the recommendation for each food group together totals 5 servings. These recommendations include fresh, frozen, canned, and dried versions of fruits and vegetables.

The 5-A-Day Program is designed to transmit healthy food messages to consumers through mass media, government agencies, community organizations, schools, worksites, and food-related industries. Research is currently being conducted in nine communities to determine if implementation of the 5-A-Day Program can indeed increase fruit and vegetable consumption within a population (Havas et al. 1994; Sorensen et al. 1998). Results from these research sites will be published in the near future.

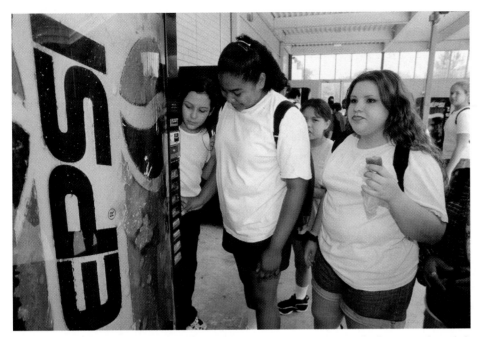

Through contracts with soft drink companies and commissions on sales, many schools earn much needed extra revenue. However, recent studies have linked childhood obesity to soft drink consumption. In response to these findings many states, including California, have banned sodas in school vending machines.

The DASH Diet Plan

The **DASH diet** resulted from a large research study funded by the National Institutes of Health (NIH). DASH stands for "Dietary Approaches to Stop Hypertension" thus, this study was designed to assess the effects of the DASH diet on high blood pressure. Table 2.7 shows the DASH eating plan for a 2,000 kcal diet. This plan is similar to the goals of Food Guide Pyramid in that it is low in fat and high in fiber. One exception is that 8 to 10 servings of fruits and vegetables are suggested daily, which is somewhat higher than the 5 to 9 servings suggested in the Food Guide Pyramid. The sodium content of the DASH diet is about 3 grams (or 3,000 mg) of sodium, which is slightly less than the average sodium intake in the United States.

The results of this study convincingly illustrated that eating the DASH diet has a very positive impact on blood pressure (Appel et al. 1997). Normal blood pressure is equal to, or lower than, 120/80 millimeters of mercury (mm Hg). For the study participants overall, systolic blood pressure (the top number) decreased by an average of 5.5 mm Hg and diastolic blood pressure (the bottom number) decreased by an average of 3.0 mm Hg. For the study participants who had high blood pressure, systolic blood pressure dropped an averge of 11.4 mm Hg and diastolic blood pressure dropped by an average of 5.5 mm Hg. These decreases occurred within the first two weeks of eating the DASH diet and were maintained throughout the duration of the study. Researchers estimated that if all Americans followed the DASH diet plan and experienced reductions in blood pressure similar to this study, then heart disease would be reduced by 15% and the number of strokes would be 27% lower.

Further study of the DASH diet has found that blood pressure decreases even more if sodium intake is reduced below 3,000 mg per day. A second study was conducted in which participants ate a DASH diet that provided either 3,300 mg (average U.S. intake), 2,400 mg (upper recommended intake), or 1,500 mg of sodium each

DASH diet The diet developed in response to research into hypertension funded by the National Institutes of Health (NIH); stands for "Dietary Approaches to Stop Hypertension."

Table 2.7 The DASH Eating Plan

Food Group	Daily Servings	Serving Size
Grains and grain products	7–8	1 slice bread 1 cup ready-to-eat cereal[1] ½ cup cooked rice, pasta, or cereal
Vegetables	4–5	1 cup raw leafy vegetables ½ cup cooked vegetable 6 fl. oz. vegetable juice
Fruits	4–5	1 medium fruit ¼ cup dried fruit ½ cup fresh, frozen, or canned fruit 6 fl. oz. fruit juice
Low-fat or fat-free dairy foods	2–3	8 fl. oz. milk 1 cup yogurt 1½ ounces cheese
Lean meats, poultry, and fish	2 or less	3 oz. cooked lean meats, skinless poultry, or fish
Nuts, seeds, and dry beans	4–5 per week	⅓ cup or 1½ oz. nuts 1 tbsp. or ½ oz. seeds ½ cup cooked dry beans
Fats and oils[2]	2–3	1 tsp. soft margarine 1 tbsp. low-fat mayonnaise 2 tbsp. light salad dressing 1 tsp. vegetable oil
Sweets	5 per week	1 tbsp. sugar 1 tbsp. jelly or jam ½ oz. jelly beans 8 fl.oz. lemonade

Note: The plan is based on 2,000 kilocalories per day. The number of servings in a food group may differ from the number listed, depending upon your own energy needs.
[1] Serving sizes vary between ½ and 1¼ cups. Check the product's nutrition label.
[2] Fat content changes serving counts for fats and oils: For example, 1 tablespoon of regular salad dressing equals 1 serving; 1 tablespoon of a low-fat dressing equals ½ serving; 1 tablespoon of a fat-free dressing equals 0 servings.
National Institutes of Health. Healthier Eating with DASH. www.nhlbi.nih.gov/health/public/heart/hbp/dash/new_dash.pdf Accessed July 2003.

day (Sacks et al. 2001). After one month on this diet, all people eating the DASH diet saw a significant decrease in their blood pressure; however, those who ate the lowest-sodium version of the DASH diet experienced the largest decrease. These results indicate that eating a diet low in sodium and high in fruits and vegetables reduces blood pressure and decreases your risk for heart disease and stroke.

Other Diet Plans

The 5-A-Day Program and the DASH diet are two programs that are linked to research studies showing healthful benefits, and both are endorsed by federal agencies. There are many other diet plans available to consumers, and many of these may or may not have been researched to determine their health benefits. Some of these plans, such as Weight Watchers, The Zone Diet, and the Ornish Program, have been marketed specifically for weight loss; many weight loss plans can be adapted to achieve healthy weight maintenance. It is inappropriate to endorse one specific diet plan for all people, as our nutritional needs and preferences are diverse and cannot be met by a single plan. Each person must make his or her own decisions about healthful diet choices based on personal preferences, ethnic considerations, activity level, cost, and convenience.

When designing a healthful diet for yourself, you need to look closely at any diet plan to determine if it meets the healthful guidelines reviewed in this book. You can use the Dietary Guidelines for Americans as a standard for comparison, and you also need to look at any diet plan to determine if it emphasizes the principles of adequacy, moderation, balance, variety, and nutrient density. For a more detailed review of various diet plans and fad diets, see Chapter 11.

> **Recap:** The 5-A-Day for Better Health Program and the DASH diet are two examples of healthy food plans. The 5-A-Day Program recommends that you eat at least 5 servings of fruits and vegetables each day. High fruit and vegetable consumption has been linked to cancer prevention and reduced risk of heart disease. The DASH diet is similar to the Food Guide Pyramid but includes 8 to 10 servings of fruits and vegetables and no more than 3,000 mg of sodium each day. The DASH diet has been shown to significantly decrease blood pressure.

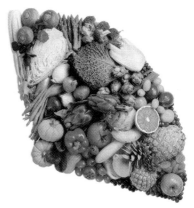

It is important to eat at least five servings of fruits and vegetables every day.

The Exchange System

The **exchange system** is another tool that can be used to plan a healthful diet. The American Dietetic Association and the American Diabetes Association originally designed the exchange system for people with diabetes. This system has also been used successfully in weight loss programs. Exchanges, or portions, are organized according to the amount of carbohydrate, protein, fat, and calories in each food. There are six food groups, or exchange lists, and these lists contain foods that are similar in calories, carbohydrate, fat, and protein content (Table 2.8). The six exchange lists are starch/bread, meat and meat substitutes, vegetables, fruits, milk, and fat. In addition to these lists, there are also other categories (not shown in Table 2.8) that can assist you in meal planning, including free foods (any food or drink with less than 20 calories per serving), combination foods (foods such as soups, casseroles, and pizza), and special occasion foods (desserts such as cakes, cookies, and ice cream).

To use the exchange system effectively, you must learn the portion sizes for each of the exchange lists. In addition, some foods are classified differently than in the Food Guide Pyramid, and you must learn which foods fit into each exchange list. For instance, starchy vegetables such as corn, potatoes, peas, beans, and lentils are placed into the starch/bread exchange list, not the vegetable exchange list. The meat and meat substitute group classifies meat in three subcategories: lean, medium-fat, and high-fat meats. While one ounce of lean meat such as turkey breast without skin is one exchange of lean meat, a high-fat meat choice such as one Ball Park frank is one high-fat meat exchange and one fat exchange.

There are many advantages of using the exchange system to plan a healthful diet. Because a portion of any food on a given exchange list has the same number of calories and macronutrients, you can easily exchange foods within each list to design a varied diet plan. In addition, the portion sizes defined in the exchange system and the distinction between meats with different fat contents help you to better control energy and fat intakes. Once you have learned how to use the exchange system, you can effectively design a healthful diet based on your energy needs. Refer to Table 2.9 for an example of how a 2,600 calorie meal plan might look using the exchange system.

> **Recap:** The exchange system is a diet plan originally designed for people with diabetes. Exchanges, or portions, are organized according to the amount of carbohydrate, protein, fat, and calories in each food. There are six exchange lists that contain foods similar in calories, carbohydrate, fat, and protein content. One advantage of the exchange system is that lean, medium-fat, and high-fat foods in the meat and dairy groups are clearly defined, which assists in controlling fat and energy intake.

exchange system Diet planning tool developed by the American Dietetic Association and the American Diabetes Association in which exchanges, or portions, are organized according to the amount of carbohydrate, protein, fat, and calories in each food.

Table 2.8   Exchange Groups and Their Energy and Macronutrient Content

Exchange List	Calories	Carbohydrate (grams)	Fat (grams)	Protein (grams)	Serving Sizes
Starch/Bread	80	15	Trace (0.5 to 1)	3	1 oz. of bread ¾ cup dry, unsweetened cereal ½ cup cooked cereal 4–5 snack crackers ½ cup pasta or starchy vegetable ⅓ cup rice, grains, stuffings 1 cup soup ⅓ cup cooked beans, peas, lentils 3 cups popcorn without added fat
Meat and Meat Substitutes					
Lean meat	55	0	3	7	1 oz. fish, poultry, lean beef (round sirloin, flank steak), processed hams, veal, cottage cheese, low-fat cheeses, lean luncheon meats
Medium-fat meat	75	0	5	7	1 oz. of most beef and pork cuts, poultry with skin, skim-milk cheeses, 1 egg
High-fat meat	100	0	8	7	1 oz. fried meats, poultry, or fish; 1 oz. prime cuts of beef, corned beef, spareribs, regular cheeses, regular luncheon meats, sausages, hot dogs, and peanut butter
Vegetables	25	5	0	2	½ cup cooked vegetables ½ cup vegetable juice 1 cup raw vegetables
Fruits	60	15	0	0	1 small to medium fresh fruit ½ cup canned fruit ¼ cup dried fruit ⅓ – ½ cup fruit juice
Milk					
Nonfat and very-low-fat milk	90	12	0–3	8	1 cup skim, ½%, or 1% milk 1 cup nonfat or low-fat buttermilk ¾ cup (6 oz.) plain nonfat yogurt 1 cup (8 oz.) nonfat or low-fat artificially sweetened fruit flavored yogurt
Low-fat milk	120	12	5	8	1 cup 2% milk ¾ cup plain low-fat yogurt
Whole milk	150	12	8	8	1 cup whole milk ½ cup evaporated whole milk
Fat	45	0	5	0	1 tsp. margarine or butter 1 tbsp. reduced-calorie margarine 1 tsp. mayonnaise or oil 1 tbsp. regular salad dressing 2 tbsp. low-calorie salad dressing 2 tbsp. sour cream

Table 2.9 Example of a One-Day Meal Plan for a 2,600 Calorie Diet Using the Exchange System

Meal	Exchanges					
	Starch/Bread	Lean Meat	Vegetable	Fruit	Nonfat Milk	Fat
Breakfast	2 slices whole wheat toast ½ cup cooked oatmeal			1 cup orange juice	1 cup skim milk	2 tsp. margarine (spread on toast)
Snack	3 cups popcorn with no added fat 5 whole wheat crackers			1 small banana		4 tsp. peanut butter (spread on crackers)
Lunch	2 slices rye bread ⅓ cup baked beans	3 oz. lean sliced turkey ham	1 cup baby carrots 1 cup raw cauliflower ½ cup V–8 juice	1 medium apple	1 cup nonfat strawberry yogurt sweetened with aspartame	2 tsp. mayonnaise (spread on rye bread) 1 tbsp. ranch dressing (for dipping vegetables)
Snack	16 animal crackers			1 small nectarine		
Dinner	1 large baked potato	4 oz. broiled skinless chicken breast	2 cups butter lettuce with ¼ cup each green onion, sweet red pepper, fresh tomatoes, and carrots		1 cup skim milk	2 tsp. butter (for potato) 2 tbsp. reduced fat Italian salad dressing (for salad)
Total exchanges/day	13	7	6	5	3	10

Can Eating Out Be Part of a Healthful Diet?

How many times each week do you eat out? A report from the National Restaurant Association states that the average American eats 4.2 commercially prepared meals every week (Ebbin 2000). Men eat an average of 4.6 meals at restaurants each week, while women eat about 3.8 meals out every week. Restaurant sales for 2003 are projected to be more than $426 billion. Over the last twenty years there has been phenomenal growth in the restaurant industry, particularly in the fast food market. During this same time period, rates of obesity have increased dramatically. In fact, the number of Americans considered overweight has increased by 61% from 1991 to 2000 (CDC 2001).

The Hidden Costs of Eating Out

Table 2.10 shows an example of foods served at McDonald's and Burger King restaurants. As you can see, a regular McDonald's hamburger has only 270 kcal, while the Big Xtra with Cheese has 810 kcal. A meal of the Quarter Pounder with Cheese, Super Size French fries, and a Super Size Coke provides 1,550 kcal. This meal has enough energy to support an entire day's needs for a small, lightly active woman! Similar meals at Burger King and other fast food chains are also very high in calories, not to mention total fat and sodium.

It is not only the fast food restaurants that serve large portions. Most sit-down restaurants also serve large meals that may include bread with butter, a salad with dressing, sides of vegetables and potatoes, and free refills of sugar-filled drinks. Combined with a high-fat appetizer like potato skins, fried onions, fried mozzarella sticks, or buffalo wings, it is easy to eat more than 2,000 kcal at one meal!

Does this mean that eating out cannot be a part of a healthful diet? Not necessarily. By becoming an educated consumer and making wise meal choices while dining out, you can enjoy both a healthful diet and the social benefits of eating out.

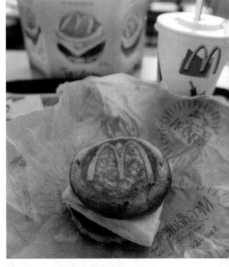

Foods served at fast food chains are often high in calories, total fat, and sodium. McDonald's popular sausage, egg, and cheese McGriddles™ breakfast sandwiches, for example, contain 550 calories, 33g of fat, and 1,290 mg of sodium.

Table 2.10 Nutritional Value of Selected Fast Foods

Menu Item	Kcal	Fat (grams)	Fat (% kcal)	Sodium (mg)
McDonald's:				
Hamburger	270	9	29.6	600
Cheeseburger	320	13	37.5	830
Quarter Pounder	430	21	44.2	840
Quarter Pounder with cheese	530	30	50.9	1310
Big Mac	570	32	49.1	1100
Big Xtra	710	46	59.2	1400
Big Xtra with cheese	810	55	60.5	1870
French fries, small	210	10	42.8	135
French fries, medium	450	22	44.4	290
French fries, large	540	26	42.6	350
French fries, Super Size	610	29	42.6	390
Burger King:				
Hamburger	320	15	43.8	520
Cheeseburger	360	19	47.2	760
Whopper	660	40	54.5	900
Whopper with cheese	760	48	56.6	1380
Double Whopper	920	59	57.6	980
Bacon Cheeseburger	400	22	50.0	940
Bacon Double Cheeseburger	620	38	54.8	1230
French fries, small	250	13	48.0	550
French fries, medium	400	21	47.5	820
French fries, King Size	590	30	45.8	1180

The Healthful Way to Eat Out

Most restaurants, even fast food restaurants, offer lower-fat menu items that you can choose. For instance, eating a regular McDonald's hamburger, a small order of French fries, and a diet beverage or water provides 480 kcal and 19 grams of fat (or 35% of kcal from fat). To provide some vegetables for the day, you could add a side salad with low-fat or nonfat salad dressing. Other fast food restaurants also offer smaller portions, sandwiches made with whole grain bread, grilled chicken or other lean meats, and side salads. Many sit-down restaurants offer "lite" menu items such as grilled chicken and a variety of vegetables, which are usually a much better choice than eating from the regular menu.

Here are some other suggestions on how to eat out in moderation. Practice some of these suggestions every time you eat out:

- Avoid whole-milk lattés and other coffee drinks with cream or whipping cream; select reduced-fat or skim milk added to your favorite coffee drink.
- Avoid eating appetizers that are breaded, fried, or filled with cheese or meat; you may want to skip the appetizer completely. Alternatively, you may want to order a healthful appetizer as an entreé instead of a larger meal.
- Share an entreé with a friend! Many restaurants serve entreés large enough for two people.
- Order broth-based soups instead of cream-based soups.
- Order any meat dish grilled or broiled, and avoid fried or breaded meat dishes.
- If you order a meat dish, select lean cuts of meat, such as chicken or turkey breast, extra-lean ground beef, pork loin chop, or filet mignon.
- Order a meatless dish filled with vegetables and whole grains. Avoid dishes with cream sauces and a lot of cheese.

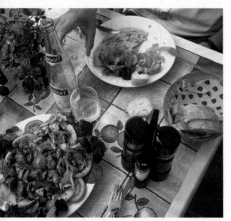

Eating out can be a part of a healthful diet, if you are careful to choose wisely.

- Order a salad with low-fat or nonfat dressing served on the side. Many restaurants smother their salads in dressing, and you will eat less by controlling how much you put on the salad.
- Order steamed vegetables on the side instead of potatoes or rice. If you order potatoes, make sure you get a baked potato (with very little butter or sour cream on the side).
- Order beverages with little or no calories, such as water, tea, or diet drinks.
- Eat no more than half of what you are served, and take the rest home for another meal.
- Skip dessert or share one dessert with a lot of friends! Another healthful alternative is to order fresh fruit for dessert.

Recap: Healthful ways to eat out include choosing menu items that are smaller in size, ordering meats that are grilled or broiled, avoiding fried foods, choosing items with steamed vegetables, avoiding energy-rich appetizers and desserts, and eating less than half of the food you are served.

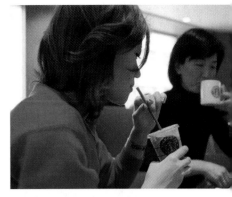

When ordering your favorite coffee drink, avoid those made with cream or whipping cream, and request reduced-fat or skim milk instead.

Chapter Summary

- A healthful diet provides adequate energy, nutrients, and fiber to maintain health.
- A healthful diet is moderate in the amounts of foods eaten. Foods that contain a lot of fat and sugar should be eaten only in moderation to maintain a healthy weight.
- A healthful diet contains the proper balance of food groups and nutrients to maintain health.
- A healthful diet provides a variety of foods every day.
- The U.S. Food and Drug Administration (FDA) regulates the content of food labels; food labels must contain a statement of identity, the net contents of the package, the contact information of the food manufacturer or distributor, an ingredient list, and nutrition information.
- The Nutrition Facts Panel on a food label contains important nutrition information about serving size, servings per package, total calories and calories of fat per serving, a list of various macronutrients, vitamins, and minerals, and the %Daily Values for the nutrients listed on the panel.
- The Dietary Guidelines are general directives about healthful eating and physical activity and include aiming for a healthy weight, being physically active each day, using the Food Guide Pyramid to select foods, eating whole grain foods, fruits, and vegetables each day, keeping food safe to eat, choosing foods lower in saturated fat and cholesterol and moderate in total

fat, moderating your intake of sugar, eating less salt, and drinking alcoholic beverages in moderation, if at all.
- The Food Guide Pyramid is a tool developed by the USDA that can be used to design a healthful diet. The groups in the pyramid include bread, cereal, rice, and pasta food group, the fruit group, the vegetable group, the milk, yogurt, and cheese group, and the meat, poultry, fish, dry beans, eggs, and nut group. The top of the pyramid emphasizes eating fats, oils, and sweets sparingly.
- Specific serving sizes are defined for foods in each group of the Food Guide Pyramid. There is no standard definition for a serving size, and the serving sizes defined in the Pyramid are generally smaller than those listed on food labels and than the servings generally sold to consumers.
- There are many ethnic and cultural variations of the Food Guide Pyramid, including the Vegetarian, Mediterranean, Latin American, and Asian Diet Pyramids.
- The Food Guide Pyramid can be used to design a diet that meets the healthful goals of adequacy, moderation, balance, variety, nutrient density.
- The limitations of the Food Guide Pyramid include relatively small serving sizes that can be confusing to consumers, failure to clearly distinguish between high-fat and low-fat food choices within the food groups, and challenges to meeting all nutrient needs even if the recommended number of servings from each food group are consumed.

- The 5-A-Day for Better Health Program is a major public health initiative promoting the intake of a combination of five fruits and vegetables every day to reduce the risk for cancer and other chronic diseases.

- The DASH diet (Dietary Approaches to Stop Hypertension) is high in fiber, low in fat, and includes 8 to 10 servings of fruits and vegetables each day.

- Eating the DASH diet can significantly decrease blood pressure, with particular benefit to people with high blood pressure.

- Eating a lower sodium version of the DASH diet improves blood pressure even more than the standard DASH diet.

- The exchange system is another tool you can use to design a healthful diet. The American Diabetes Association and the American Dietetic Association originally designed this system as a plan for individuals with diabetes.

- The exchange system includes the use of exchanges, or portions, that are organized based on amounts of carbohydrate, protein, fat, and calories.

- The six food groups, or exchange lists, contain foods that are similar in calories, carbohydrate, fat, and protein content. The six groups are starch/bread, meat and meat substitutes, vegetables, fruits, milk, and fat.

- Two advantages of using the exchange system are the ease of exchanging foods with each list, which allows for a great deal of variety, and the clear definition of portion sizes and lean, medium-fat, and high-fat food choices helps control energy and fat intake.

- Eating out is challenging because of the high fat content and large serving sizes of many fast food and sit-down restaurant menu items.

- Behaviors that can improve the quality of your diet when eating out include choosing lower fat meats that are grilled or broiled, eating vegetables and salads as side or main dishes, asking for low-fat salad dressing on the side, skipping high-fat desserts and appetizers, and drinking low- or non caloric beverages.

Review Questions

1. The Nutrition Facts Panel identifies which of the following?
   a. All of the nutrients and calories in the package of food.
   b. The recommended dietary allowance for each nutrient found in the package of food.
   c. A footnote identifying the Tolerable Upper Intake Level for each nutrient found in the package of food.
   d. The %Daily Values of select nutrients in a serving of the packaged food.

2. An adequate diet
   a. provides enough energy to meet minimum daily requirements.
   b. provides enough of the energy, nutrients, and fiber to maintain a person's health.
   c. provides a sufficient variety of nutrients to maintain a healthy weight and to optimize our body's metabolic processes.
   d. contains combinations of foods that provide healthful proportions of nutrients.

3. The USDA Food Guide Pyramid recommends eating
   a. 6 to 11 servings of whole grains, cereals, and breads each day.
   b. 6 to 11 servings of fruits and vegetables each day.
   c. 4 to 6 servings of meat, poultry, fish, dried beans, eggs, and nuts each day.
   d. 4 to 6 servings of dairy foods each day.

4. The Dietary Guidelines for Americans recommends which of the following?
   a. Choosing and preparing foods without salt.
   b. Consuming two alcoholic beverages per day.
   c. Being physically active each day.
   d. Following the Mediterranean diet.

5. What does it mean to choose foods for their nutrient density?
   a. Dense foods such as peanut butter or chicken are more nutritious choices than transparent foods such as mineral water or gelatin.
   b. Foods with a lot of nutrients per calorie such as fish are more nutritious choices than foods with less nutrients per calorie such as candy.
   c. Calorie-dense foods such as cheesecake should be avoided.
   d. Fat makes foods dense, and thus foods high in fat should be avoided.

6. **True or false?** The USDA has written a standardized definition for a serving size for most foods.

7. **True or false?** A drawback of the Food Guide Pyramid is that low-fat and low-calorie food choices are not clearly defined in each food category.

8. **True or false?** The six exchange lists are grains, meat and meat substitutes, fruits and vegetables, dairy products, sweets, and fats.

9. **True or false?** The Healthy Eating Pyramid suggests that pasta be eaten sparingly.

10. **True or false?** The 5-A-Day Program was instituted by the American Diabetes Association.

11. Defend the statement that no single diet can be appropriate for every human being.

12. Explain why the Food Guide Pyramid identifies a range in the number of suggested daily servings of each food group instead of telling us exactly how many servings of each food to eat each day.

13. Identify at least three differences between the USDA Food Guide Pyramid and the Canadian Food Guide.

14. Identify at least six differences between the USDA Food Guide Pyramid and the Healthy Eating Pyramid.

15. Defend or refute the statement that "a little glass of wine never hurt anybody."

Test Yourself Answers

1. **False.** A healthful diet can be achieved by food alone; particular attention must be paid to adequacy, variety, moderation, and balance. However, some individuals may need to take vitamin supplements under certain circumstances.

2. **True.** Food labels contain information on select nutrients found in a serving of food to assist us in selecting foods that contribute to a healthful diet.

3. **False.** Although the USDA Food Guide Pyramid does have its limitations, it can be used by most Americans to design a healthful diet. This tool is flexible and allows for modifications as needed; there are also many ethnic variations available.

4. **False.** The 5-A-Day Program encourages us to eat at least 3 servings of vegetables and 2 servings of fruit each day, totaling "5-A-Day."

5. **False.** Eating out poses many challenges to healthful eating, but it is possible to eat a healthful diet when dining out. Ordering and/or consuming smaller portion sizes, selecting foods that are lower in fat and added sugars, and selecting eating establishments that serve more healthful foods can assist you in eating healthfully while dining out.

Web Links

www.fda.gov
U.S. Food and Drug Administration (FDA)
Learn more about the government agency that regulates our food and first established regulations for nutrition information on food labels.

www.health.gov/dietaryguidelines
Dietary Guidelines for Americans
Use these guidelines to make changes in your food choices and physical activity habits to help reduce your risk for chronic disease.

www.usda.gov/cnpp
Center for Nutrition Policy and Prevention (CNPP)
Use the Interactive Healthy Eating Index provided on this Web site to assess the overall quality of your diet based on the USDA Food Guide Pyramid.

www.hc-sc.gc.ca
Health Canada
Learn more about Canadian's Food Guide to Healthy Eating and other Canadian health policies.

www.oldwayspt.org
Oldways Preservation and Exchange Trust
Find different variations of ethnic and cultural food pyramids.

www.5aday.gov
National Cancer Institute's 5-A-Day Program
Learn more about the 5-A-Day Program, a major public health initiative for nutrition and cancer prevention.

www.nih.gov
The National Institutes of Health (NIH, part of the U.S. Department of Health and Human Services)
Search this site to learn more about the DASH Diet (Dietary Approaches to Stop Hypertension).

http://hin.nhlbi.nih.gov/portion
The National Institutes of Health (NIH) Portion Distortion Quiz
Take this short quiz to see if you know how today's food portions compare to those of twenty years ago.

www.diabetes.org
The American Diabetes Association
Find out more about the nutritional needs of people living with diabetes as well as meal planning exchange lists.

www.eatright.org
The American Dietetic Association
Visit the food and nutrition information section of this Web site for additional resources to help you achieve a healthy lifestyle.

www.hsph.harvard.edu
The Harvard School of Public Health
Search this site to learn more about the Healthy Eating Pyramid, an alternative to the USDA Food Guide Pyramid.

References

Appel, L. J., T. J., Moore, E. Obarzanek, W. M. Vollmer, L. P. Svetkey, F. M. Sacks, G. A. Bray, T. M. Vogt, J. A. Cutler, M. M. Windhauser, P.-H. Lin, and N. Karanja. 1997. A clinical trial of the effects of dietary patterns on blood pressure. *New Engl. J. Med.* 336:1117–1124.

Centers for Disease Control and Prevention (CDC). 2001, November (accessed). Obesity Trends. U.S. Obesity Trends 1985 to 2000. www.cdc.gov/nccdphp/dnpa/obesity/trend/maps/index.htm.

Centers for Disease Control and Prevention. 2003, July (accessed). Overweight and Obesity. Frequently Asked Questions (FAQs). www.cdc.gov/nccdphp/dnpa/obesity/faq.htm.

Ebbin, R. 2000, November. Americans' dining-out habits. Restaurants USA. www.restaurant.org/rusa/magArticle.cfm?ArticleID=138. Accessed November 2001.

Food and Nutrition Information Center. 2002, September (accessed). Ethnic/Cultural Food Pyramids. www.nal.usda.gov/fnic/etext/000023.html.

Friedman, J. M. 2003. A war on obesity, not the obese. *Science* 299:856–858.

Greenwald, P., C. K. Clifford, and J. A. Milner. 2001. Diet and cancer prevention. *Eur. J. Cancer.* 37:948–965.

Havas, S., J. Heimendinger, K. Reynolds, T. Baranowski, T. A. Nicklas, D. Bishop, D. Buller, G. Sorensen, S. A. A. Beresford, A. Cowan, and D. Damron. 1994. 5 A Day for Better Health: a new research initiative. *J. Am. Diet. Assoc.* 94:32–36.

Heimendinger, J., M. A. Van Duyn, D. Chapelsky, S. Foerster, and G. Stables. 1996. The National 5 A Day for Better Health Program: A large-scale nutrition intervention. *J. Public Health Management Practice* 2:27–35.

Houtkooper, L. 1994. *Winning sports nutrition training manual.* Tucson: University of Arizona Cooperative Extension.

Hueter, J. S. Nutrition in schools. 2002, August 30. http://www.law.uh.edu/healthlawperspectives/Children/020830Nutrition.html (Accessed July 2003.)

Jacobson, M. F., and K. D. Brownell. 2000. Small taxes on soft drinks and snack foods to promote health. *Am. J. Public Health* 90:854–857.

Joshipura, K. J., F. B. Hu, J. E. Manson, M. J. Stampfer, E. B. Rimm, F. E. Speizer, G. Colditz, A. Ascherio, B. Rosner, D. Spiegelman, and W. C. Willett. 2001. The effect of fruit and vegetable intake on risk for coronary heart disease. *Ann. Intern. Med.* 134:1106–1114.

Kant, A. K., A. Schatzkin, T. B. Harris, R. G. Ziegler, and G. Block. 1993. Dietary diversity and subsequent mortality in the First National Health and Nutrition Examination Survey epidemiologic follow-up study. *Am. J. Clin. Nutr.* 57:434–440.

Kantor, L. S. 1998. A Dietary Assessment of the U.S. Food Supply. U.S. Department of Agriculture, Economic Research Service. Agricultural Economic Report No. 772.

Li, G., S. P. Baker, J. E. Smialek, and C. A. Soderstrom. 2001. Use of alcohol as a risk factor for bicycling injury. *JAMA* 285:893–896.

Liu, S., I.-M. L, U. Ajani, S. R. Cole, J. E. Buring, and J. E. Manson. 2001. Intake of vegetables rich in carotenoids and risk of coronary heart disease in men: The Physicians' Health Study. *Int. J. Epidemiol.* 30:130–135.

Nestle, M. Food Politics. 2002. *How the Food Industry Influences Nutrition and Health.* Berkeley, CA: University of California Press.

Renaud, S., M. de Lorgeril, J. Delaye, J. Guidollet, F. Jacquard, N. Mamelle, J.-L. Martin, I. Monjaud, P. Salen, and P. Toubol. 1995. Cretan Mediterranean diet for prevention of coronary heart disease. *Am. J. Clin. Nutr.* 61(suppl.):1360S–1367S.

Sacks, F. M., L. P. Svetkey, W. M. Vollmer, L. J. Appel, G. A. Bray, D. Harsha, E. Obarzanek, P. R. Conlin, E. R. Miller III, D. G. Simons-Morton, N. Karanja, and P.-H. Lin. 2001. Effects on blood pressure of reduced dietary sodium and the Dietary Approaches to Stop Hypertension (DASH) diet. *New Engl. J. Med.* 344:3–10.

Smith-Warner, S. A., D. Spiegelman, S.-S. Yaun, P. A. van den Brandt, A. R. Folsom, A. Goldbohm, S. Graham, L. Holmberg, G. R. Howe, J. R. Marshall, A. B. Miller, J. D. Potter, F. E. Speizer, W. C. Willett, A. Wolk, and D. J. Hunter. 1998. Alcohol and breast cancer in women. *JAMA* 279:535–540.

Sorensen, G., M. K. Hunt, N. Cohen, A. Stoddard, E. Stein, J. Phillips, F. Baker, C. Combe, J. Hebert, and R. Palombo. 1998. Worksite and family education for dietary change: the Treatwell 5-a-Day program. *Health Ed. Res.* 13:577–591.

Tavani, A., and C. La Vecchia. 1995. Fruit and vegetable consumption and cancer risk in a Mediterranean population. *Am. J. Clin. Nutr.* 61(suppl):1374S–1377S.

Tufts University. Tufts Nutrition Commentator. Accessed September 2002. Nutrition Guidelines: A modified food guide pyramid for people over 70 years. http://commentator.tufts.edu/archive/nutrition/pyramid.html. 1999.

U.S. Department of Agriculture (USDA). 1999. The Food Guide Pyramid for young children. www.usda.gov/cnpp/KidsPyra/. Accessed September 2002.

U.S. Department of Agriculture, and U.S. Department of Health and Human Services (USDHHS). 2000. Dietary Guidelines for Americans, 2000. 5th ed. Home and Garden Bulletin No. 232. (Available at www.health.gov/dietaryguidelines/dga2000/document/frontcover.htm)

Weschsler, H., G. W. Dowdall, A. Davenport, and E. B. Rimm. 1995. A gender-specific measure of binge drinking among college students. *Am. J. Public Health* 7:982–985.

Weschsler, H., J. E. Lee, M. Kuo, and H. Lee. 2000. College binge drinking in the 1990s: a continuing problem. *J. Am. Coll. Health* 48:199–210.

Wollin, S. D., and P. J. H. Jones. 2001. Alcohol, red wine and cardiovascular disease. *J. Nutr.* 131:1401–1404.

Young, L. R. and M. Nestle. 1998. Variation in perceptions of a "medium" food portion: implications for dietary guidance. *J. Am. Diet. Assoc.* 98:458–459.

Zhang, S., D. J. Hunter, M. R. Forman, B. A. Rosner, F. E. Speizer, G. A. Colditz, J. E. Manson, S. E. Hankinson, and W. C. Willett. 1999. Dietary carotenoids and vitamins A, C, and E and risk of breast cancer. *J. Nat. Cancer Inst.* 91:547–556.

Nutrition Debate:

Should the U.S. Government Regulate the Food Industry to Combat the Obesity Epidemic?

As you have learned in this chapter, obesity is now considered an epidemic in the United States and around the world. The dramatic rise in obesity is not only contributing to bulging waistlines, but is also responsible for overwhelming burdens related to health-care costs, emotional distress, and societal prejudice. What can we do to fight obesity and its extensive societal and medical consequences? Who is responsible for contributing to the obesity epidemic, and who should be held accountable to combat it?

For many years, all accountability for obesity has been placed on the obese person. These individuals have been portrayed as lazy, gluttonous, and having no will power. Losing weight has been portrayed as being as simple as eating less energy than you expend. Thus, weight loss has been viewed as the responsibility of the obese individual; they should just eat less and exercise more, and they would not be obese.

Recent research has now shown that weight loss is not quite this simple. Friedman (2003) points out that obesity has a strong genetic component. For centuries, people who were regularly exposed to famine adapted so that they could readily store fat and survive when food was scarce. When a person with a strong genetic tendency toward obesity lives in an environment with ample food and inadequate physical activity, weight gain is virtually inevitable. In addition, the drive to eat is complex and is stimulated by weight loss. Thus, it is not simply just to eat less, exercise more, and lose weight. Many believe we are now living in a "toxic" environment, one that makes living a healthful life incredibly challenging for most people and almost impossible for some.

Because of these challenges, there is a growing trend to hold someone or something accountable for this toxic environment. Recent lawsuits have targeted fast food chains and food manufacturers. Obese citizens have attempted to sue fast food restaurants for serving foods that are high in fat, energy, and sugar. Food manufacturers are being sued because of the junk foods they produce and market to children. Recent history has shown us that litigation can be a powerful tool to bring attention to a major public health problem, as has occurred with smoking and the tobacco industry. Suing food producers and restaurants may be even more challenging than suing the tobacco industry, however, as food is something we need to survive. In addition, proponents of the food and restaurant industry argue that people know that fast food and junk food is not healthful and that it is up to the individual to moderate their intake of these foods.

Another approach to combating obesity is the proposed application of taxes on unhealthful foods. The so-called "sin tax" has been applied to cigarettes and alcohol. The basic premise is to apply a small tax on soft drinks and snack foods, and then use the revenues from this tax to fund nutrition and physical activity programs across the country (Jacobson and Brownell 2000). This tax would be small enough that it would not negatively impact food sales, but it could potentially generate millions, even billions of dollars in revenue that could be used to fund a variety of health promotion programs. To date, there has been no widespread support of this proposed approach.

A growing number of people in this country believe that the U.S. government should step forward and lead

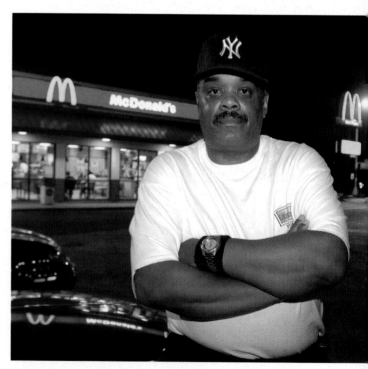

In 2002 Caesar Barber was the initial plaintiff in a class action suit against four food franchises including McDonald's. He claimed that they contributed to his weight as well as other health problems by serving fatty foods. A federal court later threw out the lawsuit.

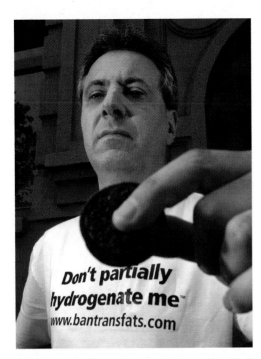

Attorney Stephen Joseph filed suit in a Marin County Superior Court seeking a ban on Oreo sales in California. He claimed that they were unhealthy because they contained trans fat. He later dropped his suit when he learned that Kraft was working on ways to reduce the trans fat in the cookie.

the way in combating obesity. The government is capable of applying taxes to foods, can regulate the types of foods sold in stores and restaurants, and controls the information listed on food labels. With obesity being such a prominent health problem in the United States, many wonder why the government does not step in and actively take a role in combating this disease.

The issues surrounding the role of government in regulating our food intake are complex and controversial. There are many who stand strongly against any governmental control over what we eat. Americans pride themselves on individuality and personal freedoms, and they are adverse to governmental control on personal behaviors. Thus, many feel that the government should play no role in what or how we eat. In addition, food companies hold a great deal of political clout, and these companies support our political candidates and contribute money to government officials, healthcare professionals, and media outlets. In fact, the politics of food make it very difficult for the federal government to place controls or demands on the food industry. The message of "eat less" does not bode well for food manufacturers and restaurant owners. These politics are discussed in detail by Marion Nestle (2002), who describes how the food industry influences nutrition and health in the United States and makes suggestions as to how we can modify public policies to promote healthier lives. Some of these suggestions include:

- mount a national campaign to "eat less, move more"
- end the sale of soft drinks, candy bars, and other foods with minimal nutrition value in schools
- require fast food restaurants to provide nutrition information labels on food wrappers and packages
- restrict television advertising of foods with minimal nutritional value
- apply taxes to soft drinks and other junk foods, and reduce the cost of fruits and vegetables

How do you feel about this debate? To what level (if any) do you feel the government should be involved in regulating the food industry? What would you be willing to give up or demand in order to fight the obesity epidemic? Are you willing to pay taxes on foods with minimal nutrition value? Should the food industry be held accountable for selling foods that are unhealthful and contribute to the obesity epidemic? These are questions that each of us may need to answer in the coming years. The obesity epidemic will not be quelled without a fight. It is up to all of us to determine whether we should fight this epidemic, and if so, just how we can fight it.

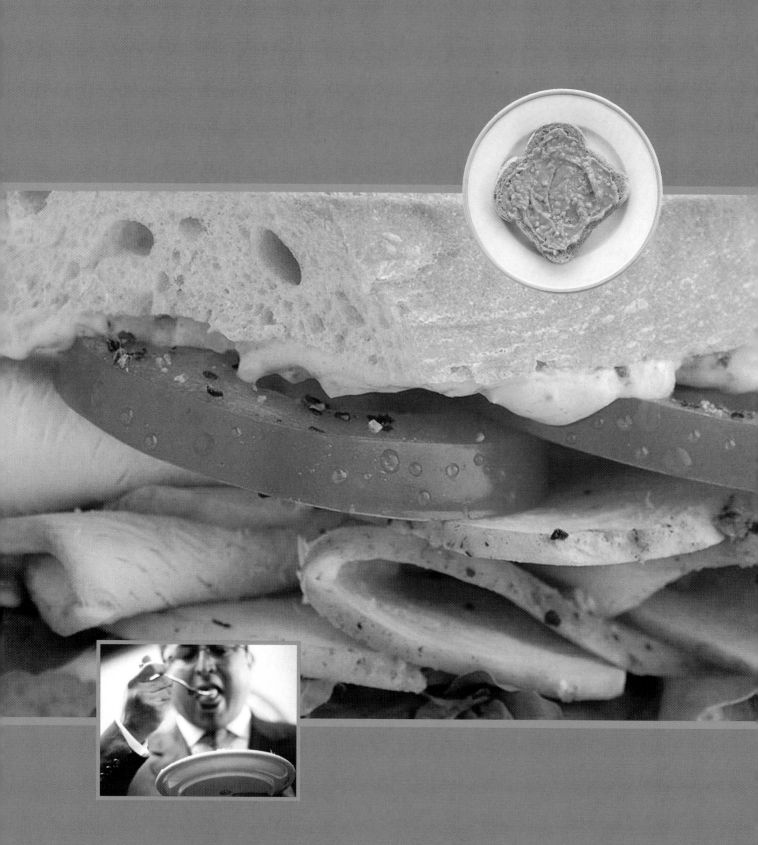

Chapter 3

The Human Body:
Are We Really What We Eat?

Chapter Objectives

After reading this chapter you will be able to:

1. Distinguish between appetite and hunger, describing the mechanisms that stimulate each, pp. 80–84.

2. Describe what is meant by the saying "We are what we eat," pp. 84–87.

3. Identify two functions of the plasma membrane, pp. 85–86.

4. Draw a picture of the gastrointestinal tract, including all major and accessory organs, pp. 87–88.

5. Describe the contribution of each organ of the gastrointestinal system to the digestion, absorption, and elimination of food, pp. 89–98.

6. Identify some of the enzymes involved in digesting foods, and list the source of these enzymes, pp. 89–94.

7. Describe the causes, symptoms, and treatments of gastroesophageal reflux disease and ulcers, pp. 100–104.

8. List three warning signs of dehydration resulting from diarrhea, p. 107.

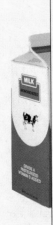
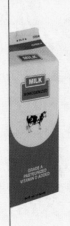

Test Yourself True or False?

1. Sometimes you may have an appetite even though you are not hungry. T or F

2. Your stomach is the primary organ responsible for telling you when you are hungry. T or F

3. The entire process of digestion and absorption of one meal takes about twenty-four hours. T or F

4. Most ulcers result from a type of infection. T or F

5. Irritable bowel syndrome is a rare disease that mostly affects older people. T or F

Test Yourself answers can be found at the end of the chapter.

Last month, Jill's life changed dramatically: She moved out of her parents' home to attend the state university three hours away, and she experienced her first bout of a mysterious and painful abdominal illness. After eating, Jill gets cramps so bad she can't stand up, and twice she has missed classes because of the pain. Because she also gets diarrhea, she thought at first that she had food poisoning or an infection; but four weeks have gone by, and she's not getting any better. The doctor at the student health center recommended Jill simply reduce her stress and avoid foods that upset her stomach, but she wants to know why she is getting sick and what she can do to get better. Jill is only eighteen years old and wonders if she is going to be this way for the rest of her life. She is even thinking of dropping out of school, if that would make her feel well again.

Do you know people who say they can't eat certain foods without experiencing upset stomach and diarrhea? Do you think these symptoms are "all in their head"? After all, how could foods that most people eat every day make someone else sick? How do we actually digest and absorb foods? If you had a food-related illness, what do you think would change in your life? How would you feel about shopping for food, dining out, or accepting an invitation to dinner with friends?

Our ability to properly digest and absorb foods is critical to health and optimal function. It is important to understand not only what happens to the foods we eat, but also why we eat and how disorders related to digestion, absorption, and elimination of food affect our health. We begin this chapter with a look at why we want to eat. We then introduce how the cells, tissues, and organs of the human body are made up of the food we eat and explore what happens to the food we eat. Finally, we look at some disorders that are related to the digestion, absorption, and elimination of food.

Why Do We Want to Eat?

Food provides us with energy, and the heat our body generates from this energy helps keep our bodies at the temperature required to maintain the proper chemical functions needed for life. Food gives us the molecular building blocks we need to manufacture new tissues for growth and repair, thereby keeping us healthy. Considering the importance of food, it makes sense that our bodies would employ a variety of mechanisms to make us want to eat.

Food Stimulates Our Senses

You've just finished eating at your favorite Thai restaurant. As you walk back to the block where you parked your car, you pass a bakery window displaying several cakes and pies, each of which looks more enticing than the last, and through the door wafts a complex aroma of coffee, cinnamon, and chocolate. You stop. Are you hungry? You must be, because you go inside and buy a slice of chocolate torte and an espresso. Later that night, when the caffeine from the chocolate and espresso keep you awake, you wonder why you succumbed.

The answer is that food stimulates our senses. Foods that are artfully prepared, arranged, or ornamented, with several different shapes and colors, appeal to our sense of sight. Advertisers know this and spend millions of dollars annually in the United States to promote and package foods in an appealing way. The aromas of foods like freshly brewed coffee and baked goods can also be powerful stimulants. Much of our ability to taste foods actually comes from our sense of smell. This is why foods are not as appealing when we are sick with a cold. Interestingly, our sense of smell is so acute that newborn babies can distinguish the scent of their own mother's breast milk from that of other mothers. Of all our senses, taste is the most important in determining what foods we choose to eat. Certain tastes, such as for sweet foods, are almost universally appealing, while others, such as the astringent taste of foods like spinach and kale, are quite individual. Texture is also important in food choices, as it stimulates nerve endings sensitive to touch in our mouth and on our tongue: do you prefer

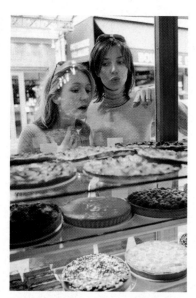

Food stimulates our senses. Foods that are artfully prepared, arranged, or ornamented, like the cakes and pies in this bakery display case, appeal to our sense of sight.

mashed potatoes, thick French fries, or rippled potato chips? Even your sense of hearing can be stimulated by foods, from the fizz of cola to the crunch of peanuts to the "snap, crackle, and pop" of Rice Krispies cereal.

> **Recap:** There are a number of factors that stimulate us to eat. Our senses of sight, smell, and taste are stimulated by foods. The texture of foods can also stimulate us to eat, or may cause some foods to be unappealing. These factors interact to motivate us to eat.

Psychosocial Factors Arouse Appetite

If it wasn't hunger that lured you into that bakery, it was probably appetite. **Appetite** is a psychological desire to consume specific foods (Figure 3.1). It is aroused by environmental cues—such as the sight of chocolate cake or the smell of coffee—and is not usually related to hunger. Appetite is generally related to pleasant sensations associated with food and is often linked to strong cravings for particular foods in the absence of hunger. **Hunger** is considered a more basic physiologic sensation, a drive that prompts us to find food and eat. Although we try to define appetite and hunger as two separate entities, many times they overlap, and symptoms of appetite and hunger are different for many people. Hunger is discussed in more detail in the following section.

In addition to environmental cues, our brain's association with certain events like birthday parties or holidays such as Thanksgiving can stimulate our appetite. At these times, society gives us permission to eat more than usual and/or to eat "forbidden" foods. For some people, being in a certain location can trigger appetite, such as at a baseball game or in a movie theater. Others may be triggered by the time of day or by an activity such as watching television or studying. Many people feel an increase in their appetite when they are under stress. Even when we feel full after a large meal, our appetite can motivate us to eat a delicious dessert.

appetite A psychological desire to consume specific foods.

hunger A physiologic sensation that prompts us to eat.

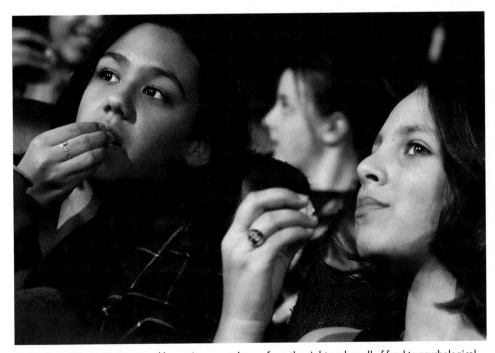

Figure 3.1   Appetite is aroused by environmental cues, from the sight and smell of food to psychological and social associations.

If you are trying to lose weight or to maintain your present weight, it is important to stay aware, as you go through a day, of whether you are truly hungry or whether you simply have an appetite. If you decide it is your appetite, try to get away from the trigger. For instance, in the previous scenario, you could have simply walked away from the bakery. By the time you'd reached your car, you would probably have forgotten the sights and smells of the bakery and would be aware of how full you felt from your Thai meal. Remember that, because appetite is a psychological mechanism, you can train yourself to stop or ignore its cues when you want to avoid its consequences.

Recap: Appetite is a psychological desire to consume certain foods and is generally related to pleasant sensations associated with food. Appetite typically involves cravings for foods in the absence of hunger. Environment and mood contribute to appetite. For people trying to lose weight, it is important to ignore the cues of appetite to avoid overeating.

Various Factors Affect Hunger and Satiation

A number of factors influence whether we experience feelings of hunger or satiation. Signals from our brain, certain chemicals produced by our bodies, and even the amount and type of food we eat interact to cause us to feel hungry or full. Let's review these factors now.

Signals From the Brain Cause Hunger and Satiation

Because *hunger* is a physiologic sensation that prompts us to find food and eat, it is more often felt as a negative or unpleasant sensation in which the physical drive to eat is very strong. The signal arises from within us, rather than in response to environmental stimuli, and is not typically associated with a specific food. A broad variety of foods appeals to us when we are really hungry.

One of the major organs affecting our sensation of hunger is the brain. That's right—it's not our stomachs, but our brains that tell us when we're hungry. The region of brain tissue that is responsible for prompting us to seek food is called the **hypothalamus** (Figure 3.2). It triggers hunger by integrating signals from nerve cells throughout our bodies. One important signal comes from special cells lining the stomach and small intestine that perceive whether these organs are empty or distended by the presence of food. These cells sense changes in pressure and fullness in the stomach and small intestine and send signals to the hypothalamus. For instance, if you have not eaten for many hours and your stomach and small intestine do not contain food, signals are sent to the hypothalamus indicating it is "time to eat," which causes you to experience the sensation of hunger.

hypothalamus A region of the forebrain below the thalamus where visceral sensations such as hunger and thirst are regulated.

Our blood glucose levels, which reflect our bodies' most readily-available fuel supply, is another primary signal affecting hunger. Falling blood glucose levels are accompanied by a change in insulin and glucagon levels. Insulin and glucagon are hormones produced in the pancreas and are responsible for maintaining blood glucose levels. These signals are relayed to the hypothalamus in the brain, where they trigger the sense that we need to eat in order to supply our bodies with more energy. Some people get irritable or feel a little faint when their blood glucose drops to a certain level. The level of blood glucose is related to when we last ate a meal, how active we are, and our individual metabolisms.

After we eat, the hypothalamus picks up the sensation of a distended stomach, other signals from the gut, and a

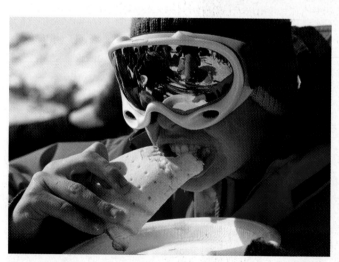

The presence of food not only initiates mechanical digestion via chewing, but also initiates chemical digestion through the secretion of various substances throughout the gastrointestinal tract.

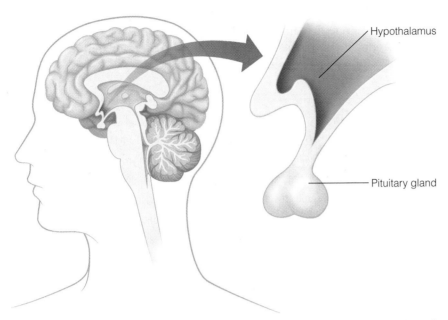

Figure 3.2 The hypothalamus triggers hunger by integrating signals from nerve cells throughout the body, as well as from messages carried by hormones.

rise in blood glucose levels. When it integrates these signals, you have the experience of feeling full, or *satiated*. However, as we saw in our previous scenario, even though our brain sends us clear signals about hunger, most of us become adept at ignoring them. . . and eat when we are not truly hungry.

Chemicals Called Hormones Affect Hunger and Satiation

A variety of hormones and hormone-like substances signal the hypothalamus to cause us to feel hungry or satiated. **Hormones** are chemical messengers that are secreted into the bloodstream by one of the many *glands* of the body. Hormones exert a regulatory effect on another organ. These glands release their secretions into the bloodstream in response to a signal. Examples of signals include falling or rising fuels within the blood, such as blood glucose, and chemical and nervous signals from the gut and the liver. The level of hormones in the blood then signal the hypothalamus to stimulate hunger or satiation. Examples of hormones and hormone-like substances that stimulate food intake include neuropeptide Y and galanin, while those that create feelings of satiety include leptin, cholecystokinin, and serotonin (Bell and Rolls 2001).

hormone Chemical messenger that is secreted into the bloodstream by one of the many glands of the body and acts as a regulator of physiological processes at a site remote from the gland which secreted it.

The Amount and Type of Food We Eat Can Affect Hunger and Satiation

Foods containing protein have the highest satiety value (Bell and Rolls 2001). This means that a ham sandwich will cause us to feel satiated for a longer period of time than will a tossed salad and toast, even if both meals have exactly the same number of calories. High fat diets have a higher satiety value than high carbohydrate diets.

Another factor affecting hunger is how bulky the meal is—that is, how much fiber and water is within the food. Bulky meals tend to stretch the stomach and small intestine, which sends signals back to the hypothalamus telling us that we are full so we stop eating. Beverages tend to be less satisfying than semisolid foods, and semi-solid foods have a lower satiety value than solid foods. For example, if you were to eat a bunch of grapes, you would feel a greater sense of fullness than if you drank a glass of grape juice (Zorrilla 1998).

Recap: In contrast to appetite, hunger is a physiologic sensation triggered by the hypothalamus in response to cues about stomach and intestinal distention, levels of energy substrates in the blood, and the release of certain hormones and hormone-like substances. High-protein foods make us feel satiated for longer periods of time, and bulky meals fill us up quickly, causing the distention that signals us to stop eating.

Nadia — *Nutri-Case*

"I'm tired of always having to watch what I eat. Now that I am pregnant and have pregnancy-induced diabetes, my doctor advised me to eat only when I am hungry and to avoid eating foods high in fat or sugar to prevent myself from gaining too much weight and to help control my diabetes. My problem is that I can't stop my cravings for foods like French fries, chocolate cake, cookies, and ice cream. These foods taste so good, and they make me feel better when I'm a little down. I want to do what is best for my baby and eat right. What can I do to stop myself from eating too many unhealthy foods?"

How would you explain to Nadia the difference between being truly hungry and just wanting foods due to stimulation of her appetite? What might you suggest to Nadia to avoid giving into her cravings? Based on what you have learned about designing a healthful diet, how might she still be able to include some of her favorite foods in a nutritious diet?

Are We Really What We Eat?

You've no doubt heard the saying over and over again that "you are what you eat." Is this scientifically true? To answer that question, and to better understand how we digest and process foods, we'll need to look at how our body is organized (Figure 3.3).

Atoms Bond to Form Molecules

Like all substances on earth, our bodies are made up of *atoms*. Atoms are the smallest units of matter, and they cannot be broken down by natural means. Atoms almost constantly bind to each other in nature. When they do, they form groups called *molecules*. For example, a molecule of water is composed of two atoms of hydrogen and an atom of oxygen, which is abbreviated H_2O.

Food Is Composed of Molecules

Molecules are critical to human life, as every particle of food we eat is composed of molecules. During digestion, we chew our food, mix it with saliva, churn it around in our stomachs, and mix it with the digestive enzymes in our small intestines. These actions result in breaking our food down into small molecules. Thus, the ultimate goal of digestion is to break the food we eat into small enough molecules that they can be easily transported through the gastrointestinal wall into the body and then travel more freely through our bloodstreams to help build the structures of our bodies and provide the energy we need to live.

Recap: Our bodies are made up of atoms, which are the smallest units of matter in nature. Atoms group together to form molecules. The food we eat is composed of molecules. The ultimate goal of digestion is to break food into small enough molecules that can be easily transported to the cells as needed.

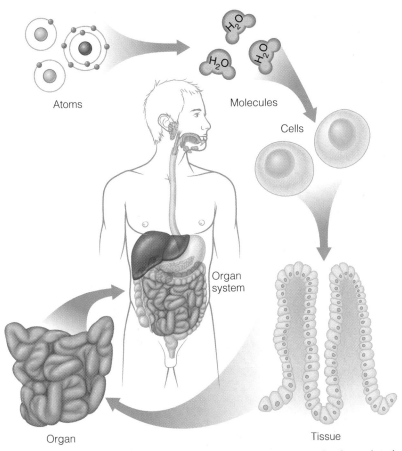

Atoms

Molecules

Cells

Organ system

Organ

Tissue

Figure 3.3   The organization of the human body. Atoms bind together to form molecules, and our body's cells are composed of molecules of the foods we eat. Cells join to form tissues, one or more types of which form organs. Body systems, such as the gastrointestinal system, are made up of several organs that perform discrete functions. For example, the stomach is the primary site of chemical breakdown of food into molecules.

Molecules Join to Form Cells

Whereas atoms are the smallest units of matter and make up both living and nonliving things, **cells** are the smallest units of life. That is, cells can grow, reproduce themselves, and perform certain basic functions, such as taking in nutrients, transmitting impulses, producing chemicals, and excreting wastes. The human body is composed of billions of cells that are constantly replacing themselves, destroying worn or damaged cells and manufacturing new ones. To support this constant demand for new cells, we need a ready supply of nutrient molecules, such as simple sugars, amino acids, and fatty acids, to serve as building blocks. These building blocks are the molecules that come from the breakdown of foods. All cells, whether of the skin, bones, or brain, are made of the same basic molecules of amino acids, sugars, and fatty acids that are also the main components of the foods we eat.

cell   The smallest unit of matter that exhibits the properties of living things, such as growth, reproduction, and metabolism.

Cells are Encased in a Functional Membrane

Cells are encased by a membrane called the **cell membrane,** or *plasma membrane* (Figure 3.4). This membrane is the outer covering of the cell and defines the cell's boundaries. It encloses the cell's contents and acts as a gatekeeper, either allowing or denying the entry and exit of molecules such as nutrients and wastes.

cell membrane   The boundary of an animal cell, composed of a phospholipid bilayer that separates its internal cytoplasm and organelles from the external environment.

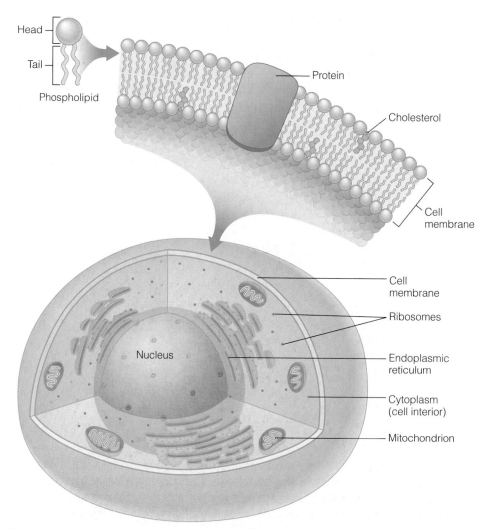

Figure 3.4   Representative cell of the small intestine, showing the cell membrane and a variety of organelles. The cell membrane is made up of phospholipid molecules, each composed of two fatty acid tails and a phosphate head. The two layers of the membrane align such that the fatty acid tails form the interior and the phosphate heads interact with the exterior aqueous environment. Inside the cell are the liquid cytoplasm and a variety of organelles.

Cell membranes are comprised of two layers. Each layer is made of molecules called *phospholipids*. Phospholipids consist of a long lipid "tail" bound to a round phospholipid "head." The phosphate head interacts with water, whereas the lipid tail repels water. In the cell membrane, the lipid tails of each layer face each other, forming the membrane interior, whereas the phosphate heads face either the extracellular environment or the cell's interior. Located throughout the membrane are molecules of another lipid, cholesterol, which help keep the membrane flexible. The membrane also contains various proteins, which assist in transport of nutrients and other substances across the cell membrane and in the manufacture of certain chemicals.

Recall that the cell membrane is the gatekeeper which, along with its proteins, determines what goes into and out of the cell. This means cell membranes are *selectively permeable*, allowing only some compounds to enter and leave the cell.

Cells Contain Organelles that Support Life

Enclosed within the cell membrane is a liquid called **cytoplasm** and a variety of **organelles** (see Figure 3.4). These tiny structures accomplish some surprisingly sophisticated functions. A full description of the roles of these organelles is beyond

cytoplasm The liquid within an animal cell.

organelle A tiny "organ" within a cell that performs a discrete function necessary to the cell.

the scope of this book, but a brief review of some of them and their functions related to nutrition are as follows:

- *Nucleus.* The *nucleus* is where our genetic information is located in the form of deoxyribonucleic acid (DNA). The cell nucleus is darkly colored because DNA is a huge molecule that is tightly packed within it. A cell's DNA contains the instructions that the cell uses to make certain proteins.
- *Ribosomes.* Ribosomes are structures the cell uses to make needed proteins.
- *Endoplasmic reticulum (ER).* The endoplasmic reticulum is important in the synthesis of proteins and lipids and storage of the mineral calcium. The ER looks like a maze of interconnected channels.
- *Mitochondria.* Often called the cell's powerhouse, mitochondria produce the energy molecule ATP (adenosine triphosphate) from basic food components. ATP can be thought of as a stored form of energy, drawn upon as we need it. Cells that have high energy needs contain more mitochondria than cells with lower energy needs.

Recap: Cells are the smallest units of life. They perform all critical body functions such as reproducing new cells, utilizing nutrients, transmitting nervous impulses, and excreting waste products. Cells are encased in a cell membrane that acts as a gatekeeper for the cell. Cells contain organelles, which are tiny structures that perform many functions such as making proteins, storing nutrients, and producing energy.

Cells Join to Form Tissues and Organs

Cells of a single type, such as muscle cells, join together to form functional groupings of cells called **tissues.** We'll introduce some of the unique tissues of our gastrointestinal tract later in this chapter. In general, several types of tissues join together to form **organs,** which are sophisticated structures that perform a unique body function. The stomach and small intestine are examples of organs.

tissue A sheet or other grouping of similar cells that performs a particular set of functions, for example, muscle tissue.

organ A body structure composed of two or more tissues and performing a specific function, for example, the esophagus.

Organs Make Up Functional Systems

Organs are further grouped into **systems** that perform integrated functions. The stomach, for example, is an organ that is part of the gastrointestinal system. It holds and partially digests a meal, but it can't perform all system functions—digestion, absorption, and elimination—by itself. These functions require several organs working together in an integrated system. In the next section, we describe how the organs of the gastrointestinal system actually work together to accomplish digestion and absorption of foods and elimination of waste products.

system A group of organs that work together to perform a unique function, for example, the gastrointestinal system.

Recap: Different cell types give rise to different tissue types and ultimately to different kinds of organs. Body systems, such as the gastrointestinal system, depend on many different organs to carry out all the varied functions they perform.

What Happens to the Food We Eat?

When we eat, the food we consume is digested, then the useful nutrients are absorbed, and finally, the waste products are eliminated. But what does each of these processes really entail? In the simplest terms, **digestion** is the process by which foods are broken down into their component molecules, either mechanically or chemically. **Absorption** is the process of taking these products of digestion through the wall of the intestine. **Elimination** is the process by which the undigested portions of food and waste products are removed from the body.

The processes of digestion, absorption, and elimination occur in the **gastrointestinal (GI) tract,** the organs of which work together to process foods. The

digestion The process by which foods are broken down into their component molecules, either mechanically or chemically.

absorption The physiologic process by which molecules of food are taken from the gastrointestinal tract into the body.

elimination The process by which the undigested portions of food and waste products are removed from the body.

gastrointestinal (GI) tract A long, muscular tube consisting of several organs: the mouth, esophagus, stomach, small intestine, and large intestine.

GI tract is a long tube: if held out straight, an adult GI tract would be about fifteen feet in length. Food within this tube is digested; in other words, food is broken down into molecules small enough to be absorbed by the cells lining the GI tract, and thereby passed into the body.

The GI tract begins at the mouth and ends at the anus (Figure 3.5). It is composed of several distinct organs, including the mouth, esophagus, stomach, small intestine, and large intestine. These organs are kept somewhat separated by muscular **sphincters,** which are tight rings of muscle that open when a nerve signal indicates that food is ready to pass into the next section. Surrounding the GI tract are several accessory organs, including the salivary glands, liver, pancreas, and gallbladder, each of which has a specific role in digestion and absorption of nutrients.

Now let's take a look at the role of each of these organs in processing the food we eat. Imagine that you ate a turkey sandwich for lunch today. It contained two slices of bread spread with mayonnaise, some turkey, two lettuce leaves, and a slice of tomato. Let's travel along with the sandwich and see what happens as it enters your GI tract and is digested into your body.

sphincter   A tight ring of muscle separating some of the organs of the GI tract and opening in response to nerve signals indicating that food is ready to pass into the next section.

Recap: Digestion is the process by which foods are broken down into molecules. Absorption is the process of taking the products of digestion across the GI tract walls and into the body. Elimination is the process by which undigested food and waste products are excreted from the body. These processes take place in the gastrointestinal (GI) tract. The organs of the GI tract include the mouth, esophagus, stomach, small intestine, and large intestine. Accessory organs such as the pancreas, gallbladder, and liver assist with digestion and absorption of nutrients.

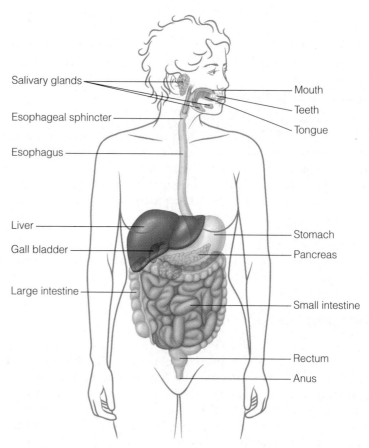

Figure 3.5   An overview of the gastrointestinal (GI) tract. The GI tract begins in the mouth and ends at the anus and is composed of numerous organs.

Digestion Begins in the Mouth

Believe it or not, the first step in the digestive process is not your first bite of that sandwich. It is your first thought about what you wanted for lunch and your first whiff of turkey and freshly baked bread as you stood in line at the deli. In this **cephalic phase** of digestion, hunger and appetite work together to prepare the GI tract to digest food. The nervous system stimulates the release of digestive juices in preparation for food entering the GI tract, and sometimes we experience some involuntary movement commonly called hunger pangs.

Now, let's stop smelling that sandwich and take a bite and chew! Chewing is very important because it moistens the food and mechanically breaks it down into pieces small enough to swallow (Figure 3.6). Thus, chewing initiates the mechanical digestion of food. The tough coating or skin surrounding the lettuce fibers and tomato seeds are also broken open, facilitating digestion. This is especially important when eating foods that are high in fiber such as grains, fruits, and vegetables.

When we chew, everything in your sandwich mixes together: the protein in the turkey, the carbohydrates in the bread, lettuce, and tomato, the fat in the mayonnaise, and the vitamins and minerals in all of the foods. The presence of food not only initiates mechanical digestion via chewing, but also initiates chemical digestion through the secretion of various substances throughout the gastrointestinal tract. As our teeth cut and grind the different foods in your sandwich, more surface area is exposed to the digestive juices in our mouth. Foremost among these is **saliva,** which you secrete from your **salivary glands.** Saliva not only moistens your food, but also begins the process of chemical breakdown. One component of saliva is *amylase*, an enzyme that starts the process of carbohydrate digestion in the mouth. Saliva also contains other components such as antibodies that protect the body from foreign bacteria entering the mouth and keep the oral cavity free from infection.

Salivary amylase is the first of many **enzymes** that assist our body in digesting and absorbing food. Since we will encounter many enzymes on our journey through the GI tract, let's discuss them briefly here. Enzymes are complex proteins that induce chemical changes in other substances to speed up bodily processes and which may be reused since they essentially are unchanged by the chemical reactions they catalyze. Imagine them as facilitators: a chemical reaction that might take an hour to occur independently might happen in a few seconds with the help of one or more enzymes. The action of enzymes can result in the production of new substances or can assist in

cephalic phase Earliest phase of digestion in which the brain thinks about and prepares the digestive organs for the consumption of food.

saliva A mixture of water, mucus, enzymes, and other chemicals that moistens the mouth and food, binds food particles together, and begins the digestion of carbohydrates.

salivary glands Group of glands found under and behind the tongue and beneath the jaw which release saliva continually as well as in response to the thought, sight, smell, or presence of food.

enzymes Small chemicals, usually proteins, that act on other chemicals to speed up body processes but are not apparently changed during those processes.

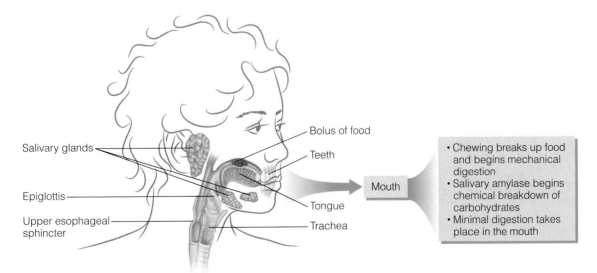

Figure 3.6 Where your food is now: the mouth. Chewing moistens food and mechanically breaks it down into pieces small enough to swallow, while salivary amylase begins chemical digestion of carbohydrates.

breaking substances apart. We make hundreds of enzymes in our bodies, and the process of digestion—as well as many other biochemical processes that go on in our body—could not happen without them. By the way, enzyme names typically end in -*ase* (as in amylase), so they are easy to recognize as we go through the digestive process.

In reality, very little digestion occurs in the mouth. This is because we do not hold food in our mouths for very long and because all of the enzymes needed to break down our food are not present in our saliva. Salivary amylase starts the digestion of carbohydrates in the mouth, and this digestion continues until food reaches the stomach. Once in the stomach, salivary amylase is no longer active because it is destroyed by the acidic environment of the stomach.

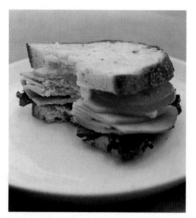

Digestion of a sandwich starts before you even take a bite.

Recap: The cephalic phase of digestion involves hunger and appetite working together before you take your first bite of food to prepare the GI tract for digestion and absorption. Chewing initiates mechanical digestion of food by breaking it into smaller components and mixing all nutrients together. Chewing also stimulates chemical digestion through the secretion of digestive juices such as saliva. Saliva moistens food and starts the process of carbohydrate digestion through the action of the enzyme salivary amylase. This action continues during the transport of food through the esophagus and stops when food reaches the acidic environment of the stomach.

The Esophagus Propels Food into the Stomach

Now that our sandwich is soft and moist in our mouths, it is time to swallow (Figure 3.7). Most of us take swallowing for granted. However, it is a very complex process involving voluntary and involuntary motion. A tiny flap of tissue called the *epiglottis* acts like a trapdoor covering the entrance to the trachea (or windpipe). The epiglottis is normally open, allowing us to breathe freely even while chewing (Figure 3.7a). As our bite of sandwich moves to the very back of the mouth, our brain is sent a signal to temporarily raise the soft palate and close the openings to our nasal passages, preventing aspiration of food or liquid into our sinuses (Figure 3.7b). The brain also signals the esophagus to close during swallowing so food and liquid cannot enter our trachea.

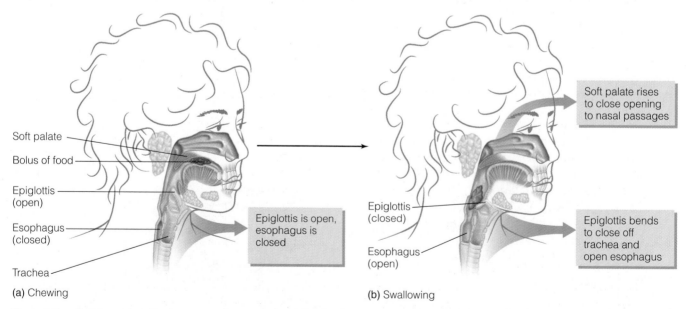

Soft palate
Bolus of food
Epiglottis (open)
Esophagus (closed)
Trachea

Epiglottis is open, esophagus is closed

Soft palate rises to close opening to nasal passages

Epiglottis (closed)
Esophagus (open)

Epiglottis bends to close off trachea and open esophagus

(a) Chewing   (b) Swallowing

Figure 3.7   Chewing and swallowing are complex processes. **(a)** During the process of chewing, the epiglottis is open and the esophagus is closed so that we can continue to breathe as we chew. **(b)** During swallowing, the epiglottis closes so that food does not enter the trachea and obstruct our breathing. The soft palate also rises to seal off our nasal passages to prevent aspiration of food or liquid into the sinuses.

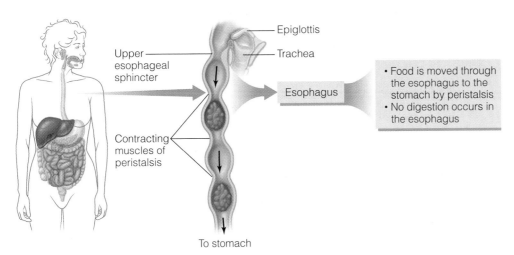

Figure 3.8   Where your food is now: the esophagus. Peristalsis, the rhythmic contraction and relaxation of both circular and longitudinal muscles in the esophagus, propels food toward the stomach. Peristalsis occurs throughout the GI tract.

Sometimes this protective mechanism goes awry, for instance when we try to eat and talk at the same time—sometimes referred to as "food going down the wrong pipe." When this happens, we experience the sensation of choking and typically cough involuntarily and repeatedly until the offending food or liquid is expelled from the trachea.

As the trachea closes, the **esophagus** opens. This muscular tube connects and transports food from the mouth to the stomach (Figure 3.8). It does this by contracting two sets of muscles: inner sheets of circular muscle squeeze the food, while outer sheets of longitudinal muscle push food along the length of the tube. Together, these rhythmic waves of squeezing and pushing are called **peristalsis.** We will see shortly that peristalsis occurs throughout the GI tract.

Gravity also helps transport food down the esophagus, which is one reason why it is wise to avoid reclining immediately after eating a meal. Together, peristalsis and gravity can transport a bite of food from our mouth to the opening of the stomach in five to eight seconds. At the end of the esophagus is a sphincter muscle, the *gastroesophageal sphincter* (*gastro-* indicates the stomach), which is normally tightly closed. When food reaches the end of the esophagus, this sphincter relaxes to allow the passage of food into the stomach. In some people, this sphincter is continually somewhat relaxed. Later in the chapter, we'll discuss this disorder and the unpleasant symptoms caused when this sphincter does not function properly.

esophagus   Muscular tube of the GI tract connecting the back of the mouth to the stomach.

peristalsis   Wave of squeezing and pushing contractions that move food in one direction through the length of the GI tract.

> **Recap:** Swallowing causes our nasal passages to close and the epiglottis to cover our trachea to prevent food from entering our sinuses and lungs. The esophagus opens as the trachea closes. The esophagus is a muscular tube that transports food from the mouth to the stomach. The rhythmic waves of muscles surrounding the esophagus, called peristalsis, push food toward the stomach. Gravity also helps move food toward the stomach. Once food reaches the stomach, the gastroesophageal sphincter opens to allow food into the stomach.

The Stomach Mixes, Digests, and Stores Food

The **stomach** is a J-shaped organ. The size of the stomach is fairly individual; in general, it's volume is about 6 fluid ounces (or ¾ cup) when it is empty. When the stomach is full, it can expand to hold about 32 fluid ounces, or about 4 cups (Kim et al. 2001). Before any food reaches the stomach, the brain sends signals telling it to be ready for the food to arrive. The hormone gastrin is secreted after ingestion of a meal;

stomach   A J-shaped organ where food is partially digested, churned, and stored until release into the small intestine.

gastric juice   Acidic liquid secreted within the stomach; it contains hydrochloric acid, pepsin, and other compounds.

denature   Term used to describe the action of unfolding proteins. Proteins must be denatured before they can be digested.

chyme   Semifluid mass consisting of partially digested food, water, and gastric juices.

this hormone acts on gastric cells and stimulates them to secrete disgestive juices. The stomach also prepares for your sandwich by secreting **gastric juice,** which contains several important compounds:

- *Hydrochloric acid (HCl)* keeps the stomach interior very acidic—more so than many citrus juices. This acid is extremely important for digestion because it starts to **denature** proteins, which means it destroys the bonds that maintain the structure of proteins. HCl also converts *pepsinogen*, an inactive substance, into the active enzyme *pepsin*, which assists in protein digestion. HCl performs another important function: it kills any bacteria and/or germs that may have entered your body with your sandwich.

- *Pepsin* begins to digest proteins into smaller components. Recall that salivary amylase begins to digest carbohydrates in the mouth. In contrast, proteins and fats enter the stomach largely unchanged. Pepsin begins the digestion of protein and activates many other GI enzymes needed to digest your meal.

- *Gastric lipase* is an enzyme responsible for fat digestion. Thus, it begins to break apart the fat in the turkey and the mayonnaise in your sandwich. Only minimal digestion of fat occurs in the stomach.

- Your stomach also secretes *mucus* that protects its lining from being digested by the HCl and pepsin.

With these gastric juices already present, chemical digestion of proteins and fats begins as soon as food enters your stomach (Figure 3.9). The stomach has several other jobs, too. One is to mix and churn the food until it becomes a liquid called **chyme.** This physical mixing and churning of food is another example of mechanical digestion that takes place in the gastrointestinal tract. Enzymes can access the liquid chyme easier than more solid forms of food. This access more easily allows chemical digestion to take place.

Although most absorption occurs in the small intestine, the stomach lining does begin absorbing a few substances. These include water, some medium chain fatty acids (Davidson 2003), and some drugs, including aspirin and alcohol.

Another of your stomach's jobs is to store your sandwich (or what's left of it!) while the next part of the digestive tract, the small intestine, gets ready for the next wave of food. Remember that the stomach can hold about 4 to 7 cups of food. If this amount suddenly moved into the small intestine all at once, it would overwhelm it. Food (chyme) stays in your stomach about two hours before it is released periodically in spurts into the duodenum, which is the first part of the small intestine. Regulating this release is the *pyloric sphincter* (see Figure 3.9).

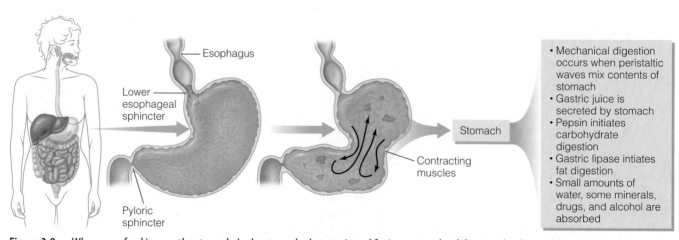

Figure 3.9   Where your food is now: the stomach. In the stomach, the protein and fat in your sandwich begin to be digested. Your meal is churned into chyme and stored until release into the small intestine.

Recap: The stomach prepares itself for digestion by secreting gastric juice. Gastric juice contains substances that assist in digestion, including, hydrochloric acid, and the enzymes pepsin and gastric lipase. The stomach also secretes mucus to protect its own lining from digestion. Digestion of proteins and fats begins in the stomach. The stomach mixes food into a liquidy substance called chyme, which is more easily digested than solid food. The stomach stores chyme and releases it periodically into the small intestine through the pyloric sphincter.

Most of Digestion and Absorption Occurs in the Small Intestine

The **small intestine** is the longest portion of the GI tract, accounting for about two-thirds (or about 10 feet) of its length. However, at only an inch in diameter, it is comparatively narrow.

The small intestine is composed of three sections (Figure 3.10). The *duodenum* is the section of the small intestine that is connected via the pyloric sphincter to the stomach. The *jejunum* is the middle portion, and the last portion is the *ileum*. It connects to the large intestine at another sphincter, called the *ileocecal valve.*

Most of digestion and absorption take place in the small intestine. Here, food is broken down into its smallest components, molecules that the body can then absorb into its internal environment. In this next section we review a variety of accessory organs, enzymes, and unique anatomical features of the small intestine that permit maximal absorption of most nutrients.

The Gallbladder and Pancreas Aid in Digestion

Now let's get back to your sandwich. As the fat from the turkey and mayonnaise enters the small intestine, a hormone-like substance called cholecystokinin (or CCK) is released in response to the presence of protein and fat. This substance signals an accessory organ, the **gallbladder,** to contract. The gallbladder is located beneath the liver (see Figure 3.5), and stores a greenish fluid, **bile,** produced by the liver. Contraction of the gallbladder sends bile through the *common bile duct* into the duodenum. Bile

small intestine The longest portion of the GI tract where most digestion and absorption takes place.

gallbladder A tissue sac beneath the liver that stores bile and secretes it into the small intestine.

bile Fluid produced by the liver and stored in the gallbladder; it emulsifies fats in the small intestine.

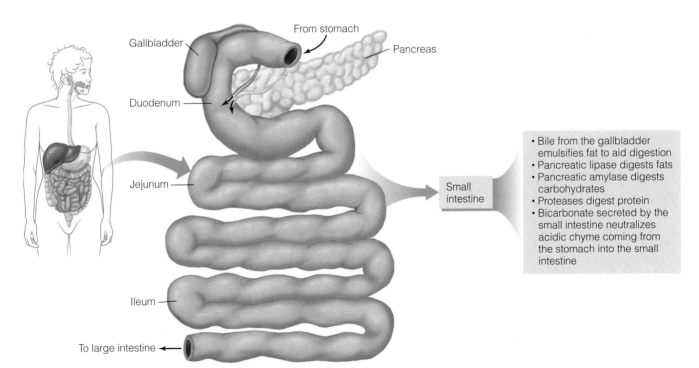

From stomach

Gallbladder

Pancreas

Duodenum

Jejunum

Small intestine

- Bile from the gallbladder emulsifies fat to aid digestion
- Pancreatic lipase digests fats
- Pancreatic amylase digests carbohydrates
- Proteases digest protein
- Bicarbonate secreted by the small intestine neutralizes acidic chyme coming from the stomach into the small intestine

Ileum

To large intestine

Figure 3.10 Where your food is now: the small intestine. Here, most digestion and absorption of the nutrients in your sandwich take place.

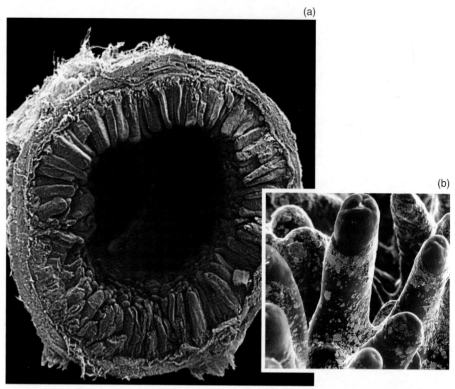

(a)

(b)

The small intestine. **(a)** The interior of the small intestine, also called the mucosal membrane. **(b)** The lining of the small intestine has thousands of folds and finger-like projections called villi that increase its surface area over 500 times, significantly increasing the small intestine's absorptive capacity.

pancreas Gland located behind the stomach; it secretes digestive enzymes.

then *emulsifies* the fat; that is, it reduces the fat into smaller globules and disperses them so they are more accessible to digestive enzymes.

The **pancreas,** another accessory organ, manufactures, holds, and secretes digestive enzymes. It is located behind the stomach (see Figure 3.5). Enzymes secreted by the pancreas include *pancreatic amylase*, which continues the digestion of carbohydrates, and *pancreatic lipase*, which continues the digestion of fats. *Proteases* secreted in pancreatic juice digest proteins. The pancreas is also responsible for manufacturing hormones that are important in metabolism. Insulin and glucagon, two hormones necessary to regulate the amount of glucose in the blood, are produced by the pancreas.

Another essential role of the pancreas is to secrete bicarbonate into the duodenum. Bicarbonate is a base and, like all bases, is capable of neutralizing acids. Recall that chyme leaving the stomach is very acidic. The pancreatic bicarbonate neutralizes this acidic chyme so that the pancreatic enzymes will work effectively and to ensure that the lining of the duodenum is not eroded.

Now the protein, carbohydrate, and fat in your sandwich have been processed into a liquid that contains molecules of nutrients small enough for absorption. This molecular "soup" continues to move along the small intestine via peristalsis, encountering the absorptive cells of the intestinal lining all along the way.

A Specialized Lining Enables the Small Intestine to Absorb Food

The lining of the GI tract is especially well-suited for absorption. If you looked at the inside of the lining, which is also referred to as the mucosal membrane, you would notice that it is heavily folded (Figure 3.11). This feature increases the surface area of the small intestine and allows it to absorb more nutrients than if it were smooth. Within these larger folds, you would notice even smaller fingerlike projections called *villi*, whose constant movement helps them to encounter and trap nutrient molecules. Inside each villus are *capillaries*, or tiny blood vessels, and a **lacteal,** which is a small lymph vessel. (The role of the lymphatic system is presented on page 96.) These vessels take up

lacteal A small lymph vessel located inside of the villi of the small intestine.

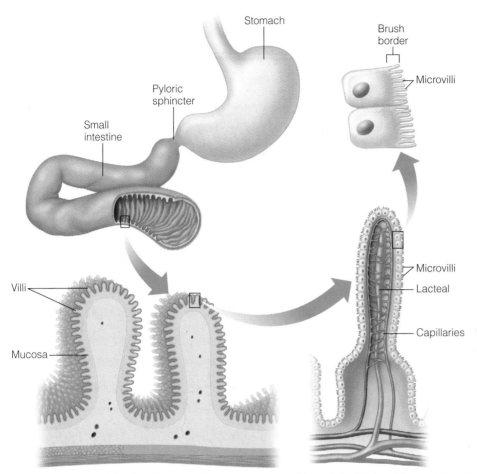

Figure 3.11   The brush border. Absorption of nutrients occurs via this specialized lining of the small intestine.

the final products of digestion. Water-soluble nutrients are absorbed directly into the bloodstream while fat-soluble nutrients are absorbed into lymph. Covering these villi are specialized cells covered with hairlike structures called *microvilli*. The microvilli look like tiny brushes and are sometimes referred to as the **brush border.** These intricate folds increase the surface area of the small intestine by more than 500 times, which tremendously increases the absorptive capacity of the small intestine.

brush border Term that describes the microvilli of the small intestine's lining. These microvilli tremendously increase the small intestine's absorptive capacity.

Intestinal Cells Readily Absorb Vitamins, Minerals, and Water

The turkey sandwich you ate contained several vitamins and minerals in addition to protein, carbohydrate, and fat. For instance, the bread contained B-complex vitamins and iron, and the tomato contained vitamin C. If you had a glass of milk with your sandwich, you also consumed the mineral calcium as well as vitamin D. The turkey contained some of the mineral zinc. Most of the sandwich also contained small amounts of sodium, potassium, and chloride.

Vitamins and minerals are not really "digested" the same way that macronutrients are. These compounds do not have to be broken down because they are small enough to be readily absorbed by the small intestine. For example, fat-soluble vitamins such as vitamins A, D, E, and K are soluble in lipids and are absorbed into the intestinal cells along with the fats in our foods. Water-soluble vitamins such as the B vitamins and vitamin C typically have some type of active transport process that helps assure the vitamin is absorbed by the small intestine.

Minerals are absorbed all along the small intestine, and in some cases in the large intestine as well, by a wide variety of mechanisms. For example, the absorption of sodium, potassium, and chloride is regulated by nerves and hormones working together to maintain water and salt balance (see Chapter 7). These minerals are absorbed in both the small and large intestines. Iron absorption increases or decreases according to the body's needs. One way the body regulates the amount of iron absorbed is by holding the iron in the mucosal cell until needed. The cells turn over every 24 to 72 hours, so any excess iron can be lost as the cell is sloughed off. There is also a specialized protein in the membrane of intestinal cells that can transport needed iron into the body (see Chapter 10). Zinc, copper, and manganese can each be absorbed with the help of a carrier protein, but they can also pass through the intestinal cells unassisted.

Finally, a large component of food is water, and of course you also drink lots of water throughout the day. Water is readily absorbed along the entire length of the GI tract because it is a small molecule that can easily pass through the cell membrane. However, as we will see shortly, a significant percentage of water is absorbed in the large intestine.

Blood and Lymph Transport Nutrients and Fluids

Our bodies have two main fluids that transport nutrients, water, and waste products throughout the body. These fluids are blood and lymph. Blood travels through the cardiovascular system, and lymph travels through the lymphatic system (Figure 3.12). The oxygen we inhale into our lungs is carried by our red blood cells. This oxygen-rich blood then travels to the heart, where it is pumped out to our body. Blood travels to all of our tissues to deliver nutrients and other materials and pick up waste products. As blood travels through the GI tract, it picks up most nutrients and fluids that are absorbed through the mucosal membrane of the small intestine. The lymphatic vessels pick up most fats and fat-soluble vitamins and fluids that have escaped from the cardiovascular system and transport them in the lymph. This lymph eventually returns to the bloodstream in an area near the heart where the lymphatic and blood vessels join together.

As the blood leaves the GI system, it is transported to the liver. The role of the liver in digestion is described in the following section. The waste products picked up by the blood as it circulates around the body are filtered and excreted by the kidneys. In addition, much of the carbon dioxide remaining in the blood once it reaches the lungs is exhaled into the outside air, making room for oxygen to attach to the red blood cells and repeat this cycle of circulation again.

The Liver Regulates Blood Nutrients

liver The largest auxillary organ of the GI tract and one of the most important organs of the body. Its functions include production of bile and processing of nutrient-rich blood from the small intestine.

Once nutrients are absorbed from the small intestine, most enter the *portal vein*, which carries them to the **liver.** The liver is a triangular wedge-shaped organ of about three pounds of tissue that rests almost entirely within the protection of the rib cage on the right side of the body (see Figure 3.5). The liver is the largest digestive organ; it is also one of the most important organs in the body, performing over five hundred discrete functions, including digestive functions. One function of the liver is to receive the products of digestion, and then release into the blood stream those nutrients needed throughout the body. The liver also processes and stores monosaccharides, triglycerides (fats), and amino acids, and plays a major role in regulating these energy nutrients. For instance, after we eat a meal, the liver picks up excess glucose from the blood and stores it as glycogen, releasing it into the bloodstream when we need energy later in the day. It also stores certain vitamins and manufactures blood proteins. The liver can even make glucose when necessary to make sure that our blood levels stay constant. Thus, the liver plays a major role in regulating the level and type of fuel or energy nutrients circulating in our blood.

Have you ever wondered why people who abuse alcohol are at risk for damaging their liver? That's because another of its functions is to filter the blood, removing wastes and toxins like alcohol, medications, and other drugs. When you drink, your liver works hard to replace the cells poisoned with alcohol, but, over time, scar tissue

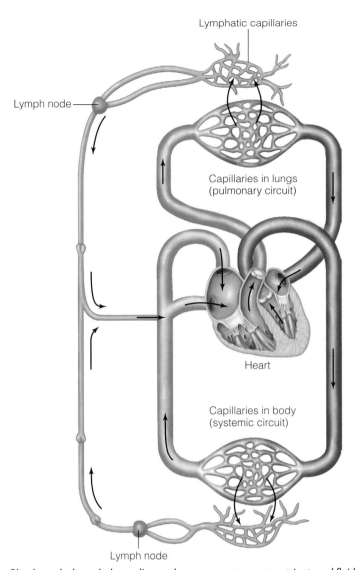

Lymphatic capillaries

Lymph node

Capillaries in lungs
(pulmonary circuit)

Heart

Capillaries in body
(systemic circuit)

Lymph node

Figure 3.12   Blood travels through the cardiovascular system to transport nutrients and fluids and pick up waste products. Lymph travels through the lymphatic system and transports most fats and fat-soluble vitamins.

forms. The scar tissue blocks the free flow of blood through the liver, so that any further toxins accumulate in the blood, causing confusion, coma, and ultimately, death.

Another important job of the liver is to synthesize many of the chemicals used by the body in carrying out metabolic processes. For example, the liver synthesizes bile, which, as we just discussed, is then stored in the gallbladder until needed to emulsify fats so they can be digested.

> **Recap:** Most digestion occurs in the small intestine. The small intestine is comprised of three sections, the duodenum, the jejunum, and the ileum. The gallbladder stores bile, which is produced by the liver. Bile emulsifies fat into pieces that are more easily digested. The pancreas synthesizes and secretes digestive enzymes that break down carbohydrates, fats, and proteins. The lining of the small intestine is heavily folded, with the surface area expanded by villi and microvilli. Nutrients are absorbed across the mucosal membrane. Vitamins and minerals can be absorbed directly into lymph or the bloodstream. The liver processes all nutrients absorbed from the small intestine and stores and regulates monosaccharides, triglycerides, and amino acids.

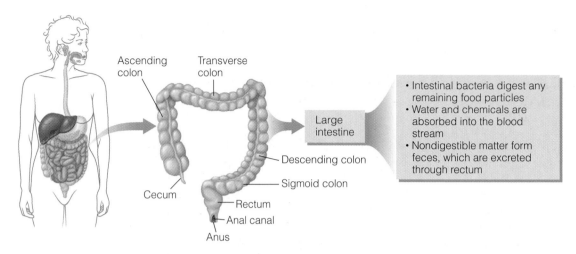

Figure 3.13   Where your food is now: the large intestine. Most water absorption occurs here, as does the formation of food wastes into semisolid feces. Peristalsis propels the feces to the body exterior.

The Large Intestine Stores Food Waste Until It Is Excreted

large intestine Final organ of the GI tract consisting of the cecum, colon, rectum, and anal canal, and in which most water is absorbed and feces are formed.

The **large intestine** is a thick tubelike structure that frames the small intestine on three-and-a-half sides (Figure 3.13). It begins with a tissue sac called the *cecum*, which explains the name of the sphincter—the *ileocecal valve*—which connects it to the ileum of the small intestine. From the cecum, the large intestine continues up along the left side of the small intestine as the *ascending colon*. The *transverse colon* runs across the top of the small intestine, and then the *descending colon* comes down on the right. The *sigmoid colon* is the last segment of the colon, and extends from the bottom right corner to the *rectum*. The last segment of the large intestine is the *anal canal*, which is about an inch and a half long.

What has happened to our turkey sandwich? The undigested food components in the chyme finally reach the large intestine. By this time, the digestive mass entering the large intestine does not resemble the chyme that left the stomach several hours before. This is because a majority of the nutrients have been absorbed, leaving mostly nondigestible food material such as fiber, bacteria, and water. The intestinal bacteria are normal and helpful residents, since they finish digesting some of the nutrients from your sandwich. The by-products of this digestion, such as short-chain fatty acids, are reabsorbed into the body where they return to the liver and are either stored or used as needed. The bacteria living in our large intestine are so helpful that, as discussed in the Nutrition Debate at the end of this chapter, many people consume them deliberately! No other digestion occurs in the large intestine. Instead, its main functions are to store the digestive mass for twelve to twenty-four hours, and during that time to absorb nutrients and water from it, leaving a semisolid mass called *feces*. Peristalsis occurs weakly to move the feces through the colon, except for one or more stronger waves of peristalsis each day that force the feces more powerfully toward the rectum for elimination.

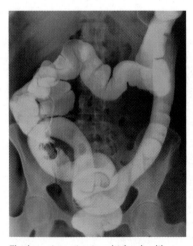

The large intestine is a thick tube-like structure that stores the undigested mass leaving the small intestine and absorbs any remaining nutrients and water.

Recap: The large intestine is comprised of six sections: the cecum, ascending colon, descending colon, sigmoid colon, rectum, and the anal canal. Small amounts of undigested food, undigestible food material, bacteria, and water enter the large intestine from the small intestine. The bacteria assist with final digestion of any remaining digestible food products. No other digestion occurs in the large intestine. The main functions of the large intestine are to store the digestive mass and absorb any remaining nutrients and water over a 12- to 24-hour period. The remaining substance, a semisolid mass called feces, is then eliminated from the body.

How Does the Body Coordinate and Regulate Digestion?

To complete your picture of the gastrointestinal system, it might help to think of your body as a manufacturing plant with the GI tract as its assembly line. Here, all the raw, unprocessed materials (foods) needed by the manufacturing plant to synthesize new products arrive. As the raw materials are processed, they are broken down into usable parts. These parts are then sent to other departments to be reassembled into new products. Wastes and unwanted parts are excreted at the end of the assembly line. Now that you can identify the organs involved in this process and the jobs they each perform, you might be wondering—who's the boss? In other words, what organ or system directs and coordinates all of these interrelated processes? The answer is the neuromuscular system. Each of its two components, the nervous and muscular systems, is an essential partner in coordinating and regulating the digestion, absorption, and elimination of food.

The Muscles of the Gastrointestinal Tract Mix and Move Food

The purpose of the muscles of the GI tract is to mix food and move it in one direction; that is, from the mouth toward the anus. When food is present, nerves respond to the stretching of the tract walls and send signals to its muscles, stimulating peristalsis. As with the assembly line, the entire GI tract functions together so that materials are moved in one direction in a coordinated manner and wastes are removed as needed.

In order to process the large amount of food we consume daily, we use both voluntary and involuntary muscles. Muscles in the mouth are primarily voluntary; that is, they are under our conscious control. Once we swallow, involuntary muscles largely take over to propel food through the rest of the GI tract. This enables us to continue digesting and absorbing our food while we're working, exercising, and even sleeping. Let's now reveal the master-controller behind these involuntary muscular actions.

The Enteric Nerves Coordinate and Regulate Digestive Activities

The nervous system in your body is like the wiring and communications system in the manufacturing plant. It enables communication between the assembly line and all other departments, allowing the transfer of messages about when to start and stop various functions, how to operate, and what is needed in other parts of the manufacturing plant. Within this communications system, the central nervous system (CNS) is like the main control desk, and each body system or region has its own branch nerves. The CNS is composed of the brain and spinal cord. As discussed earlier in this chapter, the hypothalamus of the brain plays an important role in control of hunger and satiation.

There is also an intricate system of nerves and other structures outside of the CNS; this system is called the peripheral nervous system. The nerves of the GI tract are found within the peripheral nervous system and are collectively known as the **enteric nervous system.**

enteric nervous system The nerves of the GI tract.

Enteric nerves work both independently of and in collaboration with the CNS. For example, they can respond independently to signals produced within the GI tract without first relaying them to the CNS for interpretation or assistance. On the other hand, many jobs require the involvement of the CNS. For instance, as we discussed earlier, special nerves in the GI tract pick up mechanical signals indicating how far the tract wall is stretched; that is, how full it is. These receptors signal the brain that your digestive tract is full, and then your brain sends out messages that prompt you to stop eating. Another type of enteric nerve picks up chemical signals about how acidic the digestive environment is or if there is protein or fat present. The CNS receives and responds to these signals, sending out a message to the pancreas to secrete enzymes for fat and protein digestion, for example.

All along the GI tract are a series of glands that secrete digestive juice, mucus, and water. These secretions are also under nervous system control. When food digestion products reach various locations within the GI tract, these glands are stimulated to release either digestive enzymes, mucus, or water and electrolytes. For example, as chyme moves from the stomach into the small intestine, neural signals are sent to stimulate the pancreas, gallbladder, and mucosal cells lining the intestinal tract. These signals cause these glands and cells to secrete digestive enzymes, bile, bicarbonate, and water, secretions necessary to continue digestion in the small intestine.

Recap: The coordination and regulation of digestion is directed by the neuromuscular system. The muscles of the GI tract mix food and move it from the mouth to the anus. Voluntary muscles, which are under our conscious control, assist us with chewing and swallowing. Once food is swallowed, the involuntary muscles along the entire length of the GI tract function together so that materials are moved in one direction in a coordinated manner and wastes are removed as needed. The enteric nerves of the GI tract work with the central nervous system to achieve digestion, absorption, and elimination of food.

What Disorders Are Related to Digestion, Absorption, and Elimination?

Considering the complexity of digestion, absorption, and elimination, it's no wonder that sometimes things go wrong. Disorders of the neuromuscular system, hormonal imbalances, infections, allergies, and a host of other disorders can disturb gastrointestinal functioning, as can merely consuming the wrong types or amounts of food for our unique needs. Whenever there is a problem with the GI tract, absorption of nutrients can be affected. If absorption of a nutrient is less than optimal for a long period of time, malnutrition can result. Let's look more closely at some GI tract disorders and what you might be able to do if they affect you.

Heartburn and Gastroesophageal Reflux Disease (GERD)

heartburn   The painful sensation that occurs over the sternum when hydrochloric acid backs up into the lower esophagus.

gastroesophageal reflux disease (GERD)   A painful type of heartburn that occurs more than twice per week.

When you eat food, your stomach secretes hydrochloric acid to start the digestive process. In many people, the amount of HCl secreted is occasionally excessive or the gastroesophageal sphincter opens too soon. In either case, the result is that HCl seeps back up into the esophagus (Figure 3.14). Although the stomach is protected from HCl by a thick coat of mucus, the esophagus does not have this mucus coating. Thus, the HCl burns it. When this happens, a person experiences a painful sensation in the region of his or her chest above the sternum (breastbone). This condition is commonly called **heartburn**. People often take over the counter antacids to neutralize the HCl, thereby relieving the heartburn. A non-drug approach is to repeatedly swallow: this action causes any acid within the esophagus to be swept down into the stomach, eventually relieving the symptoms.

Gastroesophageal reflux disease (GERD) is a more painful type of heartburn that occurs more than twice per week. GERD affects about nineteen million Americans and, like heartburn, occurs when HCl flows back into the esophagus. Although people who experience occasional heartburn usually have no structural abnormalities, many people with GERD have an overly relaxed or damaged esophageal sphincter or damage to the esophagus itself. Symptoms of GERD

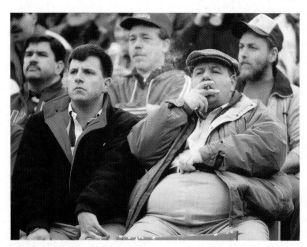

Although the exact causes of gastroesophageal reflux disease (GERD) are unknown, smoking and being overweight may be contributing factors.

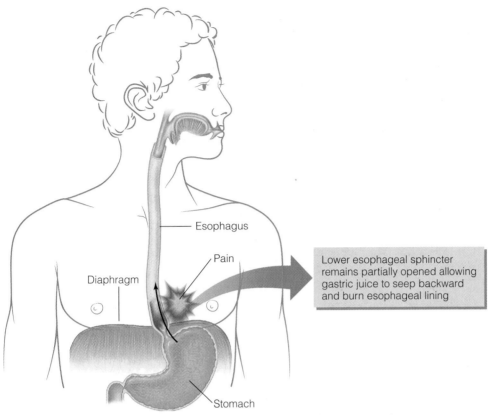

Figure 3.14 The mechanism of heartburn and gastroesophageal reflux disease is the same: acidic gastric juices seep backward through an open or relaxed sphincter into the lower portion of the esophagus, burning its lining. The pain is felt above the sternum, over the heart.

include persistent heartburn and acid regurgitation. Some people have GERD without heartburn and instead experience chest pain, trouble swallowing, burning in the mouth, the feeling that food is stuck in the throat, or hoarseness in the morning (NDDIC 2003, June).

The exact causes of GERD are unknown. However, there are a number of factors that may contribute, including the following (NDDIC 2003, June):

- A *hiatal hernia*, which occurs when the upper part of the stomach lies above the diaphragm muscle. Normally, the diaphragm muscle separates the stomach from the chest and helps keep acid from coming into the esophagus. Stomach acid can more easily enter the esophagus in people with a hiatal hernia.

- Cigarette smoking.

- Alcohol use.

- Overweight.

- Pregnancy.

- Foods such as citrus fruits, chocolate, caffeinated drinks, fried foods, garlic and onions, spicy foods, and tomato-based foods such as chili, pizza, and spaghetti sauce.

- Large, high-fat meals. These meals stay in the stomach longer and increase stomach pressure, making it more likely that acid will be pushed up into the esophagus.

- Lying down soon after a meal. This is almost certain to bring on symptoms, since it positions the body so it is easier for the stomach acid to back up into the esophagus.

There are ways to reduce the symptoms of GERD. One way is to identify the types of foods or situations that trigger episodes, and then avoid them. Eating smaller meals also helps. After a meal, waiting at least three hours before lying down is recommended. Some people relieve their nighttime symptoms by elevating the head of the bed 4 to 6 inches, for instance by placing a wedge between the mattress and the box spring. This keeps the chest area elevated and minimizes the amount of acid that can back up into the esophagus. It is also suggested that if people smoke, they should stop, and if they are overweight, that they should lose weight. Taking an antacid before a meal can help prevent symptoms if a person accidentally eats an offending food, and there are also many other medications now prescribed to treat GERD. Many of these medications are reviewed in the accompanying Highlight box.

It is important to treat GERD, as it can cause serious health problems. GERD can lead to bleeding and ulcers in the esophagus. Scar tissue can develop in the esophagus, making swallowing very difficult. Some people can also develop a condition called Barrett's esophagus, which can lead to cancer. Asthma can also be aggravated or even caused by GERD.

> **Recap:** Heartburn is caused by the seepage of gastric juices into the esophagus. Gastroesophageal reflux disease (or GERD) is a painful type of heartburn that occurs more than twice per week. Factors contributing to GERD include a hiatal hernia; cigarette smoking; overweight; alcohol use; pregnancy; spicy, acidic, and fatty foods; large meals; and lying down after a meal. GERD can be treated by changing these factors and with medications. GERD can cause serious health consequences such as esophageal bleeding, ulcers, and cancer.

Ulcers

peptic ulcer Area of the GI tract that has been eroded away by the acidic gastric juice of the stomach. The two main causes of peptic ulcers are an *H. pylori* infection or use of nonsteroidal anti-inflammatory drugs.

A **peptic ulcer** is an area of the GI tract that has been eroded away by a combination of hydrochloric acid and the enzyme pepsin (Figure 3.15). In almost all cases, it is located in the stomach area (*gastric ulcer*) or the part of the duodenum closest to the stomach (*duodenal ulcer*). It causes a burning pain in the abdominal area, typically one to three hours after eating a meal. In serious cases, eroded blood vessels bleed into the GI tract, causing vomiting of blood and/or blood in the stools, as well as anemia. If the ulcer entirely perforates the tract wall, stomach contents can leak into the abdominal cavity, causing a life-threatening infection.

The bacterium *Helicobacter pylori* (*H. pylori*) plays a key role in development of most peptic ulcers, which include both gastric and duodenal ulcers (Chan and Leung 2002). Almost all people have this bacterium in their gastrointestinal tracts. It appears that *H. pylori* infects about 20% of people younger than forty years of age and about 50% of people older than sixty years of age (NDDIC 2002, December). Most people with *H. pylori* infection do not develop ulcers, and the reason for this is not known.

Because of the role of *H. pylori* in ulcer development, treatment usually involves antibiotics and other types of medications to reduce gastric secretions. Antacids are used to weaken the gastric acid, and the same medications used to treat GERD can be used to treat peptic ulcers. Special diets are not recommended as often as they once were because they do not reduce acid secretion. In fact, we now know that ulcers are not caused by stress or eating spicy foods.

Although most peptic ulcers are caused by *H. pylori* infection, some are caused by prolonged use of nonsteroidal anti-inflammatory drugs (NSAIDs); these drugs include pain relievers such as aspirin, ibuprofen, and naproxen sodium. Acetaminophen use does not cause ulcers. The NSAIDs appear to cause ulcers by preventing the stomach from protecting itself from acidic gastric juices. Ulcers caused by NSAID use generally heal once a person stops taking the medication (NDDIC 2002, February).

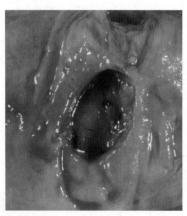

Figure 3.15   A peptic ulcer.

Medications Used to Treat Heartburn and GERD

There currently are a multitude of medications available to treat GERD. Some of these are available over-the-counter, while others can be obtained with a prescription from your doctor. These medications work in different ways, and for many people a combination of medications are needed to treat their symptoms.

Antacids have been commonly used to treat heartburn and mild symptoms of GERD. Antacids include products such as Rolaids, Tums, Alka-Seltzer, Maalox, Pepto-Bismol, and Mylanta. These products work by neutralizing stomach acid and inhibiting production of pepsin. They typically contain a combination of three salts— magnesium, aluminum, and calcium—combined with hydroxide or bicarbonate ions. One advantage of antacids is that they work relatively quickly to relieve symptoms; relief is virtually immediate upon consumption. Their action does not last very long, however, as they only work for about twenty to sixty minutes when taken on an empty stomach, or possibly up to three hours following a meal (Maton and Burton 1999). Because of their short-term action, antacids are often taken in combination with longer-acting medications that will be discussed shortly. Antacids also do not repair damage done to the esophagus.

Antacids are relatively safe for most people, but they do have potential side effects. These side effects are more common in people who take larger doses of antacids on a regular basis but are less common with occasional antacids use. Diarrhea is one of the most common side effects of magnesium-containing antacids. Constipation

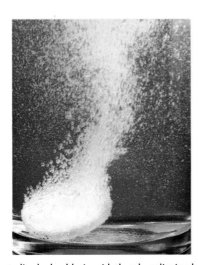

Antacids neutralize hydrochloric acid, thereby relieving heartburn.

and aluminum retention can occur with antacids containing aluminum. In fact, people with kidney disease and renal failure cannot clear the aluminum, which builds up in the brain and body tissues, causing brain damage. Long-term use of high doses of aluminum-containing antacids can also lead to bone loss and osteoporosis. Constipation, belching, intestinal gas, and excessively high blood calcium levels can result from taking calcium-containing antacids. These side effects occur more often in people with renal failure. People who consume a lot of dairy products and take vitamin D supplements should not consume large amounts of calcium-containing antacids, as these actions can lead to milk-alkali syndrome. This syndrome causes irritability, headache, distaste for milk, nausea, vomiting, weakness, and can lead to death (Maton and Burton 1999).

Another class of medications available both over-the-counter and by prescription are the H$_2$ blockers. Brand names include Tagamet HB, Pepcid AC, Axid AR, and Zantac 75. These medications work by stopping acid production before it starts. They do this by blocking the binding of histamine, a chemical produced during digestion, to H$_2$ receptor sites in the stomach. Most of these products can be taken thirty minutes to an hour before you expect to eat foods that may cause heartburn and can be taken to relieve heartburn once it has started. They do not relieve symptoms for at least 45 minutes after they are taken, as they cannot neutralize acid that is already in the stomach. Thus, antacids provide faster relief than H$_2$ blockers. However, if people are taking both antacids and H$_2$ blockers, they should stagger these and take the H$_2$ blockers at least one hour before consuming antacids. These products should also not be taken for more than two weeks continuously and are not recommended for children younger than twelve years of age. Potential side effects include diarrhea, constipation, headache, fatigue, mental confusion, drowsiness, and muscle aches (Marsh 1997).

The most effective medications currently available to treat GERD are proton pump inhibitors. These are available by prescription only and are marketed under the brand names of Prilosec, Prevacid, Protonix, Aciphex, and Nexium. These drugs block the proton pump that is responsible for secretion of gastric acid. These drugs are effective in reducing stomach acid production and in healing the damage caused as a result of GERD. Side effects are minimal and include mild dizziness, headache, nausea, rash, and diarrhea. ●

Recap: Peptic ulcers are located in the stomach or duodenum and are caused by erosion of the GI tract by hydrochloric acid and pepsin. Peptic ulcers are painful and can lead to serious health consequences such as internal bleeding, anemia, and potentially fatal infections. The two major causes of peptic ulcers are *Helicobacter pylori* infection and the use of nonsteroidal anti-inflammatory drugs. Peptic ulcers are treated with medications.

Food Allergies and Intolerances

food allergy   An allergic reaction to food, caused by a reaction of the immune system.

food intolerance   Gastrointestinal discomfort caused by certain foods that is not a result of an immune system reaction.

Food allergies and intolerances have recently received a lot of attention in the media. You may have heard of allergies to foods like peanuts, eggs, dairy, or shellfish. You have also probably heard of food intolerances such as lactose intolerance. What is the difference between a food allergy and a food intolerance? According to the National Institute of Allergy and Infectious Diseases, a **food allergy** is an actual allergic reaction to food or a hypersensitivity to a food caused by a reaction of the immune system (NIAID 2003). A **food intolerance** is GI discomfort (for example, gas, pain, diarrhea, or constipation) caused by foods. A food intolerance can lead to symptoms that mimic a food allergy, but food intolerances are not caused by an immune system reaction. An example is lactose intolerance, which is discussed in Chapter 4. Food allergies are relatively rare, affecting only 3% of children and 1% of adults. Food intolerances are much more common.

Celiac Disease

celiac disease   Genetic disorder characterized by a total intolerance for gluten that causes an immune reaction that damages the lining of the small intestine.

Celiac disease, also known as *celiac sprue*, is a genetic disorder characterized by a total intolerance for gluten, a protein found in wheat, rye, and barley. When a person with this disorder eats one of these grains, immune cells in the small intestine respond to the gluten as if it were a poison and cause an inflammatory response. The response destroys the gluten but in the process erodes the lining of the small intestine. If the person is unaware of the disorder and continues to eat gluten, repeated immune reactions cause even more damage. The villi of the small intestine become greatly decreased so there is less absorptive surface area and the enzymes located at the brush border of the small intestine become reduced. When this happens, the person becomes unable to absorb certain vitamins and minerals properly—a condition known as *malabsorption*. Over time malabsorption can lead to malnutrition (poor nutrient status). Deficiencies of vitamins A, D, E, and K, iron, folic acid, and calcium are common in those suffering from celiac disease (Murray 1999).

Symptoms of this disease often mimic those of other intestinal disturbances like irritable bowel syndrome (discussed shortly), and so the condition is often misdiagnosed. Some of the symptoms of celiac disease include fatty stools (due to poor fat absorption); frequent stools, either watery or hard, with an odd odor; cramping, anemia, pallor, weight loss, fatigue, and irritability.

Currently there is no cure for celiac disease. Treatment is with a special diet that excludes wheat, rye, and barley. Oats are allowed, but they are often contaminated with wheat flour from processing and even that small amount of wheat can cause symptoms in susceptible people. Corn, rice, tapioca, potato, arrowroot, cassava, and gluten-free breads may be used in the diet to supply the person with needed carbohydrate.

Diagnosing the disease early helps avoid growth delays in children and nutrition problems in adults. There appears to be a genetic link, as people with relatives with celiac disease are more at risk for acquiring this disease themselves. Although it is more common in Caucasians, it can develop in almost anyone at any point in his or her life. Sometimes after an illness or pregnancy, people develop celiac disease (Murray 1999).

Food Allergies

Although much less common than food intolerances, a number of people suffer from food allergies. You may have heard stories of people being allergic to something as

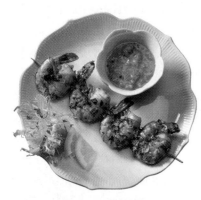

For some people, eating a meal of grilled shrimp with peanut sauce would cause a severe allergic reaction.

common as peanuts. This is the case for Liz. She was out to dinner with her parents, celebrating her birthday, when the dessert cart came around. The caramel custard looked heavenly and was probably a safe choice, but she asked the waiter just to be sure that it contained no peanuts. He checked with the chef, then returned and assured her that, no, the custard was peanut-free—but within minutes of consuming it, Liz's skin became flushed, and she struggled to breathe. As her parents were dialing 911, she lost consciousness. Fortunately, the paramedics arrived within minutes and were able to resuscitate her. It was subsequently determined that, unknown to the chef, the spoon that his prep cook had used to scoop the baked custard into serving bowls had been resting on a cutting board where he had chopped peanuts for a different dessert. Just this small exposure to peanuts was enough to cause a severe allergic reaction in Liz.

How can a food that most people consume regularly, such as peanuts, shellfish, eggs, or milk, cause some people to suffer an allergic reaction? The answer lies with the immune system. In Liz's case, a trace amount of peanut stimulated immune cells throughout her body to release their inflammatory chemicals. In celiac disease, the inflammation is localized in the small intestine, so the damage is limited. This is true of many food allergies, as well. For instance, some people's lips swell when they eat melon, whereas others develop a rash whenever they eat eggs. What made Liz's experience so terrifyingly different was that the inflammation was so widespread, affecting essentially all of her body systems and sending her into a state called *anaphylactic shock*. Left untreated, anaphylactic shock is nearly always fatal, so many people with known food allergies always carry with them a kit containing an injection of a powerful stimulant called epinephrine. This drug can reduce symptoms long enough to buy the victim time to get emergency medical care.

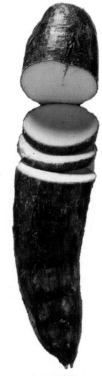

For people with celiac disease, cassava is a good gluten-free source of carbohydrates.

> **Recap:** Food allergies are a hypersensitivity to food caused by an immune reaction. Food allergies occur in 3% of children and 1% of adults in the United States. Celiac disease is a genetic disorder that causes an intolerance to gluten, a protein found in wheat, rye, and barley. People with celiac disease cannot eat gluten, as it causes an immune reaction that damages the lining of the small intestine and leads to malabsorption of nutrients and malnutrition. Other foods that may cause allergies include peanuts, milk, eggs, and shellfish. Food allergies can cause mild symptoms, such as hives and swelling, to serious consequences such as anaphylactic shock. Food allergies and celiac disease can only be treated by avoiding foods that cause the immune reactions.

Liz *Nutri-Case*

"I used to think of my peanut allergy as no big deal, but ever since my experience at that restaurant last year, I've been pretty obsessive about it. For months afterwards, I refused to eat anything that I hadn't prepared myself. I do eat out now, but I always insist that the chef prepare my food personally, with clean utensils, and I avoid most desserts. They're just too risky. Shopping is a lot harder too, because I have to check every label. The worst, though, is eating at my friends' houses. I have to ask them, do you keep peanuts or peanut butter in your house? Some of them are really sympathetic, but others look at me as if I'm a hypochondriac! I wish I could think of something to say to them to make them understand that this isn't something I have any control over."

What could Liz say in response to friends who don't understand the cause and seriousness of her food allergy? Do you think it would help Liz to share her fears with her doctor and to discuss possible strategies? If so, why? In addition to shopping, dining out, and eating at friends' houses, what other situations might require Liz to be cautious about her food choices?

Irritable Bowel Syndrome

irritable bowel syndrome A bowel disorder that interferes with normal functions of the colon. Symptoms are abdominal cramps, bloating, and constipation or diarrhea.

Irritable bowel syndrome (IBS) is a bowel disorder that interferes with normal functions of the colon. Symptoms include abdominal cramps, bloating, and either constipation or diarrhea. It is one of the most common disorders diagnosed by doctors, with approximately 20% of the U.S. population being diagnosed with IBS (NDDIC 2003, April). More women than men appear to develop IBS, which typically first appears around twenty years of age.

There is no known cause of IBS. For some people, it appears their colon is more sensitive to certain foods or stress. The immune system may also trigger symptoms of IBS. Whatever the cause, the normal movement of the colon appears to be disrupted. In some people with IBS, food moves too quickly through the colon and fluid cannot be absorbed fast enough, which causes diarrhea. In others, the movement of the colon is too slow and too much fluid is absorbed, leading to constipation.

You've probably guessed by now that Jill, in our chapter opener, has IBS. Recall that she had just moved out of her parents' home and started college. Transitions like these can be highly stressful and trigger IBS in susceptible people. In addition to stress, other factors that are linked with IBS include:

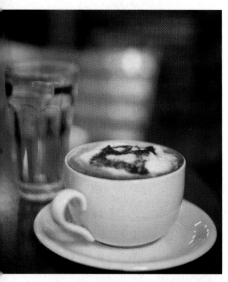

Consuming caffeinated drinks is one of several factors that have been linked with irritable bowel syndrome (IBS), a bowel disorder that interferes with normal functions of the colon.

- Caffeinated drinks, such as tea, coffee, and colas
- Foods such as chocolate, alcohol, dairy products, and wheat
- Large meals
- Certain medications

Some women with IBS find that their symptoms worsen during their menstrual period, indicating a possible link between reproductive hormones and IBS.

If you think you have IBS, it is important to have a complete physical examination to rule out any other health problems. Treatment options include certain medications to treat diarrhea or constipation, stress management, regular physical activity, eating smaller meals, avoiding foods that exacerbate symptoms, eating a higher fiber diet, and drinking at least six to eight glasses of water each day (NDDIC 2003, April). Although IBS is uncomfortable, it does not appear to endanger long-term health. However, severe IBS can be disabling and prevent people from leading normal lives; thus, accurate diagnosis and effective treatment is critical to treat this disorder.

> **Recap:** Irritable bowel syndrome (IBS) causes abdominal cramps, bloating, and constipation or diarrhea. The causes of IBS are unknown. Factors linked to IBS include stress; consumption of caffeinated drinks and foods such as chocolate, dairy, alcohol, and wheat; large meals; and certain medications. IBS can be treated with medications, stress management, regular exercise, avoiding irritating foods, eating a high-fiber diet, and drinking at least six to eight glasses of water per day.

Diarrhea and Constipation

diarrhea Condition characterized by the frequent passage of loose, watery stools.

Diarrhea is the frequent passage (more than three times in one day) of loose, watery stools. Other symptoms may include cramping, abdominal pain, bloating, nausea, fever, and blood in the stools. Diarrhea is usually caused by an infection of the gastrointestinal tract, a chronic disease, stress, food intolerances, reactions to medications, or as a result of a bowel disorder (NDDIC 2001).

Acute diarrhea lasts less than three weeks and is usually caused by an infection from bacteria, a virus, or a parasite. Chronic diarrhea, which lasts more than three weeks, affects about 3 to 5% of the U.S. population and is usually caused by allergies to cow's milk, irritable bowel syndrome, or diseases such as celiac disease.

Whatever the cause, diarrhea can be harmful if it persists for a long period of time because the person can lose large quantities of water and electrolytes and become severely dehydrated. Table 3.1 reviews the symptoms of dehydration in both adults and children. Diarrhea is particularly dangerous in infants and young children. In fact, a child can die from dehydration in just a few days. Adults, particularly the elderly, can also become dangerously ill if severely dehydrated. Table 3.2 lists warning signs that occur with diarrhea and dehydration; if you experience or observe any of these signs, a doctor should be seen immediately.

A condition referred to as *traveler's diarrhea* has become a common health concern due to the expansion in global travel. Traveler's diarrhea is discussed in the accompanying Highlight box.

In contrast, **constipation** is typically defined as a condition in which no stools are passed for two or more days; however, it is important to recognize that many people normally experience bowel movements only every second or third day. Thus, the definition of constipation varies from one person to another. In addition to being infrequent, the stools are usually hard, small, and somewhat difficult to pass.

constipation Condition characterized by the absence of bowel movements for a period of time that is significantly longer than normal for the individual. When a bowel movement does occur, stools are usually small, hard, and difficult to pass.

Constipation is frequent in people who have disorders affecting the nervous system, and in which the muscles of the large bowel do not receive the appropriate nerve signals needed for involuntary muscle movement to occur. For these individuals, drug therapy is often needed to keep the large bowel functioning.

Many people experience temporary constipation at some point in their lives in response to a variety of causes. Often people have trouble with it when they travel, when their schedule is disrupted, if they change their diet, or if they are on certain

Table 3.1 Symptoms of Dehydration in Adults and Children

Symptoms in Adults	Symptoms in Children
Thirst	Dry mouth and tongue
Light-headedness	No tears when crying
Less frequent urination	No wet diapers for 3 hours or more
Dark colored urine	High fever
Fatigue	Sunken abdomen, eyes, or cheeks
Dry skin	Irritable or listless
	Skin that does not flatten when pinched and released

Source: National Digestive Diseases Information Clearinghouse (NDDIC). 2001, January. Diarrhea. NIH Publication No. 01–2749. http://digestive.niddk.nih.gov/ddiseases/pubs/diarrhea/index.htm. Accessed August 2003.

Table 3.2 Signs Indicating the Need for a Doctor as a Result of Diarrhea

Danger Signs for Adults	Danger Signs for Children
Diarrhea lasts more than three days.	Diarrhea lasts more than 24 hours.
Severe pain is felt in abdomen or rectum.	Fever is present at a temperature of 101.4 ° Fahrenheit or higher.
Fever is present at a temperature of 102° Fahrenheit or higher.	There is blood or pus in the stools, or stools are black.
There is blood in the stools, or stools look black and tarry.	There are symptoms of dehydration.
There are symptoms of dehydration.	

Source: National Digestive Diseases Information Clearinghouse (NDDIC). 2001, January. Diarrhea. NIH Publication No. 01–2749. http://digestive.niddk.nih.gov/ddiseases/pubs/diarrhea/index.htm. Accessed August 2003.

Global Nutrition: Traveler's Diarrhea—What Is It and How Can I Prevent It?

Diarrhea is the rapid movement of fecal matter through the large intestine, often accompanied by large volumes of water. *Traveler's diarrhea* is experienced by people traveling to countries outside of their own and is usually caused by viral or bacterial infections. Diarrhea represents the body's way of ridding itself of the invasive agent. The large intestine and even some of the small intestine become irritated by the microbes and the body's defense against them. This irritation leads to increased secretion of fluid and increased motility of the large intestine, causing watery stools and a higher than normal frequency of bowel movements.

People generally get traveler's diarrhea from consuming water or food that is contaminated with fecal matter. High-risk destinations include developing countries in Africa, Asia, Latin America, and the Middle East. Low-risk destinations include the United States, most European countries, Canada, Japan, Australia, and New Zealand. Very risky foods include any raw or undercooked fish, meats, and raw fruits and vegetables. Tap water, ice made from tap water, and unpasteurized milk and dairy products are also common sources of infection.

Traveler's diarrhea usually starts about five to fifteen days after you arrive at your destination. Symptoms include fatigue, lack of appetite, abdominal cramps, and watery diarrhea. In some cases, you may also experience nausea, vomiting, and low-grade fever. Usually, this diarrhea passes within four to six days, and people recover completely. However, infants and toddlers, the elderly, and people with AIDS (acquired immunodeficiency syndrome), cancer, or other disorders that weaken their immune system are at greater risk for serious illness resulting from traveler's diarrhea, and these people do not recover as well. This is also true for people with digestive disorders such as celiac disease and ulcers (Stanley 1999).

What can you do to prevent traveler's diarrhea? Because the primary cause is contaminated water and food, avoiding the risky foods described above can help reduce your risk of contracting this illness. Table 3.3 lists foods and beverages to avoid and those that are considered relatively safe when traveling. In general, it is smart to assume that all local water and foods and beverages exposed to or cleaned with local water are contaminated and should be avoided. Brand-name bottled waters, wine, beer, and beverages made with boiling water are typically safe but beware of using ice

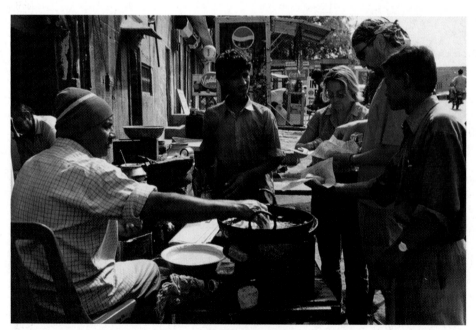

When traveling in developing countries, it is wise to avoid raw or undercooked fish, meats, and raw fruits and vegetables. Tap water, ice made from tap water, and unpasteurized milk and dairy products should also be avoided.

Table 3.3 Foods and Beverages Linked with Traveler's Diarrhea

Foods/Beverages That Can Cause Traveler's Diarrhea	Foods/Beverages Considered Safe To Consume
Tap water	Boiled tap water
Local bottled water	Brand-name bottled waters
Iced tea	Hot coffee and hot tea
Unpasteurized dairy products or juices	Wine and beer
Ice (in both alcoholic and nonalcoholic beverages)	Well-cooked foods
Undercooked or raw foods (includes meats, vegetables, and most fruits)	Fruit that can be peeled (for example, bananas and oranges)
Cooked foods that are no longer hot in temperature	
Shellfish	
Vegetables with high water content (for example, lettuce and salads)	
Food from street vendors	

Source: S. L. Stanley, Advice to travelers, in *Textbook of Gastroenterology* vol. 1, 3d ed., edited by T. Yamada (Philadelphia: Lippincott Williams & Wilkins, 1999).

made from local water. It is important to remember to wipe all bottles clean and dry them before drinking bottled beverages. To render local water safe, you need to boil it; chemicals such as chorine bleach and iodine can also be used to sterilize water, but boiling is more effective. Remember the adage "Boil it, peel it, cook it, or forget it" (Stanley 1999) when making food choices. All food should be well cooked, fruit from which the peel is removed is generally safe, and raw vegetables and those with high water content (such as lettuce) should not be eaten.

Antibiotics can also be taken prior to your trip to avoid traveler's diarrhea. This prevention option should be discussed with your physician prior to travel. Many bacteria are now resistant to antibiotic

treatment, and this option is not always safe or effective for everyone. If you do suffer from traveler's diarrhea, it is important to replace the fluid and nutrients lost as a result of the illness. There are specially formulated oral rehydration solutions available to help replenish vital nutrients that are lost; these solutions are usually available in most countries at local pharmacies or stores. Antibiotics may also be taken to kill bacteria once traveler's diarrhea sets in. Once treatment is initiated, the diarrhea should cease within two to three days. If the diarrhea persists for more than ten days after the initiation of treatment, or if there is blood in your stools, you should see a physician immediately to determine the cause of the diarrhea and get appropriate treatment to avoid serious medical consequences. ●

medications. Increasing fiber and fluid in the diet is one of the mainstays of preventing constipation. Five servings of fruits and vegetables each day and six or more servings of whole grains is helpful to most people. If you use breakfast cereal, make sure you buy a cereal containing at least 2 to 3 grams of fiber per serving. The dietary recommendation for fiber and the role it plays in maintaining healthy elimination is discussed in detail in Chapter 4. Staying well hydrated by drinking lots of water and exercising will also help you reduce the risk of constipation.

Recap: Diarrhea is the frequent passage of loose or watery stools, whereas constipation is failure to have a bowel movement for two or more days or within a time period that is normal for the individual. Diarrhea should be treated quickly to avoid dehydration or even death. Constipation can be treated with medications or by exercising and increasing your intake of fiber and water.

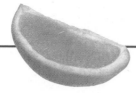

Chapter Summary

- Food stimulates our senses of smell, taste, and sight; this motivates us to eat.

- Appetite is a psychological desire to consume specific foods; this desire is motivated by the environment and pleasant thoughts about food.

- Hunger is a physiologic drive that prompts us to eat.

- The hypothalamus in the brain interacts with signals from the gastrointestinal tract and levels of blood nutrients to signal when we are hungry or satiated.

- Hormones are chemical messengers secreted by glands in the body that signal the hypothalamus to stimulate hunger or satiation.

- Foods that contain fiber, water, and large amounts of protein have the highest satiety value.

- Atoms are the smallest units of matter, and they bond together to form molecules.

- The primary goal of digestion is to break food into molecules small enough to be transported throughout the body.

- Cells are the smallest units of life, and the human body is comprised of billions of cells. We build cells from the nutrients we absorb as a result of digesting food.

- Cells are encased in a cell membrane, which acts as a gatekeeper to determine which substances go into and out of the cell.

- Cells contain organelles, which are tiny structures that perform highly sophisticated functions. The nucleus, ribosomes, and mitochondria are examples of organelles.

- Cells of a single type join together to form tissues. Several types of tissues join together to form organs, such as the liver.

- Organs group together to form systems that perform integrated functions. The gastrointestinal system and the central nervous system are examples.

- Digestion is the process of breaking down foods into molecules; absorption is the process of taking molecules of food into the body; and elimination is the process of removing undigested food and waste products from the body.

- In the mouth, chewing starts mechanical digestion of food. Saliva contains salivary amylase, which is an enzyme that initiates the chemical digestion of carbohydrates.

- Food moves down to the stomach through the esophagus via a process called peristalsis. Peristalsis involves the rhythmic waves of squeezing and pushing food through the gastrointestinal tract.

- The stomach mixes and churns food together with gastric juices. Hydrochloric acid and the enzyme pepsin initiate protein digestion, and a minimal amount of fat digestion begins through the action of gastric lipase.

- The stomach periodically releases the partially digested food, referred to as chyme, into the small intestine.

- Most digestion and absorption of nutrients occurs in the small intestine.

- The gallbladder, pancreas, and liver are examples of accessory organs.

- The gallbladder stores bile and secretes it into the small intestine to assist with the digestion of fat.

- The pancreas manufactures and secretes digestive enzymes into the small intestine. Pancreatic amylase digests carbohydrates, pancreatic lipase digests fats, and proteases digest proteins. The pancreas also synthesizes two hormones that play a critical role in carbohydrate metabolism, insulin and glucagon.

- The lining of the small intestine has thousands of folds and fingerlike projections that increase the surface area over 500 times, significantly increasing the absorptive capacity of the small intestine.

- The liver processes and stores all absorbed nutrients, alcohol, and drugs. The liver also synthesizes bile and regulates metabolism of monosaccharides, fatty acids, and amino acids.

- The large intestine digests any remaining food particles, absorbs water and chemicals, and moves feces to the rectum for elimination.

- The neuromuscular system involves coordination of the muscles, the central nervous system, and the enteric nervous system to move food along the gastrointestinal tract and to control all aspects of digestion, absorption, and elimination.

- Heartburn is caused by hydrochloric acid seeping into the esophagus and burning its lining.

- Gastroesophageal reflux disease (GERD) is a more painful type of heartburn that occurs more than twice per week. GERD can cause bleeding, ulcers, and cancer of the esophagus.

- A peptic ulcer is an area in the stomach or duodenum that has been eroded away by hydrochloric acid and pepsin. A bacterium, *Helicobacter pylori*, is the most common cause of peptic ulcers. Prolonged use of nonsteroidal anti-inflammatory drugs (NSAIDS) can also cause peptic ulcers.

- A food allergy is an allergic reaction to food that is caused by a reaction of the immune system. A food intolerance is gastrointestinal discomfort caused by foods but that is not a result of an immune system reaction.

- Celiac disease is a genetic disorder characterized by a total intolerance to gluten. This disease causes damage to the lining of the small intestine, leading to malabsorption of nutrients and to eventual malnutrition.

- Irritable bowel syndrome is a bowel disorder that interferes with normal functions of the colon, causing pain, diarrhea, and constipation.

- Diarrhea is the frequent (more than three times per day) elimination of loose, watery stools. Diarrhea should be treated promptly to avoid dehydration.

- Constipation is a condition in which no stools are passed for two or more days or for a length of time considered abnormally long for the individual. Constipation can be relieved by medications, drinking plenty of water, exercising, and eating ample fiber.

Review Questions

1. Which of the following represents the levels of organization in the human body?
   a. cells, molecules, atoms, tissues, organs, systems
   b. atoms, molecules, cells, organs, tissues, systems
   c. atoms, molecules, cells, tissues, organs, systems
   d. molecules, atoms, cells, tissues, organs, systems

2. Bile is a greenish fluid that
   a. is stored by the pancreas.
   b. is stored by the kidneys.
   c. denatures proteins.
   d. emulsifies fats.

3. The region of brain tissue that is responsible for prompting us to seek food is the
   a. pituitary gland.
   b. cephalic phase.
   c. hypothalamus.
   d. thalamus.

4. Heartburn is caused by
   a. seepage of gastric acid into the esophagus.
   b. seepage of gastric acid into the cardiac muscle.
   c. seepage of bile into the stomach.
   d. seepage of salivary amylase into the stomach.

5. Which of the following foods is likely to keep a person satiated for the longest period of time?
   a. a bean and cheese burrito
   b. a serving of full-fat ice cream
   c. a bowl of rice cereal in whole milk
   d. a tossed salad with oil and vinegar dressing

6. **True or false?** Hunger is more physiologic, and appetite is more psychologic.

7. **True or false?** The nerves of the GI tract are collectively known as the enteric nervous system.

8. **True or false?** Vitamins and minerals are digested in the small intestine.

9. **True or false?** A person with celiac disease cannot tolerate milk or milk products.

10. **True or false?** Atoms are the smallest units of life.

11. Explain why it is true that you are what you eat.

12. Discuss some factors that can help prevent or relieve constipation.

13. Imagine that the lining of your small intestine were smooth, like the inside of a rubber tube. Would this design be efficient in performing the main function of this organ? Why or why not?

14. Why doesn't the acidic environment of the stomach cause it to digest itself?

15. After dinner, your roommate lies down to rest for a few minutes before studying. When he gets up, he complains of a sharp, burning pain in his chest. Offer a possible explanation for his pain.

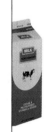

Test Yourself Answers

1. **True.** Sometimes you may have an appetite even though you are not hungry. These feelings are referred to as "cravings" and are associated with physical or emotional cues.

2. **False.** Your brain, not your stomach, is the primary organ responsible for telling you when you are hungry.

3. **True.** Although there are individual variations in how we respond to food, the entire process of digestion and absorption of one meal usually takes about twenty-four hours.

4. **True.** Most ulcers result from an infection of the bacterium *Helicobacter pylori* (*H. pylori*). Contrary to popular belief, ulcers are not caused by stress or food.

5. **False.** Irritable bowel syndrome is a relatively common disease that affects 20% of the U.S. population. The age at onset is typically around twenty years of age.

Web Links

digestive.niddk.nih.gov
National Digestive Diseases Information Clearinghouse (NDDIC)
Explore this site to learn more about diarrhea, celiac disease, irritable bowel syndrome (IBS), heartburn, and gastroesophageal reflux disease (GERD).

www.nlm.nih.gov/medlineplus
MEDLINE Plus Health Information
Search for "food allergies" to obtain additional resources as well as the latest news about food allergies.

www.healthfinder.gov
Health Finder
Search this site to learn more about disorders related to digestion, absorption, and elimination.

ific.org
International Food Information Council Foundation (IFIC)
Scroll down to "Food Safety Information" and click on the link for "Food Allergies and Asthma" for additional information on food allergies.

www.foodallergy.org
The Food Allergy and Anaphylaxis Network (FAN)
Visit this site to learn more about common food allergens.

www.gfmall.com
Gluten-Free Mall
Find out where you can buy gluten-free products.

References

Bell, E. A., and B. J. Rolls. 2001. Regulation of Energy Intake: Factors Contributing to Obesity. In *Present Knowledge in Nutrition*, 8th ed., edited by B. A. Bowman and R. M. Russell. Washington, DC: ILSI Press.

Chan, F. K. L., and W. K. Leung. 2002. Peptic-ulcer disease. *Lancet* 360:933–941.

Davidson, N. O. 2003. Intestinal lipid absorption. In *Textbook of Gastroenterology*, Volume 1. 4th ed., edited by T. Yamada, D. H. Alpers, N. Kaplowitz, L. Laine, C. Owyang, and D. W. Powell. Philadelphia: Lippincott Williams & Wilkins.

Duggan, C., J. Gannon, and W. A. Walker. 2002. Protective nutrients and functional foods for the gastrointestinal tract. *Am. J. Clin. Nutr.* 75:789–808.

Kim, D-Y, M. Camilleri, J. A. Murray, D. A. Stephens, J. A. Levine, and D. D. Burton. 2001. Is there a role for gastric accommodation and satiety in asymptomatic obese people? *Obesity Res.* 9: 655–661.

Kopp-Hoolihan, L. 2001. Prophylactic and therapeutic uses of probiotics: a review. *J. Am. Diet. Assoc.* 101:229–238, 241.

Marsh, T. D. 1997. Nonprescription H_2-receptor antagonists. *J. Am. Pharm. Assoc.* NS37:552–556.

Maton, P. N., and M. E. Burton. 1999. Antacids revisited. A review of their clinical pharmacology and recommended therapeutic use. *Drugs* 57:855–870.

Murray, J. A. 1999. The widening spectrum of celiac disease. *Am. J. Clin. Nutr.* 69:354–365.

National Digestive Diseases Information Clearinghouse (NDDIC). 2001, January. Diarrhea. NIH Publication No. 01–2749. http://digestive.niddk.nih.gov/ddiseases/pubs/diarrhea/index.htm (Accessed August 2003).

National Digestive Diseases Information Clearinghouse (NDDIC). 2002, December. H. pylori and Peptic Ulcer. NIH Publication No. 03–4225. http://digestive.niddk.nih.gov/ddiseases/pubs/hpylori/index.htm (Accessed August 2003).

National Digestive Diseases Information Clearinghouse (NDDIC). 2002, February. NSAIDs and Peptic Ulcers. NIH Publication No. 02–4644. http://digestive.niddk.nih.gov/ddiseases/pubs/nsaids/index.htm (Accessed August 2003).

National Digestive Diseases Information Clearinghouse (NDDIC). 2003, April. Irritable Bowel Syndrome. NIH Publication No. 03–693. http://digestive.niddk.nih.gov/ddiseases/pubs/ibs/index.htm (Accessed August 2003).

National Digestive Diseases Information Clearinghouse (NDDIC). 2003, June. Heartburn, Hiatal Hernia, and Gastroesophageal Reflux Disease (GERD). NIH Publication No. 03–0882. http://digestive.niddk.nih.gov/ddiseases/pubs/gerd/index.htm (Accessed August 2003).

National Institute of Allergy and Infectious Diseases (NIAID). 2003, May. Food Allergy and Intolerances. NIAID Fact Sheet. http://www.niaid.nih.gov/factsheets/food.htm (Accessed August 2003).

Roberfroid, M. D. Prebiotics and probiotics: are they functional foods? 2000. *Am. J. Clin. Nutr.* 71(suppl):1682S–1690S.

Sanders, M. E., D. C. Walker, K. M. Walker, K. Aoyama, and T. R. Klaenhammer. 1996. Performance of commercial cultures in fluid milk applications. *J. Dairy Science* 79:943–955.

Stanley, S. L. 1999. Advice to travelers. In *Textbook of Gastroenterology*, vol. 1, 3rd ed, edited by T. Yamada. Philadelphia: Lippincott Williams & Wilkins.

Zorrilla, G. 1998. Hunger and satiety: deceptively simple words for the complex mechanisms that tell us when to eat and when to stop. *J. Am. Dietetic Assoc.* 98:1111.

Nutrition Debate:

Probiotics—What Are They, Can They Improve Gastrointestinal Health, and Should I Eat Them?

There are a growing number of foods available on the market today that are touted to improve our health. These foods are called *functional foods*, a term that refers to foods that promote health beyond their basic nutritional function (Roberfroid 2000). Sport bars and beverages, calcium-fortified orange juice, and cholesterol-reducing vegetable spreads are examples of functional foods people consume on a daily basis. Probiotics are another example of a functional food. *Probiotics* are live microorganisms found in, or added to, fermented foods that optimize the bacterial environment of our intestines.

Our intestines contain an amazing number and variety of bacteria. Many of these bacteria are vital to maintaining our health and supporting digestive function. Some of these bacteria can also be harmful. Thus, it is important to maintain an environment in the intestine that can optimize the number and activity of healthful bacteria and limit the damage caused by harmful bacteria.

For more than 100 years, probiotics have been considered a means by which we can optimize the health and function of our intestines. Our interest in probiotics started in the early 1900s with the work of Elie Metchnikoff, a Nobel Prize–winning scientist. Dr. Metchnikoff linked the long, healthy lives of Bulgarian peasants with their consumption of fermented milk products. Subsequent research identified bacteria in fermented milk products that promoted health. *Probiotics* means "pro-life."

Much of the research on probiotics has been done in Europe and Asia, and foods containing probiotics are widespread in many European and Asian countries. In the United States, most foods that contain probiotics are fortified milk and fermented yogurt. Probiotics can also be found in fermented kefirs and in supplement form. The most frequently used probiotics in the food market today are species of *Lactobacillus* or *Bifidobacterium*.

How do probiotics work? When a person consumes a product containing probiotics, these bacteria adhere to the intestinal wall for a few days or until more are eaten. Once attached to the intestinal wall, the bacteria can exert their beneficial actions. The activity of these bacteria is short-lived, and they probably need to be consumed on a daily basis to benefit human health. The exact mechanism of how probiotics work is currently being researched, but one proposed benefit is enhancement of our immune system. Probiotics may increase the amount and activity of immune cells that help us fight infections. However, there is still limited research on whether probiotics can really improve immune function and overall health in humans (Kopp-Hoolihan 2001). Other conditions that may be successfully treated with probiotics include (Duggan, Gannon, and Walker 2002; Kopp-Hoolihan 2001):

- Diarrhea in children caused by a rotavirus
- Diarrhea associated with use of antibiotic medications in children and adults
- Traveler's diarrhea
- Inflammatory bowel disease
- Infection from *Helicobacter pylori*, which is the bacteria associated with conditions such as peptic ulcers, gastritis, and gastric cancer
- Food allergies
- Urinary and genital tract infections in women

Although the research supporting the potential of probiotics to successfully treat these conditions is promising, more research is needed before we can say with certainty that probiotics enhance human health.

It is important to remember that in order to be effective, there is a minimum number of bacteria that must be present in foods. While the exact number of bacteria is not known, it is estimated that a daily dose of at least one billion to ten billion (or 1×10^9 to 1×10^{10}) bacteria are needed to be effective (Sanders et al. 1996). Because these live cultures can only live for a limited period of time, foods and supplements containing probiotics have a limited shelf life, and these products must be properly stored and consumed within a relatively brief period of time to

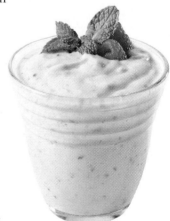

Probiotics can be found in fermented yogurt.

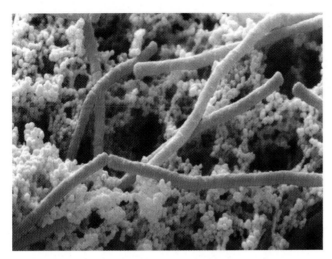

An electron micrograph of the bacteria *Lactobacillus* (pink), taken from yogurt with live active cultures.

receive maximal benefit. In general, refrigerated foods containing probiotics have a shelf life of three to six weeks, while the shelf life for supplements containing probiotics is about twelve months; however, the probiotic content of refrigerated foods is much more stable than that of supplements.

At this time, there are no national standards for identifying the level of active bacteria in foods or supplements. In the United States, the National Yogurt Association has established a "Live Active Culture" seal, which requires that refrigerated yogurt contain at least 1×10^8 viable active bacteria per gram, and that frozen yogurt contain 1×10^7 active bacteria per gram.

Can probiotics cause harm? There are many bacteria that are very harmful to humans, and it is critical that we consume only bacteria that are known to be non-toxic and to promote health. The strains of bacteria currently added to foods have been selected based on historical use in humans with no harmful side effects. In fact, to meet the definition of a probiotic, a bacterium must have a beneficial effect on humans.

Based on what you have just learned about probiotics, do you think products containing these bacteria should be consumed on a daily basis? Are you interested in adding probiotics to your diet? Do we really know enough about their role in human health to make broad-based recommendations for people across the United States? Do you think that the standards of the food and supplement industries need to be improved in regard to defining bacterial content and activity level before we can make national recommendations to consume foods that contain probiotics? How do you think food labels can be improved to assist consumers in identifying key aspects of probiotic-containing food? As the number of probiotic-containing foods increases in the U.S. market, these are just some of the questions that need to be answered to assist consumers in making healthful food choices.

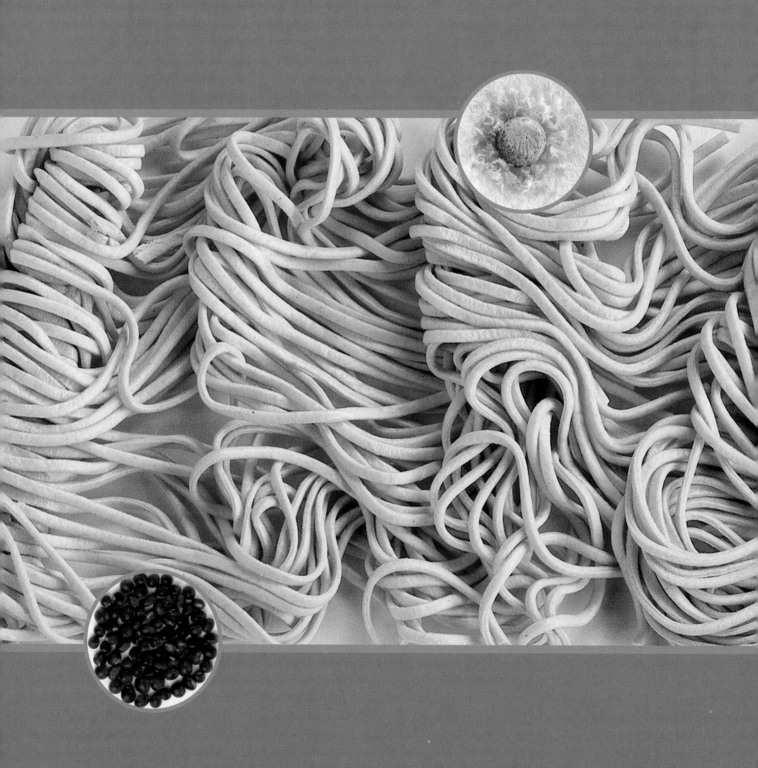

Chapter 4
Carbohydrates: Bountiful Sources of Energy and Nutrients

Chapter Objectives

After reading this chapter you will be able to:

1. Describe the difference between simple and complex carbohydrates, pp. 118–123.

2. Discuss how carbohydrates are digested and absorbed by our bodies, pp. 129–129.

3. List four functions of carbohydrates in our bodies, pp. 129–132.

4. Define the Acceptable Macronutrient Distribution Range for carbohydrates, the Adequate Intake for fiber, and the recommended intake of added sugars, p. 133.

5. Identify the potential health risks associated with diets high in simple sugars, pp. 134–135.

6. List five foods that are good sources of carbohydrates, pp. 135–140.

7. Identify at least three alternative sweeteners, pp. 140–144.

8. Describe type 1 and type 2 diabetes, and discuss how diabetes differs from hypoglycemia, pp. 145–150.

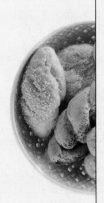
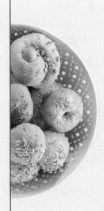

Test Yourself True or False?

1. The terms "carbohydrate" and "sugar" mean the same thing. T or F

2. Diets high in sugar cause tooth decay, diabetes, and obesity. T or F

3. Our bodies have a difficult time digesting and absorbing carbohydrates, so we should consume a diet that is low in carbohydrates. T or F

4. Carbohydrates are the primary fuel source for our brain and body tissues. T or F

5. Alternative sweeteners, such as aspartame, are safe for us to consume. T or F

Test Yourself answers can be found at the end of the chapter.

It was the final night of the fall musical at the local community college, and the actress playing the leading role had just walked off stage to thunderous applause. The curtain came down, the lights came up, and the cast assembled for the curtain call. The director counted heads. Someone was missing. Where was Maryanne, her leading lady? Stage hands ran to the women's dressing room and found her, passed out on the floor. She was rushed to the local emergency department in a coma. A friend said Maryanne had complained of feeling shaky and "spaced out" all night, with a painful headache. He also said he had seen her drinking a can of her favorite root beer at intermission, and as soon as she got off stage, another. She'd told her friend that she'd join him backstage "in a sec" but never showed up. Luckily, lab tests at the emergency department quickly revealed that Maryanne was in a diabetic coma, and prompt treatment saved her life—but Maryanne now faced the daily challenge of living with diabetes.

Does the consumption of sugary foods like soft drinks lead to diabetes—or, for that matter, to obesity or any other disorder? Several popular diets—including The Zone Diet (Sears 1995), Sugar Busters (Steward et al. 1995), and Dr. Atkins' New Diet Revolution (Atkins 1992), claim that carbohydrates are bad for your health and advocate reducing carbohydrate consumption and increasing protein and fat intake. Should we reduce our intake of carbohydrates? If you noticed that a friend regularly consumed four or five soft drinks a day, plus candy and other sweet snacks, would you say anything? Are carbohydrates a health menace, and is one type of carbohydrate as bad as another?

In this chapter, we explore the differences between simple and complex carbohydrates and learn why some carbohydrates are better than others. We also learn how the human body breaks down carbohydrates and uses them to maintain our health and to fuel our activity and exercise. Because carbohydrate metabolism sometimes does go wrong, we'll also discuss its relationship to some common health disorders.

carbohydrate One of the three macronutrients, a compound made up of carbon, hydrogen, and oxygen that is derived from plants and provides energy.

glucose The most abundant sugar molecule, a monosaccharide generally found in combination with other sugars. The preferred source of energy for the brain and an important source of energy for all cells.

photosynthesis Process by which plants use sunlight to fuel a chemical reaction that combines carbon and water into glucose, which is then stored in their cells.

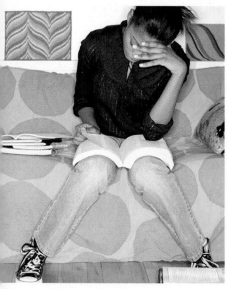

In our bodies, glucose is the preferred source of energy for the brain.

What Are Carbohydrates?

As we mentioned in Chapter 1, **carbohydrates** are one of the three macronutrients. As such, they are an important energy source for the entire body and are the preferred energy source for nerve cells, including those of the brain. We will say more about their functions later in this chapter.

The term *carbohydrate* literally means "hydrated carbon." You know that water (H_2O) is made of hydrogen and oxygen, and that when something is said to be *hydrated*, it contains water. Thus, the chemical abbreviation for carbohydrate (CHO) indicates the atoms it contains: **c**arbon, **h**ydrogen, and **o**xygen.

We obtain carbohydrates predominantly from plant foods such as fruits, vegetables, and grains. Plants make the most abundant form of carbohydrate, called **glucose,** through a process called **photosynthesis.** During photosynthesis, the green pigment of plants, called *chlorophyll,* absorbs sunlight, which provides the energy needed to fuel the manufacture of glucose. As shown in Figure 4.1, water absorbed from the earth by the plants' roots combines with carbon dioxide present in the leaves to produce the carbohydrate glucose. Plants continually store glucose and use it to support their own growth. Then, when we eat plant foods, our bodies digest, absorb, and use the stored glucose.

> **Recap:** Carbohydrates are one of the three macronutrient types that provide energy to our bodies. Carbohydrates contain carbon, hydrogen, and oxygen. Plants make one type of carbohydrate, glucose, through the process of photosynthesis.

What's the Difference Between Simple and Complex Carbohydrates?

Carbohydrates can be classified as *simple* or *complex.* Simple carbohydrates contain either one or two molecules, while complex carbohydrates contain hundreds to thousands of molecules.

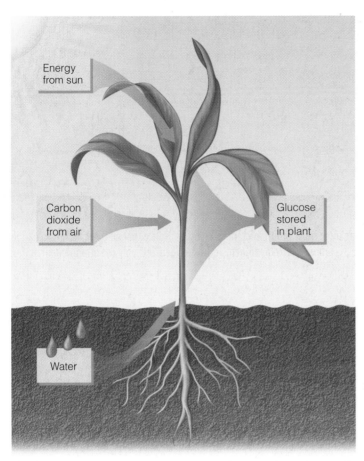

Figure 4.1 Plants make carbohydrates through the process of photosynthesis. Water, carbon dioxide, and energy from the sun are combined to produce glucose.

Simple Carbohydrates Include Monosaccharides and Disaccharides

Simple carbohydrates are commonly referred to as *sugars*. Three of these sugars are called **monosaccharides** because they consist of a single sugar molecule (*mono* meaning "one," and *saccharide* meaning "sugar"). The other three sugars are **disaccharides,** which consist of two molecules of sugar joined together (*di* meaning "two").

Glucose, Fructose, and Galactose Are Monosaccharides

Glucose, fructose, and *galactose* are the three most common monosaccharides in our diet. Each of these monosaccharides contains six carbon atoms, twelve hydrogen atoms, and six oxygen atoms (Figure 4.2). Very slight differences in the structure of the molecules in these three monosaccharides cause major differences in their level of sweetness.

Given what you've just learned about how plants manufacture glucose, it probably won't surprise you to discover that glucose is the most abundant sugar molecule found in our diets and in our bodies. Glucose does not generally occur by itself in foods but attaches to other sugars to form disaccharides and complex carbohydrates. In our bodies, glucose is the preferred source of energy for the brain, and it is a very important source of energy for all cells.

Fructose, the sweetest natural sugar, occurs naturally in fruits and vegetables. Fructose is also called *levulose*, or *fruit sugar*. In many processed foods, it comes in

simple carbohydrate Commonly called *sugar;* a monosaccharide or disaccharide such as glucose.

monosaccharide The simplest of carbohydrates. Consists of one sugar molecule, the most common form of which is glucose.

disaccharide A carbohydrate compound consisting of two sugar molecules joined together.

fructose The sweetest natural sugar; a monosaccharide that occurs in fruits and vegetables. Also called *levulose*, or *fruit sugar.*

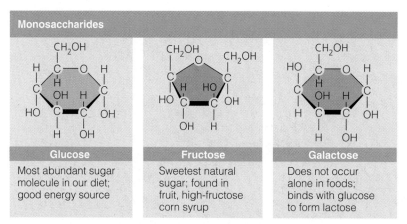

Figure 4.2 The three most common monosaccharides. Notice that all three monosaccharides contain identical atoms: six carbon, twelve hydrogen, and six oxygen. It is only the arrangement of these atoms that differs.

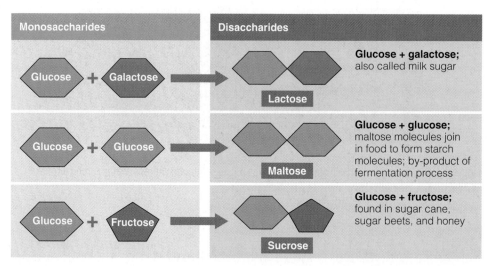

Figure 4.3 Galactose, glucose, and fructose join together to make the disaccharides lactose, maltose, and sucrose.

the form of *high-fructose corn syrup*. This syrup is made from corn and is used to sweeten soft drinks, desserts, candies, and jellies.

Galactose does not occur alone in foods. It joins with glucose to create lactose, one of the three most common disaccharides.

Lactose, Maltose, and Sucrose Are Disaccharides

The three most common disaccharides found in foods are *lactose*, *maltose*, and *sucrose* (Figure 4.3). **Lactose** (also called *milk sugar*) consists of one glucose molecule and one galactose molecule. Interestingly, human breast milk has a higher amount of lactose than cow's milk, which makes human breast milk taste sweeter.

Maltose (also called *malt sugar*) consists of two molecules of glucose. It does not generally occur by itself in foods, but rather is bound together with other molecules. As our bodies break these larger molecules down, maltose results as a by-product. Maltose is also the sugar that is fermented during the production of beer and liquor products. Contrary to popular belief, very little maltose remains in alcoholic beverages after the fermentation process; thus, alcoholic beverages are not good sources of carbohydrate.

Sucrose is composed of one glucose molecule and one fructose molecule. Because sucrose contains fructose, it is sweeter than lactose or maltose. Sucrose pro-

galactose A monosaccharide that joins with glucose to create lactose, one of the three most common disaccharides.

lactose Also called *milk sugar*, a disaccharide consisting of one glucose molecule and one galactose molecule. Found in milk, including human breast milk.

maltose A disaccharide consisting of two molecules of glucose. Does not generally occur independently in foods but results as a by-product of digestion. Also called *malt sugar*.

sucrose A disaccharide composed of one glucose molecule and one fructose molecule. Sweeter than lactose or maltose.

Forms of Sucrose Commonly Used in Foods

Brown sugar
Concentrated fruit juice
    sweetener
Confectioner's sugar
Corn sweeteners
Corn syrup
Dextrose
Fructose
Galactose

Glucose
Granulated sugar
High-fructose corn syrup
Honey
Invert sugar
Lactose
Levulose
Maltose
Mannitol

Maple sugar
Molasses
Natural sweeteners
Raw sugar
Sorbitol
Turbinado sugar
White sugar
Xylitol ●

vides much of the sweet taste found in honey, maple syrup, fruits, and vegetables. Table sugar, brown sugar, powdered sugar, and many other products are made by refining the sucrose found in sugarcane and sugar beets. See the Highlight box to learn more about the different forms of sucrose commonly used in foods. Are naturally occurring forms of sucrose more healthful than manufactured forms? The Nutrition Myth or Fact box investigates the common belief that honey is more nutritious than table sugar.

Recap: Simple carbohydrates include monosaccharides and disaccharides. Glucose, fructose, and galactose are monosaccharides; lactose, maltose, and sucrose are disaccharides.

All Complex Carbohydrates Are Polysaccharides

Complex carbohydrates, the second major type of carbohydrate, generally consist of long chains of glucose molecules. The technical name for complex carbohydrates is **polysaccharides** (*poly* meaning "many"). They include starch, glycogen, and most fibers (Figure 4.4).

complex carbohydrate A nutrient compound consisting of long chains of glucose molecules, such as starch, glycogen, and fiber.

polysaccharide A complex carbohydrate consisting of long chains of glucose.

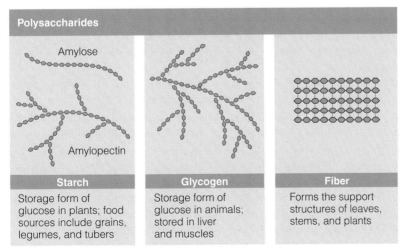

Figure 4.4 Polysaccharides, also referred to as complex carbohydrates, include starch, glycogen, and fiber.

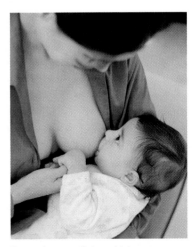

Human breast milk has a higher amount of lactose than cow's milk, which makes human breast milk taste sweeter.

Is Honey More Nutritious Than Table Sugar?

Liz's friend Tiffany is dedicated to eating healthful foods. She advises Liz to avoid sucrose and to eat foods that contain honey, molasses, or raw sugar.

Like many people, Tiffany believes these sweeteners are more natural and nutritious than refined table sugar. How can Liz sort sugar fact from fiction?

Remember that sucrose consists of one glucose molecule and one fructose molecule joined together. From a chemical perspective, honey is almost identical to sucrose, since honey also contains glucose and fructose molecules in almost equal amounts. However, enzymes in bees' "honey stomachs" separate some of the glucose and fructose molecules, resulting in honey looking and tasting slightly different from sucrose. As you know, bees store honey in combs and fan it with their wings to reduce its moisture content. This also alters the appearance and texture of honey.

Honey does not contain any more nutrients than sucrose, so it is not a more healthful choice than sucrose. In fact, per tablespoon, honey has more calories (or energy) than table sugar. This is because the crystals in table sugar take up more space on a spoon than the liquid form of honey, so a tablespoon contains less sugar. However, some people argue that honey is sweeter, so you use less.

It is important to note that honey commonly contains bacteria that can cause fatal food poisoning in infants. The more mature digestive sys-

tem of older children and adults is immune to the effects of these bacteria, but babies younger than twelve months should never be given honey.

Are raw sugar and molasses more healthful than table sugar? Actually, the "raw sugar" available in the United States is not really raw. Truly raw sugar is made up of the first crystals obtained when sugar is processed. Sugar in this form contains dirt, parts of insects, and other by-products that make it illegal to sell in the United States. The raw sugar products in American stores have actually gone through more than half of the same steps in the refining process used to make table sugar.

Molasses is the syrup that remains when sucrose is made from sugarcane. Molasses is darker and less sweet than table sugar. It does contain some iron, but this iron does not occur naturally. It is a contaminant from the machines that process the sugarcane!

The table below compares the nutrient content of white sugar, honey, molasses, and raw sugar. As you can see, none of them contain many nutrients that are important for health. This is why highly sweetened products are referred to as "empty calories." ●

Table 4.1   Nutrient Comparison of Four Different Sugars

	Table Sugar	Honey	Blackstrap Molasses	Raw Sugar
Energy (kcal)	48.8	63.8	47.0	48.8
Carbohydrate (grams)	12.6	17.3	12.2	12.6
Fat (grams)	0	0	0	0
Protein (grams)	0	0.06	0	0
Fiber (grams)	0	0.04	0	0
Vitamin C (mg)	0	0.11	0	0
Vitamin A (IU)	0	0	0	0
Thiamin (mg)	0	0	0.007	0
Riboflavin (mg)	0.003	0.008	0.01	0.003
Folate (μgrams)	0	0.42	0.20	0
Calcium (mg)	0.042	1.26	172.0	0.042
Iron (mg)	0	0.088	3.5	0
Sodium (mg)	0	0.84	11.0	0
Potassium (mg)	0.25	10.9	498.4	0.25

Source: U.S. Department of Agriculture, Agricultural Research Service. 2003. USDA National Nutrient Database for Standard Reference, Release 16. Nutrient Data Laboratory Home Page, http://www.nal.usda.gov/fnic/foodcomp.
Note: Nutrient values are identified for one tablespoon of each product.

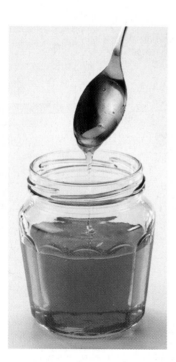

Starch Is a Polysaccharide Stored in Plants

Plants store glucose not as single molecules, but as polysaccharides in the form of **starch.** Excellent food sources of starch include grains (wheat, rice, corn, oats, and barley), legumes (peas, beans, and lentils), and tubers (potatoes and yams). Our cells cannot use the complex starch molecules exactly as they occur in plants. Instead, our bodies must break them down into the monosaccharide glucose, from which we can then fuel our energy needs.

Our bodies easily digest most starches; however, some starch in plants is not digestible and is called *resistant*. When our intestinal bacteria try to digest resistant starch, a fatty acid called *butyrate* is produced. Consuming resistant starch may be beneficial because butyrate is suggested to reduce the risk of cancer (Topping and Clifton 2001). Legumes contain more resistant starch than do grains, fruits, or vegetables. This quality, plus their high protein and fiber content, makes legumes a healthful food.

Glycogen Is a Polysaccharide Stored by Animals

Glycogen is the storage form of glucose for animals, including humans. Very little glycogen exists in food; thus, glycogen is not a dietary source of carbohydrate. We can break down glycogen very quickly into glucose when we need it for energy. We store glycogen in our muscles and liver; the storage and use of glycogen is discussed in more detail on page 125.

Fiber Is a Polysaccharide that Gives Plants Their Structure

There are currently a number of definitions of fiber. Recently, the Food and Nutrition Board of the Institute of Medicine has proposed three distinctions: *dietary fiber, functional fiber*, and *total fiber* (Institute of Medicine 2002). **Dietary fiber** is the nondigestible parts of plants that form the support structures of leaves, stems, and seeds (see Figure 4.4). In a sense, you can think of dietary fiber as the plant's "skeleton." **Functional fiber** consists of nondigestible forms of carbohydrates that are extracted from plants or manufactured in a laboratory and have known health benefits. Functional fiber is added to foods and is the form found in fiber supplements. **Total fiber** is the sum of dietary fiber and functional fiber.

Good food sources of dietary fiber include oat and wheat brans, oats, wheat, rye, barley, brown rice, seeds, legumes, fruits, and vegetables. Examples of functional fiber sources you might see on nutrition labels include cellulose, guar gum, pectin, and psyllium.

Like starch, fiber consists of long polysaccharide chains. Unlike with starch, however, the body does not easily break down the bonds that connect fiber molecules. This means that both dietary and functional fibers pass through the digestive system without being broken down and absorbed, so they contribute no energy to our diet. However, fiber offers many other health benefits, as we will see shortly (page 132).

> **Recap:** All complex carbohydrates are polysaccharides. They include starch, glycogen, and fiber. Starch is the storage form of glucose in plants, while glycogen is the storage form of glucose in animals. Fiber forms the support structures of plants; our bodies cannot digest fiber.

How Do Our Bodies Break Down Carbohydrates?

Because glucose is the form of sugar that our bodies use for energy, the primary goal of carbohydrate digestion is to break down polysaccharides and disaccharides into monosaccharides that can then be converted to glucose. Chapter 3 provided an overview of

starch A polysaccharide stored in plants; the storage form of glucose in plants.

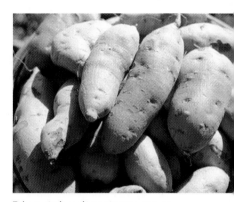

Tubers, such as these sweet potatoes, are excellent food sources of starch.

glycogen A polysaccharide stored in animals; the storage form of glucose in animals.

dietary fiber The nondigestible carbohydrate parts of plants that form the support structures of leaves, stems, and seeds.

functional fiber The nondigestible forms of carbohydrate that are extracted from plants or manufactured in the laboratory and have known health benefits.

total fiber The sum of dietary fiber and functional fiber.

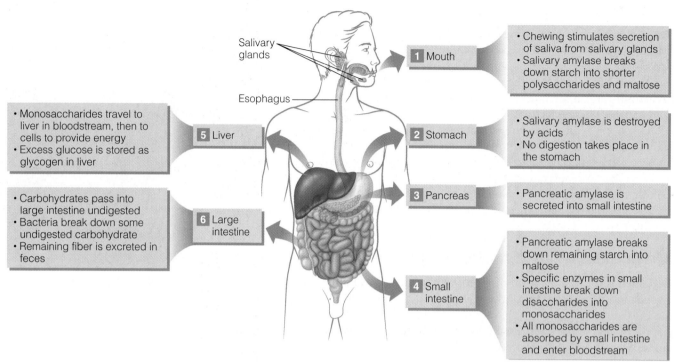

Figure 4.5   A review of carbohydrate digestion and absorption.

digestion of the three types of macronutrients, plus vitamins and minerals. Here, we focus specifically and in a bit more detail on the digestion and absorption of carbohydrates. Figure 4.5 provides a visual tour of carbohydrate digestion.

Digestion Breaks Down Most Carbohydrates into Monosaccharides

Carbohydrate digestion begins in the mouth (Figure 4.5, Step 1). As you saw in Chapter 3, the starch in the foods you eat mixes with your saliva during chewing. Saliva contains an enzyme called **salivary amylase,** which breaks starch into smaller particles and eventually into the disaccharide maltose. The next time you eat a piece of bread, notice that you can actually taste it becoming sweeter; this indicates the breakdown of starch into maltose. Disaccharides are not digested in the mouth.

As the bolus of food leaves the mouth and enters the stomach, all digestion of carbohydrates ceases. This is because the acid in the stomach inactivates most of the salivary amylase enzyme (Figure 4.5, Step 2).

The majority of carbohydrate digestion occurs in the small intestine. As the contents of the stomach enter the small intestine, an enzyme called *pancreatic amylase* is secreted by the pancreas into the small intestine (Figure 4.5, Step 3). **Pancreatic amylase** continues to digest any remaining starch into maltose. Additional enzymes found in the microvilli of the mucosal cells that line the intestinal tract work to break down disaccharides into monosaccharides. Maltose is broken down into glucose by the enzyme **maltase.** Sucrose is broken down into glucose and fructose by the enzyme **sucrase.** The enzyme **lactase** breaks lactose into glucose and galactose (Figure 4.5, Step 4). Notice that enzyme names are identifiable by the -ase suffix. All monosaccharides are then absorbed into the mucosal cells lining the small intestine, where they pass through and enter into the blood stream.

salivary amylase   An enzyme in saliva that breaks starch into smaller particles and eventually into the disaccharide maltose.

pancreatic amylase   An enzyme secreted by the pancreas into the small intestine that digests any remaining starch into maltose.

maltase   A digestive enzyme that breaks maltose into glucose.

sucrase   A digestive enzyme that breaks sucrose into glucose and fructose.

lactase   A digestive enzyme that breaks lactose into glucose and galactose.

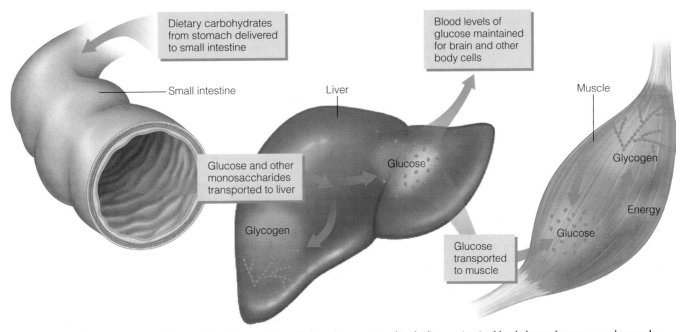

Figure 4.6   Glucose is stored as glycogen in both liver and muscle. The glycogen stored in the liver maintains blood glucose between meals; muscle glycogen provides immediate energy to the muscle during exercise.

The Liver Converts All Monosaccharides into Glucose

Once the monosaccharides enter the bloodstream, they travel to the liver. Fructose and galactose are converted to glucose in the liver (Figure 4.5, Step 5). If needed immediately for energy, the liver releases glucose into the blood stream where it can travel to the cells to provide energy. If there is no immediate demand by the body for glucose, it is stored as glycogen in our liver and muscles. Enzymes in liver and muscle cells combine glucose molecules to form glycogen (an anabolic, or building, process) and break glycogen into glucose (a catabolic, or destructive, process), depending on our bodily needs. Our liver can store 70 grams (or 280 calories) of glycogen, and our muscles can normally store about 120 grams (or 480 calories) of glycogen. Between meals, our bodies draw on liver glycogen reserves to maintain blood glucose levels and support the needs of our cells, including those of our brain, spinal cord, and red blood cells (Figure 4.6).

The glycogen stored in our muscles provides energy to the muscles during intense exercise. Endurance athletes can increase their storage of muscle glycogen from two to four times the normal amount through a process called *glycogen, or carbohydrate, loading* (see Chapter 12). Any excess glucose is stored as glycogen in the liver and muscles and saved for such future energy needs as exercise.

Fiber Is Excreted from the Large Intestine

We do not possess enzymes that can break down fiber. Thus, fiber passes through the small intestine undigested and enters the large intestine, or colon. Once in the large intestine, bacteria break down some previously undigested carbohydrates, causing the production of gas and a few fatty acids. The cells of the large intestine use these fatty acids for energy. The fiber remaining in the colon adds bulk to our stools and is excreted (Figure 4.5, Step 6) in feces. In this way, fiber assists in maintaining bowel regularity. The health benefits of fiber are discussed later in this chapter (page 132).

Recap: Carbohydrate digestion starts in the mouth and continues in the small intestine. Glucose and other monosaccharides are absorbed into the blood stream and travel to the liver, where nonglucose sugars are converted to glucose. Glucose is either used by the cells for energy or is converted to glycogen and stored in the liver and muscle for later use.

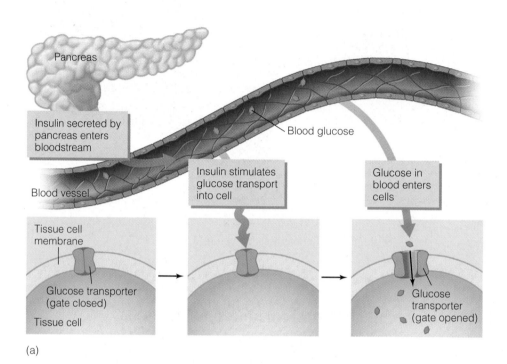

Pancreas

Insulin secreted by pancreas enters bloodstream

Blood glucose

Blood vessel

Insulin stimulates glucose transport into cell

Glucose in blood enters cells

Tissue cell membrane

Glucose transporter (gate closed)

Tissue cell

Glucose transporter (gate opened)

(a)

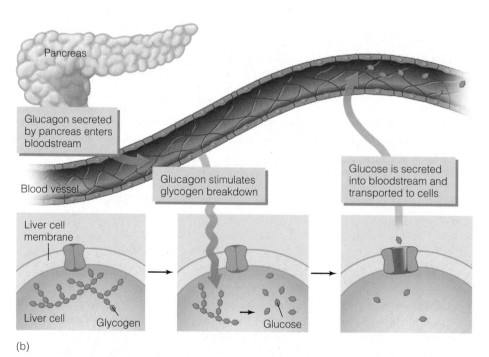

Pancreas

Glucagon secreted by pancreas enters bloodstream

Blood vessel

Glucagon stimulates glycogen breakdown

Glucose is secreted into bloodstream and transported to cells

Liver cell membrane

Liver cell   Glycogen

Glucose

(b)

Figure 4.7   Regulation of blood glucose by the hormones insulin and glucagon. **(a)** When blood glucose levels increase after a meal, the pancreas secretes insulin. Insulin opens gates in the cell membrane to allow the passage of glucose into the cell. **(b)** When blood glucose levels are low, the pancreas secretes glucagon. Glucagon enters the cell, where it stimulates the breakdown of stored glycogen into glucose. This glucose is then released into the bloodstream.

Insulin and Glucagon Regulate the Level of Glucose in Our Blood

Our bodies regulate blood glucose levels within a fairly narrow range to provide adequate glucose to the brain and other cells. Two hormones, insulin and glucagon, assist the body with maintaining blood glucose. Specialized cells in the pancreas synthesize, store and secrete both hormones.

When we eat a meal, our blood glucose level rises. But glucose in our blood cannot help the nerves, muscles, and other tissues function unless it can cross into them. Glucose molecules are too large to cross the cell membranes of our tissues independently. To get in, glucose needs assistance from the hormone **insulin,** which is secreted by the beta cells of the pancreas (Figure 4.7a). Insulin is transported in the blood to the cells of tissues throughout the body, where it stimulates special molecules located in the cell membrane to transport glucose into the cell. Insulin can be thought of as a key that opens the gates of the cell membrane, and carries the glucose into the cell interior, where it can be used for energy. Insulin also stimulates the liver and muscles to take up glucose and store it as glycogen.

When you have not eaten for some period of time, your blood glucose levels decline. This decrease in blood glucose stimulates the alpha cells of the pancreas to secrete another hormone, **glucagon** (Figure 4.7b). Glucagon acts in an opposite way to insulin: it causes the liver to convert its stored glycogen into glucose, which is then secreted into the bloodstream and transported to the cells for energy. Glucagon also assists in the breakdown of body proteins to amino acids so the liver can stimulate *gluconeogenesis*, or the production of new glucose from amino acids.

Normally the effects of insulin and glucagon balance each other to maintain blood glucose within a healthy range. If this balance is altered, it can lead to health conditions such as diabetes (page 145) or hypoglycemia (page 149).

insulin   Hormone secreted by the beta cells of the pancreas in response to increased blood levels of glucose. Facilitates uptake of glucose by body cells.

glucagon   Hormone secreted by the alpha cells of the pancreas in response to decreased blood levels of glucose. Causes breakdown of liver stores of glycogen into glucose.

Recap: Two hormones, insulin and glucagon, are involved in regulating blood glucose. Insulin lowers blood glucose levels by facilitating the entry of glucose into cells. Glucagon raises blood glucose levels by stimulating gluconeogenesis and the breakdown of glycogen stored in the liver.

The Glycemic Index Shows How Foods Affect Our Blood Glucose Levels

The **glycemic index** refers to the potential of foods to raise blood glucose levels. Foods with a high glycemic index cause sudden large increases in blood glucose. This large increase in blood glucose triggers a large increase in insulin, which may be followed by a

glycemic index   Rating of the potential of foods to raise blood glucose and insulin levels.

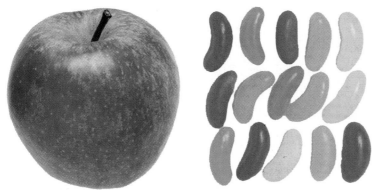

An apple (36) has a much lower glycemic index than a serving of jelly beans (78).

dramatic fall in blood glucose. Foods with a low glycemic index cause low to moderate fluctuations in blood glucose. When foods are assigned a glycemic index value, they are often compared with the glycemic effect of pure glucose.

The glycemic index of a food is not always easy to predict. Figure 4.8 ranks certain foods according to their glycemic index. Do any of these rankings surprise you? Most people assume that foods containing simple sugars have a higher glycemic index than starches, but this is not always the case. For instance, compare the glycemic index for apples and instant potatoes. Although instant potatoes are a starchy food, they have a glycemic index value of 83, while the value for an apple is only 36!

The type of carbohydrate, the way the food is prepared, and its fat and fiber content can all affect how quickly the body absorbs it. It is important to note that we eat most of our foods combined into a meal. In this case, the glycemic index of the total meal becomes more important than the ranking of each food.

Why do we care about the glycemic index? Foods or meals with a lower index are a better choice for someone with diabetes, for instance, because they will not trigger dramatic fluctuations in blood glucose. They may also reduce the risk of heart disease and colon cancer because they generally contain more fiber and help decrease fat levels in the blood. Recent studies have shown that people who eat lower glycemic index meals have higher levels of high-density lipoprotein, or HDL (which lowers their risk of heart disease) and their blood glucose values are more likely to be normal (Liu et al. 2001; Buyken et al. 2001). The easiest way to eat lower glycemic index foods and meals without having to look up the index is to consume foods such as beans and lentils, fresh vegetables, and whole wheat bread.

Despite some encouraging research findings, the glycemic index remains controversial. Many nutrition researchers feel that the evidence supporting its health benefits is weak and that we do not know enough about the impact of low glycemic index foods on long-term health. In addition, many believe the glycemic index concept is too complex for people to apply to their daily lives. Other researchers insist that helping people to choose lower glycemic index foods is critical to the prevention and treatment of many chronic diseases.

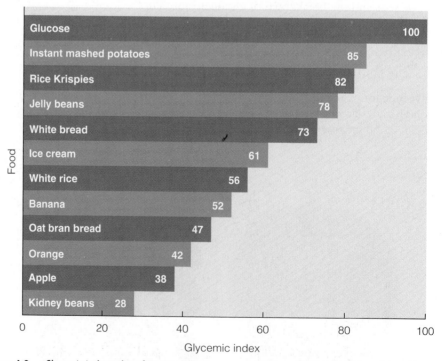

Figure 4.8 Glycemic index values for various foods as compared to pure glucose. (Values derived from K. Foster-Powell, S. H. A. Holt, and J. C. Brand-Miller. International table of glycemic index and glycemic load values. *Am. J. Clin. Nutr.* 76 (2002): 5–56.)

Recap: The glycemic index is a value that indicates the potential of foods to raise blood glucose and insulin levels. Foods with a high glycemic index cause sudden large increases in blood glucose and insulin, while foods with a low glycemic index cause low to moderate fluctuations in blood glucose.

Why Do We Need Carbohydrates?

We have seen that carbohydrates are an important energy source for our bodies. Let's now learn more about this and discuss other functions of carbohydrates.

Carbohydrates Provide Energy

Carbohydrates, an excellent source of energy for all our cells, provide 4 kilocalories (kcal) of energy per gram. Some of our cells can also use fat and even protein for energy if necessary. However, our red blood cells can utilize only glucose and our brain and other nervous tissues primarily rely on glucose. This is why you get tired, irritable, and shaky when you have not eaten for a prolonged period of time.

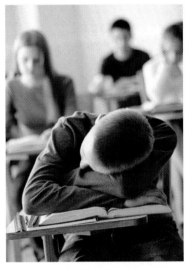

Our red blood cells can utilize only glucose and other monosaccharides, and our brain and other nervous tissues primarily rely on glucose. This is why you get tired, irritable, and shaky when you have not eaten for a prolonged period of time.

Carbohydrates Fuel Daily Activity

Many popular diets—such as Dr. Atkins' New Revolution Diet and the Sugar Busters plan—are based on the idea that our bodies actually "prefer" to use fat and/or protein for energy. They claim that current carbohydrate recommendations are much higher than we really need.

In reality, the body relies mostly on both carbohydrates and fat for energy. In fact, as shown in Figure 4.9, our bodies always use some combination of carbohydrates and fat to fuel daily activities.

Fat is the predominant energy source used by our bodies at rest and during low-intensity activities such as sitting, standing, and walking. Even during rest, however, our brain cells and red blood cells still rely on glucose.

Carbohydrates Fuel Exercise

When we exercise, whether running, briskly walking, bicycling, or performing any other activity that causes us to breathe harder and sweat, we begin to use more glucose than fat. While fat breakdown is a slow process and requires oxygen, we can

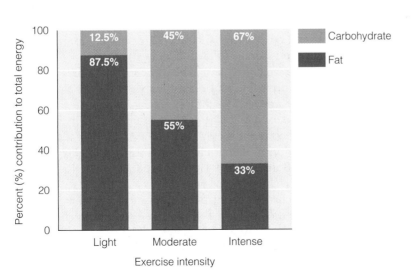

Figure 4.9   Amounts of carbohydrate and fat used during light, moderate, and intense exercise. (Adapted from J. A. Romijn, E. F. Coyle, L. S. Sidossis, A. Gastaldelli, J. F. Horowitz, E. Endert, and R. R. Wolfe. Regulation of endogenous fat and carbohydrate metabolism in relation to exercise intensity and duration. *Am. J. Physiol.* 265 (*Endocrinol. Metab.* 28) (1993): E380–E391.)

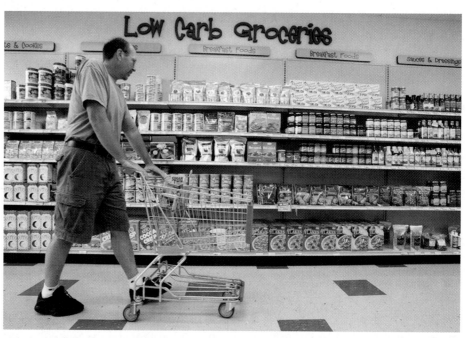

Many popular diets claim that current carbohydrate recommendations are much higher than we really need.

break down glucose very quickly either with or without oxygen. Even during very intense exercise, when less oxygen is available, we can still break down glucose very quickly for energy. That's why when you are exercising at maximal effort, carbohydrates are providing almost 100% of the energy your body requires.

If you are physically active, it is important to eat enough carbohydrates to provide energy for your brain, red blood cells, and muscles. In Chapter 12, we discuss in more detail the carbohydrate recommendations for active people. In general, if you do not eat enough carbohydrate to support regular exercise, your body will have to rely upon fat and protein as alternative energy sources. When your carbohydrate intake is insufficient, body protein is used for energy (the consequences of which are discussed beginning on page 131). In addition, you will have to reduce your amount and intensity of exercise so that you can rely more on fat for energy. One advantage of becoming highly trained for endurance-type events such as marathons and triathlons is that our muscles are able to store more glycogen, which provides us with additional glucose we can use during exercise. (See Chapter 12 for more information on how exercise improves our use and storage of carbohydrates.)

If you are trying to lose weight, you may be wondering whether you should exercise at a lower intensity so you will use more fat for energy. This is a question that researchers are still trying to answer. Weight loss studies show that, to lose weight and keep it off, it is important to exercise daily. A lower-intensity activity such as walking is generally recommended because it is easy to do and we know that fat provides much of the energy we need for walking. However, a study of highly trained athletes (Tremblay, Simoneau, and Bouchard 1994) found that they actually lost more body fat when they performed very high-intensity exercise!

Based on the evidence currently available, there is no magic formula for weight loss. It is likely that people who combine aerobic-type exercises, such as walking, jogging, or bicycling, with strength-building exercises will be more successful in losing weight and keeping it off. It is important to find activities we can do every day. The current recommendations for health suggest that people perform at least 30 minutes of activity daily; but for weight loss, it is more effective to exercise for at least one hour each day. We can help our bodies stay active and healthy by eating the proper balance of carbohydrate, fat, and protein. (For more information on weight loss, see Chapter 11.)

Low Carbohydrate Intake Can Lead to Ketoacidosis

When we do not eat enough carbohydrate, the body must find other sources of energy. While most of our body tissues can use fat and protein for energy, our brains cannot. Thus, when our carbohydrate intake is inadequate, our body seeks an alternative source of fuel for the brain and begins to break down stored fat. This process, called **ketosis,** produces an alternative fuel called **ketones.**

Ketosis is an important mechanism for providing energy to the brain during situations of fasting, low carbohydrate intake, or vigorous exercise (Pan et al. 2000). However, ketones also suppress appetite and cause dehydration and acetone breath (the breath smells like nail polish remover). If inadequate carbohydrate intake continues for an extended period of time, the body will produce excessive amounts of ketones. Because many ketones are acids, high ketone levels cause the blood to become very acidic, leading to a condition called **ketoacidosis.** The high acidity of the blood interferes with basic body functions, causes the loss of lean body mass, and damages many body tissues. People with untreated diabetes are at high risk for ketoacidosis, which can lead to coma and even death. (See page 145 for further details about diabetes.)

Carbohydrates Spare Protein

Some cells can rely on fat for energy, but other cells require glucose. If the diet does not provide enough carbohydrate, the body will make its own glucose from protein. This involves breaking down the proteins in blood and tissues into amino acids, then converting them to glucose. This process is called **gluconeogenesis** (or "generating new glucose").

When our body uses proteins for energy, the amino acids from these proteins cannot be used to make new cells, repair tissue damage, support our immune system, or perform any of their other functions. During periods of starvation or when eating a diet that is very low in carbohydrate, our body will take amino acids from the blood first, and then from other tissues like muscles, heart, liver, and kidneys. Using amino acids in this manner over a prolonged period of time can cause serious, possibly irreversible, damage to these organs. (See Chapter 6 for more details on using protein for energy.)

> **Recap:** Carbohydrates are an excellent energy source at rest and during exercise, and provide 4 kcal of energy per gram. Carbohydrates are necessary in the diet to spare body protein and prevent ketosis.

Complex Carbohydrates Have Health Benefits

The relationship between carbohydrates, heart disease, and obesity is the subject of considerable controversy. Proponents of low-carbohydrate diets claim that eating carbohydrates, not fat, makes you overweight. However, anyone who consumes extra calories, whether in the form of sugar, complex carbohydrates, protein, or fat, may eventually become obese. Studies indicate that overweight people tend to eat higher amounts of energy, including both sugar and fat, and they are not physically active enough to expend this extra energy. Thus, weight gain occurs.

Fat is more energy-dense than carbohydrate: it contains 9 kcal per gram, while carbohydrate contains only 4 kcal per gram. Thus, gram for gram, fat is twice as "fattening" as carbohydrate. In fact, eating complex carbohydrates that are high in fiber and other nutrients has been shown to reduce the overall risk for obesity, heart disease, and diabetes. Thus, all carbohydrates are not bad, and a small amount of simple carbohydrate can be included in a healthful diet. People who are very active and need more calories can eat more simple carbohydrate, while those who are older, less active, or overweight should limit their consumption and focus on complex carbohydrates.

ketosis   The process by which the breakdown of fat during fasting states results in the production of ketones.

ketones   Substances produced during the breakdown of fat when carbohydrate intake is insufficient to meet energy needs. Provide an alternative energy source for the brain when glucose levels are low.

ketoacidosis   A condition in which excessive ketones are present in the blood, causing the blood to become very acidic, which alters basic body functions and damages tissues. Untreated ketoacidosis can be fatal. This condition is found in individuals with untreated diabetes mellitus.

gluconeogenesis   The generation of glucose from the breakdown of proteins into amino acids.

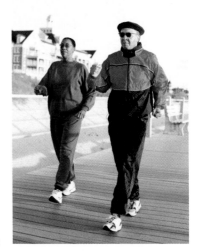

When we exercise, whether power walking or performing any other activity that causes us to breathe harder and sweat, we begin to use more glucose than fat.

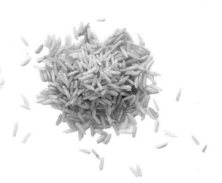

Brown rice is a good food source of dietary fiber.

Fiber Helps Us Stay Healthy

Although we cannot digest fiber, it is still an important substance in our diet. Research indicates that it helps us stay healthy and may prevent many digestive and chronic diseases. The potential benefits of fiber consumption include the following:

- May reduce the risk of colon cancer. While there is still some controversy surrounding this issue, many researchers believe that fiber binds cancer-causing substances and speeds their elimination from the colon. However, recent studies of colon cancer and fiber have shown that their relationship is not as strong as previously thought.

- Helps prevent hemorrhoids, constipation, and other intestinal problems by keeping our stools moist and soft. Fiber gives gut muscles "something to push on" and makes it easier to eliminate stools.

- Reduces the risk of *diverticulosis*, a condition that is caused in part by trying to eliminate small, hard stools. A great deal of pressure must be generated in the large intestine to pass hard stools. This increased pressure weakens intestinal walls, causing them to bulge outward and form pockets (Figure 4.10). Feces and fibrous materials can get trapped in these pockets, which become infected and inflamed. This is a painful condition that must be treated with antibiotics or surgery.

- May reduce the risk of heart disease by delaying or blocking the absorption of dietary cholesterol into the bloodstream. Fiber also contributes small fatty acids that may lower the amount of low-density lipoprotein (or LDL) to healthful levels in our bodies.

- May enhance weight loss, as eating a high fiber diet causes a person to feel more full. Fiber absorbs water, expands in our intestine, and slows the movement of food through the upper part of the digestive tract. People who eat a fiber-rich diet tend to eat fewer fatty and sugary foods.

- May lower the risk of type 2 diabetes. In slowing digestion, fiber also slows the release of glucose into the blood. It thereby improves the body's regulation of insulin production and blood glucose levels.

Recap: Complex carbohydrates contain fiber and other nutrients that can reduce the risk for obesity, heart disease, and diabetes. Fiber may reduce the risk for colon cancer, helps prevent hemorrhoids, constipation, and diverticulosis, may reduce risk of heart disease, and may assist with weight loss.

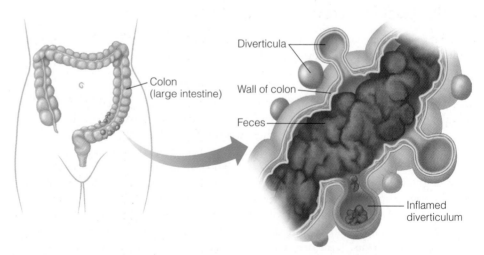

Figure 4.10 Diverticulosis occurs when bulging pockets form in the wall of the colon. These pockets become infected and inflamed, demanding proper treatment.

How Much Carbohydrate Should We Eat?

Carbohydrates are an important part of a balanced, healthy diet. The Recommended Dietary Allowance (RDA) for carbohydrate is based on the amount of glucose our brain utilizes (Institute of Medicine 2002). The current RDA for carbohydrate for adults nineteen years of age and older is 130 grams of carbohydrate per day. It is important to emphasize that this RDA does not cover the amount of carbohydrate needed to support daily activities; it only covers the amount of carbohydrate needed to supply adequate glucose to the brain.

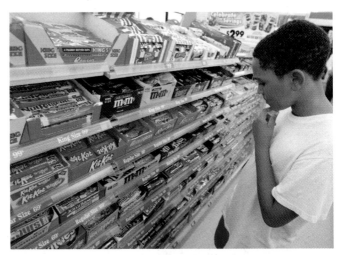

As introduced in Chapter 1, carbohydrates and the other macronutrients have been assigned an Acceptable Macronutrient Distribution Range (AMDR). This is the range of intake associated with a decreased risk of chronic diseases. The AMDR for carbohydrates is 45 to 65% of total energy intake. Table 4.2 compares the carbohydrate recommendations from the Institute of Medicine (2002) with the Dietary Guidelines for Americans related to carbohydrate-containing foods (USDA 2000). As you can see, the Institute of Medicine provides specific numeric recommendations, whereas the Dietary Guidelines for Americans are general suggestions about foods high in complex carbohydrates. Most health agencies agree that most of the carbohydrates you eat each day should be complex, or whole-grain and unprocessed carbohydrates. As recommended in the Food Guide Pyramid, eating 6 to 11 servings of whole grains and 5 to 9 servings of fruits and vegetables each day will ensure that you get

Foods with added sugars, like candy, have lower levels of vitamins and minerals than foods that naturally contain simple sugars.

enough fiber and other complex carbohydrates in your diet. Keep in mind that fruits are predominantly comprised of simple sugar and contain little or no starch. They are healthful food choices, however, as they are good sources of vitamins, some minerals, and fiber.

> **Recap:** The RDA for carbohydrate is 130 grams per day; this amount is only sufficient to supply adequate glucose to the brain. The AMDR for carbohydrate is 45 to 65% of total energy intake.

Table 4.2 Dietary Recommendations for Carbohydrates

Institute of Medicine Recommendations[1]	Dietary Guidelines for Americans[2]
Recommended Dietary Allowance (RDA) for adults 19 years of age and older is 130 grams of carbohydrate per day.	Build a healthy base: Use the Food Guide Pyramid to help make healthful food choices that you can enjoy.
The Acceptable Macronutrient Distribution Range (AMDR) for carbohydrate is 45–65% of total daily energy intake.	Build your eating pattern on a variety of plant foods, including whole grains, fruits, and vegetables.
Added sugar intake should be 25% or less of total energy intake each day.	Eat 6 or more servings of whole grains, breads, and cereals each day.
	Eat at least 2 servings of fruit and at least 3 servings of vegetables each day.
	Choose beverages and foods to moderate your intake of sugars.

[1] Institute of Medicine, Food and Nutrition Board. *Dietary Reference Intakes for Energy, Carbohydrates, Fiber, Fat, Protein and Amino Acids (Macronutrients).* (Washington, DC: The National Academy of Sciences, 2002.)
[2] U.S. Department of Agriculture (USDA). U.S. Department of Health and Human Services. *Dietary Guidelines for Americans,* 5th ed. (2000). Home and Garden Bulletin No. 232.

Most Americans Eat Too Much Simple Carbohydrate

The average carbohydrate intake in the U.S. is approximately 50%. For some people, almost half of this amount consists of simple sugars. Where does all this sugar come from? Some sugar comes from healthful food sources, such as fruit and milk. However, much of our simple sugar intake comes from *added sugars*. **Added sugars** are defined as sugars and syrups that are added to foods during processing or preparation (Institute of Medicine 2002). The most common source of added sugars in the U.S. diet is sweetened soft drinks; we drink an average of 40 gallons per person each year. Consider that one 12-ounce sugared cola contains 38.5 grams of sugar, or almost 10 teaspoons. If you drink the average amount, you are consuming more than 16,420 grams of sugar (about 267 cups) each year! Other common sources of added sugars include cookies, cakes, pies, fruit drinks, fruit punches, and candy.

added sugars Sugars and syrups that are added to food during processing or preparation.

Added sugars are not chemically different from naturally occurring sugars. However, foods and beverages with added sugars have lower levels of vitamins and minerals than foods that naturally contain simple sugars. With these nutrient limitations in mind, it is recommended that our diets contain 25% or less of our total energy from added sugars. People who are very physically active are able to consume relatively more added sugars, while smaller or less active people should consume relatively less.

Simple Carbohydrates Are Blamed for Many Health Problems

Why do simple carbohydrates have such a bad reputation? First, they are known to cause tooth decay. Second, they have been identified as a cause of hyperactivity in children. Third, eating a lot of simple carbohydrates could increase the levels of unhealthy lipids, or fats, in our blood, increasing our risk for heart disease. High intakes of simple carbohydrates have also been blamed for causing diabetes and obesity. Let's now learn the truth about these accusations related to simple carbohydrates.

Sugar Causes Tooth Decay

Simple carbohydrates do play a role in dental problems because the bacteria that cause tooth decay thrive on them. These bacteria produce acids that eat away at tooth enamel and can eventually cause cavities and gum disease (Figure 4.11). Eating sticky foods that adhere to teeth—such as caramels, crackers, sugary cereals, and licorice—and sipping sweetened beverages over a period of time increase the risk of tooth decay. This means that people shouldn't slowly sip soda or juice and that babies should not be put to sleep with a bottle unless it contains water. As we have seen, even breast milk contains sugar, which can slowly drip onto the baby's gums. As a result, infants should not routinely be allowed to fall asleep at the breast.

To reduce your risk for tooth decay, brush your teeth after each meal and especially after drinking sugary drinks and eating candy. Drinking fluoridated water and using a fluoride toothpaste also will help protect your teeth.

There is No Link Between Sugar and Hyperactivity in Children

Although many people believe that eating sugar causes hyperactivity and other behavioral problems in children, there is little scientific evidence to support this claim. Some children actually become less active shortly after a high-sugar meal! However, it is important to emphasize that most studies of sugar and children's behavior have only looked at the effects of sugar a few hours after ingestion. We know very little about the long-term effects of sugar intake on the behavior of children. Behavioral and learning problems are complex issues, most likely caused by a multitude of factors. Because of this complexity, the Institute of Medicine (2002) has stated that overall, there currently does not appear to be enough evidence that eating too much sugar causes hyperactivity or other behavioral problems in children. Thus, they have not set a Tolerable Upper Intake Level for sugar.

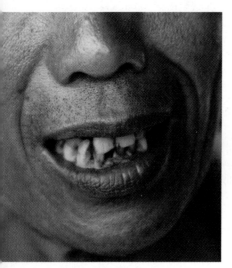

To reduce your risk for tooth decay, brush your teeth after each meal and especially after drinking sugary drinks and eating candy.

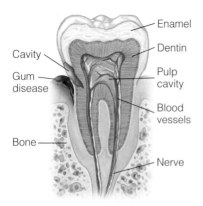

Enamel

Dentin

Cavity

Gum disease

Pulp cavity

Blood vessels

Bone

Nerve

Figure 4.11   Eating simple carbohydrates can cause an increase in cavities and gum disease. This is because bacteria in the mouth consume simple carbohydrates present on the teeth and gums and produce acids, which eat away at these tissues.

High Sugar Intake Can Lead to Unhealthful Levels of Blood Lipids

There is research evidence suggesting that consuming a diet high in simple sugars, particularly fructose, can lead to unhealthful changes in blood lipids. You will learn more about blood lipids (including cholesterol and lipoproteins) in Chapter 5. Briefly, higher intakes of simple sugars are associated with increases in triglycerides (lipids in our blood) and LDLs, which are commonly referred to as "bad cholesterol." At the same time, high simple sugar intake appears to *decrease* our HDLs, which are protective and are often referred to as "good cholesterol" (Institute of Medicine 2002; Howard and Wylie-Rosett 2002). These changes are of concern, as increased levels of triglycerides and LDL and decreased levels of HDL are known risk factors for heart disease. However, there is not enough scientific evidence at the present time to state with confidence that eating a diet high in simple sugars causes heart disease. Based on our current knowledge, it is prudent for a person at risk for heart disease to eat a diet low in simple sugars.

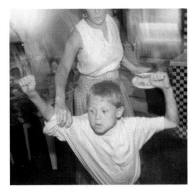

Although many people believe that eating sugar causes hyperactivity and other behavioral problems in children, there is little scientific evidence to support this claim.

High Sugar Intake Does Not Cause Diabetes But May Contribute to Obesity

There is no scientific evidence that eating a diet high in sugar causes diabetes. In fact, studies examining the relationship between sugar intake and type 2 diabetes report either no association between sugar intake and diabetes or a decreased risk of diabetes with increased sugar intake (Meyer et al. 2000; Colditz et al. 1992). However, people who have diabetes need to moderate their intake of sugar and closely monitor their blood glucose levels.

To date, there is no evidence to convincingly prove that sugar intake causes obesity; however, a recent study found that overweight children consumed more sugared soft drinks than did children of normal weight (Troiano et al. 2000). Another study found that for every extra sugared soft drink consumed by a child per day, the risk of obesity increases by 60 percent (Ludwig, Peterson, and Gortmaker 2001). We do know that if you consume more energy than you expend, you will gain weight. It makes intuitive sense that people who consume extra energy from high-sugar foods are at risk for obesity, just as people who consume extra energy from fat gain weight. In addition to the increased potential for obesity, another major concern about high-sugar diets is that they are inadequate in nutrients critical to maintain our health. Although we cannot state with certainty that consuming a high-sugar diet causes obesity, it is important to optimize your intake of nutrient-dense foods and limit added sugars. The relationship between sugared soft drinks and obesity is highly controversial, and discussed in more detail in the Nutrition Debate on page 154.

> **Recap:** Added sugars are sugars and syrups added to foods during processing or preparation. Our intake of added sugars should be 25% or less of our total energy intake each day. Sugar causes tooth decay but does not appear to cause hyperactivity in children. Higher intakes of simple sugars are associated with increases in triglycerides and low density lipoprotiens. Diets high in sugar cause unhealthy changes in blood sugar but do not cause diabetes. The relationship between added sugars and obesity is controversial.

Most Americans Eat Too Little Complex Carbohydrate

Do you get enough complex carbohydrates each day? If you are like most people in the United States, you eat only about 2 servings of fruits or vegetables each day; this is far below the 5 to 9 recommended servings. Do you eat whole grains and legumes every day? Many people eat plenty of breads, pastas, and cereals, but most do not consistently choose whole-grain products. As we explained earlier, whole-grain foods have a lower glycemic index than simple carbohydrates; thus, they prompt a more gradual release of insulin and result in less severe fluctuations in both insulin and glucose. Whole-grain foods also provide more nutrients and fiber than foods made with enriched flour (Figure 4.12).

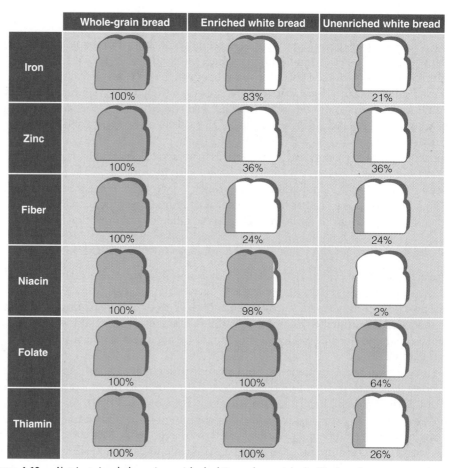

	Whole-grain bread	Enriched white bread	Unenriched white bread
Iron	100%	83%	21%
Zinc	100%	36%	36%
Fiber	100%	24%	24%
Niacin	100%	98%	2%
Folate	100%	100%	64%
Thiamin	100%	100%	26%

Figure 4.12   Nutrients in whole-grain, enriched white, and unenriched white breads.

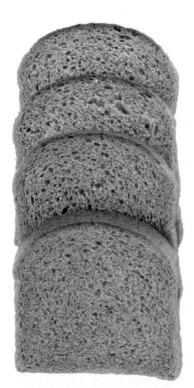

Whole-grain foods provide more nutrients and fiber than foods made with enriched flour.

Table 4.3 defines terms commonly used on nutrition labels for breads and cereals. Read the label for the breads you eat—does it list *whole-wheat flour* or just *wheat flour*? Although most labels for breads and cereals list wheat flour as the first ingredient, this term actually refers to enriched white flour, which is made when wheat flour is processed. Don't be fooled—becoming an educated consumer will help you select whole grains instead of processed foods.

We Need at Least 25 Grams of Fiber Daily

How much fiber do we need? The Adequate Intake for fiber is 25 grams per day for women and 38 grams per day for men (Institute of Medicine 2002), or 14 grams of fiber for every 1,000 kcal per day that a person eats. Most people in the United States eat only 12 to 18 grams of fiber each day, getting only half of the fiber they need. Although fiber supplements are available, it is best to get fiber from food because foods contain additional nutrients such as vitamins and minerals.

Eating the amounts of whole grains, vegetables, fruits, nuts, and legumes recommended in the Food Guide Pyramid will ensure that you eat adequate fiber. Table 4.4 lists some common foods and their fiber content. Think about how you can design your own diet to include high-fiber foods.

It is also important to drink more water as you increase your fiber intake, since fiber binds with water to soften stools. Inadequate water intake with a high-fiber diet can actually result in hard, dry stools that are difficult to pass through the colon.

Can you eat too much fiber? Excessive fiber consumption can lead to problems such as intestinal gas, bloating, and constipation. Because fiber binds with water, it causes the body to eliminate more water, so a very high fiber diet could result in

Table 4.3   Terms Used to Describe Grains and Cereals on Nutrition Labels

Term	Definition
Brown bread	Bread that may or may not be made using whole-grain flour. Many brown breads are made with white flour with brown (caramel) coloring added.
Enriched (or fortified) flour or grain	Enriching or fortifying grains involves adding nutrients back to refined foods. In order to use this term in the United States, a minimum amount of iron, folate, niacin, thiamin, and riboflavin must be added. Other nutrients can also be added.
Refined flour or grain	Refining involved removing the coarse parts of food products; refined wheat flour is flour in which all but the internal part of the kernel has been removed. Refined sugar is made by removing the outer portions of sugar beets or sugarcane.
Stone ground	Refers to a milling process in which limestone is used to grind any grain. Stone ground does not mean that bread is made with whole grain, as refined flour can be stone ground.
Unbleached flour	Flour that has been refined but not bleached; it is very similar to refined white flour in texture and nutritional value.
Wheat flour	Any flour made from wheat; includes white flour, unbleached flour, and whole-wheat flour.
White flour	Flour that has been bleached and refined. All-purpose flour, cake flour, and enriched baking flour are all types of white flour.
Whole-grain flour	A grain that is not refined; whole grains are milled in their complete form, with only the husk removed.
Whole-wheat flour	An unrefined, whole-grain flour made from whole wheat kernels.

dehydration. Since fiber binds many vitamins and minerals, a high-fiber diet can reduce our absorption of important nutrients such as iron, zinc, and calcium. In children, some elderly, the chronically ill, and other at-risk populations, extreme fiber intake can even lead to malnutrition—they feel full before they have eaten enough to provide adequate energy and nutrients. So while some societies are accustomed to a very high fiber diet, most people in the United States find it difficult to tolerate more than 50 grams of fiber per day and may end up consuming too little.

Hannah   *Nutri-Case*

"Last night, my mom made angel hair pasta. That's my favorite, and I ate a big bowl with lots of butter and cheese but no sauce. I don't like sauce! My mom said I did such a good job on my supper that I could have a popsicle for dessert. But today in school my science teacher said we shouldn't eat a lot of pasta, because that's kind of the same thing as eating a bunch of sugar. I don't get it. I mean, angel hair doesn't taste anything like sugar!"

   Was the advice that Hannah's science teacher gave her sound? How would you explain to Hannah, in ways that she could understand, what happens to the foods she eats, and why some foods that seem very different really aren't? Suppose you learned that Hannah drank a glass of apple juice with her dinner and had no vegetables. What might you propose to her mother about her food choices?

Shopper's Guide: Hunting for Complex Carbohydrates

Table 4.5 compares the food and fiber content of two diets, one rich in complex carbohydrates and the other high in simple carbohydrates. Here are some hints for selecting healthful carbohydrate sources:

Table 4.4   Fiber Content of Common Foods

Food	Fiber Content (grams)
Breads/Cereals:	
Bagel, 1 each plain, 3 ½-inch diameter	2
French bread, 1 each slice (4″ × 2½″ × 1¾″)	2
White bread, 1 slice	1
Pumpernickel bread, 1 each slice (5 × 4 × ⅜ inches)	2
Whole-wheat bread, 1 slice	2
Oatmeal, quick, 1 cup	4
Cheerios, 1 cup	1
Corn flakes, 1 ¼ cup	1
Lucky Charms, 1 cup	1
Fruits and Juices:	
Apple, 1 each (2¾-inch diameter with peel)	3
Apple juice, 1 cup	<1
Blackberries, 1 cup	6
Banana, 1 each (medium)	2
Orange, 1 each (2⅞-inch diameter, peeled)	3
Orange juice, 1 cup, from concentrate	<1
Pear, 1 each (medium with skin)	5
Strawberries, fresh, whole, 1 cup	2
Vegetables:	
Asparagus, cooked, 6 spears	2
Broccoli, raw, chopped, 1 cup	3
Broccoli, cooked, chopped, 1 cup	5
Cabbage, raw, chopped, 1 cup	1
Collard greens, cooked, ½ cup	2
Corn, canned, whole kernel, ½ cup	6
Kale, cooked, ½ cup	1
Lettuce, iceberg, shredded, 1 cup	1
Legumes:	
Black beans, cooked, ½ cup	7
Lima beans, cooked, ½ cup	7
Navy beans, cooked, ½ cup	8
Kidney beans, cooked, ½ cup	8
Lentils, cooked, ½ cup	5

Note: The Adequate Intake for fiber is 25 grams per day for women and 38 grams per day for men.

Source: U.S. Department of Agriculture, Agricultural Research Service. 2004. USDA National Nutrient Database for Standard Reference, Release 16. Nutrient Data Laboratory Home Page, http://www.nal.usda.gov/fnic/foodcomp. Values obtained from the USDA Nutrient Database for Standard Reference, Release 16.

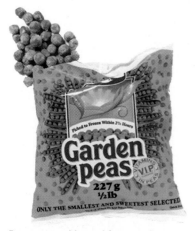

Frozen vegetables and fruits can be a healthful alternative when fresh produce is not available.

- Select breads and cereals that are made with whole grains such as wheat, oats, barley, and rye (make sure the label says "whole" before the word *grain*). Choose foods that have at least 2 or 3 grams of fiber per serving.

- Buy fresh fruits and vegetables whenever possible. When appropriate, eat foods such as potatoes, apples, and pears with the skin left on.

- Frozen vegetables and fruits can be a healthful alternative when fresh produce is not available. Check frozen selections to make sure there is no extra sugar or salt added.

- Be careful when buying canned fruits and vegetables, as many are high in sodium and added sugar. Foods that are packed in their own juice are more healthful than those packed in syrup.

- Eat legumes frequently, every day if possible. Canned or fresh beans, peas, and lentils are excellent sources of complex carbohydrates, fiber, vitamins and minerals. Add them to soups, casseroles, and other recipes—it is an easy way to eat more of them. If you are trying to consume less sodium, rinse canned beans to remove extra salt or choose low-sodium alternatives.

Table 4.5   Comparison of Two High-Carbohydrate Diets

High Complex Carbohydrate Diet	High Simple Carbohydrate Diet
Nutrient Analysis: 2150 kcal 60% of energy from carbohydrates 22% of energy from fat 18% of energy from protein 38 grams of dietary fiber	*Nutrient Analysis:* 4012 kcal 60% of energy from carbohydrates 25% of energy from fat 15% of energy from protein 18.5 grams of dietary fiber
Breakfast: 1 ½ cups Cheerios 1 cup skim milk 2 slices whole-wheat toast with 1 tbsp. light margarine 1 medium banana 8 fl. oz. fresh orange juice	*Breakfast:* 1 ½ cups Froot Loops cereal 1 cup skim milk 2 slices white bread, toasted with 1 tbsp. light margarine 8 fl. oz. fresh orange juice
Lunch: 8 fl. oz. low-fat blueberry yogurt Tuna sandwich (2 slices whole-wheat bread; ¼ cup tuna packed in water, drained; 1 tsp. Dijon mustard; 2 tsp. low-calorie mayonnaise) 2 carrots, raw, with peel 1 cup raw cauliflower 1 tbsp. peppercorn ranch salad dressing (for dipping vegetables)	*Lunch:* McDonald's Quarter Pounder—1 sandwich 1 large order French fries 16 fl. oz. cola beverage 30 jelly beans
(No Snack)	*Snack:* 1 cinnamon raisin bagel (3 ½-inch diameter) 2 tbsp. cream cheese 8 fl. oz. low-fat strawberry yogurt
Dinner: ½ chicken breast, roasted 1 cup brown rice, cooked 1 cup cooked broccoli Spinach salad (1 cup chopped spinach, 1 whole egg white, 2 slices turkey bacon, 3 cherry tomatoes, and 2 tbsp. creamy bacon salad dressing) 2 baked apples (no added sugar)	*Dinner:* 1 whole chicken breast, roasted 2 cups mixed green salad 2 tbsp. ranch salad dressing 1 serving macaroni and cheese 12 fl. oz. cola beverage Cheesecake (⅑ of cake)
(No snack)	*Late Night Snack:* 2 cups gelatin dessert (cherry flavored) 3 raspberry oatmeal no-fat cookies

Note: Diets were analyzed using Food Processor Version 7.21 (ESHA Research, Salem, OR).

Try the Nutrition Label Activity (page 140) to learn how to recognize various carbohydrates on food labels. Armed with this knowledge, you are now ready to make more healthful food choices.

Recap: The Adequate Intake for fiber is 25 grams per day for women and 38 grams per day for men. Most Americans only eat half of the fiber they need each day. Foods high in fiber and complex carbohydrates include whole grains and cereals, fruits, and vegetables. The more processed the food, the fewer complex carbohydrates it contains.

Recognizing Carbohydrates on the Label

Figure 4.13 shows labels for two breakfast cereals. The cereal on the left (a) is processed and sweetened, while the one on the right (b) is a whole-grain product with no added sugar.

- Check the center of each label to locate the amount of total carbohydrate. For the sweetened cereal, the total carbohydrate is 26 grams. For the whole-grain cereal, the total carbohydrate is almost the same, 27 grams for a smaller serving size.

- Look at the information listed as subgroups under Total Carbohydrate. The label for the sweetened cereal lists all types of carbohydrates in the cereal—dietary fiber, sugars, and other carbohydrate (which refers to starches). Notice that this cereal contains 13 grams of sugar—half of its total carbohydrates—but only 1 gram of dietary fiber.

- The label for the whole-grain cereal lists dietary fiber. In contrast to the sweetened cereal, this product contains 4 grams of fiber and only 1 gram of sugar! Notice that on this label there is no amount listed for starches (or other carbohydrates). In this case, the amount of starch is the difference between the total carbohydrate and the sum of dietary fiber and sugars, or 27 grams − 5 grams = 22 grams of starch.

- Now look at the percent values listed to the right of the Total Carbohydrate section. For both cereals (without milk), their percent contribution to daily carbohydrate is 9%. This does not mean that 9% of the calories in these cereals come from carbohydrates. Instead, this percentage refers to the Daily Values listed at the bottom of each label. For a person who eats 2,000 calories, the recommended amount of carbohydrate each day is 300 grams. One serving of each cereal contains 26–27 grams, which is about 9% of 300 grams.

- To calculate the percent of calories that comes from carbohydrate, do the following:

  a. Calculate the *calories* in the cereal that come from carbohydrate. Multiply the total grams of carbohydrate per serving by the energy value of carbohydrate:

  $$26 \text{ grams of carbohydrate} \times 4 \text{ kcal/gram} = 104 \text{ kcal from carbohydrate}$$

  b. Calculate the *percent of calories* in the cereal that come from carbohydrate. Divide the kcal from carbohydrate by the total calories for each serving:

  $$104 \text{ kcal} \div 120 \text{ kcal} = 87\% \text{ calories from carbohydrate}$$

Which cereal should you choose? Check the ingredients for the sweetened cereal. Remember that the ingredients are listed in the order from highest to lowest amount. The second and third ingredients listed are sugar and brown sugar, and the corn and oat flours are not whole-grain flours. Now look at the ingredients for the other cereal—it contains whole-grain oats. Although the sweetened product is enriched with more B vitamins, iron, and zinc, the whole grain cereal packs 4 grams of fiber per serving and contains no added sugars. Overall, it is a more healthful choice. ●

What's the Story on Alternative Sweeteners?

Most of us love sweets but want to avoid the extra calories and tooth decay that go along with eating simple sugars. Remember that all carbohydrates, including simple and complex, contain 4 kcal of energy per gram. Because sweeteners such as sucrose, fructose, honey, and brown sugar contribute calories (or energy), they are called **nutritive sweeteners.**

Other nutritive sweeteners include the *sugar alcohols* such as mannitol, sorbitol, isomalt, and xylitol. Popular in sugar-free gums and mints, sugar alcohols are less sweet than sucrose (Figure 4.14). One major advantage is that they do not promote dental problems because they do not support the bacteria that cause tooth decay. However, eating large amounts of sugar alcohols can cause diarrhea, and, because they provide 2 to 4 kcal of energy per gram, they are not calorie-free.

nutritive sweeteners Sweeteners such as sucrose, fructose, honey, and brown sugar that contribute calories (or energy).

Nutrition Facts

Serving Size: 3/4 cup (30g)
Servings Per Package: About 14

Amount Per Serving	Cereal	Cereal With 1/2 Cup Skim Milk
Calories	120	160
Calories from Fat	15	15
	% Daily Value**	
Total Fat 1.5g*	2%	2%
Saturated Fat 0g	0%	0%
Polyunsaturated Fat 0g		
Monounsaturated Fat 0.5g		
Cholesterol 0mg	0%	1%
Sodium 220mg	9%	12%
Potassium 40mg	1%	7%
Total Carbohydrate 26g	9%	11%
Dietary Fiber 1g	3%	3%
Sugars 13g		
Other Carbohydrate 12g		
Protein 1g		
Vitamin A	0%	4%
Vitamin C	0%	2%
Calcium	0%	15%
Iron	25%	25%
Thiamin	25%	25%
Riboflavin	25%	35%
Niacin	25%	25%
Vitamin B6	25%	25%
Folate	25%	25%
Zinc	25%	25%

* Amount in cereal. One-half cup skim milk contributes an additional 65mg sodium, 6g total carbohydrate (6g sugars), and 4g protein.

** Percent Daily Values are based on a 2,000 calorie diet. Your daily values may be higher or lower depending on your calorie needs:

	Calories	2,000	2,500
Total Fat	Less than	65g	80g
Sat. Fat	Less than	20g	25g
Cholesterol	Less than	300mg	300mg
Sodium	Less than	2,400mg	2,400mg
Potassium		3,500mg	3,500mg
Total Carbohydrate		300g	375g
Dietary fiber		25g	30g

Calories per gram:
Fat 9   •   Carbohydrate 4   •   Protein 4

INGREDIENTS: Corn Flour, Sugar, Brown Sugar, Partially Hydrogenated Vegetable Oil (Soybean and Cottonseed), Oat Flour, Salt, Sodium Citrate (a flavoring agent), Flavor added [Natural & Artificial Flavor, Strawberry Juice Concentrate, Malic Acid (a flavoring agent)], Niacinamide (Niacin), Zinc Oxide, Reduced Iron, Red 40, Yellow 5, Red 3, Yellow 6, Pyridoxine Hydrochloride (Vitamin B6), Riboflavin (Vitamin B2), Thiamin Mononitrate (Vitamin B1), Folic Acid (Folate) and Blue 1.

(a)

Nutrition Facts

Serving Size: 1/2 cup dry (40g)
Servings Per Container: 13

Amount Per Serving	
Calories	150
Calories from Fat	25
	% Daily Value*
Total Fat 3g	5%
Saturated Fat 0.5g	2%
Polyunsaturated Fat 1g	
Monounsaturated Fat 1g	
Cholesterol 0mg	0%
Sodium 0mg	0%
Total Carbohydrate 27g	9%
Dietary Fiber 4g	15%
Soluble Fiber 2g	
Insoluble Fiber 2g	
Sugars 1g	
Protein 5g	
Vitamin A	0%
Vitamin C	0%
Calcium	0%
Iron	10%

* Percent Daily Values are based on a 2,000 calorie diet. Your daily values may be higher or lower depending on your calorie needs:

	Calories	2,000	2,500
Total Fat	Less than	65g	80g
Sat. Fat	Less than	20g	25g
Cholesterol	Less than	300mg	300mg
Sodium	Less than	2,400mg	2,400mg
Total Carbohydrate		300g	375g
Dietary fiber		25g	30g

INGREDIENTS: 100% Natural Whole Grain Rolled Oats

(b)

Figure 4.13   Labels for two breakfast cereals. **(a)** Sweetened cereal. **(b)** Whole-grain cereal.

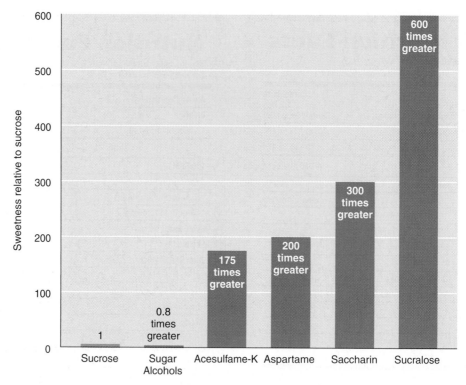

Figure 4.14 Relative sweetness of alternative sweeteners as compared to sucrose. (Values derived from International Food Information Council. Food safety and nutrition information. Sugars & low-calorie sweeteners. http://ific.org/food/sweeteners/ Accessed July 2003).

Alternative Sweeteners Are Non-Nutritive

A number of other products have been developed to sweeten foods without promoting tooth decay and weight gain. As these products provide little or no energy, they are called **non-nutritive**, or *alternative*, **sweeteners.**

non-nutritive sweeteners Also called *alternative sweeteners;* manufactured sweeteners that provide little or no energy.

Limited Use of Alternative Sweeteners Is Not Harmful

Contrary to popular belief, alternative sweeteners have been determined as safe for adults, children, and individuals with diabetes. Women who are pregnant should discuss the use of alternative sweeteners with their healthcare provider. In general, it appears safe for pregnant women to consume alternative sweeteners in amounts within the Food and Drug Administration (FDA) guidelines (Duffy and Anderson 1998). The **acceptable daily intake** (ADI) is an estimate made by the FDA of the amount of a sweetener that someone can consume each day over a lifetime without adverse effects. The estimates are based on studies conducted on laboratory animals, and they include a 100-fold safety factor. Table 4.6 lists the ADI of alternative sweeteners as set by the FDA. It is important to emphasize that actual intake by humans is typically well below the ADI.

acceptable daily intake (ADI) An estimate made by the Food and Drug Administration of the amount of a non-nutritive sweetener that someone can consume each day over a lifetime without adverse effects.

The major alternative sweeteners available on the market today are saccharin, acesulfame-K, aspartame, and sucralose.

Saccharin

Discovered in the late 1800s, *saccharin* is about 300 times sweeter than sucrose (see Figure 4.14). Evidence to suggest that saccharin may cause bladder tumors in rats surfaced in the 1970s. While subsequent research with humans did not support this

Table 4.6   Acceptable Daily Intake (ADI) Levels of Alternative Sweeteners as Set By the Food and Drug Administration (FDA)

Sweetener	ADI (mg per kg body weight per day)
Saccharin	None*
Acesulfame-K	15
Aspartame	50
Sucralose	5

*No ADI for saccharin has been set; the FDA suggests that adults not exceed a total daily saccharin intake of 1,000 mg, and that children not exceed 500 mg.

finding, the FDA felt it was prudent to ban the sweetener. The saccharin ban met with tremendous pressure from consumers and the food industry, so the U.S. government placed a moratorium on the ban. This moratorium has kept saccharin available for public consumption. More than 20 years of scientific research has shown that saccharin is not related to bladder cancer in humans. Based on this evidence, in May of 2000 the National Toxicology Program of the U.S. government removed saccharin from its list of products that may cause cancer. Saccharin is used in foods and beverages and sold as a tabletop sweetener. Saccharin is sold as Sweet n' Low in the U.S.

Acesulfame-K

Acesulfame-K (or acesulfame potassium) is marketed under the names Sunette and Sweet One. It is a calorie-free sweetener that is 175 times sweeter than sugar. It is used to sweeten gums, candies, beverages, instant tea, coffee, gelatins, and puddings. The taste of acesulfame-K does not change when it is heated, so it can be used in cooking. The body does not metabolize acesulfame-K, so it is excreted unchanged by the kidneys.

Aspartame

Aspartame, also called Equal and NutraSweet, is one of the most popular alternative sweeteners currently found in foods and beverages. Aspartame is comprised of two amino acids, phenylalanine and aspartic acid. When these amino acids are separate, one is bitter and the other has no flavor—but joined together, they make a substance that is 200 times sweeter than sucrose. Although aspartame contains 4 kcal of energy per gram, it is so sweet that only small amounts are necessary, thus it ends up contributing little or no energy. Because aspartame is made from amino acids, its taste is destroyed with heat (see Chapter 6); thus, it cannot be used in cooking.

A significant amount of research has been done to test the safety of aspartame. While a number of false claims have been published, especially on the Internet, there is no scientific evidence to support the claim that aspartame causes brain tumors, Alzheimer's disease, or nerve disorders.

Table 4.7 shows how many servings of aspartame-sweetened foods have to be consumed to exceed the ADI. Although eating less than the ADI is considered safe, note that children who consume many powdered drinks, diet sodas, and other aspartame-flavored products could potentially exceed this amount. Drinks sweetened with aspartame are extremely popular among children and teenagers, but they are very low in nutritional value and should not replace healthier beverages such as milk, water, and fruit juice.

There are some people who should not consume aspartame at all: those with the disease *phenylketonuria (PKU)*. This is a genetic disorder that prevents the breakdown of the amino acid phenylalanine. Because the person with PKU cannot metabolize

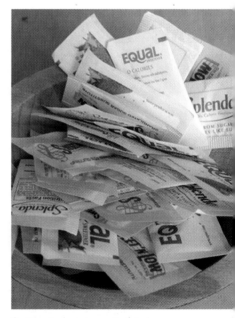

Contrary to recent reports claiming severe health consequences related to consumption of alternative sweeteners, major health agencies have determined that these products are safe for us to consume.

Table 4.7   The Amount of Food that a 50-Pound Child and a 150-Pound Adult Would Have to Consume Each Day to Exceed the ADI For Aspartame

Food	50-pound Child	150-pound Adult
12 fl. oz. carbonated soft drink	7	20
8 fl. oz. powdered soft drink	11	34
4 fl. oz. gelatin dessert	14	42
Packets of tabletop sweetener	32	97

Adapted from International Food Information Council. *Food Safety and Nutrition Information. Sweeteners. Everything you need to know about aspartame.* 2001. http://ificinfo.health.org/brochure/aspartam.htm.

phenylalanine, it builds up in the tissues of the body and causes irreversible brain damage. In the United States, all newborn babies are tested for PKU; those who have it are placed on a phenylalanine-limited diet. Some foods that are important sources of protein and other nutrients for growing children, such as meats and milk, contain phenylalanine. Thus, it is critical that children with PKU not waste what little phenylalanine they can consume on nutrient-poor products sweetened with aspartame.

Sucralose

The FDA has recently approved the use of *sucralose* as an alternative sweetener. It is marketed under the brand name Splenda. It is made from sucrose, but chlorine atoms are substituted for the hydrogen and oxygen normally found in sucrose, and it passes through the digestive tract unchanged, without contributing any energy. It is 600 times sweeter than sucrose and is stable when heated, so it can be used in cooking. It has been approved for use in many foods, including chewing gum, salad dressings, beverages, gelatin and pudding products, canned fruits, frozen dairy desserts, and baked goods. Safety studies have not shown sucralose to cause cancer or to have other adverse health effects.

Other Alternative Sweeteners

Two additional alternative sweeteners that are awaiting FDA approval in the United States are *alitame* and *D-tagatose*. Alitame is comprised of two amino acids, but unlike aspartame it remains stable when heated. D-tagatose is made from lactose. Its sweetness is equal to that of sucrose, but it contributes only half the energy.

Recap: Alternative sweeteners can be used in place of sugar to sweeten foods. Most of these products do not promote tooth decay and contribute little or no energy. The alternative sweeteners approved for use in the United States are considered safe when eaten in amounts less than the acceptable daily intake.

Nadia   *Nutri-Case*

"I used to depend on diet soda to keep my weight down. Especially at work, whenever my energy lagged and I got that urge to snack, I'd head off to the soda machine for my calorie-free 'fix.' Since I learned I was pregnant, I've been buying a carton of milk or a yogurt instead, but I keep wondering: could my diet-soda habit have harmed my baby in those first few weeks before I knew I was pregnant?"

Check out a can of calorie-free soda. Which of the sweeteners just discussed does it contain—and how much? If Nadia had been drinking three cans of your favorite soda each day during her early pregnancy, do you think she should be concerned about the possibility of harm to her fetus? Why or why not?

What Disorders Are Related to Carbohydrate Metabolism?

Health conditions that affect the body's ability to absorb and/or use carbohydrates include diabetes, hypoglycemia, and lactose intolerance.

Diabetes: Impaired Regulation of Glucose

Diabetes is a chronic disease in which the body can no longer regulate glucose within normal limits, and blood glucose levels become dangerously high or fall dangerously low. It is imperative to detect and treat the disease as soon as possible because excessive fluctuations in glucose injures tissues throughout the body. If not controlled, diabetes can lead to blindness, seizures, kidney failure, nerve disease, amputations, stroke, and heart disease. In severe cases, it is fatal.

Approximately sixteen million people in the United States—6% of the total population—are diagnosed with diabetes. It is speculated that another five million people have diabetes but do not know it. Figure 4.15 shows the percentage of adults with diabetes from various ethnic groups in the United States (National Diabetes Information Clearinghouse, 2003). As you can see, diabetes is more common in older people, African Americans, Mexican Americans, and American Indians and Alaska Natives.

There are two main forms of diabetes, type 1 and type 2. Some women develop a third form, *gestational diabetes*, during pregnancy; we will discuss this in more detail in Chapter 15.

diabetes A chronic disease in which the body can no longer regulate glucose.

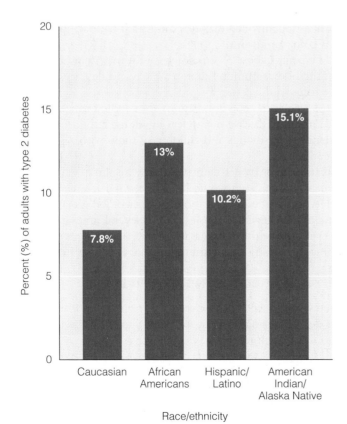

Figure 4.15   The percent of adults from various ethnic and racial groups with type 2 diabetes. (Values derived from the National Diabetes Information Clearinghouse (NDIC). National Diabetes Statistics. National Institutes of Helath (NIH) Publication No. 03-3892. May 2003. http://diabetes.niddk.nih.gov/dm/pubs/statistics/index.htm. Accessed July 2003.)

Table 4.8   Symptoms of Type 1 and Type 2 Diabetes

Type 1 Diabetes	Type 2 Diabetes*
Frequent urination	Any of the type 1 symptoms
Unusual thirst	Frequent infections
Extreme hunger	Blurred vision
Unusual weight loss	Cuts/bruises that are slow to heal
Extreme fatigue	Tingling/numbness in the hands or feet
Irritability	Recurring skin, gum, or bladder infections

*Some people with type 2 diabetes experience no symptoms.
Source: Adapted from the American Diabetes Association, Diabetes Symptoms.
www.diabetes.org. Accessed December 2003.

In Type 1 Diabetes, the Body Does Not Produce Enough Insulin

type 1 diabetes Disorder in which the body cannot produce enough insulin.

Approximately 10% of people with diabetes have **type 1 diabetes,** in which the body cannot produce enough insulin. Type 1 diabetes was once commonly referred to as juvenile-onset diabetes. When they eat a meal and their blood glucose rises, the pancreas is unable to secrete insulin in response. Glucose levels soar, and the body tries to expel the excess glucose by excreting it in the urine. In fact, the medical term for the disease is *diabetes mellitus* (from the Greek *diabainein,* "to pass through," and Latin *mellitus,* "sweetened with honey"), and frequent urination is one of its warning signs (see Table 4.8 for other symptoms). If blood glucose levels are not controlled, a person with type 1 diabetes will become confused and lethargic and have trouble breathing. This is because their brains are not getting enough glucose to properly function. As discussed earlier, uncontrolled diabetes can lead to ketoacidosis; left untreated, the ultimate result is coma and death.

The cause of type 1 diabetes is unknown, but it may be an *autoimmune disease.* This means that the body's immune system attacks and destroys its own tissues, in this case the beta cells of the pancreas.

Most cases of type 1 diabetes are diagnosed in adolescents around ten to fourteen years of age, although the disease can appear in younger children and adults. It occurs more often in families, so siblings and children of those with type 1 diabetes are at greater risk.

The only treatment for type 1 diabetes is daily insulin injections. Insulin is a hormone comprised of protein, so it would be digested in the intestine if taken as a pill. Individuals with type 1 diabetes must monitor their blood glucose levels closely, using a *glucometer,* and administer injections of insulin several times a day to maintain their blood glucose levels in a healthful range (Figure 4.16). The accompanying Highlight box describes how one young man with type 1 diabetes stays healthy.

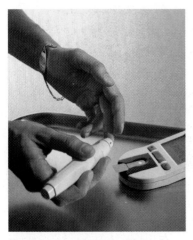

Figure 4.16   Monitoring blood glucose requires pricking the fingers each day and measuring the blood using a glucometer.

In Type 2 Diabetes, Cells Become Less Responsive to Insulin

type 2 diabetes Progressive disorder in which body cells become less responsive to insulin.

In **type 2 diabetes,** body cells become resistant, or less responsive to insulin. This type of diabetes develops progressively, meaning that the biological changes resulting in the disease occur over a long period of time.

In most cases, obesity is the trigger for a cascade of changes that eventually result in the disorder. Specifically, the cells of many obese people are less responsive to insulin, exhibiting a condition called *insulin insensitivity* (or insulin resistance). The pancreas attempts to compensate for this insensitivity by secreting more insulin. Over time, a person who is insulin insensitive will have to circulate very high levels of insulin to utilize glucose for energy. Eventually the pancreas becomes incapable of secreting these excessive amounts, and the beta cells stop producing the hormone altogether. Thus, blood glucose levels may be elevated in a person with type 2 diabetes either 1) because of insulin insensitivity, 2) because the pancreas can no

Living with Diabetes

Nadia's youngest brother, Vincent, was diagnosed with type 1 diabetes when he was ten years old. At first, Vincent and his family were frightened by the disease and found it difficult to adapt their lifestyles to provide a safe and health-promoting environment for Vincent. For example, Vincent's mother felt frustrated because her son could no longer eat the cakes, pies, and other sweets she had always enjoyed baking for her family, and Nadia found herself watching over her brother's meals and snacks, running to her parents whenever she feared that he was about to eat something that would harm him. Within a few months, though, Vincent's mother learned to adapt her recipes and cooking techniques to produce a variety of foods that Vincent could enjoy, and Nadia learned to allow Vincent the responsibility for his food choices and his health.

Vincent is now a college sophomore and has been living with diabetes for nine years, but what he still hates most about the disease is that food is always a major issue. Vincent is smart and a good student, but if his blood glucose declines, he has trouble concentrating. He has to eat three nutritious meals a day on a regular schedule, and he can't snack unless his blood sugar is low. When his friends eat candy, chips, or other snacks, he can't join them. In general he knows these dietary changes are very healthy, but sometimes he wishes he could eat like all of his friends. On the other hand, he cannot skip a meal, even if he isn't hungry. It is also important for Vincent to stay on a regular schedule for exercise and sleep.

Vincent must test his blood sugar many times each day. He has to prick his fingers to do this, and they get tender and develop calluses. During his first few years with diabetes, he had to give himself two to four shots of insulin each day. He learned to measure the insulin into a syringe, and he had to monitor where the shots were injected because each insulin shot should be given in a different place on his body to avoid damaging the skin and underlying tissue. Technological advances now offer easier alternatives than a needle and syringe. Vincent uses an insulin infusion pump, which looks like a small pager and delivers insulin into the body through a long, thin tube in very small amounts throughout the day. One of Vincent's friends also has diabetes but can't use a pump; instead, he uses an insulin pen, which includes a needle and a cartridge of insulin. Now that Vincent uses the insulin pump, he can choose to eat more of the foods he loves and deliver his insulin accordingly.

Although diabetes is challenging, it does not prevent Vincent from playing soccer and basketball almost every day. In fact, he knows that people with diabetes should be active. As long as he takes his insulin regularly, keeps an eye on his blood sugar, drinks plenty of water, and eats when he should, he knows that he can play sports and do most of the things he wants to do. There are numerous professional and Olympic athletes and other famous people who have diabetes, showing that this disease should not prevent Vincent from leading a healthful life and realizing his dreams.

Presently there is no cure for type 1 diabetes. However, there are many new treatments and potential cures being researched. The FDA has approved several devices that measure blood glucose without pricking the finger. Some of them can read glucose levels through the skin, and others insert a small needle into the body to monitor glucose continually. Tests are also being conducted on insulin nasal sprays and inhalers. Advances in genetic engineering may soon make it possible to transplant healthy beta cells into the pancreas of virtually anyone with type 1 diabetes, so that the normal cells will secrete insulin. Vincent looks forward to seeing major changes in the treatment of diabetes in the next few years. ●

longer secrete enough insulin, or 3) because the pancreas has entirely stopped insulin production.

Many factors can cause type 2 diabetes. Genetics plays a role, so relatives of people with type 2 diabetes are at increased risk (see the Highlight: Risk Factors for Type 2 Diabetes box). Obesity and physical inactivity also increase the risk. Indeed, diabetes is thought to have become an epidemic in the United States because of a combination of our poor eating habits, sedentary lifestyles, increased obesity, and an aging population. Most cases of type 2 diabetes develop after age 45, and almost 20% of Americans sixty-five years and older have diabetes. Once commonly known as *adult-onset diabetes*, type 2 diabetes in children was virtually unheard of until recently. Unfortunately, the disease

Risk Factors for Type 2 Diabetes

Age older than 45 years

Family history of diabetes

Overweight or obesity

Physically inactive lifestyle

Low HDL cholesterol (the "good" cholesterol) or high triglycerides (fat in the blood)

Certain racial and ethnic groups (e.g., African Americans, Latinos, Asian and Pacific Islanders, American Indians and Alaska Natives)

Women who had gestational diabetes or who have had a baby weighing 9 pounds or more at birth

Adapted from the American Diabetes Association, Diabetes Risk Test www.diabetes.org Accessed December 2003. ●

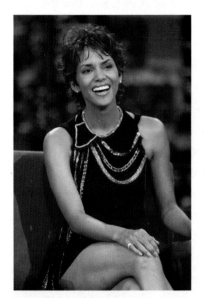

Actress Halle Berry has type 2 diabetes.

is increasing dramatically among children and adolescents (Rosenbloom, House, and Winter 1998), posing serious health consequences for them and their future children.

Type 2 diabetes can be treated in a variety of ways. Weight loss, healthful eating patterns, and regular exercise can control symptoms in some people. More severe cases may require oral medications. These drugs work in either of two ways: They improve body cells' sensitivity to insulin or reduce the amount of glucose the liver produces. If a person with type 2 diabetes can no longer secrete enough insulin, the patient must take daily injections of insulin just like a person with type 1 diabetes.

Recap: Diabetes is a disease that results in dangerously high levels of blood glucose. Type 1 diabetes typically appears at a young age; the pancreas cannot secrete sufficient insulin so insulin injections are required. Type 2 diabetes develops over time and may be triggered by obesity: body cells are no longer sensitive to the effects of insulin or the pancreas no longer secretes sufficient insulin for bodily needs. Supplemental insulin may or may not be needed to treat type 2 diabetes. Diabetes increases the risk of dangerous complications such as heart disease, blindness, kidney disease, and amputations.

Lifestyle Choices Can Help Control or Prevent Diabetes

In general, people with diabetes should follow many of the same healthy food guidelines recommended for those without diabetes. One difference is that people with diabetes may need to eat less carbohydrate and slightly more fat or protein to help regulate their blood glucose levels. Carbohydrates are still an important part of the diet, but nutritional recommendations must be developed separately based on individual responses to foods. In addition, people with diabetes should avoid alcoholic beverages, which can cause hypoglycemia (page 149). The symptoms of alcohol intoxication and hypoglycemia are very similar. The person with diabetes and his or her companions may confuse these conditions; this can result in a potentially life-threatening situation.

While there is no cure for type 2 diabetes, many cases could be prevented or onset delayed. We cannot control our family history, but we can eat a balanced diet, exercise regularly, and maintain an appropriate body weight. Studies show that losing only 10 to 30 pounds can reduce or eliminate the symptoms of type 2 diabetes (ACSM 2000). In addition, moderate daily exercise may prevent the onset of type 2 diabetes more effectively than dietary changes alone (Pan et al. 1997). By selecting plenty of whole grains, fruits, legumes and vegetables, and by staying active and maintaining a healthy body weight, our risk for diabetes should remain low.

Recap: Lifestyle plays an important role in controlling diabetes. Many cases of type 2 diabetes could be prevented or delayed with a balanced diet, regular exercise, and achieving and/or maintaining a healthful body weight.

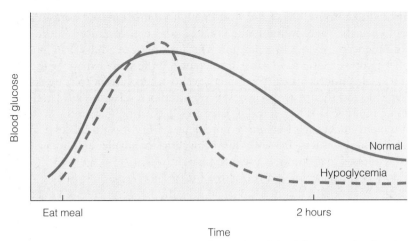

Figure 4.17 Changes in blood glucose after a meal for people with hypoglycemia and without hypoglycemia (normal).

Hypoglycemia: Low Blood Glucose

In **hypoglycemia,** blood sugar falls to lower-than-normal levels (Figure 4.17). One cause of hypoglycemia is excessive production of insulin, which lowers blood glucose too far. People with diabetes can develop hypoglycemia if they inject too much insulin or when they exercise and fail to eat enough carbohydrates. Two types of hypoglycemia can develop in people who do not have diabetes: reactive and fasting.

Reactive hypoglycemia occurs when the pancreas secretes too much insulin after a high-carbohydrate meal. The symptoms of reactive hypoglycemia usually appear about one to three hours after the meal and include nervousness, shakiness, anxiety, sweating, irritability, headache, weakness, and rapid or irregular heartbeat. Although many people believe they experience these symptoms, true hypoglycemia is rare. A person diagnosed with reactive hypoglycemia must eat smaller meals more frequently to level out blood insulin and glucose levels.

Fasting hypoglycemia occurs when the body continues to produce too much insulin, even when someone has not eaten. This condition is usually caused by another medical condition such as cancer, liver infection, alcohol-induced liver disease, or a tumor in the pancreas.

> **Recap:** Hypoglycemia refers to lower-than-normal blood glucose levels. Reactive hypoglycemia occurs when the pancreas secretes too much insulin after a high carbohydrate meal. Fasting hypoglycemia occurs when the body continues to produce too much insulin even when someone has not eaten.

Lactose Intolerance: Inability to Digest Lactose

Sometimes our bodies do not produce enough of the enzymes necessary to break down carbohydrates before they reach the colon. A common example is **lactose intolerance,** in which the body does not produce sufficient amounts of the enzyme lactase in the small intestine and therefore cannot digest foods containing lactose. Lactose intolerance should not be confused with a milk allergy. People who are allergic to milk experience an immune reaction to the proteins found in cow's milk. Symptoms of milk allergy include skin reactions such as hives and rashes; intestinal distress such as nausea, vomiting, cramping, and diarrhea; and respiratory symptoms such as wheezing, runny nose, and itchy and watery eyes. In severe cases, anaphylactic shock can occur.

Symptoms of lactose intolerance include intestinal gas, bloating, cramping, nausea, diarrhea, and discomfort. While some infants are born with lactose intolerance, it is more common to see lactase enzyme activity decrease after two years of age. In fact,

hypoglycemia A condition marked by blood glucose levels that are below normal fasting levels.

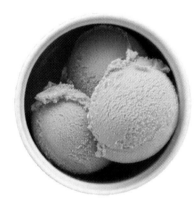

Milk products, such as ice cream, are hard to digest for people who are lactose intolerant.

lactose intolerance A disorder in which the body does not produce sufficient lactase enzyme and therefore cannot digest foods that contain lactose, such as cow's milk.

it is estimated that up to 70% of the world's adult population lose some ability to digest lactose as they age. In the United States, lactose intolerance is more common in Native American, Asian, Hispanic, and African-American adults than in Caucasians.

Not everyone experiences lactose intolerance to the same extent. Some people can digest small amounts of dairy products, while others cannot tolerate any. Suarez et al. (1998) found that many people who reported being lactose intolerant were able to consume multiple small servings of dairy products without symptoms, which enabled them to meet their calcium requirements. Thus, it is not necessary for them to avoid all dairy products; they may simply need to eat smaller amounts and experiment to find foods that do not cause intestinal distress.

It is important that people with lactose intolerance, regardless of age, find foods that can supply enough calcium for normal growth, development, and maintenance of bones. Many can tolerate specially formulated milk products that are low in lactose, while others take pills or use drops that contain the lactase enzyme when they eat dairy products (Figure 4.18). Calcium-fortified soy milk and orange juice are excellent substitutes for cow's milk. Some lactose-intolerant people can also digest yogurt and aged cheese, as the bacteria or molds used to ferment these products break down the lactose during processing.

How can you tell if you are lactose intolerant? Many people discover that they have problems digesting dairy products by trial and error. Because intestinal gas, bloating, and diarrhea may indicate other health problems too, you should consult a physician to determine the cause.

Tests for lactose intolerance include drinking a lactose-rich liquid and testing blood glucose levels over a 2-hour period. If you do not produce the normal amount of glucose, you are unable to digest the lactose present. Another test involves measuring hydrogen levels in the breath, as lactose-intolerant people breathe out more hydrogen when they drink a beverage that contains lactose.

Recap: Lactose intolerance results from the inability to digest lactose due to insufficient amounts of lactase. Symptoms include intestinal gas, bloating, cramping, diarrhea, and nausea. Lactose intolerance commonly occurs in non-Caucausian populations. The extent of lactose intolerance varies from mild to severe.

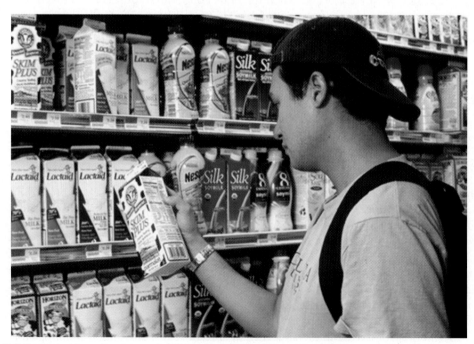

Figure 4.18 There are many products available on the market today that contain the lactase enzyme or are low in lactose. These products are developed for people with lactose intolerance.

Chapter Summary

- Carbohydrates contain carbon, hydrogen, and oxygen. Plants make the carbohydrate glucose during photosynthesis.

- Simple sugars include mono- and disaccharides. The three primary monosaccharides are glucose, fructose, and galactose.

- Two monosaccharides joined together are called disaccharides. Glucose and fructose join to make sucrose, glucose and glucose join to make maltose, and glucose and galactose join to make lactose.

- Starches are polysaccharides, and they are the storage form of glucose in plants.

- Glycogen is the storage form of glucose in humans. Glycogen is stored in the liver and in muscles. Liver glycogen provides glucose to help us maintain blood sugar levels, while muscle glycogen is used for energy during exercise.

- Dietary fiber is the nondigestible parts of plants, while functional fiber is nondigestible forms of carbohydrate extracted from plants or manufactured in the laboratory. Fiber may reduce the risk of many diseases and digestive illnesses.

- Carbohydrate digestion starts in the mouth, where chewing and an enzyme called salivary amylase start breaking down the carbohydrates in food.

- Digestion continues in the small intestine. Specific enzymes are secreted to break starches into smaller mono- and disaccharides. As disaccharides pass through the intestinal cells, they are digested into monosaccharides.

- Glucose and other monosaccharides are absorbed into the blood stream and travel to the liver, where all molecules are converted to glucose.

- Glucose is transported in the blood stream to the cells, where it is either used for energy or stored in the liver or muscle as glycogen.

- Insulin and glucagon are hormones secreted by the pancreas in response to changes in blood glucose.

- Insulin is secreted when blood glucose increases sufficiently, and it assists with the transport of glucose into cells.

- Glucagon is secreted when blood glucose levels are low, and it assists with the conversion of glycogen to glucose and with gluconeogenesis.

- The glycemic index is a value that indicates how much a food increases glucose levels. High glycemic foods can trigger detrimental increases in blood glucose for people with diabetes. The usefulness of the glycemic index for making dietary recommendations is controversial.

- All cells can use glucose for energy. The red blood cells, brain, and central nervous system prefer to use glucose exclusively for energy.

- Using glucose for energy helps spare body proteins, and glucose is an important fuel for the body during exercise. Exercising regularly trains our muscles to become more efficient at using both glucose and fat for energy.

- Fiber helps us maintain the healthy elimination of waste products. Eating adequate fiber may reduce the risk of colon cancer, type 2 diabetes, obesity, heart disease, hemorrhoids, and diverticulosis.

- The Acceptable Macronutrient Distribution Range for carbohydrate is 45 to 65% of total energy intake. Our diets should contain less than 25% of total energy from added sugars.

- High added-sugar intake can cause tooth decay, elevate triglyceride and low density lipoprotein levels in the blood, and contribute to obesity but does not appear to cause hyperactivity in children.

- The Adequate Intake for fiber is 25 grams per day for women and 38 grams per day for men, or 14 grams of fiber for every 1,000 kcal of energy consumed.

- Foods high in complex carbohydrates include whole grains and cereals, fruits, and vegetables. Eating 6 to 11 servings of breads/grains and 5 to 9 servings of fruits and vegetables help ensure that you meet your complex carbohydrate goals.

- Alternative sweeteners are added to some foods because they sweeten foods without promoting tooth decay and add little or no calories to foods.

- Sugar alcohols, saccharin, acesulfame-K, aspartame, and sucralose are examples of alternative sweeteners used in foods and beverages.

- All alternative sweeteners approved for use in the U.S. are felt to be safe when eaten at levels at or below the acceptable daily intake levels defined by the FDA.

- Diabetes is caused by insufficient insulin or by the cells becoming resistant or insensitive to insulin. Diabetes causes dangerously high blood glucose levels. There are two primary types of diabetes, type 1 and type 2.

- Lower than normal blood glucose levels is defined as hypoglycemia. There are two types, reactive and fasting. Reactive occurs when too much insulin is secreted after a high carbohydrate meal; fasting occurs when blood glucose drops even though no food has been eaten.

- Lactose intolerance results from an insufficient amount of the lactase enzyme. Symptoms include intestinal gas, bloating, cramping, diarrhea, and discomfort.

Review Questions

1. The glycemic index rates
   a. the acceptable amount of alternative sweeteners to consume in one day.
   b. the potential of foods to raise blood glucose and insulin levels.
   c. the risk of a given food for causing diabetes.
   d. the ratio of soluble to insoluble fiber in a complex carbohydrate.

2. Carbohydrates contain
   a. carbon, nitrogen, and water.
   b. carbonic acid and a sugar alcohol.
   c. hydrated sugar.
   d. carbon, hydrogen, and oxygen.

3. The most common source of added sugar in the American diet is
   a. table sugar.
   b. white flour.
   c. alcohol.
   d. sweetened soft drinks.

4. Glucose, fructose, and galactose are
   a. monosaccharides.
   b. disaccharides.
   c. polysaccharides.
   d. complex carbohydrates.

5. Aspartame should not be consumed by people who have
   a. phenylketonuria.
   b. type 1 diabetes.
   c. lactose intolerance.
   d. diverticulosis.

6. **True or false?** Sugar alcohols are non-nutritive sweeteners.

7. **True or false?** Insulin and glucagon are both pancreatic hormones.

8. **True or false?** A person with lactose intolerance is allergic to milk.

9. **True or false?** Plants store glucose as fiber.

10. **True or false?** Salivary amylase breaks down starches into galactose.

11. Describe the role of insulin in regulating blood glucose levels.

12. Identify at least four ways in which fiber helps us maintain a healthy digestive system.

13. Explain why complex carbohydrates are a superior food choice to simple carbohydrates.

14. Defend the statement that obesity can trigger type 2 diabetes.

15. Create a table listing molecular composition and food sources of each of the following carbohydrates: glucose, fructose, lactose, and sucrose.

Test Yourself Answers

1. **False.** The term *carbohydrate* refers to both simple and complex carbohydrates. The term *sugar* refers to the simple carbohydrates, monosaccharides and disaccharides.

2. **False.** Diets high in sugar do cause tooth decay. Whether high sugar diets cause obesity is still controversial. There is no evidence that diets high in sugar cause diabetes.

3. **False.** Since carbohydrates are an important energy source for our bodies, we are generally able to digest and absorb carbohydrates easily. People with health conditions such as diabetes and hypoglycemia, however, experience challenges with carbohydrate absorption and metabolism.

4. **True.** Our brains rely almost exclusively on glucose for energy, and our body tissues utilize glucose for energy both at rest and during exercise.

5. **True.** Contrary to recent reports claiming severe health consequences related to consumption of alternative sweeteners, major health agencies have determined that these products are safe for most of us to consume in limited quantities.

Web Links

www.eatright.org
American Dietetic Association
Visit this Web site to learn more about diabetes, low- and high-carbohydrates diets, and general healthful eating habits.

ific.org
International Food Information Council Foundation (IFIC)
Search this site to find out more about sugars and low-calorie sweeteners.

www.ada.org
American Dental Association
Go to this site to learn more about tooth decay as well as other oral health topics.

www.nidcr.nih.gov
National Institute of Dental and Craniofacial Research (NIDCR)
Find out more about recent oral and dental health discoveries, and obtain statistics and data on the status of dental health in the United States.

www.diabetes.org
American Diabetes Association
Find out more about the nutritional needs of people living with diabetes.

www.niddk.nih.gov
National Institute of Diabetes and Digestive and Kidney Diseases (NIDDK)
Learn more about diabetes including treatment, complications, U.S. statistics, clinical trials, and recent research.

References

American College of Sports Medicine (ACSM). 2000. Position Stand: Exercise and type 2 diabetes. *Med. Sci. Sports Exerc.* 32:1345–1360.

Atkins, R. C. 1992. *Dr. Atkins' New Diet Revolution.* New York: M. Evans & Company, Inc.

Buyken, A. E., M. Toeller, G. Heitkamp, G. Karamanos, B. Rottiers, R. Muggeo, M. Fuller. 2001. Glycemic index in the diet of European outpatients with type 1 diabetes: relations to glycated hemoglobin and serum lipids. *Am. J. Clin. Nutr.* 73:574–581.

Colditz, G. A., J. E. Manson, M. J. Stampfer, B. Rosner, W. C. Willett, and F. E. Speizer. 1992. Diet and risk of clinical diabetes in women. *Am. J. Clin. Nutr.* 55:1018–1023.

Duffy, V. B., and G. H. Anderson. 1998. Use of nutritive and nonnutritive sweeteners—Position of the ADA. *J. Am. Diet. Assoc.* 98:580–587.

Harnack, L., J. Stang, and M. Story. 1999. Soft drink consumption among U.S. children and adolescents: nutritional consequences. *J. Am. Diet. Assoc.* 99:436–441.

Howard, B. V., and J. Wylie-Rosett. 2002. Sugar and cardiovascular disease. A statement for healthcare professionals from the Committee on Nutrition of the Council on Nutrition, Physical Activity, and Metabolism of the American Heart Association. *Circulation* 106:523–527.

Institute of Medicine, Food and Nutrition Board. 2002. *Dietary Reference Intakes for Energy, Carbohydrates, Fiber, Fat, Protein and Amino Acids (Macronutrients).* Washington, DC: The National Academy of Sciences.

Liu, S., J. E. Manson, M. J. Stampfer, M. D. Holmes, F. B. Hu, S. E. Hankinson, and W. C. Willett. 2001. Dietary glycemic load assessed by food-frequency questionnaire in relation to plasma high-density-lipoprotein cholesterol and fasting plasma triacylglycerols in postmenopausal women. *Am. J. Clin. Nutr.* 73:560–566.

Ludwig, D. S., K. E. Peterson, and S. L. Gortmaker. 2001. Relation between consumption of sugar-sweetened drinks and childhood obesity: a prospective, observational analysis. *Lancet* 357:505–508.

Meyer, K. A., L. H. Kushi, D. R. Jacobs, J. Slavin, T. A. Sellers, and A. R. Folsom. 2000. Carbohydrates, dietary fiber, and incident of type 2 diabetes in older women. *Am. J. Clin. Nutr.* 71:921–930.

National Diabetes Information Clearinghouse (NDIC). National Diabetes Statistics. National Institutes of Health Publication No. 03–3892. May 2003.

http://diabetes.niddk.nih.gov/dm/pubs/statistics/index.htm. Accessed July 2003.

Nestle, M. 2002. *Food Politics: How the Food Industry Influences Nutrition and Health.* Berkeley, CA: University of California Press.

Pan, X.-P., G.-W. Li, Y.-H. Hu, J. X. Wang, W. Y. Yang, Z. X. An, Z. X. Hu, J. Lin, J. Z. Xiao, H. B. Cao, P. A. Liu, X. G. Jiang, Y. Y. Jiang, J. P Wang., H. Zheng, H. Zhang, P. H. Bennett, B. V. Howard. 1997. Effects of diet and exercise in preventing NIDDM in people with impaired glucose tolerance. *Diabetes Care* 20:537–544.

Pan, J. W., D. L. Rothman, K. L. Behar, D. T. Stein, and H. P. Hetherington. 2000. Human brain β-hydroxybutyrate and lactate increase in fasting-induced ketosis. *J. Cerebral Blood Flow Metabol.* 20:1502–1507.

Rosenbloom, A. L., D. V. House, and W. E. Winter. 1998. Non-insulin dependent diabetes mellitus (NIDDM) in minority youth: research priorities and needs. *Clin Pediatr.* 37:143–152.

Sears, B. 1995. *The Zone. A Dietary Road Map.* New York: HarperCollins Publishers.

Steward, H. L., M. C. Bethea, S. S. Andrews, and L. A. Balart. 1995. *Sugar Busters! Cut Sugar to Trim Fat.* New York: Ballantine Books.

Suarez, F. L., J. Adshead, J. K. Furne, and M. D. Levitt. 1998. Lactose maldigestion is not an impediment to the intake of 1500 mg calcium daily as dairy products. *Am. J. Clin. Nutr.* 68:1118–1122.

Topping, D. L., and P. M. Clifton. 2001. Short-chain fatty acids and human colonic function: roles of resistant starch and nonstarch polysaccharides. *Physiol. Rev.* 81:1031–1064.

Tremblay, A., J. A. Simoneau, and C. Bouchard. 1994. Impact of exercise intensity on body fatness and skeletal muscle metabolism. *Metabolism* 43:814–818.

Troiano, R. P., R. R. Briefel, M. D. Carroll, and K. Bialostosky. 2000. Energy and fat intakes of children and adolescents in the United States: Data from the National Health and Nutrition Examination Surveys. *Am. J. Clin. Nutr.* 72:1343S-1353S.

Troiano, R. P., K. M. Flegal, R. J. Kuczmarski, S. M. Campbell, and C. L. Johnson. 1995. Overweight prevalence and trends for children and adolescents. The National Health and Nutrition Examination Surveys, 1963–1991. *Arch. Pediatr. Adolesc. Med.* 149:1085–1091.

U.S. Department of Agriculture (USDA). U.S. Department of Health and Human Services. 2000. *Dietary Guidelines for Americans,* 5th ed. Washington, DC: U.S. Government Printing Office. Home and Garden Bulletin No. 232.

U.S. Department of Health and Human Services. November 2000. *Healthy People 2010: Understanding and Improving Health.* 2nd ed. Washington, DC: U.S. Government Printing Office.

Wilkinson Enns, C., S. J. Mickle, and J. D. Goldman. 2002. Trends in food and nutrient intakes by children in the United States. *Family Econ. Nutr. Rev.* 14:56–68.

Nutrition Debate:

Can Reducing Sugar Intake Be the Answer to Obesity?

Almost every day in the news we see headlines about obesity: "More Americans Overweight!", "The Fattening of America," "Obesity is a National Epidemic!" These headlines accurately reflect the state of weight in the United States. Over the past thirty years, obesity rates have increased dramatically for both adults and children. Obesity has become public health enemy number one, as many chronic diseases such as type 2 diabetes, heart disease, high blood pressure, and arthritis go hand-in-hand with obesity.

Of particular concern are the rising obesity rates in children. It is estimated that the rate of overweight in children has increased 100% since the mid-1970s, while the rate of obesity has increased 50% over this same time period (Troiano et al. 1995). Why should we concern ourselves with fighting obesity in children? First, it is well established that the treatment of existing obesity is extremely challenging, and our greatest hope of combating this disease is through prevention. Most agree that prevention should start with children at a very early age. Second, approximately 30% of children who are obese will remain obese as adults, suffering all of the health problems that accompany this disease. Young children are now experiencing type 2 diabetes, high blood pressure, and high cholesterol at increasingly younger ages, only compounding the devastating effects of these illnesses as they get older. We have reached the point where serious action must be immediately taken to curb the already growing crisis.

How can we prevent obesity? This is a difficult question to answer. One way is to better understand the factors that contribute to obesity, and then take actions to alter these factors. We know of many factors that contribute to overweight and obesity. These include genetic influences, lack of adequate physical activity, and eating foods that are high in fat, added sugar, and energy. While it is easy to blame our genetics, they cannot be held entirely responsible for the rapid rise in obesity that has occurred over the past 30 years. Our genetic make-up takes thousands of years to change; thus, humans who lived 50 or 100 years ago have essentially the same genetic make-up as humans who live now. The fact that obesity rates have risen so dramatically in recent years illustrates that we need to look more closely at how our lifestyles have changed over this same period to truly understand the factors causing obesity.

One factor that has recently come to the forefront of nutrition research and policy making is the contribution of added sugars to overweight and obesity in children. As discussed earlier in this chapter, there is still much disagreement about whether added sugar does cause, and how much it might contribute to, obesity. Many health professionals are beginning to draw attention to the potential role of added sugars, specifically sugared soft drinks, in rising obesity rates. Recent studies of soft drink consumption in children show that girls and boys ages 6 to 11 years drank about twice as many soft drinks in 1998 as compared to 1977, and consumption of milk over this same time period dropped by about 30 percent (Wilkinson Enns, Mickle, and Goldman 2002). Equally alarming is the finding that one-fourth of a group of adolescents studied were heavy consumers of sugared soft drinks, drinking at least 26 ounces of soft drinks each day.

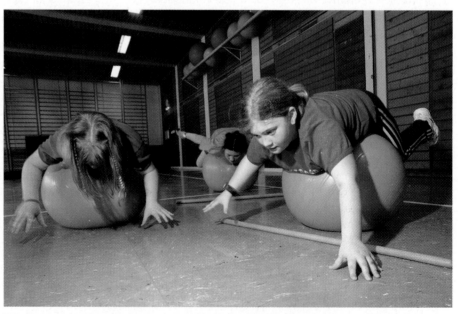

It is estimated that the rate of overweight in children has increased 100% since the mid 1970s.

This intake is equivalent to almost 400 extra calories each day, and these individuals consumed more calories from all foods than other adolescents and drank less nutritious beverages such as milk and fruit juice (Harnack, Stang, and Story 1999). A recent report found that for each extra sugared soft drink that children drink each day, the risk of obesity increases by 60% (Ludwig, Peterson, and Gortmaker 2001). Another harmful effect of soft drinks is their effect on bone density: the phosphorus available in some sodas, whether sugared or diet, binds with calcium, causing it to be drawn out of the bones. This is especially harmful during childhood and adolescence, when bones are still growing.

With all of this alarming information, you would expect dramatic changes in soft drink consumption around the country. However, this is not the case. Powerful influences are at work to not only maintain, but to increase soft drink consumption around the world. Dr. Marion Nestle highlights these influences in her book, *Food Politics: How the Food Industry Influences Nutrition and Health* (Nestle 2002). Some of these influences include:

- Large increases in advertising by soft drink companies, with an emphasis on targeting young children;

- Exclusive contracts between soft drink companies and schools, providing much needed revenues to inadequate school budgets; and

- The competition between soft drinks and other foods high in added sugar with healthful foods served at schools, with children preferring high sugar foods to those served through school nutrition programs.

The allegations brought against schools and the soft drink industry are strong. Many people feel that our schools have sold out our children's health for the sake of sports arenas and new buildings. School food service programs are expected to be self-supporting, and they cannot compete against soft drinks, chips, and candy; thus, food service programs claim that school support of soft drinks and other "junk" foods undermines their programs, and in turn, our children's health. In an effort to survive, many school food service programs have responded by serving more à la carte items, which include foods that are higher in fat, sugar, and calories than regulated school meals. Soft drink companies are under attack for pushing non-nutritious foods onto children. They are also accused of putting profits and brand loyalty ahead of our children's health.

Both schools and soft drink companies are quick to defend themselves. As adequate funding for public schools is no longer provided by state and federal governments, schools are desperate to find sources of substantial revenue to provide materials and programs to children. Thus, school administrators feel justified in accepting lucrative contracts from soft drink companies to support educational efforts. Soft drink companies argue that soft drinks and other snack foods can be part of a healthful diet and that there is no evidence to prove that soft drinks cause obesity. In a society of capitalism, they believe that they have every right to maximize profits.

This debate is growing larger and more heated every day. Health professionals, concerned citizens, and government officials are now pitting themselves against school administrators, soft drink companies, and other government officials. Many people who oppose the sales of soft drinks and other "junk" foods in schools are asking for more stringent governmental controls over what can be served and sold on school grounds. Those in favor of soft drink and junk food sales in schools are fighting for even less stringent controls. Lawsuits initiated by both sides are becoming commonplace.

This issue is extremely complex, and no easy solution is in sight. How do you feel about this issue? Should reducing soft drink consumption be up to individuals? Should schools and our government play a central role in controlling the types of foods served in schools? Should soft drink companies be allowed to pay large sums of money to schools in exchange for exclusive beverage contracts? Is there even enough evidence to suggest that soft drinks and other foods high in added sugars are linked with obesity? As this controversy grows, it is more likely that average citizens will be asked to take a stand on this issue.

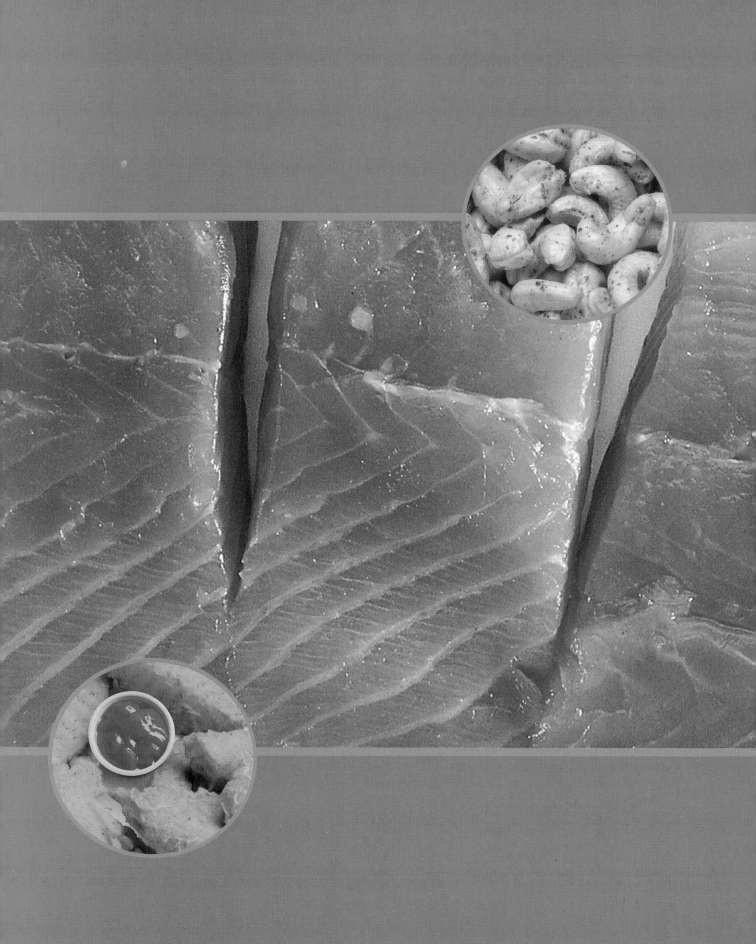

Chapter 5
Fat: An Essential
Energy-Supplying Nutrient

Chapter Objectives

After reading this chapter you will be able to:

1. List and describe the three types of lipids found in foods, pp. 158–163.

2. Discuss how the level of saturation of fatty acid affects its shape and the form it takes, pp. 159–162.

3. Identify the primary difference between a *cis* fatty acid and a *trans* fatty acid, pp. 161–162.

4. Describe the steps involved in fat digestion, pp. 164–166.

5. List three functions of fat in our bodies, pp. 166–170.

6. Define the recommended dietary intakes for total fat, saturated fat, and the two essential fatty acids, pp. 171–173.

7. Identify at least three common food sources of beneficial fats, pp. 173–177.

8. Describe the role of dietary fat in the development of cardiovascular disease, pp. 179–185.

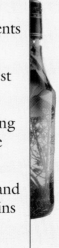

Test Yourself True or false?

1. Fat is unhealthful, and we should eat as little as possible in our diets. T or F

2. Fat does not provide any important nutrients and is only a source of excess energy. T or F

3. Fat is an important fuel source during rest and exercise. T or F

4. Fried foods are relatively nutritious as long as vegetable shortening is used to fry the foods. T or F

5. Eating a diet that is relatively low in fat and high in fruits, vegetables, and whole grains and exercising regularly can help reduce our risk for cardiovascular disease. T or F

Test Yourself answers can be found at the end of the chapter.

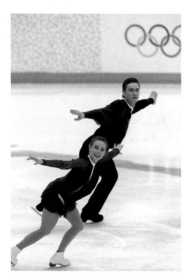

Sergei Grinkov, here skating with his partner and wife Ekaterina Gordeeva, died of a heart attack at the age of 28.

Only couch potatoes develop heart disease . . . or so we like to think. That's why the world was stunned in the fall of 1995 when 28-year-old skater Sergei Grinkov, a two-time Olympic gold medalist, collapsed and died of a fatal heart attack while training in Lake Placid, New York. An autopsy revealed that Grinkov's coronary arteries were as severely clogged as those of a 70-year-old with established heart disease. Although his widow reported that he had never complained of chest pain or shortness of breath, his family history revealed one very important clue: his father had died of a heart attack at age 52. In one recent study, a survey of U.S. public health records revealed that, from 1985 through 1995, 134 deaths of young athletes were due to heart disease.

What causes a heart attack, and how can you calculate your risk? Can a high-fat diet cause heart disease, and can a low-fat diet prevent it? When was the last time you heard anything good about dietary fat? If your best friend's father had died of a heart attack at age 44 and you noticed your friend regularly eating high-fat meals, would you say anything about it? If so, what would you say?

Although some people think of dietary fat as something to be avoided, a certain amount of fat is absolutely essential for good health. In this chapter, we'll discuss the function of fat in the human body and help you distinguish between beneficial and harmful types of dietary fat. You'll also assess how much fat you need in your diet and learn about the role of dietary fat in the development of heart disease and other disorders.

What Are Fats?

Fats are just one form of a much larger and more diverse group of substances called **lipids** that are distinguished by the fact that they are insoluble in water. Think of a salad dressing made with vinegar and olive oil—a lipid. Shaking the bottle *disperses* the oil but doesn't *dissolve* it: that's why it separates back out again so quickly. Lipids are found in all sorts of living things, from bacteria to plants to human beings. In fact, their presence on your skin explains why you can't clean your face with water alone: you need some type of soap to break down the insoluble lipids before you can wash them away. In this chapter, we focus on the small group of lipids that are found in foods.

Lipids Come in Different Forms

There are many different types of lipids in our body and in our diet. For example, butter and olive oil are two different types of lipids found in foods. Fats like butter are solid at room temperature, while oils such as olive oil are liquid at room temperature. Because most people are more comfortable with the term *fats* instead of *lipids*, we will use that term generically throughout this book, including when we are referring to oils.

Three Types of Lipids Are Present in Foods

Three types of lipids are commonly found in foods. These are triglycerides, phospholipids, and sterols. Let's take a look at each.

Triglycerides Are the Most Common Food-Based Lipid

Most of the fat we eat (95%) is in the form of triglycerides, which is the same way most of the fat in our body is stored. As reflected in the prefix *tri*, a **triglyceride** is a molecule consisting of *three* fatty acids attached to a *three*-carbon glycerol backbone. **Fatty acids** are long chains of carbon atoms bound to each other as well as to hydrogen atoms. They are acids because they contain an acid group (carboxyl group) at one end of their chain. **Glycerol,** the backbone of a triglyceride molecule, is an alcohol

lipids   A diverse group of organic substances that are insoluble in water; lipids include triglycerides, phospholipids, and sterols.

triglyceride   A molecule consisting of three fatty acids attached to a three-carbon glycerol backbone.

fatty acids   Long chains of carbon atoms bound to each other as well as to hydrogen atoms.

glycerol   An alcohol composed of three carbon atoms; it is the backbone of a triglyceride molecule.

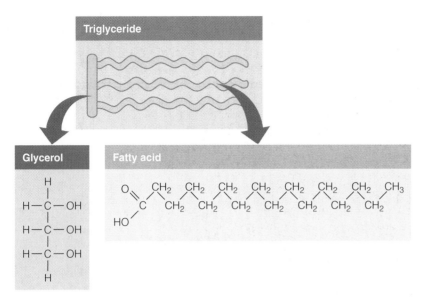

Figure 5.1   A triglyceride consists of three fatty acids attached to a three-carbon glycerol backbone.

composed of three carbon atoms. One fatty acid attaches to each of these three carbons to make the triglyceride (Figure 5.1).

Triglycerides Are Classified by Their Length, Saturation, and Shape

To understand why we want more of some fats than others, we need to know more about their properties and how they work in our body. In general, triglycerides can be classified by their chain length (number of carbons in each fatty acid), by their level of saturation (how much hydrogen, H, is attached to each carbon atom in the fatty acid chain), and their shape, which is determined in some cases by how they are commercially processed. All of these factors influence how we use the triglyceride within our bodies.

Chain Length   The fatty acids attached to the glycerol backbone can vary in the number of carbons they contain, referred to as their *chain length*.

- **Short-chain fatty acids** are usually fewer than six carbon atoms in length.
- **Medium-chain fatty acids** are six to twelve carbons in length.
- **Long-chain fatty acids** are fourteen or more carbons in length.

Fatty acid chain length is important because it determines the method of fat digestion and absorption and affects how fats function within the body. For example, short- and medium-chain fatty acids are digested and transported more quickly than long-chain fatty acids. We will discuss digestion and absorption of fats in more detail shortly.

Level of Saturation   Triglycerides can also vary by the types of bonds found in the fatty acids. If a fatty acid has no carbons bonded together with a double bond, they are referred to as **saturated fatty acids (SFA)** (Figure 5.2a). This is because every carbon atom in the chain is *saturated* with hydrogen: each has the maximum amount of hydrogen bound to it. Some foods that are high in saturated fatty acids are coconut oil, palm kernel oil, butter, cream, whole milk, and beef.

If, within the chain of carbon atoms, two are bound to each other with a double bond, then this double carbon bond excludes hydrogen. This lack of hydrogen at *one* part of the molecule results in a fat that is referred to as *monounsaturated* (recall from Chapter 4 that the prefix *mono-* means one). A monounsaturated molecule is shown in Figure 5.2a. **Monounsaturated fatty acids (MUFA)** are usually liquid at room temperature. Foods that are high in monounsaturated fatty acids are olive oil, canola oil, and cashew nuts.

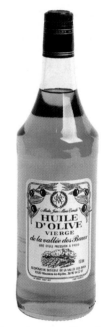

Some fats, such as olive oil, are liquid at room temperature.

short-chain fatty acids Fatty acids fewer than six carbon atoms in length.

medium-chain fatty acids Fatty acids that are six to twelve carbon atoms in length.

long-chain fatty acids Fatty acids that are fourteen or more carbon atoms in length.

saturated fatty acids (SFA) Fatty acids that have no carbons joined together with a double bond; these types of fatty acids are generally solid at room temperature.

monounsaturated fatty acids (MUFA) Fatty acids that have two carbons in the chain bound to each other with one double bond; these types of fatty acids are generally liquid at room temperature.

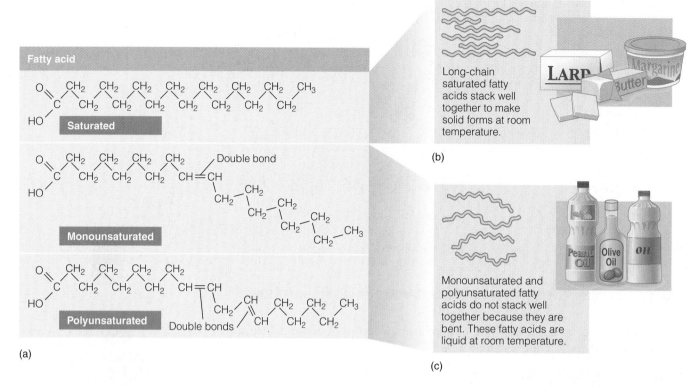

Figure 5.2 Examples of levels of saturation among fatty acids and how these levels of saturation affect the shape of fatty acids. **(a)** Saturated fatty acids are saturated with hydrogen, meaning they have no carbons bonded together with a double bond. Monounsaturated fatty acids contain two carbons bound by one double bond. Polyunsaturated fatty acids have more than one double bond linking carbon atoms. **(b)** Saturated fats have straight fatty acids packed tightly together and are solid at room temperature. **(c)** Unsaturated fats have "kinked" fatty acids at the area of the double bond, preventing them from packing tightly together; they are liquid at room temperature.

polyunsaturated fatty acids (PUFA)
Fatty acids that have more than one double bond in the chain, these types of fatty acids are generally liquid at room temperature.

If the fat molecules have *more than one* double bond, they contain even less hydrogen and are referred to as **polyunsaturated fatty acids (PUFA)** (see Figure 5.2a). Polyunsaturated fatty acids are also liquid at room temperature and include cottonseed, canola, corn, and safflower oils.

Foods vary in the types of fatty acids they contain. For example, animal fats provide approximately 40 to 60% of their energy from saturated fats, while plant fats provide 80 to 90% of their energy from monounsaturated and polyunsaturated fats (Table 5.1). You will notice that canola oil is listed as being high in both MUFA and PUFA. Most oils are a combination of fats, making them a good source of more than one type of fat. Diets higher in plant foods will usually be lower in saturated fats than diets high in animal products. The impact that various types of fatty acids have on health will be discussed later in this chapter (beginning on page 179).

Shape   Have you ever noticed how many toothpicks are packed into a small box? A hundred or more! But if you were to break a bunch of toothpicks into V shapes anywhere along their length, how many could you then fit into the same box? It would be very few because the bent toothpicks would jumble together, taking up much more space. Molecules of saturated fat are like straight toothpicks: they have no double carbon bonds and always form straight, rigid chains. As they have no kinks, these chains can pack together tightly (Figure 5.2b). That is why saturated fats, such as the fat in meats, are solid at room temperature.

In contrast, each double carbon bond of unsaturated fats gives them a kink along their length (Figure 5.2c). This means that they are unable to pack together tightly—for example, to form a stick of butter—and instead are liquid at room temperature. In addition, unsaturated fatty acids can occur in either a *cis* or a *trans* shape. The prefix *cis* means things are located on the same side or near each other,

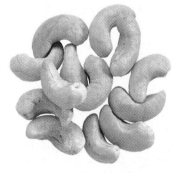

Cashew nuts are high in monounsaturated fatty acids.

Table 5.1   Major Sources of Dietary Fat

Food	Distribution of Fat by Type				
	% of total kcals from fat	*% total fat kcals as EFA*	*% total fat kcals as SFA*	*% total fat kcals as MUFA*	*% total fat kcals as PUFA*
Butter	100%	4%	65%	31%	4%
Milk, Whole (3.3% fat)	49%	4%	63%	33%	4%
Milk, 2% fat	40%	4%	66%	30%	4%
Milk, skim (non-fat)	5%	<1%	3%	10%	<1%
Beef, ground (16% fat)	54%	4%	45%	51%	4%
Chicken, breast boneless	35%	23%	32%	44%	24%
Turkey, boneless	26%	28%	32%	25%	35%
Tuna, water packed	6%	39%	32%	22%	46%
Tuna, oil-packed	37%	36%	21%	40%	39%
Salmon, Chinook	33%	16%	25%	48%	24%
Egg, large	62%	13%	37%	46%	16%
Canola oil	100%	30%	7%	59%	30%
Safflower oil	100%	74%	9%	12%	74%
Corn oil	100%	60%	13%	25%	60%
Corn oil margarine	100%	44%	2%	27%	27%
Sesame oil	100%	42%	14%	41%	42%
Olive oil	100%	10%	14%	74%	10%
Salmon oil (fish oil)	100%	34%	20%	29%	40%
Cottonseed oil	100%	50%	26%	20%	52%
Palm kernel oil	100%	2%	82%	11%	2%
Coconut oil	100%	2%	87%	6%	2%
Walnuts	86%	63%	10%	23%	64%
Cashew nuts	72%	17%	20%	59%	17%

Source: Data from Food Processor, Version 7.01 (ESHA Research, Salem, OR).
Note: EFA (essential fatty acids), SFA (saturated fatty acids), MUFA (monounsaturated fatty acids), and PUFA (polyunsaturated fatty acids).

while *trans* is a prefix that denotes across or opposite. These terms describe the positioning of the hydrogen atoms around the double carbon bond as follows:

- A *cis fatty acid* has both hydrogen atoms located on the same side of the double bond (Figure 5.3a), thus, the prefix "*cis*." This positioning gives the *cis* molecule a pronounced kink at the double carbon bond. We typically find the *cis* fatty acids in nature, and thus in foods like olive oil.

- In contrast, in a *trans fatty acid* the hydrogen atoms are attached on diagonally opposite sides of the double carbon bond (Figure 5.3b). This positioning makes *trans* fatty acids fats straighter and more rigid, just like saturated fats. Although a limited amount of *trans* fatty acids are found in cow's milk, the majority of *trans* fatty acids are produced by manipulating the fatty acid during food processing. For example, in the **hydrogenation** of oils, such as corn or safflower oil, hydrogen is added to the fatty acids. In this process, the double bonds found in the monounsaturated and polyunsaturated fatty acids in the oil are broken and additional hydrogen is inserted. This process straightens out the molecules, making the liquid fat more solid at room temperature—and also more saturated. Thus, corn oil margarine is a partially hydrogenated fat made from corn oil. The hydrogenation

hydrogenation The process of adding hydrogen to unsaturated fatty acids, making them more saturated and thereby more solid at room temperature.

cis arrangement

(a) *cis* polyunsaturated fatty acid

trans arrangement

(b) *trans* polyunsaturated fatty acid

Figure 5.3 Structure of **(a)** a *cis* and **(b)** a *trans* polyunsaturated fatty acid. *Cis* fatty acids are kinked at the area of the double bond; *trans* fatty acids are straight at the area of the double bond.

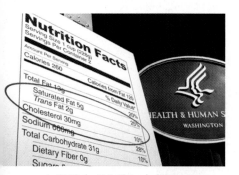

In 2003 the U.S. FDA ruled that *trans* fatty acids, or *trans* fat, must be listed as a separate line item on Nutrition Facts labels for conventional foods and some dietary supplements. Research studies show that diets high in *trans* fatty acids can increase the risk of cardiovascular disease.

phospholipids A type of lipid in which a fatty acid is combined with another compound that contains phosphate; unlike other lipids, phospholipids are soluble in water.

process is used to create a more saturated molecule; however, some of the unsaturated bonds are modified and result in the production of *trans* fatty acids. As most margarines are hydrogenated, they have more *trans* fatty acids than butter.

Does the straight, rigid shape of the saturated and *trans* fats we eat have any effect on our health? Absolutely! Research over the last two decades has shown that diets high in saturated fatty acids increase blood cholesterol and our risk of heart disease. We now know that *trans* fatty acids appear to function much like saturated fatty acids in our diet: both *trans* and saturated fatty acids raise blood cholesterol levels and appear to change cell membrane function and the way cholesterol is removed from the blood. For these reasons, many health professionals feel that diets high in *trans* fatty acids can increase the risk of cardiovascular disease, similar to diets high in saturated fat. Because of the concerns related to *trans* fatty acid consumption and heart disease, manufacturers will soon be required to list the amount of *trans* fatty acids per serving on the food label. Some margarine manufacturers are already producing products free of *trans* fatty acids, and they clearly state this claim on the label. We will talk more about *trans* fatty acids later in this chapter (page 172).

Phospholipids Combine Lipids With Phosphate

Along with the triglycerides just discussed, we also find phospholipids and sterols in the foods we eat. **Phospholipids** consist of two fatty acids and a glycerol backbone with another compound that contains phosphate (Figure 5.4). This addition of a phosphate compound makes phospholipids soluble in water, a property that enables phospholipids to assist in transporting fats in our bloodstream. We discuss this concept in more detail later in this chapter (page 165). Also, as you may recall from Chapter 3, phospholipids in our cell membrane regulate the transport of substances into and out of the cell. Note that our bodies manufacture phospholipids, so they are not essential for us to include in our diets.

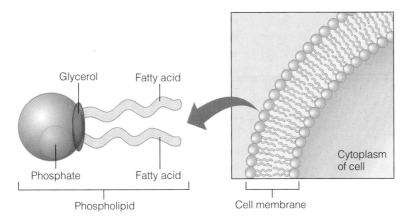

Figure 5.4   Structure of a phospholipid. Phospholipids consist of a glycerol backbone with two fatty acids and a compound that contains phosphate.

Sterols Have a Ring Structure

Sterols are also a type of lipid found in foods and in the body, but their multiple-ring structure is quite different from that of triglycerides (Figure 5.5a). Sterols are found in both plant and animal foods and are produced in the body. Plants contain some sterols, but these sterols are not very well absorbed and appear to block the absorption of dietary cholesterol, the most commonly occurring sterol in the diet (Figure 5.5b). Cholesterol is only found in the fatty part of animal products such as butter, eggs, whole milk, meats and poultry. Low- or reduced-fat animal products such as lean meats and skim milk have little cholesterol.

We don't need to consume cholesterol in our diet because our body continually synthesizes it, mostly in the liver and intestines. This continuous production is vital to our health because cholesterol is part of every cell membrane, where it works in conjunction with fatty acids to help maintain cell membrane integrity. It is particularly plentiful in the neural cells that make up our brain, spinal cord, and nerves. The body also uses cholesterol to synthesize several important sterol compounds including sex hormones (estrogen, androgen, and progesterone), adrenal hormones, and vitamin D. Thus, despite cholesterol's bad reputation, it is absolutely essential to human health.

sterols A type of lipid found in foods and the body that has a ring structure; cholesterol is the most common sterol that occurs in our diets.

> **Recap:** Fat is essential for health. There are three types of fat typically found in foods: triglycerides, phospholipids, and sterols. Triglycerides are the most common fat found in food. A triglyceride is made up of glycerol and three fatty acids. These fatty acids can be classified based on chain length, level of saturation, and shape. Phospholipids combine two fatty acids and a glycerol backbone with a phosphate-containing compound, making them soluble in water. Sterols have a multiple ring structure; cholesterol is the most commonly occurring sterol in our diets.

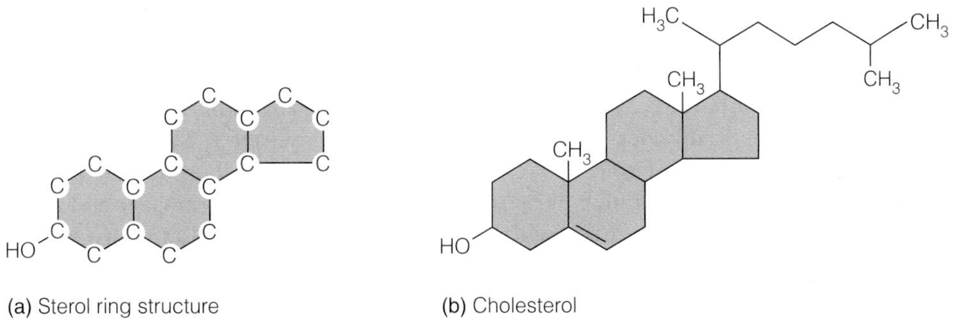

(a) Sterol ring structure

(b) Cholesterol

Figure 5.5   Sterol structure. **(a)** Sterols are lipids that contain multiple ring structures. **(b)** Cholesterol is the most commonly occurring sterol in the diet.

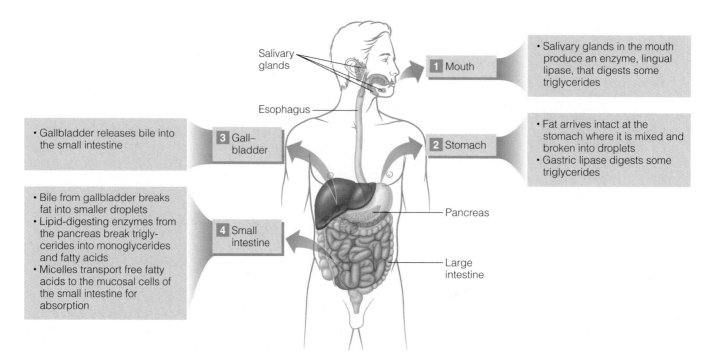

Figure 5.6   The process of fat digestion.

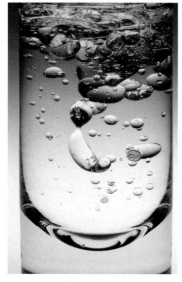

Fats and oils do not dissolve readily in water.

How Does Our Body Break Down Fats?

Because fats are not soluble in water, they cannot enter our bloodstream easily from the digestive tract. Thus, fats must be digested, absorbed, and transported within the body differently from carbohydrates and proteins, which are water-soluble substances.

The digestion and absorption of fat were discussed in detail in Chapter 3, but we briefly review the process here (Figure 5.6). Dietary fats usually come mixed with other foods in our diet, which we chew and then swallow. Salivary enzymes have a limited role in the breakdown of fats, and so fat reaches the stomach intact (Figure 5.6, step 1). The primary role of the stomach in fat digestion is to mix and break up the fat into smaller pieces or droplets. Because they are not soluble in water, these fat droplets typically float on top of the watery digestive juices in the stomach until they are passed into the small intestine (Figure 5.6, step 2).

The Gallbladder, Liver, and Pancreas Assist in Fat Digestion

Because fat is not soluble in water, its digestion requires the help of digestive enzymes from the pancreas and mixing compounds from the gallbladder. Recall from Chapter 3 that the gallbladder is a sac attached to the underside of the liver and the pancreas is an oblong-shaped organ sitting below the stomach. Both have a duct connecting them to the small intestine. As fat enters the small intestine from the stomach, the gallbladder contracts and releases a substance called bile (Figure 5.6, step 3). Bile is produced in the liver from cholesterol and is stored in the gallbladder until needed. You can think of bile acting much like soap, breaking up the fat into smaller and smaller droplets. At the same time, lipid-digesting enzymes produced in the pancreas travel through the pancreatic duct into the small intestine. Once bile has broken the fat into small droplets, these pancreatic enzymes take over, breaking the fatty acids away from their glycerol backbones. Each triglyceride molecule is broken down into two free fatty acids and one *monoglyceride,* a glycerol molecule with one fatty acid still attached.

Absorption of Fat Occurs Primarily in the Small Intestine

The majority of fat absorption occurs in the mucosal lining of the small intestine with the help of a micelle (Figure 5.6, step 4). A *micelle* is a spherical compound made up of bile and phospholipids that can trap the free fatty acids and the monoglycerides and transport them to the mucosal cells for absorption.

How does the absorbed fat get into the bloodstream? Because fats do not mix with water, most fats cannot be transported freely in the bloodstream. To solve this problem, the fatty acids are reformulated back into triglycerides and then packaged into lipoproteins before being released into the bloodstream. A **lipoprotein** is a spherical compound in which the fat clusters in the center and phospholipids and proteins form the outside of the sphere (Figure 5.7). The specific lipoprotein produced in the mucosal cell to transport fat from a meal is called a **chylomicron.** This unique compound is now soluble in water because phospholipids and proteins are water-soluble. Once chylomicrons are formed, they are transported from the intestinal lining to the lymphatic system and then into the blood. In this way, dietary fat finally arrives in your blood.

As mentioned earlier, short- and medium-chain fatty acids (those less than 14 carbons in length) can be transported in the body more readily than the long-chain fatty acids. When short and medium-chain fatty acids are digested and transported to the mucosal cell of the small intestine, they do not have to be reformed into triglycerides and incorporated into chylomicrons. Instead, they can travel in the bloodstream bound to either a transport protein or a phospholipid. For this reason, shorter-chain fatty acids can get into the system more quickly than long-chain fatty acids.

lipoprotein A spherical compound in which fat clusters in the center and phospholipids and proteins form the outside of the sphere.

chylomicron A lipoprotein produced in the mucosal cell of the intestine; transports dietary fat out of the intestinal tract.

Fat Is Stored in Adipose Tissues for Later Use

The chylomicrons, which are filled with the dietary fat you just ate, now begin to circulate through the blood looking for a place to deliver their load. There are three primary fates of this dietary fat:

1. It can immediately be taken up and used as a source of energy for the cells.
2. It can be used to make lipid-containing compounds in the body.
3. It can be stored in the muscle or adipose tissue as a triglyceride for later use.

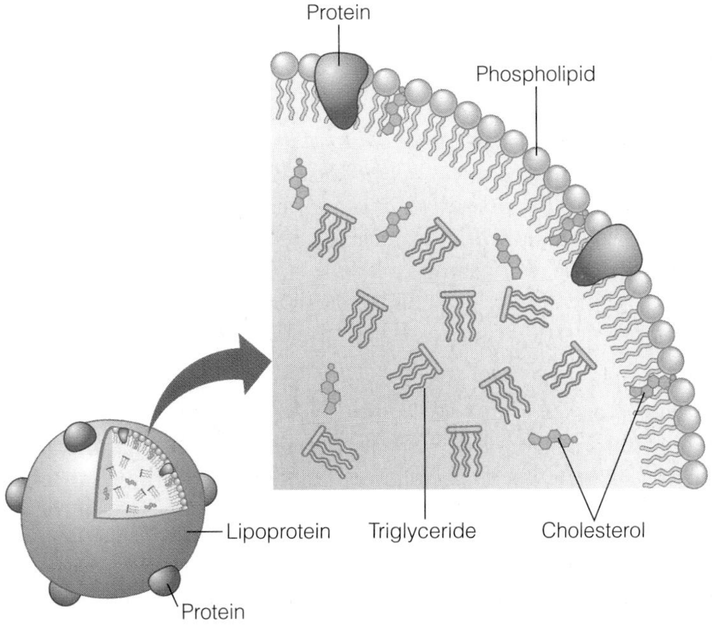

Figure 5.7   Structure of a lipoprotein. Notice that the fat clusters in the center of the molecule and the phospholipids and proteins, which are water-soluble, form the outside of the sphere. This enables lipoproteins to transport fats in the bloodstream.

lipoprotein lipase An enzyme that sits on the outside of cells and breaks apart triglycerides so that their fatty acids can be removed and taken up by the cell.

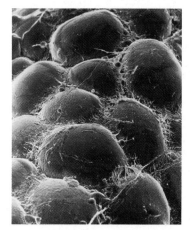

Adipose tissue. During times of weight gain, excess fat consumed in the diet is stored in the adipose tissue.

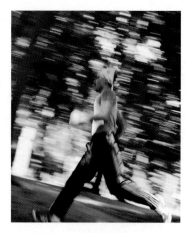

Dietary fat provides energy.

How does the fat get out of the chylomicrons and into the cell? This process occurs with the help of an enzyme called **lipoprotein lipase,** or LPL, which sits outside of our adipose cells. At the surface of the adipose cell, LPL comes in contact with the chylomicrons when they touch the surface of the adipose cell. As a result of this contact, LPL breaks apart the triglycerides in the core of the chylomicrons. This process results in the movement of individual fatty acids from within the core of the chylomicrons and out into the adipose cell. If the cell needs the fat for energy, these fatty acids will be quickly transported into the mitochondria and used as fuel. If the body doesn't need the fatty acids for immediate energy, the cell can re-create the triglycerides and store them for later use. The primary storage site for this extra energy is the adipose cell. However, if you are physically active, your body will preferentially store this extra fat in the muscle tissue first, so the next time you go out for a run, the fat is readily available to the cell for energy. Thus, people who engage in physical activity are more likely to have extra fat stored in the muscle tissue and to have less body fat—something many of us would prefer. Of course, fat stored in the adipose tissue can also be used for energy during exercise, but it must be broken down first and then transported to the muscle cells.

Recap: Fat digestion begins when fats are broken into droplets by bile. Lipid-digestive enzymes from the pancreas subsequently digest the triglycerides into two free fatty acids and one monoglyceride. These end products of digestion are then transported into the intestinal mucosal cells with the help of micelles. Once inside the mucosal cells, triglycerides are re-formed and packaged into lipoproteins called chylomicrons. Their outer layer is made up of proteins and phospholipids, which allows them to dissolve in the blood. Dietary fat is transported by the chylomicrons to cells within the body that need energy. Fat stored in the muscle tissue is used as a source of energy during physical activity. Excess fat is stored in the adipose tissue and can be used whenever the body needs energy.

Why Do We Need Fats?

Dietary fat provides energy and helps our bodies perform some essential physiologic functions.

Fats Provide Energy

Dietary fat is a primary source of energy because fat has twice the energy per gram as carbohydrate or protein. Fat provides 9 kilocalories (kcals) per gram, while carbohydrate and protein provide only 4 kilocalories (kcals) per gram. This means that fat is much more energy dense. For example, 1 tablespoon of butter or oil contains approximately 100 kcals, while it takes 2.5 cups of steamed broccoli or 1 slice of whole wheat bread to provide 100 kcals from these foods.

Fats Are a Major Fuel Source When We Are at Rest

At rest, we are able to deliver plenty of oxygen to our cells so that metabolic functions can occur. Just as a candle needs oxygen for the flame to continue burning, our cells need oxygen to use fat for energy. Thus, approximately 30 to 70% of the energy used at rest by the muscles and organs comes from fat (Jebb et al. 1996). The exact amount of energy coming from fat at rest will depend on how much fat you are eating in your diet, how physically active you are, and whether you are gaining or losing weight. If you are dieting, more fat will be used for energy than if you are gaining weight. During times of weight gain, more of the fat consumed in the diet is stored in the adipose tissue, and the body uses more dietary protein and carbohydrate as fuel sources at rest.

Fats Fuel Physical Activity

Fat is a major energy source during physical activity, and one of the best ways to lose body fat is to exercise. During exercise, fat can be mobilized from any of the following sources: muscle tissue, adipose tissue, blood lipoproteins, and/or any dietary fat consumed during exercise. A number of hormonal changes signal the body to break down stored energy to fuel the working muscles. The hormonal responses, and the amount and source of the fat used, depend on your level of fitness, the type, intensity, and duration of the exercise, and how well-fed you are before you exercise.

For example, adrenaline is a strong stimulator of breaking down stored fat. Blood levels of adrenaline rise dramatically within seconds of beginning exercise, and this action activates additional hormones within the fat cell to begin breaking down fat. Adrenaline also signals the pancreas to *decrease* insulin production. This is important, because insulin inhibits fat breakdown. Thus, when the need for fat as an energy source is high, blood insulin levels are typically low. As you might guess, blood insulin levels are high when we are eating, because during this time our need for getting energy from stored fat is low and the need for fat storage is high.

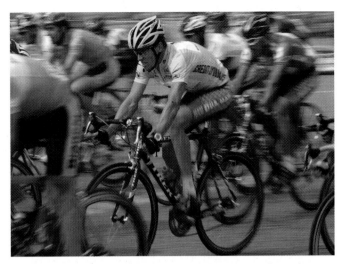

The longer you exercise, the more fat you use for energy. Cyclists in long-distance races use fat stores for energy.

Once fatty acids are released from the adipose cell, they travel in the blood attached to a protein, *albumin*, to the muscles where they enter the mitochondria and use oxygen to produce ATP, which is the cell's energy source. Becoming more physically fit means you can deliver more oxygen to the muscle to use the fat that is delivered there. In addition, you can exercise longer when you are fit. Since the body has only a limited supply of stored carbohydrate as glycogen in muscle tissue, the longer you exercise, the more fat you use for energy. This point is illustrated in Figure 5.8. In this example, an individual is running for four hours at a moderate intensity. The longer they run, the more their muscle glycogen levels become depleted and the more they must rely on fat from the adipose tissue as a fuel source for exercise.

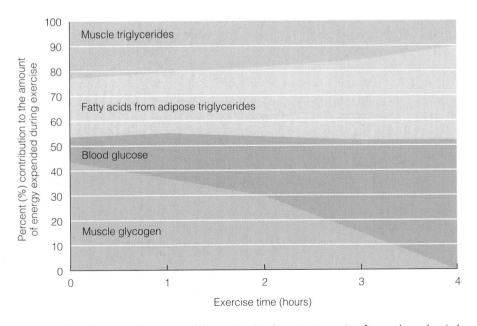

Figure 5.8 Various sources of energy used during exercise. As a person exercises for a prolonged period of time, fatty acids from adipose cells contribute relatively more energy than do carbohydrates stored in the muscle or circulating in our blood. (E. F. Coyle, Substrate utilization during exercise in active people, *Am. J. Clin. Nutr.* 61 (1995, suppl.): 968S–979S.)

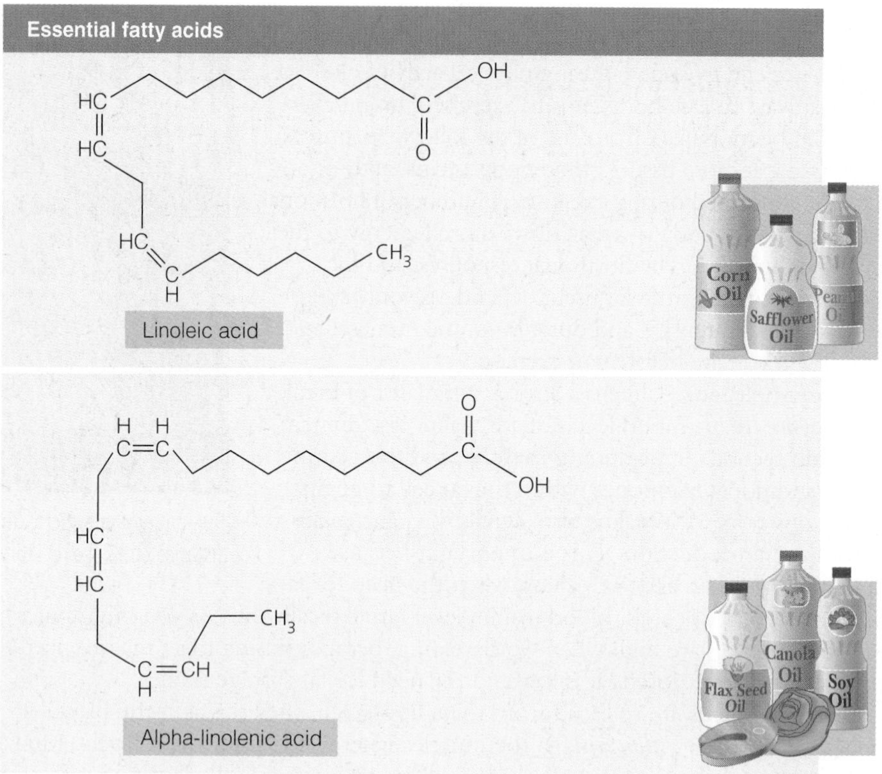

Figure 5.9   The two essential fatty acids: linoleic acid (omega-6 fatty acid) and alpha-linolenic acid (omega-3 fatty acid).

Fats Store Energy for Later Use

Our body stores extra energy in the form of body fat, which then can be used for energy at rest, during exercise, or during periods of low energy intake. Having a readily available energy source in the form of fat allows the body to always have access to energy even when we choose not to eat (or are unable to eat), when we are exercising, and while we are sleeping. Our bodies have little stored carbohydrate—only enough to last about one to two days—and there is no place that our body can store extra protein. We cannot consider our muscles and organs as a place where "extra" protein is stored! For these reasons, the fat stored in our adipose and muscle tissues is necessary to keep the body going. Although we do not want too much stored adipose tissue, some fat storage is essential to good health.

Fats Provide Essential Fatty Acids

essential fatty acids (EFA) Fatty acids that must be consumed in the diet because they cannot be made by our bodies. The two essential fatty acids are linoleic acid and alpha-linolenic acid.

Dietary fat provides the **essential fatty acids (EFA)** needed to make a number of important biological compounds. (Information on the EFA content of various foods is given in Table 5.1, page 161.) Essential fatty acids are called "essential" because they must be consumed in the diet and cannot be made in our bodies. The two essential fatty acids are linoleic acid and alpha-linolenic acid (Figure 5.9).

Linoleic Acid

linoleic acid An essential fatty acid found in vegetable and nut oils; also known as omega-6 fatty acid.

Linoleic acid, also known as *omega-6 fatty acid*, is found in vegetable and nut oils such as sunflower, safflower, corn, soy, and peanut oil. If you eat lots of vegetables, or use vegetable oil–based margarines or vegetable oils, you are probably getting adequate amounts of this essential fatty acid in your diet. Linoleic acid is metabolized in the body to arachidonic acid, which is a precursor to a number of important biological compounds that regulate body functions, such as blood clotting and blood pressure.

Alpha-Linolenic Acid

The second essential fatty acid is **alpha-linolenic acid,** an *omega-3 fatty acid*. This fatty acid is found primarily in leafy green vegetables, flax seeds and flax seed oil, soy oil and foods, canola oil, and fish products and fish oils. You may have read news reports of the health benefits of the omega-3 fatty acids found in many fish. Two of these fatty acids, **eicosapentaenoic acid (EPA)** and **docosahexaenoic acid (DHA),** are metabolic derivatives of alpha-linolenic acid, and are necessary for the synthesis of a number of regulatory compounds in the body. Research indicates that EPA and DHA tend to reduce inflammatory responses in the body, reduce blood clotting and plasma triglycerides, and thereby they reduce an individual's risk of a heart attack.

Fats Enable the Transport of Fat-Soluble Vitamins

Dietary fat enables the transport of the fat-soluble vitamins (A, D, E, and K) needed by our body for many essential metabolic functions. For example, vitamin A is especially important for normal vision and gives you the ability to see at night. Vitamin D is important for regulating blood calcium and phosphorus concentrations within normal ranges, which indirectly helps maintain bone health. If vitamin D is low, blood calcium levels will drop below normal, and the body will draw calcium from the bones to maintain blood levels. Vitamin E functions primarily as an antioxidant in our body and keeps cell membranes healthy by preventing oxidation of body fats. Finally, vitamin K is important for proteins involved in blood clotting and bone health. We discuss these vitamins in detail in Chapters 8 and 9.

Fats Help Maintain Cell Function and Provide Protection to the Body

Fats are a critical part of every cell membrane. The types of fats in cell membranes help to maintain membrane integrity, determine what substances are transported in and out of the cell, and regulate what substances can bind to the cell; thus, fats strongly influence the function of the cell. In addition, fats help maintain cell fluidity and other physical properties of the cell membrane. For example, wild salmon live in very cold water and have high levels of omega-3 fatty acids in their cell membranes. These fats stay fluid and flexible even in very cold environments, which allows the fish to swim in extremely cold water. In the same way, fats help our membranes stay fluid and flexible. For example, we want our red blood cells to be flexible enough to bend and move through the smallest capillaries in our body, delivering oxygen to all our cells. Fats help the red cells to maintain this ability. Fats, especially PUFAs, are also primary components of the tissues of the brain and spinal cord, where they facilitate the transmission of information from one cell to another. We also need fats for the development, growth, and maintenance of these tissues.

Stored body fat also plays an important role in our body. Besides being the primary site of stored energy, adipose tissue pads our body and protects our organs, such as the kidneys and liver, when we fall or are bruised. The fat under our skin acts as insulation to help us retain body heat. Although we often think of body fat as "bad," it does play an important role in keeping our body healthy and functioning properly.

Fats Contribute to the Flavor and Texture of Foods

Dietary fat plays an important role in making food taste good because it adds texture and flavor to foods. Fat makes salad dressings smooth and ice-cream "creamy," and it gives cakes and cookies their moist, tender texture. Americans like fat so much that many of us eat fried foods, such as French fries, on a daily basis.

alpha-linolenic acid An essential fatty acid found in leafy green vegetables, flax seed oil, soy oil, fish oil and fish products; an omega-3 fatty acid.

eicosapentaenoic acid (EPA) A metabolic derivative of alpha-linolenic acid.

docosahexaenoic acid (DHA) Another metabolic derivative of alpha-linolenic acid; together with EPA, it appears to reduce our risk of a heart attack.

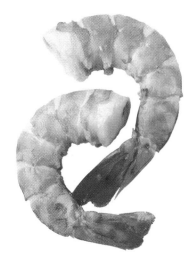

Shrimp are high in omega-3 fatty acid content.

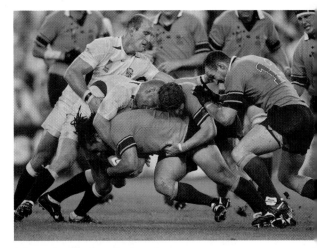

Adipose tissue pads our body and protects our organs when we fall or are bruised.

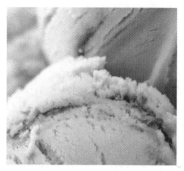

Fat adds texture and flavor to foods.

Fats Help Us to Feel Satiated

Fats in foods contribute to making us feel satiated after a meal. Two factors probably contribute to this effect: first, fat has a much higher energy density than carbohydrate or protein. For example, a pat of butter weighing 5 grams will contain 35 kcals; 5 grams of an apple contains only 3 kcals. So for every gram of fat you consume, you get 2.25 times the amount of energy that you get with the same number of grams consumed in protein or carbohydrate.

Second, fat takes longer to digest than protein or carbohydrate because more steps are involved in the digestion process, which may make you feel fuller for a longer period of time because energy is slowly being released into your body.

On the other hand, you can eat more fat in a meal without feeling overfull because fat is generally compact in its size. Going back to our apple and butter example, one medium apple weighs 117 grams (approximately 4 ounces) and has 70 calories, but the same number of calories of butter—two pats—would hardly make you feel full! Looked at another way, an amount of butter weighing the same number of grams as a medium apple would contain 840 calories!

Recap: Dietary fats play a number of important roles within the body. 1) Dietary fats provide twice the energy of protein and carbohydrate, at 9 calories per gram, and provide the majority of energy required at rest. Fats are also a major fuel source during exercise, especially endurance exercise. 2) Dietary fats provide essential fatty acids (linoleic and alpha-linolenic acid). 3) Dietary fats help transport the fat-soluble vitamins into the body. 4) Dietary fats help regulate cell function and maintain membrane integrity. 5) Stored body fat in the adipose tissue helps protect vital organs and pad the body. 6) Fats contribute to the flavor and texture of foods and the satiety we feel after a meal.

When Are Fats Harmful?

Like many things, a little can be good, but a lot can be harmful. We have just discussed why fats are an essential part of a good diet and necessary for health, but too much fat, regardless of the type, can be damaging to our bodies.

Eating Too Much of Certain Fats Can Lead to Disease

As mentioned earlier, diets high in saturated and *trans* fatty acids increase our risk of cardiovascular disease. Conversely, diets too high in omega-3 fatty acids can increase your risk of stroke, although these types of diets are rare. It is also well documented that diets that are high in fat, regardless of the type of fat, are high in calories and can contribute to weight gain and obesity. Thus, our goal is to select the right amount and types of fats to include in our diet.

Fats Limit the Shelf Life of Foods

Fats make food taste good. This is one reason most of our fast foods and convenience foods are high in fat and why they are so popular with Americans. Unfortunately, fats are susceptible to oxidation and become rancid quickly if they are not stored appropriately. This means that foods high in fat such as cookies, crackers, chips, and breads quickly become stale on the grocery store shelf. Manufacturers add preservatives to reduce the rancidity of the fats in the products and increase their shelf life because high-fat products made without preservatives spoil quickly. For example, freshly baked bread without preservatives will become stale and moldy more quickly than bread made with preservatives. The consumer has to make a decision when buying products with added fat: do I want a longer shelf life or fewer preservatives? It is important to note that not all preservatives added to increase the shelf life of high-fat products are bad. For example, vitamin E, an antioxidant, is frequently added to margarines to increase their shelf life.

Recap: The fats we eat can either contribute to health or increase our risk of disease. Selecting the right amount and type of fats in your diet is important for improving health. Because fats added to foods can be oxidized and become rancid, foods high in fat can quickly spoil. Manufacturers add preservatives to foods high in fat to increase their shelf life.

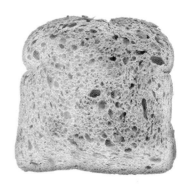

Foods containing fats, such as bread, can spoil quickly.

How Much Fat Should We Eat?

Without a doubt, Americans think dietary fat is bad! How many people have you heard say they are trying to dramatically reduce fat from their diet? Yet, because fat plays such an important role in keeping our bodies healthy, we must eat diets providing a moderate amount of energy from fat. But what, exactly, is a moderate amount? And what foods contain the most healthful fats? We'll explore these questions here.

Dietary Reference Intake for Total Fat

The Acceptable Macronutrient Distribution Range (AMDR) for fat is 20 to 35% of total energy (Institute of Medicine 2002). This recommendation is based on evidence indicating that higher intakes of fat increase the risk of obesity and its complications, especially heart disease, but that diets too low in fat and too high in carbohydrate can also increase the risk of heart disease if they cause blood triglycerides to increase (Institute of Medicine 2002). Within this range of fat intake, it is also recommended that we minimize our intake of saturated and *trans* fatty acids; these changes will lower our risk of heart disease.

Because carbohydrate is essential in replenishing glycogen, athletes and other physically active people are advised to consume less fat and more carbohydrate than sedentary people. Specifically, it is recommended that athletes consume 20 to 25% of their total energy from fat, 55 to 60% of energy from carbohydrate, and 12 to 15% of energy from protein (Manore, Barr, and Butterfield 2000). This level of fat intake represents approximately 45 to 55 grams per day of fat for an athlete consuming 2000 kcal per day, and 78 to 97 grams per day of fat for an athlete consuming 3500 kcal per day.

Although many people trying to lose weight consume less than 20% of their energy from fat, this practice may do more harm than good, especially if they are also limiting energy intake (eating fewer than 1500 kilocalories per day). Research suggests that very low fat diets, or those with less than 15% of energy from fat, do not provide additional health or performance benefits over moderate-fat diets and are usually very difficult to follow (Lichenstein and Van Horn 1998). In fact, most people find they feel better, are more successful in weight maintenance, and are less preoccupied with food if they keep their fat intakes at 20 to 25% of energy intake. Additionally, people attempting to reduce their dietary fat frequently eliminate food groups, such as meat, dairy, eggs, and nuts. Unfortunately, eliminating these food groups also eliminates potential sources of protein and many essential vitamins and minerals important for good health and maintaining an active lifestyle. Diets extremely low in fat may also be deficient in essential fatty acids.

Liz   *Nutri-Case*

"Lately I'm hungry all the time. I read on a Web site last night that if I limit my total fat intake to no more than 10% of my total calories, I can eat all the carbohydrate and protein that I want, and I won't gain weight. So I went right out to the yogurt shop down the street and ordered a large sundae with nonfat vanilla yogurt and fat-free chocolate syrup. I have to admit, though, that an hour or so after I ate it, I was hungry again. Maybe it's stress. . . ."

What do you think of Liz's approach to her persistent hunger? What have you learned in this chapter about the role of fats that might be important information to share with her?

Dietary Reference Intakes for Essential Fatty Acids

For the first time, DRIs for the two essential fatty acids were set in 2002 (Institute of Medicine 2002). The adequate intake (AI) for linoleic acid is 14 to 17 grams per day for adult men and 11 to 12 grams per day for women 19 years and older, whereas the AI for alpha-linolenic acid is 1.6 grams per day for adult men and 1.1 grams per day for adult women. Using the typical energy intakes for adult men and women, this translates into an AMDR of 5 to 10% of energy for linoleic acid and 0.6 to 1.2% for alpha-linolenic acid. For example, an individual consuming 2000 kcals per day should consume about 11 to 22 grams per day of linoleic acid and about 1.3 to 2.6 grams per day of alpha-linolenic acid.

Most Americans Eat Within the Recommended Amount of Fat but Eat the Wrong Types

Nutritionists have been recommending the reduction of dietary fat for a decade. According to the most recent data, relative fat intake has decreased from 45% of total energy intake in 1965 to 34% of energy intake in 1995 for both men and women (USDA 1998). However, this reduction in the percentage of fat consumed is misleading because Americans are consuming 15% more calories overall. As shown in Table 5.2, these additional calories have come mostly in the form of carbohydrates and proteins, and less in fats, but the end result is that daily fat consumption has not decreased; instead, it has *increased* slightly (Harnack, Jeffery, and Boutelle 2000).

Of the dietary fat we eat, saturated and *trans* fats are most highly correlated with an increased risk of heart disease because they increase blood cholesterol levels by altering the way cholesterol is removed from the blood. Thus, the recommended intake of saturated fat is less than 7% of our total energy; unfortunately, our average intake of saturated fats is between 11 and 12% of energy (Expert Panel on Detection, Evaluation, and Treatment of High Blood Cholesterol in Adults 2001). The Institute of Medicine (2002) also recommends that we keep our intake of *trans* fatty acids to an absolute minimum. Determining the actual amount of *trans* fatty acids consumed in America has been hindered by the lack of an accurate and comprehensive database of foods containing *trans* fatty acids. At the present time, a best guess as to the amount of *trans* fatty acid consumed in the United States comes from a recent national survey (Allison et al. 1999), which estimated our intake at 2.6% of our total fat intake.

Table 5.2 Trends in Energy Availability in the United States from 1970 to 1994

Nutrient	Year						Percentage change from 1970 to 1994
	1970	*1975*	*1980*	*1985*	*1990*	*1994*	
Food energy available (kcal/day)	3298	3203	3298	3489	3609	3800	+15.2
Protein (g/day)	95	93	96	101	105	110	+15.8
Carbohydrate (g/day)	386	385	406	420	458	491	+27.2
Total fat (g/day)	154	146	153	163	156	159	+3.2
Percentage (%) of total energy from fat	42	41	42	42	39	38	−9.5

Source: Adapted from L. J. Harnack, R. W. Jeffery, and K. N. Boutelle. Temporal trends in energy intake in the United States: an ecologic perspective. *Am. J. Clin. Nutr.* 71 (2000): 1478–1484.

Recap: The Acceptable Macronutrient Distribution Range (AMDR) for total fat is 20 to 35% of total energy. The adequate intake (AI) for linoleic acid is 14 to 17 grams per day for adult men and 11 to 12 grams per day for adult women. The AI for alpha-linolenic acid is 1.6 grams per day for adult men and 1.1 grams per day for adult women. Because saturated and *trans* fatty acids can increase the risk of heart disease, health professionals recommend that we reduce our intake of saturated fat to less than 7% of our total energy intake and reduce our intake of *trans* fatty acids to the absolute minimum.

Shopper's Guide: Food Sources of Fat

The last time you popped a frozen dinner into the microwave, did you stop and read the Nutrition Facts label on the box? If you had, you might have been shocked to learn how much saturated fat was in the meal. As we discuss here, many processed foods are hidden sources of fat, especially saturated fat. In contrast, many whole foods, such as oils and nuts, are rich sources of the healthful fats our bodies need.

Visible versus Invisible Fats

Americans love fat. We not only eat lots of high-fat foods, but also commonly add fat to our foods to improve their taste. There is nothing like cream in our coffee or real butter on our pancakes. These added fats, such as oils, butter, cream, shortening, margarine, or dressings (such as mayonnaise and salad dressings) are called **visible fats** because we can easily see that we are adding them to our food.

When we add fat to foods ourselves, we know how much we are adding and what kind. When fat is added in the preparation of a casserole or a fast food burger and fries, we are less aware of how much or what type of fat is actually there. In fact, unless we read food labels carefully, we might not be aware that a food contains any fat at all. We call fats in prepared and processed foods **invisible fats** because they are hidden within the food. In fact, their invisibility often tricks us into choosing them over more healthful foods. For example, a slice of yellow cake is

visible fats   Fat we can see in our foods or see added to foods, such as butter, margarine, cream, shortening, salad dressings, chicken skin, and untrimmed fat on meat.

invisible fats   Fats that are hidden in foods, such as the fats found in baked goods, regular-fat dairy products, marbling in meat, and fried foods.

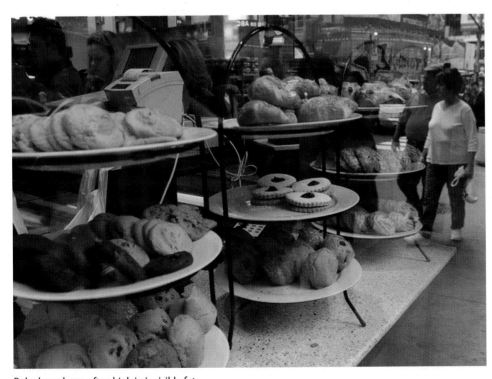

Baked goods are often high in invisible fats.

much higher in fat (40% of total energy) than a slice of angel food cake (1% of total energy). Yet many consumers just assume the fat content of these foods are the same, since they are both cake. For most of us, the majority of the fat in our diets comes from invisible fat. Foods that can be high in invisible fats are baked goods, regular-fat dairy products, processed meats or meats that are not trimmed, and most convenience and fast foods, such as hamburgers, hot dogs, chips, ice cream, French fries, and other fried foods.

As introduced in Chapter 2, one of the major limitations of the current USDA Food Guide Pyramid is that it does not clearly distinguish between higher fat and lower fat food choices. This limitation and others has led to a national campaign to revise the Food Guide Pyramid so that it can better assist consumers with making healthful food choices. Refer to the Nutrition Debate on page 192 to learn more about the controversies surrounding the Food Guide Pyramid.

Because high-fat diets have been associated with obesity, many Americans have tried to reduce their total fat intake. Food manufacturers have been more than happy to provide consumers with low-fat alternatives to their favorite foods. However, these lower-fat foods may not always have fewer calories. Read the Highlight box below and Table 5.3 to learn how to be a better consumer of reduced-fat foods.

Low-Fat, Reduced-Fat, Non-Fat . . . What's the Difference?

Although we all love high-fat foods, we also know that eating too much fat isn't good for our health or our waistlines. Because of this concern, food manufacturers have produced a host of modified fat foods—so you can have your cake and eat it too! In fact, it is now estimated that there are over 5000 different fat-modified foods on the market (Calloway 1998; Sigman-Grant 1997). This means that we have similar foods that come in a wide range of fat contents. For example, you can purchase full-fat, low-fat, or fat-free milk, ice cream, sour cream, cheese, and yogurt.

In Table 5.3, we list a number of full-fat foods with their lower-fat alternatives. These products, if incorporated in the diet on a regular basis, can significantly reduce the amount of fat consumed but may or may not reduce the amount of energy consumed. For example, drinking nonfat milk (86 kilocalories and 0.5 grams of fat per serving) instead of whole milk (150 kilocalories and 8.2 grams of fat per serving) will dramatically reduce both fat and energy intake. However, eating fat-free Fig Newton cookies (3 cookies have 204 kilocalories and 0 grams of fat) instead of regular Fig Newton cookies (3 cookies have 210 kilocalories and 4.5 grams of fat) will not reduce your energy intake, even though it will reduce your fat intake by 4.5 grams per serving.

Thus, if you think that eating fat-free-foods means you're not getting any calories and can eat all you want without gaining weight, you're mistaken. The reduced fat is often replaced with added carbohydrate, as with the Fig Newton example, resulting in a very similar total energy intake. Thus, if you want to reduce both the amount of fat and the number of calories you consume, you must read the labels of modified-fat foods carefully before you buy (Calloway 1998). ●

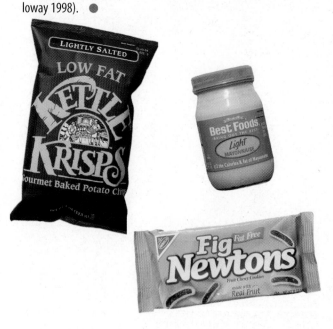

Food Sources of Beneficial Fats

Americans appear to get adequate amounts of omega-6 fatty acids, probably because of the high amount of salad dressings, vegetable oils, margarine, and mayonnaise we eat; however, our consumption of omega-3 fatty acids is more variable and can be low in the diets of people who do not eat fish or walnuts, drink soy milk, or use soybean, canola, or flax oil. Table 5.4 identifies the omega-3 fatty acid content of various foods. In general, we want to switch to healthier sources of fats without increasing our total fat intake. For example, use olive and canola oil in place of butter and margarine, and select fish more frequently instead of high fat meat sources (hot dogs, hamburgers, sausage). Dairy products can be high in saturated fats, so select low- and reduced-fat dairy products when possible and reduce the intake of hard cheeses and

Table 5.3 Comparison of Full-Fat, Reduced-Fat, and Low-Fat Foods

Product	Serving Size	Energy (kcal)	Protein (g)	Carbohydrate (g)	Fat (g)
Milk, whole (3.3% fat)	8 oz.	150	8.0	11.4	8.2
Milk, 2% fat	8 oz.	121	8.1	11.7	4.7
Milk, 1% fat	8 oz.	102	8.0	11.7	2.6
Milk, skim (nonfat)	8 oz.	86	8.4	11.9	0.5
Cheese, cheddar regular	1 oz.	111	7.1	0.5	9.1
Cheese, cheddar low-fat	1 oz.	81	9.1	0.0	5.1
Cheese, cheddar nonfat	1 oz.	41	6.8	4.0	0.0
Mayonnaise, regular	1 tbsp.	100	0.0	0.0	11.0
Mayonnaise, light	1 tbsp.	50	0.0	1.0	5.0
Mayonnaise, fat-free	1 tbsp.	10	0.0	2.0	0.0
Margarine, regular corn oil	1 tbsp.	100	0.0	0.0	11.0
Margarine, reduced-fat	1 tbsp.	60	0.0	0.0	7.0
Peanut butter, regular	1 tbsp.	95	4.1	3.1	8.2
Peanut butter, reduced-fat	1 tbsp.	81	4.4	5.2	5.4
Cream cheese, soft regular	1 tbsp.	50	1.0	0.5	5.0
Cream cheese, soft light	1 tbsp.	35	1.5	1.0	2.5
Cream cheese, soft nonfat	1 tbsp.	15	2.5	1.0	0.0
Crackers, Wheat Thins Regular	18 crackers	158	2.3	21.4	6.8
Crackers, Wheat Thins Reduced fat	18 crackers	120	2.0	21.0	4.0
Cookies, Oreo's regular	3 cookies	160	2.0	23.0	7.0
Cookies, Oreo's reduced-fat	3 cookies	130	2.0	25.0	3.5
Cookies, Fig Newton regular	3 cookies	210	3.0	30.0	4.5
Cookies, Fig Newton, fat-free	3 cookies	204	2.4	26.8	0.0
Breakfast bars, regular	1 bar	140	2.0	27.0	2.8
Breakfast bars, fat-free	1 bar	110	2.0	26.0	0.0

The Food and Drug Administration and the U.S. Department of Agriculture have set specific regulations on allowable product descriptions for reduced-fat products. The following claims are defined for one serving:
Fat-free: less than 0.5 gram of fat
Low-fat: 3 grams or less of fat
Reduced- or less fat: at least 25% less fat as compared to a standard serving
Light: one-third fewer calories or 50% less fat as compared with a standard serving size
Source: Data from Food Processor, Version 7.01 (ESHA Research, Salem, OR).

How Much Fat Is in This Food?

How do you know how much fat is in a food you buy? One simple way to determine the amount of fat in the food you eat is to read the Nutrition Facts panel on the label. By becoming a better label reader, you can make more healthful food selections. Two cracker labels are shown here; one cracker is higher in fat than the other. Let's review how you can read the label so you know what percentage of energy is coming from fat from each product. These calculations are relatively simple.

1. Divide the total calories from fat by the total calories per serving, and multiply the answer by 100.

   • For the Regular Wheat Crackers: 50 calories/150 calories = 0.33 × 100 = 33%

   Thus, for the regular crackers, the total energy coming from fat is 33%.

   • For the Reduced-Fat Wheat Crackers: 35 calories/130 calories = 0.269 × 100 = 27

   Thus, for the reduced-fat crackers, the total energy coming from fat is 27%.

   You can see that, although the total amount of energy per serving is not very different between these two crackers, the amount of fat is quite different.

2. If the total calories per serving from fat are not given on the label, you can quickly calculate this value by multiplying the grams of total fat per serving by 9 (as there are 9 calories per gram of fat).

   • For the Regular Wheat Crackers: 6 g fat × 9 calories/gram = 54 calories of fat

   • To calculate percentage of calories from fat: 54 calories/150 calories = 0.36 × 100 = 36%

   You can see that this value is not exactly the same as the 50 calories reported on the label or the 33% of calories from fat calculated in example 1. The values on food labels are rounded off, so your estimations may not be identical when you do this second calculation.

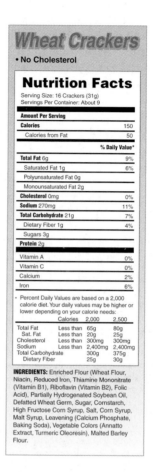

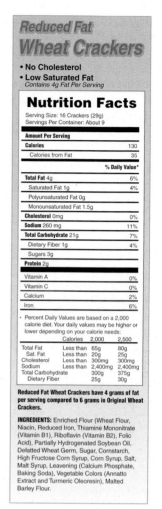

Refer to Table 5.3, which gives a list of regular, reduced-fat, and fat-free foods. You can quickly calculate the percentage of fat per serving for these foods by following the same series of steps: first multiply the grams of fat per serving by 9 calories per gram; then divide this number by the total calories per serving; and finally, multiply by 100. ●

cheese spreads. Read the Nutrition Label Activity above to learn how to calculate the amount of fat calories in the foods you buy.

It is important to recognize that there can be some risk associated with eating large amounts of fish on a regular basis. Some species of fish contain high levels of

Table 5.4   Omega-3 Fatty Acid Content of Selected Foods

Food Item	Omega-3 Fatty Acid (grams per serving)
Salmon oil (fish oil) (1 tbsp.)	4.39 g
Herring, Atlantic broiled (3 oz.)	1.52 g
Herring oil (1 tbsp.)	1.52 g
Canola oil (1 tbsp.)	1.27 g
Shrimp, broiled (3 oz.)	1.11 g
Trout, rainbow fillet baked (3 oz.)	1.05 g
Halibut, fillet baked (3 oz.)	0.58 g
Walnuts (1 tbsp.)	0.51 g
Salmon, smoked chinook (3 oz.)	0.50 g
Crab, Dungeness steamed (3 oz.)	0.34 g
Tuna, light in water (3 oz.)	0.23 g

Source: Data from Food Processor, Version 7.01 (ESHA Research, Salem, OR).

poisons such as mercury, polychlorinated biphenyls (PCBs), and other environmental contaminants. These poisons can accumulate in the bodies of individuals who regularly consume contaminated fish. Women who are pregnant or breast-feeding, women who may become pregnant, and small children are at particularly high risk for toxicity from these contaminants. Not all fish are contaminated; sport-caught fish and predator fish such as shark, swordfish, and King mackerel tend to have higher levels of contaminates. It is generally considered safe for pregnant women or women who become pregnant to consume up to 12 ounces of a variety of fish each week. Types of fish that are currently considered safe to consume include salmon (except from the Great Lakes region), farmed trout, flounder, sole, mahi mahi, and cooked shellfish. Fish that should be avoided by pregnant and breastfeeding women and small children include raw fish and shellfish of any kind, shark, swordfish, golden bass, golden snapper, marlin, bluefish, and largemouth and smallmouth bass. For more information on seafood contamination and recommendations for safe fish consumption, refer to the websites for the U.S. Environmental Protection Agency (EPA) at http://www.epa.gov/waterscience/fish/. The EPA is the agency that regulates sport-caught fish. You can also refer to the website of the U.S. Food and Drug Administration (FDA) at http://vm.cfsan.fda.gov/~dms/admehg.html. The FDA is the agency that regulates all commercial fish.

Fat Replacers

One way to lower the fat content of foods, such as chips, muffins, cakes, and cookies, is by replacing the fat in a food with a *fat replacer*. Snack foods have been the primary target for fat replacers since it is more difficult to eliminate the fat from these types of products without dramatically changing the taste. A description of the most common fat replacers used in the United States is provided in Table 5.5. Some of these products, such as olestra (brand name Olean), may cause gastrointestinal distress if used in large quantities. Until recently, foods containing olestra had to bear a label warning of potential gastrointestinal side effects. In 2003, the U.S. Food and Drug Administration (FDA) announced that this warning is no longer necessary, as recent research indicates that olestra causes only mild,

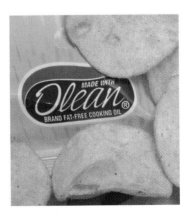

Snack foods have been the primary target for fat replacers, such as Olean, since it is more difficult to eliminate the fat from these types of foods without dramatically changing the taste.

Table 5.5 Common Fat Replacers

Types of Fat Replacers	Names of Common Fat Replacers	Description	Foods That May Contain Fat Replacers
Carbohydrate-based fat replacers that provide energy	Dextrins Maltodextrins Modified food starch	Bland, nonsweet carbohydrates made from hydrolyzed starches that can mimic the texture and mouth feel of fat due to their gel-like structure. Provides 1 to 4 kcal per gram. Can completely replace or partially replace the fat in food.	Salad dressings Puddings Spreads Dairy products Frozen desserts
	Oatrim (Beta-Trim™, TrimChoice)	A beta-glucan (type of soluble fiber) derived from oat fiber. Provides 4 kcal per gram. Can replace fat and add the additional cholesterol-lowering benefit of oat bran.	Baked goods Fillings and frostings Frozen desserts Dairy beverages Cheese Salad dressings Processed meats Confections
Carbohydrate-based fat replacers that provide negligible energy (dietary fibers)	Z-Trim	A noncaloric, bland mix of insoluble fiber made from the crushed hulls of corn, oats and rice.	Baked goods Burgers Hot dogs Cheese Ice cream Yogurt
	Polydextrose	A nonsweet starch polymer made from food-grade dextrose and small amounts of sorbitol and citric acid. Polydextrose passes through the body undigested, with only 5–10% digested, and provide only 1 kcal per gram. Can replace up to one half the fat in a product.	Baked goods Chewing gums Confections Salad dressings Frozen dairy desserts Gelatins Puddings
	Gum	Gums are a type of dietary fiber that mimic the functional properties of fat when water is used to replace fat in foods. Gums are not digested in the small intestine so add few calories to the products made with them.	Salad dressings Desserts Processed meats
Protein-based fat replacers	Microparticulated protein (Simplesse)	Made from milk or egg white proteins, water, sugar, pectin, and citric acid. Supplies 1–2 kcal per gram.	Baked goods Butter Cheese Mayonnaise spreads Salad dressings Sour cream
Fat-based fat replacers	Olestra (Olean)	The most studied fat replacer on the market. Made by binding sucrose with 6–8 long-chain fatty acids. Olestra is not sweet, has the appearance, taste, texture and mouth feel of fat, and can be used in fried, cooked and baked products. Because it is not digested, it is calorie-free, but it may reduce the absorption of fat-soluble vitamins. Foods made with olestra have vitamins A, D, E and K added.	Chips Crackers

Source: Calorie Control Council, 5775 Peachtree-Dunwoody Road, Building G, Suite 500, Atlanta, GA 30342. http://www.caloriecontrol.org

infrequent discomfort. Thus, labels for foods containing olestra will soon be revised to meet this new FDA ruling.

Since fat replacers are new to the market, the effect they have on total fat intake and the reduction of obesity and cardiovascular disease has not yet been determined. Thus, the benefit of their use for most Americans is still controversial.

Hannah   *Nutri-Case*

"Friday is my favorite day at school, because it's pizza day! Today I had two slices of pepperoni pizza, a carton of milk to drink, and banana pudding for dessert. I wish it could be pizza day every day!"

What important nutrients did Hannah consume in her lunch today? What nutrients were lacking? If Hannah has this type of lunch just once a week, do you think it presents a problem? What additional information about Hannah and her family would help you to answer this question?

Recap: Visible fats are those foods that can be easily recognized as containing fat. Invisible fats are those fats added to our food during the manufacturing or cooking process so we are not aware of how much fat was added. Fat replacers are those substances used to replace the typical fats found in foods to reduce the amount of fat in the food.

What Health Problems Are Related to Fat Intake or Metabolism?

There appears to be a generally held assumption that if you eat fat-free or low-fat foods you will lose weight and prevent chronic diseases. Certainly, we know that high-fat diets, especially those high in saturated and *trans* fatty acids, can contribute to chronic diseases, including heart disease and cancer; however, as we have explored in this chapter, unsaturated fatty acids do not have this negative effect and are essential to good health. Thus, a sensible health goal would be to eat the appropriate amounts and types of fat.

Fats Can Protect Against or Promote Cardiovascular Disease

Cardiovascular disease is a general term used to refer to any abnormal condition involving dysfunction of the heart and blood vessels. A common form of this disease occurs when blood vessels supplying the heart (the *coronary arteries*) become blocked or constricted; such blockage reduces blood flow to the heart or brain so can result in a heart attack or a stroke. According to the Centers for Disease Control and Prevention (NCCDPHP, 2002), heart disease is the leading cause of death in the United States across racial and ethnic groups and is a major cause of permanent disability (Figure 5.10). Coronary artery disease, one form of cardiovascular disease, is the leading cause of death in the United States and accounts for more than 30% of all deaths, while stroke is the third leading cause of death and accounts for about 10% of all deaths. Overall, about 61 million Americans of all ages suffer from cardiovascular diseases and it is estimated that in 2001 the cost of this disease was $300 billion.

cardiovascular disease   A general term that refers to abnormal conditions involving dysfunction of the heart and blood vessels; cardiovascular disease can result in heart attack or stroke.

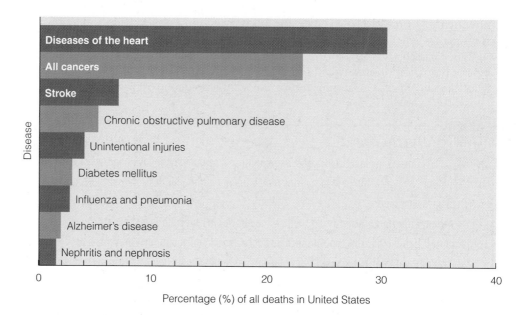

Figure 5.10 Cardiovascular disease, which includes heart disease, is the leading cause of death in the United States. (National Center for Chronic Disease Prevention and Health Promotion (NCCDPHP). 2002. Chronic Disease Prevention. Chronic Disease Overview. www.cdc.gov/nccdphp/overview.htm. Accessed February 2004.)

Risk Factors for Cardiovascular Disease

Over the last two decades, researchers have identified a number of factors that contribute to an increased risk for cardiovascular disease. Following is a brief description of each of these major risk factors, many of which have a dietary component (Hahn and Heath 1998).

- Overweight—Being overweight is associated with higher rates of death from cardiovascular disease. The risk is due primarily to a greater occurrence of high blood pressure, abnormal blood lipids (discussed in more detail on page 181), and higher rates of diabetes in overweight individuals. In general, an overweight condition develops from an energy imbalance from eating too much and exercising too little (see Chapter 11).

- Physical inactivity—Numerous research studies have shown that physical activity can reduce your risk of cardiovascular disease by improving several risk factors associated with the disease, including improved blood lipid levels, lower resting blood pressure, lower body fat and weight, and improved blood glucose levels both at rest and after eating.

- Smoking—There is strong evidence that smoking increases your risk for cardiovascular disease. Research indicates that smokers have a 70% greater chance of developing cardiovascular disease than nonsmokers. Without question, smoking cessation or never starting initially is one of the best ways to reduce your risk of cardiovascular disease. People who stop smoking live longer than those who continue to smoke, and a 15-year cessation period will reduce your risk factors for cardiovascular disease to those of a nonsmoker.

- High blood pressure—High blood pressure stresses the heart and increases the chance that blockage or rupture of a blood vessel will occur. Elevated blood pressure is associated with a number of factors, including dietary factors (e.g., high sodium intakes or low calcium intakes, high caffeine intake), elevated blood lipid levels, obesity, smoking, diabetes mellitus, and physical inactivity.

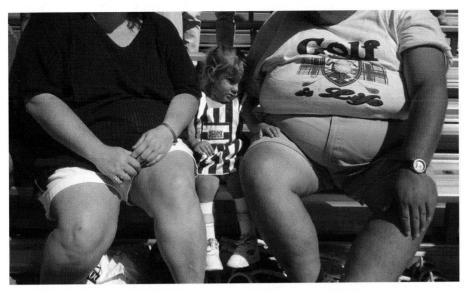

Being overweight is associated with higher rates of death from cardiovascular disease.

- Diabetes mellitus—As discussed in Chapter 4, in many individuals with diabetes, the condition is directly related to being overweight or obese, which is also associated with abnormal blood lipids and high blood pressure. The risk for cardiovascular disease is three times higher in women with diabetes and two times higher in men with diabetes compared to individuals without diabetes.

Calculating Your Risk for Cardiovascular Disease

You can estimate your risk of developing cardiovascular disease if you know your blood pressure and blood lipids levels. Your blood lipid levels are a measurement of the fat in your blood and include the measurement of total blood cholesterol and some of the lipoproteins in the blood that carry fats to and from your cells. The significance of measuring your blood lipid levels, as well as the types of lipoproteins typically measured, are discussed below. If you do not know this information about yourself, the next time you visit the doctor, ask to have your blood pressure taken and your blood lipids measured. It is especially important to do this if you have a family history of heart disease. The first step is to calculate the number of points for each risk factor in Figure 5.11, and then compare your total points to the points in the 10-year risk column. You can also do this quick assessment on family members or friends to help them become more aware of their risk factors for cardiovascular disease. There is also an online version of this risk calculator at http://hin.nhlbi. nih.gov/atpiii/calculator.asp?usertype=prof.

The Role of Dietary Fats in Cardiovascular Disease

As you recall from our discussion of fat metabolism, fats are transported in the blood by lipoproteins made up of a lipid center and a protein outer coat. These lipoproteins are soluble in our blood, and so they are commonly called *blood lipids*. At various times, whether eating or fasting, our blood contains a different mix of various types of these blood lipids. Research indicates that high intakes of saturated and *trans* fatty acids negatively alter the blood lipid assessment measures associated with heart disease. These blood lipid assessment measures are total blood cholesterol and the cholesterol found in very-low density lipoproteins (VLDLs) and low-density lipoproteins (LDLs). Conversely, omega-3 fatty acids decrease our risk of heart disease in a number of ways, one of which is by increasing high-density lipoproteins (HDLs) (Harris, 1997). We will talk about each of these blood lipid assessment measures or lipoproteins and explain how they are linked to heart disease risk.

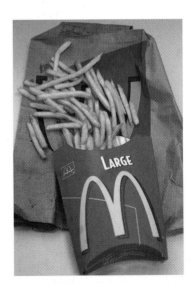

Because foods fried in hydrogenated vegetable oils, such as French fries, are high in *trans* fatty acids, these types of foods should be limited in our diet.

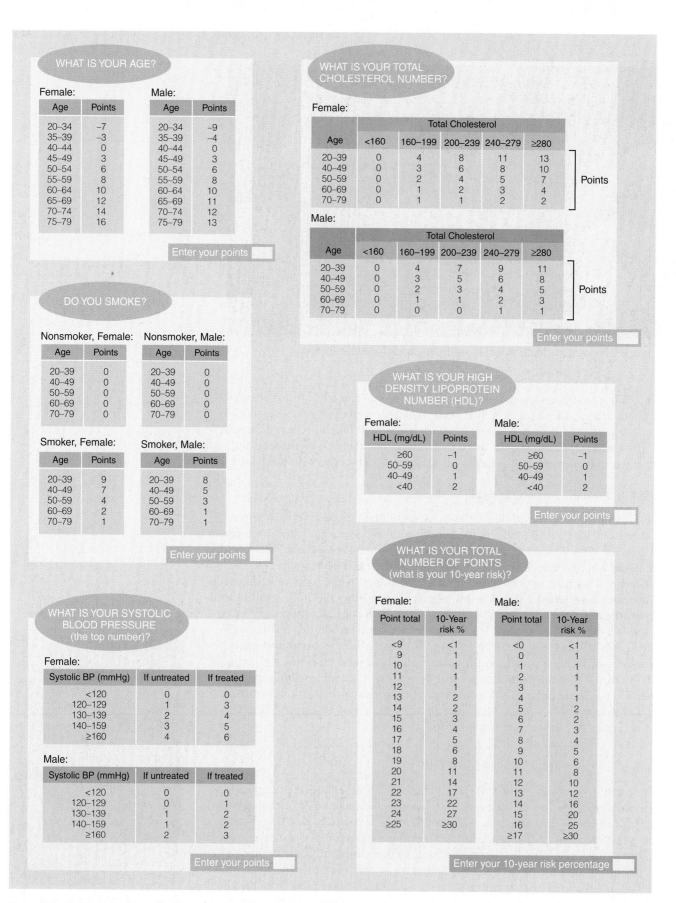

Figure 5.11   Calculation matrix to estimate the 10-year risk for cardiovascular disease for men and women.

Source: National Institutes of Health, *Third Report of the National Cholesterol Education Program: Detection, evaluation and treatment of high blood cholesterol in adults (ATP:III).* Bethesda, MD: National Cholesterol Education Program, National Heart, Lung, and Blood Institute, NIH, May 2001. Website: http://www.nhlbi.nih.gov/guideline/cholesterol/atp3xsum.pdf

We have already discussed that high blood cholesterol increases the risk of heart disease. The question is—how? Much of this blood cholesterol is packaged in the LDLs that circulate in the blood. Normally, cells that need the cholesterol take up these lipoproteins; however, diets high in saturated fat *decrease* the removal of these lipoproteins by the cells. Failure to remove the LDLs from the blood results in their continued circulation in the blood. The more cholesterol circulating in the blood, the greater the risk that some of it will adhere to the walls of the blood vessels. As more and more cholesterol builds up, it forms a fatty patch, or *plaque*, that eventually blocks the artery (Figure 5.12). Because high blood levels of LDL-cholesterol increase your risk of heart disease, it is often labeled the "bad cholesterol."

For some individuals, the level of dietary cholesterol eaten can also influence blood cholesterol levels. As you learned earlier, we consume cholesterol in our diet and make it in our body. Normally, as the dietary level of cholesterol increases, the body decreases the amount of cholesterol it makes, which keeps the body's level of cholesterol constant. Unfortunately, this feedback mechanism does not work well in everyone. For some individuals, eating dietary cholesterol doesn't decrease the amount of cholesterol produced in the body, and their total body cholesterol levels rise. This also increases the levels of cholesterol in the blood. These individuals benefit from reducing their intake of dietary cholesterol. Although this appears somewhat complicated, both dietary cholesterol and saturated fats are found in animal foods; thus, by limiting your intake of animal products or selecting low-fat animal products you will reduce your intake of both saturated fat and cholesterol.

HDLs are small lipoproteins that circulate in the blood, picking up cholesterol and returning it to the liver. The liver takes up the HDLs and the cholesterol they carry, effectively removing it from the circulatory system. The liver then uses this cholesterol to make the bile required for the digestion of fats in the small intestine. High levels of HDL-cholesterol are therefore associated with a lower risk of coronary artery disease. That's why HDL cholesterol is often referred to as the "good cholesterol." There is some evidence that diets high in omega-3 fatty acids and participating in regular physical exercise can modestly *increase* HDL-cholesterol levels.

High blood triglyceride levels can also increase your risk of heart disease. Triglycerides are primarily transported in chylomicrons and VLDLs. Normally, chylomicrons, which transport dietary triglycerides, are low in the blood except

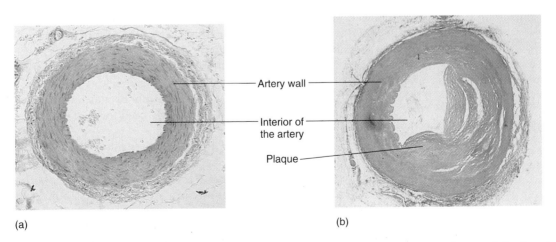

(a) (b)

Figure 5.12 These light micrographs show a cross section of **(a)** a normal artery containing little cholesterol-rich plaque and allowing adequate blood flow through the heart, and **(b)** an artery that is partially blocked with cholesterol-rich plaque, which can lead to a heart attack.

Blood Lipid Levels: Know Your Numbers!

One of the most important steps you can take to reduce your risk of heart disease is to know your "numbers"—that is, your blood lipid values. The next time you go to a physician ask to have your blood lipid levels measured. Record these numbers and have them checked every one to two years, or each time you visit your physician for a checkup. Many college and university health clinics, as well as community health fairs, offer a screening for total cholesterol as well. Based on your total cholesterol values, you can go to your physician to have a more complete testing of all your blood lipids. In this way you can know your own blood lipid levels and keep track of your risk for heart disease.

How are your blood lipids actually measured? First, a blood sample is taken, and the lipoproteins in your blood are extracted. Total cholesterol is determined by breaking apart all the lipoproteins and measuring their combined cholesterol content. You can see from Figure 5.13 that each of the lipoproteins contains some cholesterol and some triglycerides. This same process is used to determine your total blood triglycerides level. The next step is to measure the amount of cholesterol in the LDLs and HDLs, since these two lipoproteins can either raise or lower your risk of heart disease. These lipoproteins are separated, and the amount of cholesterol in each one is determined to give you an LDL-cholesterol and an HDL-cholesterol value. Once you have these values, you can compare them to the "target" level and see how you measure up.

Let's look at the blood lipid profile for Liz. Notice that each of the blood lipids discussed in this chapter is listed here, along with the normal, or target, values. How does Liz measure up? (Remember, Liz is a dancer and watches everything she eats!) We've also included space for you to write in and evaluate your own blood lipid values. ●

Liz's Blood Lipid Profile: How does she measure up?

Blood Lipid Parameter	Liz's Target Values*	Liz's Values	How Does She Measure Up?	Your Values	How Do You Measure Up?
Total blood cholesterol	<200 mg/dL	151 mg/dL			
HDL-cholesterol	>40 mg/dL	56 mg/dL			
LDL-cholesterol	<100 mg/dL	88 mg/dL			
Triglycerides	<150 mg/dL	42 mg/dL			

*Values from the National Institutes of Health, *Third Report of the National Cholesterol Education Program: Detection, evaluation and treatment of high blood cholesterol in adults (ATP:III)*. Bethesda, MD. National Cholesterol Education Program, National Heart, Lung, and Blood Institute, NIH, May 2001. Web site: http://www.nhlbi.nih.gov/guidelines/cholesterol/atp3xsum.pdf

after a meal. Therefore, we are most concerned about the triglycerides transported in the VLDLs, which are made primarily in the liver and intestines and are filled with endogenous triglycerides (triglycerides made in the body). Diets high in fat, simple sugars, and extra calories can increase the production of endogenous VLDLs, while diets high in omega-3 fatty acids can help reduce the production of endogenous triglycerides and VLDLs. In addition, exercise can reduce VLDLs because the fat produced in the body is quickly used for energy instead of remaining to circulate in the blood.

Table 5.6 contains a brief description and overview of the functions of the various blood lipoproteins. Figure 5.13 graphically shows the amount of triglycerides, phospholipids, cholesterol, and protein found in each of these lipoproteins. Finally, refer to the Highlight Box to gain more insight into understanding your blood lipid levels.

We have known for a long time that saturated fats increase our blood levels of total cholesterol and LDL-cholesterol and increase our risk of heart disease. Because saturated fat is found primarily in the fats of animal products, we can easily reduce our intake of saturated fats by eating low-fat dairy and meat products. Vegetable oils can also be converted to high-saturated fat spreads through the hydro-

Table 5.6 Descriptions and Functions of the Various Blood Lipoproteins

Lipoprotein	Description	Primary Function
Chylomicrons	Formed in the gut after a meal, these lipoproteins are released into the lymph system and then into the blood Largest of the lipoproteins, with the lowest density After triglycerides are removed from this lipoprotein, a chylomicron remnant remains and is taken up by the liver	Transports dietary fat into the blood and transports it to the tissues of the body
Very Low-density Lipoproteins (VLDLs)	Formed in the liver (80% of production) and the intestine (20% of production)	Transports endogenous lipids, especially triglycerides, to the various tissues of the body
Low-density lipoproteins (LDLs)	Formed in the blood from VLDL Transformation from VLDL to LDL occurs as the triglycerides are removed from the VLDL	Transports cholesterol to the cells of the body
High-density lipoproteins (HDLs)	Synthesized in the liver and released into the blood Move in the blood through the body, picking up free cholesterol	Transports cholesterol from tissues back to the liver

genation of the fatty acids in these oils. Once the oil has been converted to a hard spread (e.g., corn oil to corn oil margarine), the level of saturated fat dramatically increases, as does the level of *trans* fatty acids. Thus, reduction of saturated fats in our diets must include reducing intake of high-fat animal products and hydrogenated vegetable products.

Recent research indicates that *trans* fatty acids can also raise blood cholesterol levels as much as saturated fat (Oomen et al. 2001; Wootan, Lieberman, and Rosoesky 1996). Because foods fried in hydrogenated vegetable oils, such as French fries, are high in *trans* fatty acids, these types of foods should be limited in our diet. The U.S. Food and Drug Administration ruled in 2003 that *trans* fatty acid content must be listed on labels for conventional foods and some dietary supplements; food manufacturers have until January 1, 2006, to comply. Unfortunately, restaurants are not required to provide nutrition facts for any of their foods at the present time. Until all food labels are updated to give the *trans* fatty acid content on the package, use the following guidelines to help reduce your intake (Wootan, Lieberman, and Rosoesky 1996):

- Limit your intake of foods that contain "vegetable shortening" or "partially hydrogenated" oil.
- Avoid deep fried foods, especially those from fast food restaurants that re-use vegetable shortening to fry their foods.
- If you use margarine, buy tubs rather than sticks. Look for margarines that contain no *trans* fatty acids. Use olive or canola oil instead of butter, margarine, or shortening whenever possible.

Lifestyle Changes Can Prevent or Reduce Cardiovascular Disease

Diet and exercise interventions aimed at reducing the risk of cardiovascular disease center on reducing high levels of triglycerides and LDL-cholesterol while raising HDL-cholesterol. The Centers for Disease Control and Prevention (CDC) (Hahn and Heath 1998) and the Expert Panel on Detection, Evaluation, and Treatment of

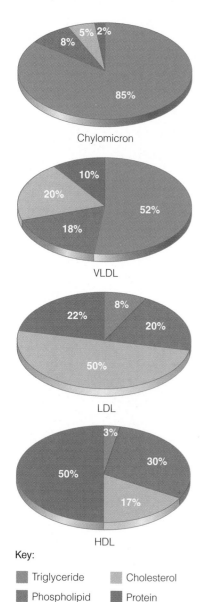

Key:

■ Triglyceride   ▨ Cholesterol
■ Phospholipid   ■ Protein

Figure 5.13 The chemical components of various lipoproteins. Notice that chylomicrons contain the highest proportion of triglycerides, making them the least dense, while high-density lipoproteins (HDL) have the highest proportion of protein, making them the most dense.

High Blood Cholesterol in Adults (APT III) (NIH 2001) have made the following dietary and lifestyle recommendations to improve blood lipid levels and reduce the risk of cardiovascular disease:

- Maintain total fat intake to within 20 to 35% of energy (Institute of Medicine 2002), and keep intake of saturated and *trans* fatty acids low. Polyunsaturated fats (e.g., soy and canola oil) can comprise up to 10% of total energy intake, while monounsaturated fats (e.g., olive oil) can comprise up to 20% of total energy intake. For some people, a lower fat intake may help to maintain a healthful body weight.

- Decrease dietary saturated fat to less than 7% of total energy intake. Decrease cholesterol intake to less than 300 mg per day, and keep *trans* fatty acid intake low. Lowering the intakes of these fats will lower your LDL-cholesterol level. Replace saturated fat (e.g., butter, margarine, vegetable shortening, or lard) with more healthful cooking oils, such as olive or canola oil.

- Increase dietary intakes of whole grains, fruits, and vegetables so that total dietary fiber is 20 to 30 grams per day, with 10 to 25 grams per day coming from fiber sources such as oat bran, beans, and fruits. Foods high in fiber decrease blood LDL-cholesterol levels.

- Maintain blood glucose and insulin concentrations within normal ranges. High blood glucose levels are associated with high blood triglycerides. Consume foods whole (such as whole-wheat breads and cereals, whole fruits and vegetables, and beans and legumes), and select low saturated-fat meats and dairy products, while limiting your intake of high-sugar and high-fat foods (e.g., cookies, high-sugar drinks and snacks, candy, fried foods, and convenience and fast foods).

- Eat throughout the day (e.g., smaller meals and snacks) instead of eating most of your calories in the evening before bed.

- Maintain an active lifestyle. Exercise most days of the week for 30 to 60 minutes if possible. Exercise will increase HDL-cholesterol while lowering blood triglyceride levels. Exercise also helps maintain a healthy body weight and a lower blood pressure and reduces your risk for diabetes.

- Maintain a healthy body weight. Blood lipids and glucose levels typically improve when obese individuals lose weight and engage in regular physical activity.

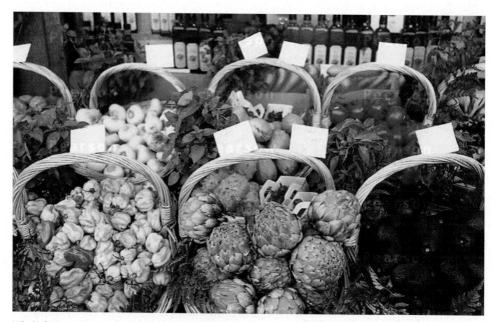

Whole fruits and vegetables can reduce your risk for cardiovascular disease.

The impact of diet on reducing the risk of cardiovascular disease was clearly demonstrated in the Dietary Approaches to Stop Hypertension (DASH) study, which is discussed in detail in Chapter 2. Although this study focused on dietary interventions to reduce hypertension (high blood pressure), the results of the study showed that eating the DASH way could dramatically improve blood lipids and lower blood pressure. The DASH diet includes high intakes of fruits, vegetables, whole grains, low-fat dairy products, poultry, fish, and nuts and reducing intake of fats, red meat, sweets, and sugar-containing beverages. Combining the DASH dietary approach with an active lifestyle significantly reduces the risk of cardiovascular disease.

Does a High-Fat Diet Cause Cancer?

Cancer develops as a result of a poorly understood interaction between the environment and genetic factors. In addition, most cancers take years to develop, so examining the impact of diet on cancer development can be a long and difficult process. Diet and lifestyle are two of the most important environmental factors that have been identified in the development of cancer (Kim 2001, 573–589). Of the dietary factors, dietary fat intake and the development of cancer have been extensively researched. There appears to be a weak relationship between type and amount of fat consumed and increased risk for breast cancer (Willett 1999, 1243–1253). Early research showed an association between animal fat intake and increased risk for colon cancer, while more recent research indicates that the association is between factors other than fat that are found in red meat. Because we now know that physical activity can reduce the risk of colon cancer, earlier diet and colon cancer studies that did not control for this factor are now being questioned. The strongest association between dietary fat intake and cancer is for prostate cancer. Research shows that there is a consistent link between prostate cancer risk and consumption of animal fats, but not other types of fats. The exact mechanism by which animal fats may contribute to prostate cancer has not yet been identified.

Recap: The types of fats we select to eat can significantly impact our health and risk of disease. Saturated and *trans* fatty acids increase our risk of heart disease, while omega-3 fatty acids can reduce our risk. Other risk factors for heart disease include being overweight, physically inactive, smoking, having high blood pressure, and having diabetes mellitus. You can calculate your 10-year risk of heart disease by knowing a few facts about yourself: your blood cholesterol and HDL-cholesterol levels, blood pressure, age, and smoking status. High levels of LDL-cholesterol and low levels of HDL-cholesterol increase your risk of heart disease. Selecting appropriate types of fat in the diet may also reduce your risk of some cancers, especially prostate cancer.

Chapter Summary

- Fats and oils are forms of a larger and more diverse group of substances called lipids; most lipids are insoluble in water.
- The three types of lipids commonly found in foods are triglycerides, phospholipids, and sterols.

- Most of the fat we eat is in the form of triglycerides; a triglyceride is a molecule that contains three fatty acids attached to a glycerol backbone.
- The various fatty acids in triglycerides are classified based on chain length, level of saturation and shape.
- Short-chain fatty acids are usually less than six carbon atoms in length; medium-chain fatty acids are six to

twelve carbons in length, and long-chain fatty acids are fourteen or more carbons in length.

- Saturated fatty acids have no carbons attached together with a double bond, which means that every carbon atom in the fatty acid chain is saturated with hydrogen.

- Monounsaturated fatty acids contain one double bond between two carbon atoms; monounsaturated fatty acids are usually liquid at room temperature.

- Polyunsaturated fatty acids contain more than one double bond between carbon atoms, and these fatty acids are also liquid at room temperature.

- Saturated fats are straight in shape, allowing the fatty acid chains to pack tightly together and making them solid at room temperature.

- Unsaturated fats (those with one or more double bonds in their fatty acid chains) have a kink along their length, which prevents them from packing tightly together and results in their being liquid at room temperature.

- A *cis* fatty acid has hydrogen atoms located on the same side of the double bond in an unsaturated fatty acid. This *cis* positioning produces a kink in the unsaturated fatty acid, and is the shape found in naturally occurring fatty acids.

- A *trans* fatty acid has hydrogen atoms located on opposite sides of the double carbon bond. This positioning causes *trans* fatty acids to be straighter and more rigid like saturated fats. This trans positioning results when oils are hydrogenated during food processing.

- Phospholipids consist of a glycerol backbone and two fatty acids with a phosphate group; phospholipids are soluble in water and assist with transporting fats in our bloodstream.

- Sterols have a ring structure; cholesterol is the most common sterol in our diets.

- The majority of fat digestion and absorption occurs in the small intestine. Fat is broken into smaller components by bile, which is produced by the liver and stored in the gallbladder.

- Because fats are not soluble in water, triglycerides are packaged into lipoproteins before being released into the bloodstream for transport to the cells.

- Dietary fat is primarily used either as an energy source for the cells or to make lipid-containing compounds in the body, or it is stored in the muscle and adipose tissue as triglyceride for later use.

- Fats are a primary energy source during rest and exercise, are our major source of stored energy, provide essential fatty acids, enable the transport of fat-soluble vitamins, help maintain cell function, provide protection for body organs, contribute to the texture and flavor of foods, and help us feel satiated after a meal.

- The AMDR for fat is 20 to 35% of total energy. Our intake of saturated fats and *trans* fatty acids should be kept to a minimum. Individuals who limit fat intake to less than 15% of energy intake need to make sure that essential fatty acid needs are met, as well as protein and energy needs.

- For the essential fatty acids, 5 to 10% of energy intake should be in the form of linoleic acid and 0.6% as alpha-linolenic acid.

- Visible fats are those we can easily see, such as butter, cream, shortening, oils, dressings, poultry skin, and fat on the edge of meats.

- Invisible fats are those hidden in foods and include fats found in cakes, cookies, marbling in meat, regular-fat dairy products, and fried foods.

- Diets high in saturated fat and *trans* fatty acids can increase our risk for cardiovascular disease. Other risk factors for cardiovascular disease are overweight or obesity, physical inactivity, smoking, high blood pressure, and diabetes mellitus.

- High levels of circulating low-density lipoproteins, or LDLs, increase total blood cholesterol and the formation of plaque on arterial walls, leading to an increased risk for cardiovascular disease. This is why LDLs are sometimes called the "bad cholesterol."

- High levels of circulating high-density lipoproteins, or HDLs, reduce our blood cholesterol level and our risk for cardiovascular disease. This is why HDLs are sometimes called the "good cholesterol."

- There are some studies showing that diets high in fat may increase our risk for prostate cancer, while the role of dietary fat in breast and colon cancer is still controversial.

Review Questions

1. Omega-3 fatty acids are
   a. a form of *trans* fatty acids.
   b. metabolized in the body to arachidonic acid.
   c. synthesized in the liver and small intestine.
   d. found in leafy green vegetables, flax seeds, soy milk, and fish.

2. One of the most sensible ways to reduce body fat is to
   a. limit intake of fat to less than 15% of total energy consumed.
   b. exercise regularly.
   c. avoid all consumption of *trans* fatty acids.
   d. restrict total calories to 1,200 per day.

3. Fats in chylomicrons are taken up by cells with the help of
   a. lipoprotein lipase.
   b. micelles.
   c. sterols.
   d. pancreatic enzymes.

4. The risk of heart disease is reduced in people who have high blood levels of
   a. triglycerides.
   b. very low-density lipoproteins.
   c. low-density lipoproteins.
   d. high-density lipoproteins.

5. Triglycerides with a double bond at one part of the molecule are referred to as
   a. monounsaturated fats.
   b. hydrogenated fats.
   c. saturated fats.
   d. sterols.

6. **True or false?** The Acceptable Macronutrient Distribution Range (AMDR) for fat is 20 to 35% of total energy.

7. **True or false?** During exercise, fat cannot be mobilized from adipose tissue for use as energy.

8. **True or false?** Triglycerides are the same as fatty acids.

9. **True or false?** *Trans* fatty acids are produced by food manufacturers; they do not occur in nature.

10. **True or false?** A serving of food labeled *reduced fat* has at least 25% less fat and 25% fewer calories than a full-fat version of the same food.

11. Explain how the straight, rigid shape of the saturated and *trans* fatty acids we eat affects our health.

12. Explain the contribution of dietary fat to bone health.

13. You have volunteered to participate in a 20-mile walk-a-thon to raise money for a local charity. You have been training for several weeks, and the event is now two days away. An athlete friend of yours advises you to "load up on carbohydrates" today and tomorrow and says you should avoid eating any foods that contain fat during the day of the walk-a-thon. Do you take this advice? Why or why not?

14. Your father returns from an appointment with his doctor feeling down. He tells you that his "blood test didn't turn out so good." He then adds, "My doctor told me I can't eat any of my favorite foods anymore. He says red meat and butter have too much fat. I guess I'll have to switch to cottage cheese and margarine!" What type of blood test do you think your father had? How would you respond to his intention to switch to cottage cheese and margarine? Finally, suggest a non-dietary lifestyle choice that might improve his health.

15. Your friend Maria has determined that she needs to consume about 2000 calories per day to maintain her healthful weight. Create a chart for Maria showing the recommended maximum number of calories she should consume in each of the following forms: unsaturated fat, saturated fat, linoleic acid, alpha-linolenic acid, and *trans* fatty acids.

Test Yourself Answers

1. **False.** Eating too much fat, or too much of unhealthful fats such as saturated and *trans* fatty acids, can increase our risk for diseases such as cardiovascular disease and obesity. However, fat is an important part of a nutritious diet, and we need to consume a certain minimum amount to provide adequate levels of essential fatty acids and fat-soluble vitamins.

2. **False.** Fats provide essential fatty acids and are important carriers of fat-soluble vitamins. Fat also provides protection for our internal organs.

3. **True.** Fat is our primary source of energy, both at rest and during low-intensity exercise. Fat is also an important fuel source during prolonged exercise.

4. **False.** Even foods fried in vegetable shortening can be unhealthful because they are higher in *trans* fatty acids. In addition, fried foods are high in fat and energy and can contribute to overweight and obesity.

5. **True.** Other lifestyle changes that can reduce our risk for cardiovascular disease include not smoking and maintaining a healthful body weight.

Web Links

www.americanheart.org
American Heart Association
Learn the best way to help lower your blood cholesterol level. Access the AHA's online cookbook for healthy-heart recipes and cooking methods.

www.caloriecontrol.org
Calorie Control Council
Go to this site to find out more about fat replacers.

www.nhlbi.nih.gov/chd
Live Healthier, Live Longer
Take a cholesterol quiz, and test your heart disease IQ. Create a diet using the Heart Healthy Diet or the TLC Diet online software.

www.nhlbi.nih.gov
National Heart, Lung, and Blood Institute
Learn how a healthful diet can lower your cholesterol levels. Use the online risk assessment tool to estimate your 10-year risk of having a heart attack.

www.cfsan.fda.gov/~dms/transfat.html
Consumer Information on the New Trans Fat Labeling Requirements
This page, created by the U.S. Food and Drug Administration, provides information about soon to be required trans fat labeling.

www.nih.gov
The National Institutes of Health (NIH)
U.S. Department of Health and Human Services
Search this site to learn more about dietary fats and the DASH Diet (Dietary Approaches to Stop Hypertension).

www.nlm.nih.gov/medlineplus
MEDLINE Plus Health Information
Search for "fats" or "lipids" to obtain additional resources and the latest news on dietary lipids, heart diseases, and cholesterol.

www.hsph.harvard.edu/nutritionsource
The Nutrition Source: Knowledge for Healthy Eating
Harvard University's Department of Nutrition
Go to this site, and click on "Fats & Cholesterol" to find out how selective fat intake can be part of a healthful diet.

http://ific.org
International Food Information Council Foundation
Access this site to find out more about fats and dietary fat replacers.

References

Allison, D. B., S. K. Egan, L. M. Barraj, C. Caughman, M. Infante, and J. T. Heimbach. 1999. Estimated intakes of *trans* fatty and other fatty acids in the U.S. population. *J. Am. Diet. Assoc.* 99:166–174.

Calloway, C. W. 1998. The role of fat-modified foods in the American diet. *Nutr. Today* 33:156–163.

Cowley, G. 2003. A better way to eat. *Newsweek*. January 20, 46–54.

Expert Panel on Detection, Evaluation, and Treatment of High Blood Cholesterol in Adults, National Institutes of Health. 2001. Executive Summary of the Third Report of the National Cholesterol Education Program (NCEP) Expert Panel on Detection, Evaluation, and Treatment of High Blood Cholesterol in Adults (Adult Treatment Panel III). *JAMA* 285(19):2486–2509.

Hahn, R. A., and G. W. Heath. 1998. Cardiovascular disease risk factors and preventive practices among adults—United States, 1994: A behavioral risk factor atlas. *Morbid. Mortal. Wkly. Rep.* 47(SS-5):35–69.

Harnack, L. J., R. W. Jeffery, and K. N. Boutelle. 2000. Temporal trends in energy intake in the United States: an ecologic perspective. *Am. J. Clin. Nutr.* 71:1478–1484.

Harris, W. S. 1997. n-3 Fatty acids and serum lipoproteins: human studies. *Am. J. Clin. Nutr.* 65 (Suppl.): 1645S–1654S.

Institute of Medicine, Food and Nutrition Board. 2002. *Dietary Reference Intakes for Energy, Carbohydrate, Fiber, Fat, Fatty Acids, Cholesterol, Protein, and Amino Acids (Macronutrients)*. Washington, DC: National Academies Press.

Jebb, S. A, A. M. Prentice, G. R. Goldberg, P. R. Murgatroyd, A. E. Black, and W. A. Coward. 1996. Changes in macronutrient balance during over- and underfeeding assessed by 12-d continuous whole-body calorimetry. *Am. J. Clin. Nutr.* 64:259–266.

Kim, Y. I. 2001. Nutrition and cancer. In *Present Knowledge in Nutrition*, 8th ed., edited by B. A. Bowman and R. M. Russell. Washington, DC: International Life Sciences Institute Press.

Lichtenstein, A. H., and L. Van Horn. 1998. Very low fat diets. *Circulation* 98:935–939.

Manore, M. M., S. I. Barr, and G. E. Butterfield. 2000. Position of the American Dietetic Association, Dietitians of Canada, and the American College of Sports Medicine: Nutrition and athletic performance. *J. Am. Diet. Assoc.* 100:1543–1556.

McCullough, M. L., D. Feskanich, M. J. Stampfer, E. L. Giovannucci, E. B. Rimm, F. B. Hu, D. Spiegelman, D. J. Hunter, G. A. Colditz, and W. C. Willett. 2002. Diet quality and major chronic disease risk in men and women: moving toward improved dietary guidance. *Am. J. Clin. Nutr.* 76(6):1261–1271.

National Center for Chronic Disease Prevention and Health Promotion (NCCDPHP). 2002. Chronic Disease Prevention. Chronic Disease Overview. www.cdc.gov/nccdphp/overview.htm. Accessed February 2004.

National Institutes of Health (NIH). *Third Report of the National Cholesterol Education Program: Detection, Evaluation and Treatment of high blood cholesterol in adults (ATP:III)*. National Cholesterol Education Program, National Heart, Lung, and Blood Institute, NIH, May 2001. Web site: http://www.nhlbi.nih.gov/guidelines/cholesterol/atp3xsum.pdf

Oomen, C. M., M. C. Ocké, E. J. Feskens, M. A. van Erp-Baart, F. J. Kok, and D. Kromhout. 2001. Association between *trans* fatty acid intake and 10-year risk of coronary heart disease in the Zutphen Elderly Study: a prospective population-based study. *Lancet* 357(9258):746–751.

Sigman-Grant, M. 1997. Can you have your low-fat cake and eat it too? The role of fat-modified products. *J. Am. Diet. Assoc.* 97(suppl):S76–S81.

USDA, Center for Nutrition Policy and Promotion (CNPP). 1998. Is total fat consumption really decreasing? *Nutrition Insights,* vol. 5, 1995. Reprinted in *Nutr. Today* 33:171–172.

Willett, W. C. 1999. Diet, nutrition and the prevention of cancer. In *Modern Nutrition in Health and Disease*, 9th ed., edited by M. E. Shils, J. A. Olsen, M. Shike, and A. C. Ross. Baltimore, MD: Williams & Wilkins, Publ.

Wootan, M., B. Lieberman, and W. Rosoesky. 1996. Trans: The phantom fat. *Nutrition Action Health Letter.* 23(7):10–13.

Nutrition Debate:

Will Revising the USDA Food Guide Pyramid Help Us Find the Perfect Diet?

In Chapter 2, we introduced the USDA Food Guide Pyramid and discussed some of its limitations. These limitations have resulted in serious criticisms about the effectiveness of the Pyramid as a tool and led nutrition experts to question its usefulness in designing a healthful diet. One major criticism is that it is overly simple and does not help consumers make appropriate food selections within each food group. For example, all the grains and cereals are grouped into one category with no distinction made between whole and refined grains or carbohydrates. A serving of Fruit Loops "counts" the same as a serving of oatmeal. Yet nutritionists know that whole-grain foods contain important nutrients, such as fiber, vitamins, and minerals—nutrients that are typically lost when grains are refined. To help make up for this loss, some of these nutrients, but not all, are added back through a process called enrichment (or fortification). Whole grains are also high in fiber, increase the feeling of fullness, and are typically digested more slowly than refined grains, gradually releasing glucose into the blood. In contrast, refined-grain foods are low in fiber and typically high in simple sugars, causing a spike in blood glucose and contributing to increased hunger shortly after their consumption.

A second criticism is that the Pyramid makes a poor distinction between healthful and unhealthful fats. All the fats are lumped together at the tip of the Pyramid, and consumers are told to use them "sparingly." As we have discussed in this chapter, not all fats have the same effect on health so they cannot be easily grouped together. We want to limit our intake of saturated and trans fats, while making sure our diets are adequate in the monounsaturated and polyunsaturated fats that are essential for good health and may protect against disease.

A third criticism is that the serving sizes suggested in the Food Guide Pyramid are unrealistic or do not coincide with typical serving sizes of foods listed on food labels. For instance, one serving of a muffin as defined in the Food Guide Pyramid is 1.5 ounces, but most muffins available to consumers range from 2 ounces to 8 ounces! The way that foods are packaged is also confusing to consumers. Unless people read food labels carefully, it is easy to consume an entire package of a food that contains multiple servings and

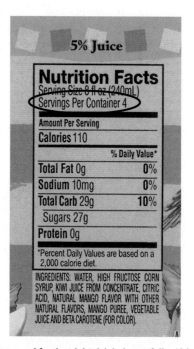

It is important to read food and drink labels carefully. Although the serving size listed on this drink label is 8 fluid ounces, the total servings per container is listed as 4.

assume that the entire package is equal to one serving. For example, it is common to find soft drinks sold in 20 fluid ounce bottles. Although the serving size listed on the label is 8 fluid ounces, and total servings per bottle is listed as 2.5, most people just drink the entire bottle in one sitting and assume they had one soft drink.

Because of these limitations and criticisms, the Food Guide Pyramid is now being identified as a contributor to the current obesity epidemic in the United States (Cowley 2003). While the Pyramid is grounded in science, new research emphasizes the importance of eating specific nutrients and whole foods that promote health and prevent disease—concepts that the Pyramid does not address. The Healthy Eating Pyramid included in Chapter 2 (page 63) has been identified as one example of a better tool for designing a healthful diet. In fact, a recent study shows that people eating a diet based on the Healthy Eating Pyramid reduced their risk for heart disease two times more than people eating a diet based on the current USDA Food Guide Pyramid (McCullough et al. 2002).

The United States government is currently in the process of redesigning the Food Guide Pyramid to address these criticisms and develop a new tool that can assist consumers in reducing their risk for obesity and other chronic diseases. It is possible that the shape of the pyramid could change; other areas the government plans to address are promoting daily physical activity, distinguishing between types of fat, promoting avoidance of *trans* fatty acids, and clarifying serving sizes that can assist in maintaining a healthful body weight. The earliest this new dietary tool will be available is 2005.

As you can see, a great deal of time, effort, and money is being invested to design a tool that the federal government and nutrition experts feel will help reduce the alarmingly high obesity rates in the United States. The primary assumption being made by these experts is that people are actually using the Food Guide Pyramid to design their diets. In fact, however, the extent to which people are using the Food Guide Pyramid in their daily lives is debatable.

Think about it; prior to taking this class, did you use the Food Guide Pyramid to help you design a healthful diet? It may be that you had not even seen this pyramid or, if you did, you had no idea how to use it. This is the case for many Americans. Our work with community members throughout the United States has shown us that some people have no idea what the Food Guide Pyramid is, and many of those who have seen it do not know how to use it. Others who have tried to use it find it confusing because of the limitations just presented. In addition, the pyramid shape does not make sense to many consumers, who do not understand why the most important or healthful foods are at the bottom of the pyramid. In their minds, the top of the pyramid should include the best, or most desirable, foods. Many others also find the Pyramid too vague, and they need specific menus and recipes to follow; these individuals prefer to buy diet books that provide this information. Still others do not use the Pyramid because they view it as another confusing mandate from experts who are out of touch with how "real" people eat and live their lives.

What do you think? Do you feel that revising the Food Guide Pyramid to address its flaws will make it a more useful tool? Do you think that the current Pyramid has significantly contributed to our obesity epidemic and that revising it will help people lose weight? It is obvious that we need to seriously address the obesity epidemic. One of the major challenges we face in this process is designing nutrition recommendations and tools that millions of Americans can, and will, use. Until new, easier-to-use guidelines are available and its impact on the rates of obesity and chronic disease are assessed, this debate will continue.

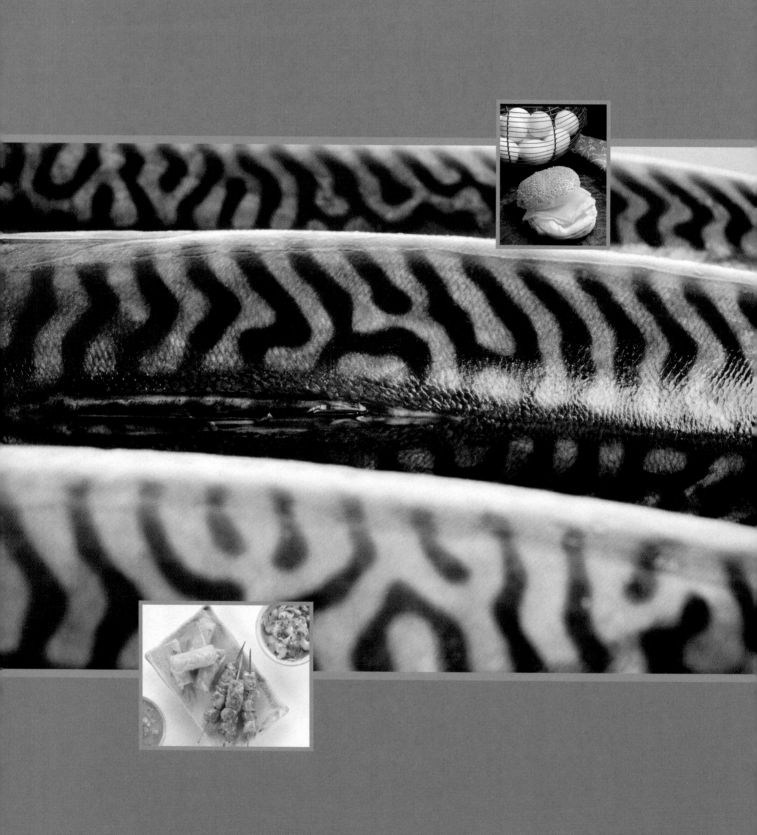

Chapter 6
Proteins: Crucial Components of All Body Tissues

Chapter Objectives

After reading this chapter you will be able to:

1. Describe how proteins differ from carbohydrates and fats, p. 196.

2. Identify nonmeat food combinations that are complete protein sources, pp. 201–202.

3. Discuss how proteins are digested and absorbed by our bodies, pp. 202–204.

4. List four functions of proteins in our bodies, pp. 204–207.

5. Calculate your recommended daily allowance for protein, pp. 207–209.

6. Identify the potential health risks associated with high protein diets, pp. 210–211.

7. List five foods that are good sources of protein, pp. 211–212.

8. Describe two disorders related to inadequate protein intake or genetic abnormalities, pp. 220–223.

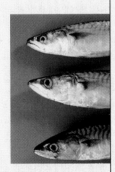

Test Yourself True or false?

1. Protein is a primary source of energy for our bodies. T or F

2. We must consume amino acid supplements in order to build muscle tissue. T or F

3. Our protein needs are calculated based on our body weight. T or F

4. Vegetarian diets are inadequate in protein. T or F

5. Most people in the United States consume more protein than they need. T or F

Test Yourself answers can be found at the end of the chapter.

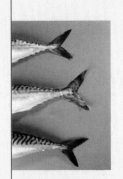

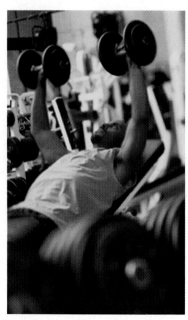

Proteins are an integral part of our body tissues, including our muscle tissue.

proteins   Large, complex molecules made up of amino acids and found as essential components of all living cells.

What do "Mr. Universe" Bill Pearl, Olympic figure skating champion Surya Bonaly, wrestler "Killer" Kowalski, and hundreds of other athletes have in common? They're all vegetarians! Olympic track icon Carl Lewis states: "A person does not need protein from meat to be a successful athlete . . . my best year of track competition was the first year I ate a vegan diet." Although precise statistics on the number of vegetarian American athletes aren't available, a total of 2.5% of the U.S. population—approximately 4 million Americans—are vegetarian.

What is a protein, and what makes it so different from carbohydrates and fats? How much protein do you really need, and do you get enough in your daily diet? What exactly is a vegetarian anyway? Do you qualify? If so, how do you plan your diet to include sufficient protein, especially if you play competitive sports? Are there real advantages to eating meat, or is plant protein just as good?

It seems as if everybody has an opinion about protein, both how much you should consume and from what sources. In this chapter, we address these and other questions to clarify the importance of protein in the diet, and dispel common myths about this crucial nutrient.

What Are Proteins?

Proteins are large, complex molecules found in the cells of all living things. While proteins are best known as a part of our muscle mass, they are in fact critical components of all tissues of the human body, including bones, blood, and hormones. As *enzymes,* proteins function in metabolism. As *antibodies,* proteins are fundamental to a healthy immune system. Without adequate proteins, the body cannot maintain its balance of fluids or its ratio of acids to bases. Although our bodies prefer to use carbohydrates and fats for energy, proteins do provide energy in certain circumstances. All of these functions of proteins will be discussed later in this chapter.

How Do Proteins Differ from Carbohydrates and Lipids?

As we saw in Chapter 1, proteins are one of the three macronutrients and are found in a wide variety of foods. Our bodies are able to manufacture, or synthesize, proteins, carbohydrates, and lipids. But unlike carbohydrates and lipids, our genetic material, or DNA, dictates the structure of each protein molecule. We'll explore how our body synthesizes proteins and the role that DNA plays in this process shortly.

Another key difference between proteins and the other macronutrients lies in their chemical makeup. In addition to the carbon, hydrogen, and oxygen also found in carbohydrates and lipids, proteins contain a special form of nitrogen that our bodies can readily use. This nitrogen is found in amino acids, which are the building blocks of proteins. By eating proteins found in plants and animals, we are able to break down these proteins into their respective amino acid components and utilize the nitrogen for many important body processes. Carbohydrates and lipids cannot provide this critical form of nitrogen.

> **Recap:** Proteins are critical components of all tissues of the human body. Like carbohydrates and lipids, they contain carbon, hydrogen, and oxygen. Unlike the other macronutrients, they also contain nitrogen and their structure is dictated by DNA.

The Building Blocks of Proteins Are Amino Acids

amino acids   Nitrogen-containing molecules that combine to form proteins.

The proteins in our bodies are made from a combination of building blocks called **amino acids,** molecules composed of a central carbon atom connected to four other groups: an amine group, an acid group, a hydrogen atom, and a side chain (Figure 6.1a). The word *amine* means *nitrogen-containing,* and nitrogen is indeed the essential component of the amine portion of the molecule.

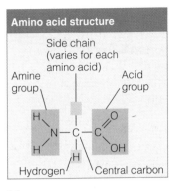

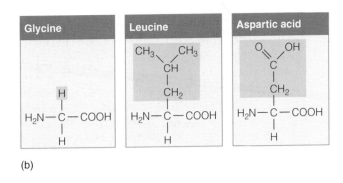

(b)

(a)

Figure 6.1   Structure of an amino acid. **(a)** All amino acids contain five parts: a central carbon atom, an amine group around the atom that contains nitrogen, an acid group, a hydrogen atom, and a side chain. **(b)** Only the side chain differs for each of the twenty amino acids, giving each its unique properties.

As shown in Figure 6.1b, the portion of the amino acid that makes each unique is its side chain. The amine group, acid group, and carbon and hydrogen atoms do not vary. Variations in the structure of the side chain give each amino acid its distinct properties.

The singular term *protein* is misleading, as there are potentially an infinite number of unique types of proteins in living organisms. Most of the proteins in our bodies are made from combinations of just twenty amino acids, identified in Table 6.1. By combining a few dozen to more than 300 copies of these twenty amino acids in various sequences, our bodies form an estimated 10,000 to 50,000 unique proteins.

We Must Obtain Essential Amino Acids from Food

Of the twenty amino acids in our bodies, nine are classified as essential. This does not mean that they are more important than the eleven nonessential amino acids. Instead, an **essential amino acid** is one that our bodies cannot produce at all or cannot produce in sufficient quantities to meet our physiological needs. Thus, we must obtain an essential amino acid from our food. Without the proper amount of essential amino acids in our bodies, we lose our ability to make the proteins and other nitrogen-containing compounds we need.

essential amino acids   Amino acids not produced by the body that must be obtained from food.

Our Body Can Make Nonessential Amino Acids

Nonessential amino acids are just as important to our bodies as essential amino acids, but our bodies can make them in sufficient quantities so we do not need to consume them in our diet. We make nonessential amino acids by transferring the

nonessential amino acids   Amino acids that can be manufactured by the body in sufficient quantities and therefore do not need to be consumed regularly in our diet.

Table 6.1   Amino Acids of the Human Body

Essential Amino Acids	Nonessential Amino Acids
These amino acids must be consumed in the diet.	*These amino acids can be manufactured by the body.*
Histidine	Alanine
Isoleucine	Arginine
Leucine	Asparagine
Lysine	Aspartic acid
Methionine	Cysteine
Phenylalanine	Glutamic acid
Threonine	Glutamine
Tryptophan	Glycine
Valine	Proline
	Serine
	Tyrosine

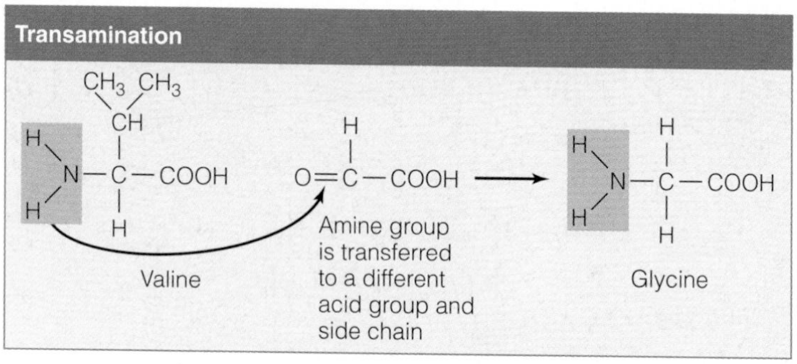

Figure 6.2   Transamination. Our bodies can make nonessential amino acids by transferring the amine group from an essential amino acid to a different acid group and side chain.

transamination The process of transferring the amine group from one amino acid to another in order to manufacture a new amino acid.

nitrogen-containing group from an essential amino acid to a different acid group and side chain. The process of transferring the amine group from one amino acid to another acid group and side chain is called **transamination,** and is shown in Figure 6.2. The acid groups and side chains can be donated by amino acids, or they can be made from the breakdown products of carbohydrates and fats. Thus, by combining parts of different amino acids, the necessary nonessential amino acid can be made.

Under some conditions, a nonessential amino acid can become an essential amino acid. In this case, the amino acid is called a *conditionally essential amino acid*. Consider what occurs in the disease known as phenylketonuria (PKU). As discussed in Chapter 4, someone with PKU cannot metabolize phenylalanine (an essential amino acid). Normally the body uses phenylalanine to produce the nonessential amino acid tyrosine, so the inability to metabolize phenylalanine results in failure to make tyrosine. If PKU is not diagnosed immediately after birth, it results in irreversible brain damage. In this situation, tyrosine becomes a conditionally essential amino acid that must be provided by the diet.

Recap: The building blocks of proteins are amino acids. The amine group of the amino acid contains nitrogen. The portion of the amino acid that changes, giving each amino acid its distinct identity, is the side chain. The body cannot make essential amino acids so we must obtain them from our diet. Our body can make nonessential amino acids from parts of other amino acids, carbohydrates, and fats.

How Are Proteins Made?

As we have stated, our bodies can synthesize proteins by selecting the needed amino acids from the pool of all amino acids available at any given time. Let's look more closely at how this occurs.

Amino Acids Bond to Form a Variety of Peptides

Figure 6.3 shows that when two amino acids join together, the amine group of one binds to the acid group of another in a unique type of chemical bond called a **peptide bond.** In the process, a molecule of water is released as a by-product.

peptide bonds Unique types of chemical bonds in which the amine group of one amino acid binds to the acid group of another in order to manufacture dipeptides and all larger peptide molecules.

Two amino acids joined together form a *dipeptide,* and three amino acids joined together are called a *tripeptide*. The term *oligopeptide* is used to identify a string of four to nine amino acids, while a *polypeptide* is ten or more amino acids bonded together. As a polypeptide chain grows longer, it begins to fold into any of a variety of complex shapes that give proteins their sophisticated structure.

Genes Regulate Amino Acid Binding

Our genetic makeup, or heredity, determines the sequence of the amino acids for each individual protein molecule. Each of us is unique because we inherited a specific

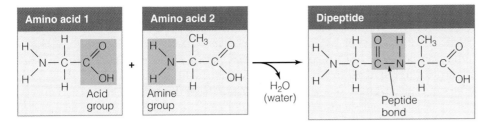

Figure 6.3   Amino acid bonding. Two amino acids join together to form a dipeptide. By combining multiple amino acids, proteins are made.

genetic code from our parents. Each person's specific genes direct minute differences in amino acid sequences, which in turn lead to slight differences in our bodies' proteins. These differences in proteins result in the unique physical and physiological characteristics each one of us possesses.

As mentioned earlier, DNA dictates the structure of each protein our body synthesizes. Figure 6.4 shows how this process occurs. **Gene expression** is a term used to refer to the process of using a gene in a cell to make a protein. A gene is a segment of DNA that serves as a template for the structure of a protein. As proteins are manufactured at

gene expression   The process of using a gene to make a protein.

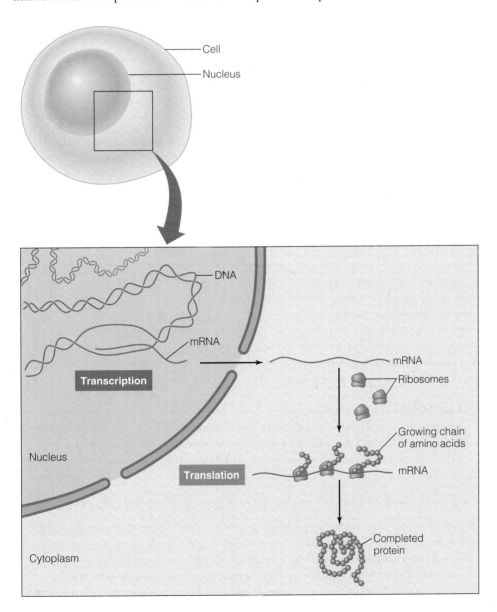

Figure 6.4   Gene expression. Messenger RNA (mRNA) transcribes the genetic information from DNA in the nucleus and carries it to the ribosomes in the cytoplasm. At the ribosome, this genetic information is translated into a chain of amino acids that eventually make a protein.

transcription The process through which messenger RNA copies genetic information from DNA in the nucleus.

translation The process that occurs when the genetic information carried by messenger RNA is translated into a chain of amino acids at the ribosome.

the site of ribosomes in the cytoplasm, and DNA never leaves the nucleus, a special molecule is needed to copy, or transcribe, the information from DNA and carry it to the ribosome. This is the job of *messenger RNA* (*messenger ribonucleic acid*, or *mRNA*); during **transcription**, mRNA copies the genetic information from DNA in the nucleus and carries it to the ribosomes in the cytoplasm. Once this genetic information is at the ribosome, **translation** occurs: genetic information from the mRNA is translated into a growing chain of amino acids that are bonded together to make a specific protein.

Although the DNA for making every protein in our bodies is contained within each cell nucleus, not all genes are expressed and each cell does not make every type of protein. For example, each cell contains the DNA to manufacture the hormone insulin. However, only the cells of the pancreas express the insulin gene so they are the only cells that can produce insulin. Our physiological needs alter gene expression, as do various nutrients. For instance, a cut in the skin that causes bleeding leads to the production of various proteins that clot the blood. If we consume more dietary iron than we need, the gene for ferritin (a protein that stores iron) is expressed so that we can store this excess iron. Our genetic makeup and how appropriately we express our genes are important factors in our health.

Amino Acid Binding and Attraction Determine Shape

The different amino acids in a polypeptide chain possess unique chemical characteristics that cause the chain to twist and turn into various shapes. The shape of each protein is also determined by how each amino acid is attracted to, or repelled by, the surrounding fluid and other amino acids. Some side chains of amino acids carry electrical charges that attract water. Others have neutral charges that repel water.

Protein Shape Determines Function

The three-dimensional shape of a protein is critically important because it determines that protein's function in the body. For example, the proteins that form tendons are much longer than they are wide. Tendons are connective tissues that attach bone to muscle, and their long, rod-like structure provides strong, fibrous connections. In contrast, the proteins that form red blood cells are globular in shape, and they result in the red blood cells being shaped like flattened discs with depressed centers, similar to a miniature doughnut (Figure 6.5). This structure and the flexibility of the proteins in the red blood cells permit them to change shape and flow freely through even the tiniest capillaries to deliver oxygen and still return to their original shape.

Proteins can uncoil and lose their shape when they are exposed to heat, acids, bases, heavy metals, alcohol, and other damaging substances. The term used to describe this change in the shape of proteins is *denaturation*. When a protein is denatured, its function is also lost. Examples of protein denaturation that we can see are stiffening of egg whites when they are whipped, the curdling of milk when lemon juice or another acid is added, and the solidifying of eggs as they cook. Denaturation also occurs when we digest proteins.

> **Recap:** Amino acids bind together to form proteins. Genes regulate the amino acid sequence, and thus the structure, of all proteins. The shape of a protein determines its function. When a protein is denatured by damaging substances such as heat and acids, it loses its shape and its function.

Protein Synthesis Can Be Limited by Missing Amino Acids

limiting amino acid The essential amino acid that is missing or in the smallest supply in the amino acid pool and is thus responsible for slowing or halting protein synthesis.

For protein synthesis to occur, all essential amino acids must be available to the cell. If this is not the case, the amino acid that is missing or in the smallest supply is called the **limiting amino acid.** Without the proper combination and quantity of essential amino acids, protein synthesis slows to the point at which proteins cannot be generated. For instance, the protein hemoglobin contains the essential amino acid histidine. If we do not

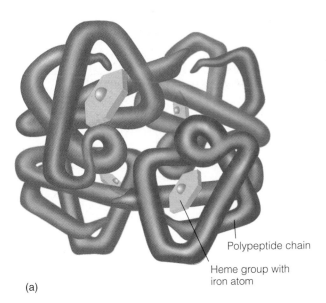

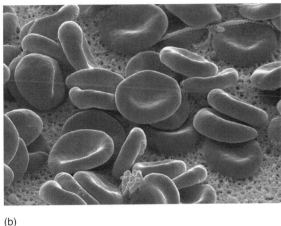

Polypeptide chain

Heme group with
iron atom

(a)

(b)

Figure 6.5 Protein shape determines function. **(a)** Hemoglobin, the protein that forms red blood cells, is globular in shape. **(b)** The globular shape of hemoglobin results in red blood cells being shaped like flattened discs.

consume enough histidine, it becomes the limiting amino acid in hemoglobin production. As no other amino acid can be substituted, our body becomes unable to make adequate hemoglobin, and we lose the ability to transport oxygen to our cells. Our cells cannot function and will eventually die if they do not receive adequate oxygen.

Inadequate energy consumption also limits protein synthesis. If there is not enough energy available from our diets, our bodies will use any accessible proteins for energy, thus preventing them from being used to build new proteins.

A protein that does not contain all of the essential amino acids in sufficient quantities to support growth and health is called an **incomplete** (or *low-quality*) **protein.** Proteins that have all nine of the essential amino acids are considered **complete** (or *high-quality*) **proteins.** The most complete protein sources are from animal sources and include egg whites, ground beef, chicken, tuna and other fish, and milk. Soybeans are the most complete source of vegetable protein. In general, the typical American diet is very high in complete proteins, as we eat proteins from a variety of food sources.

incomplete proteins Foods that do not contain all of the essential amino acids in sufficient amounts to support growth and health.

complete proteins Foods that contain all nine essential amino acids.

mutual supplementation The process of combining two or more incomplete protein sources to make a complete protein.

complementary proteins Two or more foods that together contain all nine essential amino acids necessary for a complete protein. It is not necessary to eat complementary proteins at the same meal.

Protein Synthesis Can Be Enhanced by Mutual Supplementation

Many people believe that we must consume meat or dairy products to obtain complete proteins. Not true! Consider a meal of beans and rice. Beans are low in the amino acids methionine and tryptophan but have adequate amounts of isoleucine and lysine. Rice is low in isoleucine and lysine but contains sufficient methionine and tryptophan. By combining beans and rice, a complete protein source is created.

Mutual supplementation is the process of combining two or more incomplete protein sources to make a complete protein, and the two foods involved are called complementary foods; these foods provide **complementary proteins** (Table 6.2) that, when combined, provide all nine essential amino acids. It is not necessary to eat these foods at the same meal. We maintain a free pool of amino acids in the blood; these amino acids come from food and sloughed-off cells. When we eat one complementary protein, its amino acids join those in the free amino acid pool. These free amino acids can then combine to synthesize complete proteins. However, it is wise to eat complementary-protein foods during the same day, as partially completed proteins cannot be stored and saved for a later time. Mutual supplementation is important for people eating a vegetarian diet, particularly if they consume no animal products whatsoever.

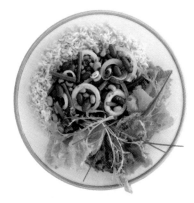

This dish of beans, rice, and vegetables is an example of mutual supplementation.

Table 6.2 Complementary Food Combinations—Turning Incomplete Proteins into Complete Proteins

Food	Limiting Amino Acid	Foods High in Limiting Amino Acid	Complementary Food Combination
Legumes	Methionine and cysteine	Grains, nuts, and seeds	Rice and lentils Red beans and rice Rice and black-eyed peas Hummus (garbanzo beans and sesame seeds)
Grains	Lysine	Legumes	Peanut butter and bread Barley and lentil soup Corn tortilla and beans
Vegetables	Lysine, methionine, cysteine	Legumes (lysine) grains, nuts, and seeds (methionine and cysteine)	Tofu and broccoli with almonds Spinach salad with pine nuts and kidney beans

Recap: When a particular amino acid is limiting, protein synthesis cannot occur. A complete protein provides all nine essential amino acids. Mutual supplementation combines two complementary-protein sources to make a complete protein.

How Do Our Bodies Break Down Proteins?

Our bodies do not directly use proteins from the foods we eat to make the proteins we need. Dietary proteins are first digested and broken into smaller particles such as amino acids, dipeptides, and tripeptides, so that they can be absorbed and transported to the cells. In this section, we will review how proteins are digested and absorbed. As you read about each step in this process, refer to Figure 6.6 for a visual tour through the digestive system.

Stomach Acids and Enzymes Break Proteins into Short Polypeptides

Virtually no enzymatic digestion of proteins occurs in the mouth. As shown in step 1 in Figure 6.6, proteins in food are chewed, crushed, and moistened with saliva to ease swallowing and to increase the surface area of the protein for more efficient digestion. There is no further digestive action on proteins in the mouth.

When proteins reach the stomach, they are broken apart by *hydrochloric acid* (Figure 6.6, step 2). Hydrochloric acid denatures the strands of protein, and converts the inactive enzyme, *pepsinogen,* into its active form, **pepsin.** Although pepsin is a protein, it is not denatured by the acid in the stomach because it has evolved to work optimally in an acidic environment. Pepsin begins breaking proteins into single amino acids and shorter polypeptides that then travel to the small intestine for further digestion.

pepsin An enzyme in the stomach that begins the breakdown of proteins into shorter polypeptide chains and single amino acids.

Enzymes in the Small Intestine Break Polypeptides into Single Amino Acids

As the polypeptides reach the small intestine, the pancreas and the small intestine secrete enzymes that digest them into oligopeptides, tripeptides, dipeptides, and single amino acids (Figure 6.6, step 3). The enzymes that digest proteins in the small intestine are called **proteases.**

The cells in the wall of the small intestine then absorb the single amino acids, dipeptides, and tripeptides. Enzymes in the intestinal cells break the dipeptides and tripeptides

proteases Enzymes that continue the breakdown of polypeptides in the small intestine.

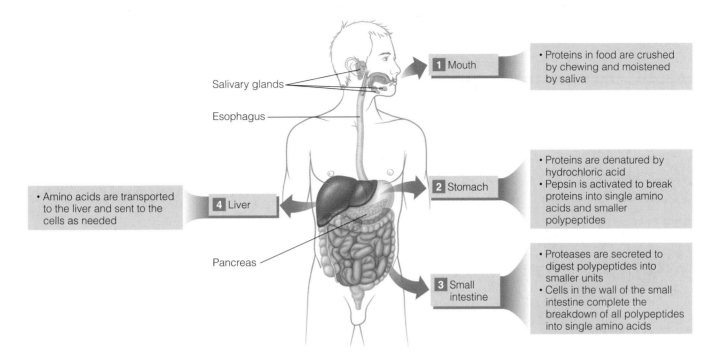

Salivary glands

Esophagus

Pancreas

1 Mouth
- Proteins in food are crushed by chewing and moistened by saliva

2 Stomach
- Proteins are denatured by hydrochloric acid
- Pepsin is activated to break proteins into single amino acids and smaller polypeptides

3 Small intestine
- Proteases are secreted to digest polypeptides into smaller units
- Cells in the wall of the small intestine complete the breakdown of all polypeptides into single amino acids

4 Liver
- Amino acids are transported to the liver and sent to the cells as needed

Figure 6.6   The process of protein digestion.

into single amino acids. The amino acids are then transported into the bloodstream to the liver and on to cells throughout our bodies as needed (Figure 6.6, step 4).

An important fact to remember is that the cells of the small intestine have different sites that specialize in transporting certain types of amino acids, dipeptides, and tripeptides. When very large doses of single amino acids are taken on an empty stomach, there is the potential of similar amino acids competing for the same absorption sites. When we consume too much of one kind, it can block the absorption of other amino acids. Some nutritionists believe that this is why it is not beneficial to consume individual amino acid supplements. In reality, people rarely take very large doses of single amino acids on an empty stomach. The primary reason people should not take single amino acids is that the amount taken is usually so small that they don't have any beneficial effect. For more information on amino acids supplements, refer to Chapter 12.

Protein Digestibility Affects Protein Quality

Earlier in this chapter we discussed how various protein sources differ in quality of protein. The quantity of essential amino acids in a protein determines its quality, as higher protein quality foods are those that contain more of the essential amino acids needed to build proteins and lower protein quality foods contain less essential amino acids.

Another factor to consider when determining protein quality is *digestibility*, or how well our bodies can digest a protein. Proteins with higher digestibility are more complete. Animal protein sources such as meat and dairy products are highly digestible, as are many soy products; we can absorb more than 90% of these proteins. Legumes are also highly digestible (about 80%). Grains and many vegetable proteins are less digestible, ranging from 60 to 90%. The **protein digestibility corrected amino acid score (PDCAAS)** uses an amino acid score and a correction factor for digestibility to calculate a value for protein quality.

Other measures of protein quality include the protein efficiency ratio and net protein utilization. The *protein efficiency ratio* assesses protein quality by comparing the weight gained by a laboratory animal consuming a test protein with the weight gained by a laboratory animal consuming a reference, or standardized protein. *Net protein utilization* is a process that compares the amount of nitrogen retained in our

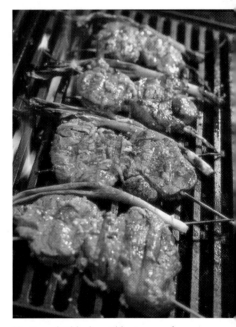

Meats are highly digestible sources of dietary protein.

protein digestibility corrected amino acid score (PDCAAS)   A measurement of protein quality that considers the balance of amino acids as well as the digestibility of the protein in the food.

bodies with the amount of nitrogen we consume in our diets. The more nitrogen we retain, the higher the quality of the protein we have consumed.

These measures of protein quality are useful when determining the quality of protein available to populations of people. However, these measures are not practical or useful for individual diet planning.

> **Recap:** In the stomach, hydrochloric acid denatures proteins and converts pepsinogen to pepsin; pepsin breaks proteins into smaller polypeptides and individual amino acids. In the small intestine, proteases break polypeptides into smaller fragments and single amino acids. The cells in the wall of the small intestine break the smaller peptide fragments into single amino acids, which are then transported to the liver for distribution to our cells.

Why Do We Need Proteins?

The functions of proteins in the body are so numerous that only a few can be described in detail in this chapter. Note that proteins function most effectively when we also consume adequate amounts of energy as carbohydrates and fat. When there is not enough energy available, the body uses proteins as an energy source, limiting their availability for the functions described below.

Proteins Contribute to Cell Growth, Repair, and Maintenance

The proteins in our body are dynamic, meaning that they are constantly being broken down, repaired, and replaced. When proteins are broken down, many amino acids are recycled into new proteins. Think about all of the new proteins that are needed to allow an embryo to develop and grow. In this case, an entirely new human body is being made! In fact, a newborn baby has more than ten trillion body cells.

Even in the mature adult, our cells are constantly turning over, meaning old cells are broken down and parts are used to create new cells. In addition, cellular damage that occurs must be repaired in order to maintain our health. Our red blood cells live for only three to four months then are replaced by new cells that are produced in our bone marrow. The cells lining our intestinal tract are replaced every three to six days. The "old" intestinal cells are treated just like the proteins in food; they are digested and the amino acids absorbed back into the body. The constant turnover of proteins from our diet is essential for such cell growth, repair, and maintenance.

Proteins Act as Enzymes and Hormones

Enzymes are proteins that speed up chemical reactions, without being changed by the chemical reaction themselves. Enzymes can act to bind substances together or break them apart and can transform one substance into another. Figure 6.7 shows how an enzyme can bind two substances together.

Each cell contains thousands of enzymes that facilitate specific cellular reactions. For example, the enzyme phosphofructokinase (PFK) increases carbohydrate metabolism during physical exercise. This enzyme is critical to driving the rate at which we break down glucose and use it for energy during exercise. Without PFK, we would be unable to generate energy at a fast enough rate to allow us to be physically active.

Hormones are substances that act as chemical messengers in the body. Some hormones are made from amino acids, while others are made from lipids (refer to Chapter 5). Hormones are stored in various glands in the body, which release them in response to changes in the body's environment. They then act on the body's organs and tissues to restore the body to normal conditions.

Insulin, a hormone made from amino acids, plays an important role in regulating blood concentrations of glucose. While glucose is an important source of energy for body cells, high blood levels can damage cells. When you digest a meal, the breakdown of the carbohydrates raises your blood glucose levels, which stimulates your pancreas to

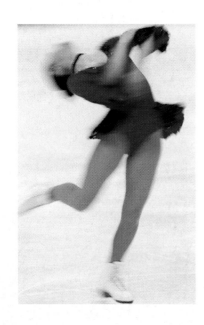

Some athletes who persistently diet are at risk for low protein intake.

enzymes Proteins that speed up chemical reactions, without being changed by the chemical reaction themselves.

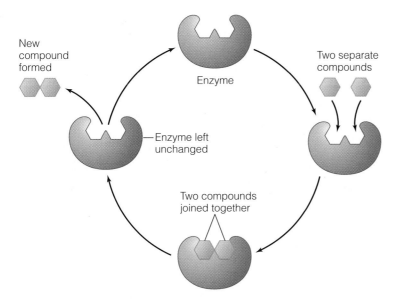

Figure 6.7   Proteins act as enzymes. Enzymes facilitate chemical reactions such as joining two compounds together.

increase its production and release of insulin. Insulin acts on cell membranes to speed up the transport of glucose into the cells and return blood glucose levels to normal.

Other examples of amino acid–containing hormones are glucagon, which responds to conditions of low blood glucose, and thyroid hormone, which helps control our resting metabolic rate.

Proteins Help Maintain Fluid and Electrolyte Balance

Electrolytes are electrically charged particles that assist in maintaining fluid balance. For our bodies to function properly, fluids and electrolytes must be maintained at healthy levels inside and outside cells and within blood vessels. Proteins attract fluids, and the proteins that are in the bloodstream, in the cells, and in the spaces surrounding the cells work together to keep fluids moving across these spaces in the proper quantities to maintain fluid balance and blood pressure. When protein intake is deficient, the concentration of proteins in the bloodstream is insufficient to draw fluid from the tissues and across the blood vessel walls; fluid then collects in the tissues, causing **edema** (Figure 6.8). In addition to being uncomfortable, edema can lead to serious medical problems.

edema A disorder in which fluids build up in the tissue spaces of the body, causing fluid imbalances and a swollen appearance.

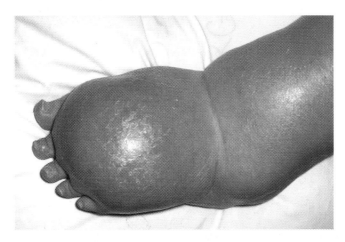

Figure 6.8   Edema can result from deficient protein intake. This foot with edema is swollen due to fluid imbalance.

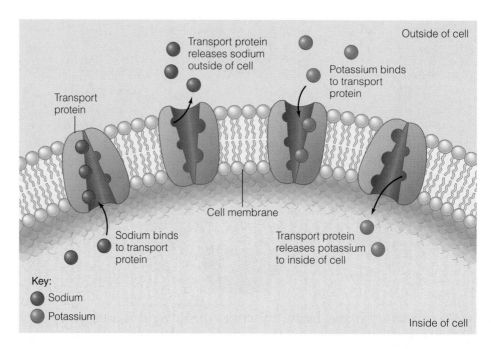

Figure 6.9 Transport proteins help maintain electrolyte balance. Transport proteins in the cell membrane pick up potassium and sodium and transport them across the cell membrane.

transport proteins Protein molecules that help to transport substances throughout the body and across cell membranes.

Sodium (Na⁺) and potassium (K⁺) are examples of common electrolytes. Under normal conditions, Na⁺ is more concentrated outside the cell, and K⁺ is more concentrated inside the cell. This proper balance of Na⁺ and K⁺ is accomplished by the action of **transport proteins** located within the cell membrane. Figure 6.9 shows how these transport proteins work to pump Na⁺ outside and K⁺ inside of the cell. Conduction of nerve signals and contraction of muscles depends on a proper balance of electrolytes. If protein intake is deficient, we lose our ability to maintain these functions, resulting in potentially fatal changes in the rhythm of the heart. Other consequences of chronically low protein intakes include muscle weakness and spasms, kidney failure, and, if conditions are severe enough, death.

Proteins Help Maintain Acid-Base Balance

pH Stands for percentage of hydrogen. It is a measure of the acidity—or level of hydrogen—of any solution, including human blood.

The body's cellular processes result in the constant production of acids and bases. These substances are transported in the blood to be excreted through the kidneys and the lungs. The human body maintains very tight control over the **pH,** or the acid-base balance of the blood. The body goes into a state called **acidosis** when the blood becomes too acidic. **Alkalosis** results if the blood becomes too basic. Both acidosis and alkalosis can be caused by respiratory or metabolic problems. Acidosis and alkalosis can cause coma and death by denaturing body proteins.

acidosis A disorder in which the blood becomes acidic; that is, the level of hydrogen in the blood is excessive. It can be caused by respiratory or metabolic problems.

alkalosis A disorder in which the blood becomes basic; that is, the level of hydrogen in the blood is deficient. It can be caused by respiratory or metabolic problems.

Proteins are excellent **buffers,** meaning they help maintain proper acid-base balance. Acids contain hydrogen ions, which are positively charged. The side chains of proteins have negative charges that attract the hydrogen ions and neutralize their detrimental effects on the body. Proteins can release the hydrogen ions when the blood becomes too basic. By buffering acids and bases, proteins maintain acid-base balance and blood pH.

buffers Proteins that help maintain proper acid-base balance by attaching to, or releasing, hydrogen ions as conditions change in the body.

Proteins Help Maintain a Strong Immune System

antibodies Defensive proteins of the immune system. Their production is prompted by the presence of bacteria, viruses, toxins, allergens, and so on.

Antibodies are special proteins that are critical components of the immune system. When a foreign substance attacks the body, the immune system produces antibodies to defend against it. Bacteria, viruses, toxins, and allergens (substances that cause allergic reactions) are examples of antigens that can trigger antibody production. (An *antigen* is any substance—but typically a protein—that our bodies recognize as foreign and that triggers an immune response.)

Each antibody is designed to destroy one specific invader. When that substance invades the body, antibodies are produced to attack and destroy the specific antigen. Once antibodies have been made, the body "remembers" this process and can respond more quickly the next time that particular invader appears. *Immunity* refers to the development of the molecular memory to produce antibodies quickly upon subsequent invasions.

Adequate protein is necessary to support the increased production of antibodies that occurs in response to a cold, flu, or allergic reaction. If we do not consume enough protein, our resistance to illnesses and disease is weakened. On the other hand, eating more protein than we need does not improve immune function.

Proteins Serve as an Energy Source

The body's primary energy sources are carbohydrate and fat. Remember that both carbohydrate and fat have specialized storage forms that can be used for energy—carbohydrate as glycogen and fat as triglycerides. Proteins do not have a specialized storage form for energy. This means that when proteins need to be used for energy, they are taken from the blood and body tissues such as the liver and skeletal muscle. In healthy people, proteins contribute very little to energy needs. Because we are efficient at recycling amino acids, protein needs are relatively low as compared to carbohydrate and fat.

To use proteins for energy, the nitrogen (or amine) group is removed from the amino acid in a process called **deamination.** The nitrogen is then transported to the kidneys where it is excreted in the urine as *urea*. The remaining fragments of the amino acid contain carbon, hydrogen, and oxygen. The body can directly metabolize these fragments for energy or use them to build carbohydrate. Certain amino acids can be converted into glucose. This is a critical process during times of low carbohydrate intake or starvation. Fat cannot be converted into glucose, but body proteins can be broken down and converted into glucose to provide needed energy to the brain.

To protect the proteins in our body tissues, it is important that we regularly eat an adequate amount of carbohydrate and fat to provide energy. We also need to consume enough dietary protein to perform the required work without using up the proteins that already are playing an active role in our bodies. Unfortunately, our body cannot store excess dietary protein. As a consequence, eating too much protein results in the removal and excretion of the nitrogen in the urine and the use of the remaining components for energy.

> **deamination** The process by which an amine group is removed from an amino acid. The nitrogen is then transported to the kidneys for excretion in the urine, while the carbon and other components are metabolized for energy or used to make other compounds.

Recap: Proteins serve many important functions, including: 1) enabling growth, repair, and maintenance of body tissues; 2) acting as enzymes and hormones; 3) maintaining fluid and electrolyte balance; 4) maintaining acid-base balance; 5) making antibodies, which strengthen our immune system; and 6) providing energy when carbohydrate and fat intake are inadequate. Proteins function best when we also consume adequate amounts of carbohydrate and fat.

How Much Protein Should We Eat?

Consuming adequate protein is a major concern of many people. In fact, one of the most common concerns among active people and athletes is that their diets are deficient in protein (see the Nutrition Myth or Fact box on page 208 for a discussion of this topic). This concern about dietary protein is generally unnecessary, as we can easily consume the protein our bodies need by eating an adequate amount of various foods.

Athletes Need More Protein Than Inactive People

At one time it was believed that the Recommended Dietary Allowance (RDA) for protein, which is 0.8 gram/kilogram body weight, was sufficient for both inactive people and athletes. Recent studies, however, show that athletes' protein needs are higher. Why do athletes need more protein? Regular exercise increases the transport of oxygen to body tissues, requiring changes in the oxygen-carrying capacity of the blood. To carry more oxygen, we need to produce more of the protein that carries oxygen in the blood (i.e., hemoglobin, which is a protein). During intense exercise, we use a small amount of protein directly for energy. We also use protein to make glucose to maintain adequate blood glucose levels and to prevent hypoglycemia (low blood sugar) during exercise. Regular exercise stimulates tissue growth and causes tissue damage, which must be repaired by additional proteins. Strength athletes (such as bodybuilders and weightlifters) need 1.8 to 2 times more protein than the current RDA, while endurance athletes (such as distance runners and triathletes) need 1.5 to 1.75 times more protein than the current RDA (Lemon 2000). Later in this chapter we will calculate the protein needs for inactive and active people.

Does this mean you should add more protein to your diet? Not necessarily. Contrary to popular belief, most Americans, including inactive people *and* athletes, already consume more than twice the RDA for protein. Thus, taking amino acid and protein supplements is not necessary. In fact, eating more protein or taking individual amino acids does not cause muscles to become bigger or stronger. Only regular strength training can achieve these goals. For healthy individuals, evidence does not support eating more than two times the RDA for protein to increase strength, build muscle, or improve athletic performance. By eating a balanced diet and consuming a variety of foods, both inactive and active people can easily meet their protein requirements. ●

Recommended Dietary Allowance (RDA) for Protein

How much protein should we eat? The RDA for sedentary people is 0.8 gram per kilogram of body weight per day. The recommended percentage of energy that should come from protein is 12–20% of total energy intake. Protein needs are higher for children, adolescents, and pregnant/lactating women because more protein is needed during times of growth and development (refer to Chapters 15 and 16 for details on protein needs during these portions of the life cycle). Protein needs can also be higher for active people and for vegetarians.

Table 6.3 lists the daily recommendations for protein for a variety of lifestyles. How can we convert this recommendation into total grams of protein for the day? In the You Do the Math box let's calculate Theo's RDA for protein.

Table 6.3   Recommended Protein Intakes

Group	Protein Intake (grams per kilogram* body weight)
Most adults[1]	0.8
Nonvegetarian endurance athletes[2]	1.2 to 1.4
Nonvegetarian strength athletes[2]	1.6 to 1.7
Vegetarian endurance athletes[2]	1.3 to 1.5
Vegetarian strength athletes[2]	1.7 to 1.8

Sources:[1]Food and Nutrition Board, Institute of Medicine, Dietary Reference Intakes for Energy, Carbohydrate, Fiber, Fat, Fatty Acids, Cholesterol, Protein, and Amino Acids (Macronutrients), (Washington, DC: National Academies Press, 2002), 465–608.
[2]American College of Sports Medicine, American Dietetic Association, and Dietitians of Canada, Joint Position Statement. Nutrition and athletic performance. *Med. Sci. Sports Exerc.* 32 (2001):2130–45.
*To convert body weight to kilograms, divide weight in pounds by 2.2.
Weight (pounds)/2.2 = Weight (kilograms)
Weight (kilograms) × protein recommendation (grams/kilograms body weight/day) = protein intake (grams/day)

Calculating Your Protein Needs

Theo wants to know how much protein he needs each day. Off season, he works out three times a week at a gym and practices basketball with friends every Friday night. He is not a vegetarian. Although Theo exercises regularly, he does not qualify as an endurance athlete or as a strength athlete. At this level of physical activity, Theo's RDA for protein probably ranges from 0.8 to 1.0 grams per kg body weight per day (see Table 6.3). To calculate the total number of grams of protein Theo should eat each day:

1. Convert Theo's weight from pounds to kilograms. Theo presently weighs 200 pounds. To convert this value to kilograms, divide by 2.2: (200 pounds) ÷ (2.2 pounds/kg) = 91 kg

2. Multiply Theo's weight in kilograms by his RDA for protein:

$$(91 \text{ kg}) \times (0.8 \text{ grams/kg}) = 72.8 \text{ grams of protein per day}$$

$$(91 \text{ kg}) \times (1.0 \text{ grams/kg}) = 91 \text{ grams of protein per day}$$

What happens during basketball season, when Theo practices or has games five to six days a week? This will probably raise his protein needs to approximately 1.0 to 1.2 grams per kg body weight per day. How much more protein should he eat?

$$91 \text{ kg} \times 1.2 \text{ grams/kg} = 109.2 \text{ grams of protein per day.}$$

Now calculate your recommended protein intake based upon your activity level.

Is it possible for Theo to eat this much protein each day? It may surprise you to discover that most Americans eat 1.5 to 2 times the RDA for protein without any effort! In the following sections, we describe the average protein intake in the United States, review foods that are good sources of protein, and give an example of calculating your daily protein intake. We will also look at potential risks of high protein diets.

Most Americans Meet or Exceed the RDA for Protein

Surveys indicate that Americans eat 16 to 17% of their total daily energy intake as protein (McDowell et al. 1994; Tillotson et al. 1997; see Figure 6.10). In these studies, women reported eating about 65 to 70 grams of protein each day, while men consumed 88 to 110 grams per day. Putting these values into perspective, let's assume that the average man weighs 75 kilograms (165 pounds) and the average woman weighs 65 kilograms (143 pounds). Their protein requirements (assuming they are not athletes or vegetarians) are 60 grams and 52 grams per day, respectively. As you can see, most adults in the United States appear to have no problems meeting their protein needs each day.

What are the typical protein intakes of active people? Table 6.4 reviews the self-reported protein intake of athletes participating in a variety of sports (Manore and Thompson 2000). As you can see, the protein intake ranges from 1.1 to 3.1 grams per kilogram body weight per day and accounts for 13 to 36% of the total daily energy intake in these active individuals. However, there are certain groups of athletes who are at risk for low protein intakes. Athletes who consume inadequate energy and limit food choices, such as distance runners, figure skaters, female gymnasts, and wrestlers who are dieting, are all at risk for low protein intakes. Unlike people who consume adequate energy, individuals who are restricting their total energy intake (kilocalories) need to pay close attention to their protein intake.

16%   **49%**   **34%**   **3%**

Key:
- Carbohydrate
- Alcohol
- Total fat
- Protein

Figure 6.10   Reported average intakes of carbohydrate, fat, protein, and alcohol for adults aged 20 years and older in the United States (adapted from M. A. McDowell, R. R. Briefel, K. Alaimo, et. al. Energy and macronutrient intakes of persons ages 2 months and over in the United States: Third National Health and Nutrition Examination Survey, Phase I 1988–1991. *Advance Data* 255 [1994]: 1–24).

Table 6.4   Self-reported Protein Intakes of Athletes

Sport Type	Gender	Protein Intake (gram/kilogram body weight/day)	Proteins Intake (% total kcal)
Football	M	1.5	15.0
Weightlifting	M	1.9	18.0
Soccer	M	2.2	14.4
Triathlon	M	2.0	13.0
Marathon running	M	2.0	14.5
Distance running	M	1.6	12.8
	F	1.1	14.1
Ultradistance running	M	1.4	16.7
	F	1.2	15.1
Bodybuilding	M	2.7–3.1	22.5–37.7
	F	1.9–2.7	22.6–35.8

Source: Adapted by permission from M. Manore and J. Thompson, 2000, *Sport Nutrition for Health and Performance,* (Champaign, IL: Human Kinetics), 118.

Recap: The RDA for protein for most nonpregnant, nonlactating, nonvegetarian adults is 0.8 grams per kg body weight. Children, pregnant women, nursing mothers, vegetarians, and active people need slightly more. Most people who eat enough kilocalories and carbohydrates have no problem meeting their RDA for protein.

Too Much Dietary Protein Can Be Harmful

High protein intake may increase the risk of health problems. Three health conditions that have received particular attention include heart disease, bone loss, and kidney disease.

High Protein Intake Is Associated with High Cholesterol

High protein diets comprised of predominantly animal sources are associated with higher blood cholesterol levels. This is probably due to the saturated fat in animal products, which is known to increase blood cholesterol levels and the risk of heart disease. One study showed that people with heart disease improved their health when they ate a diet that was high in whole grains, fruits, and vegetables and met the RDA for protein (Fleming 2000). However, some of the people in this study chose to eat a high protein diet, and their risk factors worsened. In addition, vegetarians have been shown to have a greatly reduced risk of heart disease (Fraser, Linsted, and Beeson 1995).

High Protein Intake May Contribute to Bone Loss

How might a high protein diet lead to bone loss? Until recently, nutritionists have been concerned about high protein diets because they increase calcium excretion. This may be because animal products contain more of the sulfur amino acids (methionine and cysteine). Metabolizing these amino acids makes the blood more acidic, and calcium is pulled from the bone to buffer these acids. Although eating more protein can cause you to excrete more calcium, it is very controversial whether high protein intakes actually cause bone loss. We do know that eating too little protein causes bone loss, which increases the risk of fractures and osteoporosis. Higher intakes of animal and soy protein have been shown to protect bone in middle-aged and older women

(Munger, Cerhan, and Chiu 1999; Alekel et al. 2000). There does not appear to be enough direct evidence at this time to show that higher protein intakes cause bone loss in healthy people.

High Protein Intake Can Increase the Risk for Kidney Disease

A third risk associated with high protein intakes is kidney disease. People with kidney problems are advised to eat a low protein diet because a high protein diet can increase the risk of acquiring kidney disease in people who are susceptible. People with diabetes have higher rates of kidney disease and may benefit from a lower protein diet (Kontessis et al. 1995). There is no evidence, however, that eating more protein causes kidney disease in healthy people who are not susceptible to this condition. In fact, one study found that athletes consuming up to 2.8 grams of protein per kg body weight per day experienced no unhealthy changes in kidney function (Poortmans and Dellalieux 2000). Experts agree that eating no more than 2 grams of protein per kg body weight each day is safe for healthy people.

It is important for people who consume a lot of protein to drink more water. This is because eating more protein increases protein metabolism and urea production. As we mentioned earlier, urea is a waste product that forms when nitrogen is removed during amino acid metabolism. Adequate fluid is needed to flush excess urea from the kidneys. This is particularly important for athletes, who need more fluid due to higher sweat losses.

Liz Nutri-Case

"One of my dancer friends, Silvie, was always a little pudgy, but now she's tighter than I've ever seen her. Yesterday, even our teacher commented on how great she looks! After class, I asked her secret and she said she's been on a high-protein diet for two months. She said it's pretty easy to stick to—you just have to avoid starches like bread and pasta. Oh, and most sweets, too, though you can still have ice cream. She said she never feels hungry anymore, that the meat and eggs and cheese keep her feeling full. I'm thinking to myself, heck, I'm hungry all the time. So I asked her to bring me her book about the diet so I can try it for myself."

One issue that has been a major controversy for many years is the use of high-protein diets for weight loss. Popular diets such as the Atkins' Diet, the Zone Diet, and the Sugar Busters diet support the use of high-protein or low-carbohydrate meals to achieve weight loss. The Nutrition Debate highlight at the end of the chapter (page 228) has a detailed discussion of this controversial topic. After reading it, what do you think of Liz's idea of trying the diet? Would your opinion change if you learned that Liz has high LDL cholesterol and that her father suffered a heart attack last year at age 49? How might you advise Liz to adapt the diet for her unique health concerns?

Shopper's Guide: Good Food Sources of Protein

Table 6.5 compares the protein content of a variety of foods. In general, good sources of protein include meats (beef, pork, poultry, seafood), dairy products (milk-based products and eggs), soy products, legumes, whole grains, and nuts. While most people are aware that meats are an excellent source of protein, many people are surprised to learn that the quality of the protein in some legumes is almost equal to that of meat.

Legumes include foods such as kidney beans, pinto beans, black beans, soybeans, garbanzo beans (or chickpeas), lentils, green peas, black-eyed peas, and lima beans. Interestingly, the quality of soybean protein is almost identical to that of meat, and the protein quality of other legumes is relatively high. In addition to being excellent sources of protein, legumes are also high in fiber, iron, calcium, and many of the B vitamins. They are also low in saturated fat and cholesterol. Legumes are not

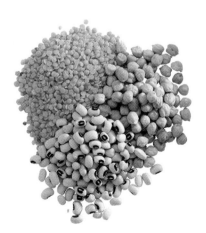

The quality of the protein in some legumes such as these black-eyed peas, lentils, and garbanzo beans, is almost equal to that of meat.

nutritionally complete, however, as they do not contain vitamins B_{12}, C, or A and are deficient in methionine, an essential amino acid. Eating legumes regularly, including foods made from soybeans, may help reduce the risk of heart disease by lowering blood cholesterol levels. Diets high in legumes and soy products are also associated with lower rates of some cancers.

Fruits and many vegetables are not particularly high in protein; however, these foods provide fiber and many vitamins and minerals and are excellent sources of carbohydrates. Thus, eating these foods can help provide the carbohydrates and energy that our body needs so that we can spare protein for use in building and maintaining our bodies rather than using it for energy. Try the Nutrition Label Activity on page 213 to determine how much protein you typically eat.

Recap: Eating too much protein may increase your risk for heart disease and kidney disease if you are already at risk for these diseases. Good sources of protein include meats, eggs, dairy products, soy products, legumes, whole grains, and nuts.

Table 6.5   Protein Content of Commonly Consumed Foods

Food	Serving Size	Protein (g)	Food	Serving Size	Protein (g)
Beef:			*Beans:*		
Ground, lean, baked (16% fat)	3.5 oz.	24	Refried	0.5 cup	7
Corned beef, brisket, cooked	3.5 oz.	18	Kidney, red	0.5 cup	9
Prime rib, broiled (½-in. trim)	3.5 oz.	21	Black	0.5 cup	8
Top sirloin, broiled (¼-in. trim)	3.5 oz.	27	Pork and beans, canned	0.5 cup	7
Poultry:			*Nuts:*		
Chicken breast, broiled, no skin	3.0 oz.	25	Peanuts, dry roasted	1 oz.	7
Chicken thigh, barbecued (BBQ) no skin	2.2 oz.	14	Peanut butter, creamy	2 tbsp.	8
Chicken drumstick, BBQ, with skin	2.5 oz.	16	Almonds, blanched	1 oz.	6
Turkey breast, roasted, Louis Rich	3.5 oz.	20	Sunflower seeds	0.25 cup	7
Turkey dark meat, roasted, no skin	3.5 oz.	29	Pecan halves	1 oz.	5
Seafood:			*Cereals, Grains, and Breads:*		
Cod, steamed	3.5 oz.	22	Barley, cooked	1 cup	4
Salmon, chinook, baked	3.5 oz.	26	Oatmeal, quick instant	1 cup	6
Shrimp, steamed	3.5 oz.	21	Cheerios	1 cup	3
Oysters, boiled	3.5 oz.	19	Corn Bran	1 cup	2
Tuna, in water, drained	3.5 oz.	29	Grape Nuts	0.5 cup	7
Pork:			Raisin Bran	1 cup	5
			Brown rice, cooked	1 cup	5
Pork loin chop, broiled	3.5 oz.	24	Whole wheat bread	1 slice	2
Spareribs, cooked, with bone	3.5 oz.	29	Rye bread	1 slice	2
Ham, roasted, lean	3.5 oz.	21	Bagel, 3½-in. diameter	1 each	7
Dairy:			*Vegetables:*		
Whole milk (3.3% fat)	8 fl. oz.	8	Carrots, raw (7.5 × 1⅛-in.)	1 each	1
1% milk	8 fl. oz.	8	Asparagus, boiled	6 spears	2
Skim milk	8 fl. oz.	8	Green beans, cooked	0.0 cup	1
Low-fat yogurt	8 fl. oz.	13	Broccoli, raw, chopped	0.0 cup	1
American cheese, processed	1 oz.	6	Collards, cooked from frozen	0.0 cup	3
Swiss cheese	1 oz.	6	Spinach, raw, chopped	1 cup	2
Cottage cheese, low-fat (2%)	1 cup	31			
Soy Products:					
Tofu	0.5 cup	10			
Tempeh, cooked	3.3 oz.	18			
Soy milk beverage	1 cup	7			

Source: Values obtained from U. S. Department of Agriculture (USDA). Nutrient Database for Standard Reference. www.nal.usda.gov/fnic/cgi-bin/nut_search.pl, Accessed July 2003.

How Much Protein Do You Eat?

Theo wants to know if his diet contains enough protein. To calculate his protein intake, he records all foods that he eats for three days in a food diary. The foods Theo consumed for one of his three days are listed below on the left, and the protein content of those foods is listed on the right. Theo recorded the protein content listed on the Nutrition Facts label for those foods with labels. For products without labels, he used the nutrient analysis program that came with this book. There is also a U.S. Department of Agriculture Web site that lists the energy and nutrient content of thousands of foods (go to www.nal.usda.gov/fnic/cgi-bin/nut_search.pl).

Foods Consumed	Protein Content (g)
Breakfast:	
Brewed coffee (2 cups) with 2 tbsp. cream	1
1 large bagel (5-in. diameter)	10
Low-fat cream cheese (1.5 oz.)	4.5
Mid-morning snack:	
Cola beverage (32 fl. oz.)	0
Low-fat strawberry yogurt (1 cup)	10
Snackwells Apple Cinnamon Bars (37 g each bar; 2 bars eaten)	2
Lunch:	
Ham and cheese sandwich:	
Whole wheat bread (2 slices)	4
Mayonnaise (1.5 tbsp.)	1
Lean ham (4 oz.)	24
Swiss cheese (2 oz.)	16
Iceberg lettuce (2 leaves)	0.5
Sliced tomato (3 slices)	0.5
Banana (1 large)	1
Triscuit crackers (20 each)	7
Bottled water (20 fl. oz.)	0
Dinner:	
Cheeseburger:	
Broiled ground beef (½-lb. cooked)	64
American cheese (1 oz.)	6
Seeded bun (1 large)	6
Ketchup (2 tbsp.)	1
Mustard (1 tbsp.)	1
Shredded lettuce (½ cup)	0.5
Sliced tomato (3 slices)	0.5
French fries (2- to 3-in. strips; 30 each)	6
Baked beans (2 cups)	28
2% low-fat milk (2 cups)	16
Evening snack:	
Chocolate chip cookies (4 each of 3-in. diameter cookie)	3
2% low-fat milk (1 cup)	8
Total Protein Intake for the Day:	**221.5 grams**

As calculated in the You Do the Math box on page 209, Theo's RDA is 72.8 to 91 grams of protein. He is consuming 2.4 to 3 times that amount! You can see that he does not need to use amino acid or protein supplements, since he has more than adequate amounts of protein to build lean tissue.

Now calculate your own protein intake using food labels and the nutrient analysis program included with this book. Do you obtain more protein from animal or non-animal sources? If you consume mostly non-animal sources, are you eating soy products and complementary foods throughout the day? If you eat animal-based products on a regular basis, notice how much protein you consume from even small servings of meat and dairy products. ●

Can a Vegetarian Diet Provide Adequate Protein?

Vegetarianism is the practice of restricting the diet to food substances of vegetable origin, including fruits, grains, and nuts. Over the last fifteen years, the number of vegetarians has increased in the United States from approximately six million to twelve million people. Many vegetarians are college students; moving away from home and taking responsibility for one's eating habits appears to influence some young adults to try it as a lifestyle choice.

vegetarianism The practice of restricting the diet to food substances of plant origin, including vegetables, fruits, grains, and nuts.

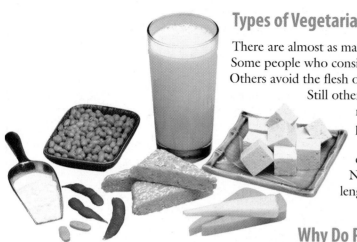

Soy products are also a good source of dietary protein.

Types of Vegetarian Diets

There are almost as many types of vegetarian diets as there are vegetarians. Some people who consider themselves vegetarians regularly eat poultry and fish. Others avoid the flesh of animals, but consume eggs, milk, and cheese liberally. Still others strictly avoid all products of animal origin, including milk and eggs, and even by-products such as candies and puddings made with gelatin.

Table 6.6 identifies the various types of vegetarian diets, ranging from the most inclusive to the most restrictive. Notice that, the more restrictive the diet, the more challenging it becomes to achieve an adequate protein intake.

Why Do People Become Vegetarians?

When discussing vegetarianism, one of the most often-asked questions is why people would make this food choice. The most common responses are included here.

Religious, Ethical, and Food-Safety Reasons

Some make the choice for religious or spiritual reasons. Several religions prohibit or restrict the consumption of animal flesh; however, generalizations can be misleading. For example, while certain sects within Hinduism forbid the consumption of meat, perusing the menu at any Indian restaurant will reveal that many other Hindus regularly consume small quantities of meat, poultry, and fish. Many Buddhists are vegetarians, as are some Christians, including Seventh Day Adventists.

Many vegetarians are guided by their personal philosophy to choose vegetarianism. These people feel that it is morally and ethically wrong to consume animals and

Table 6.6   Terms and Definitions of a Vegetarian Diet

Type of Diet	Foods Consumed	Comments
Semivegetarian (also called partial vegetarian)	Vegetables, grains, nuts, fruits, legumes; sometimes seafood, poultry, eggs, and dairy products	Typically exclude or limit red meat; may also avoid other meats
Pescovegetarian	Similar to a semivegetarian but excludes poultry	*Pesco* means fish, the only animal source of protein in this diet
Lacto-ovo-vegetarian	Vegetables, grains, nuts, fruits, legumes, dairy products (*lacto*) and eggs (*ovo*)	Excludes animal flesh and seafood
Lactovegetarian	Similar to a lacto-ovo-vegetarian but excludes eggs	Relies on milk and cheese for animal sources of protein
Ovovegetarian	Vegetables, grains, nuts, fruits, legumes, and eggs	Excludes dairy, flesh, and seafood products
Vegan (also called strict vegetarian)	Only plant-based foods (vegetables, grains, nuts, seeds, fruits, legumes)	May not provide adequate vitamin B_{12}, zinc, iron, or calcium
Macrobiotic diet	Vegan-type of diet; becomes progressively more strict until almost all foods are eliminated. At the extreme, only brown rice and small amounts of water or herbal tea are consumed.	Taken to the extreme, can cause malnutrition and death
Fruitarian	Only raw or dried fruit, seeds, nuts, honey, and vegetable oil	Very restrictive diet; deficient in protein, calcium, zinc, iron, vitamin B_{12}, riboflavin, and other nutrients

any products from animals (such as dairy or egg products) because they view the practices in the modern animal industries as inhumane. They may consume milk and eggs but choose to purchase them only from family farms where animals are treated humanely.

There is also a great deal of concern about meat handling practices, as contaminated meat is allowed into our food supply. For example, in 1982, there was an outbreak of severe bloody diarrhea that was eventually traced to hamburgers served at a fast-food restaurant. The hamburgers were contaminated with the *Escherichia coli* O157:H7 bacteria; several people became seriously ill and one child died after eating them. The Centers for Disease Control and Prevention estimate that 73,000 cases of infection and 61 deaths occur each year in the United States due to consuming foods contaminated by this bacterial strain (CDC 2001). Although many individuals feel that avoiding meat products will prevent exposure to this deadly strain this is not true, as alfalfa sprouts, lettuce, and unpasteurized milk and juice are also foods commonly contaminated with it.

One recent concern surrounding beef that has taken Europe by storm is the epidemic of **mad cow disease.** See the Highlight: Global Nutrition box on page 216 for a review of mad cow disease and its impact on the United States and other countries.

mad cow disease A fatal brain disorder prompted by consumption of food containing *prions*, which are an abnormal form of protein found in the brains and other organs of infected sheep, cows, and other livestock.

Ecological Benefits

Many people choose vegetarianism because of their concerns about the effect of meat industries on the global environment. Due to the high demand for meat in developed nations, meat production has evolved from small family farming operations into the larger system of agribusiness. Critics of agribusiness are concerned with the environmental damages that agribusiness can cause. When animals are raised on smaller farms and/or allowed to range freely, they consume grass, crop wastes, and scraps recycled from the kitchen, which is an efficient means of utilizing food sources that humans do not consume. The waste produced by these animals can be used for fertilizer and fuel.

Activists against agribusiness and meat consumption point out that animals raised in large agribusinesses consume large quantities of grain that humans could consume. Water use can also be tremendous; it is estimated that in the United States, it takes 430 gallons of water to produce one pound of pork. This is in contrast to the 151 gallons of water it takes to produce one pound of wheat. Another concern is related to the waste produced from meat production. While much of the waste produced by animals in the agribusiness system is used as fertilizer, some of it can run off into surrounding bodies of water, resulting in the pollution of neighboring streams, rivers, and lakes. Livestock are also blamed for the majority of methane production, which is a gas associated with increased global warming. There is also concern that to provide ample room to raise animals for human consumption, a great deal of land that could be used for plant food production is destroyed. It is speculated that millions of acres of rain forests around the world have been destroyed to provide enough grazing land for livestock, and that destroying the rain forests has been a major contributor to global warming.

In response to many of these claims, meat industry organizations have published information in defense of their practices. In a recent fact sheet, the National Cattlemen's Beef Association (2003) point out important facts that dispute many of the claims made by agribusiness critics:

- Virtually all of the grain consumed by livestock is unfit for human consumption.
- While it does take more water to produce a pound of beef than a pound of vegetables, the amount is much lower than claimed by many activists and is only 11% of the total amount of water used in the United States each year.

Global Nutrition: Mad Cow Disease — What's the Beef?

Mad cow disease is a fatal brain disorder caused by a *prion*, which is an abnormal form of protein. Prions influence other proteins to take on their abnormal shape, and these abnormal proteins cause brain damage. Mad cow disease is also called *bovine spongiform encephalopathy (BSE)*. The disease eats away at a cow's brain, leaving it full of spongelike holes. Eventually the brain can no longer control vital life functions, and the cow literally "goes mad." Unfortunately, people who eat infected cattle will also be infected. This disease has killed at least 100 people, most of them in Great Britain.

Scientists are not certain how the prions are introduced to cattle. They think cattle become infected by eating feed made with the brains and spinal cords of other infected cattle. In Great Britain and Europe, it was common practice to feed livestock with meal made from other animals. Even after exposure, it takes years for mad cow disease to manifest itself. Scientists speculate that older cattle are more infectious than younger animals. Since cattle are slaughtered at an older age in Europe, this increases the risk of passing the disease from one animal to another.

The effect of mad cow disease on the European beef market has been staggering, with beef consumption dropping 25 to 70% in certain countries; Great Britain, France, and Germany have been particularly affected. Even cattle that are only potentially infected must be slaughtered. To date, almost five million cattle have been destroyed.

In December 2003, the first case of mad cow disease was reported in the United States, shocking those who believed the food supply to be safe from this disease. This discovery prompted many countries to immediately ban importation of American beef. Despite this discovery, the federal government and beef industry took aggressive steps to destroy any potentially infected beef and to reassure the public that American beef is safe for consumption. Because of the protective steps taken in the United States, this case of mad cow disease is thought to be an anomaly. These protective steps include feeding U.S. cattle high protein meal made from soybeans and banning the use of animal feed made with animal by-products. In addition, cattle in the United States are slaughtered at an early age, reducing the likelihood of advanced infection. Finally, the United States has banned the import of all cattle, sheep, and goats from Europe.

Should Americans fear our beef supply? The U.S. Department of Agriculture, the FDA, the National Institutes of Health, and the Centers for Disease Control and Prevention are working together to eliminate the use of animal-based feed and to enhance technology that can track signs of the disease and act quickly if it reappears in our food supply. In addition, the U.S. beef industry is highly motivated to comply with safety regulations since reduced beef intake translates into millions of dollars in lost income.

Although it is not possible for the United States to be completely immune to mad cow disease, adherence to strict safety standards should minimize our risk and keep our beef safe for human consumption. ●

- The waste produced by cattle is very minor. In fact, the primary source of methane emissions is from landfills; only about 2% of the total methane production in the United States comes from domestic livestock.
- Much of the land used to raise livestock is not suitable for use in growing vegetable or grain crops. Interestingly, soil erosion, which is a significant problem in the United States, occurs most extensively with crops such as cotton.
- Although many countries have destroyed significant areas of rain forest to provide grazing land for domestic livestock, less than 1% of the total 2001 beef supply in the United States was imported from rain forest countries, and the largest fast-food chains have policies in place that prohibit the purchase of beef from these same countries.

This is obviously a complex emotionally and politically charged topic. While some individuals choose vegetarianism to protect the environment, it is not practical or realistic to expect every human around the world to adopt this lifestyle. Animal products provide important nutrients for our bodies, and many people on the brink of starvation cannot survive without small amounts of milk and meat. The environmental damage caused by the raising of livestock is due not only to how animals are raised but also to the large number of animals produced. There is currently a trend toward people reducing their consumption of animal products so that the overall demand for meat is considerably lessened. In this way, many hope that it may be possible to return to the system of small family farming, which is more environmentally friendly. In addition to the environmental benefits, eating less meat may also reduce our risk for chronic diseases such as heart disease and some cancers.

Health Benefits

Still others practice vegetarianism because of its health benefits. Research over several years has consistently shown that a varied and balanced vegetarian diet can reduce the risk of many chronic diseases. Health benefits include (Messina and Messina 1996):

- Reduced intake of fat and total energy, which reduces the risk for obesity. This may in turn lower a person's risk of type 2 diabetes.
- Lower blood pressure, which may be due to a higher intake of fruits and vegetables. People who eat vegetarian diets tend to be nonsmokers, drink little or no alcohol, and exercise more regularly, which are also factors known to reduce blood pressure and help maintain a healthy body weight.
- Reduced risk of heart disease, which may be due to lower saturated fat intake and a higher consumption of *antioxidants* that are found in plant-based foods. Antioxidants, discussed in detail in Chapter 8, are substances that can protect our cells from damage. They are abundant in fruits and vegetables.
- Fewer digestive problems such as constipation and diverticular disease, most likely due to the higher fiber content of vegetarian diets. Diverticular disease, discussed in Chapter 4, occurs when the wall of the bowel (large intestine) pouches and becomes inflamed.
- Reduced risk of some cancers. Research shows that vegetarians may have lower rates of cancer, particularly colon cancer (Phillips and Snowdon 1983). Many components of a vegetarian diet could contribute to reducing cancer risks, including higher fiber and antioxidant intakes, lower dietary fat intake, lower consumption of **carcinogens** (cancer-causing agents) that are formed when cooking meat, and higher consumption of soy protein, which may have anti-cancer properties (Messina 1999).
- Reduced risk of kidney disease, kidney stones, and gallstones. The lower protein contents of vegetarian diets, plus the higher intake of legumes and vegetable proteins such as soy, may be protective against these conditions.

carcinogens Cancer-causing agents, such as certain pesticides, industrial chemicals, and pollutants.

What Are the Challenges of a Vegetarian Diet?

While a vegetarian diet can be healthful, it also presents many challenges. By limiting consumption of flesh and dairy products, there is the potential for inadequate intakes of certain nutrients. Table 6.7 lists the nutrients that can be deficient in a vegan-type of diet plan and describes good nonanimal sources that can provide these nutrients.

Vegetarians who consume dairy and/or egg products obtain these nutrients more easily. However, it is important for vegetarians and nonvegetarians to consume a varied and adequate diet. Research indicates that a sign of disordered eating in some female athletes is the switch to a vegetarian diet (O'Conner et al. 1987). Instead of eating a healthy variety of nonanimal foods, people with disordered eating problems may use vegetarianism as an excuse to restrict many foods from their diets.

Can a vegetarian diet provide enough protein? Since high-quality protein sources are quite easy to obtain in developed countries, a well-balanced vegetarian diet can provide adequate protein (Figure 6.11). In fact, the American Dietetic Association (1997) endorses an appropriately planned vegetarian diet as healthful,

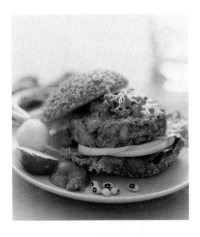

Figure 6.11   A well-balanced vegetarian diet can provide adequate protein.

Table 6.7   Nutrients of Concern in a Vegan Diet

Nutrient	Functions	Nonmeat/Nondairy Food Sources
Vitamin B_{12}	Assists with DNA synthesis; protection and growth of nerve fibers	Vitamin B_{12} fortified cereals, yeast, soy products and other meat analogs; vitamin B_{12} supplements
Vitamin D	Promotes bone growth	Vitamin D fortified cereals, margarines, and soy products; adequate exposure to sunlight; supplementation may be necessary for those who do not get adequate exposure to sunlight
Riboflavin (vitamin B_2)	Promotes release of energy; supports normal vision and skin health	Whole and enriched grains, green leafy vegetables, mushrooms, beans, nuts and seeds
Iron	Assists with oxygen transport; involved in making amino acids and hormones	Whole grain products, prune juice, dried fruits, beans, nuts, seeds, leafy vegetables such as spinach
Calcium	Maintains bone health; assists with muscle contraction, blood pressure, and nerve transmission	Fortified soy milk and tofu, almonds, dry beans, leafy vegetables, calcium-fortified juices, fortified breakfast cereals
Zinc	Assists with DNA and RNA synthesis, immune function, and growth	Whole grain products, wheat germ, beans, nuts, and seeds

nutritionally adequate, and providing many benefits in reducing and preventing various diseases. As you can see, the emphasis is on a *balanced* and *adequate* vegetarian diet; thus, it is important for vegetarians to consume soy products, eat complementary proteins, and obtain enough energy from other macronutrients to spare protein from being used as an energy source. Although the digestibility of a vegetarian diet is potentially lower than an animal-based diet, there is no separate protein recommendation for vegetarians who consume complementary plant proteins (Institute of Medicine 2002, 465–608).

Theo   *Nutri-Case*

"No way would I ever become a vegetarian! The only way to build up your muscles is to eat meat. I was reading in a bodybuilding magazine last week about some guy who doesn't eat anything from animals, not even milk or eggs, and he looked pretty buff—but I don't believe it. They can do anything to photos these days. Besides, after a game I just crave red meat. If I don't have it, I feel sort of like my batteries don't get recharged. It's just not practical for a competitive athlete to go without meat."

What two claims does Theo make here about the role of red meat in his diet? Do you think these claims are valid? Why or why not? Without trying to convert Theo to vegetarianism, what facts might you offer him about the nature of plant and animal proteins?

Using the Vegetarian Food Guide Pyramid to Achieve the RDA for Protein

The Vegetarian Food Guide Pyramid was introduced in Chapter 2, and it is illustrated again in Figure 6.12. Vegetarians can use this pyramid to design a healthful diet that contains all of the necessary nutrients. Figure 6.12a emphasizes the importance of eating whole grains, fruits, vegetables, and legumes at every meal. Daily foods include nuts and seeds, egg whites, soy milk and dairy products, and plant oils. Weekly choices include eggs and sweets. While this version provides a helpful illustration of

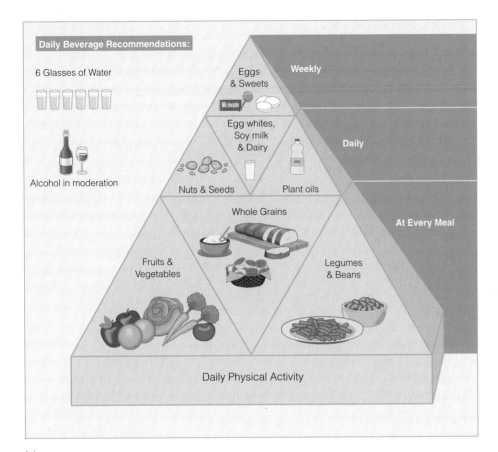

(a)

Figure 6.12 The Vegetarian Food Guide Pyramid. **(a)** This pyramid guides general food choices at each meal, daily, and weekly (© 2000 Oldways Preservation & Exchange Trust, www.oldwayspt.org). **(b)** This pyramid is similar to the standard USDA Food Guide Pyramid and illustrates the recommended number of servings of vegetarian foods that should be eaten daily from each food group. (© 1997 American Dietetic Association. "Food Guide Pyramid for Vegetarian Meal Planning." Used with permission.)

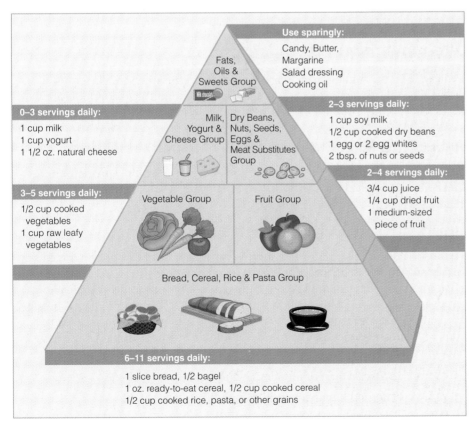

(b)

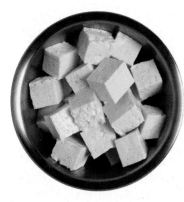

Vegetarians should eat 2–3 servings of beans, nuts, seeds, eggs, or meat substitutes daily.

the types of foods recommended for vegetarians, it does not give suggestions for daily number of servings.

Figure 6.12b provides a version of the Vegetarian Food Guide Pyramid that more closely matches the format of the standard USDA Food Guide Pyramid. This version is helpful in providing suggested numbers of servings for each food group. Notice that the bread, cereal, rice, and pasta group and the fruit and vegetable groups are identical to those shown in the standard USDA Food Guide Pyramid. It is suggested that vegetarians consume zero to three servings of foods from the milk, yogurt, and cheese group. Lacto- and lacto-ovo-vegetarians can consume low-fat or nonfat dairy products, while vegans and ovovegetarians can consume calcium-fortified soy or rice milk, yogurt, and cheese products to meet the guidelines for this food group. Another excellent source of calcium is calcium-fortified orange juice. Vegetarians should also consume two to three servings daily of foods from the dry beans, nuts, seeds, eggs, and meat substitutes group. Soy-based foods such as tempeh and tofu fit into this food group. Consistent with the standard USDA Food Guide Pyramid, it is recommended that fats, oils, and sweets be consumed sparingly.

With careful menu planning, vegetarians can meet their nutritional needs using the Vegetarian Food Guide Pyramid. Vegans need to pay special attention to consuming foods high in vitamins D, B_{12}, and riboflavin (B_2), and the minerals calcium, zinc, and iron. Supplementation of these nutrients may be necessary for certain individuals if they cannot consume adequate amounts in their diet.

> **Recap:** A balanced vegetarian diet may reduce the risk of obesity, type 2 diabetes, heart disease, digestive problems, some cancers, kidney disease, kidney stones, and gallstones. While varied vegetarian diets can provide enough protein, vegetarians who consume no animal products need to supplement their diet with good sources of vitamin B_{12}, vitamin D, riboflavin, iron, calcium, and zinc.

What Disorders Are Related to Protein Intake or Metabolism?

As we have seen, consuming inadequate protein can result in severe illness and death. Typically, this occurs when people do not consume enough total kilocalories, but a diet deficient specifically in protein can have similar effects.

Protein-Energy Malnutrition Can Lead to Debility and Death

protein-energy malnutrition A disorder caused by inadequate consumption of protein. It is characterized by severe wasting.

When a person consumes too little protein and energy, the result is **protein-energy malnutrition** (also called *protein-calorie malnutrition*). Two diseases that can follow are marasmus and kwashiorkor (Figure 6.13).

Marasmus Results from Grossly Inadequate Energy Intake

marasmus A form of protein-energy malnutrition that results from grossly inadequate intakes of protein, energy, and other nutrients.

Marasmus is a disease that results from grossly inadequate intakes of protein, energy, and other nutrients. Essentially, people with marasmus slowly starve to death. It is most common in young children (six to eighteen months of age) who are living in impoverished conditions. These children are fed diluted cereal drinks that are inadequate in energy, protein, and most nutrients. People suffering from marasmus have the look of "skin and bones" as their body fat and tissues are wasting. Consequences of marasmus include:

- Wasting and weakening of muscles, including the heart muscle
- Stunted brain development and learning impairment
- Depressed metabolism and little insulation from body fat, causing a dangerously low body temperature

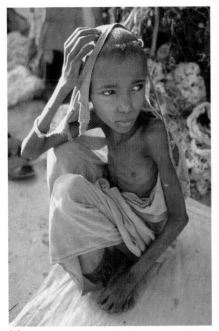

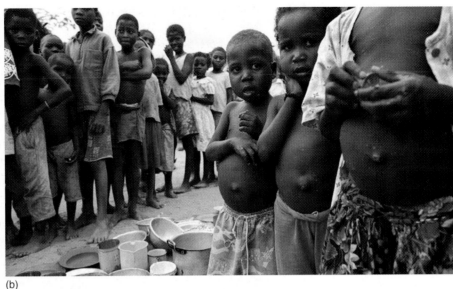

(b)

(a)

Figure 6.13   Two forms of protein-energy malnutrition are **(a)** marasmus and **(b)** kwashiorkor.

- Stunted physical growth and development
- Deterioration of the intestinal lining, which further inhibits absorption of nutrients
- *Anemia* (abnormally low levels of hemoglobin in the blood)
- Severely weakened immune system
- Fluid and electrolyte imbalances

If marasmus is left untreated, death from dehydration, heart failure, or infection will result. Treating marasmus involves carefully correcting fluid and electrolyte imbalances. Protein and carbohydrates are provided once the body's condition has stabilized. Fat is introduced much later, as the protein levels in the blood must improve to the point where they can carry fat so it can be safely metabolized by the body.

Kwashiorkor Results from a Low-Protein Diet

Kwashiorkor often occurs in developing countries where infants are weaned early due to the arrival of a subsequent baby. This deficiency disease is typically seen in young children (one to three years of age) who no longer drink breast milk. Instead, they often are fed a low protein, starchy cereal. Unlike marasmus, kwashiorkor often develops quickly and causes the person to look swollen, particularly in the belly. This is because the low protein content of the blood is inadequate to keep fluids from seeping into the tissue spaces. Other symptoms of kwashiorkor include:

- Some weight loss and muscle wasting, with some retention of body fat
- Retarded growth and development; less severe than that seen with marasmus
- Edema, which results in extreme distension of the belly and is caused by fluid and electrolyte imbalances
- Fatty degeneration of the liver
- Loss of appetite, sadness, irritability, apathy
- Development of sores and other skin problems; skin pigmentation changes
- Dry, brittle hair that changes color, straightens, and falls out easily

kwashiorkor A form of protein-energy malnutrition that is typically seen in developing countries in infants and toddlers who are weaned early because of the birth of a subsequent child. Denied breast milk, they are fed a cereal diet that provides adequate energy but inadequate protein.

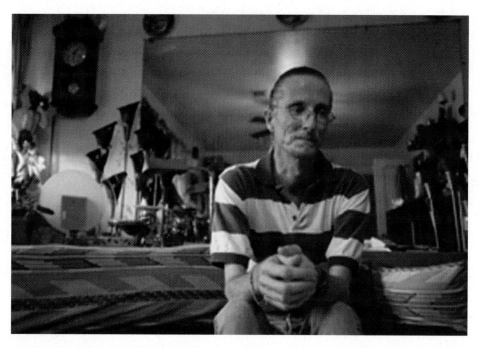

Figure 6.14   Protein-energy malnutrition occurs in several populations in the United States, including those with such wasting diseases as AIDS and cancer.

Kwashiorkor can be reversed if adequate protein and energy are given in time. Because of their severely weakened immune systems, many individuals with kwashiorkor die from diseases they contract in their weakened state. Of those who are treated, many return home to the same impoverished conditions, only to develop this deficiency once again.

Many people think that only children in developing countries suffer from these diseases. However, protein-energy malnutrition occurs in all countries and affects both children and adults. In the United States, poor people living in inner cities and isolated rural areas are affected. Others at risk include the elderly, the homeless, people with eating disorders, those addicted to alcohol and drugs, and individuals with wasting diseases such as AIDS and cancer (see Figure 6.14). Despite producing more than enough food, malnutrition can and does occur in the United States (see the Highlight: Global Nutrition box, page 223).

Disorders Related to Genetic Abnormalities

There are numerous disorders caused by defects in our DNA, or genetic material. A few of these disorders include phenylketonuria (or PKU), sickle cell anemia, and cystic fibrosis.

As discussed in Chapter 4, *phenylketonuria* is an inherited disease in which a person does not have the ability to break down the amino acid phenylalanine. As a result, phenylalanine and its metabolic by-products build up in our bodies and cause brain damage if left untreated. Individuals with PKU must eat a diet that is severely limited in phenylalanine.

Sickle cell anemia is an inherited disorder of the red blood cells in which a single amino acid present in hemoglobin is changed. As shown in Figure 6.5 (page 201), normal hemoglobin is globular in shape, which results in red blood cells having a round, doughnut-like shape. The genetic alteration that occurs with sickle cell anemia causes the red blood cells to be shaped like a sickle, or a crescent. Sickled red blood cells are hard and sticky so cannot flow smoothly through small blood vessels. These cells get clogged in the vessels and break apart, damaging the cells and

sickle cell anemia   A genetic disorder that causes red blood cells to be sickle-, or crescent-, shaped. These cells cannot travel smoothly through blood vessels, causing cell breakage and anemia.

Global Nutrition: Malnutrition in Developing Countries

At the close of the nineteenth century, infection, poverty, malnutrition, and squalid living conditions resulted in the deaths of 16% of all infants born in the United States. In fact, infant mortality rates were alarmingly high throughout the entire world at the beginning of the twentieth century, prompting serious efforts to combat this major health concern. Today, less than 1% of infants die in the United States. After 100 years, infant survival has improved dramatically in the United States and in other wealthier, developed countries; however, many developing countries continue to be plagued by high rates of malnutrition and subsequent infant mortality.

Over half (or 54%) of all deaths in children younger than 5 years of age in developing nations is due to malnutrition (Wegman 2001). Seventy percent of all childhood deaths in developing countries result from malnutrition, pneumonia, diarrhea, measles, or malaria. It is important to emphasize that malnutrition interacts with these other illnesses and diseases, leading to much higher death rates.

Millions of people in developing countries suffer from chronic malnutrition. Factors contributing to global malnutrition include:

• Famine, resulting from drought, flood, pests, war, and political sanctions that limit the importation of adequate food

• Population growth that has outpaced food production

• Deforestation, which has led to erosion and the devastation of critical water supplies

• Air pollution that has damaged crops, reduced food production, and poisoned water supplies

• Climatic changes, particularly global warming trends, have been suggested to cause heat waves and lower rainfall. Both of these changes can reduce soil moisture, impair pollination of certain crops, slow crop growth, and weaken disease resistance of crops

• Decreases in water supply, which reduces crop yield

• Unmitigated deterioration of land and water resources will eventually limit the number of animals that can be supported as potential food sources. Overgrazing and poor land management lead to rangeland deterioration, and pollution and overfishing have significantly reduced the availability of many fish, including various species of shark, sturgeon, halibut, and grouper (Musick et al. 2000).

These events eventually impact all people of the world, including those in wealthier countries. It is imperative to consider global malnutrition as a crisis that affects all of us. The causes of global malnutrition are diverse and complex, and it will take the efforts of all nations and people working together to prevent it. ●

causing anemia. This disease occurs in any person who inherits the sickle cell gene from both parents.

Cystic fibrosis is an inherited disease that primarily affects the respiratory system and digestive tract. Cystic fibrosis is caused by an abnormal protein that prevents the normal passage of chloride into and out of certain cells. This alteration in chloride transport causes cells to secrete thick, sticky mucus. The linings of the lungs and pancreas are particularly affected, causing breathing difficulties, lung infections, and digestion problems that lead to nutrient deficiencies. Symptoms include wheezing, coughing, and stunted growth. The severity of this disease varies greatly among those with it; some individuals with cystic fibrosis live relatively normal lives, while others are seriously debilitated and die in childhood.

cystic fibrosis A genetic disorder that causes an alteration in chloride transport, leading to the production of thick, sticky mucus that causes life-threatening respiratory and digestive problems.

Recap: Protein-energy malnutrition can lead to marasmus and kwashiorkor. These diseases primarily affect impoverished children in developing nations. However, residents of developed countries are also at risk, especially the elderly, homeless, alcoholics, drug addicts, and people with AIDS, cancer, and other wasting diseases. Genetic disorders that cause protein abnormalities include phenylketonuria, sickle cell anemia, and cystic fibrosis.

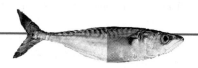

Chapter Summary

- Proteins are large, complex molecules that are critical components of all tissues, including blood, bone, and hormones.

- Unlike carbohydrates and fat, the structure of proteins is dictated by DNA, and proteins contain nitrogen.

- Amino acids are the building blocks of proteins; they are comprised of an amine group, an acid group, a hydrogen atom, and a unique side chain.

- There are twenty amino acids in our bodies: nine are essential amino acids, meaning that our bodies cannot produce them, and we must obtain them from food; eleven are nonessential, meaning our bodies can make them so they do not need to be consumed in the diet.

- Our genetic makeup determines the sequence of amino acids in our proteins. Gene expression refers to using a gene in a cell to make a protein.

- The three-dimensional shape of proteins determines their function in the body.

- When proteins are exposed to damaging substances such as heat, acids, bases, and alcohol, they are denatured, meaning they lose their shape and function.

- A limiting amino acid is one that is missing or in limited supply, preventing the synthesis of adequate proteins.

- Mutual supplementation is the process of combining two incomplete protein sources to make a complete protein. The two foods involved in this process are called complementary proteins.

- Most digestion of proteins occurs in the small intestine.

- Protein digestibility affects its quality, with proteins that are more digestible being of higher quality. Animal sources, soy protein, and legumes are highly digestible forms of protein.

- Proteins are needed to promote cell growth, repair, and maintenance. They act as enzymes and hormones; help maintain the balance of fluids, electrolytes, acids, and bases; and support healthy immune function.

- The RDA for protein for sedentary people is 0.8 g of protein per kg of body weight per day; protein should comprise 12 to 20% of total energy intake.

- Most people in the United States routinely eat 1.5 to 2 times the RDA for protein.

- High protein intakes may be harmful and can lead to increased blood cholesterol levels, increased calcium excretion, and increased risk for kidney disease in people who are susceptible to kidney problems.

- Good sources of protein include meats, dairy products, eggs, legumes, whole grains, and nuts.

- There are many forms of vegetarianism: lacto-ovo-vegetarians eat plant foods plus eggs and dairy products; pescovegetarians consume plant foods and rely on fish as the only meat source; vegans are considered strict vegetarians and consume only plant foods.

- Consuming a well-planned vegetarian diet may reduce the risk of obesity, heart disease, type 2 diabetes, and some forms of cancer.

- Vegans may need to supplement their diet with vitamins B_{12} and D, riboflavin, iron, calcium, and zinc.

- Marasmus and kwashiorkor are two forms of protein-energy malnutrition that results from grossly inadequate energy and protein intake.

- Phenylketonuria is a genetic disease in which the person cannot break down the amino acid phenylalanine. The buildup of phenylalanine and its by-products leads to brain damage.

- Sickle cell anemia is a genetic disorder of the red blood cells. Due to an alteration of one amino acid in hemoglobin, the red blood cells become sickle-shaped and cannot travel smoothly through blood vessels, thereby causing cell breakage and subsequent anemia.

- Cystic fibrosis is a genetic disease that causes an alteration in chloride transport that leads to the production of thick, sticky mucus. This mucus causes serious respiratory and digestive problems, which leads to variable levels of debilitation and, in some cases, premature death.

Review Questions

1. The process of combining peanut butter and whole wheat bread to make a complete protein is called
   a. deamination.
   b. vegetarianism.
   c. transamination.
   d. mutual supplementation.

2. Which of the following meals is typical of the vegan diet?
   a. Rice, pinto beans, acorn squash, soy butter, and almond milk
   b. Veggie dog, bun, and a banana blended with yogurt
   c. Brown rice and green tea
   d. Egg salad on whole wheat toast, broccoli, carrot sticks, and soy milk

3. The substance that breaks down polypeptides in the small intestine is called
   a. hydrochloric acid.
   b. pepsin.
   c. protease.
   d. ketones.

4. The portion of an amino acid that contains nitrogen is called the
   a. side chain.
   b. amine group.
   c. acid group.
   d. nitrate cluster.

5. Proteins contain
   a. carbon, oxygen, and nitrogen.
   b. oxygen and hydrogen.
   c. carbon, oxygen, hydrogen, and nitrogen.
   d. carbon, oxygen, and hydrogen.

6. **True or false?** After leaving the small intestine, amino acids are transported to the liver for distribution throughout the body.

7. **True or false?** When a protein is denatured, its shape is lost but its function is retained.

8. **True or false?** All hormones are proteins.

9. **True or false?** Buffers help the body maintain its fluids in proper balance.

10. **True or false?** Athletes typically require about three times as much protein as nonactive people.

11. Explain the relationship between inadequate protein intake and the swollen bellies of children with kwashiorkor.

12. Explain the relationship between excessive protein intake and an increased risk for kidney disease.

13. Identify six ways in which proteins are indispensable to human functioning.

14. Create a healthful one-day diet plan for an active twenty-year-old lacto-ovo-vegetarian.

15. Draw a sketch showing how amino acids bond to form proteins.

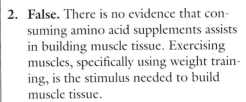 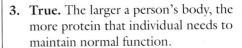 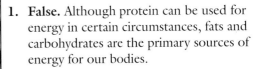

Test Yourself Answers

1. **False.** Although protein can be used for energy in certain circumstances, fats and carbohydrates are the primary sources of energy for our bodies.

2. **False.** There is no evidence that consuming amino acid supplements assists in building muscle tissue. Exercising muscles, specifically using weight training, is the stimulus needed to build muscle tissue.

3. **True.** The larger a person's body, the more protein that individual needs to maintain normal function.

4. **False.** Vegetarian diets can meet and even exceed an individual's protein needs, assuming that adequate energy-yielding macronutrients, a variety of protein sources, and complementary protein sources are consumed.

5. **True.** Most people in the United States consume 1.5 to 2 times more protein than they need.

Web Links

www.eatright.org
American Dietetic Association
Search for vegetarian diets to learn how to plan healthful meat-free meals.

http://aphis.usda.gov
Animal and Plant Health Inspection Service
Select "Hot Issues" or search for "Bovine Spongiform Encephalopathy (BSE)" to learn more about mad cow disease.

www.vrg.org
The Vegetarian Resource Group
Obtain vegetarian and vegan news, recipes, information, and additional links.

www.cdc.gov
Centers for Disease Control and Prevention
Click on "Health Topics A-Z" to learn more about *E. coli* and mad cow disease.

www.who.int/nut
World Health Organization Nutrition Site
Visit this site to find out more about the worldwide magnitude of protein-energy malnutrition and the diseases that can result from inadequate intakes of protein, energy-yielding carbohydrates and fats, and various additional nutrients.

www.nlm.nih.gov/medlineplus
MEDLINE Plus Health Information
Search for "sickle cell anemia" and "cystic fibrosis" to obtain additional resources and the latest news about these inherited diseases.

References

Alekel, D. L., A. St. Germain, C. T. Peterson, K. B. Hanson, J. W. Stewart, and T. Toda. 2000. Isoflavone-rich soy protein isolate attenuates bone loss in the lumbar spine of perimenopausal women. *Am. J. Clin. Nutr.* 72: 844–52.

Centers for Disease Control and Prevention (CDC). 2001. Division of Bacterial and Mycotic Diseases. Disease Information. *Escherichia coli* O157:H7. www.cdc.gov/ncidod/dbmd/diseaseinfo/escherichiacoli_g.htm. Accessed December 2002.

Eisenstein, J., S. B. Roberts, G. Dallal, and E. Saltzman. 2002. High-protein weight-loss diets: are they safe and do they work? A review of the experimental and epidemiologic data. *Nutr. Rev.* 60 (7): 189–200.

Fleming, R. M. 2000. The effect of high-protein diets on coronary blood flow. *Angiology* 51: 817–26.

Fraser, G. E., K. D. Linsted, and W. L. Beeson. 1995. Effect of risk factor values on lifetime risk at first coronary event. *Am. J. Epid.* 142: 746–58.

Institute of Medicine, Food and Nutrition Board. 2002. *Dietary Reference Intakes for Energy, Carbohydrate, Fiber, Fat, Fatty Acids, Cholesterol, Protein, and Amino Acids (Macronutrients)*. Washington, DC: National Academies Press.

Kontessis, P., I. Bossinakou, L. Sarika, E. Iliopoulou, A. Papantoniou, R. Trevisan, D. Roussi, K. Stipsanelli, S. Grigorakis, and A. Souvatzoglou. 1995. Renal, metabolic, and hormonal responses to proteins of different origin in normotensive, non-proteinuric type 1 diabetic patients. *Diabetes Care* 18: 1233–40.

Landers, P., M. M. Wolfe, S. Glore, R. Guild, and L. Phillips. 2002. Effect of weight loss plans on body composition and diet duration. *J. Okla. State Med. Assoc.* 95(5): 329–31.

Lemon, P. W. 2000. Beyond the zone: protein needs of active individuals. *J. Am. Coll. Nutr.* 19 (5 suppl.): 513S–521S.

Liebman, B. 2002. Big fat lies: The truth about the Atkins Diet. *Center Sci. Public Interest Nutr. Action Health Letter* 29(9): 1–7.

Manore, M., and J. Thompson. 2000. *Sport Nutrition for Health and Performance*. Champaign, IL: Human Kinetics.

McDowell, M. A., R. R. Briefel, K. Alaimo, A. M. Bischof, C. R. Caughman, M. D. Carroll, C. M. Lona, and C. L. Johnson. 1994. Energy and macronutrient intakes of persons ages 2 months and over in the United States: Third National Health and Nutrition Examination Survey, Phase I 1988–1991. *Advance Data* 255: 1–24.

Messina, M. J. 1999. Legumes and soybeans: overview of their nutritional profiles and health effects. *Am. J. Clin. Nutr.* 70 (suppl.): 439S–450S.

Messina, V. K., and K. I. Burke. 1997. Position of the American Dietetic Association: Vegetarian diets. *J. Am. Diet. Assoc.* 97: 1317–1321.

Messina, M., and V. Messina. 1996. *The Dietitian's Guide to Vegetarian Diets*. Gaithersburg, MD: Aspen Publishers.

Munger, R. G., J. R. Cerhan, and B. C.-H. Chiu. 1999. Prospective study of dietary protein intake and risk of hip fracture in postmenopausal women. *Am. J. Clin. Nutr.* 69: 147–52.

Musick, J. A., M. M. Harbin, S. A. Berkeley, G. H. Burgess, A. M. Eklund, L. Findley, R. G. Gilmore, J. T. Golden, D. S. Ha, G. R. Huntsman, J. C. McGovern, S. J. Parker, S. G. Poss, E. Sala, T. W. Schmidt, G. R. Sedberry, H. Weeks, and S. G. Wright. 2000. Marine, estuarine, and diadromous fish stocks at risk of extinction in North America (exclusive of Pacific Salmonids). *Fisheries* 25: 6–30.

National Cattlemen's Beef Association. November 2003. Beef Industry "Factoid" Fighter. www.beef.org/documents/Factoid%20Fighter%20Revisions%2011-03-03.doc. Accessed February 2004.

O'Conner, M. A., S. W. Touyz, S. M. Dunn, and P. J. V. Beaumont. 1987. Vegetarianism in anorexia nervosa? A review of 116 consecutive cases. *Med. J. Aust.* 147: 540–42.

Phillips, R. L., and D. A. Snowdon. 1983. Association of meat and coffee use with cancers of the large bowel, breast, and prostate among Seventh-Day Adventists: preliminary results. *Cancer Res.* 43 (suppl.): 2403S–2408S.

Poortmans, J. R., and O. Dellalieux. 2000. Do regular high protein diets have potential health risks on kidney function in athletes? *Int. J. Sport Nutr.* 10: 28–38.

Taubes, G. 2002. What if fat doesn't make you fat? *The New York Times Magazine,* July 7, section 6.

Tillotson, J. L., G. E. Bartsch, D. Gorder, G. A. Grandits, and J. Stamler. 1997. Food group and nutrient intakes at baseline in the Multiple Risk Factor Intervention Trial. *Am. J. Clin. Nutr.* 65 (suppl.): 228S–257S.

Wegman, M. E. 2001. Infant mortality in the 20th century, dramatic but uneven progress. *J. Nutr.* 131 (suppl.): 401S–408S.

Nutrition Debate

High Protein Diets—Are They the Key to Weight Loss?

High protein diets have been popular over the last 40 years. Very low energy, high-protein programs (200 to 400 kilocalories per day, 1.5 grams of protein per kilogram body weight) were highly popular in the 1970s. Many of these diets consisted of low-quality protein, however, and at least fifty-eight people died from heart problems while following them. As a result of these deaths, we now know that these extreme diets are only appropriate for severely obese people and must include high-quality protein sources. Supervision by a qualified physician is critical when following this type of diet plan.

Proponents of high-protein diets claim that you can eat all your favorite foods and still lose weight. Is this possible? Chapter 11 provides a detailed explanation of weight loss. However, the key to weight loss is eating less energy than you expend. If you eat more energy than you expend, you can gain weight. Thus, any type of diet, even high-protein diets, must contain fewer kilocalories than a person expends to result in weight loss.

It is important to recognize that high-protein diets are synonymous with low-carbohydrate diets, since high-protein foods typically replace those high in carbohydrates. In addition, many high-protein diets are also high in fat. It is well established that reducing carbohydrate intake causes the body to break down its stored carbohydrate (or glycogen) in the liver and muscle; this is necessary to maintain blood glucose levels and provide energy to the brain. As water is stored along with glycogen, using stored carbohydrate for energy results in the loss of water from the body, which registers on the scale as rapid weight loss.

There are many supporters of high protein diets, particularly people supporting the Atkins' Diet. A highly controversial article in support of the Atkins' Diet was published in the *New York Times Magazine* (Taubes 2002). In this article, the Atkins' Diet is touted as the most effective program for weight loss. Supporters of this diet emphasize that eating a high-carbohydrate diet (including potatoes, white bread, pasta, and refined sugars) has caused obesity in the United States. Supporters emphasize that not only does the Atkins' Diet result in substantial weight loss, but it does not cause unhealthy changes in blood cholesterol despite its high saturated fat content.

Detractors of the Atkins' Diet tell a different story. According to many nutrition and obesity experts, the U.S. population is substantially overweight because we eat too many calories, not because of eating too much carbohydrate or fat per se. There are a number of potential health risks associated with eating a low-carbohydrate (and high-fat) diet, and these risk factors have prevented many nutrition experts from endorsing the Atkins' Diet as a healthy weight loss plan. Some of these health risks include the following:

- Low blood glucose levels, or hypoglycemia, leading to low energy levels, diminished cognitive functioning, and elevated ketones. As high protein diets are low in carbohydrate, the body does not receive enough glucose to maintain brain function. This could lead to low energy levels (which could prevent some people from exercising regularly) and detrimental changes in memory and cognitive function. Because blood glucose levels are not sufficient to support brain function, the body produces ketones from body fat, as ketones are an alternative energy source for the brain and central nervous system when carbohydrate is not available. High ketone levels in the blood can be toxic, as they increase blood acidity. This state is called *ketoacidosis*, and it can be dangerous if maintained over a prolonged period of time. Left untreated, increased blood acidity causes disorientation, eventual loss of consciousness, coma, and even death. Despite this concern, there is no evidence that following the Atkins' Diet has resulted in any serious disability or death due to ketoacidosis.
- Increased risk of heart disease caused by eating foods high in saturated fat. The Atkins' Diet promotes the consumption of foods that are high in protein and saturated fat. For instance, daily intakes of cheese, whole-fat dairy products, and fatty meats such as bacon, sausage, and regular ground beef are encouraged. It is well established that eating a diet high in saturated fat increases a person's LDL cholesterol, which in turn increases the risk for heart disease.
- Increased risk of some forms of cancer due to eating a diet that is high in fat and low fiber. As the Atkins' Diet recommends few, if any, foods that contain fiber and antioxidants, many nutrition experts are concerned that eating this type of a diet over many years will increase a person's risk for some forms of cancer.

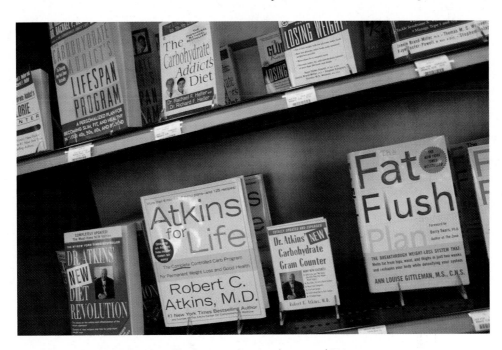

The long-term health implications of high protein diets is unknown at this time.

It appears that the Atkins' Diet will continue to be controversial for many years. After the publication of the article in the *New York Time Magazine,* the Center for Science in the Public Interest (CSPI) published a response that claimed irresponsible and inaccurate reporting (Liebman 2002). CSPI interviewed many of the experts quoted in the article as supporting the Atkins' Diet. These experts state they were misquoted or quoted out of context and that the information they shared that was contrary to supporting the Atkins' Diet was ignored.

Are there any research studies to support the contention that the Atkins' Diet is effective for weight loss? Most reports of substantial weight loss on this diet are anecdotal, meaning they come from individuals who were not participants in a controlled, scientific study. There are a few recent studies that have found that people do lose weight on the Atkins' Diet (Landers et al. 2002; Eisenstein et al. 2002). However, these studies are short-term (less than 6 months in duration), include small numbers of participants, and do not agree as to whether the Atkins' Diet results in more weight loss than other types of diet plans. Thus, at this time, it is not possible to state with any certainty that the Atkins' Diet is better than other diet plans recommending higher carbohydrate intakes. The long-term health implications of this type of a diet are also unknown at this time, and more research must be conducted in this area.

Should you adopt a high protein diet? This is not an easy question to answer. Each of us must decide on the type of diet to consume based on our own needs, preferences, health risks, and lifestyle. At the present time, there is not enough evidence to prove that the Atkins' Diet or other high-protein diets are better alternatives to higher-carbohydrate, lower-fat diets. Based on what we currently know, the healthiest weight loss plans are those that are moderately reduced in energy intake and contain ample fruits, vegetables, and whole grains, adequate carbohydrate and protein, moderate amounts of total fat, and relatively low amounts of saturated fat. It is also important to choose a food plan that you can follow throughout your lifetime. By researching the benefits and risks of various diet plans, you can make an educated decision about the type of diet that will work best to maintain a healthful weight and muscle mass and provide enough energy and nutrients to maintain your lifestyle and your long-term health.

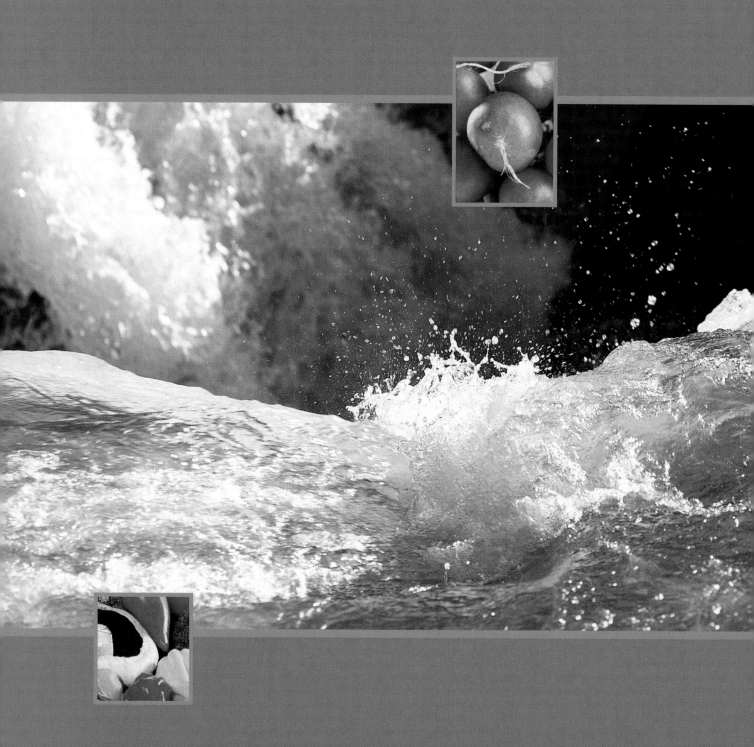

Chapter 7
Nutrients Involved in Fluid and Electrolyte Balance

Chapter Objectives

After reading this chapter you will be able to:

1. Identify four nutrients that function as electrolytes in our bodies, p. 234.

2. List three functions of water in our bodies, pp. 235–236.

3. Describe how electrolytes assist in the regulation of healthful fluid balance, pp. 236–238.

4. Discuss the physical changes that occur to trigger our thirst mechanism, p. 239.

5. Describe the avenues of fluid intake and excretion in our bodies, pp. 239–241.

6. Define hyponatremia and identify factors that can cause this condition, p. 248.

7. Identify four symptoms of dehydration, pp. 252–254.

8. Define hypertension and list three ways we can change our lifestyle to reduce hypertension, pp. 254–256.

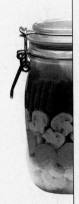

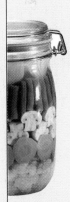

Test Yourself True or false?

1. About 50 to 70% of our body weight is made up of water. T or F

2. Sodium is an unhealthful nutrient, and we should avoid consuming it in our diets. T or F

3. Drinking until we are no longer thirsty always ensures that we are properly hydrated. T or F

4. Although persistent vomiting is uncomfortable, it does not have any long-term adverse effects on our health. T or F

5. Eating a high-sodium diet causes high blood pressure in most individuals. T or F

Test Yourself answers can be found at the end of the chapter.

In April of 2002, Cynthia Lucero, a healthy 28-year-old woman who had just completed her doctoral dissertation, was running the Boston Marathon. Although not a professional athlete, Cynthia was running in her second marathon, and, in the words of her coach, she had been "diligent" in her training. While her parents, who had traveled from Ecuador, waited at the finish line, friends in the crowd watched as Cynthia steadily completed mile after mile, drinking large amounts of fluid as she progressed through the course. They described her as looking strong as she jogged Heartbreak Hill, about six miles from the finish. But then she began to falter. One of her friends ran to her side and asked if she was okay. Cynthia replied that she felt dehydrated and rubber-legged, then she fell to the pavement. She was rushed to nearby Brigham and Women's Hospital, but by the time she got there, she was in an irreversible coma. The official cause of her death was hyponatremia, commonly called "low blood sodium." Among marathon runners seeking medical treatment after a race, as many as 10% show signs of this condition.

What is hyponatremia, and are you at risk? Even if you don't run marathons, do you or any of your friends play sports, exercise, or work a physically demanding job in hot weather? If so, do you drink sports drinks or just plain water? If at the start of football practice on a hot, humid afternoon, a friend confided to you that he had been on a drinking binge the night before, would you know how to advise him? Should you tell his coach, and why?

In this chapter, we explore the role of fluids and electrolytes in keeping our bodies properly hydrated and maintaining the functions of our nerves and muscles. We also discuss how we maintain blood pressure and take a look at some disorders that occur when our fluids and electrolytes are out of balance.

What Are Fluids and Electrolytes, and What Are Their Functions?

Of course you know that orange juice, blood, and shampoo are all fluids, but what makes them so? A **fluid** is characterized by its ability to move freely and changeably, adapting to the shape of the container that holds it. This might not seem very important, but as you'll learn in this chapter, the fluid composition of your cells and tissues is critical to your body's ability to function.

Body Fluid Is the Liquid Portion of Our Cells and Tissues

Between about 50 and 70% of a healthy adult's body weight is fluid. When we cut a finger, we can see some of this fluid dripping out as blood, but that can't account for such a large percentage. So where is all this fluid hiding?

fluid A substance composed of molecules that move past one another freely. Fluids are characterized by their ability to conform to the shape of whatever container holds them.

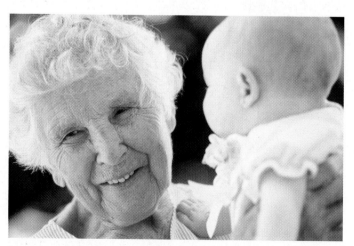

As we age, our body water content decreases: Approximately 75% of an infant's body weight is comprised of water while an elderly adult's is only 50% (or less).

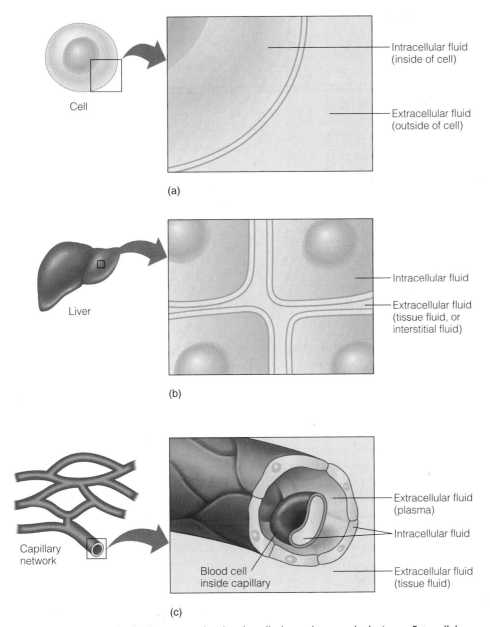

Cell

Intracellular fluid (inside of cell)

Extracellular fluid (outside of cell)

(a)

Liver

Intracellular fluid

Extracellular fluid (tissue fluid, or interstitial fluid)

(b)

Capillary network

Extracellular fluid (plasma)

Intracellular fluid

Blood cell inside capillary

Extracellular fluid (tissue fluid)

(c)

Figure 7.1   Intracellular fluid is contained within the cells that make up our body tissues. Extracellular fluid is external to cells. Tissue fluid is external to tissue cells, and plasma is external to blood cells.

About two-thirds of our body fluid is held within the walls of our cells and is therefore called **intracellular fluid** (Figure 7.1a). Every cell in our body contains fluid. When our cells lose their fluid, they quickly shrink and die. On the other hand, when cells take in too much fluid, they swell and burst apart. This is why appropriate fluid balance—which we'll discuss throughout this chapter—is so critical to life.

The remaining third of our body fluid is referred to as **extracellular fluid** because it flows outside of our cells (see Figure 7.1a). There are two types of extracellular fluid:

1. *Tissue fluid* (sometimes called *interstitial fluid*) flows between the cells that make up a particular tissue or organ, such as muscle fibers or the liver (Figure 7.1b).

2. *Plasma* is the extracellular fluid that causes your blood to drip. It is the liquid portion of blood, and it carries the red blood cells through our vessels like a river carrying ships to distant regions (Figure 7.1c).

intracellular fluid   The fluid held at any given time within the walls of the body's cells.

extracellular fluid   The fluid outside of the body's cells, either in the body's tissues, or as the liquid portion of blood, called *plasma*.

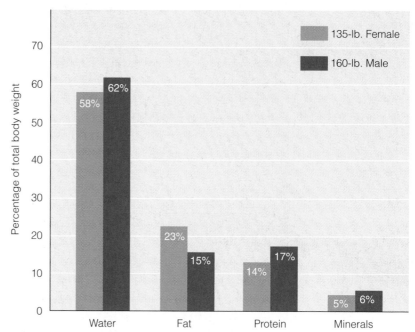

Figure 7.2 Body composition of an average adult male and female.

Not every tissue in our body contains the same amount of fluid. Lean tissues, such as muscle, are more than 70% fluid, whereas fat tissue is only between 10 and 20% fluid. This is not surprising considering the hydrophobic nature of lipid cells, which we discussed in Chapter 5.

Body fluid also varies according to gender and age. Figure 7.2 compares the body composition of a 160-pound adult male and a 135-pound adult female. As you can see, males have more lean tissue and thus more body fluid than females. Our total amount of body fluid decreases as we age. About 75% of an infant's body weight is water, whereas the total body water of an elderly person is generally less than 50% of body weight. This decrease in total body water is a result of the loss of lean tissue that occurs as we age.

Body Fluid Is Composed of Water and Dissolved Substances Called Electrolytes

As you know, pure water is made up of molecules consisting of two hydrogen atoms bound to one oxygen atom (H_2O). You might think that such pure water would be healthful, but if our cell and tissue fluids contained only pure water, we would quickly die. Instead, within our body fluids are a variety of dissolved substances (called *solutes*) critical to life. These include four major minerals: sodium, potassium, chloride, and phosphorus. We consume these minerals in compounds called *salts,* especially table salt, which is made of sodium and chloride.

These mineral salts are called **electrolytes**, because when they dissolve in water, the two component minerals separate and form electrically charged particles called **ions**, which are capable of carrying an electrical current. The electrical charge is the "spark" that stimulates nerves and causes muscles to contract, so electrolytes are critical to body functioning.

If you've ever jump-started a car, you know that electrical charges can be either positive or negative. Of the four major minerals just mentioned, sodium (Na^+) and potassium (K^+) are positively charged, whereas chloride (Cl^-) and phosphorus (in the form of hydrogen phosphate, or HPO_4^{2-}) are negatively charged. In the intracellular fluid, potassium and phosphate are the predominant electrolytes. In contrast, in the

electrolyte A substance that disassociates in solution into positively and negatively charged ions and is thus capable of carrying an electrical current.

ion Any electrically charged particle, either positively or negatively charged.

extracellular fluid, sodium and chloride predominate. There is a slight difference in electrical charge on either side of the cell's membrane that is needed in order for the cell to perform its normal functions.

Fluids Serve Many Critical Functions

Water not only quenches our thirst; it performs a number of functions that are critical to support life.

Fluids Dissolve and Transport Substances

Water is involved in almost all chemical reactions of our bodies. It is an excellent **solvent**, which means it is capable of dissolving (i.e., mixing with and breaking apart) a wide variety of substances. Since blood plasma and the interior of blood cells are mostly water, blood is an excellent vehicle for transporting these dissolved substances, or solutes, throughout our body. All water-soluble substances—such as amino acids, glucose, vitamins, minerals, and medications—are readily transported via the bloodstream. In contrast, fats do not dissolve in water. To overcome this chemical incompatibility, fatty substances such as cholesterol and fat-soluble vitamins are either attached to or surrounded by water-soluble proteins so they too can be transported in the blood to the cells.

solvent A substance that is capable of mixing with and breaking apart a variety of compounds. Water is an excellent solvent.

Fluids Account for Blood Volume

Blood volume is the amount of fluid in blood. As you might expect, appropriate fluid levels are essential to maintaining healthful blood volume. When blood volume rises, blood pressure increases; when blood volume decreases, blood pressure decreases. As you know, high blood pressure is an important risk factor for heart disease and stroke, whereas low blood pressure can cause us to feel tired, lethargic, confused, dizzy, or even to faint. The heart, blood vessels, certain blood proteins, and kidneys work together to regulate blood volume and blood pressure in a fairly complex process that we will not describe here. We discuss high blood pressure (called *hypertension*) in the disorders section at the end of this chapter.

blood volume The amount of fluid in blood.

Fluids Help Maintain Body Temperature

Just as overheating is disastrous to a car engine, a high internal temperature can cause our bodies to stop functioning. Fluids are vital to our ability to maintain our body temperature within a safe range. Two factors account for the ability of fluids to keep us cool. First, water has a relatively high heat capacity. In other words, it takes a lot of external energy to raise its temperature. Since our bodies contain a lot of water, it takes sustained high heat to increase our body temperature. Thus, the water content of our bodies protects us from high environmental temperatures.

Second, body fluids are our primary coolant. When we need to release heat from the body, we increase the flow of blood from our warm body core to the vessels lying just under the skin. This action transports the heat from the core of the body out to the periphery where it can be released from the skin. When we are hot, the sweat glands secrete more sweat from the skin. As this sweat evaporates off of the skin's surface, heat is released and the skin and underlying blood are cooled (Figure 7.3). This cooler blood flows back to the body's core and reduces internal body temperature.

Fluids Protect and Lubricate Our Tissues

Water is a major part of the fluids that protect our organs and tissues from injury. The cerebrospinal fluid that surrounds our brain and spinal column protects these vital tissues from damage, and a fetus in a mother's womb is protected by amniotic fluid. Body fluids also act as lubricants. Synovial fluid secreted by membranes surrounding our joints acts as a lubricant for smooth joint motion, and tears cleanse and lubricate

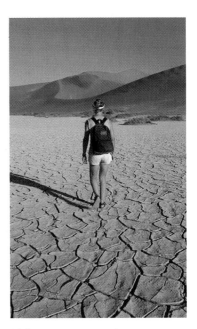

A hiker must consume adequate amounts of water to prevent heat illness in hot and dry environments.

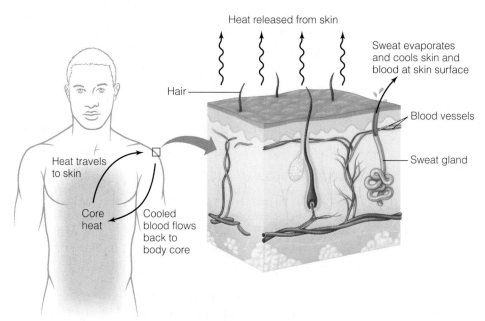

Figure 7.3   Evaporative cooling occurs when heat is transported from the body core through the bloodstream to the surface of the skin. The water evaporates into the air and carries away heat. This cools the blood, which circulates back to the body core, reducing body temperature.

our eyes. Our saliva moistens the food we eat, which helps us to effectively swallow and transport it to the stomach. The fluid-filled mucus lining the walls of our stomach and intestines facilitates the smooth movement of food and nutrients through our digestive tract, and the pleural fluid covering our lungs allows their friction-free expansion and retraction behind our chest wall.

> **Recap:** Our body fluid consists of water plus a variety of dissolved substances, including electrically charged minerals called electrolytes. Water serves many important functions in our bodies, including dissolving and transporting substances, accounting for blood volume, regulating body temperature, and cushioning and lubricating body tissues.

Electrolytes Support Many Body Functions

Now that you know why fluid is so essential to our bodies' functioning, we're ready to explore the critical role of the minerals within it.

Electrolytes Help Regulate Fluid Balance

Our cell membranes are *permeable* to water. This means that water flows easily through them. Our cells have no control over this flow of water and thus cannot actively control the overall balance of fluid between the intracellular and extracellular compartments by directly regulating water flow. In contrast, our cell membranes are *not* freely permeable to electrolytes. Sodium, potassium, and the other electrolytes stay where they are, either inside or outside of a cell, unless they are actively transported elsewhere by special proteins. So how do electrolytes help our cells maintain their fluid balance? To answer this question, we need to review a bit of chemistry.

Imagine that you have a special filter that has the same properties as our cell membranes; in other words, this filter is freely permeable to water but not permeable to electrolytes. Now imagine that you insert this filter into a glass of pure distilled water to divide the glass into two separate chambers (Figure 7.4a). The level of water on either side of the filter would of course be identical, since it is freely permeable to water. Now

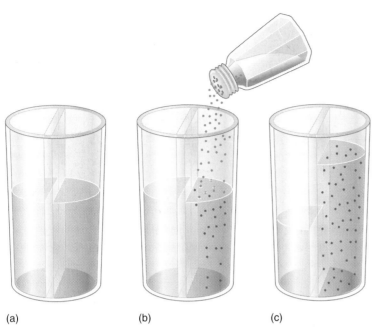

Figure 7.4 Osmosis. **(a)** A filter that is freely permeable to water is placed in a glass of pure water. **(b)** Salt is added to only one side of the glass. **(c)** Drawn by the high concentration of electrolytes, pure water flows to the "salt water" side of the filter. This flow of water into the concentrated solution will continue until the concentration of electrolytes on both sides of the membrane is equal.

imagine that you add a teaspoon of salt (which contains the electrolytes sodium and chloride) to the water on one side of the filter only (Figure 7.4b). You would see the water on the "pure water" side of the glass suddenly begin to flow through the filter to the "salt water" side of the glass (Figure 7.4c). Why would this mysterious movement of water occur? The answer is that water always moves from areas where solutes such as sodium and chloride are poorly concentrated to areas where they are highly concentrated. To put it another way, electrolytes *draw* water toward areas where they are concentrated. This movement of water toward solutes continues until the concentration of solutes is equal on both sides of the cell membrane.

Water follows the movement of electrolytes; this action provides a means to control movement of fluid into and out of the cells. Our cells can regulate the balance of fluids between their internal and extracellular environments by using special transport proteins to actively pump electrolytes across their membranes. An example of how transport proteins pump sodium and potassium across the cell membrane was illustrated in Chapter 6 (Figure 6.9). By maintaining the appropriate movement of electrolytes into and out of the cell, the proper balance of fluid and electrolytes is maintained between the intracellular and extracellular compartments (Figure 7.5a). If the concentration of electrolytes is much higher inside of the cells as compared to outside, water will flow into the cells in such large amounts that the cells can burst (Figure 7.5b). On the other hand, if the extracellular environment contains too high a concentration of electrolytes, water flows out of the cells, and they can dry up (Figure 7.5c).

Certain illnesses can threaten this delicate balance of fluid inside and outside of the cells. You may have heard of someone being hospitalized because of excessive diarrhea and vomiting. When this happens, the body loses a great deal of fluid from the intestinal tract and extracellular compartment. This heavy fluid loss causes the extracellular electrolyte concentration to become very high. In response, a great deal of intracellular fluid leaves the cells to try to balance this extracellular fluid loss. This imbalance in fluid and electrolytes changes the flow of electrical impulses through the heart, causing an irregular heart rate that can eventually lead to death if left untreated. Food poisoning

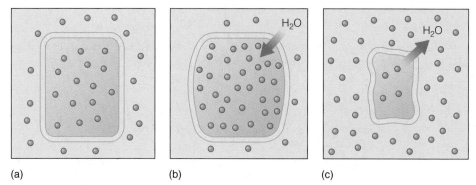

(a)   (b)   (c)

Figure 7.5 The health of our body's cells depends on maintaining the proper balance of fluids and electrolytes on either side of the cell membrane. **(a)** The concentration of electrolytes is the same on either side of the cell membrane. **(b)** The concentration of electrolytes is much greater inside the cell, drawing water into the cell and making it swell. **(c)** The concentration of electrolytes is much greater outside the cell, drawing water out of the cell and making it shrink.

and eating disorders involving repeated vomiting and diarrhea can also result in death due to these life-threatening fluid and electrolyte imbalances.

Electrolytes Enable Our Nerves to Respond to Stimuli

In addition to their role in maintaining fluid balance, electrolytes are critical in enabling our nerves to respond to stimuli. Nerve impulses are initiated at the membrane of a nerve cell due to a change in the degree of electrical charge. Changes occur that allow an influx of sodium into the cell, causing the cell to become slightly less negatively charged. This is called *depolarization*. If enough sodium enters the cell, the change in electrical charge triggers an *action potential*, an electrical signal that is propagated along nerve and muscle cells. Once this signal is complete, the cells return to their normal electrical state through the release of potassium to the outside of the cell. This return of the cell to its initial electrical state is termed *repolarization*. As you can see, both sodium and potassium play critical roles in ensuring that nerve impulses are generated in response to a variety of stimuli.

Electrolytes Signal Our Muscles to Contract

Our muscles contract due to a series of complex physiological changes that we will not describe in detail here. Simply stated, our muscles are stimulated to contract in response to stimulation of nerve cells. As described above, sodium and potassium play a key role in the generation of nerve impulses, or electrical signals. When a muscle fiber is stimulated by an electrical signal, changes occur in the cell membrane that lead to an increased flow of calcium into the muscle from the extracellular space. This release of calcium into the muscle provides the stimulus for muscle contraction. Our muscles can relax after a contraction once the electrical signal is complete and calcium has been pumped out of the muscle cell.

Recap: Electrolytes help regulate fluid balance by controlling the movement of fluid into and out of cells. Electrolytes, specifically sodium and potassium, play a key role in generating nerve impulses in response to stimuli. Calcium is an electrolyte that stimulates muscle contraction.

How Do Our Bodies Maintain Fluid Balance?

We maintain the proper balance of fluid in our bodies by a series of mechanisms that prompt us to drink and retain fluid when we are dehydrated and to excrete fluid as urine when we consume more than we need.

Our Thirst Mechanism Prompts Us to Drink Fluids

Imagine that, at lunch, you ate a ham sandwich and a bag of salted potato chips. Now it's almost time for your afternoon seminar to end, and suddenly you are very thirsty. The last five minutes of class are a torment, and when the instructor ends the session you dash to the nearest drinking fountain. What happened here? What prompted you suddenly to feel so thirsty?

Our body's command center for fluid intake is a cluster of nerve cells in a part of the brain called the *hypothalamus*. It is this group of cells, collectively referred to as the **thirst mechanism**, that causes you to consciously desire fluids. Our thirst mechanism prompts us to feel thirsty when it is stimulated by:

- Increased concentration of salt and other dissolved substances in our blood. Remember that ham sandwich and those potato chips? Both these foods are salty, and eating them causes the release of high concentrations of sodium into our blood.
- A reduction in blood volume and blood pressure. This can occur when fluids are lost due to profuse sweating, blood loss, vomiting, diarrhea, or simply when fluid intake is too low.
- Dryness in the tissues of the mouth and throat. Tissue dryness reflects a lower amount of fluid in the bloodstream, which causes a reduced production of saliva.

Once the hypothalamus detects such changes, it stimulates the release of a hormone that signals the kidneys to reduce urine flow and return more water to the bloodstream. The kidneys also secrete an enzyme that triggers blood vessels throughout our body to constrict. This helps us to retain water. Water is drawn out of the salivary glands in our mouths in an attempt to further dilute the concentration of substances in our blood; this causes our mouth and throat to become dry. Together, these mechanisms allow us to prevent a further loss of body fluid and help avoid dehydration.

Although our thirst mechanism can trigger us to drink more water, this mechanism alone is not always sufficient: we tend to drink until we are no longer thirsty, but the amount of fluid we consume may not be enough to achieve fluid balance. This is particularly true when we lose body water rapidly, such as during intense exercise in the heat. Because our thirst mechanism has some limitations, it is important that you drink regularly throughout the day and not wait to drink until you become thirsty, especially if you are active. Because our thirst mechanism becomes less sensitive as we age, elderly people can fail to drink adequate amounts of fluid and thus are at high risk for dehydration. For this reason, elderly people should be careful to drink fluids on a regular basis throughout the day. Finally, infants are also at increased risk for dehydration. A large proportion of an infant's body weight is water, so they need to drink a relatively large amount of fluid for their body size. For the same reason, fluid loss from diarrhea and vomiting are also more serious in this age group.

We Gain Fluids By Consuming Beverages and Foods and Through Metabolism

We obtain the fluid we need each day from three primary sources: beverages, foods, and the production of metabolic water by our bodies. Of course you know that beverages are mostly water, but it isn't as easy to see the water content in the foods we eat. For example, iceberg lettuce is almost 99% water, and even bacon contains a small amount of water. Table 7.1 lists the water content of commonly consumed beverages and foods.

Metabolic water is the water formed from our body's metabolic reactions. In the breakdown of fat, carbohydrate, and protein, ATP—the cell's basic energy source—and water are produced. The water that is formed during metabolic reactions contributes about 10 to 14% of the water we need each day.

thirst mechanism A cluster of nerve cells in the hypothalamus that stimulate our conscious desire to drink fluids in response to an increase in the concentration of salt in our blood or a decrease in blood pressure and blood volume.

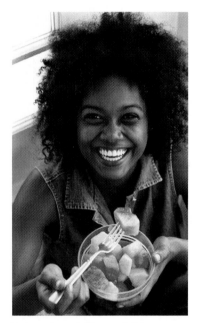

Fruits and vegetables are delicious sources of water.

metabolic water The water formed as a by-product of our body's metabolic reactions.

Table 7.1   Water Content of Common Beverages and Foods

	100%	90–99%	80–89%	60–79%	40–59%	20–39%	10–19%	1–9%[1]
Beverages	Water Plain tea Seltzer Diet soft drinks	Gatorade Clear broth Tomato juice Skim milk	Sugar-sweetened soft drinks Fruit juices 2% milk					
Fruits		Grapefruit Strawberry Tomato	Apple	Banana Avocado			Raisins	
Vegetables		Cabbage Lettuce Celery Cucumber Broccoli Squash	Carrots	Baked potato Mashed potato Boiled yams Cooked lentils				
Eggs/Dairy			Egg whites Yogurt		Egg yolk Cream cheese Jack cheese	Cheddar cheese		
Meats[2]				Lean steak Shrimp Pork chop Turkey Lean ham Salmon	Sausage Chicken Hot dog		Bacon	
Breads/ Cereals				Cooked spaghetti noodles	Pancakes Waffles	Bread Bagel Cooked oatmeal	Cooked rice	Ready-to- eat cereals
Oils/Fats				Low-calorie mayonnaise	Diet margarine		Butter Margarine Regular mayonnaise	
Other		Sugar-free gelatin	Yellow mustard	Instant pudding Ketchup		Cake Maple syrup Preserves		Peanut butter Popcorn Pretzels

[1]Cooking oils, meat fats, shortening, and white sugar have 0% water content.
[2]Value is for cooked meat.
Source: U.S. Department of Agriculture. 1999. USDA Nutrient Database for Standard Reference, Release 13. Nutrient Data Laboratory Home Page. www.nal.usda.gov/fnic/foodcomp. Accessed February 2002.

We Lose Fluids Through Urine, Sweat, Exhalation, and Feces

Our kidneys are constantly helping to maintain fluid balance by either excreting or retaining the fluid we consume. We excrete most of our water through the kidneys in the form of urine. When we consume more water than we need, the kidneys process this excess fluid and excrete it in the form of dilute urine.

During times when we need to conserve body water, the sodium concentration of our extracellular fluid increases. Special cells in the hypothalamus of the brain sense this increase in sodium levels and cause hormones to be secreted that signal the kidneys to reabsorb water instead of excreting it.

Our kidneys also respond to massive changes in fluid balance and blood pressure such as those that occur when someone suffers a large loss of blood. Major blood loss causes a significant drop in blood pressure. This drop in blood pressure signals the kidneys to retain more water and reduce urine output. In addition, the kidneys excrete certain enzymes and hormones that cause constriction of the peripheral blood vessels and also allow for the retention of water and sodium. Since water follows sodium, retaining sodium in the kidneys also helps retain water. The sodium and water can then be absorbed back into the bloodstream and cause an increase in blood volume and blood pressure.

Water is lost from our skin in the form of sweat and from our lungs during breathing. We refer to this type of water loss as **insensible water loss.** Our sweat glands produce more sweat during exercise or when we are in a hot environment. The evaporation of sweat from our skin releases heat, which cools our skin and reduces our core temperature. Under normal resting conditions, our insensible water loss is less than 1 liter of fluid each day; during heavy exercise or in hot weather, we can lose up to 2 liters of water per hour due to insensible water loss.

We excrete a relatively small amount of water in our feces. Under normal conditions, we lose only about 150 to 200 ml of water each day in our feces. Our gastrointestinal tract typically reabsorbs much of the large amounts of fluids that pass through it each day. However, when someone suffers from extreme diarrhea due to illness or from consuming excess laxatives, water loss in the feces can be as high as several liters per day.

In addition to these four avenues of regular fluid loss, certain situations can cause a significant loss of fluid from our bodies:

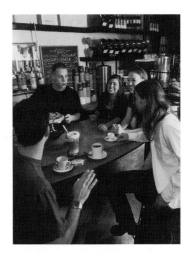

Drinking beverages that contain alcohol or caffeine causes an increase in water loss, as these drinks are diuretics.

insensible water loss The loss of water from the skin in the form of sweat and from the lungs during breathing.

- Illnesses that involve fever, coughing, vomiting, diarrhea, and a runny nose significantly increase fluid loss. This is why doctors advise people to drink plenty of fluids when they are ill.
- Traumatic injury, internal hemorrhaging, blood donation, and surgery also increase loss of fluid because of the blood loss involved.
- Exercise increases fluid loss via sweat and respiration: although urine production typically decreases during exercise, fluid losses increase through the skin and lungs.
- Environmental conditions that increase fluid loss include high altitudes, cold and hot temperatures, and low humidity such as in a desert or flying in an airplane. The water content of the environment is much lower at high altitude, in an airplane, and in the desert. Thus, water from our body more easily evaporates into the dry environment. We also breathe faster at higher altitudes due to the lower oxygen pressure, which results in greater fluid loss via the lungs. We sweat more in the heat, thus losing more water. Cold temperatures can trigger hormonal changes that result in an increased fluid loss.
- Pregnancy increases fluid loss to the mother because fluids are continually diverted to the fetus and amniotic fluid.
- Breastfeeding requires a tremendous increase in fluid intake to make up for the loss of fluid.
- Consumption of **diuretics**—substances that increase fluid loss via the urine—can result in dangerously excessive fluid loss. Diuretics include certain prescription medications, alcohol, and caffeine-containing beverages such as coffee, cola, and tea. Many over-the-counter weight-loss remedies are really just diuretics.

diuretic A substance that increases fluid loss via the urine. Common diuretics include coffee, tea, cola, and other caffeine-containing beverages, as well as prescription medications for high blood pressure and other disorders.

Recap: We maintain healthy fluid levels in our body by balancing intake with excretion. Primary sources of fluids include water and other beverages, foods, and the production of metabolic water in the body. Fluid losses occur through urination, sweating, our feces, and evaporation from our lungs.

A Profile of Nutrients Involved in Hydration and Neuromuscular Function

Nutrients that assist us in maintaining hydration and neuromuscular function include water and the minerals sodium, potassium, chloride, and phosphorus. As discussed in Chapter 1, these minerals are classified as *major minerals,* as the body needs more than

Table 7.2 Functions, Recommended Intakes, and Toxicity and Deficiency Symptoms of Primary Electrolytes

Nutrient	Primary Functions	Recommended Intake	Toxicity Symptoms	Deficiency Symptoms
Sodium	Major positively charged electrolyte in extracellular fluid Maintains proper acid-base balance Assists with transmission of nerve signals Aids muscle contraction Assists in the absorption of glucose and other nutrients	1.5 g/day[1]	Water retention High blood pressure May increase loss of calcium in urine	Muscle cramps Loss of appetite Dizziness Fatigue Nausea Vomiting Mental confusion
Potassium	Major positively charged electrolyte in intracellular fluid Regulates contraction of muscles Regulates transmission of nerve impulses Assists in maintaining healthy blood pressure levels	4.7 g/day[1]	Muscle weakness Vomiting Irregular heartbeat	Muscle weakness Muscle paralysis Mental confusion
Chloride	Assists with maintaining fluid balance Aids in preparing food for digestion (as HCl) Helps kill bacteria Assists in the transmission of nerve impulses	2.3 g/day[1]	Vomiting	Dangerous changes in pH Irregular heartbeat
Phosphorus	Major negatively charged electrolyte in intracellular fluid Maintains proper fluid balance Plays critical role in bone formation Component of ATP, which provides energy for our bodies Helps regulate biochemical reactions Major part of genetic materials (DNA, RNA) A component in cell membranes, LDL	700 mg/day[2]	Muscle spasms Convulsions Low blood calcium levels	Muscle weakness Bone pain Dizziness

[1]Adequate Intake (AI)
[2]RDA

100 milligrams of each of these minerals per day. Table 7.2 reviews the primary functions of each of these minerals. As you can see, they play many roles in the body.

Calcium and magnesium also function as electrolytes and influence our body's fluid balance and neuromuscular function. However, because of their critical importance to bone health, they are discussed in Chapter 9.

Water

Water is essential for life. Although we can live weeks without food, we can only survive one to two days without water, depending on environmental temperature. We do not have the capacity to store water, so we must continuously replace the water we lose each day.

How Much Water Should We Drink?

Our need for water varies greatly depending upon our age, body size, health status, physical activity level, and exposure to environmental conditions. It is important to pay attention to how much our need for water changes under various conditions so that dehydration can be avoided.

Recommended Intake Fluid requirements are very individualized. For example, a highly active male athlete training in a hot environment may require up to 10 liters of fluid per day to maintain healthy fluid balance, while an inactive, petite woman who lives in a mild climate and works in a temperature-controlled office building may only require about 3 liters of fluid per day. The DRI for adult men aged 19 to 50 years is 3.7 liters of total water per day. This includes approximately 3.0 liters (or 13 cups) as total beverages, which includes drinking water (Institute of Medicine 2004). The DRI for adult women aged 19 to 50 is 2.7 liters of total water per day. This includes about 2.2 (or 9 cups) as total beverages, which includes drinking water (Institute of Medicine 2004).

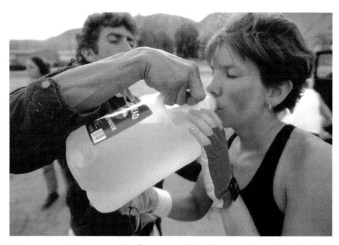

Vigorous exercise causes significant water loss that must be replenished to optimize performance and health.

Figure 7.6 shows the amount and sources of water intake and output for a woman expending 2,500 kcal per day. Based on current recommendations, this woman needs about 2,700 ml of water per day. As you can see:

- Water from metabolism provides 300 to 400 ml of water.
- The foods she eats provides her with an additional 1,000 ml of water each day.
- The beverages she drinks provide the remainder of water needed, which is equal to 1,300 ml (dotted line) to 1,400 ml.

An 8-ounce glass of water is equal to 240 ml. In this example, the woman would need to drink 5 to 6 glasses of fluid to meet her needs. You can now see why drinking 8 glasses of fluid each day is recommended for most people. Drinking this amount will provide you with enough fluid to maintain proper fluid balance. Remember that this recommendation of 8 glasses of fluid each day is a general guideline. You may need to drink a different amount to meet your fluid needs.

Athletes or people who are active, especially those working in very hot environments, may require more fluid than the current recommendations. The amount of

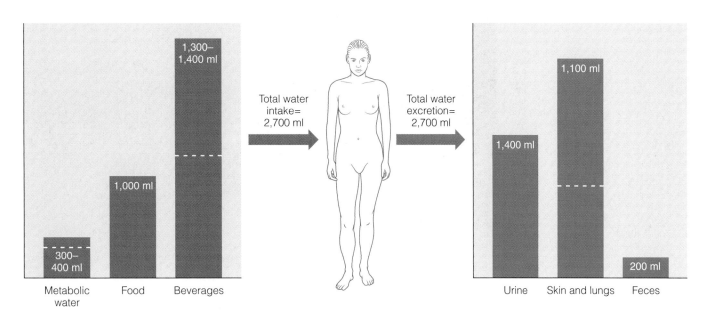

Figure 7.6 Amount and sources of water intake and output for a woman expending 2,500 kcal per day.

sweat lost during exercise is very individualized and depends on body size, exercise intensity, environmental temperature, and humidity. We do know that some people can lose as much as 4 pounds of fluid (or 1.8 kg) per hour as sweat (ACSM 1996)! Thus, these individuals need to drink more to replace the fluid they lose. One liter of sweat contains about 1 gram of sodium (ACSM 2000); we also lose some potassium and small amounts of minerals such as iron and calcium in sweat.

Because of these fluid and electrolyte losses during exercise, some athletes drink sport beverages instead of plain water to help them maintain fluid balance. Recently, sport beverages have also become popular with recreationally active people and non-athletes. Is it really necessary for people to consume these beverages? See the Nutrition Debate on sport beverages at the end of this chapter to learn whether they are right for you.

Liz *Nutri-Case*

"My dance teacher says we should be drinking at least eighty ounces (or ten cups) of fluid a day. That sounds like an awful lot, but yesterday, I kept track of how much I drank all day, and I'm pretty close: I drank a ten-ounce cup of coffee with breakfast, a sixteen-ounce bottle of spring water during dance class, and a ten-ounce diet cola at lunch. After classes, I treated myself to a skim milk latté, the twelve-ounce size, and then I had another bottle of water during rehearsal. I had half a glass of cranberry juice with dinner, probably about four ounces, and then I had an eight-ounce cup of green tea just before bed. So I'm on target. The only problem is, I have to go to the bathroom all the time!"

What do you think of Liz's dance teacher's recommendation that she drink eighty ounces of fluid a day? How is Liz doing toward that goal? Is there anything about her fluid consumption that you would advise her to change? Why do you think Liz has to go to the bathroom all the time?

Sources of Drinking Water   There are so many types of water available to drink in the United States, how can we distinguish among them? If we prefer to drink water with bubbles—carbonation—we can choose carbonated water. This type of water contains carbon dioxide gas that either occurs naturally or is added to the water. Mineral water is another beverage option. Mineral waters contain 250 to 500 parts per million

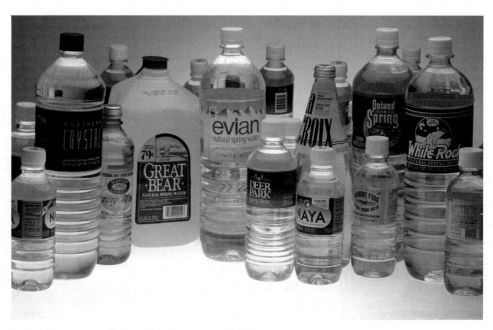

There are numerous varieties of drinking water available to consumers.

(ppm) of minerals. While many people prefer the unique taste of mineral water, a number of brands contain high amounts of sodium so should be avoided by people who are trying to reduce their sodium intake. Distilled water is processed in such a way that all dissolved minerals are removed; this type of water is often used in steam irons, as it will not clog the iron with mineral buildup. Purified water has been treated so that all dissolved minerals and contaminants are removed, making this type of water useful in research and medical procedures. Of course, we can also drink the tap water found in our homes and in public places.

One of the major changes in the beverage industry over the past twenty years is the marketing of bottled water. The meteoric rise in bottled water production and consumption is most likely due to the convenience of drinking bottled water, to the health messages related to drinking more water, and to the public's fears related to the safety of tap water. Is bottled water safer than tap water? Refer to the Nutrition Myth or Fact box on bottled water to find the answer to this question.

What Happens If We Drink Too Much Water?

Drinking too much water and becoming overhydrated is very rare, but it can occur. Some individuals suffering from certain forms of mental illness have an uncontrollable urge to consume large quantities of water. If these individuals have healthy kidneys, this condition generally does not lead to major health problems because their kidneys are able to process this excess water. Certain illnesses can cause increases in levels of a hormone that stimulates reabsorption of water by the kidneys. When this occurs, overhydration and dilution of sodium result. Dilution of sodium, also called *hyponatremia*, causes headaches, confusion, seizures, and coma. Hyponatremia is discussed in more detail in the next section.

What Happens If We Don't Drink Enough Water?

Dehydration results when we do not drink enough water. Fluid loss is one of the leading causes of death around the world, with infants and elderly individuals being particularly affected. Dehydration is generally due to some form of illness or gastrointestinal infection that causes diarrhea and vomiting. When these occur over a prolonged period of time, fluid loss is excessive and dehydration results, leading to impaired physical and mental function and even death if not treated quickly. The impact of dehydration on our health is discussed in detail on page 252.

Sodium

Over the last twenty years, researchers have linked high sodium intake to an increased risk for high blood pressure. Because of this link, many people have come to believe that sodium is harmful to the body. This simply is not true: in reality, sodium is an essential nutrient that our body needs to function optimally.

Functions of Sodium

Sodium has a variety of functions. As discussed earlier in this chapter, it is the major positively charged electrolyte in the extracellular fluid. Its exchange with potassium across cell membranes allows our cells to maintain proper fluid balance, blood pressure, and acid-base balance.

Sodium also assists with the transmission of nerve signals and aids in muscle contraction. To review, the release of sodium from inside to outside the cell stimulates the spread of nerve signals to nervous tissue and muscles. The stimulation of muscles by nerve impulses provides the impetus for muscle contraction.

Finally, sodium assists in the absorption of certain nutrients such as glucose. Glucose cannot be passively absorbed into the cell through the cell membrane. Cells transport glucose via the process of active transport, which involves assistance from a sodium-potassium pump. This pump works by acting as a carrier protein that transports glucose through the cell membrane.

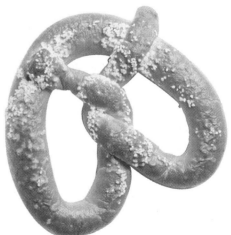

Many popular snack foods are high in sodium.

Bottled Water Is No Safer Than Tap Water

Bottled water has become increasingly popular over the past twenty years. It is estimated that Americans drink almost three billion gallons of bottled water each year (Bottled Water Web™ 2002). Many people prefer the taste of bottled water to that of tap water. They also feel that bottled water is safer than tap water. Is this true?

The water we drink in the United States generally comes from two sources: surface water and ground water. *Surface water* comes from lakes, rivers, and reservoirs. Common contaminants of surface water include runoff from highways, pesticides, animal wastes, and industrial wastes. Many of the cities across the United States obtain their water from surface water sources. *Ground water* comes from underground rock formations called *aquifers*. People who live in rural areas generally pump ground water from a well as their water source. Hazardous substances leaking from waste sites, dumps, landfills, and oil and gas pipelines can contaminate ground water.

The most common chemical used to treat and purify our water is *chlorine*. Chlorine is effective in killing many contaminants in our water supply. Water treatment plants also routinely check our water supplies for hazardous chemicals, minerals, and other contaminants. Because of these efforts, the United States has one of the safest water systems in the world.

The Environmental Protection Agency (EPA) sets and monitors the standards for our city water systems. The EPA does not monitor water from private wells, but it publishes recommendations for well owners to help them maintain a safe water supply. Local water regulatory agencies must provide an annual report on specific water contaminants to all households served by that agency.

In contrast, the Food and Drug Administration (FDA) regulates bottled water. As with tap water, bottled water is taken from either surface water or ground water sources. Bottled water is often treated and filtered differently than tap water, which changes its taste and appearance.

Although bottled water may taste better than tap water, there is no evidence that it is safer to drink. Look closely at the label of your favorite bottled water. It may come directly from the tap! Some types of bottled water may contain more minerals than tap water, but there are no other additional nutritional benefits of drinking bottled water. Most bottling plants use an ozone treatment to disinfect water instead of chlorine, and many people feel this process leaves the water tasting better than water treated with chlorine.

Should you spend money on bottled water? The answer depends on personal preference and your source of drinking water. For instance, many supermarkets have a water filtration machine in the front of the store where you can purchase and fill your own bottles of water. These machines may not be cleaned and the filters not changed on a regular basis, making this water less safe than tap water. Some people may not have access to safe drinking water where they live, making bottled water the safest alternative water source. If you choose to drink bottled water, look for brands that carry the trademark of the International Bottled Water Association (IBWA). This association follows the regulations of the FDA. If you get your water from a water cooler, make sure the cooler is cleaned once per month by running half a gallon of white vinegar through it, then rinsing thoroughly with about five gallons of clean water. If you use a special filtration system at home, be familiar with the contaminants it filters from your water and make sure that you change the filters regularly as recommended by the manufacturer. Be cautious of companies that may test your water and publish false claims about impurities in your tap water. Verify any tests conducted by a private company with your local water agency. It could save you hundreds or thousands of dollars on an unnecessary or ineffective home purifying system. For more information on drinking water safety, go to the EPA website at www.epa.gov; for information on bottled water go to www.bottledwaterweb.com. ●

How Much Sodium Should We Consume?

Many people are concerned with consuming too much sodium in the diet, as they believe it causes high blood pressure and bloating. Although this concern is warranted for certain individuals, sodium is an important nutrient that is necessary for maintaining health.

Table 7.3 High-Sodium Foods and Lower-Sodium Alternatives

High-Sodium Food	Sodium (mg)	Lower-Sodium Food	Sodium (mg)
Dill pickle (1 large, 4 in.)	1731	Low-sodium dill pickle (1 large, 4 in.)	23
Ham, cured, roasted (3 oz.)	1023	Pork, loin roast (3 oz.)	54
Chipped beef (3 oz.)	913	Beef chuck roast, cooked (3 oz.)	53
Tomato juice, regular (one cup)	877	Tomato juice, lower sodium (1 cup)	24
Tomato sauce, canned (½ cup)	741	Fresh tomato (1 medium)	11
Canned cream corn (1 cup)	730	Cooked corn, fresh (1 cup)	28
Tomato soup, canned (1 cup)	695	Lower-sodium tomato soup, canned (1 cup)	480
Potato chips, salted (1 oz.)	168	Baked potato, unsalted (1 medium)	14
Saltine crackers (4 each)	156	Saltine crackers, unsalted (4 each)	100

Source: U.S. Department of Agriculture. 1999. USDA Nutrient Database for Standard Reference, Release 13. Nutrient Data Laboratory Home Page. www.nal.usda.gov/fnic/foodcomp Accessed February 2002.

Recommended Dietary Intake for Sodium   The AI for sodium is 1.5 g/day (or 1,500 mg/day) for adult men and women aged 19 to 50 years (Institute of Nutrition 2004). Most people in the United States greatly exceed this minimum, consuming between 3,000 and 6,000 mg of sodium per day. Most health organizations recommend a daily sodium intake of no more than 2,400 mg per day.

Shopper's Guide: Good Food Sources of Sodium   Sodium is found naturally in many everyday foods, and many processed foods contain large amounts of added sodium. Because sodium is so abundant in most foods, it is easy for us to consume excess amounts in our daily diet. Try to guess which of the following foods contains the most sodium: one cup tomato juice, one ounce of potato chips, or four saltine crackers? Now look at Table 7.3 to find the answer. This table shows foods that are high in sodium and gives lower-sodium alternatives. Are you surprised to find out that of all of these food items, the tomato juice has the most sodium? When eating processed foods, such as canned soups, vegetable juices, and prepackaged rice and pasta dishes, remember to look for labels with the words "low-sodium," as these foods are lower in sodium.

What Happens If We Consume Too Much Sodium?

High blood pressure is more common in people who consume high sodium diets. This strong relationship between high-sodium diets and high blood pressure has prompted many health organizations to recommend low-sodium intakes. Whether high-sodium diets actually cause high blood pressure is unclear and controversial; this controversy is discussed on page 256. In addition, there are other less controversial reasons to consume no more than the recommended amount of sodium each day. Eating excess sodium can cause an increased excretion of calcium in some people, which in turn may increase the risk for bone loss; however, the extent to which excess sodium intake affects bone health is also the subject of controversy (Cohen and Roe 2000). Consuming excess sodium also causes bloating, as water is pulled from inside the cells into the extracellular space in an attempt to dilute the excess sodium.

Hypernatremia refers to an abnormally high blood sodium concentration (clinically defined as greater than 145 milliequivalent per liter of blood). It is usually caused by a rapid intake of high amounts of sodium, such as when a shipwrecked sailor drinks seawater. Eating too much sodium does not usually cause hypernatremia in a healthy person, as the kidneys are able to excrete excess sodium and avoid hypernatremia. But people with congestive heart failure or kidney disease are not able to excrete sodium effectively, making them more prone to the condition. Hypernatremia is dangerous because it causes an abnormally high blood volume, leading to edema (swelling) of our tissues and raising blood pressure to unhealthy levels.

hypernatremia   A condition in which blood sodium levels are dangerously high.

Can Water Be Too Much of a Good Thing? Hyponatremia in Marathon Runners

At the beginning of this chapter, we described the death of marathon runner Cynthia Lucero. Her case is only one of several that have gained attention in recent years. How can seemingly healthy, highly fit individuals competing in marathons collapse and even die during or after a race? One common issue faced by these athletes is maintaining a proper balance of fluid and electrolytes during the race.

It is well known that people participating in distance events such as marathons (26.2 miles) need to drink enough fluid to ensure proper fluid balance. Surprisingly, recent research has shown that some runners drink too much water and develop hyponatremia, or abnormally low blood sodium levels.

A recent study examined marathon runners who were treated for hyponatremia after a race (Davis et al. 2001). The major contributing factors appeared to be longer race time and drinking large amounts of water during the race. Experts speculate that less experienced athletes run more slowly, increasing the total time that they are competing; at the same time, they consume very large amounts of water to avoid potential dehydration. The longer these individuals run, the more water they drink and the more diluted their blood sodium levels become. About half of the hyponatremic runners in these studies had to be hospitalized.

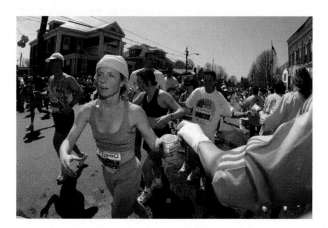

A recent study of long distance triathletes (competing in running, swimming, and cycling) found that about 18% of these athletes suffered from hyponatremia, but only one-third of these individuals had symptoms that required medical care (Speedy et al. 1999). Thus, other individuals competing in long distance events or activities are also at risk for this disorder. Hyponatremia is a dangerous and potentially fatal condition that can be prevented. Drinking sport beverages, which contain electrolytes, and moderating fluid intake during marathons and other long distance activities can help prevent the occurrence of hyponatremia. ●

What Happens If We Don't Consume Enough Sodium?

hyponatremia A condition in which blood sodium levels are dangerously low.

Because our dietary sodium intake is so high in the United States, deficiencies are extremely rare, except in individuals who sweat heavily or consume little or no sodium in the diet. Nevertheless, certain conditions can cause dangerously low blood sodium levels. **Hyponatremia,** or low blood sodium levels (clinically defined as less than 136 milliequivalent per liter of blood), can occur in active people who drink large volumes of water and fail to replace sodium. This is discussed in the above Highlight box. Severe diarrhea, vomiting, or excessive prolonged sweating can also cause hyponatremia. Symptoms include headaches, dizziness, fatigue, nausea, vomiting, and muscle cramps. If hyponatremia is left untreated it can lead to seizures, coma, and death. Treatment for hyponatremia includes replacement of the lost minerals by consuming liquids and foods high in sodium and other minerals. It may be necessary to administer electrolyte-rich solutions intravenously if the person has lost consciousness or is not able to consume beverages and foods by mouth.

> **Recap:** Sodium is the primary positively charged electrolyte in the extracellular fluid. It works to maintain fluid balance and blood pressure, assists in acid-base balance and transmission of nerve signals, aids muscle contraction, and assists in the absorption of some nutrients. We require at least 500 mg of sodium daily. Deficiencies are rare, since the typical American diet is high in sodium. Excessive sodium intake has been related to high blood pressure, bloating, and loss of bone density in some studies.

Potassium

As we discussed previously, potassium is the major positively charged electrolyte in the intracellular fluid. It is a major constituent of all living cells and is found in both plants and animals.

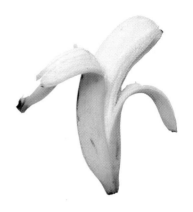

Many fresh fruits and vegetables are excellent sources of potassium.

Functions of Potassium

Potassium and sodium work together to maintain proper fluid balance. In addition to its role in maintaining fluid balance, potassium plays a major role in regulating the contraction of muscles and transmission of nerve impulses, and it assists in maintaining blood pressure. In contrast to a high-sodium diet, eating a diet high in potassium actually helps maintain a lower blood pressure.

How Much Potassium Should We Consume?

Potassium is found in abundance in many fresh foods. We can reduce our risk for high blood pressure by consuming adequate potassium in our diet.

Recommended Dietary Intake for Potassium   The AI for potassium for adult men and women aged 19 to 50 years is 4.7 g/day (or 4,700 mg/day) (Institute of Medicine 2004).

Shopper's Guide: Good Food Sources of Potassium   Processing foods generally increases their amount of sodium and decreases their amount of potassium. Thus, the best sources of potassium include fresh foods, particularly fresh fruits and vegetables. Table 7.4 identifies foods that are high in potassium. You can optimize your potassium intake and reduce your sodium intake by avoiding processed foods and eating more fresh fruits, vegetables, and whole grains. Most salt substitutes are made from potassium chloride, and these products contain relatively high amounts of potassium.

What Happens If We Consume Too Much Potassium?

People with healthy kidneys are able to excrete excess potassium effectively. However, people with kidney disease are not able to regulate their blood potassium levels. **Hyperkalemia,** or high blood potassium levels (clinically defined as greater than 5 milliequivalent per liter of blood), occurs when potassium is not excreted efficiently from the body. Because of potassium's role in cardiac muscle contraction, severe hyperkalemia can alter the normal rhythm of the heart, resulting in heart attack and death. People with kidney failure must monitor their potassium intake very carefully to prevent complications from hyperkalemia. Individuals at risk for hyperkalemia should avoid consuming salt substitutes, as these products are high in potassium.

hyperkalemia   A condition in which blood potassium levels are dangerously high.

Table 7.4   Potassium Content of Common Foods

Food	Serving Size	Potassium (mg)
Potato, baked, flesh and skin	1 medium	721
Nonfat yogurt, plain	One 8 oz. container	579
Banana	1 large, 8 to 8 7/8"	554
Tomato juice	1 cup	535
Halibut, cooked	3 oz.	490
Orange juice, from concentrate	1 cup	473
Milk, 1% fat	1 cup	443
Cantaloupe	1/4 of medium melon	426
Spinach, raw	1 cup	167

Source: U.S. Department of Agriculture. 1999. USDA Nutrient Database for Standard Reference, Release 13. Nutrient Data Laboratory Home Page. www.nal.usda.gov/fnic/foodcomp Accessed February 2002.

What Happens If We Don't Consume Enough Potassium?

Because potassium is widespread in many foods, a dietary potassium deficiency is rare. However, potassium deficiency is not uncommon among people who have serious medical disorders. Kidney disease, diabetic acidosis, and other illnesses can lead to potassium deficiency.

In addition, people with high blood pressure who are prescribed diuretic medications to treat their disease are at risk for potassium deficiency. As we noted earlier, diuretics promote the excretion of fluid as urine through the kidneys. Some diuretics also increase the body's excretion of potassium. People who are taking diuretic medications should have their blood potassium monitored regularly and should eat foods that are high in potassium to prevent **hypokalemia,** or low blood potassium levels (clinically defined as less than 3.8 milliequivalent per liter of blood). This is not a universal recommendation however, because some diuretics are specially formulated to spare potassium, and therefore, people taking this class of diuretic should not increase their dietary potassium above recommended levels.

Extreme dehydration, vomiting, and diarrhea can also cause hypokalemia. People who abuse alcohol or laxatives can also suffer from hypokalemia. Symptoms include confusion, loss of appetite, and muscle weakness. Severe cases of hypokalemia result in fatal changes in heart rate; many deaths attributed to extreme dehydration or an eating disorder are caused by abnormal heart rhythms due to hypokalemia.

hypokalemia   A condition in which blood potassium levels are dangerously low.

> **Recap:** Potassium is the major positively charged electrolyte inside of the cell. It regulates fluid balance, blood pressure, and muscle contraction, and it helps in the transmission of nerve impulses. Potassium is found in abundance in fresh foods, particularly fruits, vegetables, and meats. Both hyperkalemia, or excessive blood potassium, and hypokalemia, or low blood potassium, can result in heart failure and death.

Chloride

Chloride should not be confused with *chlorine,* which is a poisonous gas used to kill bacteria and other germs in our water supply. Chloride is a negatively charged ion that we obtain almost exclusively in our diets from consuming sodium chloride, or table salt.

Functions of Chloride

Coupled with sodium in the extracellular fluid, chloride assists with the maintenance of fluid balance. Chloride is also a part of hydrochloric acid (HCl) in the stomach, which aids in preparing food for further digestion (see Chapter 3). Chloride works with the white blood cells of our body during an immune response to help kill bacteria, and it assists in the transmission of nerve impulses.

How Much Chloride Should We Consume?

The AI for chloride for adult men and women aged 19 to 50 years is 2.3 g/day (or 2,300 mg/day) (Institute of Medicine 2004). As chloride is coupled with sodium to form table salt, our primary dietary source of chloride is salt in our foods. Chloride is also found in some fruits and vegetables.

What Happens If We Consume Too Much Chloride?

As we consume virtually all of our dietary chloride in the form of sodium chloride, consuming excess amounts of this mineral over a prolonged period leads to hypertension in salt-sensitive individuals. There is no other known toxicity symptom for chloride (National Research Council 1989).

What Happens If We Don't Consume Enough Chloride?

Because of our relatively high dietary salt intake in the United States, most people consume more than enough chloride. Even when a person consumes a low-sodium diet, chloride intake is usually adequate.

A chloride deficiency can occur, however, during conditions of severe dehydration and frequent vomiting. This occurs often in people with eating disorders who regularly vomit to rid their bodies of unwanted calories.

> **Recap:** Chloride is the major negatively charged electrolyte outside of the cell. It assists with maintaining fluid balance and aids digestion of food. It also helps our immune system fight infection and assists in the transmission of nerve impulses. Our main dietary source of chloride is sodium chloride. Excess consumption of chloride can lead to hypertension in salt-sensitive individuals. Chloride deficiencies are rare but can occur during severe dehydration and frequent vomiting.

Phosphorus

Phosphorus is the major intracellular negatively charged electrolyte. In our bodies, phosphorus is most commonly found combined with oxygen in the form of phosphate, PO_4^{3-}. Phosphorus is an essential constituent of all cells and is found in both plants and animals.

Functions of Phosphorus

Phosphorus works with potassium inside of the cell to maintain proper fluid balance. It also plays a critical role in bone formation, as it is a part of the mineral complex of bone (see Chapter 9). Indeed, about 85% of our body's phosphorus is stored in our bones.

As a primary component of adenosine triphosphate (ATP), phosphorus plays a key role in creating energy for our bodies. It also helps regulate many biochemical reactions by activating and deactivating enzymes. Phosphorus is a part of our genetic materials including deoxyribonucleic acid (DNA) and ribonucleic acid (RNA), and it is a component in cell membranes (as phospholipids) and part of the lipoproteins such as low density lipoprotein (LDL) and high density lipoprotein (HDL).

How Much Phosphorus Should We Consume?

The RDA for phosphorus is 700 mg per day (Institute of Medicine 1999). The average U.S. adult consumes about twice this amount each day; thus phosphorus deficiencies are rare. Phosphorus is widespread in many foods and is found in high amounts in foods that contain protein. Milk, meats, and eggs are good sources of phosphorus. Table 7.5 shows the phosphorus content of various foods.

It is important to note that we absorb the phosphorus from animal sources more readily than from plant sources. The phosphorus in plant foods such as beans, cereals, and nuts is found in the form of **phytic acid,** a plant storage form of phosphorus. Our bodies do not produce enzymes that can break down phytic acid, but we are still able to absorb up to 50% of the phosphorus found in plant foods because other foods and the bacteria in our large intestines can break down phytic acid. Soft drinks are another common source of phosphorus in our diet; refer to Chapter 9 to learn how heavy consumption of soft drinks may be detrimental to bone health.

What Happens If We Consume Too Much Phosphorus?

People suffering from kidney disease and people taking too many vitamin D supplements or too many phosphorus-containing antacids can suffer from high blood phosphorus levels. Severely high levels of blood phosphorus cause muscle spasms and convulsions.

What Happens If We Don't Consume Enough Phosphorus?

As mentioned previously, deficiencies of phosphorus are rare. People who may suffer from low phosphorus levels include premature infants, elderly people with poor diets, and people who abuse alcohol. People with vitamin D deficiency, hyperparathyroidism (oversecretion of parathyroid hormone), and those who overuse antacids that bind with phosphorus may also have low blood phosphorus levels.

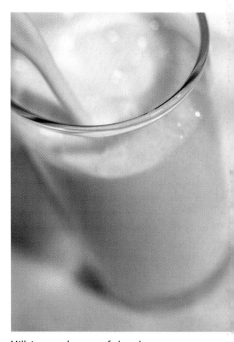

Milk is a good source of phosphorus.

phytic acid   The form of phosphorus stored in plants.

Table 7.5 Phosphorus Content of Common Foods

Food	Serving Size	Phosphorus (mg)
Cheese, cheddar	3 oz.	435
Cheese, provolone	3 oz.	423
Nonfat yogurt, plain	One 8 oz. container	356
Lentils, cooked	1 cup	356
Chicken, white meat, cooked	1 cup	323
All bran cereal	½ cup	294
Chicken, dark meat, roasted	1 cup	250
Skim milk	1 cup	247
Milk, 1% fat	1 cup	245
Milk, 2% fat	1 cup	245
Black beans, cooked	1 cup	241
Tofu, calcium processed	½ cup	239
Extra lean ground beef, broiled	3 oz.	137
Almonds	1 oz. (~24 almonds)	134
Soy milk	1 cup	120
Peanut butter, smooth style	2 tbsp.	118

Source: U.S. Department of Agriculture. 1999. USDA Nutrient Database for Standard Reference, Release 13. Nutrient Data Laboratory Home Page. www.nal.usda.gov/fnic/foodcomp Accessed February 2002.

Recap: Phosphorus is the major negatively charged electrolyte inside of the cell. It helps maintain fluid balance and bone health. It also assists us in making energy available and in regulating chemical reactions, and it is a primary component of our genetic materials. The RDA for phosphorus is 700 mg per day, and it is commonly found in high protein foods. Excess phosphorus can lead to muscle spasms and convulsion, while phosphorus deficiencies are rare.

What Disorders Are Related to Fluid and Electrolyte Imbalances?

There are a number of serious, and potentially fatal, disorders resulting from the imbalance of fluid and electrolytes in our bodies. Let's review some of these now.

Dehydration

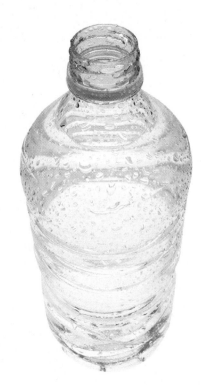

dehydration Depletion of body fluid that results when fluid excretion exceeds fluid intake.

Dehydration is a serious health problem that results when fluid excretion exceeds fluid intake. It is classified in terms of the percentage of weight loss that is exclusively due to the loss of fluid. Dehydration commonly occurs as a result of heavy exercise or exposure to high environmental temperatures because rapid weight loss is always due to losses of body water through increased sweating and breathing. However, elderly people and infants can get dehydrated even when inactive, as their risk for dehydration is much higher than that of healthy young and middle-aged adults. In the elderly it is because they have a lower total amount of body water, and their thirst mechanism is less effective than that of a younger person; they are therefore less likely to meet their higher fluid needs. Infants, on the other hand, excrete urine at a higher rate, cannot express when they are thirsty, and have a greater ratio of body surface area to body core, causing them to respond more dramatically to heat and cold and to lose more body water than an older person.

As indicated in Table 7.6, relatively small losses in body water, equal to a 1 to 2% change in body weight, result in symptoms such as thirst, discomfort, and loss of appetite. For a person weighing 160 pounds, these symptoms occur after a rapid loss of 1 to 4 pounds. More severe water losses, equal to 3 to 5% body weight, result in symptoms that include sleepiness, nausea, flushed skin, and problems with mental concentration. Severe losses of body water, greater than 8% of body weight (equal to

Table 7.6   Percentages of Body Fluid Loss Correlated with Weight Loss and Symptoms

% Body Water Loss	Weight Lost If You Weigh 160 lbs	Weight Lost If You Weigh 130 lbs	Symptoms
1–2	1.6 lbs–3.2 lbs	1.3 lbs–2.6 lbs	Strong thirst, loss of appetite, feeling uncomfortable
3–5	4.8 lbs–8.0 lbs	3.9 lbs–6.5 lbs	Dry mouth, reduced urine output, greater difficulty working and concentrating, flushed skin, tingling extremities, impatience, sleepiness, nausea, emotional instability
6–8	9.6 lbs–12.8 lbs	7.8 lbs–10.4 lbs	Increased body temperature that doesn't decrease, increased heart rate and breathing rate, dizzy, difficulty breathing, slurred speech, mental confusion, muscle weakness, blue lips
9–11	14.4 lbs–17.6 lbs	11.7 lbs–14.3 lbs	Muscle spasms, delirium, swollen tongue, poor balance and circulation, kidney failure, decreased blood volume and blood pressure

about 13 pounds of water for someone weighing 160 pounds), can result in delirium, coma, and death. Thus, a rapid loss of body fluid leads to a dangerous increase in body temperature, kidney failure, and eventual death.

Gustavo   *Nutri-Case*

"Something is going on with me this week. Every day, at work, I've been feeling weak and like I'm going to be sick to my stomach. It's been really hot, over a hundred degrees out in the fields, but I'm used to that, and besides, I've been drinking lots of water. It's probably just my high blood pressure acting up again."

What do you think might be wrong with Gustavo? If you learned that he was following a low-sodium diet prescribed to manage his high blood pressure, would this information argue for or against your theory, and why? What would you advise Gustavo to do differently at work tomorrow?

We discussed earlier the importance of fluid replacement when you are exercising. How can you tell whether you are drinking enough fluid before, during, and after your exercise sessions? First, you can measure your body weight before and after each session. If you weighed in at 160 pounds before basketball practice, and immediately afterward you weigh 158 pounds, then you have lost 2 pounds of body weight. This is equal to 1.3% of your body weight prior to practice. As you can see in Table 7.6, you are most likely feeling strong thirst, diminished appetite, and you may even feel generally uncomfortable. Your goal is to consume enough water and other fluids to bring your body weight back to 160 pounds prior to your next exercise session.

A simpler method of monitoring your fluid levels is to observe the color of your urine (Figure 7.7). If you are properly hydrated, your urine should be clear to pale yellow in color, similar to diluted lemonade. Urine that is medium to dark yellow in

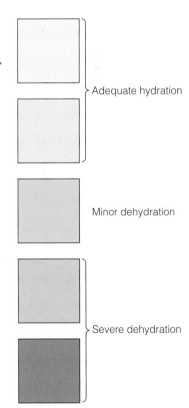

Figure 7.7   Urine color chart. Color variations indicate levels of hydration.

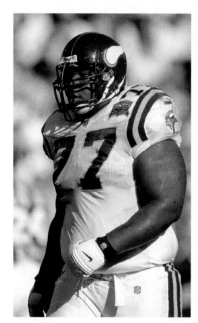

National Football League all-star Korey Stringer died in 2001 as a result of heat stroke.

heat stroke   A potentially fatal response to high temperature characterized by failure of the body's heat-regulating mechanisms. Symptoms include rapid pulse, reduced sweating, hot, dry skin, high temperature, headache, weakness, and sudden loss of consciousness. Commonly called *sunstroke*.

overhydration   Dilution of body fluid. It results when water intake or retention is excessive.

hypertension   A chronic condition characterized by above-average blood pressure readings; specifically, systolic blood pressure over 140 mm Hg or diastolic blood pressure over 90 mm Hg.

color, similar to apple juice, indicates an inadequate fluid intake. Very dark or brown colored urine, such as the color of a cola beverage, is a sign of severe dehydration and indicates potential muscle breakdown and kidney damage. People should strive to maintain a urine color that is clear or pale yellow.

Heat Stroke

Athletes who work out in hot weather are particularly vulnerable to dangerous fluid loss. In August 2001, 27-year-old National Football League all-star player Korey Stringer died of complications from **heat stroke** after working out in a hot and humid environment. Heat stroke is a potentially fatal heat illness characterized by failure of the body's heat-regulating mechanisms. Symptoms include rapid pulse, hot, dry skin, high temperature, and loss of consciousness. As illustrated in the Korey Stringer case, heat stroke can also be fatal. Despite having access to ample fluid and excellent medical assistance, Stringer's body core temperature rose to 108°F. It appears that a combination of dehydration, heat, humidity, protective clothing and headgear, and Stringer's large body size (6'4", 330 pounds) contributed to his death. Although there were suspicions that ephedra, a stimulant used by many athletes, contributed to his death, no evidence was found to support this. Our ability to sweat is extremely limited in a humid environment, and large individuals with a great deal of muscle mass produce a lot of body heat. In addition, people who have excess body fat have an extra layer of insulation that makes it even more difficult to dissipate body heat at rest and during exercise.

Similar deaths have occurred in the past with collegiate and high school football players. These deaths prompted national attention and resulted in strict guidelines encouraging regular fluid breaks and cancellation of events or changing the time of the event to avoid high heat and humidity. In addition, people who are active in a hot environment should stop exercising if they feel dizzy, light-headed, disoriented, or nauseated. Injury and death due to heat illnesses can be avoided by maintaining a healthy fluid balance before, during, and after exercise.

Water Intoxication

Is it possible to drink too much water? **Overhydration,** or *water intoxication*, can occur but it is rare. It generally only occurs in people with health problems that cause the kidneys to retain too much water, causing overhydration and hyponatremia, which were discussed earlier.

Hypertension

One of the major chronic diseases in the United States is high blood pressure, which health care professionals refer to as **hypertension.** This disease affects almost 25% of all adults in the United States and more than 50% of people over the age of 65 (CDC 2002; see Figure 7.8). Although hypertension itself is often without symptoms, it increases a person's risk for many other serious conditions including heart disease, stroke, and kidney disease; it can also reduce brain function, impair physical mobility, and cause death.

A person with hypertension is unable to maintain blood pressure in a healthy range. We measure blood pressure in two phases, systolic and diastolic. *Systolic blood pressure* represents the pressure exerted in our arteries at the moment that the heart contracts, sending blood into our blood vessels. *Diastolic blood pressure* represents the pressure in our arteries between contractions, when our heart is relaxed. You can also think of diastolic blood pressure as the resistance in our arteries that our heart must pump against every time it beats. We measure blood pressure in millimeters of mercury (mm Hg). Optimal systolic blood pressure is *less than* 120 mm Hg, while optimal diastolic blood pressure is *less than* 80 mm Hg. Prehypertension is defined as a systolic blood pressure between 120 and 139 mm Hg, or a diastolic blood pressure

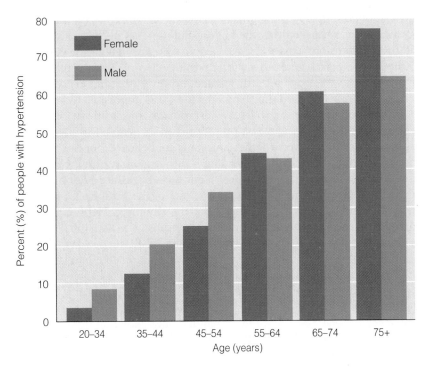

Figure 7.8   Hypertension is one of the major chronic diseases in the United States. (Centers for Disease Control and Prevention, National Center for Health Statistics, Division of Health Examination Statistics, Hypertension. www.cdc.gov/nchs/fastats/hyprtens.htm Accessed March 2002.)

between 80 and 89 mm Hg. You would be diagnosed with hypertension if your systolic blood pressure were greater than or equal to 140 mm Hg or your diastolic blood pressure were greater than or equal to 90 mm Hg.

What Causes Hypertension?

What causes hypertension? For about 95% of people who have it, the causes are unknown. This type is referred to as *primary* or *essential hypertension*. For the other 5% of people with hypertension, causes may include kidney disease, sleep apnea (a sleep disorder that affects breathing), and sensitivity to salt.

What Can Be Done to Reduce Hypertension?

Although we do not know what causes most cases of hypertension, there are five primary lifestyle changes that can help reduce it. These changes include:

- Losing weight. Blood pressure values have been shown to decrease six to seven points in people who have lost less than twenty pounds of body weight (Blumenthal et al. 2000).

- Increasing physical activity. The amount and intensity of exercise needed to improve blood pressure is easily achievable for most people. Light-intensity exercise lasting thirty to sixty minutes can reduce blood pressure, as can more intense exercise lasting twenty to thirty minutes (Lesniak and Dubbert 2001).

- Reducing alcohol intake. Because heavy alcohol consumption can worsen high blood pressure, it is suggested that people with this disease abstain from drinking alcohol or drink no more than two drinks per day.

- Reducing sodium intake in salt-sensitive individuals (people whose blood pressure increases when they eat high-sodium foods); some people who are not salt sensitive also benefit from eating lower sodium diets.

- Eating more whole grains, fruits, vegetables, and low-fat protein sources.

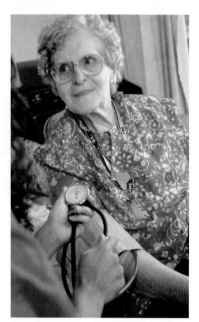

Hypertension is a major chronic disease in the United States, affecting more than 50% of adults over 65 years old.

One area of controversy is the impact that sodium intake has on our blood pressure. For years it was believed that the high sodium intakes of the typical American diet lead to hypertension. This is because people who live in countries where sodium intake is high have greater rates of hypertension than people from countries where sodium intake is low. We have recently learned, however, that not everyone with hypertension is sensitive to sodium. Unfortunately, it is impossible to know who is sensitive to sodium, as there is not an easy test for sodium sensitivity. Because lowering sodium intake does not reduce blood pressure in all people with hypertension, there is significant debate over whether everyone can benefit from eating a lower-sodium diet. Despite this debate, the leading health organizations, including the American Heart Association, the National High Blood Pressure Education Program, and the National Heart, Lung, and Blood Institute of the National Institutes of Health, continue to support a reduction in dietary sodium to 2,400 mg per day as recommended in the Dietary Guidelines for Americans (USDA 2000). Currently the average sodium intake in the United States is about 3,300 mg per day.

In contrast to sodium, other minerals such as calcium, magnesium, and potassium have been shown to help reduce hypertension. As discussed in Chapter 2, the DASH (Dietary Approaches to Stop Hypertension) diet is an eating plan that is high in these minerals, moderately low in sodium, low in saturated fat, and it includes ten servings of fruits and vegetables each day. The DASH diet has been shown to significantly reduce blood pressure in people with and without hypertension, with even greater reductions occurring in a lower-sodium version of the DASH diet (Appel et al. 1997; Sacks et al. 2001). Thus, eating a healthful diet that contains plenty of fruits, vegetables, whole grains, and low-fat dairy products has been proven to reduce blood pressure levels.

For some individuals, lifestyle changes are not completely effective in normalizing hypertension. When this is the case, there are a variety of medications that can be prescribed to bring a person's blood pressure into the normal range. Individuals taking medications to control blood pressure should also continue to practice the healthful lifestyle changes listed earlier in this section, as these changes will continue to benefit their long-term health.

Hypertension is called "the silent killer," because often there are no obvious symptoms of this disease. For this reason, it is important that people get their blood pressure checked on a regular basis. Tragically, many people with hypertension fail to take their prescribed medication because they do not feel sick. Many of these people eventually suffer the consequences of their actions by experiencing a heart attack or stroke.

Neuropsychiatric Disorders

Electrolyte imbalances can cause changes in nervous function that result in psychiatric disorders. Low levels of magnesium, hypokalemia, and chronic hyponatremia may be associated with conditions of apathy and depression. High blood levels of calcium can also cause depression. A variety of electrolyte imbalances can cause confusion, delirium, and psychosis, including hyponatremia, excessive blood calcium, and low blood calcium. Electrolyte disorders can also impair cognitive function, diminishing a person's capacity to think, concentrate, solve problems, and remember information.

Muscle Disorders

seizures Uncontrollable muscle spasms caused by increased nervous system excitability that can result from electrolyte imbalances.

Muscle function is altered by electrolyte imbalances because of the changes in nervous system function that occur with these imbalances. Seizures are an example of a muscle disorder that can occur with electrolyte imbalances. **Seizures** are uncontrollable muscle spasms that may be localized to one area of the body, such as the face, or can violently wrack a person's entire body. Some people lose consciousness during seizures, while others may experience hallucinations, flashbacks, or emotional outbursts. Severe seizures can result in bone fractures, loss of bowel and bladder function, and severe biting of the tongue.

Muscle cramps are involuntary, spasmodic, and painful muscle contractions that last for many seconds or even minutes. Hypernatremia that occurs with dehydration is known to cause cramps, as are other electrolyte imbalances. Muscle weakness and paralysis can also occur with various electrolyte imbalances such as hypokalemia, hyperkalemia, and low blood phosphorus levels.

muscle cramps Involuntary, spasmodic, and painful muscle contractions that last for many seconds or even minutes; electrolyte imbalances are often the cause of muscle cramps.

Recap: Dehydration, heat stroke, and even death can occur when water loss exceeds water intake. Since our thirst mechanism is not always sufficient, it is important to drink water regularly throughout the day to promote adequate fluid intake. High blood pressure is a major chronic illness in the United States; it can be controlled by losing weight, increasing physical activity, decreasing alcohol intake, and making specific dietary changes. Electrolyte imbalances can lead to neuropsychiatric disorders such as depression, delirium, and psychosis; they can also lead to muscle disorders such as seizures and muscle cramps.

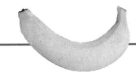

Chapter Summary

- Between approximately 50 and 70% of a healthy adult's body weight is fluid. Two-thirds of this fluid is intracellular fluid, and the remainder is extracellular fluid.

- Electrolytes are electrically charged particles found in our body fluid that assist in maintaining fluid balance and the normal functioning of our cells and nervous system.

- Water acts as a solvent in our bodies, provides protection and lubrication for our organs and tissues, and acts to maintain blood volume, body temperature, and blood pressure.

- The three primary sources of fluid intake are beverages, foods, and metabolic water produced by our bodies.

- The three primary avenues of fluid excretion are urine, insensible water loss (via sweat and exhalation), and feces.

- Conditions that significantly increase water loss from our bodies include fever, vomiting, diarrhea, hemorrhage, blood donation, heavy exercise, and exposure to heat, cold, and altitude.

- Fluid intake needs are highly variable and depend upon body size, age, physical activity, health status, and environmental conditions.

- Drinking too much water can lead to overhydration and hyponatremia, or dilution of blood sodium, whereas drinking too little water leads to dehydration, one of the leading causes of death around the world.

- Sodium assists in maintaining fluid balance, blood pressure, nervous function, and muscle contraction.

- Consuming excess sodium can cause high blood pressure or hypernatremia. Sodium deficiencies are rare,

but hyponatremia can occur from excessive fluid intake not accompanied by adequate sodium intake.

- Potassium assists in maintaining fluid balance, healthy blood pressure, transmission of nerve impulses, and muscle function.

- Hyperkalemia is excess blood potassium, which occurs due to kidney disease or malfunction. Hypokalemia is low blood potassium and can occur as a result of kidney disease, diabetic acidosis, and through the use of some diuretic medications.

- Chloride assists in maintaining fluid balance, normal nerve transmission, and the digestion of food via the action of HCl.

- Excessive chloride intake occurs with excessive sodium intake, leading to hypertension in salt-sensitive people. Chloride deficiency is rare but can occur with prolonged dehydration and vomiting.

- Phosphorus assists in maintaining fluid balance and transferring energy via ATP. It is also a component of bone, phospholipids, genetic material, and lipoproteins.

- High blood phosphorus levels can occur with kidney disease and when individuals consume too many vitamin D supplements or phosphorus-containing antacids. Phosphorus deficiencies are rare but can occur with vitamin D deficiency and in premature infants or people with poor diets.

- Dehydration occurs when water excretion exceeds water intake. Individuals at risk include the elderly, infants, people exercising heavily for prolonged periods in the heat, and individuals suffering from prolonged vomiting and diarrhea.

- Heat stroke occurs when the body's core temperature rises above 100°F. Heat stroke can lead to death if left untreated.

- Overhydration, or water intoxication, is caused by consuming too much water. Hyponatremia can also result from water intoxication.
- Hypertension, or high blood pressure, increases the risk for heart disease, stroke, and kidney disease. Consuming excess sodium is associated with hypertension in some people.
- Electrolyte imbalances can cause neuropsychiatric disorders such as apathy, depression, confusion, and psychosis. These imbalances can also cause seizures, muscle cramps, muscle weakness, and paralysis.

Review Questions

1. Which of the following is a characteristic of potassium?
   a. It is the major positively charged electrolyte in the extracellular fluid.
   b. It can be found in fresh fruits and vegetables.
   c. It is a critical component of the mineral complex of bone.
   d. It is the major negatively charged electrolyte in the extracellular fluid.

2. Which of the following people probably has the greatest percentage of bodily fluid?
   a. A female adult who is slightly overweight and vomits nightly after eating dinner.
   b. An elderly male of average weight who has low blood pressure.
   c. An overweight football player who has just completed a practice session in high heat.
   d. A healthy infant of average weight.

3. Plasma is one example of
   a. extracellular fluid.
   b. intracellular fluid.
   c. tissue fluid.
   d. metabolic water.

4. Which of the following is true of the cell membrane?
   a. It is freely permeable to most solutes except fats.
   b. It is freely permeable to water and all solutes.
   c. Is freely permeable only to fats.
   d. It is freely permeable to water but impermeable to solutes.

5. Which of the following lifestyle changes has been shown to reduce hypertension in all people?
   a. Consuming a low-sodium diet.
   b. Losing weight.
   c. Getting at least eight hours of sleep nightly.
   d. Consuming at least two glasses of red wine daily.

6. **True or false?** Drinking lots of purified water throughout a marathon will prevent fluid imbalances.

7. **True or false?** A decreased concentration of electrolytes in our blood stimulates the thirst mechanism.

8. **True or false?** Hypernatremia commonly occurs when we are dehydrated.

9. **True or false?** Absence of thirst is a reliable indicator of adequate hydration.

10. **True or false?** Conditions that increase fluid loss include constipation, blood transfusions, and high humidity.

11. Explain why chronic diarrhea in a young child can lead to death from abnormal heart rhythms.

12. After winning a cross-country relay race, you and your teammates celebrate with a trip to the local tavern for a few beers. That evening, you feel shaky and disoriented, and you have a "pins and needles" feeling in your hands and feet. What could be going on that is contributing to these feelings?

13. For lunch today, your choices include: (a) chicken soup, a ham sandwich, and a can of tomato juice; or (b) potato salad, a tuna-fish sandwich, and a bottle of mineral water. You have hockey practice in mid-afternoon. Which lunch should you choose, and why?

14. Your cousin, who is breastfeeding her 3-month-old daughter, confesses to you that she has resorted to taking over-the-counter weight loss pills to help her lose the weight she gained during pregnancy. What would you advise her?

Test Yourself Answers

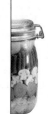

1. **True.** Between approximately 50 and 70% of our body weight consists of water.

2. **False.** Sodium is a nutrient necessary for health, but we should not consume more than recommended amounts.

3. **False.** Our thirst mechanism signals that we need to replenish fluids, but it is not sufficient to ensure we are completely hydrated.

4. **False.** Persistent vomiting can lead to long-term health consequences and even death.

5. **False.** We do not know the cause of high blood pressure in most people. A high-sodium diet can cause high blood pressure in people who are sensitive to sodium.

Web Links

www.epa.gov/OW
U.S. Environmental Protection Agency
Go to the EPA's water site for more information about drinking water quality, standards, and safety.

www.bottledwaterweb.com
Bottled Water Web
Find current and accurate information about bottled water.

www.mayoclinic.com
MayoClinic.com
Search for "hyponatremia" to learn more about this potentially fatal condition.

www.nlm.nih.gov/medlineplus
MEDLINE Plus Health Information
Search for "dehydration" and "heat stroke" to obtain additional resources and the latest news about the dangers of these heat-related illnesses.

www.nhlbi.nih.gov
National Heart, Lung, and Blood Institute
Go to this site to learn more about heart and vascular diseases including how to prevent high blood pressure and hypertension.

www.americanheart.org
American Heart Association
Discover the best way to help lower your blood pressure.

www.nih.gov
The National Institutes of Health (NIH)
Search this site to learn more about the DASH diet (Dietary Approaches to Stop Hypertension).

digestive.niddk.nih.gov
National Digestive Diseases Information Clearinghouse (NDDIC)
Go to this site to find out more about the causes, symptoms, and treatment of diarrhea.

References

American College of Sports Medicine (ACSM). 2000. Nutrition and athletic performance. *Med. Sci. Sports Exerc.* 32:2130–2145.

American College of Sports Medicine (ACSM). 1996. Exercise and fluid replacement. *Med. Sci. Sports Exerc.* 28:i–vii.

Appel L. J., T. J. Moore, E. Obarzanek, W. M. Vollmer, L. P. Svetkey, F. M. Sacks, G. A. Bray, T. M. Vogt, J. A. Cutler, M. M. Windhauser, P.-H. Lin, and N. Karanja. 1997. A clinical trial of the effects of dietary patterns on blood pressure. *New Engl. J. Med.* 336:1117–1124.

Bilzon J. L., A. J. Allsopp, and C. Williams. 2000. Short-term recovery from prolonged constant pace running in a warm environment: The effectiveness of a carbohydrate-electrolyte solution. *Eur. J. Appl. Physiol.* 82:305–312.

Blumenthal J. A., A. Sherwood, E. C. D. Gullette, M. Babyak, R. Waugh, A. Georgiades, L. W. Craighead, D. Tweedy, M. Feinglos, M. Applebaum, J. Hayano, and A. Hinderliter. 2000. Exercise and weight loss reduce blood pressure in men and women with mild hypertension. *Arch. Intern. Med.* 160:1947–1958.

Bottled Water Web™: Facts. www.bottledwaterweb.com/indus.html Accessed March 2002.

Centers for Disease Control and Prevention (CDC), National Center for Health Statistics, Division of Health Examination Statistics, Hypertension. www.cdc.gov/nchs/fastats/hyprtens.htm Accessed March 2002.

Cohen A. J., and F. J. Roe. 2000. Review of risk factors for osteoporosis with particular reference to a possible aetiological role of dietary salt. *Food Chem. Toxicol.* 38:237–253.

Davis D. P., J. S. Videen, A. Marino, G. M. Vilke, J. V. Dunford, S. P. Van Camp, and L. G. Maharam. 2001. Exercise-associated hyponatremia in marathon runners: a two-year experience. *J. Emerg. Med.* 21:47–57.

Galloway S. D., and R. J. Maughan. 2000. The effects of substrate and fluid provision on thermoregulatory and metabolic responses to prolonged exercise in a hot environment. *J. Sports Sci.* 18:339–351.

Institute of Medicine. 2004. *Dietary Reference Intakes for Water, Potassium, Sodium, Chloride, and Sulfate.* Washington, DC: The National Academics Press.

Institute of Medicine. Food and Nutrition Board. 1999. *Dietary Reference Intakes for Calcium, Phosphorus, Magnesium, Vitamin D, and Fluoride.* Washington, DC: National Academies Press.

Lesniak K. T., and P. M. Dubbert. 2001. Exercise and hypertension. *Current Opinion Cardiol.* 16:356–359.

Manore M., and J. Thompson. 2000. *Sport Nutrition for Health and Performance.* Champaign, IL: Human Kinetics.

National Research Council. Food and Nutrition Board. 1989. *Recommended Dietary Allowances.* 10th ed. Washington, DC: National Academy Press.

Sacks F. M., L. P. Svetkey, W. M. Vollmer, L. J. Appel, G. A. Bray, D. Harsha, E. Obarzanek, P. R. Conlin, E. R. Miller III, D. G. Simons-Morton, N. Karanja, and P.-H. Lin. 2001. Effects on blood pressure of reduced dietary sodium and the Dietary Approaches to Stop Hypertension (DASH) diet. *New Engl. J. Med.* 344:3–10.

Speedy D. B., T. D. Noakes, I. R. Rogers, J. M. Thompson, R. G. Campbell, J. A. Kuttner, D. R. Boswell, S. Wright, and M. Hamlin. 1999. Hyponatremia in ultra-distance triathletes. *Med. Sci. Sports Exerc.* 31:809–815.

U.S. Department of Agriculture (USDA). U.S. Department of Health and Human Services. 2000. *Dietary Guidelines for Americans.* 5th ed. Home and Garden Bulletin No. 232. (Available at www.health.gov/dietaryguidelines/dga2000/DIETGD.PDF Accessed March 2002)

Nutrition Debate:

Sport Beverages: Help or Hype?

Once considered specialty items used exclusively by elite athletes, sport beverages have become popular everyday beverage choices for both active and non-active people. The market for these drinks has become so lucrative that many of the large soft drink companies now produce these drinks. This surge in popularity of sport beverages leads us to ask three important questions:

- Do these beverages benefit highly active athletes?
- Do these beverages benefit recreationally active people?
- Do non-athletes need to consume sport beverages?

The first question is relatively easy to answer. Sport beverages were originally developed to meet the unique fluid, electrolyte, and carbohydrate needs of competitive athletes. As you learned in this chapter, highly active people need to replenish both fluids and electrolytes to avoid either dehydration or hyponatremia. Sport beverages can especially benefit athletes who exercise in the heat and are thus at an even greater risk for loss of water, electrolytes, and carbohydrates through respiration and sweat. The carbohydrates in sport beverages provides critical fuel during relatively intense (more than 60% of maximal effort) exercise bouts lasting more than one hour. Thus, endurance athletes are able to exercise longer, maintain a higher intensity, and improve performance times when they drink a sport beverage during exercise (Manore and Thompson 2000). Sport beverages may help athletes consume more energy than they could by eating solid foods and water alone. Some athletes, such as endurance bicyclists, train or compete for six to eight hours each day on a regular basis. It is virtually impossible for these athletes to consume enough solid foods to support this intense level of exercise.

Do recreationally active people need to consume sport beverages? Most probably do not, but if they exercise for periods longer than one hour at more than 60% maximal effort, they can benefit from consuming the carbohydrate and electrolytes in sport beverages during exercise. In addition, recent laboratory studies found that healthy people who are active but not elite athletes are able to exercise longer in high temperatures when they consume sport beverages (Bilzon, Allsopp, and Williams 2000; Galloway and Maughan 2000). These beverages can also be beneficial when exercising in an indoor environment, since many times the temperature in indoor areas is relatively high and results in a large volume of fluid being lost during the activity.

It is not always easy to determine whether someone should consume a sport beverage. However, keep in mind that these beverages were orginally formulated for people who exercise. Whether these beverages are needed depends on the duration and intensity of exercise, the environmental conditions, and on the characteristics of the individual. Here are some situations in which drinking a sport beverage is appropriate (Manore and Thompson 2000):

- Before exercise where dehydration can occur, especially if someone is already dehydrated prior to exercise.
- During exercise or physical work in high heat and/or high

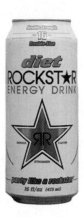
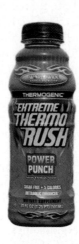
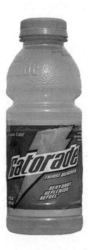
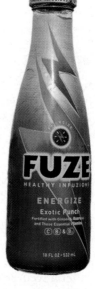

Table 7.7   Nutrient Content of Sport Beverages and Other Common Beverages*

Beverage	Energy (kcal)	Carbohydrate (g)	Sodium (mg)	Potassium (mg)
Cola, regular	153	39	15	4
Ginger ale	124	32	26	4
Beer, regular	146	9	18	89
Gatorade	90	22.5	144	39
All Sport	80	22.5	55.5	55.5
Beer, light	8	<1	1	5
Coffee, brewed	7.5	1.5	7.5	192
Cola, diet	4	<1	21	0
Tea, brewed	3	<1	7	88
Water, bottled	0	0	2	0
Water, tap	0	0	7	0

*Amounts compared are 12 fluid ounces (1.5 cups)

humidity, or if someone has recently had diarrhea or vomiting; may also be appropriate for someone who is not accustomed to activity in the heat.

- During exercise at high altitude and in cold environments; these conditions increase fluid and electrolyte losses.
- After exercise for rapid rehydration or between exercise bouts when it is difficult to consume food, such as between multiple soccer matches during a tournament.
- During long-duration exercise when blood glucose levels get low. For bouts of continuous, vigorous exercise lasting longer than sixty minutes, sport beverages may be needed to maintain energy levels and to provide both the fluid necessary to prevent dehydration.
- During exercise in people who may have poor glycogen stores prior to exercise or who are not well-fed due to illness or inability to eat enough solid food prior to exercise.

Interestingly, sport beverages have become very popular with people who do little or no regular exercise. Are there any benefits or negative consequences for inactive or lightly active people who regularly consume these drinks? There does not appear to be any evidence that people who do not exercise derive any benefits from consuming

sport beverages. Even if these individuals live in a hot environment, they should be able to replenish the fluid and electrolytes they lose during sweating by drinking water and other beverages and eating a normal diet.

Negative consequences could result when inactive people drink sport beverages. The primary consequence is weight gain, which could lead to obesity. As you can see in Table 7.7, sport beverages contain not only fluid and electrolytes, but they also contain energy. Drinking 12 fluid ounces (1.5 cups) of Gatorade adds 90 kcal to a person's daily energy intake. Many inactive people consume two to three times this amount each day, which contributes an additional 180 to 270 kcal of energy to one's diet. An inactive person has much lower energy needs than someone who is physically active. As with any other food, sport beverages could contribute to excess energy consumption, especially if these drinks are consumed in addition to alcoholic beverages and sugared drinks. With obesity rates at an all-time high, it is important that we attempt to consume only the foods and beverages necessary to support our health. Sport beverages are not designed to be consumed by inactive people, and they do not contribute to the overall health of inactive or lightly active people. What do you think—are there any reasons why an inactive person might benefit from drinking sport beverages? Should these drinks be used exclusively by athletes and highly active people?

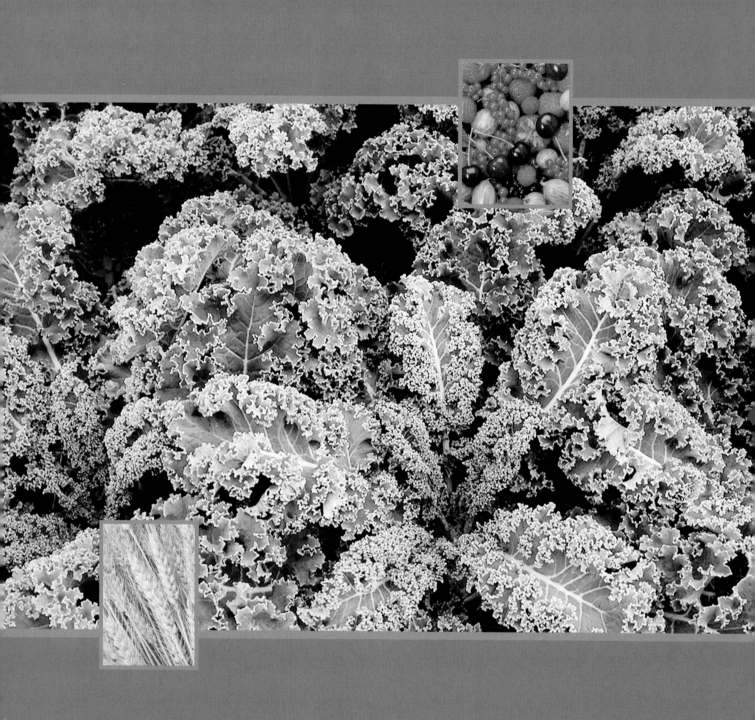

Chapter 8
Nutrients Involved in Antioxidant Function

Chapter Objectives

After reading this chapter you will be able to:

1. Define free radicals and discuss how they can damage our cells, pp. 265–267.

2. Describe how antioxidants protect our cells from the oxidative damage caused by free radicals, p. 268.

3. List three vitamins and two minerals that have antioxidant properties, pp. 268–286.

4. List three antioxidant enzyme systems and describe how these systems help fight oxidative damage, p. 268.

5. Identify food sources that are high in nutrients with antioxidant properties, pp. 271, 275, 278, 282.

6. Describe the relationship between antioxidant nutrients and our risk for cancer, pp. 287–294.

7. Define phytochemicals and describe their relationship with our risk for cancer, pp. 293–294.

8. Discuss how consuming nutrients with antioxidant properties can reduce our risk for cardiovascular disease, pp. 295–296.

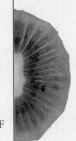

Test Yourself True or false?

1. Consuming antioxidant nutrients can help cure cancer. T or F

2. Taking vitamin C supplements does not reduce our risk of suffering from the common cold. T or F

3. Consuming large amounts of vitamin E supplements can lead to serious illness. T or F

4. We cannot consume enough antioxidant nutrients in our diets, so we should take supplements containing these nutrients. T or F

5. There is no scientific evidence supporting the contention that antioxidants can prolong life and reduce the effects of aging. T or F

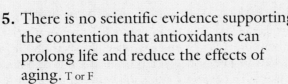

Test Yourself answers can be found at the end of the chapter.

Baseball greats Eric Davis and Darryl Strawberry have a special bond that goes beyond their childhood friendship and amiable rivalry in the major leagues. At the height of their careers, each began experiencing the same symptoms: extreme weight loss, debilitating fatigue, rectal bleeding, and severe abdominal pain. Davis was diagnosed in the spring of 1997, and Strawberry's diagnosis came in the fall of 1998—both had colon cancer. But wait a minute! Doesn't colon cancer only strike elderly people of European ancestry? Davis says, "It's not a white disease. It's not a young, it's not an old. It's a deadly disease."

What exactly is colon cancer anyway? Does any aspect of your lifestyle increase your risk? Can a poor diet cause cancer, and can a healthful diet prevent it? What are antioxidants, and why do some people claim they fight cancer? If your health food store were promoting an antioxidant supplement, would you buy it?

It isn't easy to sort fact from fiction when it comes to antioxidants. Fitness and health magazines, supplement companies, and even food manufacturers tout their benefits. In contrast, some researchers claim that antioxidants do not give any added protection from diseases and in some cases may even be harmful. In this chapter, you will learn what antioxidants are and how they work in our bodies. We will also profile the antioxidant nutrients and discuss their relationship to health. Finally, you'll learn about the role antioxidants may play in preventing cancer and heart disease and in slowing the aging process.

What Are Antioxidants, and How Do Our Bodies Use Them?

Antioxidants are compounds that protect our cells from the damage caused by oxidation. *Anti* means "against," and antioxidants work *against*, or *prevent* oxidation. Before we can go further in our discussion of antioxidants, we need to learn what oxidation is and how it does damage.

Oxidation Is a Chemical Reaction in Which Atoms Lose Electrons

A review of some basic chemistry will help us understand the process of oxidation.

Molecules Are Composed of Atoms

Molecules are the smallest *physical unit* of an element or compound. They consist of one or more of the same atoms in an element (e.g., hydrogen gas, or H_2) and two or more different atoms in a compound (such as water, H_2O). Our bodies are constantly breaking down molecules of food and air into their component atoms, and then rearranging these freed atoms to build the different types of molecules our body needs. But what, really, are atoms? Simply put, an **atom** is an infinitely small but *unique* unit of matter. Elements such as carbon or hydrogen are unique because their atoms are unique. Every atom of carbon, for example, is identical to every other atom of carbon. The same is true for hydrogen and for every other element of matter. All of the matter in the universe breaks down into just ninety-two elements, each consisting of one unique type of atom. Even more surprisingly, just six elements make up 99% of the matter in our bodies.

Atoms Are Composed of Particles

During the twentieth century, physicists learned how to split atoms into even smaller particles. As you can see in Figure 8.1, their research revealed that all atoms have a central core, called a **nucleus,** which is positively charged. Orbiting around this nucleus at close to the speed of light are one or more **electrons,** which are negatively charged. The opposite attraction between the positive nucleus and the negative electrons keeps an atom together by making the atom stable, so that its electrons remain with it and do not veer off toward other atoms.

antioxidant   A compound that has the ability to prevent or repair the damage caused by oxidation.

atom   A discrete, irreducible unit of matter. It is the smallest unit of an element and is identical to all other atoms of that element.

nucleus   The positively charged, central core of an atom. It is made up of two types of particles—protons and neutrons—bound tightly together. The nucleus of an atom contains essentially all of its atomic mass.

electron   A negatively charged particle orbiting the nucleus of an atom.

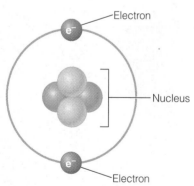

Figure 8.1   An atom consists of a central nucleus and orbiting electrons. The nucleus exerts a positive charge, which keeps the negatively charged electrons in its vicinity. Notice how electrons are paired with each other in a ring. This pairing of electrons results in the atom being chemically stable.

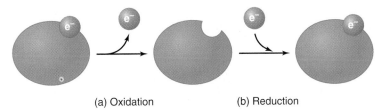

(a) Oxidation   (b) Reduction

Figure 8.2   The exchange reaction. Exchange reactions consist of two parts. **(a)** During oxidation, molecules *lose* electrons. **(b)** In the second part of the reaction, molecules *gain* electrons, which is called reduction.

During Metabolism, Atoms Exchange Electrons

As you recall from Chapter 3, the process by which our bodies break down and build up molecules is called *metabolism*. During metabolism, atoms may lose electrons (Figure 8.2a). We call this loss of electrons **oxidation,** because it is fueled by oxygen. Atoms are capable of gaining electrons during metabolism as well. We call this process *reduction* (Figure 8.2b). This loss and gain of electrons typically results in an even exchange of electrons. Scientists call this loss and gain of electrons an *exchange reaction.*

> **Recap:** An atom is an infinitely small and unique unit of matter having a nucleus and orbiting electrons. Atoms exist together with other atoms as molecules. During metabolism, molecules break apart and their atoms lose electrons; this process is fueled by oxygen and is called oxidation.

oxidation   A chemical reaction in which molecules of a substance are broken down into their component atoms. During oxidation, the atoms involved lose electrons.

Oxidation Sometimes Results in the Formation of Free Radicals

Stable atoms have an even number of electrons orbiting in pairs at successive distances (called *shells* or *rings*) from the nucleus. When a stable atom loses an electron during oxidation, it is left with an odd number of electrons in its outermost shell. In other words, it now has an *unpaired electron.* As we have seen, in most exchange reactions, unpaired electrons immediately pair up with other unpaired electrons, making newly stabilized atoms, but in rare cases, atoms with unpaired electrons in their outermost shell remain unpaired. Such atoms are highly unstable and are called **free radicals.**

free radical   A highly unstable atom with an unpaired electron in its outermost shell.

Energy Metabolism Involves Oxidation and Gives Rise to Free Radicals

Free radicals are formed as a by-product of many of our bodies' fundamental physiologic processes. Although some free radicals are a necessary part of our bodily functions, others cause serious damage to our cells and other body components. Let's look at the most common way they arise. As you know, our bodies use oxygen and hydrogen to generate the energy (ATP) that is needed by the body (Figure 8.3). We are constantly inhaling air into our bodies, thereby providing the oxygen needed to fuel this reaction. At the same time, we generate the necessary hydrogen as a result of digesting food. As shown in Figure 8.4, occasionally during metabolism, oxygen accepts a single electron that was released during this process. When it does so, the newly unstable oxygen molecule becomes a free radical because of the added unpaired electron.

Other Factors Can Also Cause Free Radical Formation

Free radicals are also formed from other metabolic processes, such as when our immune systems fight infections. Other factors that cause free radical formation include pollution, overexposure to the sun, toxic substances, radiation exposure, tobacco smoke, and asbestos. Continual exposure to these factors leads to uncontrollable free radical formation.

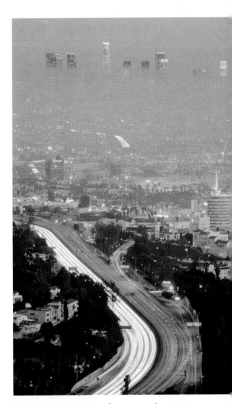

Exposure to pollution from car exhaust and industrial waste increases our production of free radicals.

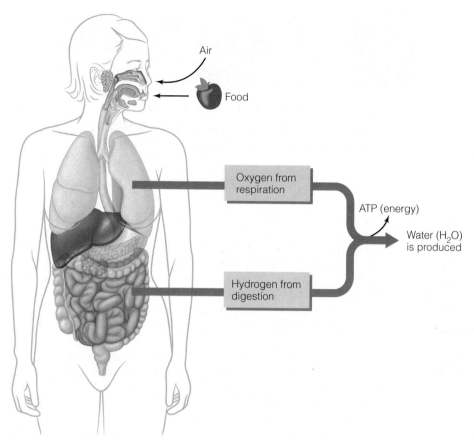

Figure 8.3   Oxygen (O) is consumed by inhaling air. Through the process of metabolizing food, hydrogen (H) is produced. As these substances undergo exchange reactions during metabolism, electrons are freed to contribute their energy to the production of ATP, which occurs throughout the body at the cellular level. The hydrogen and oxygen then recombine to form water (H_2O).

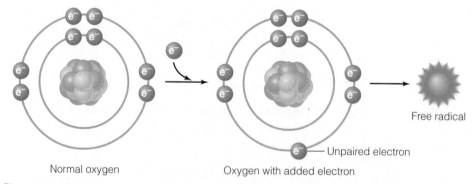

Figure 8.4   Normally, an oxygen molecule contains eight electrons. Occasionally oxygen will accept an unpaired electron during the oxidation process. This acceptance of a single electron causes oxygen to become an unstable molecule called a free radical.

Free Radicals Can Destabilize Other Molecules and Damage Our Cells

Why are we concerned with the formation of free radicals? Simply put, it is because of their destabilizing power. If you were to think of paired electrons as a married couple, a free radical would be an extremely seductive outsider. Its unpaired electron exerts a powerful attraction toward all stable molecules around it. In an attempt to stabilize

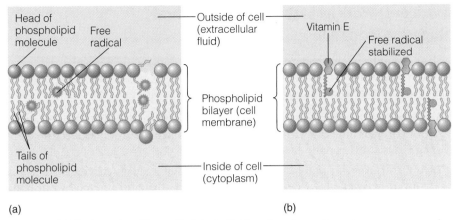

Figure 8.5 **(a)** The formation of free radicals in the lipid portion of our cell membranes can cause a dangerous chain reaction that damages the integrity of the membrane and can cause cell death. **(b)** Vitamin E is stored in the lipid portion of our cell membranes. By donating an electron to free radicals, it protects the lipid molecules in our cell membranes from themselves being oxidized and stops the chain reaction of oxidative damage.

itself, a free radical will "steal" an electron from stable compounds, in turn generating more unstable free radicals. This is a dangerous chain reaction, since the free radicals generated can damage or destroy our cells.

One of the most significant sites of free radical damage is the cell membrane. As shown in Figure 8.5a, free radicals that form within the lipid layer of cell membranes steal electrons from these stable lipid molecules. When the lipid molecules, which are hydrophobic, are destroyed, they no longer repel water. With the cell membrane's integrity lost, the ability to regulate the movement of fluids and nutrients into and out of the cell is also lost. This loss of cell integrity causes damage to the cell and to all systems affected by this cell.

Other sites of free radical damage include low-density lipoproteins (LDLs), cell proteins, and our genetic material (DNA, or deoxyribonucleic acid). Damage to these sites disrupts the transport of substances into and out of cells, alters protein function, and can disrupt cell function because of defective DNA. These changes may increase our risk for heart disease and cancer and can cause our cells to die prematurely.

Not surprisingly, many diseases are linked with free radical production, including:

- cancer
- heart disease
- diabetes
- arthritis
- cataracts
- kidney disease
- Alzheimer's disease
- Parkinson's disease

Recap: Free radicals are formed during oxidation when a stable atom loses or gains an electron and this electron remains unpaired. Free radicals can be produced during the formation of ATP, when our immune system fights infections, and when we are exposed to pollution, toxic substances, radiation, the sun, and tobacco smoke. Free radicals are highly unstable entities that cause the production of more free radicals. They can damage our LDLs, cell proteins, and DNA and are associated with many diseases including heart disease, cancer, and diabetes.

Antioxidants Work by Stabilizing Free Radicals or Opposing Oxidation

How do our bodies fight free radicals and repair the damage they cause? These actions are performed by antioxidants which are vitamins, minerals, and other compounds that perform their antioxidant role in either of two ways:

1. Certain antioxidant *vitamins* work independently by donating their electrons or hydrogen molecules to free radicals to stabilize them and reduce the damage caused by oxidation (Figure 8.5b).

2. Antioxidant *minerals* function within complex antioxidant enzyme systems that convert free radicals to less damaging substances that are excreted by our bodies. These enzymes also work to break down fatty acids that have become oxidized. In breaking down the fatty acids, they destroy the free radicals associated with the oxidized fatty acids. The antioxidant enzyme system makes more vitamin antioxidants available to fight other free radicals. Examples of antioxidant enzymes systems are superoxide dismutase, catalase, and glutathione peroxidase.

   - Superoxide dismutase converts free radicals to less damaging substances, such as hydrogen peroxide.
   - Catalase removes hydrogen peroxide from our bodies by converting it to water and oxygen.
   - Glutathione peroxidase also removes hydrogen peroxide from our bodies, and stops the production of free radicals in lipids.

3. Other compounds such as *beta-carotene* and *phytochemicals* help stabilize free radicals and prevent damage to cells and tissues.

Many enzyme systems require minerals as cofactors to help them perform their work. A **cofactor** is a compound required to activate an enzyme. In the case of antioxidant enzymes, the minerals selenium, copper, iron, zinc, and manganese act as cofactors, helping fight the damage caused by free radicals.

In summary, free radical formation is generally kept safely under control by the protective antioxidant systems in our body. When our natural antioxidant defenses are not sufficient, free radical damage can be quite significant.

cofactor A compound that is needed to allow enzymes to function properly.

> **Recap:** Antioxidant vitamins donate electrons or hydrogens to free radicals to stabilize them and reduce oxidative damage. Antioxidant minerals are part of antioxidant enzyme systems that convert free radicals to less damaging substances, which our bodies then excrete. Other compounds stabilize free radicals, which prevent them from damaging cells and tissues. Selenium, copper, iron, zinc, and manganese act as cofactors for the antioxidant enzyme systems, allowing the enzymes to function properly. Superoxide dismutase, catalase, and glutathione peroxidase are examples of antioxidant enzymes.

A Profile of Nutrients That Function As Antioxidants

Our bodies cannot form antioxidants spontaneously. Instead, we must consume them in our diet. Table 8.1 reviews the antioxidant vitamins and minerals and the way they work in our bodies. Nutrients that appear to have antioxidant properties or are part of our protective antioxidant enzyme systems include vitamins E, C, and A, beta-carotene (a precursor to vitamin A), and the mineral selenium. The minerals copper, iron, zinc, and manganese play a peripheral role in fighting oxidation and are only briefly introduced in this chapter. Let's review each of these nutrients now and learn more about their functions in the body.

Table 8.1 Antioxidant Substances and Their Mechanisms of Action

Antioxidant	Mechanism of Action
Vitamin E	Protects lipids from free radical damage
Vitamin C	Scavenges free radicals, regenerates vitamin E after it has been oxidized
Beta-carotene	Scavenges free radicals, protects our LDLs from oxidation
Vitamin A	Under investigation as an antioxidant
Selenium	Part of the glutathione peroxidase antioxidant enzyme system

Vitamin E

As reviewed in Chapter 1, vitamin E is one of the fat-soluble vitamins, which means that dietary fats carry it from our intestines through the lymph system and eventually transport it to our cells. As you remember, our bodies store the fat-soluble vitamins. The liver serves as a storage site for vitamins A and D, and about 90% of the vitamin E in our bodies is stored in our adipose tissue. The remaining vitamin E is found in cell membranes.

Vitamin E is actually two separate compounds, **tocotrienol** and **tocopherol.** The tocotrienol compounds do not appear to play an active role in our bodies. The tocopherol compounds are the biologically active forms of vitamin E in our bodies. Four different tocopherol compounds have been discovered: alpha, beta, gamma, and delta. Of these, the most active, or potent, vitamin E compound found in food and supplements is *alpha-tocopherol*. The RDA for vitamin E is expressed as alpha-tocopherol in milligrams per day (α-tocopherol, mg per day). Food labels and vitamin and mineral supplements may express vitamin E in units of alpha-tocopherol equivalents (α-TE), milligrams, and as International Units (IU). For conversion purposes, 1 α-TE is equal to 1 mg of active vitamin E. In supplements, 1 IU is equal to 0.67 mg α-TE if the vitamin E in the supplement is from natural sources. If synthetic vitamin E is used in the supplement, 1 IU is equal to 0.45 mg α-TE.

tocotrienol A form of vitamin E that does not play an important biological role in our bodies.

tocopherol The active form of vitamin E in our bodies.

Functions of Vitamin E

The primary function of vitamin E is as an antioxidant. As described earlier in this chapter, this means that vitamin E donates an electron to free radicals, stabilizing them, and preventing them from destabilizing other molecules. Once vitamin E is oxidized, it is either excreted from the body or recycled back into active vitamin E through the help of other antioxidant nutrients, such as vitamin C.

Because vitamin E is prevalent in our adipose tissues and cell membranes, its action specifically protects *polyunsaturated fatty acids* (PUFAs) and other fatty components of our cells and cell membranes from being oxidized (see Figure 8.5b). Vitamin E also protects our low-density lipoproteins (LDLs) from being oxidized, which lowers our risk for heart disease. (The relationship between antioxidants and heart disease is reviewed later in this chapter.) In addition to protecting our PUFAs and LDLs, vitamin E protects the membranes of our red blood cells from oxidation and plays a critical role in protecting the cells of our lungs, which are constantly exposed to oxygen and the potentially damaging effects of oxidation.

Vitamin E serves many other roles essential to human health. Vitamin E is critical for normal fetal and early childhood development of nerves and muscles, as well as for maintenance of their functions. It enhances our immune function by protecting white blood cells and other components of our immune system, thereby helping to defend our bodies against illness and disease. Vitamin E also improves the absorption of vitamin A if the dietary intake of vitamin A is low. A full list of the functions, requirements, and toxicity and deficiency symptoms associated with vitamin E is provided in Table 8.2.

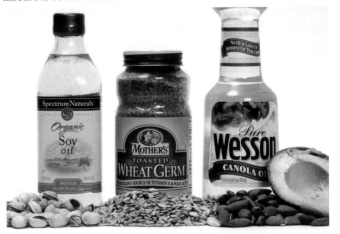

Vegetable oils, nuts, seeds, and avocados are good sources of vitamin E.

Table 8.2   Functions, Recommended Intakes, and Toxicity and Deficiency Symptoms of Antioxidant Substances

Antioxidant	Primary Functions	Recommended Intake	Toxicity Symptoms/ Side Effects	Deficiency Symptoms/ Side Effects
Vitamin E (fat-soluble)	Protects cell membranes from oxidation Protects polyunsaturated fatty acids (PUFAs) from oxidation Protects vitamin A from oxidation Protects white blood cells and enhances immune function Improves absorption of vitamin A	RDA: Men = 15 mg alpha-tocopherol Women = 15 mg alpha-tocopherol	Inhibition of blood clotting Increased risk of hemorrhagic stroke Intestinal discomfort	Red blood cell hemolysis Anemia Impairment of nerve transmission Muscle weakness and degeneration Leg cramps Difficulty walking Fibrocystic breast disease
Vitamin C (water-soluble)	Antioxidant in extracellular fluid and lungs Regenerates oxidized vitamin E Reduces formation of nitrosamines in stomach Assists with collagen synthesis Enhances immune function Assists in the synthesis of hormones, neurotransmitters, and DNA Enhances absorption of iron	RDA: Men = 90 mg Women = 75 mg Smokers = 35 mg more per day than RDA	Nausea and diarrhea Nosebleeds Abdominal cramps Increased oxidative damage Increased formation of kidney stones in those with kidney disease	Scurvy Bleeding gums and joints Loose teeth Weakness Hemorrhaging of hair follicles Poor wound healing Swollen ankles and wrists Diarrhea Bone pain and fractures Depression Anemia
Beta-carotene (fat-soluble provitamin for vitamin A)	Protects cell membranes and LDLs from oxidation Enhances immune system Protects skin from sun's ultraviolet rays Protects eyes from oxidative damage	None at this time	Carotenosis or carotenodermia (yellowing of skin)	Unknown
Vitamin A * (fat-soluble)	Necessary for our ability to adjust to changes in light Protects color vision Cell differentiation Necessary for sperm production in men and fertilization in women Contributes to healthy bone growth	RDA: Men = 900 µg Women = 700 µg	Spontaneous abortions and birth defects in fetus of pregnant women Loss of appetite Blurred vision Hair loss Abdominal pain, nausea, diarrhea Liver and nervous system damage	Night blindness Xerophthalmia which leads to permanent blindness Impaired immunity and increased risk of illness and infection Inability to reproduce Failure of normal growth
Selenium (trace mineral)	Part of glutathione peroxidase, an antioxidant enzyme Indirectly spares vitamin E from oxidation Assists in production of thyroid hormone Assists in maintaining immune function	RDA: Men = 55 µg Women = 55 µg	Brittle hair and nails Skin rashes Vomiting, nausea Weakness Cirrhosis of liver	Keshan disease: a specific form of heart disease Kashin-Beck disease: deforming arthritis Impaired immune function Increased risk of viral infections Infertility Depression, hostility Muscle pain and wasting

* Vitamin A is still under investigation as a potential antioxidant.

How Much Vitamin E Should We Consume?

Considering the importance of vitamin E to our health, you might think that you need to consume a huge amount daily. In fact, the RDA is modest and the food sources plentiful.

Recommended Dietary Allowance for Vitamin E   The RDA for vitamin E for men and women is 15 mg alpha-tocopherol per day. The tolerable upper intake level (UL) is 1,000 mg alpha-tocopherol per day. Remember that one of the primary roles of vitamin E is to protect PUFAs from oxidation. Thus, our need for vitamin E increases as we eat more oils and other foods that contain PUFAs. Fortunately these foods also contain vitamin E, so we typically consume enough vitamin E within them to protect their PUFAs from oxidation.

Shopper's Guide: Good Food Sources of Vitamin E   Vitamin E is very widespread in the foods we eat. Much of the vitamin E that we consume comes from vegetable oils and the products made from them (Figure 8.6). Safflower oil, sunflower oil, canola oil, and soybean oil are good sources of vitamin E. Mayonnaise and salad dressings made from these oils also contain vitamin E. Nuts, seeds, and some vegetables also contribute vitamin E to our diet. Although no single fruit or vegetable contains very high amounts of vitamin E, eating 5 to 9 servings of fruits and vegetables each day will help ensure adequate intake of this nutrient. Cereals are often fortified with vitamin E, and other grain products contribute modest amounts of vitamin E to our diet. Wheat germ and soybeans are also good sources of vitamin E. Animal and dairy products are poor sources of vitamin E.

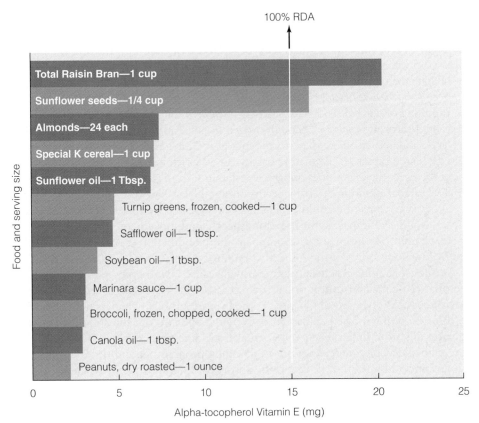

Figure 8.6   Common food sources of vitamin E. The RDA for vitamin E is 15 mg alpha-tocopherol per day for men and women. (Data from U.S. Department of Agriculture, Agricultural Research Service, 2002. USDA Nutrient Database for Standard Reference, Release 15. Nutrient Data Laboratory Home Page, www.nal.usda.gov/fnic/foodcomp Accessed August 2002.)

Vitamin E is destroyed by exposure to oxygen, metals, ultraviolet light, and heat. Although raw (uncooked) vegetable oils contain vitamin E, heating these oils destroys vitamin E. Thus, foods that are deep-fried and processed contain little vitamin E. This includes most fast foods and convenience foods.

What Happens If We Consume Too Much Vitamin E?

Vitamin E toxicity is uncommon, and there is little evidence to support significant health problems with vitamin E supplementation. Standard supplemental doses (1 to 18 times the RDA) are not associated with any adverse health effects. Interestingly, it appears that taking even much higher doses of vitamin E may be safe. Daily intakes of up to 800 mg alpha-tocopherol (or about 53 times the RDA) are known to be tolerable.

As with any nutrient, however, it is important to exercise caution when supplementing. Some individuals do report side effects such as nausea, intestinal distress, and diarrhea, with vitamin E supplementation. Certain medications interact negatively with vitamin E. The most important of these are the *anticoagulants*, substances that stop blood from clotting excessively. Aspirin is an anticoagulant, as is the prescription drug Coumadin. Vitamin E supplements can augment the action of these substances, causing uncontrollable bleeding. In addition, new evidence suggests that in some people, long-term use of standard vitamin E supplements may cause hemorrhaging in the brain, leading to a type of stroke called *hemorrhagic stroke*.

What Happens If We Don't Consume Enough Vitamin E?

True vitamin E deficiencies are uncommon in humans. This is primarily because vitamin E is fat-soluble, which allows us to store ample amounts in our fatty tissues. Thus, we typically have adequate amounts of vitamin E available even when our diet is low in this nutrient. However, it is common for people in the United States to consume suboptimal amounts of vitamin E in their diets. Results from the NHANES III survey show that the dietary intake of vitamin E of many Americans is low enough that 27 to 41% of these individuals have blood levels of vitamin E putting them at increased risk for cardiovascular disease (Ford and Sowell 1999).

Despite the rarity of vitamin E deficiencies, they do occur. One vitamin E deficiency symptom is *erythrocyte hemolysis*, or the rupturing (*lysis*) of red blood cells (*erythrocytes*). The rupturing of our red blood cells leads to *anemia*, a condition in which our red blood cells cannot carry and transport enough oxygen to our tissues, leading to fatigue, weakness, and a diminished ability to perform physical and mental work. We discuss anemia in more detail in Chapter 10. Premature babies can suffer from vitamin E–deficiency anemia; if born too early, the infant does not receive vitamin E from its mother, since the transfer of this vitamin from mother to baby occurs during the last few weeks of the pregnancy.

Other symptoms of vitamin E deficiency include loss of muscle coordination and reflexes, leading to impairments in vision, speech, and movement. As you might expect, vitamin E deficiency can also impair immune function especially if accompanied by low body stores of the mineral selenium.

In adults, vitamin E deficiencies are usually caused by diseases, particularly diseases that cause malabsorption of fat, such as those that affect the liver, gallbladder, and pancreas. As reviewed in Chapter 3, the liver makes bile, which is necessary for the absorption of fat. The gallbladder delivers the bile into our intestines, where it facilitates digestion of fat. The pancreas makes fat-digesting enzymes. Thus, when the liver, gallbladder, or pancreas are not functioning properly, fat and the fat-soluble vitamins, including vitamin E, cannot be absorbed, leading to their deficiency.

Recap: Vitamin E protects our cell membranes from oxidation, enhances immune function, and improves our absorption of vitamin A if dietary intake is low. The RDA for vitamin E is 15 mg alpha-tocopherol per day for men and women. Vitamin E is found primarily in vegetable oils and nuts. Toxicity is uncommon, but taking very high doses can cause excessive bleeding. Deficiency is rare, but symptoms include anemia and impaired vision, speech, and movement.

Vitamin C

Vitamin C is a water-soluble vitamin. We must therefore consume it on a regular basis, since any excess is excreted (primarily in our urine) rather than stored. There are two active forms of vitamin C: ascorbic acid and dehydroascorbic acid. Interestingly, most animals can make their own vitamin C from glucose. Humans and guinea pigs are two groups that cannot synthesize their own vitamin C and must consume it in the diet.

Functions of Vitamin C

Vitamin C is probably most well known for its role in preventing scurvy, a disease that ravaged sailors on long sea voyages centuries ago. It was characterized by bleeding tissues, especially of the gums, and over half of the deaths that occurred at sea were attributable to scurvy. During these long voyages the crew ate all of the fruits and vegetables early in the trip then had only grain and animal products available until they reached land to resupply. In 1740 in England, Dr. James Lind discovered that citrus fruits could prevent scurvy. This is due to their high vitamin C content. Fifty years after the discovery of the link between citrus fruits and prevention of scurvy, the British Navy finally required all ships to provide daily lemon juice rations for each sailor to prevent the onset of scurvy. A century later, sailors were given lime juice rations, earning them the nickname "limeys." It wasn't until 1930 that vitamin C was discovered and identified as a nutrient.

One important role of vitamin C is to assist in the synthesis of **collagen.** Collagen, a protein, is a critical component of all connective tissues in our bodies, including bone, teeth, skin, tendons, and blood vessels. Collagen assists in preventing bruises, and it ensures proper wound healing, as it is a part of scar tissue and a component of the tissue that mends broken bones. Without adequate vitamin C, our bodies cannot form collagen, and tissue hemorrhage, or bleeding, is a major symptom of vitamin C deficiency.

Vitamin C also acts as an antioxidant. Like vitamin E, it donates electrons to free radicals, thus preventing the damage of cells and tissues. Since it is water-soluble, vitamin C primarily acts as an antioxidant in the extracellular fluid. Vitamin C acts as an important antioxidant in the lungs, protecting us from the damage caused by ozone and cigarette smoke. Vitamin C also regenerates vitamin E after it has been oxidized by donating an electron. This enables vitamin E to continue to protect our cell membranes and other tissues. In the stomach, vitamin C reduces the formation of *nitrosamines,* cancer-causing agents found in foods such as cured and processed meats. We discuss the role of vitamin C and other antioxidants in preventing some forms of cancer later in this chapter (page 286).

Vitamin C also enhances our immune response, protecting us from illness and infection. But contrary to popular belief, it is not a miracle cure (see the accompanying Nutrition Myth or Fact box on vitamin C page 274). Vitamin C also assists in the synthesis of DNA, neurotransmitters such as serotonin (which helps regulate mood) and various hormones. Vitamin C helps ensure that appropriate levels of thyroxine, a hormone produced by the thyroid gland, are produced to support our basal metabolic rate and to maintain body temperature.

Vitamin C also enhances the absorption of iron. It is recommended that people with low iron stores consume vitamin C–rich foods along with iron sources to improve absorption. For people with high iron stores, this practice can be dangerous and lead to iron toxicity (discussed on page 274). Refer to Table 8.2 for a review of the functions, requirements, and toxicity and deficiency symptoms associated with vitamin C.

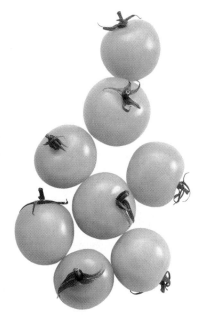

Many fruits, like these yellow tomatoes, are high in vitamin C.

collagen   A protein found in all connective tissues in our body.

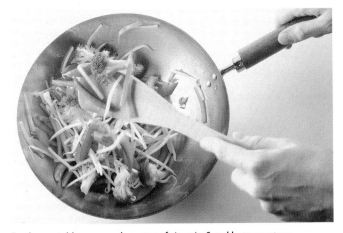

Fresh vegetables are good sources of vitamin C and beta-carotene.

Can Vitamin C Prevent the Common Cold?

What happens when you feel a cold coming on? If you are like many people, you will drink a lot of orange juice or take vitamin C supplements to ward off a cold. Do these tactics really help prevent a cold?

It is well known that vitamin C is important for a healthy immune system. A vitamin C deficiency can seriously weaken our immune cells' ability to detect and destroy invading microbes, increasing our susceptibility to many diseases and illnesses—including the common cold. Many people have taken vitamin C supplements to prevent the common cold, basing their behavior on its actions of enhancing our immune function. Interestingly, scientific studies do not support this action. A recent review of many of the studies of vitamin C and the common cold found that people taking vitamin C experienced as many colds as people who took a placebo (Hemila 1997). The amount of vitamin C taken in these studies was quite high, at least 1,000 mg per day (over 10 times the RDA). Thus, despite their popularity, vitamin C supplements do not appear to enhance our ability to fight the common cold. Consuming a healthful diet that includes excellent sources of vitamin C will assist us with maintaining a strong immune system, but vitamin C supplements do not appear to be effective in enhancing the immune system of an already well-nourished individual. So next time you feel yourself getting a cold, you may want to think twice before taking extra vitamin C. ●

How Much Vitamin C Should We Consume?

Although popular opinion suggests our needs for vitamin C are high, we really only require amounts that are easily obtained when we eat 5 to 9 servings of fruits and vegetables daily.

Recommended Dietary Allowance for Vitamin C The RDA for vitamin C is 90 mg per day for men and 75 mg per day for women. The tolerable upper intake level (UL) is 2,000 mg per day for adults. Smoking increases a person's need for vitamin C. Thus, the RDA for smokers is 35 mg more per day than for nonsmokers. This equals 125 mg per day for men and 110 mg per day for women.

Shopper's Guide: Good Food Sources of Vitamin C Fruits and vegetables are the best sources of vitamin C. Because heat and oxygen destroy vitamin C, fresh sources of these foods have the highest content of vitamin C. Cooking foods, especially boiling them, leaches their vitamin C, which is then lost when we strain them. Forms of cooking that are least likely to compromise the vitamin C content of foods includes steaming, microwaving, and stir-frying.

As indicated in Figure 8.7, many fruits and vegetables are high in vitamin C. Citrus fruits (such as oranges, lemons, and limes), potatoes, strawberries, tomatoes, kiwi fruit, broccoli, spinach and other leafy greens, cabbage, green and red peppers, and cauliflower are excellent sources of vitamin C. Fortified beverages and cereals are also sources of vitamin C. Dairy foods, meats, and nonfortified cereals and grains provide little or no vitamin C. By eating the recommended 5 to 9 servings of fruits and vegetables daily, we can easily meet our body's requirement for vitamin C. Remember that a serving of vegetables is ½ cup of cooked or 1 cup of raw vegetables or 6 ounces of vegetable juice, while a serving of fruit is one medium fruit, ½ cup of chopped or canned fruit or 6 ounces of fruit juice.

What Happens If We Consume Too Much Vitamin C?

Because vitamin C is water-soluble, we usually excrete any excess. Consuming excess amounts in food sources does not lead to toxicity, and only supplements can lead to toxic doses. Doses of a nutrient that are ten or more times greater than

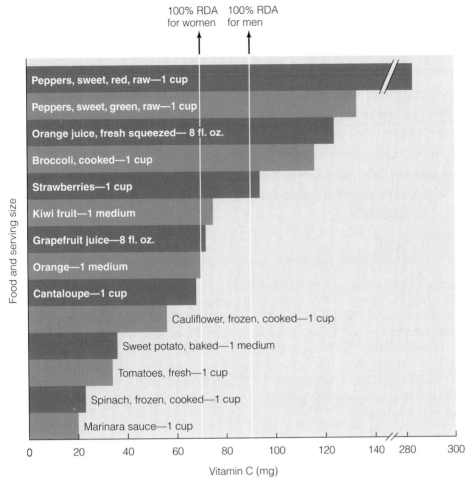

Figure 8.7   Common food sources of vitamin C. The RDA for vitamin C is 90 mg per day for men and 75 mg per day for women. (Data from U.S. Department of Agriculture, Agricultural Research Service, 2002. USDA Nutrient Database for Standard Reference, Release 15. Nutrient Data Laboratory Home Page, www.nal.usda.gov/fnic/foodcomp Accessed August 2002.)

the recommended amount are referred to as **megadoses.** Taking megadoses of vitamin C is not fatally harmful. However, side effects of doses exceeding 2,000 mg per day for a prolonged period include nausea, diarrhea, nosebleeds, and abdominal cramps.

There are rare instances in which consuming even moderately excessive doses of vitamin C can be harmful. As mentioned earlier, vitamin C enhances the absorption of iron. This action is beneficial to people who need to increase iron absorption. It can be harmful, however, to people with a disease called *hemochromatosis,* which causes an excess accumulation of iron in our bodies. Such iron toxicity can damage our tissues and lead to a heart attack. In people who have preexisting kidney disease, taking excess vitamin C can lead to the formation of kidney stones. This does not appear to occur in healthy individuals. Critics of vitamin C supplementation claim that taking the supplemental form of the vitamin is "unbalanced" nutrition and leads vitamin C to act as a prooxidant. A **prooxidant,** as you might guess, is a nutrient that promotes oxidation. It does this by pushing the balance of exchange reactions toward oxidation, which promotes the production of free radicals. Although the results of a few studies suggested that vitamin C acts as a prooxidant, these studies were found to be flawed or irrelevant for humans. At the present time, there appears to be no strong scientific evidence that vitamin C, either from food or dietary supplements, acts as a prooxidant in humans.

megadose   A dose of a nutrient that is ten or more times greater than the recommended amount.

prooxidant   A nutrient that promotes oxidation and oxidative cell and tissue damage.

Nadia   *Nutri-Case*

"When I went for my monthly check-up yesterday, my doctor told me I'm anemic and prescribed an iron supplement. She said that I need to take it because iron is very important to my growing baby. Then she recommended that I take the supplement with orange juice. After I got home, I remembered that my nutritionist had told me that I'm not supposed to have sweet things like juices, because of my diabetes. I feel like I don't know which way to turn. All of these recommendations are driving me crazy!"

Why did Nadia's doctor advise her to take her iron supplement with orange juice? Was the advice sound? Given what you learned about diabetes in Chapter 4, what action might you suggest that Nadia take?

What Happens If We Don't Consume Enough Vitamin C?

Vitamin C deficiencies are rare in developed countries but can occur in underdeveloped countries. Scurvy is the most common vitamin C deficiency disease. The symptoms of scurvy appear after about one month of a vitamin C–deficient diet. Symptoms include bleeding gums and joints, loose teeth, weakness, hemorrhages around the hair follicles of the arms and legs, wounds that fail to heal, swollen ankles and wrists, bone pain and fractures, diarrhea, and depression. Anemia can also result from vitamin C deficiency. People most at risk of deficiencies include those who eat few fruits and vegetables, including impoverished or home-bound individuals, and people who abuse alcohol and drugs.

Recap: Vitamin C scavenges free radicals and regenerates vitamin E after it has been oxidized. Vitamin C prevents scurvy and assists in the synthesis of collagen, hormones, neurotransmitters, and DNA. Vitamin C also enhances iron absorption. The RDA for vitamin C is 90 mg per day for men and 75 mg per day for women. Many fruits and vegetables are high in vitamin C. Toxicity is uncommon; symptoms include nausea, diarrhea, and nosebleeds. Deficiency symptoms include scurvy, anemia, diarrhea, and depression.

Beta-Carotene

provitamin An inactive form of a vitamin that the body can convert to an active form. An example is beta-carotene.

carotenoids Fat-soluble plant pigments that the body stores in the liver and adipose tissues. The body is able to convert certain carotenoids to vitamin A.

Although beta-carotene is not considered an essential nutrient, it is a *provitamin* found in many fruits and vegetables. **Provitamins** are inactive forms of vitamins that the body cannot use until they are converted to their active form. Our bodies convert beta-carotene to the active form of vitamin A, or *retinol;* thus, beta-carotene is a precursor of retinol.

Beta-carotene is classified as a **carotenoid,** one of a group of plant pigments that are the basis for the red, orange, and deep yellow colors of many fruits and vegetables. (Even dark green leafy vegetables contain plenty of carotenoids, but the green pigment, chlorophyll, masks their color!) Although there are over 600 carotenoids found in nature, only about 50 are found in the typical human diet. The six most common carotenoids found in human blood are alpha-carotene, beta-carotene, cryptoxanthin, lutein, lycopene, and zeaxanthin. Notice, however, that our bodies can convert only alpha-carotene, beta-carotene, and beta-cryptoxanthin to retinol. These are referred to as provitamin A carotenoids. We are just beginning to learn more about how carotenoids function in our body and how they may impact our health. Most of our discussion will focus on beta-carotene, as the majority of research on carotenoids to date have focused on this substance.

It takes two units of beta-carotene to make one unit of active vitamin A. Not surprisingly, nutritionists express the units of beta-carotene in a food as Retinol Equivalents, or RE. This measurement tells us how much active vitamin A is available to the body after it has converted the beta-carotene in the food.

Functions of Beta-Carotene

Beta-carotene and some other carotenoids are nutrients recognized to have antioxidant properties. Like vitamin E, they are fat-soluble and fight the harmful effects of oxidation in the lipid portions of our cell membranes and in our LDLs; but, compared with vitamin E, beta-carotene is a relatively weak antioxidant. In fact, other carotenoids, such as lycopene and lutein, may be stronger antioxidants than beta-carotene. Research is currently being conducted to elucidate how many carotenoids are found in foods and which ones are effective antioxidants.

Carotenoids play other important roles in our bodies. Specifically, they:

- Enhance our immune system and boost our ability to fight illness and disease.
- Protect our skin from the damage caused by the sun's ultraviolet rays.
- Protect our eyes from damage, preventing or delaying age-related vision impairment.

Carotenoids are also associated with a decreased risk of certain types of cancer. We discuss the roles of carotenoids and other antioxidants in cancer later in this chapter. Refer to Table 8.2 for a review of the functions, requirements, and toxicity and deficiency symptoms associated with beta-carotene.

How Much Beta-Carotene Should We Consume?

While there is evidence in the research laboratory that beta-carotene is an antioxidant, its importance to health is not known. Beta-carotene is not defined as a nutrient, so no formal DRI for beta-carotene has been determined.

Recommended Dietary Allowance for Beta-Carotene Nutritionists do not consider beta-carotene and other carotenoids to be essential nutrients, as they play no known essential roles in our body and are not associated with any deficiency symptoms. Thus, no RDA for these compounds has been established. It has been suggested that consuming 6 to 10 mg of beta-carotene per day from food sources can increase the beta-carotene levels in our blood to amounts that may reduce our risks for some diseases such as cancer and heart disease (Burri 1997). Supplements containing beta-carotene have become very popular, and supplementation studies have prescribed doses of 15 to 30 mg of beta-carotene. Refer to the accompanying Nutrition Myth or Fact box on beta-carotene, page 279, to learn more about how supplementation with this compound may affect your risk for cancer.

Shopper's Guide: Good Food Sources of Beta-Carotene Fruits and vegetables that are red, orange, yellow, and deep green are generally high in beta-carotene and other carotenoids such as lutein and lycopene. Tomatoes, carrots, cantaloupe, sweet potatoes, apricots, leafy greens such as kale and spinach, and pumpkin are good sources of beta-carotene. Eating 5 to 9 fruits and vegetables each day ensures an adequate intake of beta-carotene and other carotenoids. Also, because of its color, beta-carotene is used as a natural coloring agent for many foods including margarine, cereal, cake mixes, gelatins, and soft drinks. However, these foods are not significant sources of beta-carotene. Figure 8.8 identifies common foods that are high in beta-carotene.

We generally absorb only between 20 and 40% of the carotenoids present in the foods we eat. In contrast to vitamins E and C, heating foods high in carotenoids improves our ability to digest and absorb these compounds. Carotenoids are bound in the cells of plants, and the process of lightly cooking these plants breaks chemical bonds and can rupture cell walls, which humans don't digest. These actions result in more of the carotenoids being released from the plant. For instance, 100 grams of raw carrots contain approximately 7.3 mg of beta-carotene, while the same amount of cooked carrots contains approximately 8.0 mg (U.S. Department of Agriculture 1998).

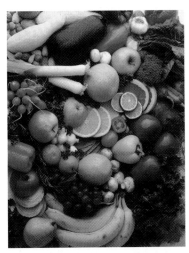

Foods that are high in carotenoids are easy to recognize by their bright colors.

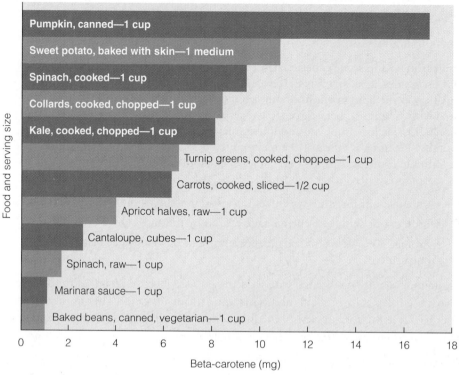

Figure 8.8   Common food sources of beta-carotene. There is no RDA for beta-carotene. (Data from U.S. Department of Agriculture, Agricultural Research Service. USDA – NCC Carotenoid Database for U.S. Foods, 1998. Nutrient Data Laboratory Home Page, www.nal.usda.gov/fnic/foodcomp Accessed August 2002.)

What Happens If We Consume Too Much Beta-Carotene?

Consuming large amounts of beta-carotene or other carotenoids in foods does not appear to cause toxic symptoms. However, your skin can turn yellow or orange if you consume large amounts of foods that are high in beta-carotene. This condition is referred to as *carotenosis* or *carotenoderma*, and it appears to be both reversible and harmless. Taking beta-carotene supplements is not generally recommended, as we can get adequate amounts of this nutrient by eating more fruits and vegetables.

What Happens If We Don't Consume Enough Beta-Carotene?

There are no known deficiency symptoms of beta-carotene or other carotenoids apart from beta-carotene's function as a precursor for vitamin A. Although studies have shown that eating foods high in carotenoids is associated with reduced risks of diseases such as heart disease and cancer, taking carotenoid supplements is not linked with any health benefits, and in some cases may be harmful, as illustrated in the Nutrition Myth or Fact box concerning beta-carotene supplements and cancer rates.

Recap: Beta-carotene is a carotenoid and a provitamin of vitamin A. It protects the lipid portions of our cell membranes and LDL-cholesterol from oxidative damage. It also enhances our immune function and protects our vision. There is no RDA for beta-carotene. Orange, red, and deep green fruits and vegetables are good sources of beta-carotene. There are no known toxicity or deficiency symptoms, but yellowing of the skin can occur if too much beta-carotene is consumed.

Beta-Carotene Supplements Can Cause Cancer

Beta-carotene is one of many carotenoids known to have antioxidant properties. Because there is substantial evidence that people eating foods high in antioxidants have lower rates of cancer, large-scale studies are being conducted to determine if taking antioxidant supplements can decrease our risk for cancer. One such study is the Alpha-Tocopherol Beta-Carotene (ATBC) Cancer Prevention Study (Albanes et al. 1995).

The ATBC Cancer Prevention Study was conducted in Finland from 1985 to 1993. The primary purpose of this study was to determine the effects of beta-carotene and vitamin E supplements on the rates of lung cancer and other forms of cancer. The study focused on the benefit of these antioxidants on a group of male smokers, who are considered to be at high risk for lung and other cancers. Almost 30,000 men between the ages of 50 and 69 years participated in the study. The participants were given daily either a beta-carotene supplement, a vitamin E supplement, a supplement containing both beta-carotene and vitamin E, or a placebo.

The average length of time people participated in this study was six years. Contrary to what was expected, the male smokers who took beta-carotene supplements experienced an *increased* number of deaths during the study. More men in this group died of lung cancer, heart disease, and stroke. There was also a trend in this group for higher rates of prostate and stomach cancers. This negative effect appeared to be particularly strong in men who had a higher alcohol intake.

The reasons why beta-carotene increased lung cancer risk in this population are not clear. It is possible that the supplementation period was too brief to benefit these high-risk individuals, although studies of shorter duration have found beneficial effects. There may be other components in foods besides beta-carotene that are protective against cancer, making supplementation with an isolated nutrient ineffective. In any case, the results of this study suggest that for certain people, supplementation with beta-carotene may be harmful. There is still much to learn about how people of differing risk levels respond to antioxidant supplementation. ●

Vitamin A

Vitamin A is a fat-soluble vitamin. We store about 90% of the vitamin A we absorb in our liver, with the remainder stored in our adipose tissue, kidneys, and lungs. Because fat-soluble vitamins cannot dissolve in our blood, they require proteins that can bind with and transport them through the bloodstream to target tissues and cells. *Retinol-binding protein* is one such carrier protein for vitamin A. Retinol-binding protein carries retinol from the liver to the cells that require it.

There are three active forms of vitamin A in our bodies: **retinol** is the alcohol form; **retinal** is the aldehyde form; and **retinoic acid** is the acid form. These three forms are collectively referred to as the *retinoids* (Figure 8.9). Of the three, retinol has the starring role in maintaining our bodies' physiologic functions. Remember from the previous section that beta-carotene is a precursor to vitamin A. When we eat foods with beta-carotene, it is converted to retinol in the wall of our small intestine.

The unit of expression for vitamin A is retinol activity equivalents (RAE). You may still see the expression Retinol Equivalents (RE) or International Units (IU) for vitamin A on food labels or dietary supplements. The conversions to RAE from various forms of retinol and from the units IU and RE are as follows:

- 1 RAE = 1 microgram (μg) retinol
- 1 RAE = 12 μg beta-carotene
- 1 RAE = 24 μg alpha-carotene or beta-cryptoxanthin
- 1 RAE = 1 RE
- 1 RAE = 3.3 IU

retinol An active, alchohol form of vitamin A that plays an important role in healthy vision and immune function.

retinal An active, aldehyde form of vitamin A that plays an important role in healthy vision and immune function.

retinoic acid An active, acid form of vitamin A that plays an important role in cell growth and immune function.

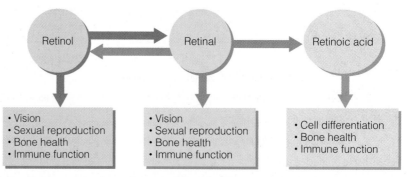

Figure 8.9   The three active forms of vitamin A in our bodies are retinol, retinal, and retinoic acid. Retinol and retinal can be converted interchangeably; retinoic acid is formed from retinal, and this process is irreversible. Each form of vitamin A contributes to many of our bodily processes.

Functions of Vitamin A

The known functions of vitamin A are numerous, and researchers speculate that many are still to be discovered.

Vitamin A Acts As an Antioxidant   Limited research indicates that vitamin A may act as an antioxidant (Livrea et al. 1995; Gutteridge and Halliwell 1994). Like vitamins E and C, it appears to scavenge free redicals and protect our LDLs from oxidation. As you might expect, adequate vitamin A levels in the blood are associated with lower risks of some forms of cancer and heart disease. However, the role of vitamin A as an antioxidant is not strongly established and is still under investigation.

Vitamin A Is Essential to Sight   Vitamin A's most critical role in our bodies is certainly in the maintenance of healthy vision. Specifically, vitamin A affects our sight in two ways: it enables us to react to changes in the brightness of light, and it enables us to distinguish between different wavelengths of light—in other words, to see different colors. Let's take a closer look at this process.

Light enters our eyes through the cornea, travels through the lens, and then hits the **retina,** which is a delicate membrane lining the back of the inner eyeball (see Figure 8.10). You might already have guessed how *retinal* got its name: it is found

retina   The delicate light-sensitive membrane lining the inner eyeball and connected to the optic nerve. It contains retinal.

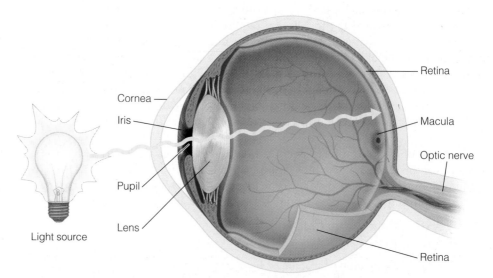

Figure 8.10   Vitamin A is necessary to maintain healthy vision. Light enters the eye through the cornea, travels through the lens, and hits the retina located in the back of the eye. The light reacts with the retinal stored in the retina, which allows us to see black and white images.

in—and integral to—the retina. When light hits the retina, retinal is used to effect a chemical transformation in the light-sensitive *rod cells*, causing the transmission of a signal to the brain which is interpreted as a black and white image. This process goes on continually, allowing our eyes to adjust moment-to-moment to subtle changes in our surroundings or in the level of light. At the same time, the *cone cells* of the retina, which are only effective in bright light, use retinal to interpret different wavelengths of light as different colors.

In summary, our abilities to adjust to dim light, recover from a bright flash of light, and see in color are all critically dependent on adequate levels of retinal in our eyes.

Vitamin A Contributes to Cell Differentiation   Another important role of vitamin A is its contribution to **cell differentiation,** the process by which cells mature into highly specialized cells that perform unique functions. Obviously, this process is critical to the development of healthy organs and effectively functioning body systems. As an example of cell differentiation, let's look at the development of the mucus-producing cells in our epithelial tissues. Epithelial tissues include our skin and the protective linings of the lungs, vagina, intestines, stomach, bladder, urinary tract, and eyes. The mucus that epithelial tissues produce lubricates the tissue and helps us to propel microbes, dust particles, foods, or fluids out of our body tissues (e.g., when we cough up secretions or empty our bladder). When vitamin A levels are insufficient, the epithelial cells fail to differentiate appropriately, and we lose these protective barriers against infection and irritants. Vitamin A is also critical to the differentiation of specialized immune cells called *T-lymphocytes,* or *T-cells,* which help us fight infections. You can now see why vitamin A deficiency can lead to a breakdown of our immune responses and to infections and other disorders of the lungs and respiratory tract, urinary tract, vagina, and eyes.

cell differentiation The process by which immature, undifferentiated stem cells develop into highly specialized functional cells of discrete organs and tissues.

Other Functions of Vitamin A   Vitamin A is involved in reproduction. Although its exact role is unclear, it appears necessary for sperm production in men and for fertilization to occur in women.

Vitamin A contributes to healthy bone growth. It assists in breaking down old bone so that new, longer, and stronger bone can develop. As a result of a vitamin A deficiency, children suffer from stunted growth and wasting.

Two popular treatments for acne contain derivatives of vitamin A. Retin-A, or tretinoin, is a treatment applied to the skin. Accutane is taken orally. These medications should be used carefully and only under the supervision of a licensed physician. Although they are relatively less toxic forms of vitamin A, they can cause birth defects in infants if used while a woman is pregnant and can lead to other toxicity problems in some individuals. It is recommended that these medications be stopped at least two years prior to conceiving. Interestingly, vitamin A itself has no effect on acne; thus, vitamin A supplements are not recommended in its treatment. See Table 8.2 for the functions, requirements, toxicity and deficiency symptoms associated with vitamin A.

How Much Vitamin A Should We Consume?

Vitamin A toxicity can occur readily because it is a fat-soluble vitamin, so it is important to consume only the amount recommended, as this amount is known to be safe.

Recommended Dietary Intake for Vitamin A   The RDA for vitamin A is 900 µg per day for men and 700 µg per day for women. The UL is 3000 µg per day of preformed vitamin A in women (including those pregnant and lactating) and men.

Shopper's Guide: Good Food Sources of Vitamin A   We consume vitamin A from both animal and plant sources. About half of the vitamin A in our diets is the preformed vitamin A found in animal foods such as beef liver, chicken liver, eggs, and whole-fat dairy products. Vitamin A is also found in fortified reduced-fat milks, margarine, and some breakfast cereals (Figure 8.11).

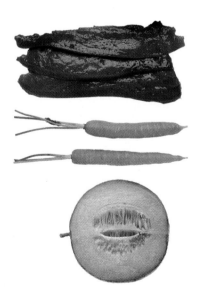

Liver, carrots, and cantaloupe all contain vitamin A.

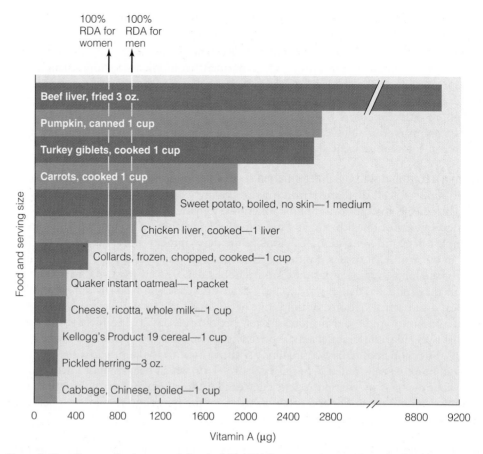

Figure 8.11 Common food sources of vitamin A. The RDA for vitamin A is 900 µg per day for men and 700 µg per day for women. (Data from U.S. Department of Agriculture, Agricultural Research Service, 2002. USDA Nutrient Database for Standard Reference, Release 15. Nutrient Data Laboratory Home Page, www.nal.usda.gov/fnic/foodcomp Accessed August 2002.)

The other half of the vitamin A we consume comes from foods high in beta-carotene and other carotenoids that can be converted to vitamin A. As discussed earlier in this chapter, dark green, orange, and deep yellow fruits and vegetables are good sources of beta-carotene, and thus of vitamin A. Carrots, spinach, mango, cantaloupe, and tomato juice are excellent sources of vitamin A because they contain beta-carotene.

What Happens If We Consume Too Much Vitamin A?

Vitamin A is highly toxic, and toxicity symptoms develop after consuming only three to four times the RDA. Toxicity rarely results from food sources, but vitamin A supplements are known to have caused severe illness and even death. Consuming excess vitamin A while pregnant can cause serious birth defects and spontaneous abortions. Other toxicity symptoms include loss of appetite, blurred vision, hair loss, abdominal pain, nausea, diarrhea, and damage to the liver and nervous system. If caught in time, many of these symptoms are reversible once vitamin A supplementation is stopped. However, permanent damage can occur to the liver, eyes, and other organs. Because liver contains such a high amount of vitamin A, children and pregnant women should not consume liver on a daily or weekly basis.

What Happens If We Don't Consume Enough Vitamin A?

Night blindness is the condition that results from vitamin A deficiency. It results in the inability to adjust to dim light and can also result in the failure to regain sight quickly after a bright flash of light. As we discussed earlier, since the cone

night blindness A vitamin A–deficiency disorder that results in loss of the ability to see in dim light.

Global Nutrition: Combating Vitamin A Deficiency Around the World

Vitamin A deficiency and its resultant illness, night blindness, is a major health concern in lower income nations. Approximately 118 nations are affected, particularly African and Southeast Asian countries. According to the World Health Organization (WHO 2002), between 100 and 140 million children suffer from vitamin A deficiency. Of the children affected, 250,000 to 500,000 become permanently blinded every year. At least half of these children will die within one year of losing their sight. Death is due to infections and illnesses, including measles and diarrhea, that are easily treated in wealthier countries.

Vitamin A deficiency is also a tragedy for pregnant women in these countries. These women suffer from night blindness, are more likely to transmit HIV to their child if HIV-positive, and run a greater risk of maternal mortality.

What is being done to combat this tragedy? WHO has partnered with the United Nations International Children's Emergency Fund (UNICEF), the Canadian International Development Agency, the U.S. Agency for International Development, and the Micronutrient Initiative to bring the Vitamin A Global Initiative into high-risk countries. This initiative provides support to deliver vitamin A supplements through immunization programs. Providing high-dose vitamin A sup-

plements has reduced overall mortality by 23%, and it has reduced mortality from measles by 50%. While this is an important short-term solution, longer-term interventions include:

- Encouraging breastfeeding, since breast milk is a critical source of vitamin A for infants.

- Fortification with vitamin A of food sources that are readily available to high-risk groups.

- Assisting in the development and maintenance of home and community gardens that provide a diverse supply of vitamin A–rich fruits and vegetables.

Significant progress has been made in the fight against vitamin A deficiency and night blindness. Despite this progress, there are still too many people suffering from this preventable disorder. A recent study of children in Bangladesh found that although the rates of night blindness in preschool children is decreasing, a significant number of children and pregnant women still show low serum retinol levels (Ahmed 1999). Children in Ethiopia also show alarmingly high rates of night blindness and low serum retinol levels (Haider and Demissie 1999). These findings illustrate that many people are still at risk for vitamin A deficiency and that the supplementation programs already employed must be strengthened with the intervention strategies listed above. ●

cells of the retina process colors, color blindness can also result from a vitamin A deficiency.

How severe a problem is night blindness? Although less common among people of developed nations, vitamin A deficiency is a severe public health concern in low-income nations. Refer to the accompanying Highlight: Global Nutrition for a more complete discussion of this health issue.

If vitamin A deficiency progresses, it can result in irreversible blindness due to hardening of the cornea (the transparent membrane covering the front of the eye), a condition called *xerophthalmia*. The prefix of this word, *xero-*, comes from a Greek word meaning "dry." Lack of vitamin A causes the epithelial cells of the cornea to lose their ability to produce mucus, causing the eye to become very dry. This leaves the cornea susceptible to damage, infection, and hardening. Once the cornea hardens in this way, the resulting blindness is irreversible. This is why it is critical to catch vitamin A deficiency in its early stages and treat it with either the regular consumption of fruits and vegetables that contain beta-carotene or with vitamin A supplementation.

Other deficiency symptoms include impaired immunity, increased risk of illness and infections, reproductive system disorders, and failure of normal growth. Individuals who are at risk for vitamin A deficiency include elderly people with poor diets, young children with inadequate vegetable and fruit intakes, and alcoholics. Any condition that results in fat malabsorption can also lead to vitamin A deficiency. Children with cystic fibrosis, individuals with diseases of the liver, pancreas, or gallbladder, and people who consume large amounts of the fat substitute Olestra are at risk for vitamin A deficiency.

> **Recap:** The role of vitamin A as an antioxidant is still under investigation. Vitamin A is critical for maintaining our vision. It is also necessary for cell differentiation, reproduction, and growth. The RDA for vitamin A is 900 µg per day for men and 700 µg per day for women. Animal livers, dairy products, and eggs are good animal sources of vitamin A; fruits and vegetables are high in beta-carotene, which is used to synthesize vitamin A. Supplementation can be dangerous, as toxicity is reached at levels of only three to four times the RDA. Toxicity symptoms include birth defects, spontaneous abortions, blurred vision, and liver damage. Deficiency symptoms include night blindness, impaired immune function, and growth failure.

Selenium

Selenium is a trace mineral, and it is found in varying amounts in soil. As reviewed in Chapter 1, trace minerals are needed by our bodies in amounts less than 100 mg per day. Keep in mind that, although we need only minute amounts of trace minerals, they are just as important to our health as the vitamins and the major minerals.

Functions of Selenium

Keshan disease A heart disorder caused by selenium deficiency. It was first identified in children in the Keshan province of China.

It is only recently that we have learned about the critical role of selenium as a nutrient in human health. In 1979, Chinese scientists reported an association between a heart disorder called **Keshan disease** and selenium deficiency. This disease occurs in children in the Keshan province of China, where the soil is depleted of selenium. The scientists found that Keshan disease can be prevented with selenium supplementation.

The selenium in our bodies is contained in proteins, or more specifically, amino acids. Two amino acid derivatives contain the majority of selenium in our bodies: *selenomethionine* is the storage form for selenium, while *selenocysteine* is the active form of selenium.

Selenium is a critical component of the antioxidant system, functioning as part of the glutathione peroxidase enzyme system mentioned earlier (page 268). Thus, selenium helps spare vitamin E and prevents oxidative damage to our cell membranes.

Selenium is also needed for the production of *thyroxine*, or thyroid hormone. By this action, selenium is involved in the maintenance of our basal metabolism and body temperature. Selenium appears to play a role in immune function, and poor selenium status is associated with higher rates of some forms of cancer. The functions, requirements, and toxicity and deficiency symptoms associated with selenium are listed in Table 8.2.

How Much Selenium Should We Consume?

Selenium content is highly variable in our foods. As it is a trace mineral, we need only minute amounts to maintain health.

Recommended Dietary Allowance for Selenium   The RDA for selenium is 55 µg per day for both men and women. The UL is 400 µg per day.

Shopper's Guide: Good Food Sources of Selenium   Selenium is present in both plant and animal food sources but in variable amounts. Because it is stored in the tissues of animals, selenium is found in reliably consistent amounts in animal foods. Organ meats, such as liver, kidney, pork, and seafood, are particularly good sources of selenium (see Figure 8.12).

In contrast, the amount of selenium in plants is dependent upon the selenium content of the soil in which the plant is grown. Thus, the amount of selenium in the

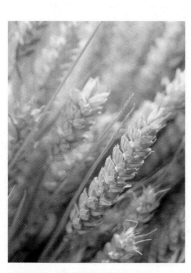

Wheat is a rich source of selenium.

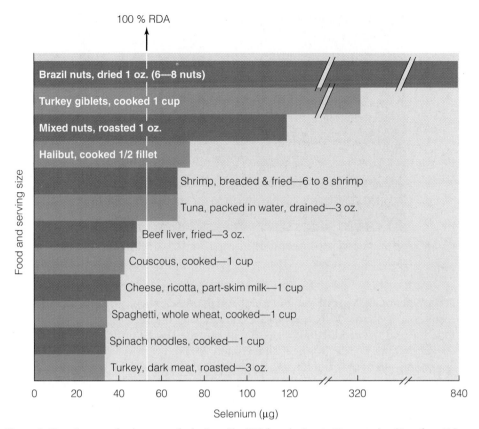

Figure 8.12   Common food sources of selenium. The RDA for selenium is 55 µg per day. (Data from U.S. Department of Agriculture, Agricultural Research Service, 2002. USDA Nutrient Database for Standard Reference, Release 15. Nutrient Data Laboratory Home Page, www.nal.usda.gov/fnic/foodcomp. Accessed August 2002.)

fruits and vegetables you eat can vary widely depending on what part of the world or region of the United States in which the plant is grown. Many companies marketing selenium supplements warn that the agricultural soils in the United States are depleted of selenium and inform us that we need to take selenium supplements. In reality, the selenium content of soil varies greatly across North America, and because we obtain our food from a variety of geographic locations, few people in the United States suffer from selenium deficiency. This is especially true for people who eat even small quantities of meat or seafood. As indicated in Figure 8.12, nuts, wheat, and rice are particularly rich sources of selenium.

What Happens If We Consume Too Much Selenium?

Selenium toxicity does not result from eating foods high in selenium. However, supplementation with selenium can cause toxicity. Toxicity symptoms include brittle hair and nails that can eventually break and fall off. Other symptoms of toxicity include skin rashes, vomiting, nausea, weakness, and cirrhosis of the liver.

What Happens If We Don't Consume Enough Selenium?

As discussed previously, selenium deficiency is associated with a special form of heart disease called Keshan disease. Selenium deficiency does not cause the disease, but selenium is necessary to help the immune system effectively fight the virus that causes the disease. Another deficiency disease is *Kashin-Beck disease,* a deforming arthritis also found in selenium-depleted areas in China and in Tibet. Other deficiency symptoms include impaired immune responses, increased risk of viral infections, infertility, depression, hostility, impaired cognitive function, and muscle pain and wasting.

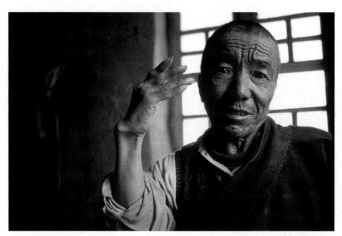

Selenium deficiency can lead to deforming arthritis called Kashin-Beck disease.

Recap: Selenium is part of the glutathione peroxidase enzyme system. It indirectly spares vitamin E from oxidative damage, and it assists with immune function and the production of thyroid hormone. The RDA for selenium is 55 micrograms per day for men and women. Organ meats, pork, and seafood are good sources of selenium, as are nuts, wheat, and rice. The selenium content of plants is dependent upon the amount of selenium in the soil in which they are grown. Toxicity symptoms include brittle hair and nails, vomiting, nausea, and liver cirrhosis. Deficiency symptoms and side effects include Keshan disease, Kashin-Beck disease, impaired immune function, infertility, and muscle wasting.

Copper, Iron, Zinc, and Manganese Play a Peripheral Role in Antioxidant Function

As discussed earlier, there are numerous antioxidant enzyme systems in our bodies. Copper, zinc, and manganese are a part of the superoxide dismutase enzyme complex. Iron is part of the structure of catalase. In addition to their role in protecting us from oxidative damage, copper, iron, manganese, and zinc play major roles in the optimal functioning of many other enzymes in our bodies. Copper, iron, and zinc help us maintain the health of our blood, and manganese is an important cofactor in carbohydrate metabolism. The functions, requirements, food sources, and deficiency and toxicity symptoms of these nutrients are discussed in detail in Chapter 10, which focuses on the nutrients involved in energy metabolism and blood formation.

Recap: Copper, zinc, and manganese are cofactors for the superoxide dismutase antioxidant enzyme system. Iron is a cofactor for the catalase antioxidant enzyme. These minerals play critical roles in blood health and energy metabolism.

What Disorders Are Related to Oxidation?

Through your experiences you may have found that there are a plethora of claims related to the functions of antioxidants. These claims include the slowing of aging and age-related diseases and the prevention of cancer and heart disease. In opposition to these claims, there is some evidence that taking antioxidant supplements may be harmful for certain people (refer back to the Nutrition Myth or Fact box on beta-carotene, page 279).

In this section, we will review what is currently known about the role of antioxidant nutrients in cancer, heart disease, and aging.

Cancer

Before we explore how antioxidants affect our risk for cancer, let's take a closer look at precisely what cancer is and how it spreads. **Cancer** is actually a group of diseases that are all characterized by cells that grow "out of control." By this we mean that cancer cells reproduce spontaneously and independently, and they are not inhibited by the boundaries of tissues and organs. Thus, they can aggressively invade tissues and organs far away from those in which they originally formed.

Most forms of cancer result in one or more **tumors,** which are newly formed masses of undifferentiated cells that are immature and have no physiologic function. Although the word "tumor" sounds frightening, it is important to note that not every tumor is *malignant,* or cancerous. Many are *benign* (not harmful to us) and are made up of cells that will not spread widely.

Figure 8.13 shows how changes to normal cells prompt a series of other changes that can progress into cancer. There are three primary steps of cancer development: initiation, promotion, and progression. These steps occur as follows:

1. **Initiation**—The initiation of cancer occurs when a cell's DNA is *mutated* (or changed). This mutation causes permanent changes in the cell.

2. **Promotion**—During this phase the genetically altered cell is stimulated to repeatedly divide. The mutated DNA is locked into each new cell's genetic instructions. Since the enzymes that normally work to repair damaged cells cannot detect alterations in the DNA, the cells can continue to divide uninhibited.

3. **Progression**—During this phase, the cancerous cells grow out of control and invade surrounding tissues. These cells then *metastasize* (spread) to other sites of the body. In the early stages of progression, our immune system can sometimes detect these cancerous cells and destroy them. However, if the cells continue to grow, they develop into malignant tumors, and cancer results.

Genetic, Lifestyle, and Environmental Factors Can Increase Our Risk for Cancer

Cancer is the second leading cause of death in the United States, and researchers estimate that about half of all men and one-third of all women will develop cancer during their lifetime. But what factors cause cancer? Are you and your loved ones at risk? The answer depends on several factors, including your family history of cancer, your exposure to environmental agents, and various lifestyle choices.

The American Cancer Society identifies five primary factors that have been shown to have the greatest impact on an individual's cancer risk (American Cancer Society 2002):

- **Tobacco use**—It is an established and well-known fact that smoking cigars and cigarettes and using smokeless tobacco significantly increase your risk for cancer. Over 4,000 compounds have been identified in tobacco and tobacco smoke, and over 40 of these compounds are **carcinogens,** or substances that can cause cancer. Using tobacco increases your risk for cancers of the lung, larynx, mouth, and esophagus, and can also cause heart disease, stroke, and emphysema. (See the Highlight box on disorders linked to tobacco use, page 289.) Smoking significantly increases the risk for lung and other forms of cancer (Figure 8.14), and almost 90% of all lung cancer deaths are due to smoking. The positive news is that tobacco use is a modifiable risk factor. If you smoke or use smokeless tobacco, you can reduce your risk for cancer considerably by quitting.

cancer A group of diseases characterized by cells that reproduce spontaneously and independently and may invade other tissues and organs.

tumor Any newly formed mass of undifferentiated cells.

carcinogen Any substance capable of causing the cellular mutations that lead to cancer.

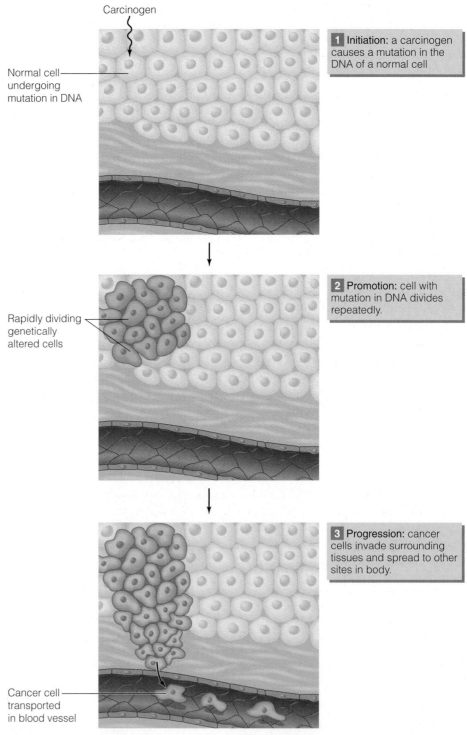

Carcinogen

1 **Initiation:** a carcinogen causes a mutation in the DNA of a normal cell

Normal cell undergoing mutation in DNA

2 **Promotion:** cell with mutation in DNA divides repeatedly.

Rapidly dividing genetically altered cells

3 **Progression:** cancer cells invade surrounding tissues and spread to other sites in body.

Cancer cell transported in blood vessel

Figure 8.13 Cancer cells develop as a result of a genetic mutation in the DNA of a normal cell. The mutated cell replicates uncontrollably, eventually resulting in a tumor. If not destroyed or removed, the cancerous tumor metastasizes and spreads to other parts of the body.

- **Sun exposure**—Skin cancer is the most common form of cancer in the United States and accounts for over half of all cancers diagnosed each year. Most cases of skin cancer are linked to sun exposure. The ultraviolet (UV) rays of the sun can damage the DNA of your skin cells and increase your risk for skin cancer. Your risk for skin cancer increases even if you do not get sunburned. Skin can-

Disorders Linked to Tobacco Use

 Many people smoke cigarettes or cigars, or use smokeless tobacco. The use of these products can lead to serious health consequences. Tobacco use is a risk factor in development of all of the following health problems and diseases:

1. Cancers:

   - Lung
   - Larynx
   - Mouth
   - Pharynx
   - Esophagus
   - Bladder
   - Pancreas
   - Uterus
   - Kidney
   - Stomach
   - Some leukemias

2. Heart disease
3. Bronchitis
4. Emphysema
5. Stroke
6. Erectile dysfunction
7. Conditions related to maternal smoking:

   - Miscarriage
   - Preterm delivery
   - Stillbirth
   - Infant death
   - Low birth weight

Figure 8.14 illustrates how significantly cigarette smoking increases our risks for early mortality due to various forms of cancer. ●

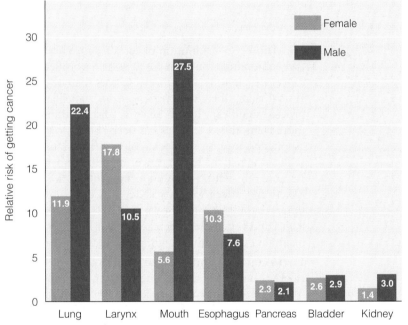

Figure 8.14   Cigarette smoking significantly increases our risk for lung and other types of cancer. The risk of lung cancer is 22.4 times higher in men who smoke and 12 times higher in women who smoke. The risk of mouth cancer is 28 times and 6 times higher for male and female smokers, respectively. (Data from P.A. Newcomb and P.P. Carbone. The health consequences of smoking: cancer. In *Cigarette Smoking: A Clinical Guide to Assessment and Treatment,* edited by M.C. Fiore. Philadelphia: W.B. Saunders, 1992, *Medical Clinics of North America,* pp. 305–331.)

cer includes the nonmelanoma cancers (basal cell and squamous cell cancers) and melanoma, the latter of which is the most deadly. Skin cancer can be cured if caught early. Wearing sunscreen with at least a 15 SPF (sun protection factor) rating and protective clothing and avoiding the sun between 10 A.M. and 4 P.M. can help reduce your risk for skin cancer.

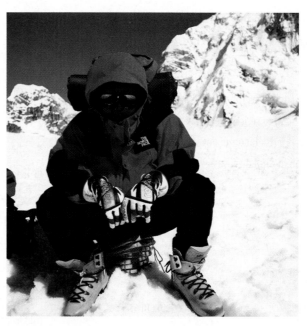

Artic explorers wear special clothing to protect themselves from the cold as well as the high levels of ultraviolet rays from the sun.

- **Nutrition**—Consumption of certain substances, including alcohol, dietary fat, and compounds found in cured and charbroiled meats, can increase our risk for cancer (Table 8.3). Nutritional factors that are protective against cancer include antioxidants, fiber, and *phytochemicals*, which are chemicals in plants that may provide significant health benefits (discussed in detail on page 293). Eating more fruits and vegetables has been shown to reduce the risk for cancers of the esophagus, mouth, stomach, colon, rectum, lung, and prostate, and it may also reduce the risk for breast cancer in premenopausal women (Zhang et al. 1999). Because our diet plays an important role in the prevention of many cancers, the American Cancer Society has developed recommendations for cancer prevention (see the Highlight box, page 292). Increasing your intake of whole grains, fruits, and vegetables, decreasing your intake of red meats and fatty meats, and maintaining a healthy weight are keys to cancer prevention.

- **Environmental and occupational exposures**—These include such things as cigarette and cigar smoke, chemicals in our food and water supply, sun exposure, infectious diseases, radiation, and chemicals found in the workplace. Proven carcinogens found in various worksites include benzene, asbestos, vinyl chloride, arsenic, coal tars, radon, wood dust, and aflatoxins (produced by molds in agricultural products such as peanuts). Only two forms of radiation have been linked to cancer: ionizing radiation and ultraviolet radiation. Ionizing radiation sources include x-rays, gamma rays, cosmic rays, radon, and particles given off by radioactive materials. Our primary source of ultraviolet rays is from the sun.

- **Level of physical activity**—Studies conducted over the past ten years have shown a possible link between lower cancer risk and higher levels of physical activity. A recent review of these studies has found that higher levels of leisure and occupational physical activity are associated with a 20 to 30% reduction in our overall risk for cancer (Thune and Furberg 2001). A clear protective effect of exercise was found specifically for breast and colon cancers. The intensity of physical activity appears important, as the reduction in risk was found only for moderate or vigorous intensity activity. At this time, we do not know how exercise reduces the overall risk for cancer or for certain types of cancers. Suggested

Table 8.3   Nutritional Factors That Can Influence Our Risk for Cancer

Factors That May Increase Cancer Risk	Factors That May Be Protective Against Cancer*	Factors Falsely Claimed to Cause Cancer
Heterocyclic amines in cooked meat: carcinogenic chemicals formed when meat is cooked at high temperatures, such as during broiling, barbecuing, and frying.	Antioxidants: includes vitamins E, C, A, beta-carotene, and other carotenoids, and minerals such as selenium. Supplementation with individual antioxidants does not show consistant benefits.	Artificial sweeteners: there are claims that aspartame (brand name Nutrasweet) is carcinogenic. There is no evidence to support the claim that aspartame causes brain or any other form of cancer; these unsubstantiated claims continue to resurface on the Internet.
Nitrates in drinking water: a carcinogenic chemical found in fertilizers that is proven to increase the risk of non-Hodgkin's lymphoma. People drinking contaminated tap water in agricultural areas may be at risk.	Dietary fiber: some studies show reduced risks for breast, colon, and rectal cancer with increased fiber intake, although findings are not consistent.	Coffee: there are no studies to support that drinking coffee increases the risk for cancer. Some of the chemicals used to make decaffeinated coffee are now known to be carcinogenic; most companies now use safer chemicals for this process.
Nitrites and nitrates: compounds found in cured meats such as sausage, ham, bacon, and some lunch meats. These compounds bind with amino acids to form nitrosamines, which are potent carcinogens.	Phytoestrogens: compounds found in soy-based foods and some vegetables and grains that may decrease the risk for breast, endometrial, and prostate cancers.	Fluoridated water: studies conducted over the past 40 years show no association between drinking fluoridated water and increased cancer risk.
Obesity: appears to increase the risk of cancers of the breast, colon, prostate, endometrium (the lining of the uterus), cervix, ovary, kidney, gallbladder, liver, pancreas, rectum, and esophagus. The exact link between obesity and increased cancer risk is not clear but may be linked with hormonal changes that occur with having excess body fat.	Omega-3 fatty acids: includes alpha-linolenic acid, eicosapentaenoic acid (EPA), and docosahexaenoic acid (DHA). These fatty acids are found in fish and fish oils. Consuming foods high in omega-3 fatty acids is associated with reduced rates of breast, colon, and rectal cancers.	Food additives: it is estimated that over 15,000 substances are added to our foods during growth, processing, and packaging. To date, there is no evidence that food additives contribute significantly to cancer risk.
High fat diet: these have been associated with increased risk of many cancers, including prostate and breast. However, not all studies support this association.		
Alcohol: use is linked with an increased risk of cancers of the esophagus, pharynx, and mouth. Alcohol use may also increase the risk for cancers of the liver, breast, colon, and rectum. Alcohol may impair the cell's ability to repair damaged DNA, increasing the possibility of cancer initiation.		

*Eating a diet high in whole grains, fruits, and vegetables: such a diet is associated with lower cancer risks.
Source: Information gathered from The American Cancer Society (www.cancer.org, accessed July 2002), The National Cancer Institute (www.cancer.gov, accessed July 2002), and P. Greenwald, C. K. Clifford, and J. A. Milner, Diet and cancer prevention, *Eur. J. Cancer* 37 (2001): 948–965.

mechanisms include: 1) improved circulation; 2) increased ventilation and shortened bowel transit time, which reduces the time our lungs and bowels are exposed to potential carcinogens; 3) maintenance of healthier weight; 4) improved immune function; 5) modulation of sex hormones such as estrogen and testosterone, which could reduce the risk of breast, endometrial, ovarian, testicular, and prostate cancers; and 6) enhanced repair of damaged DNA. None of these mechanisms have been sufficiently studied to allow us to draw any firm conclusions about how physical activity may be protective against cancer. However, these findings have prompted the American Cancer Society and the National Cancer Institute to promote increased physical activity as a way to reduce our risk for cancer.

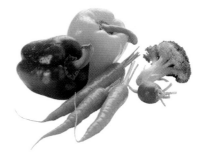

Eating more fruits and vegetables has been shown to reduce the risk of several cancers.

Antioxidants Play a Role in Preventing Cancer

There is a large and growing body of evidence that antioxidants play an important role in cancer prevention. How do antioxidants work to reduce our risk for cancer? Some proposed mechanisms include:

- Enhancing our immune system, which assists in the destruction and removal of precancerous cells from our bodies.

Cancer Prevention Recommendations from the American Cancer Society

1. Eat a variety of healthful foods, with an emphasis on plant sources.
   - Eat five or more servings of a variety of vegetables and fruits each day.
   - Choose whole grains in preference to processed (refined) grains and sugars.
   - Limit consumption of red meats, especially those high in fat and processed.
   - Choose foods that maintain a healthful weight.
2. Adopt a physically active lifestyle.
   - Adults: Engage in at least moderate activity for 30 minutes or more on five or more days of the week; 45 minutes or more of moderate to vigorous activity on five or more days per week may further enhance reductions in the risk of breast and colon cancer.
   - Children and adolescents: Engage in at least 60 minutes per day of moderate-to-vigorous physical activity at least five days per week.
3. If you drink alcoholic beverages, limit consumption.

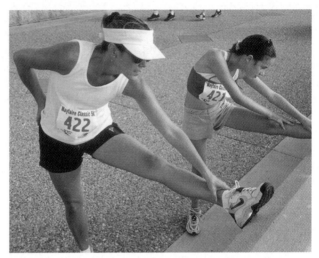

Staying physically active may help reduce our risk for some cancers.

Source: The American Cancer Society. ACS recommendations for nutrition and physical activity for cancer prevention. www.cancer.org Accessed July 2002. Reprinted by permission of The American Cancer Society, Inc. ●

- Inhibiting the growth of cancer cells and tumors.
- Preventing oxidative damage to our cells' DNA by scavenging free radicals and stopping the formation and subsequent chain reaction of oxidized molecules.

While very few studies show benefits of individual antioxidant nutrients such as vitamins E, C, beta-carotene, and selenium, eating whole foods that are high in these nutrients—especially fruits, vegetables, and whole grains—is consistently shown to be associated with decreased cancer risk (Greenwald, Clifford, and Milner 2001). Additional studies show that populations eating diets low in antioxidant nutrients have a higher risk for cancer. These studies show a strong association between eating whole foods high in antioxidants and lower cancer risk, but they do not prove cause and effect. Nutrition experts agree that there are important interactions between antioxidant nutrients and other substances in foods, such as fiber and phytochemicals, which work together to reduce the risk for many types of cancers. Studies are now being conducted to determine whether eating foods high in antioxidants directly cause lower rates of cancer.

The link between taking antioxidant supplements and reducing cancer risk is not very clear. Laboratory animal and test tube studies show that the individual nutrients reviewed in this chapter act as antioxidants in various situations. However, supplementation studies in humans do not consistently show benefits of taking antioxidant supplements in the prevention of cancer and other diseases. For example, in the Alpha-Tocopherol Beta-Carotene Cancer Prevention Study discussed earlier (Albanes et al. 1995), supplementation with vitamin E resulted in a lower risk for cancers of the prostate, colon, and rectum, but was related to more cancers of the stomach. In this same study, beta-carotene supplements increased risk for cancers of the lung, prostate, and stomach in current and former smokers (Heinonen et al. 1998). In the Nutritional Prevention of Cancer Trial (Clark et al. 1998), selenium supplementation was found to reduce the risk of prostate, colon, and lung cancers, but it did not reduce the risk of nonmelanoma skin cancers. The Linxian intervention trials, named for the region of China where the studies were conducted, found that a supplement containing beta-carotene, vitamin E, and selenium reduced mortality from overall cancer, specifically reducing the risk for cancers of the esophagus and stomach (Blot et al. 1995).

Why do antioxidant supplements appear to work in some studies and for some cancers but not in others? The human body is very complex, as is the development and progression of the numerous forms of cancer. People differ substantially in their susceptibility for cancer and in their response to protective factors and to cancer-causing agents. These complexities cloud the relationship between nutrition and cancer. It is impossible to control all factors that may increase our risk for cancer in any research study. Thus, there are many unknown factors that can affect study outcomes. It has also been speculated that antioxidants taken in supplemental form may act as prooxidants in some situations, but consuming antioxidants in the form of food may provide these nutrients in a more balanced state. There are many studies currently being conducted to determine the impact of whole foods and antioxidant supplements on our risk for various forms of cancers. The results of these studies will provide important insights into the link between whole foods, individual nutrients, and cancer. Refer to the Nutrition Debate box at the end of the chapter to gain a better understanding of situations that may warrant vitamin and mineral supplementation.

Gustavo Nutri-Case

"Last night, there was an actress on TV talking about having colon cancer and saying everybody over age fifty should get tested. It brought back all the memories of my father's cancer, how thin and weak he got before he went to the doctor, so that by the time they found the cancer it had already spread too far. But I don't think I'm at risk. I only eat red meat two or three times a week, and I eat a piece of fruit or a vegetable at every meal. I don't smoke, and I get plenty of exercise, sunshine, and fresh air working in the vineyard."

What lifestyle factors reduce Gustavo's risk for cancer? What factors increase his risk? Think especially about possible occupational risk factors. Would you recommend he increase his consumption of fruits and vegetables? Why or why not? If Gustavo were your father, would you ask him to have the screening test for colon cancer that the actress on television recommended?

Phytochemicals Contribute to Cancer Prevention

Phytochemicals are naturally occurring chemicals in plants that may reduce our risk for diseases such as cancer and heart disease. Phytochemicals are found in abundance in fruits, vegetables, whole grains, legumes, seeds, soy products, garlic, onion, and green and black teas. Table 8.4 lists many of the phytochemicals that are linked to cancer prevention.

Phytochemicals have been studied in the laboratory, and they exhibit clear cancer prevention properties under this condition. At this time, our knowledge of phytochemicals and their effect on cancer in humans is in its infancy stage. We do not know the specific phytochemical content of most foods, and a marker (or markers) of phytochemical intake in humans has not yet been discovered. Progress is being made in this area of research, however. There is growing evidence that phytochemicals such as lycopene (found in tomato products), organosulphur compounds (found in garlic, onions, and cruciferous vegetables), flavonoids (found in fruits, vegetables, tea and red wine), and phytoestrogens (found in whole grains, vegetables, and soy products) may reduce the risk for some forms of cancer (Greenwald et al. 2001). Future studies will shed insight into how phytochemicals work to reduce our risk for cancer, how these substances work in conjunction with other nutrients to improve health, and whether supplementing our diets with phytochemicals is protective against chronic diseases.

phytochemicals Chemicals found in plants (*phyto-* is from the Greek word for plant,) such as pigments and other substances, that may reduce our risk for diseases such as cancer and heart disease.

Table 8.4   Food Sources of Various Phytochemicals

Phytochemical	Example	Food Sources
Carotenoids	Alpha-carotene, beta-carotene, lycopene, lutein	Yellow-red, red, orange, and deep green vegetables and fruit such as carrots, cantaloupe, sweet potatoes, apricots, kale, spinach, pumpkin, and tomatoes
Glucosinolates, isothiocyanates, indoles	Glucobrassicin, indole-3-carbinol	Cruciferous vegetables such as broccoli, cabbage, cauliflower, and Brussels sprouts
Organosulphur compounds	Diallyl sulfide, allyl methyl trisulfide, dithiolthiones	Allium vegetables, including onion and garlic, and cruciferous vegetables such as broccoli, cabbage, cauliflower, and Brussels sprouts
Polyphenols	Flavonoids and phenolic acids	Apple skins, berries, broccoli, citrus fruit, red wine, black and green tea
Phytoestrogens	Isoflavones, lignans	Soybeans and soy-based foods, vegetables, rye

Source: Adapted from P. Greenwald C. K. Clifford, and J. A. Milner. Diet and cancer prevention. *Eur. J. Cancer* 37 (2001): 948–965. Copyright © 2001, with permission from Elsevier.

Recap: Cancer is a group of diseases in which genetically mutated cells grow out of control. Tobacco use, sun exposure, nutritional factors, radiation and chemical exposures, and low physical activity levels are related to a higher risk for some cancers. Eating foods high in antioxidants is associated with lower rates of cancer, but studies of antioxidant supplements and cancer are equivocal. Phytochemicals are recently discovered substances in plants that may reduce our risk for cancer.

Cardiovascular Disease

The details of *cardiovascular disease* (CVD) and its relationship to cholesterol and lipoproteins were presented in Chapter 5. A brief review of CVD is presented in this section, and an explanation is provided on how antioxidants may reduce our risk for CVD.

CVD is the leading cause of death for adults in the United States. CVD encompasses all diseases of the heart and blood vessels, including coronary heart disease, hypertension (or high blood pressure), and atherosclerosis (or hardening of the arteries). The two primary manifestations of CVD are heart attack and stroke. Almost one million people die each year from CVD, and about sixty-one million people (or 25% of the U.S. population) live with this disease. It is estimated that CVD costs our country $298 billion in health care costs and lost work revenue (NCCDPHP 2002).

Remember that the major risks for CVD are:

- smoking
- hypertension (high blood pressure)
- high blood levels of low-density lipoprotein (LDL) cholesterol
- obesity
- sedentary lifestyle

Other risk factors include a low level of high-density (HDL) lipoprotein cholesterol, impaired glucose tolerance or diabetes, family history (CVD in males younger than 55 years of age and females younger than 65 years of age), being a male older than 45 years of age, and menopause in women. While we cannot alter our gender, family history, or age, we can change our nutrition and physical activity habits to reduce our risk for CVD.

Research has recently identified a risk factor for CVD that may be even more important than elevated cholesterol levels. This risk factor is a condition called *low-grade inflammation* (de Ferranti and Rifai 2002). This condition weakens the plaque in the blood vessels, making it more fragile. You may remember from Chapter 5 that plaque is the fatty material that builds on the inside of our arteries and causes hardening of the arteries. As the plaque becomes more fragile, it is more likely to burst and break away from the sides of our arteries. It may then form a blood clot that closes off the vessels of the heart or brain, leading to a heart attack or stroke, respectively. The marker in our bodies that indicates the degree of inflammation is C-reactive protein. Having higher levels of C-reactive protein increases our risk for a heart attack even if we do not have elevated cholesterol levels. For people with high levels of C-reactive protein and cholesterol, their risk of a heart attack is almost nine times higher than that of someone with normal cholesterol and C-reactive protein levels. These findings have prompted the medical community to develop standards for testing C-reactive protein along with cholesterol as a test for CVD risk.

How can antioxidants decrease our risk for CVD? There is growing evidence that certain antioxidants, specifically vitamin E and lycopene, work in a variety of ways that reduce the damage to our vessels, which in turn, reduces our risk of a heart attack or stroke. Some of the ways these nutrients decrease our risk for CVD include:

- **Scavenging free radicals**—This action prevents oxidative damage to the LDLs. Remember from Chapter 5 that oxidized LDL particles stimulate the buildup of plaque in the blood vessel walls.

- **Reducing low-grade inflammation**—This action can prevent the rupture of plaque in the blood vessels, thus preventing the release of clots that can cause a heart attack or stroke.

- **Reducing blood coagulation and the formation of clots**—Vitamin E has known anticoagulant properties. This means that it acts to prevent excessive thickening and clotting of the blood, preventing the formation of clots that can block blood vessels.

As with the research conducted on cancer, the studies of antioxidants and CVD show inconsistent results. Two large-scale surveys conducted in the United States show that men and women who eat more fruits and vegetables have a significantly reduced risk of CVD (Joshipura et al. 2001; Liu et al. 2001). However, few intervention studies have been conducted to determine the effect of antioxidant supplements on risk for CVD. Vitamin E was found to lower the number of heart disease deaths in smokers in the Alpha-Tocopherol Beta-Carotene Cancer Prevention Study (The ATBC Study Group 1994) but had no overall effect on the risk of stroke. In the HOPE study (The HOPE Investigators 2000), vitamin E had no impact on the risk for CVD in people who are at high risk for heart attack and stroke. Additional studies are currently being conducted, and their results should provide more information on whether or not antioxidant supplements can reduce our risk for CVD.

It is important to note that there are other compounds (besides antioxidants) are found in fruits, vegetables, and whole grains that can reduce our risk for CVD. For instance, soluble fiber has been shown to reduce elevated LDL-cholesterol and total cholesterol. The most successful effects have been found in people eating oatmeal and oat bran cereals. Dietary fiber in general has been shown to reduce blood pressure, lower total cholesterol levels, and improve blood glucose and insulin levels. Folate, a B-vitamin, is found in fortified cereals, green leafy vegetables, bananas, legumes, and orange juice. Folate is known to reduce homocysteine levels in the blood, and a high concentration of homocysteine in the blood is a known risk factor for CVD. A recent study from the Netherlands showed that individuals who drank more than three cups of black tea (which is high in flavonoids) had a lower rate of heart attacks than non-tea drinkers (Geleijnse et al. 2002). Thus, it appears that there are a plethora of nutrients and other components in fruits, vegetables, and whole grain foods that may be protective against CVD.

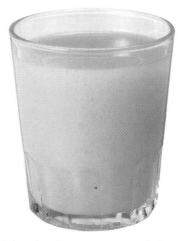

Folate, found in orange juice, can help reduce the risk of CVD.

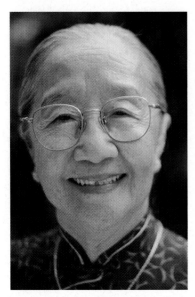

Aging is a natural and inevitable process of life.

Recap: Cardiovascular disease (CVD) is the leading cause of death in the United States. Risk factors for CVD include smoking, hypertension, high LDL-cholesterol, obesity, and a sedentary lifestyle. Antioxidants may help reduce our risk for heart disease by preventing oxidative damage to LDL cholesterol, reducing inflammation in our vessels, and reducing the formation of blood clots.

Vision Impairment and Other Results of Aging

In most Eastern and nonindustrialized cultures, aging is viewed as a natural and desirable process that begins with conception and ends with death. The aged are respected and valued for their wisdom and experience and are often the decision-makers in their communities. In contrast, for centuries, many people in Western countries have searched to find an elixir of eternal youth. Today, in the United States and Europe, researchers continue this search, developing skin creams, supplements, botulism toxin injections, and new techniques of plastic surgery to conceal or fight the effects of aging. Despite these efforts, aging is inevitable.

Antioxidant supplements have gotten a great deal of attention as potential substances to reverse the effects of aging. This is because the process of aging is associated with increased oxidative damage and reduced activity of antioxidant enzymes in most body tissues. Despite this link between antioxidants and aging, there is no scientific evidence to support the contention that taking antioxidant supplements can prolong our lives.

However, we know that our ability to digest, absorb, and metabolize many nutrients is impaired as we age (refer to Chapter 16 for more detailed information on aging). These nutritional limitations have prompted some experts to suggest that specific RDAs be increased for adults according to new, narrower age brackets, such as 51 to 60 years, 61 to 70 years, 71 to 80 years, and 81 to 90 years. Currently, the RDAs are defined for adults 51 to 70 years and 71 years and older. A great deal more will be learned about optimal nutrition for older adults over the next decade as people live longer and we learn more about how our nutritional needs change as we age.

There are some diseases associated with aging that may be preventable by consuming antioxidants. Two of these diseases are macular degeneration and cataracts, both of which impair vision in older adults.

Macular degeneration is the leading cause of blindness of adults 55 years and older in the United States. The macula is the central part of the retina (Figure 8.15a), and it is responsible for our central vision and our ability to see details. When a person has macular degeneration, he or she loses the ability to see details, such as small print, small objects, and facial features. Objects seem to fade or disappear, straight lines or edges appear wavy, and the ability to read standard print type is lost (Figure 8.15b). Macular degeneration does not affect our peripheral vision.

There is no known cure for macular degeneration. The causes of this disease are unknown, but proposed causes include:

- Lack of nutrients to the retina, including antioxidant nutrients
- Poor circulation in the retina
- Untreated health problems that cause undue pressure to the eye, such as high blood pressure; other health problems such as high cholesterol and diabetes may degenerate the macula over time
- Excessive exposure to ultraviolet rays
- Genetic susceptibility

A **cataract** is a damaged portion of the eye's lens, the portion of the eye through which we focus entering light. Cataracts cause cloudiness in the lens that impairs vision (Figure 8.16). People with cataracts have a very difficult time seeing in bright light; for instance, they see halos around lights, glare, and scattering of light. Having cataracts also impairs a person's ability to adjust from dark to bright light. It is estimated that over one-half of all people over the age of 65 years in the United States have some cataract development.

macular degeneration A vision disorder caused by deterioration of the central portion of the retina and marked by loss or distortion of the central field of vision.

cataract A damaged portion of the eye's lens, which causes cloudiness that impairs vision.

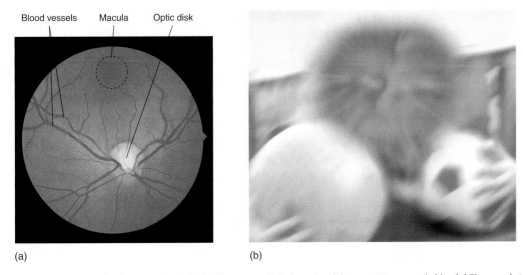

(a)

(b)

Figure 8.15   Macular degeneration is the leading cause of blindness in adults ages 55 years and older. **(a)** The macula is the central part of the retina that allows us to see details and small print. **(b)** This simulation of the vision loss typical in patients with macular degeneration illustrates the loss of central vision. *Source:* National Eye Institute, National Institutes of Health. November 2003. Photos, Images, and Videos. Ref # EDS05. www.nei.nih.gov/photo/search/ref_num.asp?ref = EDS05&Submit = Go Accessed February 2004.

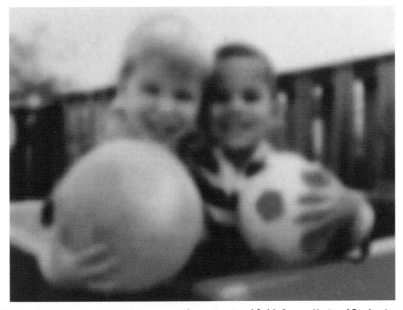

Figure 8.16   Cataracts can impair vision across the entire visual field. *Source:* National Eye Institute, National Institutes of Health. November 2003. Photos, Images, and Videos. Ref # EDS03. www.nei.nih.gov/photo/search/ref_num.asp?ref = EDS03&Submit = Go. Accessed February 2004.

Cataracts can be treated with surgery. As with macular degeneration, the causes of cataracts are unknown. However, some possible causes of cataracts include:

- Free radical damage caused by exposure to oxygen, ultraviolet light, and x-rays
- Inflammation caused by some eye diseases
- Use of certain drugs such as corticosteroids
- Complications of diabetes

Current research findings are showing some promise of reducing the risk for macular degeneration and cataracts through the use of antioxidant supplements. A recent study conducted with individuals who had early signs of macular degeneration found that consuming an antioxidant supplement reduced the progression of this disease (Age-Related Eye Disease Study Research Group 2001a). Earlier studies have also shown that higher blood levels of antioxidants and consuming more antioxidants in the diet are associated with a lower risk of macular degeneration (Delcourt et al. 1999; West et al. 1994). The effects of antioxidant supplements and cataracts are mixed, with some studies showing a reduced rate of cataract development in people taking antioxidant supplements or having higher blood levels of antioxidants (Chylack et al. 2002; Gale et al. 2001), but other studies show no benefit of antioxidants (Age-Related Eye Disease Study Research Group 2001b).

At this time, it is not possible to reach a conclusion regarding the effectiveness of antioxidant supplements to prevent these two diseases of aging. However, there is enough evidence that consuming a healthful diet that includes fruits, vegetables, and whole grains is associated with improved quality of life as we age.

Recap: There is no evidence that antioxidants can reverse or prevent aging or significantly prolong our lives. Macular degeneration and cataracts are two diseases of vision that are associated with aging. Antioxidant nutrients have been found to reduce the risk of these diseases in some studies.

Chapter Summary

- Antioxidants are compounds that protect our cells from oxidative damage.

- Free radicals are produced under many situations, including when our body generates ATP, when our immune system fights infection, and when we are exposed to environmental toxins such as pollution, overexposure to the sun, radiation, and tobacco smoke.

- Free radicals are dangerous because they can damage the lipid portion of our cell membranes, destroying the integrity of our cell membranes. Free radicals also damage LDLs, cell proteins, and DNA.

- Antioxidant vitamins donate their electrons or hydrogen molecules to free radicals to neutralize them. Antioxidant minerals are cofactors in antioxidant enzyme systems, which convert free radicals to less damaging substances that our body excretes.

- Vitamin E is an antioxidant that protects the fatty components of cell membranes from oxidation. It also protects LDLs, vitamin A, and our lungs from oxidative damage. Other functions of vitamin E are the development of nerves and muscles, enhancement of the immune function, and improvement of the absorption of vitamin A if intake of vitamin A is low.

- Vitamin C is an antioxidant that is oxidized by free radicals and prevents the damage of cells and tissues. Vitamin C also regenerates vitamin E after it has been oxidized. Other functions of vitamin C include helping the synthesis of collagen, various hormones, neurotransmitters, and DNA; enhancing immune function; and increasing the absorption of iron.

- Beta-carotene is one of about 600 carotenoids identified to date. Beta-carotene is a provitamin, or precursor, to vitamin A, meaning it is an inactive form of vitamin A that is converted to vitamin A in the body.

- Beta-carotene protects the lipid portions of our membranes and the LDL-cholesterol from oxidative damage. Other functions of beta-carotene include enhancing our immune system, protecting our skin from sun damage, and protecting our eyes from oxidative damage. The carotenoids may help reduce our risk for some forms of cancer.

- Vitamin A is a fat-soluble vitamin. The three active forms of vitamin A are retinol, retinal, and retinoic acid. Beta-carotene is converted to vitamin A in our small intestine.

- Vitamin A is extremely important for healthy vision. It ensures our ability to adjust to changes in the brightness of light, and it also helps us maintain color vision. Vitamin A may also act as an antioxidant, as it protects LDL-cholesterol from oxidative damage. Other functions of vitamin A include assistance in cell differentiation, sexual reproduction, and proper bone growth.

- Selenium is a trace mineral. Selenium is part of the structure of glutathione peroxidases, a family of antioxidant enzymes. These enzymes break down fatty acids that have become oxidized, which indirectly spares vitamin E from oxidation and helps prevent oxidative damage to our cell membranes and fatty tissues. Other functions of selenium include assisting in the production of thyroid hormone and enhancing immune function.

- Copper, iron, zinc, and manganese are minerals that act as cofactors for antioxidant enzyme systems. Cofactors are necessary to allow enzymes to function properly. Copper, zinc, and manganese are part of the superoxide dismustase complex, while iron is part of catalase. These minerals also play critical roles in energy metabolism and blood formation.

- Antioxidants play a role in cancer prevention. Eating foods high in antioxidants results in lower rates of some cancers, but supplementing with antioxidants can cause cancer in some situations.

- Phytochemicals are naturally occurring components in food that may reduce our risk for diseases such as cancer and heart disease. Phytochemicals are found in fruits, vegetables, nuts, seeds, whole grains, soy products, garlic, onion, and tea. The impact of phytochemicals on reducing our risk for cancer is still under investigation.

- Antioxidants may help reduce our risk for CVD by scavenging free radicals and preventing oxidative damage to LDL-cholesterol, reducing low-grade inflammation (which in turn, prevents the rupture of plaque in our blood vessels), and preventing the formation of blood clots.

- Antioxidants may help prevent two age-related diseases of vision, macular degeneration and cataracts. Macular degeneration causes us to lose the ability to see details, small print, and facial features. A cataract is a damaged portion of the eye's lens. This damage leads to cloudiness and impairs vision. Cataracts impair our ability to adjust from dark to bright light. Antioxidant supplements have been found to reduce the risk for macular degeneration and cataracts in some studies.

Review Questions

1. Which of the following is a characteristic of vitamin E?
   a. It enhances the absorption of iron.
   b. It can be manufactured from beta-carotene.
   c. It is a critical component of the glutathione peroxidase system.
   d. It is destroyed by exposure to high heat.

2. Oxidation is best described as a process in which
   a. a carcinogen causes a mutation in a stem cell's DNA.
   b. an atom loses an electron.
   c. an element loses an atom of oxygen.
   d. a compound loses a molecule of water.

3. Which of the following disorders is linked with the production of free radicals?
   a. cardiovascular disease
   b. carotenosis
   c. ulcers
   d. malaria

4. Which of the following are known carcinogens?
   a. phytochemicals
   b. antioxidants
   c. carotenoids
   d. nitrates

5. Taking daily doses of three to four times the RDA of which of the following nutrients may cause death?
   a. vitamin A
   b. vitamin C
   c. vitamin E
   d. selenium

6. **True or false?** Tocopherol is the biologically active form of vitamin E in our bodies.

7. **True or false?** Free radical formation can occur as a result of normal cellular metabolism.

8. **True or false?** Vitamin C helps regenerate vitamin A.

9. **True or false?** Reliable food sources of selenium include beef liver, pork, and seafood.

10. **True or false?** Pregnant women are advised to consume plentiful quantities of beef liver.

11. Explain how free radicals damage cell membranes and lead to cell death.

12. Describe the process by which cancer occurs, beginning with initiation and ending with metastasis of the cancer to widespread body tissues.

13. Explain why people taking anticoagulents should avoid vitamin E supplementation.

14. Discuss the contribution of trace minerals such as selenium to the prevention of oxidation.

15. Explain how vitamin E reduces our risk for heart disease.

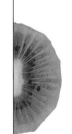

Test Yourself Answers

1. **False.** Currently, there is no known dietary cure for cancer. However, eating a diet that is plentiful in fruits and vegetables and exercising regularly may help reduce our risk for some forms of cancer.

2. **True.** Overall, the research on vitamin C and colds does not show strong evidence that taking vitamin C supplements reduces our risk of suffering from the common cold.

3. **False.** We can consume up to 50 times the RDA for vitamin E with no serious health consequences.

4. **False.** By eating at least five servings of fruits and vegetables each day, we can consume enough antioxidants in our diets.

5. **True.** In general, there is little support for the contention that consuming antioxidants prolongs life or reduces the impact of aging.

Web Links

www.who.int
World Health Organization (WHO)
Click on Health Topics and select "deficiency diseases" to find out more about vitamin A deficiency around the world.

www.americanheart.org
American Heart Association
Discover the best way to lower your risk for cardiovascular disease.

www.cancer.org
The American Cancer Society
Get ACS recommendations for nutrition and physical activity for cancer prevention.

www.cancer.gov
The National Cancer Institute
Learn more about the nutritional factors that can influence your risk for cancer.

www.nei.nih.gov
National Eye Institute
Visit this site to find out more about how macular degeneration and cataracts can impair vision.

www.fda.gov
U.S. Food and Drug Administration (FDA)
Select Dietary Supplements on the pull-down menu for more information on how to make informed decisions and evaluate information related to dietary supplements.

www.nal.usda.gov/fnic
The Food and Nutrition Information Council (FNIC)
Click on the Dietary Supplements button to obtain information on vitamin and mineral supplements, including consumer reports and industry regulations.

http://dietary-supplements.info.nih.gov
Office of Dietary Supplements
Go to this site to obtain current research results and reliable information about dietary supplements.

References

Age-Related Eye Disease Study Research Group. 2001a. A randomized, placebo-controlled, clinical trial of high-dose supplementation with vitamins C and E, beta-carotene, and zinc for age-related macular degeneration and vision loss: AREDS Report No. 8. *Arch. Ophthalmol.* 119:1417–1436.

Age-Related Eye Disease Study Research Group. 2001b. A randomized, placebo-controlled, clinical trial of high-dose supplementation with vitamins C and E and beta-carotene for age-related cataract and vision loss: AREDS Report No. 9. *Arch. Ophthalmol.* 119:1439–1452.

Ahmed F. 1999. Vitamin A deficiency in Bangladesh: a review and recommendations for improvement. *Public Health Nutr.* 2:1–14.

Albanes D., O. P. Heinonen, J. K. Huttunen, P. R. Taylor, J. Virtamo, B. K. Edwards, J. Haapakoski, M. Rautalahti, A. M. Hartman, J. Palmgren, and P. Greenwald. 1995. Effects of α-tocopherol and β-carotene supplements on cancer incidence in the Alpha-Tocopherol Beta-Carotene Cancer Prevention Study. *Am. J. Clin. Nutr.* 62 (suppl.):1427S–1430S.

Alpha-Tocopherol, Beta-Carotene Cancer Prevention Study Group, The. (The ATBC Study Group). 1994. The effect of vitamin E and beta carotene on the incidence of lung cancer and other cancers in male smokers. *N. Engl. J. Med.* 330:1029–1035.

American Cancer Society. 2002. *Cancer Prevention.* www.cancer.org. Accessed July 2002.

American Dietetic Association. 2001. Position of the American Dietetic Association: food fortification and dietary supplements. *J. Am. Diet. Assoc.* 101:115–125.

Anonymous. 2000. Sports supplement sales rise to $1.4 billion. *Nutrition Business Journal* 12:5–6.

Blendon R. J., C. M. DesRoches, J. M. Benson, M. Brodie, and D. E. Altman. 2001. Americans' views on the use and regulation of dietary supplements. *Arch. Intern. Med.* 26:805–810.

Blot W. J., J.-Y. Li, P. R. Taylor, W. Guo, S. M. Dawsey, and B. Li. 1995. The Linxian trials: mortality rates by vitamin-mineral intervention group. *Am. J. Clin. Nutr.* 62 (suppl.):1424S–1426S.

Burri B. J. 1997. Beta-carotene and human health: a review of current research. *Nutr. Res.* 17:547–580.

Chylack L. T. Jr., N. P. Brown, A. Bron, M. Hurst, W. Kopcke, U. Thien, and W. Schalch. 2002. The Roche European American Cataract Trial (REACT): a randomized clinical trial to investigate the efficacy of an oral antioxidant micronutrient mixture to slow progression of age-related cataract. *Ophthalmic Epidemiol.* 9:49–80.

Clark L. C., B. Dalkin, A. Krongrad, G. F. Combs Jr., B. W. Turnbull, E. H. Slate, R. Witherington, J. H. Herlong, E. Janosko, D. Carpenter, C. Borosso, S. Falk, and J. Rounder. 1998. Decreased incidence of prostate cancer with selenium supplementation: results of a double-blind cancer prevention trial. *Br. J. Urol.* 81:730–734.

Dancho C., and M. M. Manore. 2001. Dietary supplement information on the World Wide Web. Sorting fact from fiction. *ACSM's Health and Fitness J.* 5:7–12.

de Ferranti S., and N. Rifai. 2002. C-reactive protein and cardiovascular disease: a review of risk prediction and interventions. *Clinica Chimica Acta* 317:1–15.

Delcourt C., J. P. Cristol, F. Tessier, C. L. Léger, B. Descomps, and L. Papoz. 1999. Age-related macular degeneration and antioxidant status in the POLA study. POLA Study Group. Pathologies Oculaires Liées à l'Age. *Arch. Ophthalmol.* 117:1384–1390.

Ford, E. S. and A. Sowell. 1999. Serum alpha-tocopherol status in the United States population: findings from the Third National Health and Nutrition Examination Survey. *Am. J. Epidemiol.* 150(3): 290–300.

Gale C. R., N. F. Hall, D. I. Phillips, and C. N. Martyn. 2001. Plasma antioxidant vitamins and carotenoids and age-related cataract. *Ophthalmology* 108:1992–1998.

Geleijnse J. M., L. J. Launer, D. A. M. van der Kuip, A. Hofman, and J. C. M. Witteman. 2002. Inverse association of tea and flavonoid intakes with incident myocardial infarction: the Rotterdam Study. *Am. J. Clin. Nutr.* 75:880–886.

Greenwald P., C. K. Clifford, and J. A. Milner. 2001. Diet and cancer prevention. *Eur. J. Cancer* 37:948–965.

Gutteridge J. M. C., and B. Halliwell. 1994. *Antioxidants in Nutrition, Health, and Disease.* Oxford, UK: Oxford University Press.

Haider J., and T. Demissie. 1999. Malnutrition and xerophthalmia in rural communities of Ethiopia. *East Afr. Med. J.* 76:590–593.

Heart Outcomes Prevention Evaluation Study Investigators, The (The HOPE Investigators). 2000. Vitamin E supplementation and cardiovascular events in high-risk patients. *N. Engl. J. Med.* 342:154–160.

Heinonen O. P., D. Albanes, J. Virtamo, P. R. Taylor, J. K. Huttunen, A. M. Hartman, J. Haapakoski, N. Malila, M. Rautalahti, S. Ripatti, H. Maepaa, L. Teerenhovi, L. Koss, M. Virolainen, and B. K. Edwards. 1998. Prostate cancer and supplementation with α-tocopherol and β-carotene: incidence and mortality in a controlled trial. *J. Natl. Cancer Inst.* 90:440–446.

Hemila H. 1997. Vitamin C intake and susceptibility to the common cold. *Br. J. Nutr.* 77:59–72.

Joshipura, K. J., F. B. Hu, J. E. Manson, M. J. Stampfer, E. B. Rimm, F. E. Speizer, G. Colditz, A. Ascherio, B. Rosner, D. Spiegelman, and W. C. Willett. 2001. The effect of fruit and vegetable intake on risk for coronary heart disease. *Ann. Intern. Med.* 134:1106–1114.

Liu S., I.-M. Lee, U. Ajani, S. R. Cole, J. E. Buring, and J. E. Manson. 2001. Intake of vegetables rich in carotenoids and risk of coronary heart disease in men: the Physicians' Health Study. *Intl. J. Epidemiol.* 30:130–135.

Livrea M. A., L. Tesoriere, A. Bongiorno, A. M. Pintaudi, M. Ciaccio, and A. Riccio. 1995. Contribution of vitamin A to the oxidation resistance of human low density lipoproteins. *Free Radic. Biol. Med.* 18:401–409.

National Cancer Institute. 2002. Cancer Causes and Risk Factors. www.cancer.gov. Accessed July 2002.

National Center for Chronic Disease Prevention and Health Promotion (NCCDPHP). 2002. Chronic Disease Prevention. Chronic Disease Overview. www.cdc.gov/nccdphp/overview. Accessed February 2004.

Thune I., and A. S. Furberg. 2001. Physical activity and cancer risk: dose-response and cancer, all sites and site-specific. *Med. Sci. Sports Exerc.* (suppl.) 33:S530–S550.

U.S. Department of Agriculture (USDA), Agricultural Research Service. 1998. USDA–NCC Carotenoid Database for U.S. Foods. Nutrient Data Laboratory Home Page, www.nal.usda.gov/fnic/foodcomp. Accessed August 2002.

U.S. Food and Drug Administration (FDA). 1998. An FDA guide to dietary supplements. *FDA Consumer Magazine.* September/October. www.fda.gov/fdac/features/1998/598_guid.html. Accessed August 2002.

U.S. Food and Drug Administration (FDA). Center for Food Safety and Applied Nutrition. 2001, January 3. Overview of dietary supplements. www.cfsan.fda.gov/~dms/ds-oview.html. Accessed August 2002.

West S., S. Vitale, J. Hallfrisch, B. Munoz, D. Muller, S. Bressler, and N. M. Bressler. 1994. Are antioxidants or supplements protective for age-related macular degeneration? *Arch. Ophthalmol.* 112:222–227.

World Health Organization (WHO). 2002. Vitamin A. www.who.int/vaccines/en/vitaminamain.shtml. Accessed October 2002.

Zhang S., D. J. Hunter, M. R. Forman, B. A. Rosner, F. E. Speizer, G. A. Colditz, J. E. Manson, S. E. Hankinson, and W. C. Willett. 1999. Dietary carotenoids and vitamins A, C, and E and risk of breast cancer. *J. Natl. Cancer Inst.* 91:547–556.

Nutrition Debate:

Vitamin and Mineral Supplementation: Necessity or Waste?

Ben, Hannah's father, has type 2 diabetes and high blood cholesterol and is worried about his health. He attended a nutrition seminar in which the health benefits of various vitamin and mineral supplements were touted. After attending this seminar, Ben was convinced that he needed to take a series of supplements that contain more than 200% of the RDA for many vitamins and minerals. After a few months of taking these supplements on a daily basis, Ben started to experience headaches, nausea, diarrhea, and tingling in his hands and feet. Although Ben was not an expert in nutrition, he suspected that he might be experiencing side effects related to nutrient toxicity. He decided to talk to his doctor about the supplements he was taking to determine if they could be causing his symptoms.

Ben's story is not unique. The use of dietary supplements in the United States has skyrocketed in recent years. Americans spend almost $18 billion dollars each year on dietary supplements (Anonymous 2000). A recent review of national opinion surveys found that a significant number of Americans regularly take dietary supplements, but they do not report the use of these products to their physicians because they feel their physicians have little knowledge of these products and may harbor a bias toward their use (Blendon et al. 2001). Interestingly, many supplement users stated that they would continue to use these products even if scientific studies found them to be ineffective!

Why do so many people take dietary supplements? Many people believe they cannot consume adequate nutrients in their diet, and they take a supplement as extra nutritional insurance. Others have been advised by their health care provider to take a supplement due to a given health condition. There are people, like Ben, who believe that certain supplements can be used to treat illness or disease. There are also people who believe supplements are necessary to enhance their physical looks or athletic performance.

Although many people believe taking dietary supplements benefits their health, this is not always the case. Who should be taking supplements? This question is not simple. Before deciding whether you may benefit from taking dietary supplements, a review of the definition of dietary supplements and their regulation is necessary to gain a more complete understanding of how these products are marketed and regulated for safety.

Dietary Supplements Include Vitamins, Minerals, and Other Products

According to the U.S. Food and Drug Administration (FDA), a dietary supplement is "a product taken by mouth that contains a 'dietary ingredient' intended to supplement the diet" (FDA 2001, p. 1). Ingredients in supplements may include vitamins, minerals, herbs or other botanicals, amino acids, enzymes, tissues from animal organs or glands, or a concentrate, metabolite, constituent, or extract. Supplements come in many forms, including pills, capsules, liquids, or powders.

How Are Dietary Supplements Regulated?

As presented in the Dietary Supplement Health and Education Act (DSHEA) of 1994, dietary supplements are categorized within the general group of foods, not drugs. This means that the regulation of supplements is much less rigorous than the regulation of drugs. As an informed consumer, you should know that:

- Supplements do not need approval from the FDA before they are marketed.
- The company that manufactures the supplements is responsible for determining that the supplement is safe; the FDA does not test any supplement for safety prior to marketing.
- Supplement companies do not have to provide the FDA with any evidence that its supplements are safe unless the company is marketing a new dietary ingredient that was not sold in the United States prior to 1994.
- There are at present no federal guidelines on practices to ensure the purity, quality, safety, and composition of dietary supplements.
- There are no rules to limit the serving size or amount of a nutrient in any dietary supplement.
- Once a supplement is marketed, the FDA must prove it unsafe before the product will be removed from the market.

Despite these limitations in supplement regulations, supplement manufacturers are required to follow dietary supplement labeling guidelines. The figure in this box shows a label from a multivitamin and mineral supplement. As you can see, there are specific requirements for the information that must be included on the supplement label.

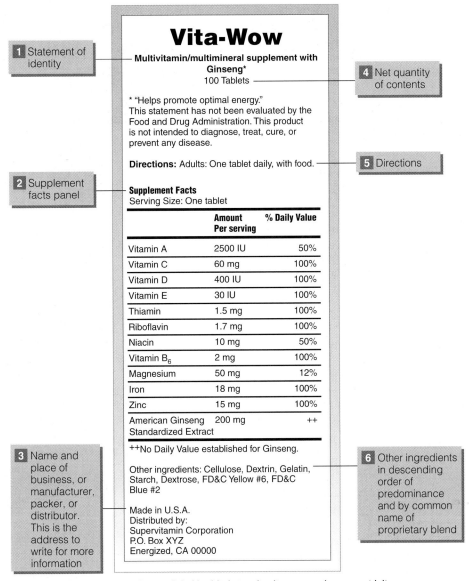

Vita-Wow

1 Statement of identity

Multivitamin/multimineral supplement with Ginseng*
100 Tablets

4 Net quantity of contents

* "Helps promote optimal energy."
This statement has not been evaluated by the Food and Drug Administration. This product is not intended to diagnose, treat, cure, or prevent any disease.

Directions: Adults: One tablet daily, with food.

5 Directions

2 Supplement facts panel

Supplement Facts
Serving Size: One tablet

	Amount Per serving	% Daily Value
Vitamin A	2500 IU	50%
Vitamin C	60 mg	100%
Vitamin D	400 IU	100%
Vitamin E	30 IU	100%
Thiamin	1.5 mg	100%
Riboflavin	1.7 mg	100%
Niacin	10 mg	50%
Vitamin B$_6$	2 mg	100%
Magnesium	50 mg	12%
Iron	18 mg	100%
Zinc	15 mg	100%
American Ginseng Standardized Extract	200 mg	++

++No Daily Value established for Ginseng.

3 Name and place of business, or manufacturer, packer, or distributor. This is the address to write for more information

Other ingredients: Cellulose, Dextrin, Gelatin, Starch, Dextrose, FD&C Yellow #6, FD&C Blue #2

Made in U.S.A.
Distributed by:
Supervitamin Corporation
P.O. Box XYZ
Energized, CA 00000

6 Other ingredients in descending order of predominance and by common name of proprietary blend

A multivitamin–mineral supplement label highlighting the dietary supplement guidelines.

Federal advertising regulations also require that any advertising on the label must be truthful and not misleading and that advertisers must have adequate substantiation of all product claims before disseminating the advertisement. Any products not meeting these labeling and advertising guidelines can be removed from the market.

How Can We Protect Ourselves from Fraudulent or Dangerous Supplements?

Although many of the supplement products sold today are safe, there are many products that are not. In addition, some companies are less than forthright about the true content of ingredients in their supplements. How can we avoid purchasing fraudulent or dangerous supplements? The FDA suggests that consumers can do the

following to protect themselves from fraudulent or dangerous supplements (FDA 1998):

1. Look for the U.S.P. (U.S. Pharmacopoeia) symbol or notation on the label. This symbol indicates that the manufacturer followed the standards established by U.S.P. for drugs for features such as purity, strength, quality, packaging, labeling, and acceptable length of storage.

2. Consider buying recognized brands of supplements. Although not guaranteed, products made by nationally recognized companies more likely have well-established manufacturing standards.

3. Do not assume that the word "natural" on the label means that the product is safe. Arsenic, lead, and mercury are all natural substances that can kill you if consumed in large enough quantities.

4. Do not hesitate to contact a company about how it makes its products. Reputable companies have nothing to hide and are more than happy to inform their customers about the safety and quality of their products.

Many supplements are also sold today over the Internet. Dancho and Manore (2001) suggest six criteria that can be used to evaluate dietary supplement Web sites. Keep these criteria in mind each time you consider buying a dietary supplement over the Web:

1. What is the purpose of the site? Is the Web site trying to sell a product or educate the consumer? Keep in mind that the primary purpose of supplement companies is to make money. Look for sites that provide educational information about a specific nutrient or product and don't just focus on selling the products.

2. Does the site contain accurate information? Accuracy of the information on the Web site is the most difficult thing for a consumer to determine. Testimonials (claims by athletes or other famous people) are *not* reliable and accurate; claims supported by scientific research are most desirable. If what the company claims about their product sounds too good to be true, it probably is.

3. Does the site contain reputable references? References should be from articles published in peer-reviewed scientific journals. The reference should be complete and contain author names, title of article, journal title, date, volume, and page numbers. This information allows the consumer to check original research for the validity of a company's claims about their product. Be cautious of sites that refer to claims that are proven by research studies but fail to provide a complete reference.

4. Who owns or sponsors the site? Full disclosure regarding sponsorship and possible sources of bias or conflict of interest should be included in the site's information.

5. Who wrote the information? Web sites should clearly identify the author of the article and include the credentials of the author. Recognized experts include individuals with relevant health-related credentials such as R.D., Ph.D., M.D., or M.S. Keep in mind that this person is responsible for the information posted in the article but may not be the creator of the Web site.

6. Is the information current and updated regularly? As information about supplements changes regularly, Web sites should be updated regularly, and the date should be clearly posted. All Web sites should also include contact information to allow consumers to ask questions about the information posted.

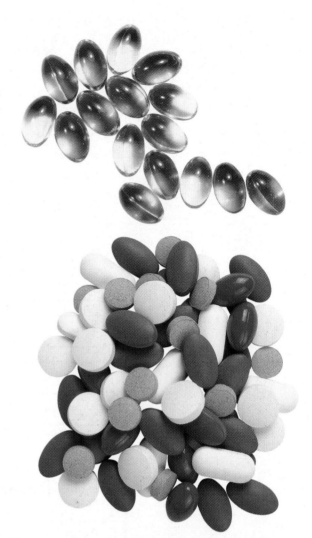

Always research supplements and supplement manufacturers before purchasing.

For more information on how to make informed decisions and evaluate information related to dietary supplements, go to the Dietary Supplements Web site of the U.S. FDA Center for Food Safety and Applied Nutrition at www.cfsan.fda.gov/~dms.ds-savvy.html. Other Web sites that contain reliable information about dietary supplements include The National Institutes of Health (NIH) Office of Dietary Supplements at dietary-supplements.info.nih.gov, and The Food and Nutrition Information Council (FNIC) at www.nal.usda.gov/fnic/.

Dietary Supplements Can Be Both Helpful and Harmful

As mentioned earlier in this debate, it is not always easy to determine who should take dietary supplements. Our nutritional needs change throughout our lifespan, and some of us may need to take supplements

Table 8.5   Individuals Who May Benefit from Dietary Supplementation

Example of Individual	Specific Supplements That May Help
Newborns	Routinely given a single dose of vitamin K at birth
Infants	Depends on condition; may need iron or other nutrients
Children not drinking fluoridated water	Fluoride supplements
Children on strict vegetarian diets	Vitamin B_{12}, iron, zinc, vitamin D (if not exposed to sunlight)
Children with poor eating habits or overweight children on an energy-restricted diet	Multivitamin-mineral supplement that does not exceed the RDA for the nutrients it contains
Pregnant teenagers	Iron and folic acid; other nutrients may be necessary if diet is very poor
Women who may become pregnant	Multivitamin or multivitamin-mineral supplement that contains 0.4 mg of folic acid
Pregnant or lactating women	Multivitamin-mineral supplement that contains iron, folic acid, zinc, copper, calcium, vitamin B_6, vitamin C, vitamin D
People on prolonged weight reduction diets	Multivitamin-mineral supplement
People recovering from serious illness or surgery	Multivitamin-mineral supplement
People with HIV/AIDS or other wasting diseases; people addicted to drugs or alcohol	Multivitamin-mineral supplement or single-nutrient supplements
Women	Calcium supplements: women need to consume 1000 to 1300 mg of calcium per day through food, and supplements may also be necessary
People eating a vegan diet	Vitamin B_{12}, riboflavin, calcium, vitamin D, iron, and zinc
People who have had portions of the intestinal tract removed; people who have a malabsorptive disease	Depends upon the exact condition; may include various fat-soluble and/or water-soluble vitamins and other nutrients.
People with lactose intolerance	Calcium supplements
Elderly people	Multivitamin-mineral supplement, vitamin B_{12}

at certain times for various conditions. For instance, some athletes can benefit from consuming foods formulated to provide carbohydrate and other nutrients necessary to support intense exercise. Women at risk for osteoporosis may benefit from taking calcium and vitamin D supplements. Dietary supplements include hundreds of thousands of products sold for many purposes, and it is impossible to discuss here all of the various situations in which these supplements may be needed. To simplify this discussion, let's focus on describing who may or may not benefit from taking vitamin and mineral supplements.

Who Might Benefit from Taking Vitamin and Mineral Supplements?

Contrary to what some people believe, the U.S. food supply is not void of nutrients, and all people do not need to supplement all of the time. In fact, we now know that foods contain a diverse combination of compounds that are critical to our health, and vitamin and

mineral supplements do not contain the same amount or variety of substances found in foods. Thus, dietary supplements are not substitutes for whole foods.

However, there are certain individuals who may benefit from taking vitamin and mineral supplements. Table 8.5 lists various individuals who may benefit from supplementation. It is important to remember that analyzing your total diet is an important first step in determining whether you might need to take a vitamin and mineral supplement. It is always a good idea to check with your healthcare provider or a Registered Dietitian (RD) before taking any supplements, as supplements can interfere with some prescription and over-the-counter medications.

When Can Taking a Vitamin and Mineral Supplement Be Harmful?

You can see from Table 8.5 that there are many people who can benefit from taking vitamin and mineral supplements in certain situations. There are also many

Table 8.6   Ingredients Found in Supplements That Are Associated with Illnesses and Injuries

Ingredient	Potential Risks
Herbal Ingredients:	
Chaparral	Liver disease
Comfrey	Obstruction of blood flow to liver, possible death
Slimming/dieter's teas	Nausea, diarrhea, vomiting, stomach cramps, constipation, fainting, possible death
Ephedra (also known as ma huang, Chinese ephedra, and epitonin)	High blood pressure, irregular heart beat, nerve damage, insomnia, tremors, headaches, seizures, heart attack, stroke, possible death
Germander	Liver disease, possible death
Lobelia	Breathing problems, excessive sweating, rapid heart beat, low blood pressure, coma, possible death
Magnolia-Stephania preparation	Kidney disease, can lead to permanent kidney failure
Willow bark	Reyes syndrome (a potentially fatal disease that may occur when children take aspirin), allergic reaction in adults
Wormwood	Numbness of legs and arms, loss of intellectual processing, delirium, paralysis
Vitamins and Essential Minerals:	
Vitamin A (when taking 25,000 IU or more per day)	Birth defects, bone abnormalities, severe liver disease
Vitamin B_6 (when taking more than 100 mg per day)	Loss of balance, injuries to nerves that alter our touch sensation
Niacin (when taking slow-release doses of 500 mg or more per day, or when taking immediate-release doses of 750 mg or more per day)	Stomach pain, nausea, vomiting, bloating, cramping, diarrhea, liver disease, damage to the muscles, eye, and heart
Selenium (when taking 800 to 1,000 micrograms per day)	Tissue damage
Other Ingredients:	
Germanium (a nonessential mineral)	Kidney damage, possible death
L-tryptophan (an amino acid)	Eosinophilia-myalgia syndrome (a potentially fatal blood disorder that causes high fever, joint and muscle pain, swelling of legs and arms, skin rash, and weakness)

Source: U.S. Food and Drug Administration. 1998. Supplements associated with illnesses and injuries. *FDA Consumer Magazine.* September/October. www.fda.gov/fdac/features/1998/dietchrt.html Accessed August 2002.

people who do not need to take supplements but do so anyway. Instances in which taking vitamin and mineral supplements is unnecessary or harmful include:

1. Providing fluoride supplements to children who already drink fluoridated water.

2. Taking supplements in the belief that they will cure a disease such as cancer, diabetes, or heart disease.

3. Taking supplements with certain medications. For instance, people who take the blood-thinning drug, Coumadin, should not take vitamin E supplements, as this can cause excessive bleeding. People who take aspirin daily should check with their physician before taking vitamin E supplements, as aspirin also thins the blood.

4. Taking nonprescribed supplements if you have liver or kidney diseases. A physician may prescribe vitamin and mineral supplements for their patients because many nutrients are lost during treatment for these diseases. However, these individuals cannot properly metabolize certain supplements and should not take any that are not prescribed by their physician because of a high risk for toxicity.

5. Taking beta-carotene supplements if you are a smoker. As already mentioned, there is evidence

that beta-carotene supplementation increases the risk of lung and other cancers in smokers.

6. Taking vitamins and minerals in an attempt to improve physical appearance or athletic performance. There is no evidence that vitamin and mineral supplements enhance appearance or athletic performance in healthy adults who consume a varied diet with adequate energy.

7. Taking supplements to increase your energy level. Vitamin and mineral supplements do not provide energy, because they do not contain fat, carbohydrate, or protein (sources of calories). Although many vitamins and minerals are necessary for us to produce energy, taking dietary supplements in place of eating food will not provide us with the energy necessary to live a healthy and productive life.

8. Taking single-nutrient supplements, unless a qualified healthcare practitioner prescribes a single-nutrient supplement for a diagnosed medical condition (for example, prescribing iron supplements for someone with anemia). These products contain very high amounts of the given nutrient, and taking these types of products can quickly lead to toxicity.

As advised by the American Dietetic Association (2001), the ideal nutritional strategy for optimizing health is to eat a healthful diet that contains a variety of foods. This way, you will not need to take vitamin and mineral supplements. However, some people may still need to take supplements despite their best efforts. If you do supplement your diet, select a supplement that contains no more than 100% of the recommended levels for the nutrients it contains. Avoid taking single-nutrient supplements unless advised by your healthcare practitioner. Finally, avoid taking supplements that contain substances that are known to cause illness or injuries. Some of these substances are listed in Table 8.6.

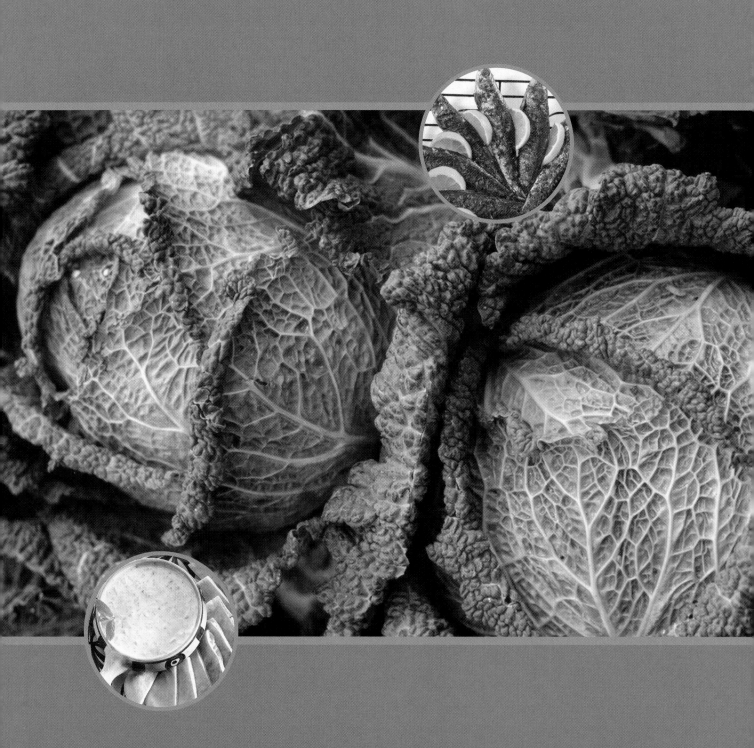

Chapter 9
Nutrients Involved in Bone Health

Chapter Objectives

After reading this chapter you will be able to:

1. Describe the differences between cortical bone and trabecular bone, p. 311.

2. Discuss the processes of bone growth, modeling, and remodeling, pp. 312–313.

3. Describe three methods used to measure bone density, pp. 314–315.

4. List two vitamins and three minerals that play important roles in maintaining bone health, pp. 315–333.

5. Identify foods that are good sources of calcium, pp. 318–319.

6. Describe three potential reasons why consumption of soft drinks may be detrimental to bone health, pp. 328–329.

7. Define osteoporosis, and discuss how it impacts a person's health, pp. 333–334.

8. List three factors that influence our risk for osteoporosis, pp. 334–338.

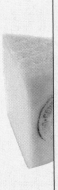

Test Yourself True or False?

1. Most people are unable to consume enough calcium in their diets; therefore, they must take calcium supplements. T or F

2. Osteoporosis is a disease that affects only elderly women. T or F

3. We are capable of making vitamin D within our bodies by using energy obtained from exposure to sunlight. T or F

4. In addition to most dairy products, many green leafy vegetables are good sources of calcium. T or F

5. Cigarette smoking increases a person's risk for osteoporosis. T or F

Test Yourself answers can be found at the end of the chapter.

As a young woman, Erika Goodman leapt across the stage in leading roles with the Joffrey Ballet, one of the premier dance companies in the world. Now in her mid-fifties, she cannot cross a room without assistance. Goodman has a disease called *osteoporosis,* which means "porous bone." As you might suspect, the less dense the bone, the more likely it is to break; indeed, osteoporosis can cause bones to break during even minor weight-bearing activities, such as carrying groceries. In advanced cases, bones in the hip and spine fracture spontaneously, merely from the effort of holding the body erect.

If you are age 20 or older, your bones are already at or close to their peak density. But just how dense are your bones, and what changes can you make right now, no matter what your age, to keep them as strong as possible? What foods build bone? Are there foods that break it down? In this chapter, we discuss the nutrients and lifestyle factors that play a critical role in maintaining bone health.

How Does Our Body Maintain Bone Health?

Contrary to what most people think, our skeleton is not an inactive collection of bones that simply holds our body together. Bones are living organs that contain several tissues, including bone tissue, nerves, cartilage, and connective tissue. Blood vessels supply nutrients to bone to support its activities. Bones have many important functions in our bodies, some of which might surprise you (Table 9.1). For instance, did you know that most of your blood cells are formed deep within your bones?

Given the importance of bones, it is critical that we maintain their health. Bone health is achieved through complex interactions between nutrients, hormones, and environmental factors. To better understand these interactions, we first need to learn about how bone structure and the constant activity of bone tissue influence bone health throughout our lifetime.

Bone Composition and Structure Provide Strength and Flexibility

We tend to think of bones as totally rigid, but if they were, how could we twist and jump our way through a basketball game or even carry an armload of books up a flight of stairs? Our bones need to be both strong and flexible so they can resist the compression, stretching, and twisting that occurs throughout our daily activities. Fortunately, the composition of bone is ideally suited for its complex job: about 65% of bone tissue is made up of an assortment of minerals (mostly calcium and phosphorus) that provide hardness, but the remaining 35% is a mixture of organic substances that provide strength, durability, and flexibility. The most important of these substances is a fibrous protein called **collagen.** You might be surprised to learn that collagen fibers are actually stronger than steel fibers of similar size. Within our bones, the minerals form

collagen A protein that forms strong fibers in bone and connective tissue.

Table 9.1 Functions of Bone in the Human Body

Functions Related to Structure and Support	Functions Related to Metabolic Processes
Bones provide physical support for our organs and body segments.	Bone tissue acts as a storage reservoir for many minerals, including calcium, phosphorus, and fluoride. The body draws upon such deposits when these minerals are needed for various body processes; however, this can reduce bone mass.
Bones protect our vital organs; for example, the rib cage protects our lungs, the skull protects our brains, and the vertebrae in our spine protect our spinal cord.	Most of the blood cells needed by our bodies are produced in the marrow of our bones.
Bones provide support for muscles that allow movement—muscles attach to bones via tendons, and we are able to move all of our joints because of the connections between our muscles and our bones.	

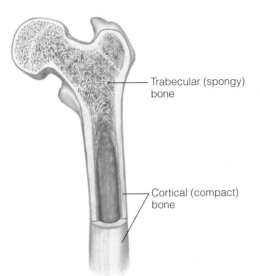

Figure 9.1   The structure of bone. Notice the difference in density between the trabecular (spongy) bone and the cortical (compact) bone.

Trabecular (spongy) bone

Cortical (compact) bone

tiny crystals (called *hydroxyapatite*) that cluster around the collagen fibers. This design enables bones to bear our weight while responding to our demands for movement.

Bone strength and flexibility is also affected by its structure. If you examine a bone very closely, you will notice two distinct types of tissue (Figure 9.1): cortical bone and trabecular bone. **Cortical bone,** which is also called *compact bone,* is very dense. It comprises approximately 80% of our skeleton. The outer surface of all bones is cortical; plus many small bones of the body, such as the bones of the wrists, hands, and feet, are made entirely of cortical bone. Although cortical bone looks solid to the naked eye, it actually contains many microscopic openings that serve as passageways for blood vessels and nerves.

In contrast, **trabecular bone** makes up only 20% of our skeleton. It is found within the ends of the long bones (such as the bones of the arms and legs), inside the spinal vertebrae, inside the flat bones (breastbone, ribs, and most bones of the skull) and inside the bones of the pelvis. Trabecular bone is sometimes referred to as *spongy* (or *cancellous*) *bone* because to the naked eye it looks like a sponge, with no clear organization. The microscope reveals that trabecular bone is in fact aligned in a precise network of columns that protects the bone from extreme stress. You can think of trabecular bone as the scaffolding of the inside of the bone, as it supports the outer cortical bone much like the interior scaffolding of a building supports its outer walls.

Cortical and trabecular bone also differ in their rate of turnover; that is, in how quickly the bone tissue is broken down and replenished. Trabecular bone has a faster turnover rate than cortical bone, meaning that more of the trabecular bone is being broken down and replenished at any given time as compared to cortical bone. This makes trabecular bone more sensitive to changes in hormones and nutritional factors, and we can more easily detect a loss of trabecular bone than we can of cortical bone. It also accounts for the much higher rate of age-related fractures in the spine and pelvis (including the hip)—all of which contain a significant amount of trabecular bone. Let's now investigate how bone turnover, or the constant activity of bone, influences our bone health.

cortical bone (compact bone)   A dense bone tissue that makes up the outer surface of all bones as well as the entirety of most small bones of the body.

trabecular bone (spongy or cancellous bone)   A porous bone tissue that makes up only 20% of our skeleton and is found within the ends of the long bones, inside the spinal vertebrae, inside the flat bones (breastbone, ribs, and most bones of the skull) and inside the bones of the pelvis.

Recap: Bones are organs that contain metabolically active tissues composed primarily of minerals and a fibrous protein called collagen. We have two types of bone, cortical and trabecular. Cortical bone is dense and comprises about 80% of our bone. Trabecular bone is porous in nature and comprises about 20% of our bone. Trabecular bone is more sensitive to hormonal and nutritional factors and turns over more rapidly than cortical bone.

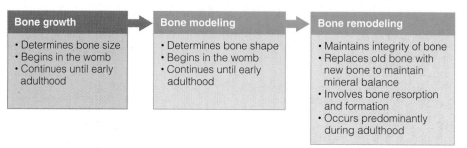

Figure 9.2 Bone develops through three processes: bone growth, bone modeling, and bone remodeling.

The Constant Activity of Bone Tissue Promotes Bone Health

Our bones develop through a series of three processes: bone growth, bone modeling, and bone remodeling (Figure 9.2). Bone growth and modeling begin during the early months of fetal life when our skeleton is forming and continue through infancy, childhood, and adolescence. As a result of this constant activity, the shape and size of our bones is well defined by the time we reach puberty. Bone remodeling predominates during adulthood; this process helps us to maintain a healthy skeleton as we age.

Bone Growth and Modeling Determine the Size and Shape of Our Bones

Through the process of *bone growth,* the size of our bones increases. The first period of rapid bone growth is from birth to age two, but growth continues in spurts throughout childhood and into adolescence. Most girls reach their adult height by age 14, and boys generally reach adult height by age 17 (Ball and Bindler 2003). In the later decades of life, some loss in height usually occurs because of decreased bone density in the spine, as will be discussed shortly.

Bone modeling is the process by which the shape of our bones is determined, from the round "pebble" bones that make up our wrists, to the uniquely shaped bones of our face, to the long bones of our arms and legs. Although our bones stop growing in length by the time we are 18 to 21 years of age, bones can still increase in thickness if they are stressed by excessive or repetitive exercise such as weight training or by being overweight or obese.

Bone Remodeling Maintains a Balance Between Breakdown and Repair

Although the shape and size of our bones do not significantly change after puberty, our **bone density,** or the strength of our bones, continues to develop into early adulthood. *Peak bone density* is the point at which our bones are strongest because they are at their highest density. About 90% of a woman's bone density is built by 17 years of age, whereas the majority of a man's bone density is built during his twenties. However, male or female, before we reach the age of 30 years, our bodies have reached peak bone mass, and we can no longer significantly add to our bone density. In our thirties, our bone density remains relatively stable, but by age 40, it begins its irreversible decline.

Although our bones cannot increase their peak density after our twenties, bone tissue still remains very active throughout adulthood. To preserve bone density to the extent possible, our bodies attempt to achieve a balance between the breakdown of older bone tissue and the formation of new bone tissue. Thus, our bone mass is regularly recycled in a process called **remodeling.** We also use remodeling to repair bone that has been broken or damaged and to strengthen bone regions that are exposed to higher physical stress. The process of remodeling involves two steps: the breakdown of existing bone and the formation of new bone.

bone density The degree of compactness of bone tissue, reflecting the strength of the bones. *Peak bone density* is the point at which a bone is strongest.

remodeling The two-step process by which bone tissue is recycled; includes the breakdown of existing bone and the formation of new bone.

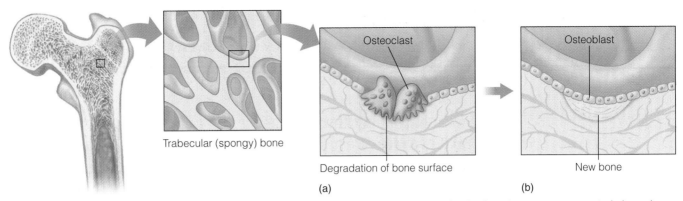

Trabecular (spongy) bone

Osteoclast

Degradation of bone surface

(a)

Osteoblast

New bone

(b)

Figure 9.3 Bone remodeling involves resorption and formation. (**a**) Osteoclasts erode the bone surface by degrading its components, including calcium, other minerals, and collagen; these components are then transported to the bloodstream. (**b**) Osteoblasts work to build new bone by filling the pit formed by the resorption process with new bone.

Bone is broken down through a process referred to as **resorption** (Figure 9.3a). During resorption, cells called **osteoclasts** erode the bone surface by secreting enzymes and acids that dig grooves into the bone matrix. Their ruffled surface also acts much like a scrubbing brush to assist in the erosion process. But why would we ever want to break down our bones? One of the primary reasons is to release calcium into our bloodstream. As discussed in more detail later in this chapter, calcium is critical for many physiological processes, and our bone is an important source of calcium needed to support these processes. We also want to break down bone when we fracture (or break) a bone and need to repair it. Breaking down the damaged bone at the injury site smoothes the rough edges created by the break. We may also break down bone in areas away from the damaged site to obtain the minerals, or raw materials, that are needed to repair the damage caused by the break. Regardless of the reason, once bone is broken down, the resulting products of this breakdown process are transported into the bloodstream and utilized for various body functions.

New bone is formed through the action of cells called **osteoblasts,** or "bone builders" (see Figure 9.3b). These cells work to synthesize new bone matrix by laying down the collagen-containing organic component of bone. Within this substance, the hydroxapatite crystallizes and packs together to create new bone where it is needed.

In young healthy adults, the processes of bone resorption and formation are equal, so that just as much bone is broken down as is built, resulting in bone mass being maintained. Around forty years of age, bone resorption begins to occur more rapidly than bone formation, and this imbalance results in an overall loss in bone density. Because this affects the vertebrae of the spine, we also tend to lose height as we age. As we discuss shortly, achieving a high peak bone mass through proper nutrition and exercise when we are young provides us with a stronger skeleton before we begin to lose bone as we age, and it can be protective against the debilitating effects of osteoporosis.

Recap: The three types of bone activity are growth, modeling, and remodeling. Our bones reach their peak bone mass by our late teenage years and into our twenties; bone mass begins to decline around age 40. Bone is constantly being recycled through a process called remodeling. Remodeling of bone involves the resorption of bone through the action of osteoclasts, and the formation of bone through the action of osteoblasts.

resorption The process by which the surface of bone is broken down by cells called osteoclasts.

osteoclasts Cells that erode the surface of bones by secreting enzymes and acids that dig grooves into the bone matrix.

osteoblasts Cells that prompt the formation of new bone matrix by laying down the collagen-containing component of bone that is then mineralized.

How Do We Assess Bone Health?

Until relatively recently, we had no way to measure the health of bone tissue. Over the past thirty years, however, technologic advancements have led to the development of a number of affordable methods for measuring bone health.

Dual Energy X-Ray Absorptiometry Provides a Measure of Bone Density

dual energy x-ray absorptiometry (DXA or DEXA) Currently the most accurate tool for measuring bone density.

Dual energy x-ray absorptiometry, also referred to as DXA (or DEXA), is considered the most accurate assessment tool for measuring bone density. This method can measure the density of the bone mass over the entire body. Special software is also available that provides an estimation of percent body fat.

The DXA procedure is simple, painless, safe, and non-invasive. The person participating in the test remains fully clothed but must remove all jewelry or other metal objects. The participant lies quietly on a table, and bone density is assessed through the use of a very low level of x-ray (Figure 9.4). The test takes less than 15 minutes for a scan of the hip and lower spine, while a whole-body scan takes about 30 minutes. The level of radiation exposure during a DXA test is much lower than the exposure during a dental x-ray.

DXA is a very important tool to determine a person's risk for osteoporosis. Once someone's bone mineral density is determined, his or her number is compared to the average peak bone density of a 30-year-old healthy adult. Doctors use this comparison, which is known as the **T-score,** to assess the risk of fracture and determine whether or not this person has osteoporosis. A negative T-score indicates lower than normal bone mass. For instance, if the T-score is between –1 and –2.5, this person has low bone mass and is at an increased risk for fractures. If the T-score is more negative than –2.5, this person has osteoporosis. If bone density is normal, the T-score will range between +1 and –1 of the 30-year-old healthy adult value.

T-score A comparison of an individual's bone density to the average peak bone density of a 30-year-old healthy adult.

DXA tests are generally recommended for postmenopausal women because they are at highest risk for osteoporosis and fracture. Men and younger women may also

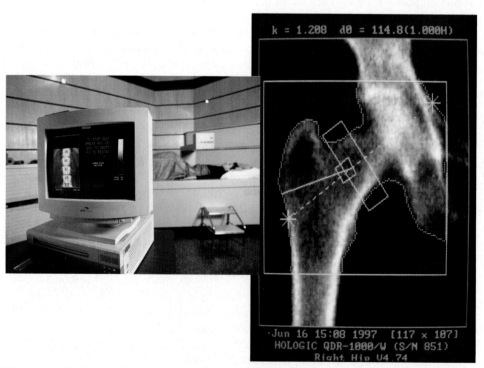

Figure 9.4 Dual energy x-ray absorptiometry is a safe and simple procedure that assesses bone density.

be recommended for a DXA test if they have significant risk factors for osteoporosis (see page 334).

> **Recap:** Dual energy x-ray absorptiometry (DXA or DEXA) is the gold standard measurement of bone mass. It is a simple, safe, and painless procedure. DXA can measure bone mass throughout the entire body. The results of a DXA include a T-score, which is a comparison of your bone density with that of a 30-year-old healthy adult. A T-score between +1 and −1 is normal; a score between −1 and −2.5 indicates poor bone density; and a score more negative than −2.5 indicates osteoporosis.

Other Bone Density Measurement Tools

Three other technologies have been developed to measure bone density. The quantitative ultrasound technique uses sound waves to measure the density of bone in the heel, shin, and kneecap. Peripheral dual energy x-ray absorptiometry, or pDXA, is a form of DXA that measures bone density in the peripheral regions of our bodies including the wrist, heel, or finger. Single energy x-ray absorptiometry is a method that measures bone density at the wrist or heel. These technologies are frequently used at health fairs because the machines are portable and provide scores faster than the traditional DXA. If your results from these tests indicate low bone density, you should contact your physician to schedule a DXA to determine the bone density status of your hip and spine or your full body.

> **Recap:** Quantitative ultrasound, peripheral dual energy x-ray absorptiometry, and single energy x-ray absorptiometry are additional methods that can be used to measure bone density. These methods typically measure the bone density of peripheral sites such as the heel, wrist, or finger.

A Profile of Nutrients That Maintain Bone Health

Calcium is the most recognized nutrient associated with bone health; however, vitamins D and K, phosphorus, magnesium, and fluoride are also essential for strong bones. Let's now learn more about these nutrients and their functions in our bodies.

Calcium

Remember from Chapter 1 that major minerals are those required in our diet in amounts greater than 100 mg per day. Calcium is by far the most abundant major mineral in our body, comprising about 2% of our entire body weight! Not surprisingly, it plays many critical roles in maintaining overall function and health.

Functions of Calcium

One of the primary roles of calcium is to provide structure to our bones and teeth. About 99% of the calcium found in our bodies is stored in our bones. As discussed earlier in this chapter, calcium and phosphorus crystallize to form hydroxyapatite. These crystals pack themselves tightly together and build up on the collagen foundation of bone. This combination of crystals and collagen provide both the characteristic hardness of bone and the flexibility needed to support various activities. Thus, one major role of calcium is to form and maintain bones and teeth.

The remaining 1% of calcium in our bodies is found in the blood and soft tissues. Calcium is alkaline, or basic, and because of this property it plays a critical role in assisting with acid-base balance. We cannot survive for long if our blood calcium level

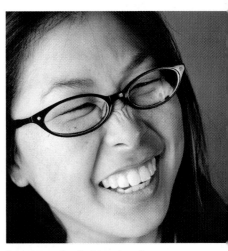

One major role of calcium is to form and maintain bones and teeth.

rises above or falls below a very narrow range; therefore, our body maintains the appropriate blood calcium level at all costs. This means that if we do not consume or absorb enough calcium from our diet, osteoclasts will erode our bones so that calcium can be released into our blood. Thus, our skeleton not only provides physical support to our bodies, but it also acts as a storehouse for calcium to assist in the regulation of blood calcium. However, we need to consume enough calcium in our diet to make sure it balances the calcium we take from our bones so that we can maintain a healthy bone density.

Calcium is also critical for the normal transmission of nerve impulses. Calcium flows into nerve cells and stimulates the release of molecules called neurotransmitters, which transfer the nerve impulses from one nerve cell (neuron) to another. Without adequate calcium, our nerves' ability to transmit messages is inhibited. Not surprisingly, when blood calcium levels fall dangerously low, a person can experience convulsions.

A fourth role of calcium is to assist in muscle contraction. Our muscles are relaxed when calcium levels in the muscle are low. Contraction of our muscles is stimulated by calcium flowing into the muscle cell; conversely, our muscles relax when calcium is pumped back outside of the muscle cell. If calcium levels are inadequate, normal muscle contraction and relaxation is inhibited, and the person may suffer from twitching and spasms. This problem affects the function not only of skeletal muscles, but also of heart muscle, and can cause heart failure.

Other roles of calcium include the maintenance of healthy blood pressure, the initiation of blood clotting, and the regulation of various hormones and enzymes. A summary of the functions, recommended intakes, and toxicity and deficiency symptoms associated with calcium is provided in Table 9.2.

How Much Calcium Should We Consume?

Much attention has recently been given to the fact that many people, particularly women, do not consume enough calcium to maintain bone health. In response to these findings, new DRI values have recently been published for calcium (Institute of Medicine 1997).

Recommended Dietary Intake for Calcium   Calcium requirements, and thus recommended intakes, vary according to age, gender, and whether a woman is pregnant or breastfeeding. There are no RDA values for calcium. The adequate intake (AI) value for adult men and women aged 19 to 50 years is 1,000 mg of calcium per day. For men and women older than 50 years of age, the AI increases to 1,200 mg of calcium per day. The AI for boys and girls aged 15 to 18 years is even higher, being 1,300 mg per day. The upper limit (UL) for calcium is 2,500 mg for all age groups.

bioavailability The degree to which our bodies can absorb and utilize any given nutrient.

The term **bioavailability** refers to the degree to which our bodies can absorb and utilize any given nutrient. The bioavailability of calcium depends in part upon our age and our need for calcium. For example, infants and children can absorb more than 60% of the calcium they consume, as calcium needs are very high during these stages of life. In addition, pregnant and lactating women can absorb about 50% of dietary calcium. In contrast, healthy young adults only absorb about 30% of the calcium consumed in the diet. When our calcium needs are high, the body can generally increase its absorption of calcium from the small intestine. Although older adults have a high need for calcium, the ability to absorb calcium diminishes as we age and can be as low as 25%. Our reduced ability to absorb calcium as we age is primarily due to changes in absorption capacity from the small intestine. This change in calcium absorption with aging was taken into account when calcium recommendations were determined.

The bioavailability of calcium also depends on how much calcium we consume throughout the day or at any one time. When our diets are generally high in calcium, our absorption of calcium is reduced. In addition, our body cannot absorb more than

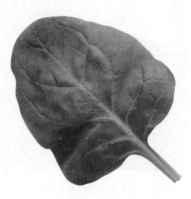

Spinach is a good source of calcium.

Table 9.2 Nutrients Essential to Bone Health

Nutrient	Primary Functions	Recommended Intake	Toxicity Symptoms or Related Diseases	Deficiency Symptoms or Related Diseases
Calcium (major mineral)	Primary component of bone and teeth structure Helps maintain optimal acid-base balance Maintains normal nerve transmission Supports muscle contraction and relaxation Regulates blood pressure, blood clotting, and various hormones and enzymes	Adequate Intake (AI): Men and women aged 19 to 50 years = 1,000 mg/day Men and women aged > 50 years = 1,200 mg/day	Potential mineral imbalances; calcium can interfere with absorption of iron, zinc, and magnesium; shock; kidney failure; fatigue; mental confusion	Osteoporosis: bone fractures; convulsions and muscle spasms; heart failure; bleeder's disease
Vitamin D (fat-soluble vitamin)	Regulates blood calcium levels Maintains bone health Cell differentiation	AI*: Men and women aged 19 to 50 = 5 μg/day Men and women aged 50 to 70 = 10 μg/day Men and women aged > 70 = 15 μg/day	Hypercalcemia, including weakness, loss of appetite, diarrhea, mental confusion, vomiting, excessive urine output, extreme thirst, and formation of calcium deposits in kidney, liver, and heart Increased bone loss	Rickets (in children), leading to bone weakness and deformities Osteomalacia (in adults), leading to bone weakness and increased rate of fractures Osteoporosis, leading to increased rate of fractures
Vitamin K (fat-soluble vitamin)	Serves as a coenzyme during production of specific proteins that assist in blood coagulation and bone metabolism	AI: Men = 120 μg/day Women = 90 μg/day	No known side effects or toxicity symptoms from consuming excess vitamin K	Reduced ability to form blood clots, leading to excessive bleeding and easy bruising Effect on bone health is controversial
Phosphorus (major mineral)	Part of hydroxyapatite crystals, which are the mineral complex of bone Assists in maintaining fluid balance Primary component of ATP Helps activate and inactivate enzymes Component of DNA and RNA Component of cell membranes and lipoproteins	Recommended Dietary Allowance (RDA): Men and women = 700 mg/day	High blood phosphorus levels, causing muscle spasms and convulsions	Low blood phosphorus levels, causing dizziness, bone pain, muscle weakness, and muscle damage
Magnesium (major mineral)	An essential component of bone tissue Influences formation of hydroxyapatite crystals and bone growth Cofactor for over 300 enzyme systems, including ATP, DNA and protein synthesis, vitamin D metabolism and action Supports muscle contraction and blood clotting	RDA: Men aged 19 to 30 = 400 mg/day Men aged > 30 = 420 mg/day Women aged 19 to 30 = 310 mg/day Women aged > 30 = 320 mg/day	No known toxicity symptoms of consuming excess in diet Toxicity from pharmacological use includes diarrhea, nausea, abdominal cramps; in severe cases, massive dehydration, cardiac arrest, and death can result	Hypomagnesemia, resulting in low blood calcium levels, muscle cramps, spasms or seizures, nausea, weakness, irritability, and confusion Chronic diseases such as heart disease, high blood pressure, osteoporosis, and type 2 diabetes
Fluoride (trace mineral)	Maintains health of teeth and bones Protects teeth against dental caries Stimulates new bone growth	Adequate Intake (AI): Men = 4 mg/day Women = 3 mg/day	Teeth fluorosis, which causes staining and pitting of teeth Skeletal fluorosis, which ranges from mild to severe; causes joint pain and stiffness, and in extreme cases can cause crippling, wasting of muscles, and osteoporosis of the extremities	High occurence of dental caries and tooth decay Low fluoride intakes may also be associated with lower bone density

*Based on the assumption that a person does not get adequate sun exposure.

500 mg of calcium at any one time, and as the amount of calcium in a single meal or supplement goes up, the fraction that we absorb goes down. This explains why it is critical to consume calcium-rich foods throughout the day, rather than relying on a single high-dose supplement. Conversely, when dietary intake of calcium is low, we increase our absorption of calcium.

Dietary factors can also affect our absorption of calcium. Binding factors such as phytates and oxalates occur naturally in some calcium-rich seeds, nuts, grains, and vegetables such as spinach and Swiss chard. Such factors bind to the calcium in these foods and prevent their absorption from the intestine. Additionally, consuming calcium at the same time as iron, zinc, magnesium, or phosphorus has the potential to interfere with the absorption and utilization of all of these minerals. Despite these potential interactions, the Institute of Medicine (1997) concluded that at the present time, there is not sufficient evidence to suggest that these interactions cause deficiencies of calcium or other minerals in healthy individuals. However, there are people who are vulnerable to mineral deficiencies, such as elderly or people consuming very low mineral intakes, and more research needs to be done in these populations to determine the health risks associated with interactions between calcium and other minerals.

Finally, because vitamin D is necessary for the absorption of calcium, lack of vitamin D severely limits the bioavailability of calcium. We discuss this and other contributions of vitamin D to bone health shortly (page 322).

Shopper's Guide: Good Food Sources of Calcium   Dairy products are the most common sources of calcium in the United States diet. Skim milk, low-fat cheeses, and nonfat yogurt are excellent sources of calcium, and they are low in fat and calories (Figure 9.5). Ice cream, regular cheese, and whole milk also contain a relatively high amount of calcium, but these foods should be eaten in moderation because of their high fat and energy content. Cottage cheese is one dairy product that is a relatively poor source of calcium, as the processing of this food removes a great deal of the calcium. One cup of low-fat cottage cheese contains approximately 150 mg of calcium, while the same serving of low-fat milk contains almost 300 mg.

Other good sources of calcium are green leafy vegetables such as kale, turnip greens, broccoli, cauliflower, green cabbage, Brussels sprouts, and Chinese cabbage (bok choy). The bioavailability of the calcium in these vegetables is relatively high compared to spinach, as these vegetables contain low levels of oxalates. Many packaged foods are now available fortified with calcium. For example, you can buy calcium-fortified orange juice, soy milk, and tofu processed with calcium. Some dairies have even boosted the amount of calcium in their brand of milk! When you are selecting foods that are good sources of calcium, it is important to remember that we do not absorb 100% of the calcium contained in our foods. For example, although a serving of milk contains approximately 300 mg of calcium, we do not actually absorb this entire amount into our bodies. To learn more about how calcium absorption rates vary for select foods, see the Nutrition Label Activity (page 320).

In general, meats and fish are not good sources of calcium. An exception is canned fish with bones (for example, sardines or salmon), providing you eat the bones. Fruits (except dried figs) and nonfortified grain products are also poor sources of calcium.

Although there are many foods in the U.S. diet that are good sources of calcium, many people in the United States do not consume adequate amounts because they consume very few dairy-based foods. At particular risk are women and young girls. For example, a large national survey conducted by the U.S. Department of Agriculture found that teenage girls consume less than 60% of the recommended amount of calcium (Nusser et al. 1996). If you do not consume enough dietary calcium, you will probably benefit from taking calcium supplements. Refer to the Highlight box on page 321 to learn how to choose a calcium supplement that is right for you.

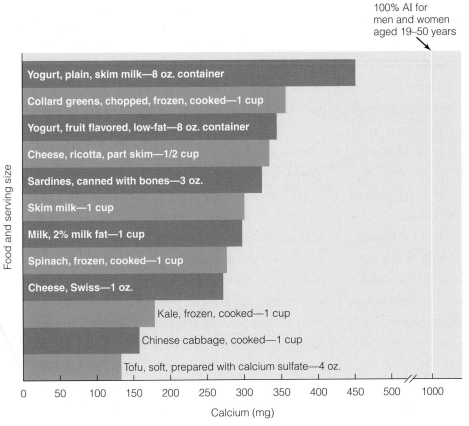

Figure 9.5   Common food sources of calcium. (Nutrient data from U.S. Department of Agriculture, Agricultural Research Service, 2002, USDA Nutrient Database for Standard Reference, Release 15. Nutrient Data Laboratory Home Page, www.nal.usda.gov/fnic/foodcomp Accessed May 2003.)

What Happens If We Consume Too Much Calcium?

In general, consuming too much calcium in the diet does not lead to significant toxicity symptoms in healthy individuals. Much of the excess calcium we consume is not absorbed from the intestine but instead is excreted in our urine and feces. However, excessive intake of calcium from supplements can lead to health problems. As mentioned earlier, one concern with consuming too much calcium is that it can lead to various mineral imbalances because calcium interferes with the absorption of other minerals, including iron, zinc, and magnesium. This interference may only be of major concern in individuals vulnerable to mineral imbalance, such as elderly and people who consume very low amounts of minerals in their diets. In some people, the formation of kidney stones is associated with high intakes of calcium, oxalates, protein, and vegetable fiber (Massey et al. 1993). However, more studies need to be done to determine whether high intakes of calcium actually cause kidney stones.

Various diseases and metabolic disorders can alter our ability to regulate blood calcium. **Hypercalcemia** is a condition in which our blood calcium levels reach abnormally high concentrations. Hypercalcemia can be caused by cancer and also by the overproduction of a hormone called parathyroid hormone (PTH). PTH stimulates the osteoclasts to break down bone and release more calcium into the bloodstream. Symptoms of hypercalcemia include fatigue, loss of appetite, constipation, and mental confusion and can lead to coma and possibly death. Hypercalcemia can also result in an accumulation of calcium deposits in the soft tissues such as the liver and kidneys, causing failure of these organs.

hypercalcemia   A condition marked by an abnormally high concentration of calcium in the blood.

How Much Calcium Am I Really Consuming?

As you have learned in this chapter, we do not absorb 100% of the calcium contained in our foods. This is particularly true for individuals who eat a diet predominated by foods that are high in fiber, oxalates, and phytates, such as whole grains and certain vegetables. Thus it is important to understand how the rate of calcium absorption differs for various foods as you design an eating plan that contains adequate calcium to optimize bone health.

How do you determine the amount of calcium you are absorbing from various foods? Unfortunately, the absorption rate of calcium has not been determined for most foods. However, estimates have been established for a variety of common foods that are considered good sources of calcium. The table below shows some of these foods, their calcium content per serving, the calcium absorption rate, and the estimated amount of calcium absorbed from each food:

Food	Serving Size	Calcium per Serving (mg)[1]	Absorption Rate (%)[2]	Estimated Amount of Calcium Absorbed (mg)
Yogurt, plain skim milk	8 fl. oz.	452	32	145
2% milk	1 cup	298	32	95
Skim milk	1 cup	301	32	95
Kale, frozen cooked	1 cup	179	59	106
Broccoli, frozen, chopped, cooked	1 cup	61	61	37
Spinach, frozen	1 cup	290	5	15

[1]*Source:* U.S. Department of Agriculture, Agricultural Research Service. 2002. USDA Nutrient Database for Standard Reference, Release 15. Nutrient Data Laboratory Home Page. www.nal.usda.gov/fnic/foodcomp Accessed May 2003.

[2]*Sources:* C. M. Weaver, W. R. Proulx, and R. Heaney, Choices for achieving adequate dietary calcium with a vegetarian diet, *Am. J. Clin. Nutr.* 70, 1999, (suppl.) 543S–548S. C. M. Weaver, and K. L. Plawecki, Dietary calcium: adequacy of a vegetarian diet, *Am. J. Clin. Nutr.* 59 1994, (suppl.) 1238S–1241S.

As you can see from this table, many dairy products have a similar calcium absorption rate, just over 30%. Interestingly, many green leafy vegetables have a higher absorption rate of around 60%; however, because a serving of these foods many times contains less calcium than dairy foods, you would have to eat more vegetables to get the same calcium as you would from a standard serving of dairy foods. Note the relatively low calcium absorption rate for spinach, even though it contains a relatively high amount of calcium.

Remember that the DRIs for calcium take these differences in absorption rate into account. Thus, the 300 mg of calcium in a glass of milk counts as 300 mg toward your daily calcium goal. In general, you can trust that dairy products such as milk and yogurt (but not cottage cheese) are good, absorbable sources of calcium, as are most dark green leafy vegetables. Other good sources of calcium with good absorption rates include calcium-fortified orange juice, tofu processed with calcium, and fortified breakfast cereals such as Total and Special K (Keller, Lanou, and Barnard 2002). Armed with this knowledge, you will be better able to select food sources that can optimize your calcium intake and support bone health. ●

What Happens If We Don't Consume Enough Calcium?

There are no short-term symptoms associated with consuming too little calcium. Even when we do not consume enough dietary calcium, our bodies continue to tightly regulate blood calcium levels by taking the calcium from bone. The long-term repercussion of inadequate calcium intake is osteoporosis. This disease is discussed in more detail beginning on page 333.

Hypocalcemia is a term that describes an abnormally low level of calcium in the blood. Hypocalcemia does not result from consuming too little dietary calcium, but is caused by various diseases. Some of the causes of hypocalcemia include kidney disease, vitamin D deficiency, and diseases that inhibit the production of PTH. Symptoms of hypocalcemia include muscle spasms and convulsions.

hypocalcemia A condition characterized by an abnormally low concentration of calcium in the blood.

Calcium Supplements: Which Ones Are Best?

We know that calcium is a critical nutrient for bone health. Ideally, people should try to consume the recommended amount of calcium in their daily diet. But for vegans and other people who avoid dairy products, it may be difficult to get sufficient calcium from the diet. Small or inactive people who eat less to maintain a healthy weight may not be able to consume enough food to provide adequate calcium, and elderly people may need more calcium than they can obtain in their normal diets. In these circumstances, calcium supplements may be warranted.

There are an abundance of calcium supplements available to consumers, but which one is best? Most supplements come in the form of calcium carbonate, calcium citrate, calcium lactate, or calcium phosphate. Our bodies are able to absorb about 30% of the calcium from these various forms. Calcium citrate malate, which is the form of calcium used in fortified juices, is slightly more absorbable at 35%. Many antacids are also good sources of calcium, and it appears these are safe to take as long as you only consume enough to get the recommended level of calcium.

What is the most cost-effective form of calcium? In general, supplements that contain calcium carbonate tend to have more calcium per pill than other types. Thus, you are getting more calcium for your money when you buy this type. However, be sure to read the label of any calcium supplement you are considering taking to determine just how much calcium it contains. Some very expensive calcium supplements do not contain a lot of calcium per pill, and you could be wasting your money. Often, chelated forms of calcium supplements are touted as the best supplements available. Chelate refers to a claw-shaped protein that protects the calcium. Chelated calcium is easier to absorb, as the chelate protects the calcium from inhibitors such as phytates and oxalates that can bind with calcium in our intestine and make it harder to absorb. However, chelated calcium products are typically much more expensive and improve the absorption of calcium only by about 5 to 10%.

The lead content of calcium supplements is an important public health concern. Calcium supplements made from "natural" sources such as oyster shell, bone meal, and dolomite are known to be higher in lead. In fact, many of these products can contain dangerously high levels of lead and should be avoided. We have typically considered calcium supplements that include refined sources of calcium carbonate to be very low in lead. However, a recent study conducted on twenty-two calcium supplements found that eight (or 36%) of the supplements tested were unacceptably high in lead; this was true for oyster shell supplements and refined calcium carbonate (Ross, Szabo, and Tebbett 2000). Shockingly, the supplement with the highest lead content was a popular, nationally recognized brand name supplement! How can we avoid taking supplements that contain too much lead? Unfortunately, the lead content of supplements is not reported on the label. However, there are some supplements available that claim to be lead-free; in the study by Ross et al. (2000), the supplements claiming to be lead-free were found to have no detectable levels of lead. In addition, most supplements not made from oyster shell and other natural products are generally very low in lead. Look for the words "purified" on the label, and make sure the label contains the U.S.P. (U.S. Pharmacopoeia) symbol.

How should we take our supplements? Remember that our bodies cannot absorb more than 500 mg of calcium at any given time. Thus, taking a supplement that contains 1000 mg will be no more effective than one that contains 500 mg calcium. If at all possible, try to consume calcium supplements in small doses throughout the day. In addition, we absorb calcium better with meals, as the calcium stays in our intestinal tract longer during a meal and more calcium can be absorbed. However, it is better to take one calcium supplement outside of meals than to do nothing.

By consuming foods high in calcium every day, we can minimize our need for calcium supplements. When we cannot consume enough calcium in our diets, there are many inexpensive, safe, and effective supplements available. The best supplement for you is the one that you can tolerate, is affordable, and is readily available when you need it.

Recap: Calcium is the most abundant mineral in our bodies. It is a significant component of our bones. Blood calcium is maintained within a very narrow range, and we use our bone calcium to maintain normal blood calcium if dietary intake is inadequate. Calcium is necessary for normal nerve and muscle function. The AI for calcium is 1,000 mg per day for adults aged 19 to 50; the AI increases to 1,200 mg per day for older adults and 1,300 mg per day for adolescents. Dairy products, canned fish with bones, and some green leafy vegetables are good sources of calcium. The most common long-term effect of inadequate calcium consumption is osteoporosis. Hypercalcemia causes fatigue and mental confusion, while hypocalcemia causes muscle spasms and convulsions.

Vitamin D

Vitamin D is like other fat-soluble vitamins in that we store excess amounts in the liver and adipose tissue. But vitamin D is different from other nutrients in two ways. First, vitamin D does not always need to come from the diet. This is because our bodies can synthesize vitamin D using energy from exposure to sunlight. However, when we do not get enough sunlight, we must consume vitamin D in our diet. Second, in addition to being a nutrient, vitamin D is considered a *hormone* because it is made in one part of the body, yet regulates various activities in other parts of the body.

Figure 9.6 illustrates how our body makes vitamin D by converting a cholesterol compound in our skin to the active form of vitamin D that we need to function properly. When the ultraviolet rays of the sun hit our skin, they react with 7-dehydrocholesterol. This cholesterol compound is converted into a precursor of vitamin D, cholecalciferol, which is also called provitamin D_3. This inactive form is then converted to calcidiol in the liver. Calcidiol travels to the kidney where it is converted into **calcitriol,** which is considered the primary active form of vitamin D in our bodies. Calcitriol then circulates to various parts of the body, performing its many functions.

calcitriol   The primary active form of vitamin D in the body.

Functions of Vitamin D

Vitamin D, PTH, and another hormone called *calcitonin* all work together continuously to regulate blood calcium levels, which in turn maintains bone health. They do this by regulating the absorption of calcium and phosphorus from the small intestine, causing more to be absorbed when our needs for them are higher and less when our needs are lower. They also decrease or increase blood calcium levels by signaling the

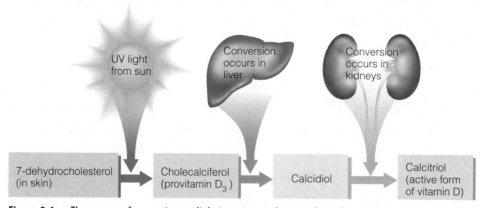

Figure 9.6   The process of converting sunlight into vitamin D in our skin. When the ultraviolet rays of the sun hit our skin, they react with 7-dehydrocholesterol. This compound is converted to cholecalciferol, an inactive form of vitamin D also called provitamin D_3. Cholecalciferol is then converted to calcidiol in the liver. Calcidiol travels to the kidney where it is converted into calcitriol, which is considered the primary active form of vitamin D in our bodies.

kidneys to excrete more or less calcium in our urine. Finally, vitamin D works with PTH to stimulate osteoclasts to break down bone when calcium is needed elsewhere in the body.

Vitamin D is also necessary for the normal calcification of bone; this means it assists the process by which minerals such as calcium and phosphorus are crystallized. Vitamin D may also play some role in decreasing the formation of some cancerous tumors, as it can prevent certain types of cells from growing out of control. Similar to vitamin A, vitamin D appears to play a role in cell differentiation in various tissues. A review of the functions, recommended intakes, and toxicity and deficiency symptoms associated with vitamin D is provided in Table 9.2 (page 317).

How Much Vitamin D Should We Consume?

If your exposure to the sun is adequate, then you do not need to consume any vitamin D in your diet. How do you know whether or not you are getting enough sun?

Recommended Dietary Intake for Vitamin D   As with calcium, there is no RDA for vitamin D. The AI is based on the assumption that an individual does not get adequate sun exposure. Of the many factors that affect our ability to synthesize vitamin D from sunlight, latitude and time of year are most significant (Table 9.3). Individuals living in very sunny climates relatively close to the equator, such as the southern United States and Mexico, may synthesize enough vitamin D from the sun to meet their needs throughout the year—as long as they spend time outdoors. However, vitamin D synthesis from the sun is not possible during most of the winter months for people living in places located at a latitude of more than 40°N or more than 40°S. This is because at these latitudes the sun never rises high enough in the sky during the winter to provide the direct sunlight needed. The 40°N latitude runs like a belt across the United States from northern Pennsylvania in the East to northern California in the West. Thus, people living in New England, New York, the Great Lakes region, or the upper Midwestern to Pacific Northwestern states need to consume vitamin D in the winter. In addition, entire countries such as Canada and the United Kingdom are affected, as of course are countries in the far southern hemisphere. Thus, there are many people around the world who need to consume vitamin D in their diets, particularly during the winter months.

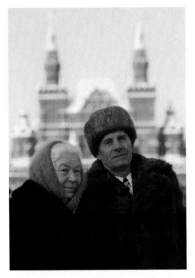

Vitamin D synthesis from the sun is not possible during most of the winter months for people living in high latitudes. Therefore, many people around the world, such as this couple in Russia, need to consume vitamin D in their diets, particularly during the winter.

Table 9.3   Factors Affecting Sunlight-Mediated Synthesis of Vitamin D in the Skin

Factors That Enhance Synthesis of Vitamin D	Factors That Inhibit Synthesis of Vitamin D
Season—Most vitamin D produced during summer months, particularly June and July	Season—Winter months (October through February) result in little or no vitamin D production
Latitude—Locations closer to the equator get more sunlight throughout the year	Latitude—Locations that are more north of 40°N and more south than 40°S get inadequate sun
Time of Day—Generally between the hours of 9 AM and 3 PM (dependent upon latitude and time of year)	Time of Day—Early morning, late afternoon, and evening hours
Age—younger age	Age—older age, particularly elderly (due to reduced skin thickness with age)
Limited or no use of sunscreen	Use of sunscreen with SPF 8 or greater
Sunny weather	Cloudy weather
Exposed skin	Clothing or dark skin pigmentation
	Glass and plastics—windows or other barriers made of glass or plastic (such as Plexiglas) block the sun's rays

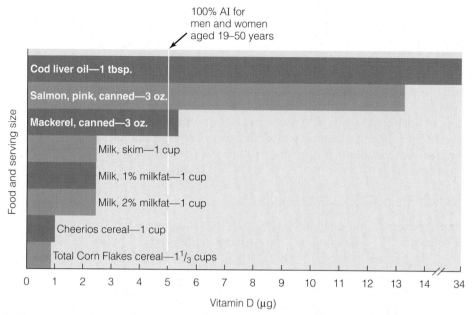

Figure 9.7   Common food sources of vitamin D. (Nutrient data from U.S. Department of Agriculture, Agricultural Research Service, 2002, USDA Nutrient Database for Standard Reference, Release 15. Nutrient Data Laboratory Home Page, www.nal.usda.gov/fnic/foodcomp Accessed May 2003.)

Other factors influencing vitamin D synthesis include time of day and level of exposure. More vitamin D can be synthesized during the time of day when the sun's rays are strongest, generally between 9 AM and 3 PM. Vitamin D synthesis is severely limited or may be non-existent on overcast days. Individuals with darker skin have a more difficult time synthesizing vitamin D from the sun than do light-skinned people. Wearing protective clothing and sunscreen (with an SPF greater than 8) limits sun exposure, so it is suggested that we expose our hands, face, and arms to the sun two to three times per week for a period of time that is one-third to one-half of the amount needed to get sunburned (Holick 1994). This means that if you normally sunburn in one hour, you should expose yourself to the sun for 20 to 30 minutes two to three times per week to synthesize adequate amounts of vitamin D. Again, this guideline does not apply to people living in more northern climates during the winter months; they can only get enough vitamin D by consuming it in their diet.

Because not everyone is able to get adequate sun exposure throughout the year, an AI has been established for vitamin D. For men and women aged 19 to 50 years, the AI for vitamin D is 5 μg per day. Beyond age 50, our need for vitamin D increases: it is estimated that we experience a four-fold decrease in our capacity to synthesize vitamin D from the sun by the time we reach 65 years of age or older (Holick, Matsuoka, and Wortsman 1989; Need et al. 1993). Thus, the AI for vitamin D for men and women aged 50 to 70 years is 10 μg per day, and the AI increases to 15 μg per day for adults over the age of 70 years. The UL for vitamin D is 50 μg per day for all age groups.

You will see the amount of vitamin D expressed on food and supplement labels in units of either μg or IU. For conversion purposes, 1 μg of vitamin D is equal to 40 IU of vitamin D.

ergocalciferol   Vitamin D$_2$, a form of vitamin D found exclusively in plant foods.

cholecalciferol   Vitamin D$_3$, a form of vitamin D found in animal foods and the form we synthesize from the sun.

Shopper's Guide: Good Food Sources of Vitamin D
There are many forms of vitamin D, but only two are active in our bodies. These two forms are vitamin D$_2$, also called **ergocalciferol,** and vitamin D$_3$, or **cholecalciferol.** Vitamin D$_2$ is found exclusively in plant foods, while vitamin D$_3$ is found in animal foods and is also the form of vitamin D we synthesize from the sun.

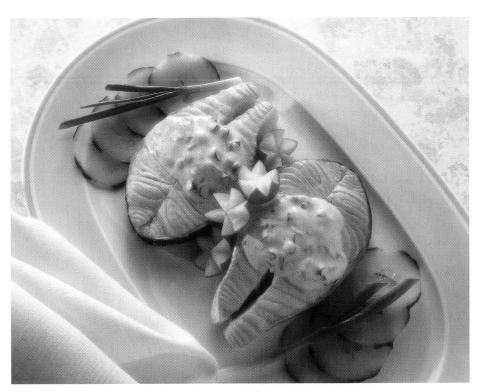

Salmon is one type of food that contains high amounts of vitamin D.

Most foods naturally contain very little vitamin D. Thus, our primary source of vitamin D in the diet is from fortified foods such as milk (Figure 9.7). In the United States, milk is fortified with 10 μg of vitamin D per quart. Interestingly, studies examining the actual vitamin D content of fortified milk found that the amount of vitamin D varies widely. It has been reported that up to 70% of various fortified milks that were sampled did not contain 8 to 12 μg per quart of milk, over half of various samples contained less than 8 μg per quart, while 14% of skim milk samples had no traceable amounts of vitamin D (Chen et al. 1993; Holick et al. 1992). Because of these findings, the USDA now monitors dairies to make sure they meet the mandated vitamin D fortification guidelines.

Other foods that contain high amounts of vitamin D include cod liver oil, fatty fish (such as salmon, mackerel, and sardines), and certain fortified cereals. Eggs, butter, some margarines, and liver contain small amounts of vitamin D, but we would have to eat very large amounts of these foods to consume enough vitamin D. In addition, since plants contain very little vitamin D, vegetarians who consume no dairy products need to obtain their vitamin D from sun exposure, fortified soy or cereal products, or supplements.

What Happens If We Consume Too Much Vitamin D?

We cannot get too much vitamin D from sun exposure, as our skin has the ability to limit its production. The only way we can consume too much vitamin D is through supplementation.

Toxicity symptoms can occur when eating as little as five to ten times the AI. Consuming too much vitamin D causes hypercalcemia, or high blood calcium concentrations. As discussed in the section on calcium, symptoms of hypercalcemia include weakness, loss of appetite, diarrhea, mental confusion, vomiting, excessive urine output, and extreme thirst. Hypercalcemia also leads to the formation of calcium deposits in soft tissues such as the kidney, liver, and heart. In addition, toxic levels of vitamin D lead to increased bone loss because calcium is then pulled from the bones and excreted more readily from the kidneys.

What Happens If We Don't Consume Enough Vitamin D?

The primary deficiency associated with inadequate vitamin D is loss of bone mass. In fact, when vitamin D levels are inadequate, our intestines can only absorb 10 to 15% of the calcium we consume. Vitamin D deficiencies occur most often in individuals who have diseases that cause intestinal malabsorption of fat, and thus the fat-soluble vitamins. People with liver disease, kidney disease, Crohn's disease, celiac disease, cystic fibrosis, or Whipple's disease suffer from vitamin D deficiencies and require supplements.

Vitamin D deficiency disease in children, called **rickets,** is caused by inadequate mineralization or demineralization of the skeleton. The symptoms of rickets include deformities of the skeleton such as bowed legs and knocked knees (Figure 9.8). Rickets is not common in the United States because of fortification of milk products with vitamin D. However, it is still a significant nutritional problem for children outside of the United States.

Vitamin D deficiency disease in adults is called **osteomalacia,** a term meaning "soft bones." With osteomalacia, bones become weak and prone to fractures. Osteoporosis, discussed in detail later in the chapter (page 333), can also result from a vitamin D deficiency.

Vitamin D deficiencies have recently been found to be more common among American adults than previously thought. This may be partly due to jobs and lifestyle choices that keep us indoors for most of the day. Not surprisingly, the population at greatest risk is older institutionalized individuals who get little or no sun exposure.

Various medications can also alter the metabolism and activity of vitamin D. For instance, glucocorticoids, which are medications used to reduce inflammation, can cause bone loss by inhibiting our ability to absorb calcium through the actions of vitamin D. Anti-seizure medications such as phenobarbital and Dilantin alter vitamin D metabolism. Thus, people who are taking such medications may need to increase their vitamin D intake.

> **Recap:** Vitamin D is a fat-soluble vitamin and a hormone. Vitamin D can be made in our skin from the sun. Vitamin D regulates blood calcium levels and maintains bone health. The AI for vitamin D is 5 μg per day for adult men and women aged 19 to 50 years; the AI increases to 15 μg per day for adults over the age of 70 years. Foods contain little vitamin D, with fortified milk being the primary source. Vitamin D toxicity causes hypercalcemia. Vitamin D deficiency causes poor bone density; rickets is vitamin D deficiency in children, while osteomalacia describes vitamin D deficiency in adults. Osteoporosis can also result from vitamin D deficiency.

rickets Vitamin D deficiency disease in children. Symptoms include deformities of the skeleton such as bowed legs and knocked knees.

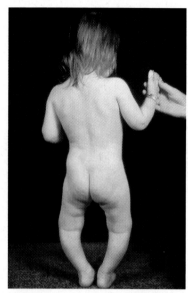

Figure 9.8 A vitamin D deficiency causes a bone-deforming disease in children called rickets.

osteomalacia Vitamin D deficiency disease in adults, in which bones become weak and prone to fractures.

Vitamin K

Vitamin K, a fat-soluble vitamin stored primarily in the liver, is actually a family of compounds known as quinones. **Phylloquinone** is the plant form of vitamin K, while **menaquinone** is the form of vitamin K produced by bacteria found in our large intestine.

Functions of Vitamin K

The primary function of vitamin K is to serve as a coenzyme during the production of specific proteins that play important roles in the coagulation of our blood and in bone metabolism. A **coenzyme** is an organic compound that combines with an inactive enzyme to form an active enzyme. In the case of vitamin K, it assists in the production of *prothrombin,* a protein that plays a critical role in the clotting of our blood. It also assists in the production of *osteocalcin,* a protein that is associated with bone turnover. A summary of the functions, recommended intakes, and toxicity and deficiency symptoms associated with vitamin K is provided in Table 9.2 (page 317).

phylloquinone The form of vitamin K found in plants.

menaquinone The form of vitamin K produced by bacteria in the large intestine.

coenzyme An organic compound that combines with an inactive enzyme to form an active enzyme.

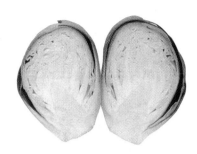

How Much Vitamin K Should We Consume?

We can obtain vitamin K from our diets, and we also produce vitamin K in our large intestine. These two sources of vitamin K usually provide adequate amounts of this nutrient to maintain health.

Recommended Dietary Intake for Vitamin K   There is no RDA for vitamin K. AI recommendations for adult men and adult women are 120 μg per day and 90 μg per day, respectively. No upper limit (UL) has been set for vitamin K.

Shopper's Guide: Good Food Sources of Vitamin K   Only a few foods contribute substantially to our dietary intake of vitamin K. Green leafy vegetables including spinach, collard greens, turnip greens, and lettuce are good sources, as are broccoli, Brussels sprouts, and cabbage. Vegetable oils, such as soybean oil and canola oil, are also good sources of vitamin K. Figure 9.9 identifies the μg per serving for these foods.

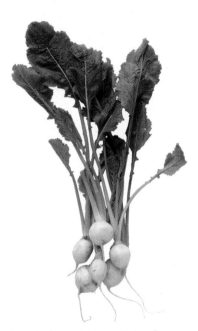

What Happens If We Consume Too Much Vitamin K?

Based on our present knowledge, for healthy individuals there appear to be no side effects associated with consuming large amounts of vitamin K (Institute of Medicine 2002). This appears to be true for both supplements and food sources. In the past, a synthetic form of vitamin K was used for therapeutic purposes and was shown to cause liver damage; thus, this form is no longer used.

What Happens If We Don't Consume Enough Vitamin K?

Vitamin K deficiency is associated with a reduced ability to form blood clots, leading to excessive bleeding; however, primary vitamin K deficiency is rare in humans. People with diseases that cause malabsorption of fat, such as celiac disease, Crohn's disease, and cystic fibrosis, can suffer secondarily from a deficiency of vitamin K. Newborns are typically given an injection of vitamin K at birth, as they lack the intestinal bacteria necessary to produce this nutrient.

The impact of vitamin K deficiency on bone health is controversial. A recent study of vitamin K intake and risk of hip fractures found that women who consumed

Green leafy vegetables, including Brussels sprouts and turnip greens are good sources of vitamin K.

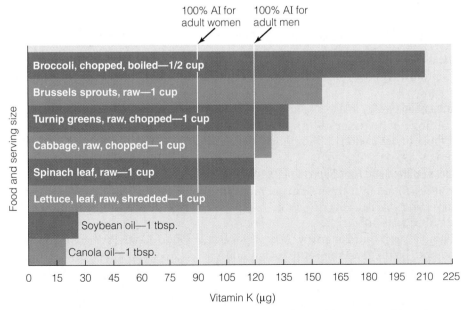

Figure 9.9   Common food sources of vitamin K. (Nutrient data from U.S. Department of Agriculture, Agricultural Research Service, 2002, USDA Nutrient Database for Standard Reference, Release 15. Nutrient Data Laboratory Home Page, www.nal.usda.gov/fnic/foodcomp Accessed May 2003.)

the least amount of vitamin K had a higher risk of bone fractures than women who consumed relatively more vitamin K (Feskanich et al. 1999). Despite the results of this study, there is not enough scientific evidence to support the contention that vitamin K deficiency leads to osteoporosis (Institute of Medicine 2002). In fact, there is no significant impact on overall bone density in people who take anticoagulant medications that result in a relative state of vitamin K deficiency.

> **Recap:** Vitamin K is a fat-soluble vitamin and coenzyme that is important for blood clotting and bone metabolism. We obtain vitamin K largely from bacteria in our large intestine. The AIs for adult men and adult women are 120 µg per day and 90 µg per day, respectively. Green leafy vegetables and vegetable oils contain vitamin K. There are no known toxicity symptoms for vitamin K in healthy individuals. Vitamin K deficiency is rare and may lead to excessive bleeding.

Phosphorus

As discussed in Chapter 7, phosphorus is the major intracellular negatively charged electrolyte. In our bodies, phosphorus is most commonly found combined with oxygen in the form of phosphate (or PO_4^{3-}). Phosphorus is an essential constituent of all cells and is found in both plants and animals.

Functions of Phosphorus

Phosphorus plays a critical role in bone formation, as it is a part of the mineral complex of bone. As discussed earlier in this chapter, calcium and phosphorus crystallize to form hydroxyapatite crystals, which provide the hardness of bone. About 85% of our body's phosphorus is stored in our bones, with the rest stored in soft tissues such as muscles and organs.

The role of phosphorus in maintaining proper fluid balance was discussed in detail in Chapter 7. Phosphorus is also a primary component of adenosine triphosphate (ATP), the energy molecule that fuels body functions. It helps activate and deactivate enzymes, is a component of the genetic material in the nuclei of our cells (including both DNA and RNA), and is a component of our cell membranes and lipoproteins. A summary of the functions, recommended intakes, and toxicity and deficiency symptoms associated with phosphorus is provided in Table 9.2 (page 317).

How Much Phosphorus Should We Consume?

The details of phosphorus recommendations, food sources, and deficiency and toxicity symptoms were discussed in Chapter 7 (page 251). A brief review is provided here.

Recommended Dietary Intake for Phosphorus   The RDA for phosphorus is 700 mg per day (Institute of Medicine 1997). Because the average U.S. adult consumes about twice this amount each day, phosphorus deficiencies are rare.

Shopper's Guide: Good Food Sources of Phosphorus   Phosphorus is widespread in many foods and is found in high amounts in foods that contain protein. Milk, meats, and eggs are good sources. Refer to Table 7.5 (page 252) for a review of the phosphorus content of various foods.

Phosphorus is found in many processed foods as a food additive, where it enhances smoothness, binding, and moisture retention. In the form of phosphoric acid, it is also a major component of soft drinks. Our society has increased its consumption of processed foods and soft drinks substantially over the past twenty years, resulting in an estimated 10 to 15% increase in phosphorus consumption (Institute of Medicine 1997).

Nutrition and medical professionals have become increasingly concerned that the heavy consumption of soft drinks may be detrimental to bone health. Studies have shown that consuming soft drinks is associated with reduced bone mass or an increased risk of fractures in both youth and adults (Wyshak et al. 1989; Wyshak and Frisch 1994; Wyshak 2000). Researchers have proposed three theories to explain why consumption of soft drinks may be detrimental to bone health. These include the following:

- consuming soft drinks in place of calcium-containing beverages, such as milk, leads to a deficient intake of calcium;
- the acidic properties and high phosphorus content of soft drinks cause an increased loss of calcium because calcium is drawn from bone into the blood to neutralize the excess acid; and
- the caffeine found in many soft drinks causes increased calcium loss through the urine.

A recent study of this problem tried to tease out which component of soft drinks may be detrimental to bone health (Heaney and Rafferty 2001). Four different carbonated soft drinks were tested: two that contained phosphoric acid and two that contained citric acid. Two of these drinks also contained caffeine and two did not. Calcium loss was measured as the amount of calcium excreted in the participants' urine. Interestingly, the results showed that the contents of soft drinks had little effect on calcium status. Although the two beverages that contained caffeine caused some loss of calcium during the 5-hour testing period, this effect of caffeine on calcium tends to taper off throughout the day and night, leading to no overall impact on calcium status over a 24-hour period. The researchers concluded that the most likely explanation for the link between soft drink consumption and poor bone health is the *milk-displacement effect;* that is, soft drinks take the place of milk in our diets, depriving us of calcium and vitamin D. Additional nutritional and lifestyle factors that affect bone health are discussed later in this chapter (page 336).

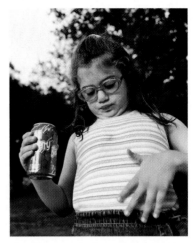

Phosphorus, in the form of phosphoric acid, is a major component of soft drinks.

What Happens If We Consume Too Much Phosphorus?

As discussed in Chapter 7, people with kidney disease and those who take too many vitamin D supplements or too many phosphorus-containing antacids can suffer from high blood phosphorus levels; severely high levels of blood phosphorus can cause muscle spasms and convulsions.

What Happens If We Don't Consume Enough Phosphorus?

Phosphorus deficiencies are rare but can occur in people who abuse alcohol, in premature infants, and in elderly people with poor diets. People with vitamin D deficiency, hyperparathyroidism (oversecretion of parathyroid hormone), and those who overuse antacids that bind with phosphorus may also have low blood phosphorus levels.

Recap: Phosphorus is the major negatively charged electrolyte inside of the cell. It helps maintain fluid balance and bone health. It also assists in regulating chemical reactions, and it is a primary component of ATP, DNA, and RNA. The RDA for phosphorus is 700 mg per day, and it is commonly found in high-protein foods. Excess phosphorus can lead to muscle spasms and convulsion, while phosphorus deficiencies are rare.

Hannah *Nutri-Case*

"After they took the soda vending machines out of my school, they replaced them with ones that sell bottled water and milk. I don't know who they think is going to buy that stuff. As soon as school's out, my friends and I go to the market across the street and buy our sodas and snacks there. Diet cola doesn't have any calories, and it tastes a whole lot better than water or milk!"

From what you know about Hannah, is her habit of drinking a diet cola after school a problem? Why or why not? Imagine that you were her nutrition teacher: what arguments could you use to try to persuade her and her friends to buy a carton of plain or chocolate milk instead of a diet cola?

Magnesium

Magnesium is a major mineral. Our total body magnesium content is approximately 25 grams. About 50 to 60% of the magnesium in our bodies is found in our bones, with the rest located in our soft tissues.

Functions of Magnesium

Magnesium is one of the minerals that make up the structure of bone. It is also important in the regulation of bone and mineral status. Specifically, magnesium influences the formation of hydroxyapatite crystals through its regulation of calcium balance and its interactions with vitamin D and parathyroid hormone.

cofactor Any organic or inorganic compound that combines with an enzyme to make that enzyme active.

Magnesium is a critical *cofactor* for over 300 enzyme systems. A **cofactor** is a compound that is needed for an enzyme to be active. As discussed earlier in this book, a coenzyme is an organic compound that combines with an enzyme to make it active. The term *cofactor* refers to both organic compounds (coenzymes) and inorganic compounds (such as minerals) that combine with enzymes to make them active. Magnesium is necessary for the production of ATP, and it plays an important role in DNA and protein synthesis. Magnesium supports normal vitamin D metabolism and action and is necessary for normal muscle contraction and blood clotting. A review of the functions, recommended intakes, and toxicity and deficiency symptoms associated with magnesium is provided in Table 9.2 (page 317).

How Much Magnesium Should We Consume?

As magnesium is found in a wide variety of foods, people who are adequately nourished generally consume adequate magnesium in their diets.

Recommended Dietary Intake for Magnesium   The RDA for magnesium changes across age groups and genders. For adult men 19 to 30 years of age, the RDA for magnesium is 400 mg per day; the RDA increases to 420 mg per day for men 31 years of age and older. For adult women 19 to 30 years of age, the RDA for magnesium is 310 mg per day; this value increases to 320 mg per day for women 31 years of age and older. There is no UL for magnesium for food and water; the UL for magnesium from pharmacological sources is 350 mg per day.

Shopper's Guide: Good Food Sources of Magnesium   Magnesium is found in green leafy vegetables such as spinach. It is also found in whole grains, seeds, and nuts. Other good food sources of magnesium include seafood, beans, and some dairy products. Figure 9.10 shows many foods that are good sources of magnesium. Refined and processed foods are low in magnesium.

The magnesium content of drinking water varies considerably. The "harder" the water, the higher its content of magnesium. This large variability in the magnesium content of water makes it impossible to estimate how much our drinking water may contribute to the magnesium content of our diets.

The ability of our small intestine to absorb magnesium is reduced when we consume diets that are very high in fiber and phytates because these substances bind with magnesium. Beans, seeds, nuts, and whole grains are high in both fiber and phytates. Our absorption of magnesium should be sufficient if we consume the recommended amount of fiber each day (20 to 35 grams per day). In contrast, higher dietary protein intakes enhance the absorption and retention of magnesium.

What Happens If We Consume Too Much Magnesium?

There are no known toxicity symptoms related to consuming excess magnesium in the diet. The toxicity symptoms that result from pharmacological use of magnesium include diarrhea, nausea, and abdominal cramps. In extreme cases, large doses can result in acid-base imbalances, massive dehydration,

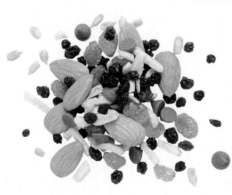

Trail mix with chocolate chips, salted nuts, and seeds is one common food source of magnesium.

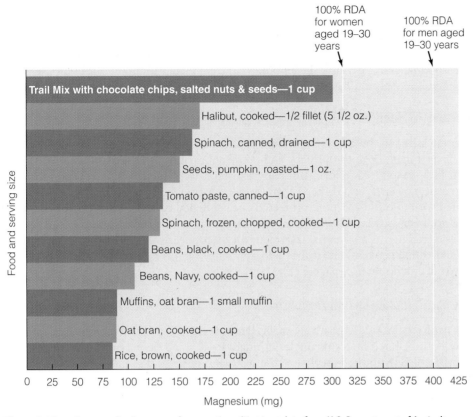

Figure 9.10 Common food sources of magnesium. (Nutrient data from U.S. Department of Agriculture, Agricultural Research Service, 2002, USDA Nutrient Database for Standard Reference, Release 15. Nutrient Data Laboratory Home Page, www.nal.usda.gov/fnic/foodcomp Accessed May 2003.)

cardiac arrest, and death. High blood magnesium levels, or **hypermagnesemia,** occur in individuals with impaired kidney function who consume large amounts of non-dietary magnesium, such as antacids. Side effects include impairment of nerve, muscle, and heart function.

What Happens If We Don't Consume Enough Magnesium?

Hypomagnesemia, or low blood magnesium, results from magnesium deficiency. This condition may result from kidney disease, chronic diarrhea, or chronic alcohol abuse. Elderly people seem to be at particularly high risk of low dietary intakes of magnesium because they have a reduced appetite and blunted senses of taste and smell. In addition, elderly face challenges related to shopping and preparing meals that contain foods high in magnesium, and their ability to absorb magnesium is reduced.

Low blood calcium levels are a side effect of hypomagnesemia. Other symptoms of magnesium deficiency include muscle cramps, spasms or seizures, nausea, weakness, irritability, and confusion. Considering magnesium's role in bone formation, it is not surprising that long-term magnesium deficiency is associated with osteoporosis. Magnesium deficiency is also associated with many other chronic diseases, including heart disease, high blood pressure, and type 2 diabetes (Institute of Medicine 1997).

Recap: Magnesium is a major mineral found in fresh foods, including spinach, nuts, seeds, whole grains, and meats. Magnesium is important for bone health, energy production and muscle function. The RDA for magnesium is a function of age and gender. Hypermagnesemia can result in diarrhea, muscle cramps, and cardiac arrest. Hypomagnesemia causes hypocalcemia, muscle cramps, spasms, and weakness. Magnesium deficiencies are also associated with osteoporosis, heart disease, high blood pressure, and type 2 diabetes.

hypermagnesemia A condition marked by an abnormally high concentration of magnesium in the blood.

hypomagnesemia A condition characterized by an abnormally low concentration of magnesium in the blood.

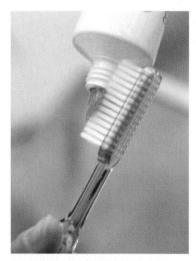

Fluoride is readily available in many communities in the United States through fluoridated water and dental products.

fluorohydroxyapatite A mineral compound in human teeth which contains fluoride, calcium, and phosphorus and is more resistant to destruction by acids and bacteria than hydroxyapatite.

Fluoride

Fluoride is the ionic form of the element fluorine, and it is also a trace mineral. As discussed in Chapter 1, trace minerals are minerals that our body needs in amounts less than 100 milligrams per day; the amount of trace minerals found in our bodies is less than 5 grams. About 99% of the fluoride in our bodies is stored in our teeth and bones.

Functions of Fluoride

Fluoride assists in the development and maintenance of our teeth and bones. During the development of both our baby and permanent teeth, fluoride combines with calcium and phosphorus to form **fluorohydroxyapatite,** which is more resistant to destruction by acids and bacteria than hydroxyapatite. Thus, teeth that have been treated with fluoride are more protected against dental caries (cavities) than teeth that have not been treated. Fluoride also stimulates new bone growth, and it is currently being researched as a potential treatment for osteoporosis. A review of the functions, recommended intakes, and toxicity and deficiency symptoms associated with fluoride is provided in Table 9.2 (page 317).

How Much Fluoride Should We Consume?

Our need for fluoride is relatively small. Fluoride is readily available in many communities in the United States through fluoridated water and dental products. Fluoride is absorbed directly in the mouth into the teeth and gums and can also be absorbed from the gastrointestinal tract once it is ingested. In the early 1990s, there was considerable concern that our intake of fluoride was too high and could be contributing to an increased risk for cancer, bone fractures, kidney and other organ damage, infertility, and Alzheimer's disease. After reviewing the potential health hazards of fluoride, the U.S. Department of Health and Human Services (1991) found that there is no reliable scientific evidence available to indicate that fluoride increases our risk for these illnesses. Currently there are concerns that individuals who consume bottled water exclusively may be consuming too little fluoride and increasing their risk for dental caries, as most bottled waters do not contain fluoride.

Recommended Dietary Intake for Fluoride   There is no RDA for fluoride. The AI for fluoride for children aged 4 to 8 years is 1 mg per day; this value increases to 2 mg per day for boys and girls aged 9 to 13 years. The AI for boys and girls aged 14 to 18 years is 3 mg per day. The AI for adults is 4 mg per day for adult men and 3 mg per day for adult women. The UL for fluoride is 2.2 mg per day for children aged 4 to 8 years; the UL for everyone older than 8 years of age is 10 mg per day

fluorosis A condition marked by staining and pitting of the teeth; caused by an abnormally high intake of fluoride.

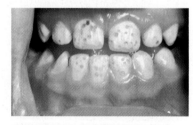

Figure 9.11   Consuming too much fluoride causes fluorosis, leading to staining and pitting of the teeth.

Shopper's Guide: Good Food Sources of Fluoride   The two primary sources of fluoride for people in the United States are fluoridated dental products and fluoridated water. People who live in communities that do not have fluoridated water may still consume fluoride through beverages that contain fluoridated water and through fluoridated dental products. Toothpastes and mouthwashes that contain fluoride are widely marketed and used by the majority of consumers in the United States, and these products can contribute as much if not more fluoride to our diets than fluoridated water. Fluoride supplements are available only by prescription, and these are generally only given to children who do not have access to fluoridated water.

What Happens If We Consume Too Much Fluoride?

Consuming too much fluoride increases the protein content of tooth enamel, resulting in a condition called **fluorosis.** Because increased protein makes the enamel more porous, the teeth become stained and pitted (Figure 9.11). Teeth seem to be at highest risk for fluorosis during the first eight years of life. Mild fluorosis generally causes white patches on the teeth, and it has no effect on tooth function. Although moderate and severe fluorosis cause greater discoloration of the teeth, there appears to be no adverse effect on tooth function (Institute of Medicine 1997).

Excess consumption of fluoride can also cause fluorosis of our skeleton. Mild skeletal fluorosis results in an increased bone mass and stiffness and pain in the joints. Moderate and severe skeletal fluorosis can be crippling, leading to severe joint pain and stiffness, abnormal hardening of the bones in the pelvis and vertebrae, osteoporosis in the extremities, and wasting of the muscles. Severe skeletal fluorosis is extremely rare in the United States, with only five confirmed cases in the last thirty-five years (Institute of Medicine, 1997).

What Happens If We Don't Consume Enough Fluoride?

The primary result of fluoride deficiency is dental caries. Adequate fluoride intake appears necessary at an early age and throughout our adult life to reduce our risk for tooth decay. Inadequate fluoride intake may also be associated with lower bone density, but there is not enough research currently available to support the widespread use of fluoride to prevent osteoporosis. Studies are currently being done to determine the role fluoride might play in reducing our risk for osteoporosis and fractures.

> **Recap:** Fluoride is a trace mineral whose primary function is to support the health of teeth and bones. The AI for fluoride is 4 and 3 mg per day for adult men and women, respectively. Primary sources of fluoride are fluoridated dental products and fluoridated water. Fluoride toxicity causes fluorosis of the teeth and skeleton, while fluoride deficiency causes an increase in tooth decay.

What Disorders Can Result from Poor Bone Health?

Of the many disorders associated with poor bone health, the most prevalent in the United States is osteoporosis. In addition to osteoporosis, a few other disorders related to poor bone health are introduced in this section.

Osteoporosis

Osteoporosis is a disease characterized by low bone mass and deterioration of bone tissue, leading to enhanced bone fragility and increase in fracture risk. The bone tissue of a person with osteoporosis is more porous and thinner than that of a person with healthy bone. These structural changes weaken the bone, leading to a significantly reduced ability of the bone to bear weight (Figure 9.12).

As mentioned earlier in this chapter, the hip and the vertebrae of the spinal column are common sites of osteoporosis; thus, it is not surprising that osteoporosis is the single most important cause of fractures of the hip and spine in older adults. These fractures are extremely painful and can be debilitating, with many individuals requiring nursing home care. In addition, they cause an increased risk of infection and other related illnesses that can lead to premature death. In fact, it is estimated that in the United States and Europe up to 130,000 people will die each year as a direct result of osteoporosis-related hip fractures (International Osteoporosis Foundation 2003). Osteoporosis of the spine also causes a generalized loss of height and can be disfiguring: gradual compression fractures in the vertebrae of the upper back lead to a shortening and hunching of the spine, commonly referred to as *dowager's hump*.

Unfortunately, osteoporosis is a common disease: worldwide, one in three women and one in eight men are affected (International Osteoporosis Foundation 2003), and in the United States, more than 10 million people have been diagnosed (National Osteoporosis Foundation 2002). Factors that influence our risk for osteoporosis include age, gender, genetics, nutrition, and physical activity (Table 9.4).

osteoporosis A disease characterized by low bone mass and deterioration of bone tissue, leading to increased bone fragility and fracture risk.

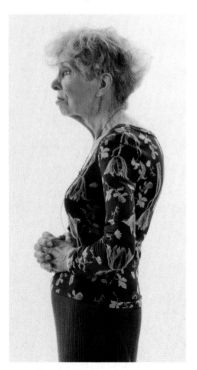

80% of Americans with osteoporosis are women.

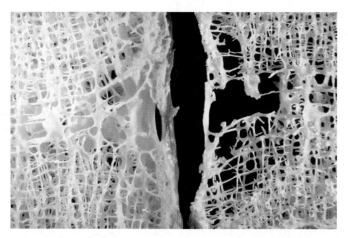

Figure 9.12 The vertebrae of a person with osteoporosis (right) are thinner and more collapsed than the vertebrae of a healthy person, in which the bone is more dense and uniform (left).

Table 9.4 Risk Factors for Osteoporosis

Modifiable Risk Factors	Nonmodifiable Risk Factors
Smoking	Older age (elderly)
Low body weight	Caucasian or Asian race
Low calcium intake	History of fractures as an adult
Low sun exposure	Family history of osteoporosis
Alcohol abuse	Female
History of amenorrhea (failure to menstruate) in women with inadequate nutrition	History of amenorrhea (failure to menstruate) in women with no recognizable cause
Estrogen deficiency (females)	
Testosterone deficiency (males)	
Repeated falls	
Sedentary lifestyle	

Source: Table adapted from J. L. Milott, S. S. Green, and M. M. Schapira, Osteoporosis: evaluation and treatment, *Comp. Ther.* 26 (2000):183–189. Copyright © 2000 American Society of Contemporary Medicine and Surgery. Reprinted with permission.

Let's review these factors and discuss how we can change our lifestyle to reduce our risk for osteoporosis.

The Impact of Aging on Osteoporosis Risk

As discussed previously in this chapter, bone density declines as we age. Low bone mass and osteoporosis are therefore significant health concerns for both older men and women. Figure 9.13 illustrates how the prevalence of osteoporosis and low bone mass are predicted to increase in the United States over the next 20 years. This is primarily due to increased longevity: as the U.S. population ages, more people will live long enough to suffer from osteoporosis.

Hormonal changes that occur with aging have a significant impact on bone loss. Average bone loss approximates 0.3 to 0.5% per year after 30 years of age; however, during menopause in women, levels of the hormone estrogen decrease dramatically and cause bone loss to increase to about 3% per year during the first five years of menopause. Both estrogen and testosterone play important roles in promoting the deposition of new bone and limiting the activity of osteoclasts. Thus, men can also

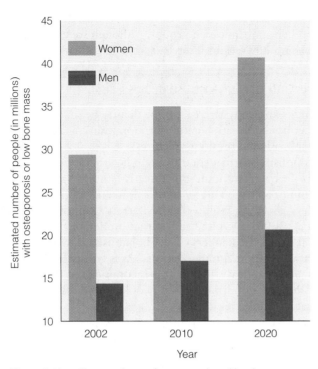

Figure 9.13   The prevalence of osteoporosis and low bone mass are predicted to steadily increase over the next twenty years in both men and women in the United States. (Adapted from National Osteoporosis Foundation, www.nof.org/advocacy/prevalence/ index.htm Accessed November 2002.)

suffer from osteoporosis caused by age-related decreases in testosterone. In addition, reduced levels of physical activity in older people and a decreased ability to metabolize vitamin D with age exacerbate the hormone-related bone loss.

Gender and Genetics Affect Osteoporosis Risk

Osteoporosis disproportionately affects women: 80% of Americans with osteoporosis are women. There are three primary reasons for this.

- Adult women have a lower absolute bone density than men. From birth through puberty, bone mass is the same in girls as in boys. But during puberty, bone mass increases more in boys, probably because of their prolonged period of accelerated growth. Thus, when bone loss begins around age 40, women have less bone stored in their skeleton than men. Since a woman's skeleton is already less dense, the loss of bone that occurs with aging causes osteoporosis sooner and to a greater extent in women than in men.

- As we have discussed, the hormonal changes that occur in men as they age do not have as dramatic an effect on bone density as those for women.

- Women live longer than men, and since risk increases with age, more elderly women suffer from this disease.

Secondary factors that are gender-specific include social pressure on girls to be extremely thin. Extreme dieting is particularly harmful in adolescence, when bone mass is building and adequate consumption of calcium and other nutrients is critical. In many girls, weight loss causes both a loss of estrogen and reduced weight-bearing stress on the bones. In contrast, men experience pressure to "bulk up," typically by lifting weights. This puts healthful stress on the bones, resulting in increased density.

Some individuals have a family history of osteoporosis, which increases their risk for this disease. Particularly at risk are Caucasian women of low body weight who have

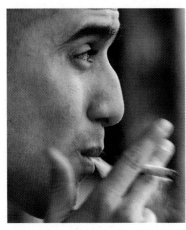

Smoking increases our risk for osteoporosis and resulting fractures.

a first degree relative (mother or sister) with osteoporosis. Asian women are also at higher risk than other non-Caucasian groups. Although we cannot change our gender or genetics, we can modify various lifestyle factors that affect our risk for osteoporosis.

Smoking and Poor Nutrition Increase Osteoporosis Risk

Cigarette smoking is known to decrease bone density because of its effects on hormones that impact bone formation and resorption; thus, cigarette smoking increases our risk for osteoporosis and resulting fractures.

Chronic alcoholism is detrimental to bone health and is associated with high rates of fractures. In contrast, numerous research studies have shown that bone density is higher in people who are *moderate* drinkers (Laitinen, Valimaki, and Keto 1991; Feskanich et al. 1999; Holbrook and Barrett-Connor 1993; Felson et al. 1995; Rapuri et al. 2000). Despite the fact that moderate alcohol intake may be protective for our bone, the dangers of alcohol abuse on overall health warrant caution in making any dietary recommendations. As is consistent with the alcohol recommendations related to heart disease, it is recommended that people should not start drinking if they are nondrinkers, and people who do drink should not consume more than two drinks per day.

Some researchers consider excess caffeine consumption to be detrimental to bone health. Caffeine is known to increase calcium loss in our urine, at least over a brief period of time. Younger people are able to compensate for this calcium loss by increasing absorption of calcium from the intestine. However, older people are not always capable of compensating to the same degree. Although the findings have been inconsistent, recent research now indicates that the relative amounts of caffeine and calcium consumed are critical factors affecting bone health. In general, elderly women do not appear to be at risk for increased bone loss if they consume adequate amounts of calcium and moderate amounts of caffeine (equal to less than two cups of coffee, four cups of tea, or six 12-ounce cans of caffeine-containing soft drinks per day) (Massey 2001). Elderly women who consume high levels of caffeine (more than three cups of coffee per day) have much higher rates of bone loss than women with low intakes (Rapuri et al. 2001). Thus, it appears important to bone health that we moderate our caffeine intake and ensure adequate consumption of calcium in our diets.

The effect of high dietary protein intake on bone health is controversial. While it is well established that high protein intakes increase calcium loss, protein is a critical component of bone tissue and is necessary for bone health. High protein intakes have been shown to have both a negative and positive impact on bone health. Similar to caffeine, the key to this mystery appears to be adequate calcium intake. Elderly individuals taking calcium and vitamin D supplements and eating higher protein diets were able to significantly increase bone mass over a 3-year period, while those eating more protein and not taking supplements lost bone mass over this same time period (Dawson-Hughes and Harris 2002). Low protein intakes are also associated with bone loss and increased risk for osteoporosis and fractures in elderly people. Thus, there appears to be an interaction between dietary calcium and protein, in that adequate amounts of each nutrient are needed together to support bone health.

As you've learned, a multitude of nutrients play critical roles in maintaining bone health. Of these nutrients, calcium and vitamin D have received the most attention regarding their role in the prevention of osteoporosis. Research studies conducted with older individuals have shown that their risk of bone fractures is reduced by taking calcium and vitamin D supplements. We know that if people do not consume enough of these two nutrients over a prolonged period of time, their bone density is lower and they have a higher risk of bone fractures. Because our bones reach peak density when we are young, it is very important that children and adolescents consume a high-quality diet that contains the proper balance of calcium, vitamin D, protein, and other nutrients to allow for optimal bone growth. Young adults also require a proper balance of these nutrients to maintain bone mass. In older adults, diets rich in calcium and vitamin D can help minimize bone loss.

In addition to their role in reducing our risk for heart disease and cancer, diets high in fruits and vegetables are also associated with improved bone health (Tucker et al. 1999; Tucker et al. 2002). This is most likely due to the fact that fruits and vegetables are good sources of nutrients that play a role in bone and collagen health, including magnesium, vitamin C, and vitamin K.

The Impact of Physical Activity on Osteoporosis Risk

Regular exercise is highly protective against bone loss and osteoporosis. Athletes are consistently shown to have more dense bones than non-athletes, and regular participation in weight-bearing exercises such as walking, jogging, tennis, and strength training can help us increase and maintain our bone mass. When we exercise, our muscles contract and pull on our bones; this stresses our bone tissue in a healthful way that stimulates increases in bone density. In addition, carrying our weight during activities such as walking and jogging stresses the bones of our legs, hips, and lower back, resulting in a healthier bone mass in these areas. It appears that people of all ages can improve and maintain bone health by consistent physical activity.

Can exercise ever be detrimental to bone health? Yes, when the body is not receiving the nutrients it needs to rebuild the hydoxyapatite and collagen broken down in response to physical activity. Thus, active people who are chronically malnourished, including people who are impoverished and those who suffer from eating disorders, are at increased fracture risk. Research has confirmed this association between nutrition, physical activity, and bone loss in the **female athlete triad,** a condition characterized by the coexistence of three (or a *triad* of) disorders in some athletic females: an eating disorder, amenorrhea, and osteoporosis. In the female athlete triad, inadequate food intake and regular strenuous exercise together result in a state of severe energy drain that causes a multitude of hormonal changes that impact menstrual function, including a reduction in estrogen production. These hormonal changes can result in the complete loss of menstrual function, called *amenorrhea*. As you have learned, estrogen is also important to maintaining healthy bone in women, so the loss of estrogen leads to osteoporosis in young women. The female athlete triad is discussed in more detail in Chapter 13.

female athlete triad A condition characterized by the co-existence of three disorders in some athletic females: an eating disorder, amenorrhea, and osteoporosis.

Gustavo *Nutri-Case*

"When my wife, Antonia, fell and broke her hip, I was shocked. You see, the same thing happened to her mother, but she was an old lady by then! Antonia's only 68, and she still seems young and beautiful—at least to me! As soon as she's better, her doctor wants to do some kind of scan to see how thick her bones are. But I don't think she has that disease everyone talks about! She's always watched her weight and keeps active with our kids and grandchildren. It's true she likes her coffee and diet colas, and doesn't drink milk, but that's not enough to make a person's bones fall apart, is it?"

Study Table 9.4 (page 334). What risk factors do *not* apply to Antonia? What risk factors do? Given what Gustavo has said about his wife's nutrition and lifestyle, would you suggest he encourage her to have a DXA test? Why or why not?

Treatments for Osteoporosis

While there is no cure for osteoporosis, a variety of treatments can slow and even reverse bone loss. First, individuals with osteoporosis are encouraged to consume adequate calcium and vitamin D and to exercise regularly. Studies have shown that the most effective exercise programs include weight-bearing exercises such as jogging, stair climbing, and resistance training (South-Pal 2001).

In addition, several **anti-resorptive** medications are available; such medications slow or stop bone resorption but do not affect bone formation. This results in an

anti-resorptive Characterized by an ability to slow or stop bone resorption without affecting bone formation. Anti-resorptive medications are used to reduce the rate of bone loss in people with osteoporosis.

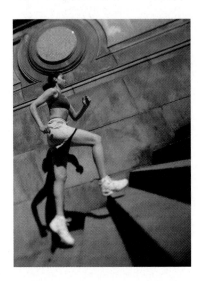

Regular weight-bearing exercises such as jogging can help us increase and maintain our bone mass.

overall reduction or cessation in the rate of bone loss in people with osteoporosis. As various side effects are associated with each of these medications, patients must work closely with their physician to decide which is most appropriate.

Estrogen replacement therapy (ERT) and *hormone replacement therapy (HRT)* can be used for the prevention of osteoporosis in women. There are many brand names associated with these drugs, including Premarin and Prempro. ERT reduces bone loss, increases bone density, and reduces the risk of hip and spinal fractures. One major drawback of ERT is that taking estrogen alone increases a woman's risk for endometrial cancer, which is a cancer of the lining of the uterus. HRT combines estrogen with a hormone called progestin, greatly reducing the risk of endometrial cancer. Side effects of both ERT and HRT include breast tenderness, changes in mood, vaginal bleeding, and an increased risk for gallbladder disease.

Until recently, it was believed that HRT protected women against heart disease. A recent study found that one type of HRT actually increases a woman's risk for heart disease, stroke, and breast cancer. As a result, hundreds of thousands of women in the United States have recently quit taking HRT as a means to prevent or treat osteoporosis. The controversy surrounding HRT is discussed in detail in the Nutrition Debate Box at the end of this chapter.

Alendronate (brand name Fosamax) and risedronate (brand name Actonel) are approved for the prevention and treatment of osteoporosis. These drugs decrease bone loss, increase bone density, and reduce the risk of spinal and nonspinal fractures. Side effects are not common and include abdominal or musculoskeletal pain, nausea, diarrhea, constipation, gas, heartburn, and irritation of the esophagus. These drugs must be taken in the morning on an empty stomach, at least 30 minutes before eating, drinking, or taking any other medications, and must be taken with 8 ounces of water and no other liquid. In addition, the person taking these drugs must stay upright during the 30 minutes following drug administration.

Raloxifene (brand name Evista) is a drug that was developed to mimic the beneficial effects of estrogen without the potential risks and is used for the prevention and treatment of osteoporosis. It increases bone mass and reduces the risk of spinal fractures while apparently reducing the risk of some forms of breast cancer. It may even reduce the risk of heart disease and stroke in women who have a high risk for these diseases. Side effects are not common and include hot flashes and the formation of blood clots in the veins.

Calcitonin (brand name Miacalcin) is a hormone that occurs naturally in our bodies and assists in the regulation of calcium and in bone metabolism. When used in the treatment of osteoporosis, calcitonin slows bone loss, increases the bone density of the spine, and reduces the risk for spinal fractures. Calcitonin is a protein; thus, it cannot be taken orally or it would be digested in our intestinal tract. It therefore must be injected or inhaled through a nasal spray. Side effects of injected calcitonin include allergic reactions, flushing of the face and hands, skin rash, increased need to urinate, and nausea. Side effects of nasal calcitonin include nasal irritation, bloody nose, headaches, and backaches.

Recap: Osteoporosis is a major disease of concern for elderly in the United States. Osteoporosis increases our risk for fractures and premature death from subsequent illness. Factors that increase our risk for osteoporosis include genetics, being female, being of the Caucasian or Asian race, cigarette smoking, alcohol abuse, sedentary lifestyle, and diets low in calcium and vitamin D. Medications are available for the prevention and treatment of osteoporosis.

Other Bone Health Disorders

In addition to osteoporosis, there are other disorders of bone that are debilitating and increase the risk for fractures. Two of these disorders, Paget's disease and osteogenesis imperfecta, are discussed briefly here.

Paget's disease is characterized by excessive breakdown and formation of bone tissue, causing bones to enlarge, weaken, become deformed, and eventually fracture. It typically occurs in people over the age of forty who have family members with this disease. Symptoms of Paget's disease include bone pain that is often localized in areas near the joints, loss of hearing, headaches, increased head size, bowed limbs, curvature of the spine, hip pain, and damage to the cartilage of the joints that leads to arthritis. In many cases, people do not know they have Paget's disease because they have a mild form or they confuse their symptoms with those of arthritis or other disorders. Paget's disease can lead to other diseases such as arthritis, loss of hearing, heart disease, kidney stones, loosening of the teeth, some loss of vision, and in rare cases, a form of bone cancer called osteogenic sarcoma. Paget's disease does not cause osteoporosis, but a person can suffer from both diseases.

The disease is treatable but not curable. Medications such as bisphosphonates and calcitonin are used to treat Paget's disease, and some individuals also require surgery. For more information on Paget's disease, refer to the Web site of the Osteoporosis and Related Bone Diseases—National Resource Center (National Institutes of Health) at www.osteo.org.

Osteogenesis imperfecta (OI), or "brittle bones" is a genetic disorder affecting 20,000 to 50,000 people in the U.S. It is caused by a genetic defect that affects collagen production. People with OI either have less collagen, or their collagen is of a poorer quality. The result is bones that break very easily, often from no apparent cause. The severity of this disorder is highly variable: one person may suffer only a few broken bones, while another person may have hundreds of fractures throughout his or her life. In addition to fractures, other symptoms may include bone deformity, hearing loss, triangular-shaped face, and brittle teeth.

There is no cure for OI. Treatments include surgery to correct bone deformities, dental restoration, and physical therapy to improve movement; people with severe OI may need to use a wheelchair, braces, or other forms of equipment to assist in movement. Regular exercise is encouraged, and common forms include swimming and water therapy. People with OI can lead productive lives with proper treatment. For more information on OI refer to the Web site of the Osteogenesis Imperfecta Foundation at www.oif.org.

Paget's disease A bone disease characterized by excessive breakdown and formation of bone tissue, causing bones to enlarge, weaken, become deformed, and eventually fracture.

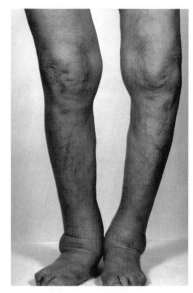

One symptom of Paget's disease is bowed limbs.

osteogenesis imperfecta (OI) A bone disease caused by a genetic defect that affects collagen production, resulting in a significantly increased rate of fractures, often from no apparent cause.

Recap: Paget's disease involves excessive breakdown and formation of bone tissue, which causes bones to weaken, become deformed, and eventually fracture. Osteogenesis imperfecta is caused by a genetic defect that affects collagen formation. A person with OI suffers from multiple fractures, bone deformities, and other health problems. Neither Paget's disease nor OI can be cured, but both can be treated with medications.

Chapter Summary

- Bones are organs that are constantly active, building new bone and breaking down old bone.

- Bone develops through three processes: growth, modeling, and remodeling. Bone size is determined during growth, bone shape is determined during modeling and remodeling, and bone remodeling also affects the density of bone.

- Bone health can be assessed by measuring bone density. Dual energy x-ray absorptiometry (DXA) is the most accurate tool for measuring bone density.

- Calcium is a major mineral that is an integral component of bones and teeth. Calcium levels are maintained in our blood at all times; calcium is also necessary for normal nerve transmission, muscle contraction, healthy blood pressure, and blood clotting.

- The AI for calcium is 1,000 mg per day for adult men and women aged 19 to 50 years, and 1,200 mg per day for adult men and women older than 50 years of age.

- Consuming excess calcium leads to mineral imbalance, while consuming inadequate calcium causes osteoporosis.

- Vitamin D is a fat-soluble vitamin that we can produce from the cholesterol in our skin using the energy from sunlight. Vitamin D regulates blood calcium levels, regulates absorption of calcium and phosphorus from our intestines, and helps us maintain bone health.

- The AI for vitamin D is 5 μg per day for adult men and women aged 19 to 50 years; the AI increases to 10 μg per day for men and women aged 51 to 70 years, and to 15 μg per day for adults over the age of 70 years.

- Hypercalcemia results from consuming too much vitamin D, causing weakness, loss of appetite, diarrhea, vomiting, and formation of calcium deposits in soft tissues. Vitamin D deficiency leads to loss of bone mass, causing rickets in children or osteomalacia and osteoporosis in adults.

- Vitamin K is a fat-soluble vitamin that we obtain in the diet; it is also produced in our large intestine by normal bacteria. Vitamin K serves as a coenzyme for blood clotting and bone metabolism.

- The AI for vitamin K is 120 μg per day for men and 90 μg per day for women.

- There are no side effects of excess vitamin K intake for healthy individuals; vitamin K deficiency is rare and leads to excessive bleeding.

- Phosphorus is a major mineral that is an important part of the structure of bone; phosphorus is also a component of ATP, DNA, RNA, cell membranes, and lipoproteins.

- The RDA for phosphorus is 700 mg per day for all adults.

- Consuming too much phosphorus causes high blood phosphorus levels, leading to muscle spasms and convulsions; phosphorus deficiencies are rare and cause dizziness, bone pain, and muscle damage.

- Magnesium is a major mineral that is part of the structure of bone, influences the formation of hydroxyapatite crystals and bone health through its regulation of calcium balance and the actions of vitamin D and parathyroid hormone, and is a cofactor for over 300 enzyme systems.

- The RDA for magnesium is 400 mg for men aged 19 to 30 years of age; 420 mg for men older than 30 years of age; 310 mg per day for women aged 19 to 30 years of age; and 320 mg per day for women older than 30 years of age.

- There are no known toxicity symptoms of consuming excess magnesium in the diet, though pharmacological excesses can result in such problems as diarrhea, cramping, dehydration, and cardiac arrest. Hypomagnesemia results from magnesium deficiency, resulting in low blood calcium levels, muscle cramps, seizures, confusion, and increased risk of some chronic diseases such as heart disease and type 2 diabetes.

- Fluoride is a trace mineral that strengthens our teeth and bones and reduces our risk for dental caries.

- The AI for fluoride is 4 mg per day for men and 3 mg per day for women.

- Consuming too much fluoride causes fluorosis of the teeth and bones. Consuming too little fluoride increases our risk for dental caries and tooth decay and can weaken bones.

- Osteoporosis is a major bone disease in the United States, affecting over 10 million Americans. About 80% of people with this disease are women.

- Osteoporosis leads to increased risk of bone fractures and premature disability and death due to subsequent illness.

- Factors that increase our risk for osteoporosis include increased age, being female, being of the Caucasian or Asian race, cigarette smoking, alcohol abuse, low calcium and vitamin D intakes, and a sedentary lifestyle.

- Paget's disease is a bone disorder that causes enlarged and deformed bones, leading to increased fractures. Bone and joint pain are common symptoms.

- Osteogenesis imperfecta is a genetic disorder that affects collagen formation. Due to either inadequate or poor quality collagen, bones are weak and break easily. This disease also causes bone deformities, hearing loss, and tooth damage.

Review Questions

1. Hydroxyapatite crystals are predominantly made up of
   a. calcium and phosphorus.
   b. hydrogen, oxygen, and titanium.
   c. calcium and vitamin D.
   d. calcium and magnesium.

2. On a DXA test, a T-score of −0.5 indicates that the patient
   a. has osteoporosis.
   b. is at greater risk of fractures than an average, healthy person of the same age.
   c. has normal bone density as compared to an average, healthy 30-year-old.
   d. has slightly lower bone density than an average, healthy person of the same age.

3. Which of the following statements about trabecular bone is true?
   a. It accounts for about 80% of our skeleton.
   b. It forms the core of almost all of the bones of our skeleton.
   c. It is also called compact bone.
   d. It provides the scaffolding for cortical bone.

4. Which of the following individuals is most likely to require vitamin D supplements?
   a. a dark-skinned child living and playing outdoors in Hawaii
   b. a fair-skinned construction worker living in Florida
   c. a fair-skinned retired teacher living in a nursing home in Ohio
   d. none of the above

5. Calcium is necessary for several body functions, including
   a. demineralization of bone, nerve transmission, and immune responses.
   b. cartilage structure, nerve transmission, and muscle contraction.
   c. structure of bone, nerve, and muscle tissue, immune responses, and muscle contraction.
   d. structure of bone, nerve transmission, and muscle contraction.

6. **True or false?** The process by which bone is formed through the action of osteoblasts and resorbed through the action of osteoclasts is called remodeling.

7. **True or false?** Moderate consumption of alcohol has been associated with increased bone density.

8. **True or false?** Although osteoporosis can lead to painful and debilitating fractures, it is not associated with an increased risk of premature death.

9. **True or false?** The amount of calcium we absorb depends upon our age, our calcium intake, the types of calcium-rich foods we eat, and our body's supply of vitamin D.

10. **True or false?** Our body absorbs vitamin D from sunlight.

11. Explain why people with diseases that cause a malabsorption of fat may suffer from deficiency of vitamins D and K.

12. Most people reach their peak height by the end of adolescence, maintain that height for several decades, and then start to lose height in their later years. Describe the two processes behind this phenomenon.

13. The morning after reading this chapter, you are eating your usual breakfast cereal when you notice that the Nutrition Facts panel on the box states that one serving contains 100% of your DRI for calcium. In addition, you're eating the cereal with about ½ cup of skim milk. Does this meal ensure that your calcium needs for the day are met? Why or why not?

14. Your best friend has light skin and lives in Buffalo, New York. How much time does your friend need to spend out of doors with exposed skin on winter days

to avoid the need for consuming vitamin D in the diet or from supplements?

15. Look back at the information you learned about Liz in the Nutri-Case introductions in Chapter 1, as well as in Chapters 5, 6, and 7. Identify aspects of Liz's nutrition and lifestyle that put her at increased risk for osteoporosis.

Test Yourself Answers

1. **False.** By selecting foods that are good sources of calcium each day, most people can consume enough calcium in their diets to maintain bone health. People at risk for low calcium intakes include elderly people, people who do not consume enough minerals in their diets, and people who do not consume enough food to maintain a healthful weight.

2. **False.** Osteoporosis is more common among elderly women, but elderly men are also at increased risk for osteoporosis. Young women who suffer from an eating disorder and menstrual cycle irregularity, referred to as the female athlete triad, may also have osteoporosis.

3. **True.** Our bodies can convert a cholesterol compound in our skin into vitamin D.

4. **True.** Kale, broccoli, and collard greens are good sources of calcium.

5. **True.** Cigarette smoking has an unhealthy impact on the hormones that influence the density of our bones. People who smoke have an increased risk for osteoporosis and fractures.

Web Links

www.nlm.nih.gov/medlineplus
MEDLINE Plus Health Information
Search for rickets or osteomalacia to learn more about these vitamin D–deficiency diseases.

www.ada.org
American Dental Association
Look under "oral health topics" to learn more about the fluoridation of community water supplies and the use of fluoride-containing products.

www.nof.org
National Osteoporosis Foundation
Learn more about the causes, prevention, detection, and treatment of osteoporosis.

www.osteofound.org
International Osteoporosis Foundation
Find out more about this foundation and its mission to increase awareness and understanding of osteoporosis worldwide.

www.osteo.org
National Institutes of Health
Osteoporosis and Related Bone Diseases—National Resource Center
Access this site for additional resources and information on metabolic bone diseases including osteoporosis, Paget's disease, and osteogenesis imperfecta.

www.oif.org.
Osteogenesis Imperfecta (OI) Foundation
Go to this site for more information on OI and related health and medical issues.

References

Ball, J. W., and R. C. Bindler. 2003. *Pediatric Nursing: Caring for Children*. Upper Saddle River, NJ: Pearson Education.

Chen, T. C., A. Shao, H. Heath III, and M. F. Holick. 1993. An update on the vitamin D content of fortified milk from the United States and Canada. *N. Engl. J. Med.* 329:1507.

Dawson-Hughes, B., and S. S. Harris. 2002. Calcium intake influences the association of protein intake with rates of bone loss in elderly men and women. *Am. J. Clin. Nutr.* 75:773–779.

Felson, D. T., Y. Zhang, M. T. Hannan, W. B. Kannel, and D. P. Kiel. 1995. Alcohol intake and bone mineral density in elderly men and women. The Framingham Study. *Am. J. Epidemiol.* 142:485–492.

Feskanich, D., S. A. Korrick, S. L. Greenspan, H. N. Rosen, and G. A. Colditz. 1999. Moderate alcohol consumption and bone density among postmenopausal women. *J. Women's Health* 8:65–73.

Heaney, R. P., and K. Rafferty. 2001. Carbonated beverages and urinary calcium excretion. *Am. J. Clin. Nutr.* 74:343–347.

Holbrook, T. L., and E. Barrett-Connor. 1993. A prospective study of alcohol consumption and bone mineral density. *BMJ* 306:1506–1509.

Holick, M. F. 1994. McCollum Award Lecture, 1994: Vitamin D: New Horizons for the 21st Century. *Am. J. Clin. Nutr.* 60:619–630.

Holick, M. F., L. Y. Matsuoka, and J. Wortsman. 1989. Age, vitamin D, and solar ultraviolet. *Lancet* 2:1104–1105.

Holick, M. F., Q. Shao, W. W. Liu, and T. C. Chen. 1992. The vitamin D content of fortified milk and infant formula. *N. Engl. J. Med.* 326:1178–1181.

Institute of Medicine, Food and Nutrition Board. 1997. *Dietary Reference Intakes for Calcium, Phosphorus, Magnesium, Vitamin D, and Fluoride*. Washington, DC: National Academy Press.

Institute of Medicine, Food and Nutrition Board. 2002. *Dietary Reference Intakes for Vitamin A, Vitamin K, Arsenic, Boron, Chromium, Copper, Iodine, Iron, Manganese, Molybdenum, Nickel, Silicon, Vanadium, and Zinc*. Washington, DC: National Academy Press.

International Osteoporosis Foundation. 2003. The facts about osteoporosis and its impact. www.osteofound.org/press_centre/fact_sheet.html (Accessed December 15, 2003.)

Keller, J. L., A. J. Lanou, and N. D. Barnard. 2002. The consumer cost of calcium from food and supplements. *J. Am. Diet. Assoc.* 102:1669–1671.

Laitinen, K., M. Valimaki, and P. Keto. 1991. Bone mineral density measured by dual-energy x-ray absorptiometry in healthy Finnish women. *Calcif. Tissue Int.* 48:224–231.

Massey, L. K. 2001. Is caffeine a risk factor for bone loss in the elderly? *Am. J. Clin. Nutr.* 74:569–570.

Massey, L. K., H. Roman-Smith, and R. A. Sutton. 1993. Effect of dietary oxalate and calcium on urinary oxalate and risk of formation of calcium oxalate kidney stones. *J. Am. Diet. Assoc.* 93:901–906.

National Osteoporosis Foundation. 2003. Advocacy: News & Updates. www.nof.org/advocacy/prevalence/index.htm (Accessed November, 2003.)

Need, A. G., H. A. Morris, M. Horowitz, and C. Nordin. 1993. Effects of skin thickness, age, body fat, and sunlight on serum 25-hydroxyvitamin D. *Am. J. Clin. Nutr.* 58:882–885.

Nusser, S. M., A. L. Carriquiry, K. W. Dodd, and W. A. Fuller. 1996. A semiparametric transformation approach to estimating usual daily intake distributions. *J. Am. Stat. Assoc.* 91:1440–1449.

Rapuri, P. B., J. C. Gallagher, K. E. Balhorn, and K. L. Ryschon. 2000. Alcohol intake and bone metabolism in elderly women. *Am. J. Clin. Nutr.* 72:1206–1213.

Rapuri, P. B., J. C. Gallagher, H. K. Kinyamu, and K. L. Ryschon. 2001. Caffeine intake increases the rate of bone loss in elderly women and interacts with vitamin D receptor genotypes. *Am. J. Clin. Nutr.* 74:694–700.

Ross, E. A., N. J. Szabo, and I. R. Tebbett. 2000. Lead content of calcium supplements. *JAMA* 284:1425–1433.

South-Pal, J. E. 2001. Osteoporosis: Part II. Nonpharmacologic and Pharmacologic Treatment. *Am. Fam. Physician* 63:1121–1128.

Tucker, K. L., H. Chen, M. T. Hannan, L. A. Cupples, P. W. F. Wilson, D. Felson, and D. P. Kiel. 2002. Bone mineral density and dietary patterns in older adults: the Framingham Osteoporosis Study. *Am. J. Clin. Nutr.* 76:245–252.

Tucker, K. L., M. T. Hannan, H. Chen, L. A. Cupples, P. W. F. Wilson, and D. P. Kiel. 1999. Potassium, magnesium, and fruit and vegetable intakes are associated with greater bone mineral density in elderly men and women. *Am. J. Clin. Nutr.* 69:727–736.

U.S. Department of Health and Human Services. Public Health Service. 1991. Review of fluoride: Benefits and risks. Report of the Ad Hoc Subcommittee on Fluoride of the Committee to Coordinate Environmental Health and Related Programs. www.health.gov/environment/ReviewofFluoride/ default.htm. (Accessed November 2003.)

Writing Group for the Women's Health Initiative Investigators. 2002. Risks and benefits of estrogen plus progestin in healthy postmenopausal women. Principal results from the Women's Health Initiative randomized control trial. *JAMA* 288:321–332.

Wyshak, G. 2000. Teenaged girls, carbonated beverage consumption, and bone fractures. *Arch. Pediatr. Adolesc. Med.* 154:610–613.

Wyshak, G., and R. E. Frisch. 1994. Carbonated beverages, dietary calcium, the dietary calcium/phosphorus ratio, and bone fractures in girls and boys. *J. Adolesc. Health* 15:210–215.

Wyshak, G., R. E. Frisch, T. E. Albright, N. L. Albright, I. Schiff, and J. Witschi. 1989. Nonalcoholic carbonated beverage consumption and bone fractures among women former college athletes. *J. Orthop. Res.* 7:91–99.

Nutrition Debate:

Hormone Replacement Therapy—Is It Safe?

Research has consistently shown that hormone replacement therapy (HRT) and estrogen replacement therapy (ERT) are effective in preventing and treating osteoporosis. They have also been shown to reduce the less serious symptoms some menopausal women experience, including hot flashes, vaginal dryness, sleep disturbances, and memory loss. As a result, the use of these medications skyrocketed in the last twenty years, and it became standard medical practice to prescribe either HRT or ERT to any menopausal woman who requested it. HRT in particular has been viewed as a safe and effective medication option for millions of women in the United States. But is it?

ERT contains estrogen, a female sex hormone that is responsible for many of a woman's sexual characteristics. Because ERT is known to significantly increase a woman's risk for endometrial cancer if her uterus is intact, HRT was developed. HRT is a combination of estrogen and the hormone progestin. This combination of hormones appears to treat the symptoms of menopause and minimize postmenopausal bone loss without increasing a woman's risk for endometrial cancer.

Research had also suggested that HRT lowered cholesterol levels and reduced a woman's risk for heart disease. However, much of the evidence supporting the benefits of HRT had been observational in nature, meaning that these studies were not actually designed to administer HRT and test its direct effect on health risks and benefits. In 1991, researchers involved in the Women's Health Initiative began designing clinical trials that would test the direct effects of HRT and ERT on risks for heart disease, various cancers, and bone fractures. The researchers hypothesized that women taking these hormones would have a lower risk of heart disease and hip fracture but higher rates of breast cancer. More than 160,000 women ranging in age from 50 to 79 years were recruited into this study, and researchers planned to follow these women over an average of 8.5 years.

Much to the surprise of many researchers and health professionals, the trials testing HRT had to be stopped early because the health risks to women on HRT exceeded the health benefits over an average follow-up of only five years (Writing Group for the Women's Health Initiative Investigators 2002). Women taking HRT were found to have increased risk for breast cancer, heart disease, stroke, and pulmonary embolism, which is a clot that forms in the arteries of the lungs. These results became news headlines throughout the United States and around the world. Within weeks, hundreds of thousands of women had either stopped taking HRT or rushed to meet with their physicians to discuss their options.

Although these findings appear to be sensational, the risks of taking HRT may not be as high as many fear. In addition to the negative findings of HRT, the Women's Health Initiative trials found positive health effects of HRT, in that this treatment decreased the number of hip, spine, and other osteoporosis-related fractures, and it also decreased the risk for colorectal cancer. In general, the risk of taking HRT is relatively low. The investigators report that over one year, 10,000 women taking HRT may experience seven more heart-disease related events, eight more strokes, eight more cases of breast cancer, and eight more pulmonary emboli then women taking no hormone therapy. Women on HRT will also experience six less cases of colorectal cancer and five less fractures of the hip than women not taking HRT.

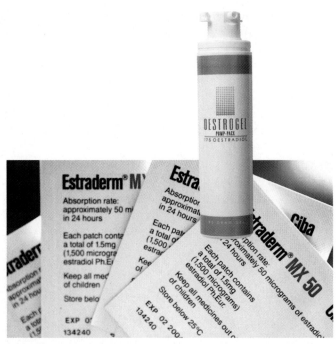

Estrogen replacement medications come in a variety of forms for use by postmenopausal women.

Based on this discussion, should a woman take HRT to combat osteoporosis and treat menopausal symptoms? This question can only be answered by the woman herself after consulting with her physician. HRT is still an effective treatment and prevention option for osteoporosis, and women at low risk for breast cancer and heart disease may decide to use this therapy. Women at high risk for breast cancer and heart disease may decide to avoid taking HRT and may select some other medication approved for the prevention or treatment of osteoporosis. In summary, working with their physician, women must weigh the benefits of reducing fracture risk with the increased risks of breast cancer and heart disease when considering HRT as a treatment option for osteoporosis and low bone density.

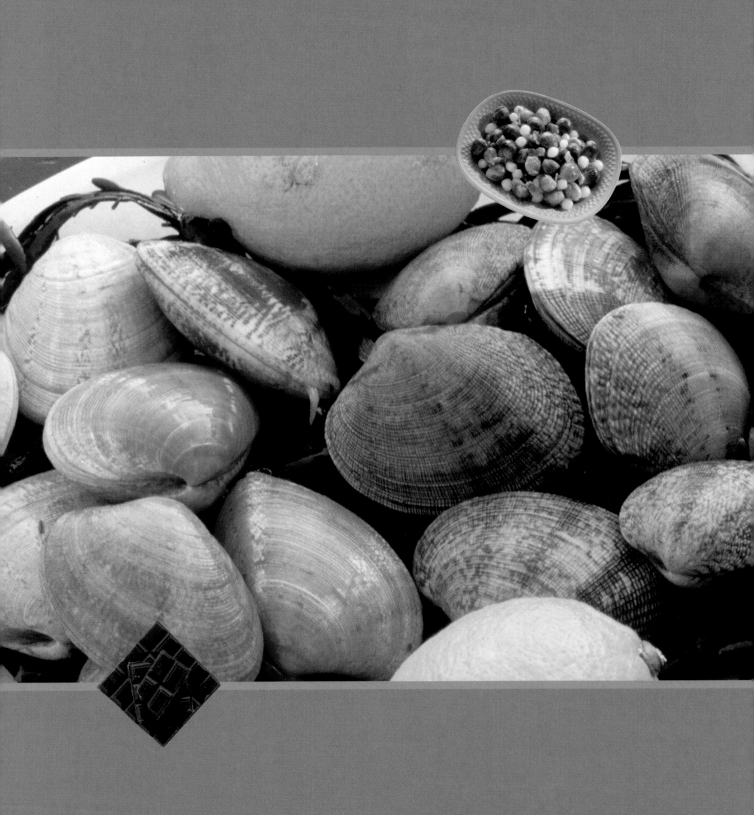

Chapter 10
Nutrients Involved in Energy Metabolism and Blood Health

Chapter Objectives

After reading this chapter you will be able to:

1. Describe how coenzymes enhance the activities of enzymes, pp. 348–349.

2. Name the eight B-complex vitamins and describe how they are involved in energy metabolism, pp. 350–355.

3. Identify the deficiency disorders of three B-complex vitamins, pp. 351–352.

4. List at least two minerals that function as coenzymes in energy metabolism, pp. 360 and 368–370.

5. Describe the four components of blood, pp. 361–362.

6. Discuss the role that iron plays in oxygen transport, pp. 364–365.

7. Distinguish between iron-deficiency anemia, pernicious anemia, and macrocytic anemia, pp. 373–374.

8. Describe the association between folate, vitamin B_{12}, and vascular disease, p. 373.

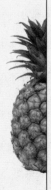 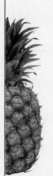

Test Yourself True or False?

1. The B-complex vitamins are an important source of energy for our bodies. T or F

2. People consuming a vegan diet are at greater risk for micronutrient deficiencies than are people who eat foods of animal origin. T or F

3. Chromium supplements are consistently effective in reducing body fat and enhancing muscle mass. T or F

4. Iron deficiency is the most common nutrient deficiency in the world. T or F

5. Taking a daily multivitamin/mineral supplement is a waste of money. T or F

Test Yourself answers can be found at the end of the chapter.

Dr. Leslie Bernstein looked in astonishment at the 80-year-old man in his office. A leading gastroenterologist and professor of medicine at Albert Einstein College of Medicine in New York City, he had admired Pop Katz for years as one of his most healthy patients, a strict vegetarian and athlete who just weeks before had been going on three-mile runs as if he were forty years younger. Now he could barely stand. He was confused, cried easily, was wandering away from the house partially clothed, and had lost control of his bladder. Tests showed that he was not suffering from Alzheimer's disease, had not had a stroke, did not have a tumor or infection, and had no evidence of exposure to pesticides, metals, drugs, or other toxins. Blood tests were normal except that his red blood cells were slightly enlarged. Bernstein consulted with a neurologist, who diagnosed "rapidly progressive dementia of unknown origin."

Bernstein was unconvinced: "In a matter of weeks, a man who hadn't been sick for eighty years suddenly became demented. . . . 'Holy smoke!,' I thought, 'I'm an idiot! The man's been a vegetarian for thirty-eight years. No meat. No fish. No eggs. No milk. He hasn't had any animal protein for decades. He has to be B_{12} deficient!'" Bernstein immediately tested Katz's blood, then gave him an injection of B_{12}. The blood test confirmed Bernstein's hunch: the level of B_{12} in Katz's blood was too low to measure. The morning after his injection, Katz could sit up without help. Within a week of continuing treatment, he could read, play card games, and hold his own in conversations. Unfortunately, the delay in diagnosis left some permanent neurological damage, including alterations in his personality and an inability to concentrate. Bernstein notes, "A diet free of animal protein can be healthful and safe, but it should be supplemented periodically with B_{12} by mouth or by injection." (Bernstein, 2000).

It was not until 1906, when the English biochemist F. G. Hopkins discovered what he called *accessory factors,* that scientists began to appreciate the many critical roles of micronutrients in maintaining human health. Vitamin B_{12}, for instance, was not even isolated until 1948! In Chapters 7 through 9, we explored several key roles of vitamins and minerals, including regulation of fluids and nerve-impulse transmission, protection against the damage caused by oxidation, and maintenance of healthy bones. In this chapter, we conclude our exploration of the micronutrients with a discussion of two final roles: their contribution to the metabolism of carbohydrates, fats, and proteins, and their role in the formation and maintenance of our blood.

How Do Our Bodies Regulate Energy Metabolism?

We explored the digestion and metabolism of carbohydrates, fats, and proteins in Chapters 3 through 6 of this text. In those chapters, you learned that the regulation of energy metabolism is a complex process involving numerous biological substances and chemical pathways. Here, we describe how the micronutrients we consume in our diet assist us in generating energy from the carbohydrates, fats, and proteins we eat along with them.

Our Bodies Require Vitamins and Minerals to Produce Energy

Although vitamins and minerals do not directly provide energy, we are unable to generate energy from the macronutrients without them. The B-complex vitamins are particularly important in assisting us with energy metabolism. Also referred to as the B vitamins, this group includes thiamin, riboflavin, vitamin B_6, niacin, folate, vitamin B_{12}, pantothenic acid, and biotin.

The primary role of the B-complex vitamins is to act as coenzymes. Remember from Chapter 6 that an *enzyme* is a protein that accelerates the rate of chemical reactions but is not used up or changed during the reaction. A **coenzyme** is a molecule that combines with an enzyme to activate it and help it do its job. Figure 10.1 illustrates how coenzymes work. Without coenzymes, we would be unable to produce the energy necessary for sustaining life and supporting daily activities.

coenzyme A molecule that combines with an enzyme to activate it and help it do its job.

Figure 10.2 provides an overview of how some of the B-complex vitamins act as coenzymes to promote energy metabolism. For instance, thiamin is part of the coenzyme thiamin pyrophosphate, or TPP, which assists in the breakdown of glucose. Riboflavin is a part of two coenzymes, flavin mononucleotide (FMN) and flavin adenine dinucleotide (FAD), which help break down both glucose and fatty acids. The specific functions of each B-complex vitamin are described in detail shortly.

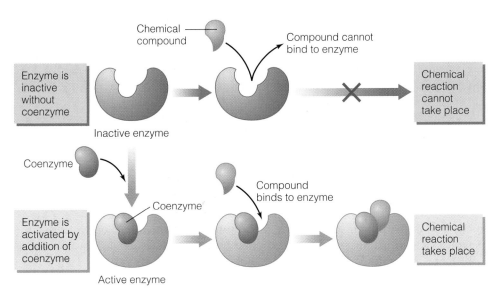

Figure 10.1   Coenzymes combine with enzymes to activate them, ensuring that the chemical reactions that depend upon these enzymes can occur.

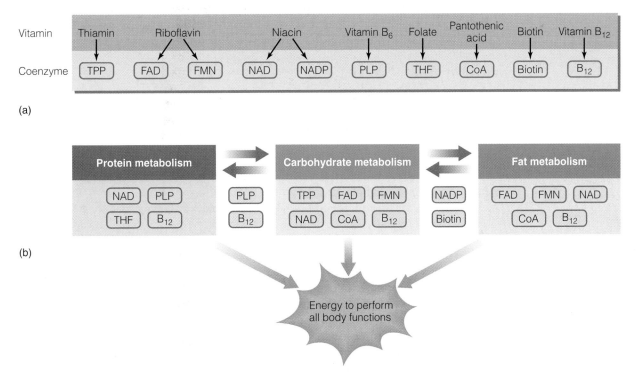

Figure 10.2   The B-complex vitamins play many important roles in the reactions involved in energy metabolism. **(a)** B-complex vitamins and the coenzymes they are a part of. **(b)** This chart illustrates many of the coenzymes essential for various metabolic functions; however, this is only a small sample of the thousands of roles that the B-complex vitamins serve in our bodies.

Some Micronutrients Assist with Nutrient Transport and Hormone Production

Some micronutrients promote energy metabolism by facilitating the transport of nutrients into the cells. For instance, the mineral chromium helps improve glucose uptake into cells. Other micronutrients assist in the production of hormones that regulate metabolic processes; the mineral iodine, for example, is necessary for synthesis of thyroid hormones, which regulate our metabolic rate and promote growth and development. The details of these processes and their related nutrients are discussed in the following section.

> **Recap:** Vitamins and minerals are not direct sources of energy, but they help generate energy from carbohydrates, fats, and proteins. Acting as coenzymes, nutrients such as the B-complex vitamins assist enzymes in metabolizing nutrients to produce energy. Minerals such as chromium and iodine assist with nutrient uptake into the cells and with regulating energy production and cell growth.

A Profile of Nutrients Involved in Energy Metabolism

In addition to the B-complex vitamins, other nutrients involved in energy metabolism include a vitamin-like substance called choline and the minerals iodine, chromium, manganese, and sulfur. Let's take a closer look at these nutrients.

B-Complex Vitamins Act as Coenzymes in Energy Metabolism

Thiamin (vitamin B_1), riboflavin (vitamin B_2), niacin (nicotinamide and nicotinic acid), vitamin B_6 (pyridoxine), folate (folic acid), vitamin B_{12} (cobalamin), pantothenic acid, and biotin are the nutrients identified as the B-complex vitamins. In this section we discuss the functions, recommended intakes, toxicity, and deficiency symptoms for these vitamins. For a summary of this discussion, see Table 10.1.

Thiamin (Vitamin B_1)

Thiamin was the first B-complex vitamin discovered, hence its designation as vitamin B_1. Thiamin is part of the coenzyme thiamin pyrophosphate, or TPP. As a part of TPP, thiamin plays a critical role in the breakdown of glucose for energy and acts as a coenzyme in the metabolism of the branched–chain amino acids, which include leucine, isoleucine, and valine. TPP assists in producing DNA and RNA, and plays a role in the synthesis of neurotransmitters, or chemicals that transmit messages throughout our central nervous system.

The RDA for thiamin for adults aged 19 and older is 1.2 mg/day for men and 1.1 mg/day for women. Good food sources of thiamin include enriched cereals and grains, whole-grain products, ready-to-eat cereals, and ham and other pork products.

As the B-complex vitamins are involved in most energy-generating processes, many of the deficiency symptoms include a combination of fatigue, apathy, muscle weakness, and detriments in cognitive function (see Table 10.1). Thiamin-deficiency disease is called **beriberi.** In this disease, the body's inability to metabolize energy leads to muscle wasting and nerve damage; in later stages, patients may be unable to move at all. The heart muscle may also be affected, and the patient may die of heart failure. Beriberi is seen in countries in which unenriched, processed grains are a primary food source; for instance, beriberi was widespread in China when rice was processed and refined, and it still occurs in refugee camps and other settlements dependent on poor-quality food supplies. Beriberi is also seen in industrialized countries in people with heavy alcohol consumption and limited food intake. There are no known adverse effects from consuming excess amounts of thiamin.

beriberi   A disease caused by thiamin deficiency.

Table 10.1 Functions, Recommended Intakes, and Toxicity and Deficiency Symptoms of B Vitamins and Choline

Nutrient	Primary Functions	Recommended Intake	Toxicity Symptoms/Side Effects	Deficiency Symptoms/Side Effects
Thiamin (vitamin B_1)	Part of the coenzyme thiamin pyrophosphate (TPP) involved in carbohydrate metabolism Coenzyme involved in branched–chain amino acid metabolism	RDA for 19 years and older: Men = 1.2 mg/day Women = 1.1 mg/day	None known at this time	Beriberi Anorexia and weight loss Apathy Decreased short-term memory Confusion and irritability Muscle weakness Enlarged heart
Riboflavin (vitamin B_2)	Coenzymes including flavin mononucleotide (FMN) and flavin adenine dinucleotide (FAD), involved in oxidation-reduction reactions for metabolism of carbohydrates and fats	RDA for 19 years and older: Men = 1.3 mg/day Women = 1.1 mg/day	None known at this time	Ariboflavinosis Sore throat Swelling of mouth and throat Cheilosis—dry, cracked lips Angular stomatitis—inflammation of the mucous membranes of the mouth Glossitis—magenta tongue Seborrheic dermatitis—inflammation of oil glands in the skin Anemia—lower than normal amount of red blood cells
Niacin (nicotinamide and nicotinic acid)	Coenzymes in carbohydrate and fatty acid metabolism, including nicotinamide adenine dinucleotide (NAD$^+$ and NADH) and nicotinamide adenine dinucleotide phosphate (NADP$^+$) Plays role in DNA replication and repair and cell differentiation	RDA for 19 years and older: Men = 16 mg/day Women = 14 mg/day	Excessive supplementation causes: Flushing Liver dysfunction and damage Glucose intolerance Blurred vision and edema of eyes	Pellagra Pigmented rash Vomiting Constipation or diarrhea Bright red tongue Depression Apathy Headache Fatigue Loss of memory
Vitamin B_6 (pyridoxine)	Part of coenzyme (pyridoxal phosphate, or PLP) involved in amino acid metabolism, synthesis of blood cells, and carbohydrate metabolism	RDA for 19 to 50 years of age: Men and women = 1.3 mg/day RDA for 51 years and older: Men = 1.7 mg/day Women = 1.5 mg/day	Excessive supplementation causes: Sensory neuropathy Lesions of the skin	Seborrheic dermatitis Microcytic anemia Convulsions Depression and confusion
Folate (folic acid)	Coenzyme tetrahydrofolate (THF), (or tetrahydrofolic acid, THFA) involved in DNA synthesis and amino acid metabolism Involved in the metabolism of homocysteine	RDA for 19 years and older: Men and women = 400 µg/day	Excessive supplementation causes: A masking of symptoms of vitamin B_{12} deficiency Neurological damage	Macrocytic anemia Weakness and fatigue Difficulty concentrating Irritability Headache Palpitations Shortness of breath Elevated levels of homocysteine in the blood Neural tube defects in the developing fetus

(continued)

Table 10.1 Continued

Nutrient	Primary Functions	Recommended Intake	Toxicity Symptoms/ Side Effects	Deficiency Symptoms/ Side Effects
Vitamin B$_{12}$ (cobalamin)	Part of coenzymes that assist with formation of blood, nervous system function, and homocysteine metabolism	RDA for 19 years and older: Men and women = 2.4 µg/day	None known at this time	Pernicious anemia Pale skin Diminished energy and low exercise tolerance Fatigue Shortness of breath Palpitations Tingling and numbness in extremities Abnormal gait Memory loss Poor concentration Disorientation Dementia
Pantothenic acid	Component of coenzymes (coenzyme A, or CoA) that assist with fatty acid metabolism	AI for 19 years and older: Men and women = 5 mg/day	None known at this time	Rare; only seen in people fed diets with virtually no pantothenic acid
Biotin	Component of coenzymes involved in carbohydrate, fat, and protein metabolism	AI for 19 years and older: Men and women = 30 µg/day	None known at this time	Red, scaly skin rash Depression Lethargy Hallucinations Burning, tingling, tickling Paresthesia of the extremities
Choline	Assists with homocysteine metabolism Accelerates the synthesis and release of the neurotransmitter acetylcholine Assists in synthesis of phospholipids and other components of cell membranes Assists in the transport and metabolism of fats and cholesterol	AI for 19 years and older: Men = 550 mg/day Women = 425 mg/day	Excessive supplementation causes: Fishy body odor Vomiting Excess salivation Sweating Diarrhea Low blood pressure	Increased fat accumulation in the liver, leading to liver damage

Riboflavin (Vitamin B$_2$)

Riboflavin is an important component of coenzymes that are involved in oxidation-reduction reactions occurring within the energy-producing metabolic pathways. These coenzymes, flavin mononucleotide (FMN) and flavin adenine dinucleotide (FAD) are involved in the metabolism of carbohydrates and fat. Riboflavin is also a part of the antioxidant enzyme glutathione peroxidase, thus assisting in the fight against oxidative damage.

The RDA for riboflavin for adults aged 19 and older is 1.3 mg/day for men and 1.1 mg/day for women. Note that milk is a good source of riboflavin; however, riboflavin is destroyed when it is exposed to light. Thus, milk is generally stored in opaque containers to prevent the destruction of riboflavin. Other good food sources include yogurt, enriched bread and grain products, ready-to-eat cereals, and organ meats.

There are no known adverse effects from consuming excess amounts of riboflavin. Riboflavin deficiency is referred to as **ariboflavinosis.** Symptoms of ariboflavinosis include sore throat, swelling of the mucous membranes in the mouth and throat, lips that are dry and scaly, a purple-colored tongue, and inflamed, irritated patches on the skin. Severe riboflavin deficiency can impair the metabolism of vitamin B_6 (or pyridoxine).

ariboflavinosis A condition caused by riboflavin deficiency.

Niacin

Niacin refers to the compounds nicotinamide and nicotinic acid. Interestingly, our bodies can make niacin from the amino acid tryptophan. Niacin is a coenzyme that assists in the metabolism of carbohydrates and fatty acids, and it also plays an important role in DNA replication and repair and in the process of cell differentiation.

The RDA for niacin for adults aged 19 and older is 16 mg/day for men and 14 mg/day for women. The UL for niacin is 35 mg/day. Good food sources include meat, fish, poultry, enriched bread products, and ready-to-eat cereals.

Niacin can cause toxicity symptoms when taken in supplement form. These symptoms include *flushing,* which is defined as burning, tingling, and itching sensations accompanied by a reddened flush primarily on the face, arms, and chest. Liver damage, glucose intolerance, blurred vision, and edema of the eyes can be seen with very large doses of niacin taken over long periods of time.

Pellagra results from severe niacin deficiency. Pellagra commonly occurred in the United States and parts of Europe in the early twentieth century in areas where corn or maize was the dietary staple. These foods are low in niacin and the amino acid tryptophan. At the present time, pellagra is rarely seen in industrialized countries, except in cases of chronic alcoholism. Pellagra is still found in countries such as India, China, and Africa. (For more information on pellagra, see the Highlight: Solving the Mystery of Pellagra, page 5.)

pellagra A disease that results from severe niacin deficiency.

Vitamin B_6 (Pyridoxine)

Vitamin B_6 is actually a group of six related compounds: pyridoxine, pyridoxal, pyridoxamine, and the phosphate forms of these compounds which include PNP, PLP, and PMP (respectively). Vitamin B_6 is part of a coenzyme for more than 100 enzymes involved in the metabolism of amino acids. It plays a critical role in transamination, which is the key process in making nonessential amino acids; without adequate vitamin B_6, all amino acids become essential, as our bodies cannot make them in sufficient quantities. Vitamin B_6 also assists in the metabolism of carbohydrate and the amino acid homocysteine and plays a role in the synthesis of hemoglobin and in oxygen transport.

The RDA for vitamin B_6 for adult men and women aged 19 to 50 years is 1.3 mg/day. For adults 51 years of age and older, the RDA increases to 1.7 mg/day for men and 1.5 mg/day for women. The UL for vitamin B_6 is 100 mg/day. Good food sources include enriched ready-to-eat cereals, meat, fish, poultry, white potatoes and other starchy vegetables, organ meats, and fortified soy-based meat substitutes.

Vitamin B_6 supplements have been used to treat conditions such as premenstrual syndrome and carpal tunnel syndrome. You need to use caution, however, when using such supplements. Whereas consuming excess vitamin B_6 from food sources does not cause toxicity, supplementing can result in nerve damage and lesions of the skin. The symptoms of vitamin B_6 deficiency include anemia, convulsions, depression, confusion, and inflamed, irritated patches on the skin.

Folate

Folate is involved in DNA synthesis and amino acid metabolism. Its role in assisting with cell division makes it a critical nutrient during the first few weeks of pregnancy when the combined sperm-egg cell multiplies rapidly to form the primitive tissues and structures of the human body. Folate, vitamin B_{12}, and vitamin B_6 are closely interrelated in some metabolic functions, including homocysteine metabolism.

The RDA for folate for adult men and women aged 19 years and older is 400 µg/day. The UL for folate is 1,000 µg/day. Because of its critical role during the first few weeks of pregnancy and the fact that many women of childbearing age do not consume adequate folate, this nutrient has been added to ready-to-eat cereals and bread products. Thus, these two foods are among the primary sources of folate in the United States. Other good food sources include liver, spinach, lentils, oatmeal, asparagus, and romaine lettuce.

Toxicity can occur when taking supplemental folate. One especially frustrating problem with folate toxicity is that it can mask a simultaneous vitamin B_{12} deficiency. This often results in failure to detect the B_{12} deficiency and, as you saw in the chapter-opening case, a delay in diagnosis of B_{12} deficiency can contribute to severe damage to the nervous system. There do not appear to be any clear symptoms of folate toxicity independent from its interaction with vitamin B_{12} deficiency.

A folate deficiency can cause many adverse health effects, including *macrocytic anemia*. Folate and vitamin B_{12} deficiencies can cause elevated levels of homocysteine in the blood, a condition that is associated with heart disease. When folate intake is inadequate in pregnant women, *neural tube defects* (major malformations of the central nervous system that occur during the growth and development of the fetus) can occur. All of these conditions are discussed in more detail in the disorders section at the end of this chapter.

Vitamin B_{12} (Cobalamin)

Vitamin B_{12} is part of coenzymes that assist with formation of our blood. Also, as you saw in the chapter-opening scenario, B_{12} is essential for healthy functioning of the nervous system because it helps maintain the sheath that coats nerve fibers. When this sheath is damaged or absent, the conduction of nervous signals is altered, causing numerous neurological problems.

homocysteine An amino acid that requires adequate levels of folate, vitamin B_6, and vitamin B_{12} for its metabolism. High levels of homocysteine in the blood are associated with an increased risk for vascular diseases such as cardiovascular disease.

Adequate levels of folate and vitamin B_{12} are also necessary to break down the amino acid **homocysteine.** This amino acid is produced as a byproduct during the metabolism of another amino acid, methionine. When folate and vitamin B_{12} consumption is inadequate, homocysteine levels rise. A high level of homocysteine in the blood is related to an increased risk of heart disease. We discuss the relationship between homocysteine and heart disease in more detail on page 373.

The RDA for vitamin B_{12} for adult men and women aged 19 and older is 2.4 µg/day. Vitamin B_{12} is only found in dairy products, meats, and poultry; as discussed in Chapter 6, individuals consuming a vegan diet need to eat vegetable-based foods that are fortified with vitamin B_{12} or take vitamin B_{12} supplements or injections to ensure that they maintain adequate blood levels of this nutrient.

atrophic gastritis A condition that results in low stomach-acid secretion; is estimated to occur in about 10 to 30% of adults older than 50 years of age.

As we age, our sources of vitamin B_{12} may need to change. Individuals younger than 51 years are generally able to meet the RDA for vitamin B_{12} by consuming it in foods. However, it is estimated that about 10 to 30% of adults older than 50 years have a condition referred to as **atrophic gastritis** (Institute of Medicine, 1998) that results in low stomach-acid secretion. Since stomach acid separates food-bound vitamin B_{12} from dietary proteins, if the acid content of the stomach is inadequate, then we cannot free up enough vitamin B_{12} from food sources alone. Because atrophic gastritis can affect almost one-third of the older adult population, it is recommended that people older than 50 years of age consume foods fortified with vitamin B_{12}, take a vitamin B_{12}–containing supplement, or have periodic B_{12} injections.

Vitamin B_{12} deficiency causes general symptoms of anemia, including pale skin, diminished energy and exercise tolerance, fatigue, and shortness of breath. Neurological symptoms include tingling and numbness of extremities, abnormal gait, memory loss, dementia, disorientation, visual disturbances, insomnia, and impaired bladder and bowel control. One of the primary causes of vitamin B_{12} deficiency is a condition called *pernicious anemia*. People with pernicious anemia lack adequate amounts of a specialized protein secreted by the stomach that binds with vitamin B_{12} and allows for its absorption into the bloodstream. Pernicious anemia is discussed in more detail with other micronutrient-related disorders on page 374.

There are no known adverse effects from consuming excess amounts of vitamin B_{12}.

Pantothenic Acid

Pantothenic acid is a component of coenzymes that assist with the metabolism of fatty acids. It is also critical for building new fatty acids.

The AI for pantothenic acid for adult men and women aged 19 years and older is 5 mg/day. Food sources include chicken, beef, egg yolk, potatoes, oat cereals, tomato products, whole grains, and organ meats. There are no known adverse effects from consuming excess amounts of pantothenic acid. Deficiencies of pantothenic acid are very rare.

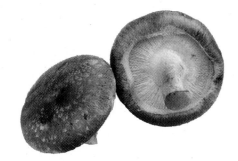

Shiitake mushrooms contain pantothenic acid.

Biotin

Biotin is a component of coenzymes involved in the various steps of carbohydrate, fat, and protein metabolism. It also plays an important role in gluconeogenesis.

The AI for biotin for adult men and women aged 19 and older is 30 µg/day. The biotin content has been determined for very few foods, and these values are not reported in food composition tables or dietary analysis programs. Biotin appears to be widespread in foods. There are no known adverse effects from consuming excess amounts of biotin. Biotin deficiencies are typically only seen in people who consume a large number of raw egg whites over long periods of time. This is because raw egg whites contain a protein that binds with biotin and prevents its absorption. Biotin deficiencies are also seen in people fed total parenteral nutrition (nutrients are administered by a route other than the GI tract) that is not supplemented with biotin. Symptoms include thinning of hair; loss of hair color; development of red, scaly rash around the eyes, nose, and mouth; depression; lethargy; and hallucinations.

Consuming Adequate B-Complex Vitamins Is Easy for Most People

In general, foods such as whole grains, enriched breads and ready-to-eat cereals, meat, poultry, milk and dairy products, some fruits and vegetables are good sources of the B-complex vitamins. Figure 10.3 shows the B-complex vitamin content of two enriched ready-to-eat cereals. Although there are other food sources that contain more of these vitamins, these kinds of cereals are regularly eaten by adults and children in the United States and are consequently a consistently good source of the B-complex vitamins. Table 10.2 summarizes other good sources of B-complex vitamins.

Because most of the B-complex vitamins are so widespread in foods, consuming adequate quantities from food sources is relatively easy for people who consume a varied diet and are able to adequately absorb these vitamins. Notice that, as shown in Table 10.1, most of the B vitamins have an RDA value. At the present time, tolerable upper intake levels (UL) can only be set for niacin, vitamin B_6, and folate (Institute of Medicine, 1998).

> **Recap:** The B-complex vitamins include thiamin, riboflavin, niacin, vitamin B_6 (pyridoxine), folate, vitamin B_{12} (cobalamin), pantothenic acid, and biotin. These vitamins primarily act as coenzymes in the metabolism of carbohydrates, fats, and protein. They are commonly found in whole grains, enriched breads, ready-to-eat cereals, meats, dairy products, and some fruits and vegetables. B-complex vitamin toxicity is rare unless a person consumes large doses as supplements. Thiamin deficiency causes beriberi, niacin deficiency causes pellagra, folate deficiency causes macrocytic anemia and can lead to neural tube defects in the developing fetus, and vitamin B_{12} deficiency leads to anemia and nervous system damage.

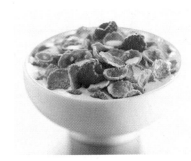

Ready-to-eat cereals are a good source of B-complex vitamins.

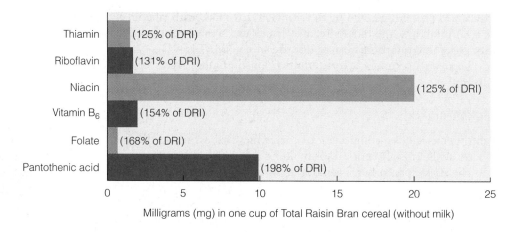

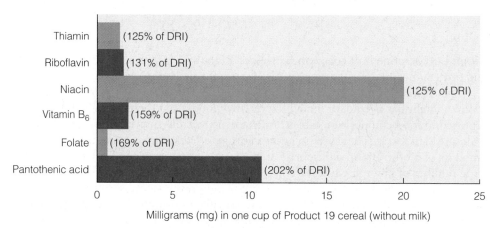

Figure 10.3 Enriched ready-to-eat cereals are a consistently good source of B-complex vitamins. (Data from U.S. Department of Agriculture, Agricultural Research Service, 2003, USDA Nutrient Database for Standard Reference, Release 16. Nutrient Data Laboratory Home Page, http://www.nal.usda.gov/fnic/foodcomp Accessed January 2004.)

Liz Nutri-Case

"Ever since my dance company folded after Christmas, I've been feeling exhausted. I know I should start auditioning for other companies, but it just seems too overwhelming right now. I'm cranky and spaced-out, and the least little thing makes me cry. Besides, I'm too fat to audition anywhere these days, because I'm so tired I've been skipping dance class. When I was still in bed at eleven o'clock this morning, my roommate told me I needed to start taking some B vitamins. She says that they give you energy. Maybe I'll ask her to drive me down to the health food store to buy some. It's only a mile away, but I don't think I have the energy to walk."

Is Liz's roommate correct when she asserts that B-complex vitamins "give you energy"? Considering what you've learned about Liz in previous Nutri-Case episodes, do you think it is likely that she'd benefit from taking B-complex vitamin supplements? Why or why not? What other concerns does her situation raise, and what additional advice might you give her?

Choline

acetylcholine A neurotransmitter that is involved in many functions, including muscle movement and memory storage.

Choline is a vitamin-like substance found in many foods. It is typically grouped with the B-complex vitamins because of its role in assisting homocysteine metabolism (see Table 10.1). Choline also accelerates the synthesis and release of **acetylcholine,** a

Table 10.2   Common Foods That Contain at Least 50% of the DRI for Select B-Complex Vitamins

Food Group	Thiamin	Riboflavin	Niacin	Vitamin B$_6$	Folate	Vitamin B$_{12}$	Pantothenic Acid
Meat, Poultry, Fish, Legumes	Pork loin, fried — 3 oz. Pork ham, canned — 3 oz.	Beef liver, fried — 3 oz. Shrimp, breaded and fried — 6–8 shrimp	Beef liver, fried — 3 oz. Chicken breast, breaded and fried — ½ breast Halibut, baked — ½ fillet Tuna fish, canned in oil, drained — 3 oz.	Beef liver, fried — 3 oz. Halibut, baked — ½ fillet Garbanzo beans, canned — 1 cup	Turkey giblets, simmered — 1 cup Lentils, boiled — 1 cup Pinto beans, boiled —1 cup	Clams, canned — 3 oz. Beef liver, fried — 3 oz. New England clam chowder soup — 1 cup Salmon, baked — ½ fillet Tuna fish, canned in water, drained — 3 oz.	Beef liver, fried – 3 oz.
Dairy	No dairy source	Chocolate milk-shake — 16 fl. oz.	No dairy source	No dairy source	No dairy source	New England clam chowder soup — 1 cup (a milk- or cream-based soup)	Yogurt, plain, skim milk — 8 oz. container
Grains	Trail mix, with chocolate chips, salted nuts and seeds — 1 cup	No grain source	No grain source	Long grain white rice, dry — 1 cup	Long grain white rice, dry — 1 cup	No grain source	Sunflower seeds, dry roasted — ¼ cup Long grain white rice, dry—1 cup
Vegetables and Fruits	Sweet potato, baked with skin — 1 potato	No vegetable or fruit source	Tomato paste, 1 cup	Hashed brown potatoes – 1 cup	No vegetable or fruit source	No vegetable or fruit source	Shiitake mushrooms, cooked — 1 cup

Source: Data from U.S. Department of Agriculture. Agricultural Research Service. 2003. USDA Nutrient Database for Standard Reference, Release 16. Nutrient Data Laboratory Home Page. http://www.nal.usda.gov/fnic/foodcomp Accessed January 2004.

neurotransmitter that is involved in many functions, including muscle movement and memory storage. Choline is also necessary for the synthesis of phospholipids and other components of cell membranes; thus, choline plays a critical role in the structural integrity of cell membranes. Finally, choline plays an important role in the transport and metabolism of fats and cholesterol.

Choline has an AI of 550 mg/day for men aged 19 and older and an AI of 425 mg/day for women ages 19 and older. The choline content of foods is not typically reported in nutrient databases. However, we do know that choline is widespread in foods, especially milk, liver, eggs, and peanuts. Inadequate intakes of choline can lead to increased fat accumulation in the liver, which eventually leads to liver damage. Excessive intake of supplemental choline results in various toxicity symptoms, including a fishy body odor, vomiting, excess salivation, sweating, diarrhea, and low blood pressure. The UL for choline for adults 19 years of age and older is 3.5 grams/day.

Iodine

Iodine is a trace mineral needed to support energy regulation. In our foods, iodine is mostly found in the form of iodide.

Iodine is critical for the synthesis of thyroid hormones. Our bodies require thyroid hormones to regulate body temperature, maintain resting metabolic rate, and support reproduction and growth.

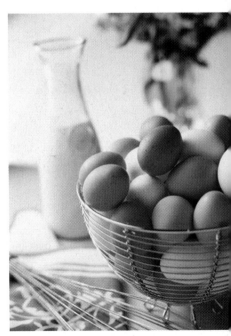

Choline is widespread in foods and can be found in eggs and milk.

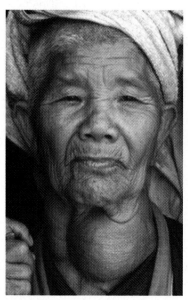

Figure 10.4   Goiter, or enlargement of the thyroid gland, occurs with both iodine toxicity and deficiency.

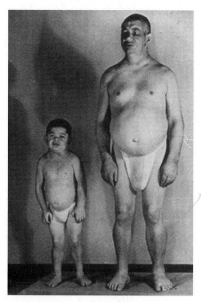

Figure 10.5   Cretinism is a special form of mental retardation that occurs in an infant when the pregnant mother suffers from iodine deficiency.

goiter   Enlargement of the thyroid gland; can be caused by either iodine toxicity or deficiency.

cretinism   A special form of mental retardation that occurs in infants when the mother experiences iodine deficiency during pregnancy.

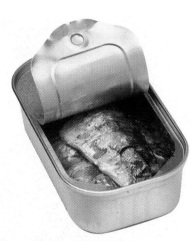

Saltwater fish, fresh or canned, contain iodine.

While our bodies need relatively little iodine, adequate amounts are necessary to maintain health. The RDA for adults 19 years of age and older is 150 µg/day. The UL for iodine is 1,100 µg/day.

Very few foods naturally contain iodine. Saltwater foods tend to have higher amounts of iodine because marine animals concentrate iodine from seawater. Good food sources include saltwater fish, shrimp, iodized salt, white and whole-wheat breads made with iodized salt and bread conditioners, and milk and other dairy products. Interestingly, iodine is added to dairy cattle feed and used in sanitizing solutions in the dairy industry, making dairy foods an important source of iodine. Iodine has been added to salt in the United States since the twentieth century to combat iodine deficiency resulting from poor iodine content of soils in this country. For many people, iodized salt is their only source of iodine, and approximately one-half a teaspoon of iodized salt meets the entire adult RDA for iodine.

Too much iodine blocks the synthesis of thyroid hormones. As the thyroid attempts to produce more hormones, it may enlarge, a condition known as **goiter** (Figure 10.4). (Goiter refers only to the enlarged thyroid gland, regardless of its cause.) Iodine toxicity generally occurs due to excessive supplementation.

Paradoxically, goiter is also the primary symptom of iodine deficiency. Iodine deficiency suppresses the production of thyroid hormones, leading to *hypothyroidism* (low levels of thyroid hormones) and goiter. Other symptoms of hypothyroidism are decreased body temperature, inability to tolerate cold environmental temperatures, weight gain, fatigue, and sluggishness. If a woman experiences iodine deficiency during pregnancy, her infant has a high risk of being born with a special form of mental retardation referred to as **cretinism.** In addition to mental retardation, these infants may suffer from stunted growth, deafness, and muteness (Figure 10.5).

Chromium

Chromium is a trace mineral that plays an important role in carbohydrate metabolism. You may be interested to learn that the chromium in our bodies is the same metal used in the chrome plating for cars.

Can Chromium Supplements Enhance Body Composition?

Because athletes are always looking for a competitive edge, there are a multitude of supplements marketed and sold to enhance exercise performance and body composition. Chromium supplements, predominantly in the form of chromium picolinate, are popular with body builders and weight lifters. This popularity stems from the claims that chromium increases muscle mass and muscle strength and decreases body fat.

An early study of chromium supplementation was promising, in that chromium use in both untrained men and football players was found to decrease body fat and increase muscle mass (Evans 1989). These findings caused a surge in popularity of chromium supplements, and motivated many scientists across the United States to test the reproducibility of these early findings. The next study of chromium supplementation found no effects of chromium on muscle mass, body fat, or muscle strength (Hasten et al. 1992).

These contradictory reports led experts to closely examine the two studies and to design more sophisticated studies to assess the effect of chromium on body composition. There were a number of flaws in the methodology of these early studies. One major concern was that the chromium status of the research participants prior to the study was not measured or controlled. It was possible that the participants were deficient in chromium; this deficiency could cause a more positive reaction to chromium than would be expected in people with normal chromium status.

A second major concern was that body composition was measured in these studies using the skinfold technique, in which calipers are used to measure the thickness of the skin and fat at various sites on the body. While this method gives a good general estimate of body fat in young, lean, healthy people, it is not sensitive to small changes in muscle mass. Thus, subsequent studies of chromium used more sophisticated methods of measuring body composition.

The results of research studies conducted over the past ten years consistently show that chromium supplementation has no effect on muscle mass, body fat, or muscle strength in a variety of groups, including untrained college males and females, obese females, collegiate wrestlers, and older men and women (Lukaski et al. 1996; Hallmark et al. 1996; Pasman, Westerterp-Plantenga, and Saris 1997; Walker et al. 1998; Campbell et al. 1999; Volpe et al. 2001; and Campbell et al. 2002). Despite the overwhelming evidence to the contrary, many supplement companies still claim that chromium supplements enhance strength and muscle mass and reduce body fat. These claims result in millions of dollars of sales of supplements to consumers each year. Armed with this information, you will be able to avoid being fooled by such an expensive nutrition myth. ●

Chromium enhances the ability of insulin to transport glucose from the bloodstream into cells. Chromium also plays important roles in the metabolism of RNA and DNA, in immune function, and in growth. Chromium supplements are marketed to reduce body fat and enhance muscle mass and have become popular with body builders and other athletes interested in improving their body composition. The Nutrition Myth or Fact box (above) investigates whether taking supplemental chromium is effective in improving body composition.

We have only very small amounts of chromium in our bodies. Whether the U.S. diet provides adequate chromium is controversial; our bodies appear to store less chromium as we age.

The AI for chromium for adults aged 19 to 50 years is 35 µg/day for men and 25 µg/day for women. For adults 51 years of age and older, the AI decreases to 30 µg/day and 20 µg/day for men and women, respectively.

Foods that have been identified as good sources of chromium include mushrooms, prunes, dark chocolate, nuts, whole grains, cereals, asparagus, brewer's yeast, some beers, and red wine. Dairy products are typically poor sources of chromium.

There appears to be no toxicity related to consuming chromium in the diet or in supplement form. Chromium deficiency appears to be uncommon in the United States. When induced in a research setting, chromium deficiency inhibits the uptake

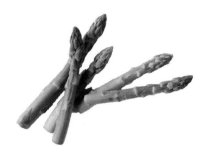

Our bodies contain very little chromium. Asparagus is a good dietary source of this trace mineral.

of glucose by the cells, causing a rise in blood glucose and insulin levels. Chromium deficiency can also result in elevated blood lipid levels and in damage to the brain and nervous system.

Manganese

A trace mineral, manganese is a cofactor involved in energy metabolism and in the formation of urea, the primary component of our urine. It also assists in the synthesis of the protein matrix found in bone tissue and in building cartilage, a tissue supporting our joints. As reviewed in Chapter 8, manganese is also an integral component of superoxide dismutase, an antioxidant enzyme. Thus, manganese assists in the conversion of free radicals to less damaging substances, protecting our bodies from oxidative damage.

The AI for manganese for adults 19 years of age and older is 2.3 mg/day for men and 1.8 mg/day for women. The UL for manganese is 11 mg/day for adults 19 years of age and older. Manganese requirements are easily met as this mineral is widespread in foods and is readily available in a varied diet. Whole-grain foods such as oat bran, wheat flour, whole-wheat spaghetti, and brown rice are good sources of manganese (Figure 10.6). Other foods that are good sources of manganese include pineapple, pine nuts, okra, spinach, and raspberries.

Manganese toxicity can occur in occupational environments in which people inhale manganese dust and can also result from drinking water high in manganese. Toxicity results in impairment of the neuromuscular system, causing symptoms similar to those seen in Parkinson's disease, such as muscle spasms and tremors. Manganese deficiency is rare in humans. Symptoms of manganese deficiency include impaired growth and reproductive function, reduced bone density and impaired skeletal growth, impaired glucose and lipid metabolism, and skin rash.

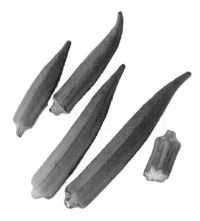

Okra is one of the many foods that contain manganese.

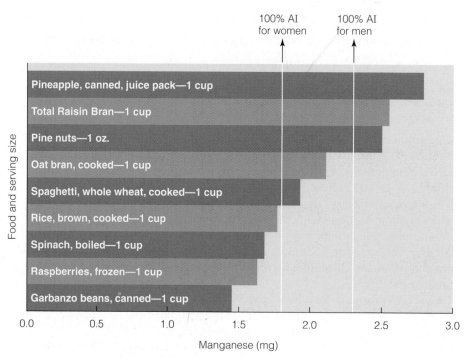

Figure 10.6   Common food sources of manganese. The AI for manganese is 2.3 mg/day for men and 1.8 mg/day for women. (Data from U.S. Department of Agriculture, Agricultural Research Service, 2003, USDA Nutrient Database for Standard Reference, Release 16. Nutrient Data Laboratory Home Page, http://www.nal.usda.gov/fnic/foodcomp Accessed January 2004.)

Sulfur

Sulfur is a major mineral and a component of the B-complex vitamins thiamin and biotin. In addition, as part of the amino acids methionine and cysteine, sulfur helps stabilize the three-dimensional shapes of proteins in our bodies. Our liver requires sulfur to assist in the detoxification of alcohol and various drugs, and sulfur assists us in maintaining acid-base balance.

We are able to synthesize ample sulfur from the protein-containing foods we eat; as a result, we do not need to consume sulfur in the diet, and there is no DRI for sulfur. There are no known toxicity or deficiency symptoms associated with sulfur.

> **Recap:** Choline is a vitamin-like substance that assists in homocysteine metabolism and the production of acetylcholine. Iodine is necessary for the synthesis of thyroid hormones, which regulate metabolic rate and body temperature. Chromium enhances the transport of glucose into the cell, is important in the metabolism of RNA and DNA, and plays a role in immune function and growth. Manganese is involved in energy metabolism, the formation of urea, the synthesis of bone protein matrix and cartilage, and protection against free radicals. Sulfur is part of the B-complex vitamins thiamin and biotin and also part of the amino acids methionine and cysteine.

What Is the Role of Blood in Maintaining Health?

Blood is critical to maintaining life, as it transports virtually everything in our bodies. No matter how efficiently we metabolize carbohydrates, fats, and proteins, without healthy blood to transport those nutrients to our cells, we could not survive. In addition to transporting nutrients and oxygen to our cells to support life, blood removes the waste products generated from metabolism so that they can be properly excreted. Our health and our ability to perform daily activities are compromised if the quantity and quality of our blood is diminished.

Blood is actually a tissue, the only fluid tissue in our bodies. Blood is comprised of four components (Figure 10.7). **Erythrocytes,** or red blood cells, are the cells that transport oxygen. **Leukocytes,** or white blood cells, are the key to our immune

erythrocytes The red blood cells, which are the cells that transport oxygen in our blood.

leukocytes The white blood cells, which protect us from infection and illness.

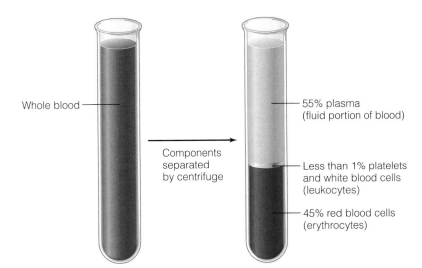

Figure 10.7   Blood has four components, which are visible when the blood is drawn into a test tube and spun in a centrifuge. The bottom layer is the erythrocytes, or red blood cells. The milky layer above the erythrocytes contains the leukocytes and platelets. The yellow fluid on top is the plasma.

platelets   Cell fragments that assist in the formation of blood clots and help stop bleeding.

plasma   The fluid portion of the blood; is needed to maintain adequate blood volume so that the blood can flow easily throughout our bodies.

function and protect us from infection and illness. **Platelets** are cell fragments that assist in the formation of blood clots and help stop bleeding. **Plasma** is the fluid portion of the blood, and it is needed to maintain adequate blood volume so that the blood can flow easily throughout our bodies.

Certain micronutrients play important roles in the maintenance of blood health through their actions as cofactors, coenzymes and regulators of oxygen transport. These nutrients are discussed in detail in the following section.

A Profile of Nutrients That Maintain Healthy Blood

The nutrients recognized as playing a critical role in maintaining blood health include vitamin K, iron, zinc, and copper. A summary of the functions, requirements, and toxicity and deficiency symptoms of these nutrients is provided in Table 10.3.

Vitamin K

Vitamin K is a fat-soluble vitamin important for both bone and blood health. The role of vitamin K in the synthesis of proteins involved in maintaining bone density was discussed in detail on page 312 in Chapter 9. In this section we focus primarily on its role in blood health.

Functions of Vitamin K

Vitamin K acts as a coenzyme that assists in the synthesis of a number of proteins that are involved in the coagulation of blood, including *prothrombin* and the *procoagulants, factors VII, IX,* and *X.* Without adequate vitamin K, our blood does not clot properly: clotting time can be delayed, or clotting may even fail to occur. The failure of our blood to clot can lead to increased bleeding from even minor wounds, as well as internal hemorrhaging.

How Much Vitamin K Should We Consume?

Our needs for vitamin K are relatively small, but intakes of this nutrient in the United States are highly variable because vitamin K is found in few foods (Booth and Suttie 1998). Healthful intestinal bacteria produce vitamin K in our large intestine, providing us with an important non-dietary source of vitamin K.

The AI for vitamin K for adults 19 years of age and older is 120 µg/day and 90 µg/day for men and women, respectively. There is no UL established for vitamin K at this time (Institute of Medicine 2001).

Green, leafy vegetables are good sources of vitamin K. Examples include collard greens, spinach, broccoli, brussels sprouts, and cabbage. Soybean and canola oils are also good sources. Refer to Figure 9.9 (page 327) for a description of the vitamin K content of these foods.

What Happens if We Consume Too Much Vitamin K?

There are no known side effects associated with consuming large amounts of vitamin K from supplements or from food (Institute of Medicine 2001). In the past, a synthetic form of vitamin K was used for therapeutic purposes and was shown to cause liver damage; this form is no longer used.

What Happens If We Don't Consume Enough Vitamin K?

Vitamin K deficiency inhibits our ability to form blood clots, resulting in excessive bleeding and even severe hemorrhaging in some cases. Vitamin K deficiency is rare in humans. People with diseases that cause malabsorption of fat, such as celiac disease, Crohn's disease, and cystic fibrosis, can suffer secondarily from a deficiency of vitamin K. Newborns are typically given an injection of vitamin K at birth, as they lack the intestinal bacteria necessary to produce this nutrient.

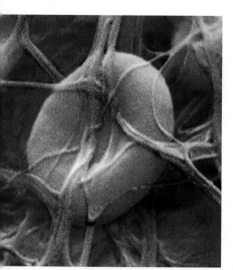

Blood clotting. Without enough vitamin K our blood will not clot properly.

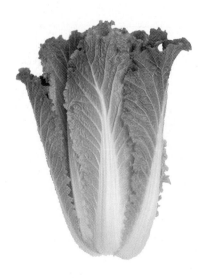

Green, leafy vegetables are a good source of vitamin K.

Table 10.3   Nutrients Involved in Maintaining Blood Health

Nutrient	Primary Functions	Recommended Intake	Toxicity Symptoms/ Side Effects	Deficiency Symptoms/ Side Effects
Vitamin K (fat-soluble vitamin)	Coenzyme that assists in the synthesis of proteins involved in the coagulation of blood Coenzyme involved in the synthesis of proteins that assist in maintaining bone density	AI for 19 years and older: Men = 120 µg/day Women = 90 µg/day	None known at this time	Excessive bleeding or severe hemorrhaging due to inability to form blood clots Effect on bone health is controversial
Iron (trace mineral)	As a component of hemoglobin, assists with oxygen transport in our blood As a component of myoglobin, assists in the transport of oxygen into muscle cells Cofactor for enzymes involved in energy metabolism Part of the antioxidant enzyme system that combats free radicals	RDA for 19 to 50 years: Men = 8 mg/day Women = 18 mg/day RDA for 51 years and older: Men = 8 mg/day Women = 8 mg/day RDA for pregnant females = 27 mg/day	Nausea Vomiting Diarrhea Dizziness, confusion Rapid heart beat Damage to heart, central nervous system, liver, kidneys Death	First stage of iron deficiency is marked by a decrease in iron stores with no physical symptoms Second stage of iron deficiency is marked by a decrease in iron transport, causing reduced work capacity Third stage of iron deficiency is marked by anemia, causing impaired work performance, general fatigue, pale skin, depressed immune function, impaired cognitive and nerve function, and impaired memory
Zinc (trace mineral)	Cofactor that assists with hemoglobin production Part of superoxide dismutase antioxidant enzyme system that combats free radicals Assists enzymes in metabolizing carbohydrates, fats, and proteins and in activating vitamin A to facilitate vision Facilitates folding of proteins which assists in gene regulation Plays role in cell replication and normal growth and sexual maturation Plays a role in proper development and function of immune system	RDA for 19 years and older: Men = 11 mg/day Women = 8 mg/day	Intestinal pain and cramps Nausea Vomiting Loss of appetite Diarrhea Headaches Depressed immune function Decreased concentration of high-density lipoprotein Reduced absorption of copper	Growth retardation Diarrhea Delayed sexual maturation and impotence Eye and skin lesions Hair loss Impaired appetite Increased incidence of illness and infections
Copper (trace mineral)	Cofactor in metabolic pathways that produce energy Coenzyme that assists in production of collagen and elastin Part of superoxide dismutase antioxidant enzyme system that combats free radicals Component of ceruloplasmin, which facilitates the proper transport of iron	RDA for 19 years of age and older: Men and Women = 900 µg/day	Abdominal pain and cramps Nausea Diarrhea Vomiting Liver damage occurs in extreme cases that result from Wilson's disease and other rare disorders	Anemia Reduced levels of white blood cells Osteoporosis in infants and growing children

As discussed in Chapter 9, the impact of vitamin K deficiency on bone health is controversial. Although a recent study found that low intakes of vitamin K were associated with a higher risk of bone fractures in women (Feskanich et al., 1999), there is not enough scientific evidence to strongly illustrate that vitamin K deficiency causes osteoporosis (Institute of Medicine 2001).

> **Recap:** Vitamin K is a fat-soluble vitamin and coenzyme that is important for blood clotting and bone metabolism. Bacteria manufacture vitamin K in our large intestine. The AIs for adult men and adult women are 120 µg per day and 90 µg per day, respectively.

Iron

Iron is a trace mineral that is needed in very small amounts in our diets. Despite our relatively small need for iron, iron deficiency is the most common nutrient deficiency in the world.

Functions of Iron

hemoglobin   The oxygen-carrying protein found in our red blood cells; almost two-thirds of all of the iron in our bodies is found in hemoglobin.

heme   The iron-containing molecule found in hemoglobin.

Iron is a component of many proteins in our bodies, including various enzymes and **hemoglobin,** which is the oxygen-carrying protein found in our red blood cells. In fact, almost two-thirds of all of the iron in our bodies is found in hemoglobin. As shown in Figure 10.8, the hemoglobin molecule consists of four polypeptide chains studded with four iron-containing **heme** groups. You know that we cannot survive for more than a few minutes without oxygen. Thus, hemoglobin's ability to transport oxygen throughout the body is absolutely critical to life. To carry oxygen, hemoglobin depends on the iron in its heme groups. Iron is able to bind with and release atoms such as oxygen, nitrogen, and sulfur very easily. It does this by transferring electrons to and from the other atoms as it moves between various oxidation

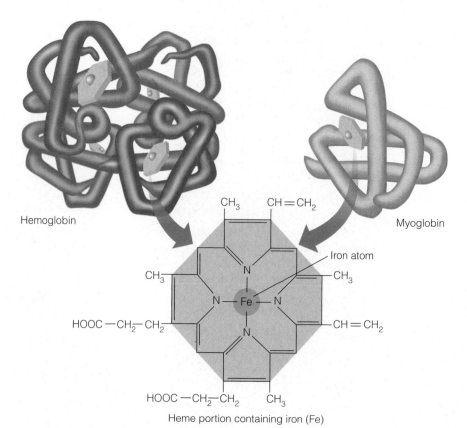

Heme portion containing iron (Fe)

Figure 10.8   Iron is contained in the heme portion of hemoglobin and myoglobin.

states. In the bloodstream, iron acts as a shuttle, picking up oxygen from the environment, binding it during its transport in the bloodstream, and then dropping it off again in our tissues.

In addition to being a part of hemoglobin, iron is a component of **myoglobin,** a protein similar to hemoglobin but found in muscle cells. As a part of myoglobin, iron assists in the transport of oxygen into muscle cells.

Finally, iron is found in the body in certain enzymes. As a component of *cytochromes,* iron is a cofactor involved in energy production. Cytochromes are electron carriers within the metabolic pathways that result in the production of energy from carbohydrates, fats, and protein. Also, as you learned in Chapter 8, iron is a part of the antioxidant enzyme system that assists in fighting free radicals. Interestingly, excess iron can also act as a prooxidant and promote the production of free radicals.

How Much Iron Should We Consume?

Our bodies contain relatively little iron; men have less than 4 grams of iron in their bodies, while women have just over 2 grams. Our bodies are capable of storing excess iron in two storage forms, **ferritin** and **hemosiderin.** The most common areas of iron storage in our bodies are the liver, bone marrow, intestinal mucosa, and spleen.

Our ability to absorb iron from the diet is influenced by a number of factors, including iron status, stomach acid content, the amount and type of iron in foods, and the presence of dietary factors that can either enhance or inhibit the absorption of iron. Absorption of iron is highest when our iron stores are low. Thus, people who have poor iron status, such as those with iron deficiency, pregnant women, or people who have recently experienced blood loss (including menstruation), have the highest iron absorption rates. In addition, adequate amounts of stomach acid are necessary for iron absorption. People with low levels of stomach acid, including many older adults, have a decreased ability to absorb iron.

The total amount of iron in your diet influences your absorption rate. People who consume low levels of dietary iron absorb more iron from their foods than those with higher dietary iron intakes. Our bodies can also detect when iron stores are high; when this occurs, less iron is absorbed from food.

The type of iron in the foods you eat is a major factor influencing your iron absorption. There are two types of iron found in foods: heme iron and non-heme iron. **Heme iron** is a part of hemoglobin and myoglobin and is found only in animal-based foods such as meat, fish, and poultry. **Non-heme iron** is the form of iron that is not a part of hemoglobin or myoglobin. It is found in both plant-based and animal-based foods. Heme iron is much more absorbable than non-heme iron. Since the iron in animal-based foods is about 40% heme iron and 60% non-heme iron, animal-based foods are good sources of absorbable iron. In contrast, all of the iron found in plant-based foods is non-heme iron. Meat, fish, and poultry also contain a special factor, **MPF factor,** (meat protein factor) that enhances the absorption of non-heme iron. Vitamin C (or ascorbic acid) also enhances the absorption of non-heme iron.

Dietary factors that impair iron absorption include phytates, polyphenols, vegetable proteins, and calcium. Phytates are found in legumes, rice, and whole grains. Polyphenols include tannins found in tea and coffee, and polyphenols are also present in oregano and red wine. Soybean protein and calcium inhibit iron absorption. Due to the variability of iron absorption as a result of these dietary factors, it is estimated that the bioavailability of iron from a vegan diet is approximately 10%, while it averages 18% for a mixed Western diet (Institute of Medicine 2001).

To optimize our absorption of iron, it is important to consume either foods rich in heme iron or iron-rich foods with food that is high in vitamin C. For instance, eating meat with beans or vegetables enhances the absorption of the non-heme iron found in the beans and vegetables. Drinking a glass of orange juice with your breakfast cereal will increase the absorption of the non-heme iron in the cereal. Cooking foods in cast-iron pans will also significantly increase the iron content of foods, as the iron in the pan is absorbed into the food during the cooking process.

myoglobin An iron-containing protein similar to hemoglobin except that it is found in muscle cells.

ferritin A storage form of iron in our bodies found primarily in the intestinal mucosa, spleen, bone marrow, and liver.

hemosiderin A storage form of iron in our bodies found primarily in the intestinal mucosa, spleen, bone marrow, and liver.

heme iron Iron that is a part of hemoglobin and myoglobin; found only in animal-based foods such as meat, fish, and poultry.

non-heme iron The form of iron that is not a part of hemoglobin or myoglobin; found in animal- and plant-based foods.

MPF factor (meat protein factor) A special factor found in meat, fish, and poultry that enhances the absorption of non-heme iron.

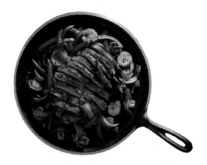

Cooking foods in cast-iron pans significantly increases their iron content.

It is best to avoid taking calcium supplements or drinking milk when eating iron-rich foods, as iron absorption will be impaired.

Recommended Dietary Intakes for Iron   The variability of iron availability from food sources was taken into consideration when estimating dietary recommendations for iron. The RDA for iron for men aged 19 years and older is 8 mg/day. The RDA for iron for women aged 19 to 50 years is 18 mg/day and decreases to 8 mg/day for women 51 years of age and older. The higher iron requirement for younger women is due to the excess iron and blood lost during menstruation. Pregnancy is a time of very high iron needs, and the RDA for pregnant women is 27 mg/day. The UL for iron for adults aged 19 and older is 45 mg/day.

There are a number of special circumstances that significantly affect iron requirements. These are identified in Table 10.4.

Shopper's Guide: Good Food Sources of Iron   Good food sources of heme iron include meats, poultry, and fish (Figure 10.9). Clams, oysters, and beef liver are particularly good sources of iron. Many breakfast cereals and breads are enriched with iron; although this iron is the non-heme type and less absorbable, it is still significant because these foods are a major part of the U.S. diet. Some vegetables and legumes are also good sources of iron, and the absorption of their non-heme iron can be enhanced by eating them with foods that contain MPF factor and heme iron or with vitamin-C rich foods.

What Happens if We Consume Too Much Iron?

Accidental iron overdose is the most common cause of poisoning deaths in children younger than six years of age in the United States (U.S. Food and Drug Administration 1997). It is important for parents to take the same precautions with dietary supplements as they would with other drugs, keeping them in a locked cabinet or well out of reach of children. Symptoms of iron toxicity include nausea, vomiting, diarrhea, dizziness, confu-

Table 10.4   Special Circumstances Affecting Iron Status

Circumstances That Improve Iron Status	Circumstances That Diminish Iron Status
Use of oral contraceptives — use of oral contraceptives reduces menstrual blood loss in women.	Use of hormone replacement therapy — use of hormone replacement therapy in postmenopausal women can cause uterine bleeding, increasing iron requirements.
Breastfeeding — breastfeeding delays resumption of menstruation in new mothers so reduces menstrual blood loss. It is therefore an important health measure, especially in developing nations.	Eating a vegetarian diet — vegetarian diets, particularly vegan diets, contain no sources of heme iron or MFP. Due to the low absorbability of non-heme iron, vegetarians have iron requirements that are 1.8 times higher than nonvegetarians.
Consumption of iron-containing foods and supplements.	Intestinal parasitic infection — approximately one billion people suffer from intestinal parasite infection. Many of these parasites cause intestinal bleeding and occur in countries in which iron intakes are inadequate. Iron deficiency anemia is common in people with intestinal parasitic infection.
	Blood donation — blood donors have lower iron stores than nondonors; people who donate frequently, particularly premenopausal women, may require iron supplementation to counter the iron losses that occur with blood donation.
	Intense endurance exercise training — people engaging in intense endurance exercise appear to be at risk for poor iron status due to many factors, including suboptimal iron intake and increased iron loss due to rupture of red blood cells and increased fecal losses.

Source: Data from Institute of Medicine, Food and Nutrition Board. *Dietary Reference Intakes for Vitamin A, Vitamin K, Arsenic, Boron, Chromium, Copper, Iodine, Iron, Manganese, Molybdenum, Nickel, Silicon, Vanadium, and Zinc.* © 2000 by the National Academy of Sciences. (Washington, DC: National Academies Press, 2000.)

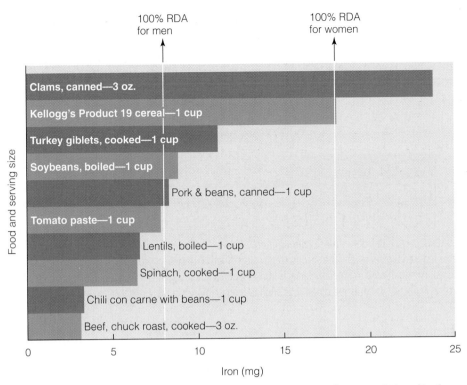

Figure 10.9   Common food sources of iron. The RDA for iron is 8 mg/day for men and 18 mg/day for women aged 19 to 50 years. (Data from U.S. Department of Agriculture, Agricultural Research Service, 2003, USDA Nutrient Database for Standard Reference, Release 16. Nutrient Data Laboratory Home Page, http://www.nal.usda.gov/fnic/foodcomp Accessed January 2004.)

sion, and rapid heart beat. If iron toxicity is not treated quickly, significant damage to the heart, central nervous system, liver, and kidneys can result in death.

Adults who take iron supplements even at prescribed doses commonly experience constipation. Taking vitamin C with the iron supplement not only enhances absorption but also can help reduce constipation. Other gastrointestinal symptoms include nausea, vomiting, and diarrhea.

As introduced in Chapter 8, some individuals suffer from a hereditary disorder called hemochromatosis. This disorder affects between 1 in 200 and 1 in 400 individuals of northern European descent (Bacon et al. 1999). Hemochromatosis is characterized by excessive absorption of dietary iron and altered iron storage. The accumulation of iron in these individuals over many years causes cirrhosis of the liver, liver cancer, heart attack and heart failure, diabetes, and arthritis. Men are more at risk for this disease than women due to the higher losses of iron in women through menstruation. Treatment includes reducing dietary intake of iron, avoiding high intakes of vitamin C, and withdrawing blood occasionally.

What Happens if We Don't Consume Enough Iron?

Iron deficiency is the most common nutrient deficiency in the world. People at particularly high risk for iron deficiency include infants and young children, adolescent girls, premenopausal women, and pregnant women. Refer to the Highlight box on page 369 to learn more about the impact of iron deficiency on people around the world.

Iron deficiency progresses through three stages (Figure 10.10). The first stage of iron deficiency causes a decrease in iron *stores*, resulting in reduced levels of ferritin. During this first stage, there are generally no physical symptoms because hemoglobin levels are not yet affected. The second stage of iron deficiency causes a decrease in the *transport* of iron. This manifests as a reduction in the transport protein for iron, called **transferrin**. The production of heme also starts to decline during this stage,

transferrin   The transport protein for iron.

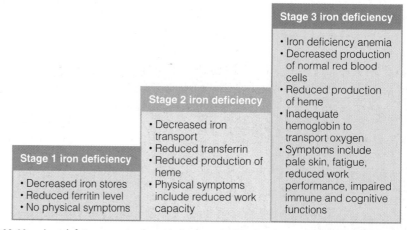

Figure 10.10 Iron deficiency passes through three stages. The first stage is identified by decreased iron stores, or reduced ferritin levels. The second stage is identified by decreased iron transport, or a reduction in transferrin. The final stage of iron deficiency is iron-deficiency anemia, which is identified by decreased production of normal, healthy red blood cells and inadequate hemoglobin levels.

iron-deficiency anemia A form of anemia that results from severe iron deficiency.

leading to symptoms of reduced work capacity. During the third and final stage of iron deficiency, **iron-deficiency anemia** results. In iron-deficiency anemia, the production of normal, healthy red blood cells decreases and hemoglobin levels are inadequate. Iron-deficiency anemia is discussed in detail on page 373.

> **Recap:** Iron is a trace mineral that, as part of the hemoglobin protein, plays a major role in the transportation of oxygen in our blood. Iron is also a coenzyme in many metabolic pathways involved in energy production. The RDA for adult men aged 19 years and older is 8 mg/day. The RDA for adult women aged 19 to 50 years is 18 mg/day. Meat, fish, and poultry are good sources of heme iron, which is more absorbable than non-heme iron. Toxicity symptoms for iron range from nausea and vomiting to organ damage and potentially death. If left untreated, iron deficiency eventually leads to iron deficiency anemia.

Zinc

Zinc is a trace mineral that acts as a cofactor for approximately a hundred different enzymes. It thereby plays an important role in many physiologic processes in nearly every body system.

Functions of Zinc

As a cofactor, zinc assists in the production of hemoglobin, indirectly supporting the adequate transport of oxygen to our cells. Zinc is also part of the superoxide dismutase antioxidant enzyme system and thus helps fight the oxidative damage caused by free radicals. It assists enzymes in generating energy from carbohydrates, fats, and protein and in activating vitamin A in the retina of the eye.

Zinc also plays a role in facilitating the folding of proteins into biologically active molecules used in gene regulation. Zinc is critical for cell replication and normal growth. In fact, zinc deficiency was discovered in the early 1960s when researchers were trying to determine the cause of severe growth retardation, anemia, and poorly developed testicles in a group of Middle Eastern men. These symptoms of zinc deficiency illustrate its critical role in normal growth and sexual maturation.

Zinc is vital for the proper development and functioning of the immune system. In fact, zinc has received so much attention for its contribution to immune system health that zinc lozenges have been formulated to fight the common cold. The Nutrition Debate at the end of this chapter explores the question of whether or not these lozenges are effective in combating the common cold.

Global Nutrition: Iron Deficiency Around the World

Iron deficiency is the most common nutritional deficiency in the world. According to the World Health Organization (2003), approximately four to five billion people, or 66 to 80% of the world's population, are iron deficient. Because of its high prevalence worldwide, iron deficiency is considered an epidemic.

As you have learned in this chapter, severe iron deficiency results in anemia. Iron deficiency appears to be the main cause of anemia around the world. Other factors that can cause anemia include deficiencies of folate, vitamin B₁₂, and vitamin A, and infections such as hookworm and malarial parasites. In fact, it is estimated that two billion people suffer from worm infections, while 300 to 500 million people suffer from malaria.

Those who are particularly susceptible to iron deficiency include people living in developing countries, pregnant women, and young children. But iron deficiency does not only hurt individuals. Because it results in increased healthcare needs, premature death and resultant family breakdown, and lost work productivity, it also damages communities and entire nations.

Among children, the health consequences of iron deficiency anemia are particularly devastating. They include:

- Premature birth

- Low birth weight

- Increased risk of infections

- Increased risk of premature death

- Impaired cognitive and physical development

- Behavioral problems and poor school performance

To date, it is still unclear if iron supplementation in children already suffering from iron deficiency anemia can effectively and consistently reverse the cognitive and behavioral damage that has occurred (Grantham-McGregor and Ani 2001).

The World Health Organization (2003) has developed a comprehensive plan to address all aspects of iron deficiency and anemia. This plan is being implemented in developing countries that suffer high rates of iron deficiency and anemia. This plan involves:

1. Increasing iron intake with iron supplements, iron-rich foods, and with foods that enhance iron absorption;
2. Controlling infections that cause anemia, including hookworm infections and malaria; and
3. Improving overall nutritional status by controlling major nutrient deficiencies and improving the quality and diversity of people's diets.

By implementing this plan around the world, it is hoped that the devastating effects of iron deficiency can be reduced and potentially even eliminated. ●

How Much Zinc Should We Consume?

As with iron, our need for zinc is relatively small, but our intakes are variable and absorption is influenced by a number of factors. Overall, zinc absorption is similar to that of iron, ranging from 10 to 35% of dietary zinc. People with poor zinc status absorb more zinc than individuals with optimal zinc status, and zinc absorption increases during times of growth, sexual development, and pregnancy.

Several dietary factors influence zinc absorption. High non-heme iron intakes can inhibit zinc absorption, which is a primary concern with iron supplementation (which are non-heme) particularly during pregnancy and lactation. High intakes of heme iron appear to have no effect on zinc absorption. Although calcium is known to inhibit zinc absorption in animals, this has not been demonstrated to occur in humans. The phytates and fiber found in whole grains and beans strongly inhibit iron absorption. In contrast, dietary protein enhances zinc absorption, with animal-based proteins increasing the absorption of zinc to a much greater extent than plant-based proteins. It's not surprising, then, that the primary cause of the zinc deficiency in the Middle Eastern men just mentioned was their low consumption of meat and high consumption of beans and unleavened breads (also called *flat breads*). In leavening bread, the baker adds yeast to the dough. This not only makes the bread rise, but also helps reduce the phytate content of the bread.

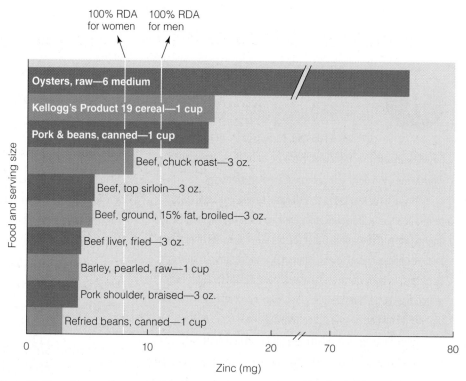

Figure 10.11   Common food sources of zinc. The RDA for zinc is 11 mg/day for men and 8 mg/day for women. (Data from U.S. Department of Agriculture, Agricultural Research Service, 2003, USDA Nutrient Database for Standard Reference, Release 16. Nutrient Data Laboratory Home Page, http://www.nal.usda.gov/fnic/foodcomp Accessed January 2004.)

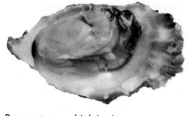

Raw oysters are high in zinc.

The RDA values for zinc for adult men and women aged 19 and older are 11 mg/day and 8 mg/day, respectively. The UL for zinc for adults aged 19 and older is 40 mg/day.

Good food sources of zinc include red meats, some seafood, whole grains, and enriched grains and cereals. The dark meat of poultry has a higher content of zinc than white meat. As zinc is significantly more absorbable from animal-based foods, zinc deficiency is a concern for people eating a vegan diet. Figure 10.11 shows various foods that are relatively high in zinc.

What Happens if We Consume Too Much Zinc?

Eating high amounts of dietary zinc does not appear to lead to toxicity. Zinc toxicity can occur from consuming zinc in supplement form and in fortified foods. Toxicity symptoms include intestinal pain and cramps, nausea, vomiting, loss of appetite, diarrhea, and headaches. Excessive zinc supplementation has also been shown to depress immune function and decrease high-density lipoprotein concentrations. High intakes of zinc can also reduce copper status, as zinc absorption interferes with the absorption of copper.

What Happens if We Don't Consume Enough Zinc?

Zinc deficiency is uncommon in the United States but occurs more often in countries in which people consume predominantly grain-based foods. Symptoms of zinc deficiency include growth retardation, diarrhea, delayed sexual maturation and impotence, eye and skin lesions, hair loss, and impaired appetite. As zinc is critical to a healthy immune system, zinc deficiency also results in increased incidence of infections and illnesses.

Copper

Copper is a trace mineral that functions as a cofactor in many physiologic reactions. Copper is widely distributed in foods, and copper deficiency is rare.

Copper functions as a cofactor in the metabolic pathways that produce energy, in the production of the connective tissues collagen and elastin, and as part of the superoxide dismutase enzyme system that fights the damage caused by free radicals. Copper is a component of *ceruloplasmin,* a protein that is critical for the proper transport of iron. If ceruloplasmin levels are inadequate, iron accumulation results, causing symptoms similar to those described with the genetic disorder hemochromatosis (page 367). Copper is also necessary for the regulation of certain neurotransmitters important to brain function.

Copper needs are very small, and people who eat a varied diet can easily meet their requirements. As we saw with iron and zinc, people with low dietary copper intakes absorb more copper than people with high dietary intakes. Also recall that high zinc intakes can reduce copper absorption, and subsequently, copper status. In fact, zinc supplementation is used as a treatment for a rare disorder called Wilson's disease, in which copper toxicity occurs. High iron intakes can also interfere with copper absorption in infants.

The RDA for copper for men and women aged 19 years and older is 900 µg/day. The UL for adults ages 19 years and older is 10 mg/day.

Good food sources of copper include organ meats, seafood, nuts, and seeds. Whole-grain foods are also relatively good sources. Figure 10.12 reviews some foods relatively high in copper.

The long-term effects of copper toxicity are not well studied in humans. Toxicity symptoms include abdominal pain and cramps, nausea, diarrhea, and vomiting. Liver damage occurs in the extreme cases of copper toxicity that occur with Wilson's disease and other health conditions associated with excessive copper levels.

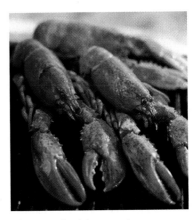

Lobster is a food that contains copper.

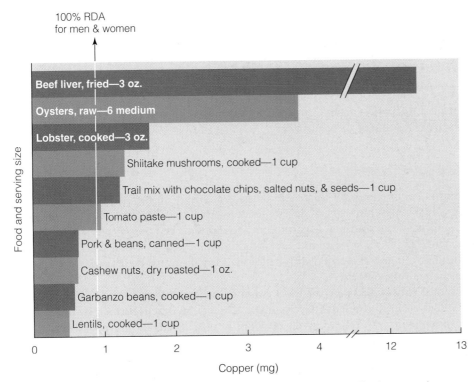

Figure 10.12 Common food sources of copper. The RDA for copper is 900 µg/day for men and women. (Data from U.S. Department of Agriculture, Agricultural Research Service, 2003, USDA Nutrient Database for Standard Reference, Release 16. Nutrient Data Laboratory Home Page, http://www.nal.usda.gov/fnic/foodcomp Accessed January 2004.)

Copper deficiency is rare but can occur in premature infants fed milk-based formulas and in adults fed prolonged formulated diets that are deficient in copper. Deficiency symptoms include anemia, reduced levels of white blood cells, and osteoporosis in infants and growing children.

> **Recap:** Zinc is a trace mineral that is a part of almost a hundred enzymes that impact virtually every body system. Zinc plays a critical role in hemoglobin synthesis, physical growth and sexual maturation, immune function, and assists in fighting the oxidative damage caused by free radicals. Copper is a trace mineral that is a cofactor in the metabolic pathways that produce energy, in the production of the connective tissues collagen and elastin, and as part of the superoxide dismutase enzyme system that fights the damage caused by free radicals. Copper is also a component of ceruloplasmin, a protein that is critical for the proper transport of iron.

Theo *Nutri-Case*

"You know, I never thought I needed to take a multivitamin because I'm healthy and I eat lots of different kinds of foods. But now I've learned in my nutrition course about what all these vitamins and minerals do in the body, and I'm thinking, heck, maybe I should take one just for insurance. I mean, I use up a lot of fuel playing basketball and working out. Maybe if I popped a pill every day, I'd have an easier time keeping my weight up!"

Do you think Theo should take a multivitamin-mineral supplement "just for insurance"? Why or why not? Would taking one be likely to have any effect on Theo's weight?

What Disorders Can Result from Inadequate Intakes of Nutrients Involved in Energy Metabolism and Blood Health?

There are a number of illnesses and disorders that can occur if our intake of the nutrients related to energy metabolism and blood health are inadequate. Following is a brief review of some of these disorders.

Neural Tube Defects

A woman's requirement for folate substantially increases during pregnancy. This is because of the high rates of cell development needed for enlargement of the uterus, development of the placenta, expansion of the mother's red blood cells, and growth of the fetus. Inadequate folate intake during pregnancy can not only cause macrocytic anemia, but it is also associated with major malformations in the fetus that are classified as neural tube defects.

neural tube defects The most common malformations of the central nervous system that occur during fetal development. A folate deficiency can cause neural tube defects.

Neural tube defects are the most common malformations of the central nervous system that occur during fetal development. The neural tube is formed by the fourth week of pregnancy, and it eventually develops into the brain and the spinal cord of the fetus. In a folate-deficient environment, the tube will fail to fold and close properly. The resultant defect in the newborn depends on the degree of failure and can range from protrusion of the spinal cord outside of the spinal column to a partial absence of brain tissue. Some forms of neural tube defects are minor and can be surgically repaired, while other forms are fatal. Neural tube defects are described in more detail in Chapter 15.

The challenging aspect of neural tube defects is that they occur very early in a woman's pregnancy, almost always before a woman knows she is pregnant. Thus, adequate folate intake is extremely important for all sexually active women of child-bearing age, whether or not they intend to become pregnant. To prevent neural tube defects, it is recommended that all women capable of becoming pregnant consume 400 μg of folate daily from supplements, fortified foods, or both in addition to the folate they consume in their standard diet (Institute of Medicine 1998). The importance of folate in early pregnancy is also discussed in more detail on page 544.

Vascular Disease and Homocysteine

Folate and vitamin B_{12} are necessary for the metabolism of the amino acid homocysteine. When intakes of these two nutrients are insufficient, homocysteine cannot be properly metabolized, and it becomes more concentrated in our blood. A thorough review of recent studies on this topic showed that elevated levels of homocysteine are associated with a 1.5 to 2 times greater risk for cardiovascular, cerebrovascular, and peripheral vascular diseases (Beresford and Boushey 1997). These diseases substantially increase a person's risk for a heart attack or stroke.

The exact mechanism by which elevated homocysteine levels increase the risk for vascular diseases is currently unknown. It has been speculated (Mayer, Jacobsen, and Robinson 1996) that homocysteine may damage the lining of our blood vessels and stimulate the accumulation of plaque, which can lead to hardening of the arteries. Homocysteine also increases the clotting of our blood, which could lead to an increased risk of blocked arteries.

Although there is growing research evidence to suggest that low intakes of folate and vitamin B_{12} are associated with elevated homocysteine levels, the Institute of Medicine (1998) states that the DRI values for these two nutrients cannot be established based on this evidence at the present time. However, the importance of consuming adequate amounts of folate and vitamin B_{12} cannot be minimized. By eating foods that contain ample amounts of these nutrients, we not only reduce our risk for macrocytic and pernicious anemias, but we may also decrease our risk for a heart attack or stroke.

Anemia

The term *anemia* literally means "without blood"; it is used to refer to any condition in which hemoglobin levels are low. Some anemias are caused by genetic problems. For instance, you've probably also heard of *sickle cell anemia*, a genetic disorder in which the red blood cells have a sickle shape. Another inherited anemia is *thalassemia*, a condition characterized by red blood cells that are small and short-lived. Other anemias are due to micronutrient deficiencies. Earlier in this chapter, we introduced three common deficiency-related anemias: iron-deficiency anemia, pernicious anemia, and macrocytic anemia. We discuss these in more detail here.

Iron-Deficiency Anemia

Red blood cells that are produced in an iron-deficient environment are smaller than normal and do not contain enough hemoglobin to transport adequate oxygen or to allow the proper transfer of electrons to produce energy. As normal cellular death occurs over time, more and more healthy red blood cells are replaced by these deficient cells, and the classic symptoms of oxygen and energy deprivation develop. These symptoms include impaired work performance, general fatigue, pale skin, depressed immune function, impaired cognitive and nerve function, and impaired memory. Pregnant women with severe anemia are at higher risk for low-birth-weight infants, premature delivery, and increased infant mortality.

Pernicious Anemia

pernicious anemia A special form of anemia that is the primary cause of a vitamin B_{12} deficiency; occurs at the end stage of an autoimmune disorder that causes the loss of various cells in the stomach.

intrinsic factor A protein secreted by cells of the stomach that binds to vitamin B_{12} and aids its absorption in the small intestine.

As mentioned earlier in this chapter, **pernicious anemia** is a special form of anemia that is the primary cause of a vitamin B_{12} deficiency. Pernicious anemia occurs at the end stage of an autoimmune disorder that causes the loss of various cells in the stomach. The most common cause of the vitamin B_{12} deficiency seen with pernicious anemia is lack of a protein called **intrinsic factor,** which is normally secreted by these particular cells in the stomach. Intrinsic factor binds to vitamin B_{12} and aids its absorption in the small intestine. Pernicious anemia results in a reduction or complete cessation of intrinsic factor production. Without intrinsic factor, vitamin B_{12} cannot cross the intestinal lining. Inadequate production of intrinsic factor occurs more commonly in older people, making them at higher risk for vitamin B_{12} deficiency and pernicious anemia. Pernicious anemia can also occur in people who consume little or no vitamin B_{12} in their diets, such as people following a vegan diet. It is also commonly seen in people with malabsorption disorders, as well as in people with tapeworm infestation of the gut, as the worms take up the vitamin B_{12} before it can be absorbed by the intestines.

Symptoms of pernicious anemia include pale skin, reduced energy and exercise tolerance, fatigue, and shortness of breath. In addition, because nerve cells are destroyed, patients with pernicious anemia lose the ability to perform coordinated movements and maintain their body's positioning. Central nervous system involvement can lead to irritability, confusion, depression, and even paranoia. As we saw in the case of Mr. Katz in the chapter opener, even with prompt administration of vitamin B_{12} after onset of CNS-involved symptoms, such symptoms are only partially reversible.

Macrocytic Anemia

macrocytic anemia A form of anemia manifested as the production of larger than normal red blood cells containing insufficient hemoglobin, which inhibits adequate transport of oxygen; also called megaloblastic anemia. Macrocytic anemia can be caused by a severe folate deficiency.

A severe folate deficiency results in a condition called **macrocytic anemia.** Folate deficiency impairs DNA synthesis, which impairs the normal production of red blood cells. Macrocytic anemia is manifested as the production of larger than normal red blood cells containing insufficient hemoglobin, thus inhibiting adequate transport of oxygen. Because larger than normal red blood cells are produced in this situation, another term for macrocytic anemia is *megaloblastic anemia.* Symptoms of macrocytic anemia are similar to the symptoms that occur with other types of anemia, including weakness, fatigue, difficulty concentrating, irritability, headache, shortness of breath, and reduced exercise tolerance.

Recap: Neural tube defects are potentially serious and even fatal malformations of the central nervous system in a developing fetus that can result from folate deficiency in the first few weeks of pregnancy. Low intakes of folate and vitamin B_{12} are associated with elevated blood homocysteine levels, which increase the risk of cardiovascular, cerebrovasular, and peripheral vascular disease. Anemia refers to any condition in which hemoglobin levels are low. Inadequate intake of iron causes iron-deficiency anemia, an autoimmune disorder causes pernicious anemia, and an inadequate intake of folate causes macrocytic anemia.

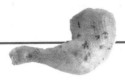

Chapter Summary

- The B-complex vitamins include thiamin, riboflavin, vitamin B_6, niacin, folate, vitamin B_{12}, pantothenic acid, and biotin.

- The primary role of the B-complex vitamins is to act as coenzymes. In this role, they activate enzymes and assist them in: the metabolism of carbohydrates, fats, and amino acids; the repair and replication of DNA; cell differentiation; the formation and maintenance of the central nervous system; and the formation of blood.

- Deficiencies of the B-complex vitamins can cause beriberi (thiamin), pellagra (niacin), neural tube defects (folate), and elevated homocysteine levels (folate and vitamin B_{12}).

- Choline is a vitamin-like substance that assists with homocysteine metabolism. Choline also accelerates the synthesis and release of acetylcholine, a neurotransmitter that is involved in a variety of functions such as muscle function and memory storage.

- Iodine is a trace mineral needed for the synthesis of thyroid hormones. Thyroid hormones are integral to the regulation of body temperature, maintenance of resting metabolic rate, and healthy reproduction and growth.

- Chromium is a trace mineral that enhances the ability of insulin to transport glucose from the bloodstream into the cell. Chromium is also necessary for the metabolism of RNA and DNA, and supports normal growth and immune function.

- Manganese is a trace mineral that acts as a cofactor in energy metabolism and in the formation of urea. Manganese also assists in the synthesis of the protein matrix found in bone, assists in building cartilage, and is a component of the superoxide dismutase antioxidant enzyme system.

- Sulfur is a major mineral that is a component of the B-complex vitamins thiamin and biotin. It is also a part of the amino acids methionine and cysteine. Sulfur helps stabilize the three-dimensional shapes of proteins and helps the liver detoxify alcohol and various drugs.

- Blood is the only fluid tissue in our bodies. It has four components: erythrocytes, or red blood cells; leukocytes, or white blood cells; platelets; and plasma, or the fluid portion of our blood.

- Blood is critical for transporting oxygen and nutrients to our cells and for removing waste products from our cells so they can be properly excreted.

- Vitamin K is a fat-soluble vitamin that acts as a coenzyme assisting in the coagulation of blood. Vitamin K is also a coenzyme in the synthesis of proteins that assist in maintaining bone density.

- Iron is a trace mineral. Almost two-thirds of the iron in our bodies is found in hemoglobin, the oxygen-carrying protein in our blood. One of the primary functions of iron is to assist with the transportation of oxygen in our blood. Iron is a cofactor for many of the enzymes involved in the metabolism of carbohydrates, fats, and protein. It is also a part of the superoxide dismutase antioxidant enzyme system that fights free radicals.

- Zinc is a trace mineral that acts as a cofactor in the production of hemoglobin, in the superoxide dismutase antioxidant enzyme system, in the metabolism of carbohydrates, fats, and proteins, and in activating vitamin A in the retina. Zinc is also critical for cell reproduction and growth and for proper development and functioning of the immune system.

- Copper is a trace mineral that functions as a cofactor in the metabolic pathways that produce energy, in the production of collagen and elastin, and as part of the superoxide dismutase antioxidant enzyme system. Copper is also a component of ceruloplasmin, a protein needed for the proper transport of iron.

- Neural tube defects, which can result from inadequate folate intake during the first four weeks of pregnancy, are the most common malformations of the fetal central nervous system. Some neural tube defects are minor and can be treated with surgery; other neural tube defects are fatal.

- Inadequate intakes of folate and vitamin B_{12} are associated with elevated homocysteine levels. Elevated homocysteine levels are associated with a greater risk of suffering from cardiovascular, cerebrovascular, and peripheral vascular diseases. These diseases significantly increase one's risk for a heart attack or stroke.

- *Anemia* is a term that means "without blood". Severe iron deficiency results in iron-deficiency anemia, in which the production of normal, healthy red blood cells decreases and hemoglobin levels are inadequate. Iron deficiency is the most common nutrient deficiency in the world.

- Pernicious anemia is caused by a deficit of intrinsic factor, which in turn results in vitamin B_{12} deficiency. Pernicious anemia causes reduced energy and exercise tolerance, as well as signs of nervous system damage, including impaired movement and cognitive and personality changes.

- Macrocytic anemia results from folate deficiency and causes the formation of excessively large red blood cells that have reduced hemoglobin. Symptoms are similar to those of iron-deficiency anemia.

Review Questions

1. The B-complex vitamins include
   a. niacin, folate, and iodine.
   b. cobalamin, iodine, and chromium.
   c. manganese, riboflavin, and pyridoxine.
   d. thiamin, pantothenic acid, and biotin.

2. The micronutrient most closely associated with blood clotting is
   a. iron.
   b. vitamin K.
   c. zinc.
   d. vitamin B_{12}.

3. Which of the following statements about iron is true?
   a. Iron is stored primarily in the liver, the blood vessel walls, and the heart muscle.
   b. Iron is a component of hemoglobin, myoglobin, and certain enzymes.
   c. Iron is a component of red blood cells, platelets, and plasma.
   d. Excess iron is stored primarily in the form of ferritin, cytochromes, and intrinsic factor.

4. Homocysteine is
   a. a byproduct of glycolysis.
   b. a trace mineral.
   c. an amino acid.
   d. a B-complex vitamin.

5. Which of the following statements about choline is true?
   a. Choline is found exclusively in foods of animal origin.
   b. Choline is a B-complex vitamin that assists in homocysteine metabolism.
   c. Choline is a neurotransmitter that is involved in muscle movement and memory storage.
   d. Choline is necessary for the synthesis of phospholipids and other components of cell membranes.

6. **True or false?** Blood has four components: erythrocytes, leukocytes, platelets, and plasma.

7. **True or false?** There is no DRI for sulfur.

8. **True or false?** Iron deficiency causes pernicious anemia.

9. **True or false?** The best way for a pregnant woman to protect her fetus against neural tube defects is to begin taking a folate supplement as soon as she learns she is pregnant.

10. **True or false?** Wilson's disease occurs when copper deficiency allows accumulation of iron in the body.

11. In the chapter-opening story, Mr. Katz was given an injection of vitamin B_{12}. Why didn't his physician simply give him the vitamin in pill form?

12. Cassandra is eleven years old and has just begun menstruating. She and her family members are vegans (that is, they consume only plant-based foods). Explain why Cassandra's parents should be careful that their daughter consume not only adequate iron, but also adequate vitamin C.

13. Avery is a lacto-ovo-vegetarian. His typical daily diet includes milk, yogurt, cheese, eggs, nuts, seeds, legumes, whole grains, and a wide variety of fruits and vegetables. He does not take any supplements. What, if any, micronutrients are likely to be inadequate in his diet?

14. Janine is 23 years old and engaged to be married. She is forty pounds overweight, has hypertension, and her mother suffered a mild stroke recently, at age 45. For all these reasons, Janine is highly motivated to lose weight and has put herself on a strict low-carbohydrate diet recommended by a friend. She now scrupulously avoids breads, pastries, pasta, rice, and "starchy" fruits and vegetables. Identify two reasons why Janine should consider taking a folate supplement.

15. Create a simple flow chart showing how loss of intrinsic factor in an older adult can lead to symptoms of dementia.

Test Yourself Answers

1. **False.** B-complex vitamins do not directly provide energy for our bodies. However, they play critical roles in ensuring that our bodies are able to generate energy from carbohydrates, fats, and proteins.

2. **True.** People who consume a vegan diet need to pay particularly close attention to consuming enough vitamin B_{12}, iron, and zinc. In some cases, these individuals may need to take supplements to consume adequate amounts of these nutrients.

3. **False.** Research studies have failed to show any consistent effects of chromium supplements on reducing body fat or enhancing muscle mass.

4. **True.** This deficiency is particularly common in infants, children, and women of childbearing age.

5. **True and false!** For an individual who consumes a varied diet that provides adequate energy and nutrients, this statement is true. However, many people do not consume a varied diet that provides adequate levels of micronutrients, and others have health issues that increase their requirements or affect their ability to absorb micronutrients from food. For these individuals, a daily multivitamin-mineral supplement is not a waste of money and is important to optimize health.

Web Links

www.nal.usda.gov/fnic/foodcomp
Nutrient Data Laboratory Home Page
Click on Reports for Single Nutrients to find reports listing food sources for selected nutrients.

www.bbc.co.uk/health/complementary/vitamins.shtml
BBC Healthy Living: Complementary Medicine: Vitamins
This page provides information on vitamins and minerals, signs of deficiency, therapeutic uses, and food sources.

www.cdc.gov/nceh/dls/factsheets/folate.htm
Assessing Levels of Folate, B Vitamins, and Related Metabolites in the U.S. Population
The U.S. Centers for Disease Control provide information on the effects of folate and B vitamin deficiencies and the agency's plan to assess the public's intake of these nutrients.

www.anemia.com
Anemia Lifeline
Visit this site to learn about anemia and its various treatments.

www.unicef.org/nutrition/index
UNICEF-Nutrition
This site provides information about micronutrient deficiencies in developing countries and the efforts to combat them.

www.thearc.org
The Arc
Search this site for "neural tube defects" and find a wealth of information on the development and prevention of these conditions.

References

Bacon, B. R., J. K. Olynyk, E. M. Brunt, R. S. Britton, and R. K. Wolff. 1999. HFE genotype in patients with hemochromatosis and other liver diseases. *Ann. Intern. Med.* 130: 953–962.

Beresford, S. A., and C. J. Boushey. 1997. Homocysteine, folic acid, and cardiovascular disease risk. In *Preventive Nutrition: The Comprehensive Guide for Health Professionals* edited by A. Bendich and R. J. Deckelbaum. Totowa, NJ: Humana Press.

Bernstein, L. 2000, February. Dementia without a cause: Lack of vitamin B_{12} can cause dementia. *Discover.* (Available at www.discover.com/issues/feb–00/departments/featdementia Accessed March 2004.)

Booth, S. L., and J. W. Suttie. 1998. Dietary intake and adequacy of vitamin K. *J. Nutr.* 128: 785–788.

Campbell, W. W., L. J. O. Joseph, R. A. Anderson, S. L. Davey, J. Hinton, and W. J. Evans. 2002. Effects of resistive training and chromium picolinate on body composition and skeletal muscle size in older women. *Int. J. Sports Nutr. Ex. Metab.* 12: 125–135.

Campbell, W. W., L. J. Joseph, S. L. Davey, D. Cyr-Campbell, R. A. Anderson, and W. J. Evans. 1999. Effects of resistance training and chromium picolinate on body composition and skeletal muscle in older men. *J. Appl. Physiol.* 86: 29–39.

Evans, G. W. 1989. The effect of chromium picolinate on insulin controlled parameters in humans. *Int. J. Biosoc. Med. Res.* 11: 163–180.

Feskanich, D., S. A. Korrick, S. L. Greenspan, H. N. Rosen, and G. A. Colditz. 1999. Moderate alcohol consumption and bone density among post-menopausal women. *J. Women's Health* 8: 65–73.

Grantham-McGregor, S., and C. Ani. 2001. A review of studies on the effect of iron deficiency on cognitive development in children. *J. Nutr.* 131: 649S–668S.

Hallmark, M. A., T. H. Reynolds, C. A. DeSouza, C. O. Dotson, R. A. Anderson, and M. A. Rogers. 1996. Effects of chromium and resistive training on muscle strength and body composition. *Med. Sci. Sports Exerc.* 28: 139–144.

Hasten, D. L., E. P. Rome, D. B. Franks, and M. Hegsted. 1992. Effects of chromium picolinate on beginning weight training students. *Int. J. Sports Nutr.* 2: 343–350.

Institute of Medicine, Food and Nutrition Board. 1998. *Dietary Reference Intakes for Thiamin, Riboflavin, Niacin, Vitamin B$_6$, Folate, Vitamin B$_{12}$, Pantothenic Acid, Biotin, and Choline.* Washington, DC: National Academy Press.

Institute of Medicine, Food and Nutrition Board. 2001. *Dietary Reference Intakes for Vitamin A, Vitamin K, Arsenic, Boron, Chromium, Copper, Iodine, Iron, Manganese, Molybdenum, Nickel, Silicon, Vanadium, and Zinc.* Washington, DC: National Academy Press.

Jackson, J. L., E. Lesho, and C. Peterson. 2000. Zinc and the common cold: A meta-analysis revisited. *J. Nutr.* 130: 1512S–1515S.

Lukaski, H. C., W. W. Bolonchuk, W. A. Siders, and D. B. Milne. 1996. Chromium supplementation and resistance training: effects on body composition, strength, and trace element status of men. *Am. J. Clin. Nutr.* 63: 954–965.

Mayer, E. L., D. W. Jacobsen, and K. Robinson. 1996. Homocysteine and coronary atherosclerosis. *J. Am. Coll. Cardiol.* 27: 517–527.

National Institute of Allergy and Infectious Diseases. National Institutes of Health. 2001. The Common Cold. www.niaid.nih.gov/factsheets/cold.htm Accessed January 2004.

Pasman, W. J., M. S. Westerterp-Plantenga, and W. H. Saris. 1997. The effectiveness of long-term supplementation of carbohydrate, chromium, fibre and caffeine on weight maintenance. *Int. J. Obesity Related Metab. Disorders* 21: 1143–1151.

Prasad, A. 1996. Zinc: the biology and therapeutics of an ion. *Ann. Intern. Med.* 125: 142–143.

U.S. Food and Drug Administration. 1997. Preventing Iron Poisoning in Children. FDA Backgrounder. http://www.fda.gov/opacom/backgrounders/ironbg.html Accessed January 2004.

Volpe, S. L., H. W. Huang, K. Larpadisorn, and I. I. Lesser. 2001. Effect of chromium supplementation and exercise on body composition, resting metabolic rate and selected biochemical parameters in moderately obese women following an exercise program. *J. Am. Coll. Nutr.* 20: 293–306.

Walker, L. S., M. G. Bemben, D. A. Bemben, and A. W. Knehans. 1998. Chromium picolinate effects on body composition and muscular performance in wrestlers. *Med. Sci. Sports Exerc.* 30: 1730–1737.

World Health Organization. 2003. Nutrition. Micronutrient Deficiencies. Battling iron deficiency anemia. www.who.int/nut/ida.htm Accessed January 2004.

Nutrition Debate:

Do Zinc Lozenges Help Fight the Common Cold?

The common cold has plagued human beings since the beginning of time. It is estimated that approximately one billion colds occur in the United States each year (National Institute of Allergy and Infectious Diseases 2001). Children suffer from six to ten colds each year, and adults average two to four per year. Although colds are typically benign, they result in significant absenteeism from work and cause discomfort and stress. Finding a cure for the common cold has been at the forefront of modern medicine for many years.

The most frequent causes of the adult colds are viruses called coronaviruses; rhinovirus is another virus that causes about one-third of all adult colds. It is estimated that there are more than two hundred viruses that can cause a cold. Because a cold can be caused by so many different viruses, finding treatments or potential cures for a cold is extremely challenging.

The role of zinc in the health of our immune system is well known. Zinc has been shown to inhibit the replication of rhinovirus and other viruses that cause the common cold (Prasad 1996), thus leading to speculation that taking zinc supplements may reduce the length and severity of colds. Consequently, zinc lozenges were formulated as a means of providing potential relief from cold symptoms. These lozenges are readily found in most drugstores.

Does taking zinc in lozenge form actually reduce the length and severity of a cold? Over the past twenty years, numerous research studies have been conducted to try to answer this question. Unfortunately, the results of these studies are inconclusive because about half have found that zinc lozenges do reduce the length and severity of a cold, while about half find that zinc lozenges have no effect on cold symptoms or duration (Jackson, Lesho, and Peterson 2000). Some reasons that various studies report different effects of zinc on a cold include:

- Inability to truly "blind" participants to the treatment — Because zinc lozenges have a unique taste, it may be difficult to keep the research participants uninformed as to whether they are getting zinc lozenges or a placebo. Knowing which lozenge they are taking could lead participants to report biased results.
- Self-reported symptoms are subject to inaccuracy — Many studies had the research participants self-report changes in symptoms, which may be inaccurate and influenced by mood and other emotional factors.

- Wide variety of viruses that cause a cold — Because over two hundred viruses can cause a cold, it is highly unlikely that zinc can combat all of these viruses. It is possible that people who do not respond favorably to zinc lozenges are suffering from a cold virus that cannot be treated with zinc.
- Differences in zinc formulations and dosages — The type of zinc formulation and the dosages of zinc consumed by study participants differed across studies. These differences most likely contributed to various responses across studies. It is estimated that for zinc to be effective, at least 80 mg of zinc should be consumed each day, and that people should begin using zinc lozenges within 48 hours of onset of cold symptoms. Also, sweeteners and flavorings found in many zinc lozenges, such as citric acid, sorbitol, and mannitol, may bind the zinc and inhibit its ability to be absorbed into the body, limiting its effectiveness.

Based on what you have learned here, do you think taking zinc lozenges can be effective in fighting the common cold? Have you ever tried zinc lozenges, and did you find them effective? Even if you only have about a 50% chance of reducing the length and severity of your cold by taking zinc lozenges, would you take these to combat your cold? Because there is no conclusive evidence supporting or refuting the effectiveness of zinc lozenges on the common cold, the debate on whether people should take them to treat their colds will most likely continue for many years.

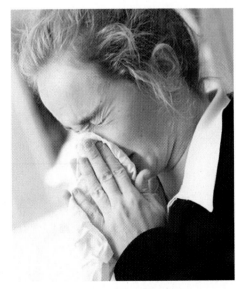

Zinc lozenges may help fight cold symptoms.

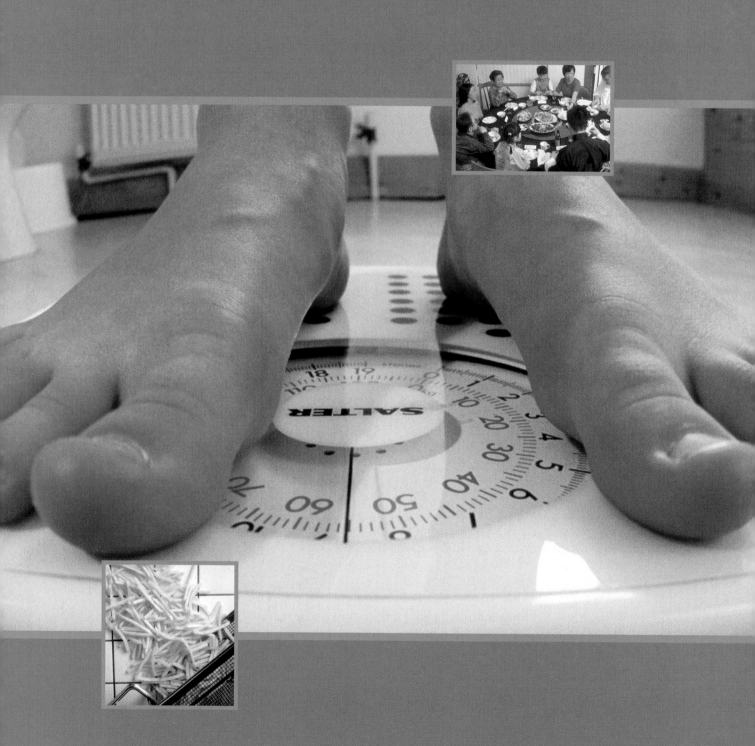

Chapter 11
Achieving and Maintaining a Healthful Body Weight

Chapter Objectives

After reading this chapter you will be able to:

1. Define what is meant by a healthful weight, pp. 382–383.

2. Define the terms *underweight*, *overweight*, *obesity*, and *morbid obesity* and discuss the health risks of each of these conditions, pp. 382–383 and 408–409.

3. List at least three methods that can be used to assess your body composition or risk for overweight, pp. 385–388.

4. Identify and discuss the three components of energy expenditure, pp. 389–393.

5. List and describe at least two theories that link genetic influences to control of body weight, pp. 393–395.

6. Describe how childhood experiences influence adult weight and the risk for obesity in adulthood, p. 395.

7. Discuss at least two societal factors that influence our body weight, pp. 397–398.

8. List and describe three treatment options for obesity, pp. 400–404.

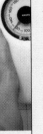

Test Yourself True or False?

1. Being underweight can be just as detrimental to our health as being obese. T or F

2. Obesity is a condition that is simply caused by people eating too much food and not getting enough exercise. T or F

3. Getting my body composition measured at the local fitness club will give me an accurate assessment of my body fat level. T or F

4. By staying physically active as we get older, we can prevent some of the decline in our muscle mass and our basal metabolic rate. T or F

5. People who are moderately overweight and physically active should not be considered healthy. T or F

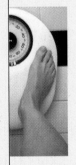

Test Yourself answers can be found at the end of the chapter.

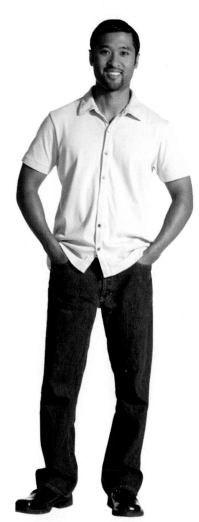

A healthful body weight varies from person to person.

As a teenager, she won a full athletic scholarship to Syracuse University, where she was honored for her "significant contribution to women's athletics and to the sport of rowing." After graduating, she became a television reporter and anchor for an NBC station in Flagstaff, Arizona. Then she went into modeling, and soon her face smiled out from the covers of fashion magazines, cosmetics ads, even a billboard in Times Square. Now considered a "supermodel," she hosts her own television show, has her own Web site, her own clothing line, and even a collection of dolls. *People* magazine has twice selected her as one of the "50 Most Beautiful People" and *Glamour* magazine named her "Woman of the Year." So who is she? Her name is Emme Aronson. . . and by the way, her average weight is 190 pounds.

Emme describes herself as "very well-proportioned." She focuses not on maintaining a certain weight, but instead on keeping healthy and fit. So she eats when she's hungry and works out regularly. Observing that "We live in a society that is based on the attainment of unrealistic beauty," Emme works hard to get out the message that self-esteem should not be contingent on size. In fact, she says, "I don't know if I'll ever be perfect, but I'm happy with who I am" (Emme 2004; PBS 2004).

Are you happy with your weight, shape, body composition, and fitness? If not, what needs to change—your attitude, your diet, your level of physical activity? What role do diet and physical activity play in maintaining a healthful body weight? How much of your body size and shape is due to genetics? What influence does society—including food advertising—have on your weight? And if you decide that you do need to lose weight, what's the best way to do it? In this chapter, we will explore these questions and provide some answers.

What Is a Healthful Body Weight?

As you begin to think about achieving and maintaining a healthful weight, it's important to make sure you understand what a healthful body weight actually means. We can define a healthful weight as all of the following (Manore and Thompson 2000):

- A weight that is appropriate for your age and physical development
- A weight that you can achieve and sustain without severely curtailing your food intake or constantly dieting
- A weight that is acceptable to you
- A weight that is based upon your genetic background and family history of body shape and weight
- A weight that promotes good eating habits and allows you to participate in regular physical activity

As you can see, a healthful weight is not one in which a person must be extremely thin or overly muscular. In addition, there is no one particular body type that can be defined as healthful. Thus, achieving a healthful body weight should not be dictated by the latest fad or current societal expectations of what is acceptable.

Now that we know what a healthful body weight is, let's look at some terms applying to underweight and overweight. Physicians, nutritionists, and other scientists define **underweight** as having too little body fat to maintain health, causing a person to have a weight that is below an acceptably defined standard for a given height. **Overweight** is defined as having a moderate amount of excess body fat, resulting in a person having a weight that is greater than some accepted standard for a given height but is not considered obese. **Obesity** is defined as having an excess body fat that adversely affects health, resulting in a person having a weight that is substantially greater than some accepted standard for a given height. People can also suffer from **morbid obesity**; in this case, their body weights exceed 100% of normal, putting them at very high risk for serious health consequences. In the next section we discuss how these terms are defined using certain indicators of body weight and body fat.

underweight Having too little body fat to maintain health, causing a person to have a weight that is below an acceptably defined standard for a given height.

overweight Having a moderate amount of excess body fat, resulting in a person having a weight that is greater than some accepted standard for a given height but is not considered obese.

obesity Having an excess body fat that adversely affects health, resulting in a person having a weight that is substantially greater than some accepted standard for a given height.

morbid obesity A condition in which a person's body weight exceeds 100% of normal, putting him or her at very high risk for serious health consequences.

Recap: A healthful body weight is one that is appropriate for your age and physical development, can be achieved and sustained without constant dieting, is acceptable to you, is based upon your genetic background and family history of body shape and weight, promotes good eating habits, and allows for regular physical activity. Underweight is having too little body fat to maintain health. Overweight occurs when someone has a moderate amount of excess body fat, while obesity occurs when someone has excess body fat that adversely affects health. Morbid obesity occurs when a person's weight exceeds 100% of normal.

How Can You Evaluate Your Body Weight?

Various methods are available to help you determine whether or not you are currently maintaining a healthful body weight. Let's review a few of these methods.

Determine Your Body Mass Index (BMI)

Body mass index (**BMI,** or *Quetelet's index*) is a commonly used index representing the ratio of a person's body weight to the square of his or her height. You can calculate your BMI using the following equation:

$$BMI = weight\ (kg)\ /\ height\ (m)^2$$

A less exact but often useful method is to use the graph in Figure 11.1, which shows approximate BMIs for your height and weight and whether your BMI is in a

body mass index (BMI) A measurement representing the ratio of a person's body weight to his or her height.

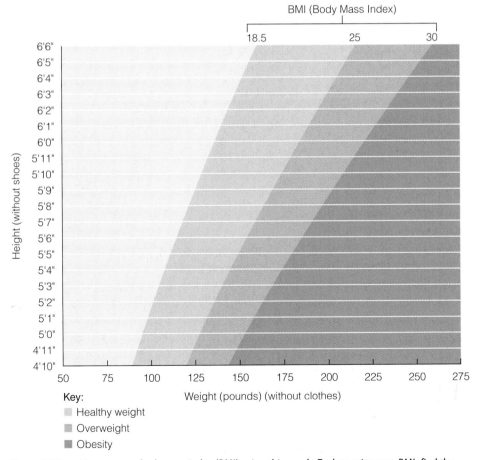

Figure 11.1 Measure your body mass index (BMI) using this graph. To determine your BMI, find the value for your height on the left and follow this line to the right until it intersects with the value for your weight on the bottom axis. The area on the graph where these two points intersect is your BMI.

healthful range. You can also calculate your BMI on the Internet using the BMI calculator found at http://www.nhlbisupport.com/bmi/.

Why Is BMI Important?

Your body mass index provides an important clue to your overall health. Research studies show that a person's risk for type 2 diabetes, high blood pressure, heart disease, and other diseases largely increases when BMI is above a value of 30. On the other hand, having a very low BMI, defined as a value below 18.5, is also associated with increased risk of health problems and death.

Figure 11.2 shows how the *mortality rate,* or death rate, from all diseases increases significantly above a value of 30. Having a BMI value within the healthful range means that your risk of dying prematurely is within the expected average. If your BMI value falls outside of this range, either higher or lower, your risk of dying prematurely becomes greater than the average risk. For example, men with a BMI equal to or greater than 35 kg/m^2 have a risk of dying prematurely that is more than twice that of men with a BMI value in the range of 22 to 25 kg/m^2.

Theo always worries about being too thin, and he wonders if he is underweight. Theo calculates his BMI (see the calculations in the You Do the Math box on p. 386) and is surprised to find that it is 22 kg/m^2 and falls within the healthy range.

Limitations of BMI

While calculating your BMI can be very helpful in estimating your health risk, this method is limited when used with people who have a disproportionately higher muscle mass for a given height. For example, one of Theo's friends, Randy, is a 23-year-old weight lifter who is 5'7" and weighs 210 pounds. According to our BMI calculations, Randy's BMI is 32.9, placing him in the obese and high-risk category for

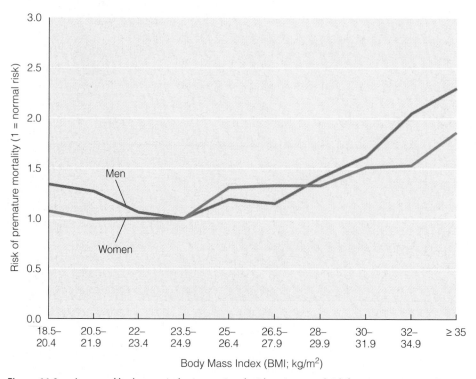

Figure 11.2 Increased body mass index is associated with an increased risk for premature mortality. These results pertain only to U.S. adults who have never smoked and have no history of disease. (Adapted from E. E. Calle, M. J. Thun, J. M. Petrelli, C. Rodriguez, and C. W. Heath, Jr., Body-mass index and mortality in a prospective cohort of U.S. adults, *N. Engl. J. Med.* 341 [1999]:1097–1105.)

many diseases. Is Randy really obese? In cases such as his, an assessment of body composition is necessary.

Measure Your Body Composition

There are many methods available to assess your **body composition,** or the amount of body fat (or *adipose tissue*) and lean body mass (or *lean tissue*) you have. Table 11.1 lists some of the more common methods used to assess body composition. It is important to remember that measuring body composition provides only an estimate of your body fat and lean body mass, meaning that we cannot measure your exact level of these tissues. Because the range of error of these methods can be from 3% to more than 20%, body composition results should not be used as the only indicator of health status.

body composition The ratio of a person's body fat to lean body mass.

Underwater Weighing Method

In underwater weighing, a technician submerges a person underwater, the person exhales fully while underwater, and then the technician measures the person's weight. Although this method is available in most exercise physiology laboratories across the United States, it is not readily available or affordable for many people. It is therefore used mostly for research purposes.

If you have access to a laboratory performing underwater weighing, it is worth having the procedure done, as this method of determining body composition is considered to be one of the most accurate. Under the best of circumstances, underwater weighing can estimate body fat within a 2 to 3% margin of error. This means that if your underwater weighing test shows you have 20% body fat, this value could be no lower than 17% nor higher than 23%. This test can only be done with people who are

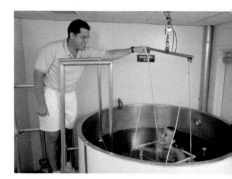
Underwater weighing.

Table 11.1   Overview of Various Body Composition Assessment Methods

Method	Strength	Limitations
Underwater weighing	Fairly accurate Inexpensive	Must be comfortable in water Requires trained technician and specialized equipment
Skinfolds	Fairly accurate if technician is well trained Inexpensive Easy for person being measured Can be done anywhere	Less accurate unless technician is well trained Proper prediction equation must be used to improve accuracy Person being measured may not want to be touched or may not want to expose their skin Cannot be used to measure obese people
Bioelectrical impedance analysis (BIA)	Inexpensive Easy for person being measured Can be done anywhere May be more accurate for obese people	Less accurate Body fluid levels must be normal Proper prediction equation must be used to improve accuracy
Near infrared reactance (NIR)	Inexpensive Easy for person being measured Can be done anywhere	Accuracy is very low Only one equation is used to compute body fat, which limits its use with a wide variety of people
Bod Pod	Easy for the person being measured Does not require a trained technician	Expensive Less accurate

Calculating Your Body Mass Index

Calculate your personal BMI value based on your height and weight. Let's use Theo's values as an example:

$$\text{BMI} = \text{weight (kg)} / \text{height (m)}^2$$

1. Theo's weight is 200 pounds. To convert his weight to kg, divide his weight in pounds by 2.2 pounds per kg:
   200 pounds/2.2 pounds per kg = 90.91 kg

2. Theo's height is 6 feet 8 inches, or 80 inches. To convert his height to meters, multiply his height in inches by 0.0254 meters/inch:
   80 inches × 0.0254 meters/inch = 2.03 meters

3. Find the square of his height in meters:
   2.03 m × 2.03 m = 4.13 m^2

4. Then, divide his weight in kg by his height in m^2 to get his BMI value:
   90.91 kg/4.13 m^2 = 22.01 kg/m^2

Is Theo underweight according to this BMI value? As you can see in Figure 11.1, this value shows that he is maintaining a normal, healthful weight! ●

---

comfortable in water and does not work well with obese people. Before participating in this test, you must abstain from food for at least 8 hours, and you should not have exercised during the previous 12 hours.

Skinfold Measurements

Measuring skinfolds involves "pinching" a person's fold of skin (with it's underlying layer of fat) at various locations of the body. The fold is measured using a specially designed caliper. This method cannot be used with many obese people, as their skin-folds are too large to be measured by the caliper. Himes (2001) found that almost 25% of women aged 50 years and older have skinfolds that are too large to measure. When we consider that the U.S. population is getting heavier each year, it is possible that this method will soon be useless for more than half of the population.

Another major challenge of measuring body fat using skinfolds is that this method relies on a technician predicting a person's body fat using one of over 400 equations developed in research studies, and it is only accurate if the correct prediction equation is applied. Many places that offer this measurement have untrained technicians performing the measurement, and they use only one equation for their entire client base, which severely limits the accuracy of this method.

When performed by a skilled technician, skinfold measurement can estimate your body fat with an error of 3 to 4%. This means that if your skinfold test shows you have 20% body fat, your actual value could be as low as 16% or as high as 24%.

Bioelectrical Impedance Analysis

Bioelectrical impedence analysis (BIA) is a method of determining body composition that involves sending a very low level of electrical current through a person's body. As water is a good conductor of electricity and lean body mass is made up of mostly water, the rate at which the electricity is conducted gives an indication of a person's lean body mass and body fat. This method can be done while lying down, with electrodes attached to the feet, hands, and the BIA machine. There are also hand-held and standing models (that look like bathroom scales) now available, where only half of the body's impedance to electricity is measured, and total body fat is determined by estimating the impedance of the remainder of the body.

One of the challenges of the BIA method is that the person being measured must follow certain guidelines to improve accuracy of the test. This includes no eating for 4

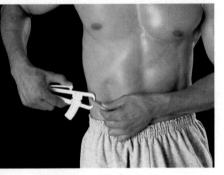

Skinfold measurement.

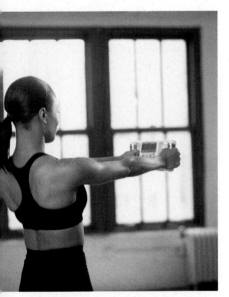

Bioelectrical impedance analysis.

hours and no exercise for 12 hours prior to the test and no alcohol consumption within 48 hours of the test. Females should not be measured if they are retaining water because of menstrual cycle changes. Another challenge is that, as with the skinfold method, most places that offer BIA only use one prediction equation for all clients; this limits the accuracy of the BIA method. When done under the best of circumstances, BIA can estimate your body fat with an error of 3 to 4%.

Near Infrared Reactance

The brand name of the machine most commonly used to estimate body fat using *near infrared reactance (NIR)* technology is the Futrex 5000. The technology is based on the principles of light absorption and reflection. A probe, or wand, is attached to the biceps (upper arm) using a velcro-type strip. An infrared beam then penetrates the arm and is reflected back into the probe.

Although this method is widely used at the present time, especially in health clubs, its accuracy has been shown to be very poor, and there is no way to know if the results you obtain from this test are of any real value. The few studies done with this method show that the margin of error for predicting a person's body fat ranges from 2% to as high as 10% (Panotopoulos et al. 2001; Heyward and Stolarczyk 1996). Most researchers consider this wide range of potential error unacceptable.

Bod Pod

The Bod Pod is the brand name of a machine that uses air displacement to measure body composition. This machine is a large, egg-shaped chamber made from fiberglass. The person being measured sits in the machine wearing a swimsuit, and the door to the machine is closed. The machine measures how much air is displaced once the person being measured enters the chamber, and this value is used to calculate body composition. The Bod Pod is expensive and is currently used mostly in research settings. While this method appears to be fairly accurate in Caucasians, a recent study indicates that it overestimates body fat in some African American men (Wagner, Heyward, and Gibson 2000). Despite these limitations, this technology appears promising as an easier and equally accurate alternative to underwater weighing in many populations.

Let's return to Randy, whose BMI of 32.9 kg/m^2 places him in the obese category. Is he overweight? Randy trains with weights four days per week, rides the exercise bike for about 30 minutes per session three times per week, and does not take drugs, smoke cigarettes, or drink alcohol. Through his local gym, Randy contacted a technician who assesses body composition. The results of his skinfold measurements show that his body fat is 9%. See Table 11.2 for a list of the percent body fat standards that are appropriate for health. According to this table, Randy's body

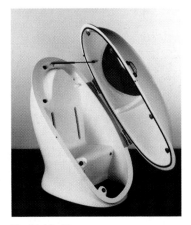

The Bod Pod®.

Table 11.2   Percent Body Fat Standards for Health

Body Fat Levels					
	Unhealthfully Low	Low	Mid	Upper	Obesity
Men:					
Young adult	<8	8	13	22	>22
Middle adult	<10	10	18	25	>25
Elderly	<10	10	16	23	>23
Women:					
Young adult	<20	20	28	35	>35
Middle adult	<25	25	32	38	>38
Elderly	<25	25	30	35	>35

Source: Reprinted from T. G. Lohman, L. Houtkooper, and S. B. Going. Body fat measurement goes high-tech: not all are created equal. *ACSM's Health Fit. J.* 7 (1997):30–35. Used by permission.

Table 11.3 Strengths and Limitations of Various Tools for Defining Overweight

	Strengths	Limitations
BMI	Gives ratio of weight to height Accurately predicts health risks related to obesity in large groups of people	Cannot indicate pattern of fat or amount of fat or lean body mass Does not account for differences in gender, frame size, or activity level
Body Composition	If done properly, most accurate way to measure body fat	Can be expensive Equipment not always available
Fat Patterning	Tells us about a person's body shape Can indicate if a person has a higher risk of certain chronic diseases	Does not directly measure body fat content

fat values are within the healthful (low to mid) range. Randy is an example of a person whose BMI appears very high but who is not actually obese.

Assess Your Fat Distribution Patterns

To evaluate the health of your current body weight, it is also helpful to consider the way fat is distributed throughout your body. This is because your fat distribution pattern is known to affect your risk for various diseases. Figure 11.3 shows two types of fat patterning. *Apple-shaped fat patterning*, or upper-body obesity, is known to significantly increase a person's risk for many chronic diseases such as type 2 diabetes, heart disease, and high blood pressure. It is thought that the apple-shaped patterning causes problems with the metabolism of fat and carbohydrate, leading to unhealthful changes in blood cholesterol, insulin, glucose, and blood pressure. In contrast, *pear-shaped fat patterning*, or lower-body obesity, does not seem to significantly increase your risk for chronic diseases. Women tend to store fat in their lower body, and men in their abdominal region. In 2004, a study involving more than 10,000 people found that 64% of women are pear-shaped and 38% of men are apple-shaped (Zernike, 2004).

Two methods, the waist-to-hip ratio and the waist circumference, can determine type of fat patterning. The *waist-to-hip ratio* is determined by measuring the waist circumference at the level of the natural waist (or the narrowest part of the torso as observed from the front). The hip circumference is measured at the maximal circumference (includes the maximal width of the buttocks as observed from the side). The waist value is divided by the hip value. If a man's waist-to-hip ratio is higher than 0.90 or a woman's is higher than 0.80, then they are considered to have a higher risk for chronic diseases. For the waist circumference, a man's risk is increased above 40 in. (or 102 cm.), and a woman's risk is increased above 35 in. (or 88 cm.).

It is important to understand how BMI, body composition assessment, and fat distribution patterning differ in their ability to define a person's overweight status. Table 11.3 lists the strengths and limitations of these techniques in determining whether or not you are maintaining a healthful weight. There is no single best way to determine overweight or obesity, and each technique has its own advantages and disadvantages.

> **Recap:** Body mass index, body composition, and the waist-to-hip ratio and waist circumference are tools that can help you evaluate the health of your current body weight. None of these methods is completely accurate, but most may be used appropriately as general health indicators.

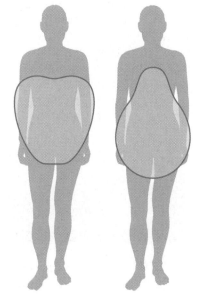

(a) Apple-shaped fat patterning   (b) Pear-shaped fat patterning

Figure 11.3 Fat distribution patterns. **(a)** An apple-shaped fat distribution pattern increases an individual's risk for many chronic diseases. **(b)** A pear-shaped distribution pattern does not seem to be associated with an increased risk for chronic disease.

What Makes Us Gain and Lose Weight?

Have you ever wondered why some people are thin and others are overweight, even though they seem to eat about the same diet? If so, you're not alone. For hundreds of years, researchers have puzzled over what makes us gain and lose weight. In this section, we explore some information and current theories that may shed some light on this question.

We Gain or Lose Weight When Our Energy Intake and Expenditure Are Out of Balance

Fluctuations in body weight are a result of changes in our **energy intake** (the food we eat) and our **energy expenditure** (or the amount of energy we expend at rest and during physical activity). This relationship between what we eat and what we do is defined by the energy balance equation:

Energy balance occurs when energy intake = energy expenditure

This means that our energy is balanced when we consume the same amount of energy that we burn each day. Figure 11.4 shows how our weight changes when we change either side of this equation. From this figure, you can see that in order

energy intake The amount of food a person eats; in other words, it is the number of kilocalories consumed.

energy expenditure The energy the body expends to maintain its basic functions and to perform all levels of movement and activity.

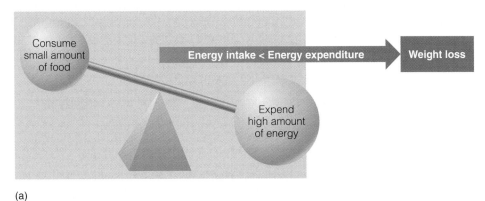

(a)

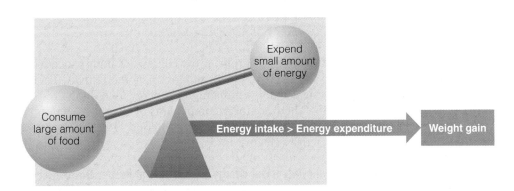

(b)

Figure 11.4 Energy balance describes the relationship between the food we eat and the energy we burn each day. **(a)** Weight loss occurs when food intake is less than energy output. **(b)** Weight gain occurs when food intake is greater than energy output. **(c)** We maintain our body weight when food intake equals energy output.

(c)

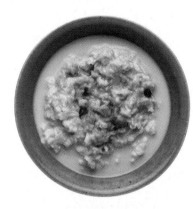

The energy provided by a bowl of oatmeal is derived from its protein, carbohydrate, and fat content.

to lose body weight, we must expend more energy than we consume. In contrast, to gain weight, we must consume more energy than we expend. Finding the proper balance between energy intake and expenditure allows us to maintain a healthful body weight.

Energy Intake Is the Food We Eat Each Day

Energy intake is equal to the amount of energy in the food we eat each day. This value includes all foods and beverages. Daily energy intake is expressed as *kilocalories per day* (*kcal/day*, or *kcal/d*). Energy intake can be estimated manually using food composition tables or by using computerized dietary analysis programs. The energy content of each food is a function of the amount of carbohydrate, fat, protein, and alcohol that each food contains; vitamins and minerals have no energy value, so they contribute zero kilocalories to our energy intake.

Remember that the energy value of carbohydrate and protein is 4 kcal/g and the energy value of fat is 9 kcal/g. The energy value of alcohol is 7 kcal/g. By multiplying the energy value (in kcal/g) times the amount of the nutrient (in grams), you can calculate how much energy is in a particular food. For instance, 1 cup of quick oatmeal has an energy value of 142 kcal. How is this energy value derived? One cup of oatmeal contains 6 grams of protein, 25 grams of carbohydrate, and 2 grams of fat. Using the energy values for each nutrient, you can calculate the total energy content of oatmeal:

$$6 \text{ grams protein} \times 4 \text{ kcal/gram} = 24 \text{ kcal from protein}$$

$$25 \text{ grams carbohydrate} \times 4 \text{ kcal/gram} = 100 \text{ kcal from carbohydrate}$$

$$2 \text{ grams fat} \times 9 \text{ kcal/gram} = 18 \text{ kcal from fat}$$

$$\text{Total kcal for 1 cup oatmeal} = 24 \text{ kcal} + 100 \text{ kcal} + 18 \text{ kcal} = 142 \text{ kcal}$$

When someone's total daily energy intake exceeds the amount of energy they expend, then weight gain results. An excess intake of approximately 3,500 kcal will result in a gain of one pound. Without exercise, this gain will likely be fat.

Energy Expenditure Includes More Than Just Physical Activity

basal metabolic rate (BMR) The energy the body expends to maintain its fundamental physiologic functions.

Energy expenditure (also known as energy output) is the energy our body expends to maintain its basic functions and to perform all levels of movement and activity. Total 24-hour energy expenditure is calculated by estimating the energy used during rest and as a result of physical activity. There are three components of energy expenditure: basal metabolic rate (BMR), thermic effect of food (TEF), and energy cost of physical activity (Figure 11.5).

Our Basal Metabolic Rate Is Our Energy Expenditure at Rest Basal metabolic rate, or **BMR,** is the energy we expend just to maintain our body's *basal*, or *resting*, functions. These functions include respiration, circulation, maintaining body temperature, synthesis of new cells and tissues, secretion of hormones, and nervous system activity. The majority of our energy output each day (about 60–70%) is a result of our BMR. This means that 60 to 70% of our energy output goes to fuel the basic activities of staying alive, aside from any physical activity.

BMR varies widely among people. The primary determinant of our BMR is the amount of lean body mass that we have. People with a higher lean body mass have a higher BMR, as lean body mass is more metabolically active than body fat. Thus, it takes more energy to support this active tissue. One common assumption is that obese people have a depressed BMR. This is usually not the case. Most studies of obese people show that the amount of energy they expend for every kilogram of lean body mass is similar to that of a non-obese person. In

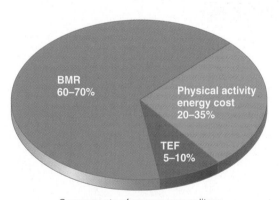

Components of energy expenditure

Figure 11.5 The components of energy expenditure include basal metabolic rate (BMR), the thermic effect of food (TEF), and the energy cost of physical activity. BMR accounts for 60–70% of our total energy output, whereas TEF and physical activity together account for 25–45%.

Key:
■ Lean body mass
▨ % body fat

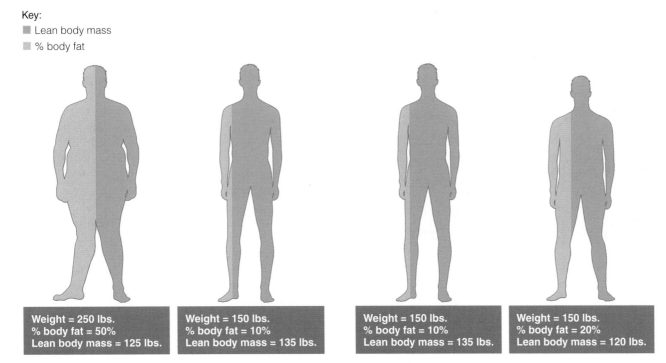

(a) Variation in lean body mass in individuals of different weights

(b) Variation in lean body mass in individuals of same weight

Figure 11.6 Lean body mass varies in people with different body weights and body fat levels. **(a)** The person on the left has a higher body weight, body fat, and lean body mass than the person on the right, who is very lean. **(b)** Both people are the same weight but the person on the right has more body fat and less lean body mass than the person on the left.

general, people who weigh more also have more lean body mass and consequently have a *higher* BMR. See Figure 11.6 for an example of how lean body mass can vary for people with different body weights and body fat levels.

BMR decreases with age, approximately 3 to 5% per decade after age 30. This age-related decrease results partly from hormonal changes, but much of this change is due to the loss of lean body mass resulting from physical inactivity. Thus, a large proportion of this decrease may be prevented with regular physical activity. There are other factors that can affect a person's BMR, and some of these are listed in Table 11.4.

How can you estimate the amount of energy you expend for your BMR? Of the many equations that can be used, one of the simplest ways to estimate your BMR is to multiply your body weight in kilograms (kg) by 1.0 kcal per kg of body weight per hour for men or by 0.9 kcal per kg of body weight per hour for women. A little later

Table 11.4 Factors Affecting Basal Metabolic Rate (BMR)

Factors that Increase BMR	Factors that Decrease BMR
Higher lean body mass	Lower lean body mass
Greater height (more surface area)	Lower height
Younger age	Older age
Elevated levels of thyroid hormone	Depressed levels of thyroid hormone
Stress	Starvation or fasting
Male gender	Female gender
Pregnancy and lactation	
Certain drugs such as stimulants, caffeine, and tobacco	

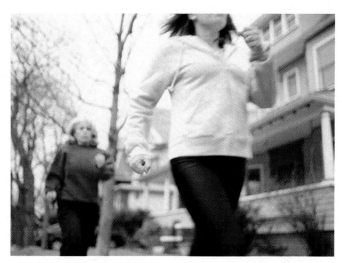

Brisk walking expends energy.

thermic effect of food (TEF) The energy expended as a result of processing food consumed.

energy cost of physical activity The energy that is expended on body movement and muscular work above basal levels.

in this chapter you will have an opportunity to calculate BMR and determine your total daily energy needs.

The Thermic Effect of Food Is the Energy Expended to Process Food

The **thermic effect of food (TEF)** is the energy we expend as a result of processing the food we eat. A certain amount of energy is needed to digest, absorb, transport, metabolize, and store the nutrients we eat. The TEF is equal to about 5 to 10% of the energy content of a meal, a relatively small amount. Thus, if a meal contains 500 kcal, the thermic effect of processing that meal is about 25 to 50 kcal. These values apply to eating what is referred to as a mixed diet, or a diet containing a mixture of carbohydrate, fat, and protein. Most of us eat some combination of these nutrients throughout the day. Individually, the processing of each nutrient takes a different amount of energy. While fat requires very little energy to digest, transport, and store in our cells, protein and carbohydrate require relatively more energy to process.

At one time, it was thought that obese people had a blunted (or reduced) TEF, which was identified as an important contributor to obesity. We now know that there are a lot of errors associated with measuring the TEF. These errors make our previous assumptions about the link between obesity and the thermic effect of food questionable. One of the most important contributors to obesity in industrialized countries is having an inactive lifestyle, which significantly reduces the energy output due to physical activity, our next topic.

The Energy Cost of Physical Activity Is Highly Variable

The **energy cost of physical activity** represents about 20 to 35% of our total energy output each day. This is the energy that we expend due to any movement or work above basal levels. This includes lower intensity activities such as sitting, standing, and walking, and higher intensity activities such as running, skiing, and bicycling. One of the most obvious ways to increase how much energy we expend as a result of physical activity is to do more activities for a longer period of time.

Table 11.5 lists the energy costs for certain activities. As you can see, the activities such as running, swimming, and cross-country skiing that involve moving our larger muscle groups (or more parts of the body) require more energy. The amount of energy we expend during activities is also affected by our body size, the intensity of the activity, and how long we perform the activity. This is why the values in Table 11.5 are expressed as kcal of energy per kg of body weight per minute.

Using the energy value for running at 6 miles per hour (or a 10-minute per mile running pace) for 30 minutes, let's calculate how much energy Theo would expend doing this activity:

- Theo's body weight (in kg) = 200 pounds/2.2 pounds per kg = 90.91 kg
- Energy cost of running at 6 mph = 0.175 kcal/kg body weight/minute
- At Theo's weight, the energy cost of running per minute = 0.175 kcal/kg body weight/min × 90.91 kg = 15.91 kcal/minute
- If Theo runs this pace for 30 minutes, his total energy output = 15.91 kcal/minute × 30 minutes = 477 kcal

Recap: The energy balance equation relates food intake to energy expenditure. Eating more energy than you expend causes weight gain, while eating less energy than you expend causes weight loss. The three components of energy expenditure are basal metabolic rate, the thermic effect of food, and the energy cost of physical activity.

Table 11.5   Energy Costs of Various Physical Activities

Activity	Intensity	Energy Cost (kcal/kg body weight/min)
Sitting, knitting/sewing	Light	0.026
Cooking or food preparation (standing or sitting)	Light	0.035
Walking, shopping	Light	0.04
Walking, 2 mph (slow pace)	Light	0.044
Cleaning (dusting, straightening up, vacuuming, changing linen, carrying out trash)	Moderate	0.044
Stretching — Hatha Yoga	Moderate	0.044
Weight lifting (free weights, Nautilus, or universal type)	Light or moderate	0.052
Bicycling < 10 mph	Leisure (work or pleasure)	0.07
Walking, 4 mph (brisk pace)	Moderate	0.088
Aerobics	Low impact	0.088
Weight lifting (free weights, Nautilus, or universal type)	Vigorous	0.105
Bicycling 12 to 13.9 mph	Moderate	0.14
Running, 5 mph (12 minutes per mile)	Moderate	0.14
Running, 6 mph (10 minutes per mile)	Moderate	0.175
Running, 8.6 mph (7 minutes per mile)	Vigorous	0.245

Source: B. E. Ainsworth, W. L. Haskell, M. C. Whitt, M. L. Irwin, A. M. Swartz, S. J. Strath, W. L. O'Brien, D. R. Bassett, Jr., K. H. Schmitz, P. O. Emplaincourt, D. R. Jacobs, Jr., and A. S. Leon. Compendium of physical activities: an update of activity codes and MET intensities. *Med. Sci. Sports Exerc.* 32 (2000): S498–S516.

Genetic Factors Affect Body Weight

Our genetic background influences our height, weight, body shape, and metabolic rate. A classic study shows that the body weights of adults who were adopted as children are similar to the weights of their biological parents, not their adoptive parents (Stunkard et al. 1986). Figure 11.7 shows that about 25% of our body fat is accounted for by genetic influences. Some proposed theories linking genetics with our body weight are the thrifty gene theory, the set-point theory, and the leptin theory.

The Thrifty Gene Theory

The **thrifty gene theory** suggests that some people possess a gene (or genes) that causes them to be energetically thrifty. This means that at rest and even during active times these individuals expend less energy than people who do not possess this gene. The proposed purpose of this gene is to protect a person from starving to death during times of extreme food shortages. This theory has been applied to some Native American tribes, as these societies were exposed to centuries of feast and famine. Those with a thrifty metabolism survived when little food was available, and this trait was passed on to future generations. Although an actual thrifty gene (or genes) has not yet been identified, researchers continue to study this explanation as a potential cause of obesity.

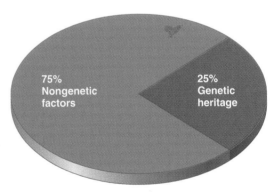

75% Nongenetic factors

25% Genetic heritage

Percent (%) contribution to body fat

Figure 11.7   Research indicates that about 25% of our body fat is accounted for by our genetic heritage. However, nongenetic factors such as diet and exercise play a much larger role.

thrifty gene theory   A theory that suggests that some people possess a gene (or genes) that causes them to be energetically thrifty, resulting in them expending less energy at rest and during physical activity.

If this theory is true, think about how people who possess this thrifty gene might respond to today's environment. Low levels of physical activity, inexpensive food sources that are high in fat and energy, and excessively large serving sizes are the norm in our society. A person with a thrifty metabolism will experience a great amount of weight gain, and their bodies are more resistant to weight loss. Theoretically, having thrifty genetics appears advantageous during times of minimal food resources; however, this state could lead to very high levels of obesity in times of plenty.

The Set-Point Theory

set-point theory A theory that suggests that the body raises or lowers energy expenditure in response to increased and decreased food intake and physical activity. This action serves to maintain an individual's body weight within a narrow range.

The **set-point theory** suggests that our bodies are designed to maintain our weight within a narrow range, or at a "set point." In many cases, our bodies appear to respond in such a way as to maintain our present weight. When we dramatically reduce energy intake (such as with fasting or strict diets), our body responds with physiologic changes that cause our BMR to drop. This causes a significant slowing of our energy output. In addition, being physically active while fasting or starving is difficult because we just don't have the energy for it. These two mechanisms of energy conservation may contribute to some of the rebound weight gain many dieters experience after they quit dieting.

Conversely, overeating in some people may cause an increase in BMR, and is thought to be associated with an increased thermic effect of food as well as an increase in spontaneous movements, or fidgeting. This in turn increases energy output and prevents weight gain. These changes may explain how some people fail to gain all of the weight expected from eating excess food. We don't eat the exact same amount of food each day; some days we overeat, other days we eat less. When you think about how much our daily energy intake fluctuates (about 20% above and below our average monthly intake), our ability to maintain a certain weight over long periods of time suggests that there is some evidence to support the set-point theory.

Can we change our weight set point? It appears that, when we maintain changes in our diet and activity level over a long period of time, weight change does occur. This is obvious in the case of obesity, since many people become obese during middle adulthood, and they are not able to maintain the lower body weight they had as a younger adult. Also, many people do successfully lose weight and maintain that weight loss over long periods of time. Thus, the set-point theory cannot entirely account for our body's resistance to weight loss. An interesting study on weight gain in twins demonstrates how genetics may affect our tendency to maintain a set point; this study is reviewed in the accompanying Highlight box.

The Leptin Theory

leptin A hormone that is produced by body fat that acts to reduce food intake and to decrease body weight and body fat.

Leptin, first discovered in mice, is a hormone that is produced by body fat. Leptin acts to reduce food intake, and it causes a decrease in body weight and body fat. Obese mice were found to have genetic mutations in the *ob gene,* or obesity gene, and these mutations caused overeating, decreased energy output, and extreme obesity in these animals. When the *ob* gene is functioning normally, it produces leptin. When there is a genetic mutation of the *ob* gene, leptin is not secreted in sufficient amounts, food intake increases dramatically, and energy output is reduced.

A great deal of excitement was generated about how leptin might decrease obesity in humans. Unfortunately, studies have shown that although obese mice respond positively to leptin injections, obese humans tend to have very high amounts of leptin in their bodies and are insensitive to leptin's effects. In truth, we have just begun to learn about leptin and its role in the human body. Researchers are currently studying its role during starvation and overeating, and it appears it might play a role in cardiovascular and kidney complications that result from obesity and related diseases.

Overfeeding Responses of Identical Twins

A classic study done by researchers at Laval University in Quebec, Canada, shows how genetics plays a role in our responses to overeating (Bouchard et al. 1990). Twelve pairs of male identical twins volunteered to stay in a dormitory where they were supervised 24 hours a day for 120 consecutive days. Researchers measured how much energy each man needed to maintain his body weight at the beginning of the study. For 100 days, the subjects were fed 1,000 kcal more per day than they needed to maintain body weight. Daily physical activity was limited, but each person was allowed to walk outdoors for 30 minutes each day, read, watch television and videos, and play cards and video games. The research staff stayed with these men to ensure that they did not stray from the study protocol.

The average weight gain experienced by this group of men was almost 18 pounds. Although they were all overfed enough energy to gain about 26 pounds, the average weight gain was 8 pounds less than expected. These men gained mostly fat but also gained about 6 pounds of lean body mass. Interestingly, there was a very wide range of weight gained. One man only gained about 9.5 pounds, while another man gained over 29 pounds! Keep in mind that the food these men ate and the activities they performed were tightly controlled.

This study shows that when people overeat by the same amount of food, they can gain very different amounts of weight and body fat. While each twin gained a similar amount of weight to his twin pair, there was a lot of difference in how each set of twins responded. It is suggested that those more resistant to weight gain when they overeat have the ability to increase BMR, store more excess energy as lean body mass instead of fat, and increase spontaneous movements such as fidgeting. Thus, genetic differences may explain why some people have a better ability to maintain a certain weight set point than others. ●

Recap: There are many factors that affect our ability to gain and lose weight. Our genetic background influences our height, weight, body shape, and metabolic rate. The thrifty gene theory suggests that some people possess a thrifty gene, or set of genes, that causes them to expend less energy at rest and during physical activity than people who do not have this gene. The set-point theory suggests that our bodies are designed to maintain weight within a narrow range, also called a set point. Leptin is a hormone produced by body fat that reduces food intake and decreases body weight and fat. The role of leptin in weight regulation and obesity is still under investigation.

Childhood Weight Influences Adult Weight

In addition to genetic factors, the environmental factors present in our childhood can influence our food choices, activity level, and other behaviors as adults and cause us to weigh more or less than others of similar body type. For example, children who are very physically active and eat healthful diets that do not contain a lot of excess fat and sugar are less likely to be overweight or obese as children. In contrast, children who spend most of their time on the computer or watching television and who eat a lot of foods that contain excess fat and sugar are more likely to be overweight or obese as children. These patterns can very likely be carried into adulthood and result in adult overweight and obesity. We know that being overweight or obese as a child can be detrimental to our health as we age, as childhood overweight has been shown to significantly increase a person's risk of heart disease and premature death in adulthood (Gunnell et al. 1998).

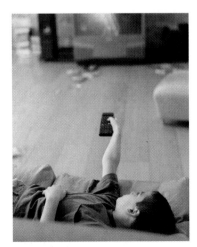

Behaviors learned as a child can affect adulthood weight and physical activity patterns.

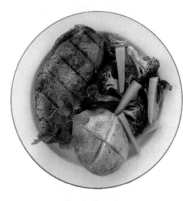

A balanced diet contains protein, carbohydrate, and fat.

Behavioral Factors Affect Food Choices and Body Weight

We know that there are a number of behavioral factors that can contribute to obesity. Behavioral factors include such things as how we select the carbohydrate, fat, and protein composition of our diet and which motivators drive us to eat, including hunger and appetite.

Composition of the Diet

As we have said, when we eat more energy than we expend, we gain weight. Most people eat what is referred to as a "mixed" diet, meaning it contains a mix of carbohydrate, fat, and protein. Scientists used to think that people would gain the same amount of weight if they ate too much food of any type, but now there is evidence to support the theory that when we overeat dietary fat, we store it much more easily as adipose tissue than we do either carbohydrate or protein (Hellerstein, Christiansen, and Kaempfer 1991). This may be due to the fact that eating fat doesn't cause much of an increase in metabolic rate, and the body stores fat in the form of adipose tissue quite easily. In contrast, when we overeat protein or carbohydrate, our body's initial response is to use this extra food for energy, storage, or the building of tissues, with a smaller amount of the excess stored as fat. This does not mean, however, that you can eat as many low-fat foods as you want and not gain weight! Consistently overeating protein or carbohydrate will also lead to weight gain. Instead, maintain a balanced diet combining fat, carbohydrate, and protein, and reduce your dietary fat to less than 30% of total energy. This strategy may help reduce your storage of fat energy as adipose tissue.

Hunger Versus Appetite

As introduced in Chapter 3, *hunger* is our innate, physiological drive or need to eat. We can tell when we are hungry by paying attention to our body's signals, such as a growling stomach and lightheadedness. This need for food is triggered by physiologic changes such as low blood glucose that affect the chemicals in our brain. The hypothalamus is the part of the brain that plays an important role in hunger regulation. Special cells referred to as *feeding cells* in the hypothalamus respond to conditions of low blood glucose, causing us to be hungry and to eat.

Once we have eaten and our bodies respond accordingly, other centers in the hypothalamus are triggered, and our desire to eat is reduced. The state we reach in which we no longer desire to eat is referred to as *satiety*. It may be that some people have an insufficient satiety mechanism, which prevents them from feeling full after a meal, allowing them to overeat. Some of the factors that increase satiety (or decrease food intake) include:

- Stomach expansion
- Nutrient absorption from the small intestine
- Increased blood glucose
- Hormones such as leptin, serotonin, and cholecystokinin (CCK). Leptin is produced by adipose tissue; serotonin is made from the amino acid tryptophan; and CCK is produced by the intestinal cells and stimulates the gallbladder to secrete bile.

There are also many factors that can decrease satiety (or increase food intake). These include:

- Hormones such as beta-endorphins. Beta-endorphins increase a sense of pleasure while eating, which can increase food intake
- Neuropeptide Y, which is an amino-acid containing compound produced in the hypothalamus, stimulates appetite
- Decreased blood glucose

We explored in Chapter 3 the concept that *appetite* can be experienced in the absence of hunger. Appetite may therefore be considered a psychological drive to eat, being stimulated by learned preferences for food and particular situations that promote eating. For instance, some people learn as children to love or hate certain foods. This may explain why foods such as frogs' legs, cactus, and cultured yeast extract (Marmite) appeal to people in certain cultures who were raised on them but are almost never adopted into the diet as new foods by an adult. Others may follow learned behaviors related to timing and size of meals. In addition, the sight and fragrance of certain foods stimulate the pleasure centers of the brain, whether or not we happen to be hungry at the time. Mood can also affect appetite, as some people will eat more or less if they feel depressed or happy. As you can imagine, appetite leads many people to overeat.

Social Factors Influence Behavior and Body Weight

Social factors can encourage us to overeat or choose high-calorie foods. For example, pressure from family and friends to eat the way they do and easy access to large servings of inexpensive and high-fat foods contribute to overeating. Think about how you might eat differently when you attend a birthday celebration with family or friends. You are offered hot dogs, pizza, birthday cake, ice cream, and many other dishes that taste great but are relatively high in fat and energy. The pressure to overeat during holidays is also high, with constant encouragement to eat extra servings of your favorite holiday foods and to finish a very large meal with dessert.

We also have numerous opportunities to overeat because of easy access to foods high in fat and energy throughout our normal daily routine. Vending machines selling junk foods are everywhere: at schools, in business offices, and even at laundromats. Shopping malls are filled with fast-food restaurants, where inexpensive, large serving sizes are the norm. Even foods we have traditionally considered healthful, such as peanut butter, yogurt, and milk, are filled with added sugars and other ingredients that are high in energy and fat. We don't even have to spend time or energy preparing our food anymore, as everything is either ready-to-serve or requires just a few minutes to cook in a microwave oven. This easy access to high-fat and high-energy foods leads many of us to overeat.

Similarly, social factors can cause people to be less physically active. Social factors restricting physical activity include living in an unsafe community, watching a lot of television, maintaining a busy lifestyle that does not include a lot of physical activity, coping with family responsibilities, and living in an area with harsh weather conditions. Many overweight people identify such factors as major barriers to maintaining a healthful body weight, and research seems to confirm their influence. There is growing evidence that sedentary behaviors such as television watching are associated with obesity in both children and adults. A study of 11- to 13-year-old schoolchildren found that children who watched more than 2 hours of television per night were more likely to be overweight or obese than children who watched less than 2 hours of television per night. Interestingly, adults who reported an increase in television watching of 20 hours per week (approximately 3 hours per day) over a 9-year period had a significant increase in waist circumference (Koh-Banerjee et al. 2003), indicating significant weight gain in these adults.

On the other hand, social pressures to maintain a lean body are great enough to encourage many of us to undereat or to avoid foods we perceive as "bad," especially fats. Our society ridicules and often ostracizes overweight people, many of whom even face job discrimination. Media images of waiflike fashion models and men in tight jeans with washboard abdomens and muscular chests encourage many people—especially adolescents and young adults—to skip meals, resort to crash diets, and exercise obsessively. Even some people of normal body weight push themselves to achieve an unrealistic and unattainable weight goal, in the process threatening their health and even their life (see Chapter 13 for consequences of disordered eating).

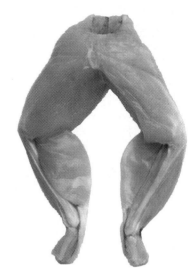

Food preferences often depend on culture. Some cultures enjoy foods such as frogs' legs, while others do not.

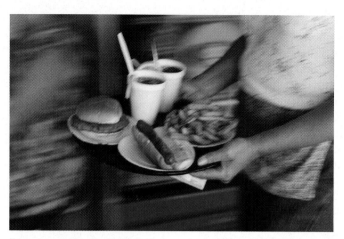

Easy access or fast foods may be inexpensive and filling, but are often high in fat and sugar.

It should be clear that how we gain, lose, and maintain our body weight is a complex matter. Most people who are overweight have tried several weight-loss programs but have been unsuccessful in maintaining long-term weight loss. A significant number of these people have consequently given up all weight-loss attempts. Some even suffer from severe depression related to their body weight. Should we condemn these people as failures and continue to pressure them to lose weight? Should people who are overweight but otherwise healthy (e.g., low blood pressure, cholesterol, and glucose levels) feel compelled to lose weight? The Nutrition Debate at the end of this chapter addresses these issues and provides an opportunity to discuss how we should deal with the growing concerns and prejudices related to obesity in our society.

Recap: Our diet and activity patterns as children influence our body weight as adults. Behavioral factors such as the amount of dietary fat, carbohydrate, and protein, and alterations in satiety and appetite also influence our body weight. Social factors influencing our weight include ready availability of high-calorie foods, lack of physical activity, and too much television watching. There are prejudices and social pressures against those who are overweight and obese, and these pressures can even drive many normal weight individuals to use unhealthful and even dangerous approaches in an attempt to achieve an unrealistic body weight.

How Many Kilocalories Do You Need?

Given everything we've discussed so far, you're probably asking yourself, "How much should I eat?" This question is not always easy to answer, as our energy needs fluctuate from day to day according to our activity level, environmental conditions, and other factors such as the amount and type of food we eat and our intake of caffeine. However, you can get a general estimate of how much energy your body needs to maintain your present weight.

One potential way to estimate how much energy you need each day is to record your total food and beverage intake for a defined period of time, such as three or seven days. You can then use a food composition table or computer dietary assessment program to estimate the amount of energy you eat each day. Assuming that your body weight is stable over this period of time, your average daily energy intake should represent how much energy you need to maintain your present weight.

Unfortunately, many studies of energy intake in humans have shown that dietary records estimating energy needs are not very accurate. Most studies show that humans underestimate the amount of energy they eat by 10 to 30%. Overweight people tend to underestimate by an even higher margin, at the same time overestimating the amount of activity they do. This means that someone who really eats about 2000 kcal/day may only record eating 1400 to 1800 kcal/day. So one reason why many people are confused about their ability to lose weight is that they are eating more than they realize.

A simpler and more accurate way to estimate your total daily energy needs is to calculate your BMR, and then add the amount of energy you expend as a result of your activity level. Refer to the You Do the Math Box, "Calculating BMR and Total Daily Energy Needs" (page 399), for an example of how to do this. As the energy cost for the thermic effect of food is very small, you don't need to include it in your calculations.

Calculating BMR and Total Daily Energy Needs

1. *Calculate your BMR:* If you are a man, you will need to multiply your body weight in kg by 1 kcal per kg body weight per hour. Assuming you weigh 175 pounds, your body weight in kg would be 175 pounds/2.2 pounds per kg = 79.5 kg. Next, multiply your weight in kg by 1 kcal per kg body weight per hour:

   1 kcal per kg body weight per hour
   × 79.5 kg = 79.5 kcal per hour

   Calculate your BMR for the total day (or 24 hours):

   79.5 kcal per hour × 24 hours per day
   = 1,909 kcal per day

   (If you are a woman, multiply your body weight in kg by 0.9 kcal per kg body weight per hour.)

2. *Estimate your activity level by selecting the description that most closely fits your general lifestyle.* The energy cost of activities is expressed as a percentage of your BMR. Refer to these values when estimating your own energy output:

	Men	Women
Sedentary/inactive Involves mostly sitting, driving, or very low levels of activity.	25–40%	25–35%
Lightly Active Involves a lot of sitting; may also involve some walking, moving around, and light lifting.	50–70%	40–60%
Moderately Active Involves work plus intentional exercise such as an hour of walking or walking four to five days per week; may have a job requiring some physical labor.	65–80%	50–70%
Heavily Active Involves a great deal of physical labor, such as roofing, carpentry work, and/ or regular heavy lifting and digging.	90–120%	80–100%
Exceptionally Active Involves a lot of physical activities for work and intentional exercise. Also applies to athletes who train for many hours each day, such as triathletes and marathon runners or other competitive athletes performing heavy, regular training.	130–145%	110–130%

3. *Multiply your BMR by the decimal equivalent of the lower and higher percentage values for your activity level.* Let's use the man referred to in step 1 above. He is a college student who lives on campus. He walks to classes located throughout campus, carries his book bag, and spends most of his time reading and writing. He does not exercise on a regular basis. His lifestyle would be defined as lightly active, meaning he expends 50 to 70% of his BMR each day in activities. You want to calculate how much energy he expends at both ends of this activity level. How many kcal does this equal?

   1,909 kcal/day × 0.50 (or 50%) = 955 kcal/day

   1,909 kcal/day × 0.70 (or 70%)
   = 1,336 kcal/day

   These calculations show that this man expends about 955 to 1,336 kcal/day doing daily activities.

4. *Calculate total daily energy output by adding together BMR and the energy needed to perform daily activities.* In this man's case, his total daily energy output is:

   1,909 kcal/day + 955 kcal/day
   = 2,864 kcal/day

   OR

   1,909 kcal/day + 1,336 kcal/day
   = 3,245 kcal/day

   Assuming this man is maintaining his present weight, he requires between 2,864 and 3,245 kcal/day to stay in energy balance! ●

Recap: Accurately determining daily energy needs is difficult due to the limitations of currently available estimation methods. A less accurate way to estimate energy needs is to record food intake for three to seven days; if body weight is stable, average energy intake should be representative of daily energy needs. A simpler and more accurate way to estimate daily energy needs is to calculate your BMR and then add your estimated daily activity level to that value.

How Can You Achieve and Maintain a Healthful Body Weight?

Achieving and maintaining a healthful body weight involves many factors including healthful dietary approaches and participation in regular physical activity. In this section we discuss these factors and review the use of prescribed medications and dietary supplements in losing or gaining body weight.

Healthful Weight Change Involves Moderation and Consistency

There are an unlimited number of weight loss and weight gain programs available. How can you know which plan or program is based on sound dietary principles and whether it will result in long-term weight change? There are three primary components of a sound weight change plan:

- Gradual changes in energy intake
- Incorporation of regular and appropriate physical activity
- Application of behavior modification techniques

Following a lifestyle plan that includes each of these components will help insure a healthful approach to weight change.

Beware of fad diets! They are simply what their name implies — fads that do not result in long-term, healthful weight changes. Most of these programs will "die" only to be born again as a "new and improved" fad diet. See the Highlight box, "The Anatomy of Fad Diets" to learn more about this issue.

Safe and Effective Weight Loss

Setting realistic weight loss goals is an important part of a weight loss plan. Although making gradual changes in body weight is frustrating for most people, this slower change is much more effective in maintaining weight loss over the long-term. Ask yourself the question, "How long did it take me to gain this extra weight?" A fair expectation for weight loss is that it should take about the same amount of time to lose the weight as it took to gain it. In general, a sound weight loss plan involves a modest reduction in energy intake, incorporating physical activity into each day, and practicing changes in behavior that can assist you in meeting your weight loss goals. The guidelines for a sound weight loss plan are outlined in the accompanying Highlight box.

Eat Smaller Portions of Lower-Fat Foods

What changes can you make to reduce your energy intake and stay healthy? Here are some helpful suggestions:

1. Follow the serving sizes recommended in the Food Guide Pyramid (page 51). Making this change involves understanding what constitutes a serving size and measuring foods to determine if they meet or exceed the recommended serving

The Anatomy of Fad Diets

Fad diets are programs that enjoy short-term popularity and are sold based on a marketing gimmick that appeals to the public's desires and fears. There are hundreds of these types of diets on the market today, and the goal of the person or company designing and marketing these diets is to make money. How can you tell if the program you are interested in is a fad diet? Here are some pointers to help you:

- The promoters of the diet claim that the program is new, improved, or based on some new discovery; however, no scientific data are available to support these claims.

- The program is touted for its ability to result in rapid weight loss or body fat loss, usually more than 2 pounds per week, and may include the claim that weight loss can be achieved with little or no physical exercise.

- The diet includes special foods and supplements, many of which are expensive and/or difficult to find or can only be purchased from the diet promoter. Common recommendations for these diets include avoiding certain foods, only eating a special combination of certain foods, or including magic foods in the diet that "burn" fat and speed up metabolism.

- The diet may include a rigid menu that must be followed daily or may limit participants to eating a few select foods each day. Variety and balance are discouraged, and restriction of certain foods (such as fruits and vegetables) is encouraged.

- Many programs include supplemental foods and/or nutritional supplements that are identified as substances critical to the success of the diet and usually include claims that these supplements can cure or prevent a variety of health ailments or that the diet can stop the aging process.

The success of fad diets lies in their ability to appeal to the concerns of many people: being overweight or not being muscular enough; reducing the effects of aging such as wrinkles, loose skin, and tissue damage; and eating anything you want or desire and still losing weight. It is estimated that we currently spend more than $33 billion on fad diets each year (American Dietetic Association 2001). In a world where many of us feel we have to meet a certain physical standard to be attractive and "good enough," these types of diets flourish. Unfortunately, the only people who usually benefit from them are their marketers, who can become very wealthy promoting programs that are highly ineffectual. ●

---

size. Remember that one pound of fat is equal to about 3,500 kcal; to lose one pound of fat, you must eat less food and expend more energy.

2. Reduce the amount of foods that are high in fat and energy from your daily diet. Dietary fat intake should be 20 to 25% of total energy. This goal can be achieved by eliminating extra fats such as butter, margarine, and mayonnaise and snack foods such as ice cream, doughnuts, and cakes. Save these foods as occasional special treats. Select lower-fat versions of the foods listed in the Food Guide Pyramid. This means selecting leaner cuts of meat (such as the white meat of poultry and extra-lean ground beef) and reduced-fat or skim dairy products, and selecting lower-fat preparation methods (baking and broiling instead of frying).

By following these suggestions, you can make simple changes that are effective in reducing energy intake and help contribute to a more healthful diet overall.

Participate in Regular Physical Activity

The forthcoming revision of the USDA Food Guide Pyramid will place far greater emphasis on the role of physical activity in maintaining a healthful weight. Why is being physically active so important for achieving changes in body weight and for maintaining a healthful body weight? Of course we expend extra energy during physical activity, but there's more to it than that because exercise alone (without a reduction of energy intake) does not result in dramatic decreases in body weight. Instead, one of the most important reasons for being regularly active is that it helps

Recommendations for a Sound Weight Loss Plan

Dietary Recommendations:

- Reasonable weight loss is defined as 0.5 to 2 pounds per week. To achieve this rate of weight loss, energy intake should be reduced approximately 250 to no more than 1,000 kcal/day of present intake. A weight loss plan should never provide less than a total of 1,200 kcal/day.

- Total fat intake should be 15 to 25% of total energy intake.

  - Saturated fat intake should be 5 to 10% of total energy intake.

  - Monounsaturated fat intake should be 10 to 15% of total energy intake.

  - Polyunsaturated fat intake should be no more than 10% of total energy intake.

- Cholesterol intake should be less than 300 mg/day.

- Protein intake should be approximately 15 to 20% of total energy intake.

- Carbohydrate intake should be around 55% of total energy intake, with less than 10% of energy intake coming from simple sugars.

- Fiber intake should be 25 to 35 grams/day.

- Calcium intake should be 1,000 to 1,500 mg/day.

Physical Activity Recommendations:

- A long-term goal for physical activity should be a minimum of 30 minutes of moderate physical activity most, or preferably all, days of the week.

- Doing 45 minutes or more of an activity such as walking at least five days per week is ideal.

Behavior Modification Recommendations:

- Eliminate inappropriate behaviors by shopping when you are not hungry, only eating at set times in one location, refusing to buy problem foods, and avoiding vending machines, convenience stores, and fast-food restaurants.

- Suppress inappropriate behaviors by taking small food portions, eating foods on smaller serving dishes so they appear larger, and avoiding feelings of deprivation by eating regular meals throughout the day.

- Strengthen appropriate behaviors by sharing food with others, learning appropriate serving sizes, planning healthful snacks, scheduling walks and other physical activities with friends, and keeping clothes and equipment for physical activity in convenient places.

- Repeat desired behaviors by slowing down eating, always using utensils, leaving food on your plate, moving more throughout the day, and joining groups who are physically active.

- Reward yourself for positive behaviors by getting a massage, buying new clothes or tickets to nonfood amusements, taking a walk, or reading a book (for fun).

- Using the "buddy" system by exercising with a friend or relative and/or calling this support person when you need an extra boost to stay motivated.

- Don't punish yourself if you deviate from your plan (and you will—everyone does). Ask others to avoid responding to any slips you make.

Source: Adapted from National Heart, Lung, and Blood Institute Expert Panel, National Institutes of Health. *Clinical Guidelines on the Identification, Evaluation, and Treatment of Overweight and Obesity in Adults.* Washington, DC: Government Printing Office, 1998. ●

us maintain or increase our lean body mass and our BMR. In contrast, energy restriction alone causes us to lose lean body mass. As you've learned, the more lean body mass we have, the more energy we expend over the long-term.

The National Weight Control Registry is an ongoing project documenting the habits of people who have lost at least 30 pounds and kept their weight off for at least one year. Of the 784 people studied thus far, average weight loss was 66 pounds, and the group maintained the minimum weight loss criteria of 30 pounds for more than five years (Klem et al. 1997). Virtually all of the people (89%) reported changing both physical activity and dietary intake to lose weight and maintain weight loss. No one form of exercise seems to be most effective, but many people report doing some form of aerobic exercise (such as bicycling, walking, running, aerobic dance, step aerobics, or hiking) and weight lifting at least 45 minutes most days of the week. In fact, on average, this group expended more than 2,800 kcal each week through physical activity! While very few weight loss studies have documented long-term maintenance of weight loss, those that have find that only people who are regularly active are able to maintain most of their weight loss.

In addition to expending energy and maintaining lean body mass and BMR, regular physical activity improves our mood, results in a higher quality of sleep, increases self-esteem, and gives us a sense of accomplishment (see Chapter 12 for more benefits of regular physical activity). All of these changes enhance our ability to engage in long-term healthful lifestyle behaviors.

Weight Loss Can Be Enhanced With Prescribed Medications

The biggest complaint about the recommendations for healthful weight loss is that they are too difficult for most people to follow. Many people are looking for a "magic bullet" that will allow them to lose weight quickly and easily, requiring little sustained effort on their part to achieve their weight goals. Other people have tried to follow healthful weight-loss suggestions for years and have not been successful. In response to these challenges, prescription drugs have been developed to assist people with weight loss. These drugs typically act as appetite suppressants and may also increase satiety.

Weight loss medications should be used only with proper supervision from a physician. One reason physician involvement is so critical is that many drugs developed for weight loss have side effects. Some have even proven deadly. Fenfluramine (brand name Pondimin), dexfenfluramine (brand name Redux) and a combination of phentermine and fenfluramine (called "phen-fen") are appetite-suppressing drugs that were banned from the market in 1996. These drugs, while resulting in more weight loss than diet alone, were found to cause two life-threatening conditions: primary pulmonary hypertension and valvular heart disease. Use of the drugs resulted in several deaths and caused an increased risk for heart and lung disease.

Two relatively new prescription weight loss drugs are available, and their long-term safety and efficacy are still being explored. Sibutramine (brand name Meridia) is an appetite suppressant that can cause increased blood pressure in some people. Orlistat (brand name Xenical) is a drug that acts to inhibit the absorption of dietary fat from the intestinal tract, which can result in weight loss in some people. A one-year study of orlistat found that it was effective in minimizing weight regain in obese people who lost weight using a low calorie diet (Hill et al. 1999). The side effects of these drugs are identified in Table 11.6.

Table 11.6   Side Effects of Two Prescription Weight Loss Drugs

Sibutramine (Brand name Meridia)	Orlistat (Brand name Xenical)
Increased blood pressure	Abdominal pain
Dry mouth	Fatty and loose stools
Anorexia	Leaky stools
Constipation	Flatulence
Insomnia	Decreased absorption of fat-soluble nutrients such as vitamins E and D
Dizziness	
Nausea	

Source: G. A. Bray. Drug treatment of obesity. *Baillière's Clin. Endocrinol. Metab.* 13 (1999):131–148.

Using Dietary Supplements to Lose Weight Is Controversial

Over-the-counter dietary supplements and medications are also marketed for weight loss. Many of these products can increase metabolic rate and decrease appetite because they contain caffeine, ephedrine, and phenylpropanolamine (PPA), which is a substance also found in many cold medications. Use of these substances is controversial and may be dangerous, as abnormal increases in heart rate and blood pressure can occur. It is important to remember that the Food and Drug Administration (FDA) regulates prescription drugs and over-the-counter medications, but they do not have control over dietary supplements. Thus, dangerous or ineffective supplements can be marketed and sold without meeting strict safety guidelines and are unlikely to be pulled from the shelves.

In the year 2000, PPA was banned from the market in response to the deaths of several women caused by brain hemorrhage after taking the prescribed dose. Consumers were instructed to throw away any cold medications and allergy products in their homes that contained PPA. Ephedrine use has also been associated with dangerous elevations in heart rate, blood pressure, and death; for this reason, the United States has banned the use of ephedrine in over-the-counter products. However, some herbal supplement producers still include ma huang, the so-called "herbal ephedra," in their weight loss products. Some herbal weight-loss supplements contain a combination of ma huang, caffeine, and aspirin. Because heart problems and deaths have also been associated with this herb, the FDA banned the manufacture and sale of ephedra in the United States in 2004.

As you can see, using weight loss supplements can have dangerous consequences. Even the use of prescribed weight loss medications is associated with side effects and a certain level of risk. So for whom are such medications justified? The answer is, for people who are severely obese. That's because the health risks of severe obesity override the risks of the medications. Specifically, prescription weight-loss medications are advised for people who have:

- a BMI greater than or equal to 30 kg/m²
- a BMI greater than or equal to 27 kg/m² who also have other significant health risk factors such as heart disease, high blood pressure, and type 2 diabetes.

These medications should only be used while under a physician's supervision so that progress and health risks can be closely monitored. They are most effective when combined with a program that supports energy restriction, regular exercise, and increasing physical activity throughout the day.

> **Recap:** Maintaining a healthful body weight involves healthful dietary approaches and participation in regular physical activity. Weight loss can be accomplished by eating smaller portion sizes, eating less dietary fat, incorporating regular physical activity, and applying appropriate behavioral modification techniques. Maintenance of weight loss is enhanced by healthful eating habits and regular physical activity. When necessary, drugs can be used to reduce obesity with a doctor's prescription and supervision. Using dietary supplements to lose weight is controversial and can be dangerous in some instances.

Safe and Effective Weight Gain

With so much emphasis in the United States on obesity and weight loss, some find it surprising that many people are trying to gain weight. People looking to gain weight include those who are underweight to the extent that it is compromising their health, and it also includes many athletes who are attempting to increase strength and power for competition.

Eat More Energy Than Expended

To gain weight, people must eat more energy than they expend. While overeating large amounts of high saturated-fat foods (such as bacon, sausage, and cheese) can cause weight gain, doing this without exercising is not considered healthful because most of the weight gained is fat, and high-fat diets increase our risks for cardiovascular and other diseases. Unless there are medical reasons to eat a high-fat diet, it is recommended that people trying to gain weight eat a diet that is relatively low in dietary fat (less than 30% of total calories) and relatively high in complex carbohydrates (55% of total calories). Recommendations for weight gain include:

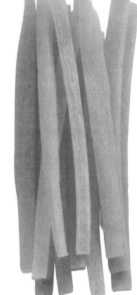

- Eat a diet that includes about 500 to 1,000 kcal/day more than is needed to maintain present body weight. Although we don't know exactly how much extra energy is needed to gain one pound, estimates range from 3,000 to 3,500 kcal. Thus, eating 500 to 1,000 kcal/day in excess should result in a gain of 1 to 2 pounds of weight each week.

- Eat a diet that contains about 55% of total energy from carbohydrate, 25 to 30% of total energy from fat, and 15 to 20% of total energy from protein.

- Eat frequently, including meals and numerous snacks throughout the day. Many underweight people do not take the time to eat often enough.

- Avoid the use of tobacco products, as they depress appetite and increase metabolic rate, which prevent weight gain. They also cause lung, mouth, and esophageal cancers.

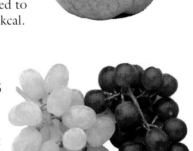

Eating frequent nutrient-dense snacks can help promote weight gain.

- Exercise regularly and incorporate weight-lifting or some other form of resistance training into your exercise routine. This form of exercise is most effective in increasing muscle mass. Performing aerobic exercise (such as walking, running, bicycling, or swimming) at least 30 minutes for three days per week will help maintain a healthy cardiovascular system.

The key to gaining weight is to eat frequent meals throughout the day and to select energy-dense foods. When selecting foods that are higher in fat, make sure you select foods higher in polyunsaturated and monounsaturated fats (such as peanut butter, olive and canola oils, and avocados). For instance, smoothies and milkshakes made with low-fat milk or yogurt are a great way to take in a lot of energy. Eating peanut butter with fruit or celery and including salad dressings on your salad are other ways to increase the energy density of foods. The biggest challenge to weight gain is setting aside time to eat; by packing a lot of foods to take with you throughout the day, you can enhance your opportunities to eat more.

Theo

Nutri-Case

"I'm sick and tired of everybody everywhere complaining about how they can't lose weight even though they're starving themselves and feel hungry all the time. Nobody talks about people like me, who have exactly the opposite problem. I keep super-busy, I'm almost never hungry, and I can't keep weight on! It's especially bad right now because its basketball season: no matter what I do, the pounds peel off! For breakfast this morning, I had bacon and eggs. For lunch, I'll probably eat a couple of ham sandwiches. Then a protein bar after practice, and for dinner, I'll probably go out for burgers with my friends. What more can I do? Don't tell me to eat between meals because, like I said, I'm just not that hungry."

Given what you've learned about energy balance and weight management, what if any problems do you perceive with Theo's food intake today? What might you advise him to change about his food choices that might help stimulate his appetite? What else might he do to gain weight?

Global Nutrition: Overweight and Wasting Among Preschool Children

We know that wealthy, developed countries are experiencing significant upward trends of obesity in adults and children. In contrast, in developing countries, wasting (or starvation) has generally been considered one of the most significant health concerns. Recently, however, poverty and low socioeconomic status have been linked with higher rates of obesity worldwide. In fact, the United Nations now estimates that over one billion people are overweight or obese worldwide, including 22 million children under age 5 (Arnst 2004). So, is childhood obesity on the rise in developing countries, too?

A recent study documents the prevalence and trends of overweight among children aged 0 to 6 years in developed and developing countries (de Onis and Blössner (2000)). Figure 11.8 shows a graph of some of the countries studied. Of the 94 countries surveyed, 76% reported less than 5% of their young children to be overweight.

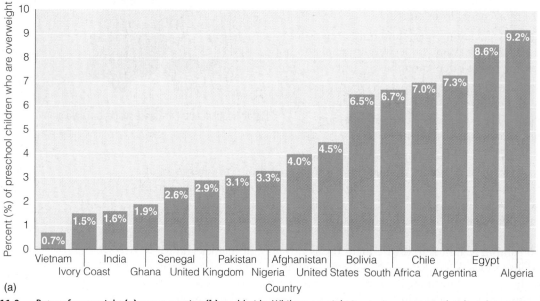

(a)

Figure 11.8 Rates of overweight **(a)** versus wasting **(b)** worldwide. While overweight is a major concern in developed countries, wasting is still a major concern in developing countries. (Adapted from M. de Onis and M. Blössner. Prevalence and trends of overweight among preschool children in developing countries. *Am. J. Clin. Nutr.* 72 (2000):1032–1039.)

Protein Supplements Do Not Increase Muscle Growth or Strength

As with weight loss, there are many products marketed for weight gain. One of the most common claims is that these products are *anabolic;* that is, that they increase muscle mass. These products include protein supplements and *androstenedione,* which is a substance that became very popular after baseball player Mark McGuire claimed he used this product during the time he was breaking home run records. Do these substances really work?

A growing body of evidence exists to show that amino acid and protein supplements do not enhance muscle gain or result in improvements in strength (Kreider, Miriel, and Bertun 1993). Although the case of Mark McGuire may seem to suggest that androstenedione is an extremely effective product for building muscle mass, gaining strength, and improving performance, recent studies report that this product did not have any benefits (Joyner 2000; Broeder et al. 2000; Brown et al. 2000). Protein supplements and androstenedione are legal to sell in the United States, but these and other potentially anabolic substances are banned by the National Football League, the National Collegiate Athletic Association, and the International Olympic Committee.

In contrast, 21% of these countries reported that 5 to 10% of their children were overweight, and 2% reported over 10% of their children as overweight. As you might suspect, the countries with the least amount of overweight were developing countries such as those in Africa and Asia. The countries with the highest rates of overweight were developed countries such as the United States.

Although overweight appears to be on the rise in some developing countries, it is important to note that wasting rates are much higher in these countries than are rates of overweight. Forty-five of the countries studied reported greater than 5% of their children as malnourished. These findings show that while the overall global rate of obesity may be increasing, we must not focus on reducing overweight in young children at the expense of solving problems with wasting. ●

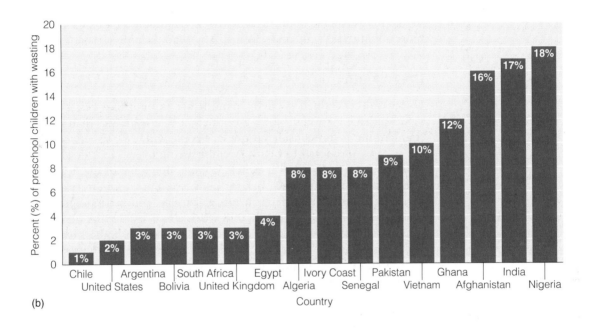

(b)

The health consequences of using protein supplements are unknown. Androstenedione caused unhealthy changes in high-density and low-density lipoprotein (HDL and LDL) levels in middle-aged men, potentially increasing their risk for heart disease (Broeder et al. 2000). The use of anabolic steriods is known to cause major health problems. These include unhealthy changes in blood cholesterol, mood disturbances (such as anger leading to violence), testicular shrinkage and breast enlargement in men, and irreversible clitoral enlargement in women (see Chapter 12 for a more detailed discussion of anabolic steroid use). We also know that buying these substances can have a substantial impact on your wallet and, at least in the case of protein supplements and androstenedione, is most likely a waste of money.

Recap: Weight gain can be achieved by eating more and performing weight lifting and aerobic exercise. Protein and amino acid supplements and androstenedione do not increase muscle growth or strength, and their potential side effects are unknown. Anabolic steroid use can increase body weight and muscle mass but is known to cause major health problems.

What Disorders Are Related to Energy Intake?

At the beginning of this chapter, we provided some definitions of underweight, overweight, obesity, and morbid obesity. Let's take a closer look at these disorders.

Underweight

As defined earlier in this chapter, underweight occurs when a person has too little body fat to maintain health. People with a BMI of less than 18.5 kg/m^2 are typically considered underweight. Being underweight can be just as unhealthful as being obese. Many people are underweight due to heavy smoking, an underlying disease such as cancer or HIV infection, or an eating disorder such as anorexia nervosa (see Chapter 13). Being underweight increases the risk for infections and illness, and can even be fatal.

Although childhood overweight and obesity are major health concerns in most developed countries, wasting (or starvation) is still a critical health crisis for children in many developing countries. Refer to the Highlight box on global nutrition to learn more about overweight and wasting in preschool children around the world.

Overweight

Overweight is defined as having a moderate amount of excess body fat, resulting in a person having a weight for a given height that is greater than some accepted standard but is not considered obese. People with a BMI between 25 and 29.9 kg/m^2 are considered to be overweight. Being overweight does not appear to be as detrimental to our health as being obese, but some of the health risks of overweight include an increased risk for high blood pressure, heart disease, type 2 diabetes, sleep disorders, osteoarthritis, gallstones, and gynecological abnormalities (National Institutes of Health 1998). It is also possible that people who are overweight will become obese, which can lead to an even higher risk for these diseases and for premature death. Because of these concerns, health professionals recommend that overweight individuals adopt a lifestyle that incorporates healthful eating and regular physical activity in an attempt to prevent additional weight gain, to reduce body weight to the normal level, and/or to support long-term health even if body weight is not significantly reduced.

Hannah   *Nutri-Case*

"My mom says the YMCA is having a swim camp at the lake during spring break and I can go if I want, but I told her "no thanks." When she asked why not, I said "cause it's for little kids," but that's not the real reason. The real reason is that, when I went last year, the other kids picked on me so bad the whole time. I had a real pretty swimsuit, but one of the boys said it was bigger than his grandma's. The girls were even meaner, especially when I was changing in the locker room, calling me "fatty" and "elephant" and even worse stuff I won't repeat. I'd just as soon stay home and watch television during spring break."

Think back to your own childhood. Were you ever teased for some aspect of yourself that you felt unable to change? Can Hannah change her weight? What strategies might she try, and what obstacles does she face? If you were her parent, would you encourage her to attend the swim camp despite her feelings? Why or why not? How might organizations that work with children, such as YMCAs, scout troops, and church-based groups, increase their leaders' awareness of social stigmatization of overweight children and reduce incidents of teasing and other insensitivity?

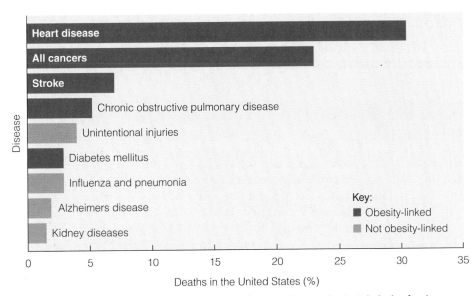

Figure 11.9   Of the nine leading causes of death in the United States, obesity is linked to five (see areas shaded in red). (Adapted from National Center for Chronic Disease Prevention and Health Promotion (NCCDPHP), 2002, Chronic Disease Prevention, Chronic Disease Overview, www.cdc.gov/nccdphp/overview.htm. Accessed February 2004.)

Obesity and Morbid Obesity

Obesity is defined as having an excess body fat that adversely affects health, resulting in a person having a weight for a given height that is substantially greater than some accepted standard. People with a BMI between 30 and 39.9 kg/m^2 are considered obese. Morbid obesity occurs when a person's body weight exceeds 100% of normal; people who are morbidly obese have a BMI greater than or equal to 40 kg/m^2.

Both overweight and obesity are now considered an epidemic in the United States. It is estimated that about 64% of adults in the United States are either overweight or obese (CDC 2004). Obesity rates have increased more than 50% over the past 20 years. This alarming rise in obesity is a major health concern because it is linked to many chronic diseases, including heart disease, high blood pressure, type 2 diabetes, some cancers, and osteoarthritis. At least five of the nine leading causes of death in the United States are associated with obesity (see Figure 11.9).

It has been estimated that the financial costs associated with obesity total more than $99 billion. These costs affect not just the person with obesity, but all of society, as they increase the costs of health care and medications, reduce productivity because of days of lost work, and reduce future earnings because of premature death.

Ironically, up to 40% of women and 25% of men are dieting at any given time. How can obesity rates be so high when there are so many people dieting? Certainly some people dieting at any given time are actually at a normal or even below-normal weight, and these people account for a small percentage of this total; however, many obese people who are dieting are somehow failing to lose weight or to maintain long-term weight loss.

What Causes Obesity?

Obesity is known as a **multifactorial disease,** meaning that there are many things that cause it. This makes obesity extremely difficult to treat. Although it is certainly true that obesity, like overweight, is caused by eating more energy than is expended, it is also true that some people are more susceptible to becoming obese than others. In addition, as we saw with the twin study, some people are more resistant to weight loss and maintaining weight loss than others. Research on the causes and best treatments of obesity is ongoing, but let's explore some current theories.

multifactorial disease   Any disease which may be attributable to one or more of a variety of causes.

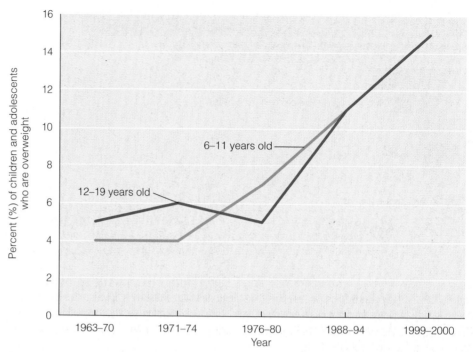

Figure 11.10 Increases in childhood and adolescent overweight from 1963 to 2000. (Adapted from Centers for Disease Control and Prevention. National Center for Health Statistics, 2002, Prevalence of overweight among children and adolescents: United States, 1999–2000, http://www.cdc.gov/nchs/products/pubs/pubd/hestats/overwght99.htm Accessed February 2004.)

Genetic Factors Because our genetic background influences our height, weight, body shape, and metabolic rate, it also affects our risk for obesity. The thrifty gene theory (page 393) suggests that some people possess a thrifty gene (or genes), which causes them to expend less energy at rest and during physical activity. This theory has been used to try to explain the high rates of obesity among Native Americans and other indigenous peoples. The set-point theory (page 394) suggests that our bodies work to maintain our weight at a set point, which could partially explain why most obese people are very resistant to weight loss. Although we know that leptin (page 394) plays a role in energy intake and metabolism, it is still not clear exactly how, or if, leptin directly contributes to obesity. As we learn more about genetics, we will gain a greater understanding of the role that our genetic background plays in the development and treatment of obesity.

Childhood Overweight and Obesity Are Linked to Adult Obesity The prevalence of overweight in children and adolescents is increasing at an alarming rate in the United States (Figure 11.10). There was a time when having extra "baby fat" was considered good for the child. We assumed that childhood overweight and obesity were temporary and that the child would grow out of it. While it is important for children to have a certain minimum level of body fat to maintain health and to grow properly, researchers are now concerned that overweight and obesity are harmful to children's health and increase their risk of overweight and obesity in adulthood.

Health data demonstrate that obese children are already showing signs of disease while they are young, including elevated blood pressure, high cholesterol levels, and changes in insulin and glucose metabolism that may increase the risk for type 2 diabetes (formerly known as *adult onset diabetes*). In some communities, children as young as 6 years of age have been diagnosed with type 2 diabetes. Unfortunately, many of these children are maintaining these disease risk factors into adulthood.

Does being an obese child guarantee that obesity will be maintained during adulthood? Not all obese adults were obese as children, and some children who are obese grow up to have a normal body weight. However, it has been estimated that about 50% of children who are obese will maintain their higher weight as adults. This has important consequences for their health.

What factors contribute to obesity in children? For young people, it has been suggested that there are three critical periods during which weight gain can increase the risk of obesity and related diseases in adulthood:

- Gestation and early infancy
- The period of weight gain (called *adiposity rebound*) that occurs between 5 and 7 years of age
- Adolescence (or puberty)

Substantial weight gain during these periods can increase the risk for adult obesity and related diseases. Having either one or two overweight parents increases the risk of obesity two to four times (Dietz 1994).

An additional important contributor to childhood obesity includes low physical activity levels. There was a time when children played outdoors regularly and when physical education was offered daily in school. In today's society, many children cannot play outdoors due to safety concerns and lack of recreational facilities, and few schools have the resources to regularly offer physical education to children. In addition, many popular activities for children today are sedentary in nature, including playing video games, watching television, using the computer, and playing with hand-held game toys. As childhood and adolescence are critical times for forming activity habits, many young people today are not getting an opportunity to be physically active, which will likely have a significant impact on their physical activity levels and potential for obesity as adults.

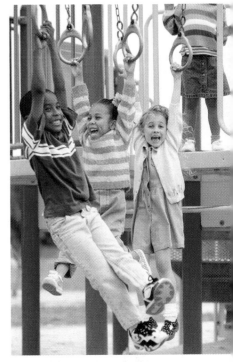

Adequate physical activity is instrumental in preventing childhood obesity.

How Is Obesity Treated?

The first line of defense in treating obesity is a low-calorie diet and regular physical activity. Overweight and obese individuals should work with their health care practitioner to design and maintain a low-fat diet (less than 30% of total energy from fat) that has a deficit of 500 to 1,000 kcal/day (National Institutes of Health 1998). Physical activity should be increased gradually so that the person can build a program in which they are exercising at least 30 minutes per day, five times per week.

As discussed earlier in this chapter, prescription medications are used to treat some cases of obesity. Again, these medications should only be used while under a physician's supervision, and they appear to be most effective when combined with energy restriction and regular physical activity.

For people who are morbidly obese, surgery may be recommended. Generally, surgery is advised in people with a BMI greater than or equal to 35 kg/m^2 who have not been able to lose weight with energy restriction and exercise. The three most common types of weight loss surgery performed are gastroplasty, gastric bypass, and gastric banding (Figure 11.11).

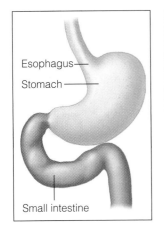

Esophagus
Stomach

Small intestine

(a) Normal anatomy

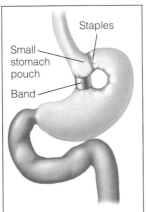

Small stomach pouch

Band

Staples

(b) Vertical banded gastroplasty

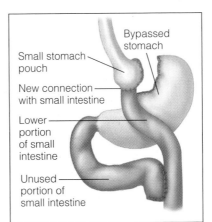

Small stomach pouch

New connection with small intestine

Lower portion of small intestine

Unused portion of small intestine

Bypassed stomach

(c) Gastric bypass

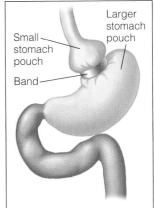

Small stomach pouch

Band

Larger stomach pouch

(d) Gastric banding

Figure 11.11   Various forms of surgery alter the normal anatomy of the gastrointestinal tract **(a)** to result in weight loss. Vertical banded gastroplasty **(b)**, gastric bypass **(c)**, and gastric banding **(d)** are three surgical procedures used to reduce morbid obesity.

- *Gastroplasty* involves partitioning or "stapling" a small section of the stomach to reduce total food intake.
- *Gastric bypass surgery* involves attaching the lower part of the small intestine to the stomach, so that most of the food bypasses the stomach and small intestine. This results in significantly less absorption of food in the intestine.
- *Gastric banding* is a relatively new procedure is which stomach size is reduced using a constricting band, thus restricting food intake.

The risks of surgery in people with obesity are extremely high and include increased infections, higher formation of blood clots, and more adverse reactions to anesthesia.

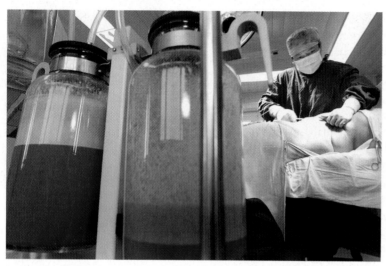

Liposuction removes fat cells from specific areas of the body.

After the surgery, these people may face a lifetime of problems with chronic diarrhea, vomiting, intolerance to dairy products and other foods, dehydration, and nutritional deficiencies resulting from alterations in nutrient digestion and absorption. Thus, the potential benefits of the procedure must outweigh the risks. It is critical that each surgery candidate is carefully screened by a trained medical professional. If the immediate threat of serious disease and death is more dangerous than the risks associated with surgery, then the procedure is justified.

Are these surgical procedures successful in reducing obesity? About one-third to one-half of people who received obesity surgery lose significant amounts of weight and keep this weight off for at least five years. The reasons that one-half to two-thirds do not experience long-term success include that some are unable to eat less over time, even with a smaller stomach. For others, staples and gastric bands loosen and stomach pouches enlarge. Some individuals do not survive the surgery. Although these surgical procedures may seem extremely risky, those who lose weight, keep it off, and improve their health feel that the eventual benefits are worth the risks.

Liposuction is a cosmetic surgical procedure that removes fat cells from localized areas in the body. It is not recommended or typically used to treat obesity or morbid obesity. This procedure is not without risks; blood clots, skin and nerve damage, adverse drug reactions, and perforation injuries can and do occur as a result of liposuction. It can also result in deformations in the area where the fat is removed. This procedure is not the solution to long-term weight loss, as the millions of fat cells that remain in the body after liposuction enlarge if the person continues to overeat.

Recap: Obesity is caused by many factors. Genetic theories about obesity include the thrifty gene theory, set-point theory, and leptin theory. In addition, childhood obesity is strongly associated with adult obesity. Treatments for overweight, obesity, and morbid obesity include low-calorie, low-fat diets in combination with regular physical activity, weight loss prescription medications, and/or weight loss surgery.

Chapter Summary

- Definitions of a healthful body weight include one that is appropriate for someone's age and level of development, that can be achieved and sustained without constant dieting, and that promotes good eating habits and allows for regular physical activity.
- Underweight is defined as having too little body fat to maintain health, causing a person to have a weight for a given height that is below an acceptably defined standard.

- Overweight is defined as having a moderate amount of excess body fat, resulting in a person having a weight for a given height that is greater than some accepted standard but is not considered obese.

- Obesity is defined as having excess body fat that adversely affects health, resulting in a person having a weight for a given height that is substantially greater than some accepted standard. Morbid obesity occurs when a person's body weight exceeds 100% of normal, which puts him or her at very high risk for serious health consequences.

- Body mass index (BMI) is an index of weight/height^2. It is useful to indicate health risks associated with overweight and obesity in groups of people.

- Body composition assessment involves estimating the proportions of a person's body fat (or adipose tissue) and lean body mass. Methods include underwater weighing, skinfold measures, bioelectrical impedance analysis, near infrared reactance, and the Bod Pod.

- The waist-to-hip ratio and waist circumference are used to determine patterns of fat storage. People with large waists (as compared to hips) have an apple-shaped fat pattern. People with large hips (as compared to the waist) have a pear-shaped fat pattern. Having an apple-shaped pattern increases your risk for heart disease, type 2 diabetes, and other chronic diseases.

- We lose or gain weight based on changes in our energy intake, the food we eat, and our energy expenditure (both at rest and when physically active).

- Basal metabolic rate (BMR) is the energy needed to maintain our body's resting functions. BMR accounts for 60 to 70% of our total daily energy needs.

- The thermic effect of food is the energy we expend to process the food we eat. It accounts for 5 to 10% of the energy content of a meal and is higher for processing proteins and carbohydrates than for fats.

- The energy cost of physical activity represents energy that we expend for physical movement or work we do above basal levels. It accounts for 20 to 35% of our total daily energy output.

- Our genetic heritage influences our risk for obesity, and factors such as possessing a thrifty gene (or genes), maintaining a weight set point, and genetic alterations in the hormone leptin may affect a person's risk for obesity.

- Being overweight or obese as a child can lead to adult obesity, and childhood obesity is linked with the risk for heart disease and premature death later in adulthood.

- Behavioral factors contributing to obesity include eating a high-fat diet and alterations in the cues for hunger, appetite, and satiety. Social factors that may contribute to obesity include pressure to eat from family and peers, easy access to inexpensive and high-fat foods, watching too much television, and not taking time to exercise. Mood and emotional state also affect appetite.

- A sound weight change plan involves a modest change in energy intake, incorporating physical activity into each day, and practicing changes in behavior that can assist in meeting realistic weight change goals.

- Prescription drugs can be used to assist with weight loss when the risks of obesity override the risks associated with the medications.

- Various dietary supplements are marketed as weight loss products. Many of these products cause dangerous changes in heart rate and blood pressure. Unlike prescription drugs, these products are not strictly regulated by the Food and Drug Administration.

- Most of the products marketed for weight gain have been shown to be ineffective. The risks associated with these products are not well documented; many of these may have no effect on a person's weight and are simply a waste of money. Healthful weight gain involves consuming more calories than expended by selecting ample servings of nutritious, high-energy foods and exercising regularly by including resistance training and aerobic exercise.

- Being underweight can be dangerous to one's health, and wasting (or starvation) among children is still a health crisis in many developing countries.

- Overweight is not as detrimental to health as obesity, but it is associated with an increased risk for high blood pressure, heart disease, type 2 diabetes, sleep disorders, osteoarthritis, gallstones, and gynecological abnormalities.

- Obesity and morbid obesity are associated with significantly increased risks for many diseases and for premature death. Obesity can be treated with low-calorie diets and regular physical activity, prescription medications, and surgery when necessary.

Review Questions

1. The ratio of a person's body weight to height is represented as his or her
   a. body composition.
   b. basal metabolic rate.
   c. bioelectrical impedance.
   d. body mass index.

2. The body's total daily energy expenditure includes
   a. basal metabolic rate, thermal effect of food, and effect of physical activity.
   b. basal metabolic rate, movement, standing, and sleeping.
   c. effect of physical activity, standing, and sleeping.
   d. body mass index, thermal effect of food, and effect of physical activity.

3. All people gain weight when they
   a. eat a high-fat diet (>30% fat).
   b. take in more energy than they expend.
   c. fail to exercise.
   d. take in less energy than they expend.

4. The set-point theory proposes that
   a. obese people have a gene not found in slender people that regulates their weight so that it always hovers near a given set-point.
   b. obese people have a gene that causes them to be energetically thrifty.
   c. all people have a genetic set-point for their body weight.
   d. all people have a hormone that regulates their weight so that it always hovers near a given set-point.

5. Our innate, physiologic drive to eat is called
   a. hunger.
   b. appetite.
   c. satiety.
   d. our basal metabolic rate.

6. **True or false?** Pear-shaped fat patterning is known to increase a person's risk for many chronic diseases, including diabetes and heart disease.

7. **True or false?** One pound of fat is equal to about 3,500 kcalories.

8. **True or false?** Weight-loss medications are typically prescribed for people who have a body mass index greater than or equal to 18.5 kg/m^2.

9. **True or false?** Recommendations for weight gain include avoiding both aerobic and resistance exercise for the duration of the weight-gain program.

10. **True or false?** More than half of the people in the United States are currently either overweight or obese.

11. Identify at least four characteristics of a healthful weight.

12. Describe a sound weight-loss program, including recommendations for diet, physical activity, and behavioral modifications.

13. Can you increase your basal metabolic rate? Is it wise to try? Defend your answer.

14. Identify at least four societal factors that may have influenced the rise in obesity rates in the United States since 1963. Think especially of the effect of advances in technology that have occurred in the last forty years.

15. Your friend Misty joins you for lunch and confesses that she is discouraged about her weight. She says that she has been trying "really hard" for three months to lose weight, but that no matter what she does, she cannot drop below 148 pounds. Based on her height, you know Misty is not overweight, and she exercises regularly. What questions would you suggest she think about? How would you advise her?

Test Yourself Answers

1. **True.** Being underweight increases our risk for illness and premature death and in many cases can be just as unhealthful as being obese.

2. **False.** Obesity is a multifactorial disease with many contributing factors. Although eating too much food and not getting enough exercise can lead to being overweight and obese, the disease of obesity is complex and is not simply caused by overeating.

3. **False.** Body composition assessments can help give us a general idea of our body fat levels, but most methods are not extremely accurate.

4. **True.** Staying physically active helps us maintain our muscle mass, which in turn assists us in preventing a dramatic drop in our basal metabolic rate. These changes can help reduce our risk for becoming obese as we get older.

5. **False.** Health can be defined in many ways. An individual who is overweight, but who exercises regularly and has no additional risk factors for various diseases such as heart disease and type 2 diabetes, is considered a healthy person.

Web Links

www.nhlbisupport.com/bmi
National Heart, Lung, and Blood Institute BMI calculator
Calculate your body mass index (BMI) on the Internet.

www.ftc.gov
Federal Trade Commission
Click on For Consumers and then Diet Health and Fitness to find how to avoid false weight loss claims.

www.consumer.gov/weightloss
Partnership for Healthy Weight Management
Visit this site to learn about successful strategies for achieving and maintaining a healthy weight.

www.eatright.org
American Dietetic Association
Go to this site to learn more about fad diets.

www.niddk.nih.gov/health/nutrit/nutrit.htm
National Institute of Diabetes and Digestive and Kidney Diseases
Find out more about healthy weight loss.

www.sne.org
Society for Nutrition Education
Click on Resources and Relationships and then Weight Realities Division for additional resources related to positive attitudes about body image and healthful alternatives to dieting.

References

American Dietetic Association. 2001. Send fad diets down the drain. www.eatright.org. (Accessed February 2004.)

Arnst, C. 2004. Let them eat cake—if they want to. *Business Week.* February 23, 110–111.

Bouchard, C., A. Tremblay, J. P. Després, A. Nadeau, P. J. Lupien, G. Thériault, J. Dussault, S. Moorjani, S. Pinault, and G. Fournier. 1990. The response to long-term overfeeding in identical twins. *N. Engl. J. Med.* 322: 1477–1482.

Broeder, C. E., J. Quindry, K. Brittingham, L. Panton, J. Thomson, S. Appakondu, K. Breuel, R. Byrd, J. Douglas, C. Earnest, C. Mitchell, M. Olson, T. Roy, and C. Yarlagadda. 2000. The Andro Project: physiological and hormonal influences of androstenedione supplementation in men 35 to 65-years-old participating in a high-intensiy resistance training program. *Arch. Int. Med.* 160: 3093–3104.

Brown, G. A., M. D. Vukovich, T. A. Reifenrath, N. L. Uhl, K. A. Parsons, R. L. Sharp, and D. S. King. 2000. Effects of anabolic precursors on serum testosterone concentrations and adaptations to resistance training in young men. *Intl. J. Sport Nutr. Ex. Metab.* 10: 340–359.

Centers for Disease Control and Prevention (CDC). 2004. National Center for Health Statistics. Prevalence of overweight and obesity among adults: United States, 1999–2000. www.cdc.gov/nchs/products/pubs/pubd/hestats/obese/obse99.htm. (Accessed May 2004.)

de Onis M., and M. Blössner. 2000. Prevalence and trends of overweight among preschool children in developing countries. *Am. J. Clin. Nutr.* 72: 1032–1039.

Dietz, W. H. 1994. Critical periods in childhood for the development of obesity. *Am. J. Clin. Nutr.* 59: 955–959.

Emme. 2004. Bio profile. http://www.safesearching.com/officialemme/allaboutemme/bio.shtml (Accessed February 2004.)

Gaesser, G. A. 1999. Thinness and weight loss: beneficial or detrimental to longevity? *Med. Sci. Sports Exerc.* 31: 1118–1128.

Gunnell, D. J., S. J. Frankel, K. Nanchahal, T. J. Peters, and G. Davey Smith. 1998. Childhood obesity and adult cardiovascular mortality: a 57-y follow-up study based on the Boyd Orr cohort. *Am. J. Clin. Nutr.* 67: 1111–1118.

Hellerstein, M., K. Christiansen, and S. Kaempfer. 1991. Measurement of de novo hepatic lipogenesis in humans using stable isotopes. *J. Clin. Invest.* 87: 1841–1852.

Heyward, V. H., and L. M. Stolarczyk. 1996. *Applied Body Composition Assessment.* Champaign, IL: Human Kinetics.

Hill, J. O., J. Hauptman, J. W. Anderson, K. Fujioka, P. M. O'Neil, D. K. Smith, J. H. Zavoral, and L. J. Aronne. 1999. Orlistat, a lipase inhibitor, for weight maintenance after conventional dieting: a 1-y study. *Am. J. Clin. Nutr.* 69: 1108–1116.

Himes, J. H. 2001. Prevalence of individuals with skinfolds too large to measure. *Am. J. Public Health* 91: 154–155.

Joyner, M. J. 2000. Over-the-counter supplements and strength training. *Exerc. Sport Sci. Rev.* 28:2–3.

Klem, M. L., R. R. Wing, M. T. McGuire, H. M. Seagle, and J. O. Hill. 1997. A descriptive study of individuals successful at long-term maintenance of substantial weight loss. *Am. J. Clin. Nutr.* 66: 239–246.

Koh-Banerjee, P., N. F. Chu, D. Spiegelman, B. Rosner, G. Colditz, W. Willett, and E. Rimm. 2003. Prospective study of the association of changes in dietary intake, physical activity, alcohol consumption, and smoking with 9-y gain in waist circumference among 16,587 U.S. men. *Am. J. Clin. Nutr.* 78: 719–27.

Kreider, R. B., V. Miriel, and E. Bertun. 1993. Amino acid supplementation and exercise performance. *Sports Med.* 16: 190–209.

Manore, M. M., and J. Thompson. 2000. *Sport Nutrition for Health and Performance.* Champaign, IL: Human Kinetics.

National Institutes of Health. National Heart, Lung, and Blood Institute. 1998. Clinical Guidelines on the Identification, Evaluation, and Treatment of Overweight and Obesity in Adults. Executive Summary. www.nhlbi.nih.gov/guidelines/obesity/ob_exsum.pdf (Accessed February 2004.)

Panotopoulos, G., J. C. Ruiz, B. G. Grand, A. Basdevant. 2001. Dual x-ray absorptiometry, bioelectrical impedance, and near infrared interactance in obese women. *Med. Sci. Sports Exerc.* 33: 665–670.

PBS. 2004. Beyond the scale. *Healthweek.* http://www.pbs.org/healthweek/featurep3_428.htm (Accessed February 2004.)

Stunkard, A. J., T. I. A. Sørensen, C. Hanis, T. W. Teasdale, R. Chakraborty, W. J. Schull, and F. Schulsinger. 1986. An adoption study of human obesity. *N. Engl. J. Med.* 314: 193–198.

Wagner, D. R., V. H. Heyward, and A. L. Gibson. 2000. Validation of air displacement plethysmography for assessing body composition. *Med. Sci. Sports Exerc.* 32: 1339–1344.

Zernike, K. 2004. U.S. body survey, head to toe, finds signs of expansion. *the New York Times.* March 1, 1, 12.

Nutrition Debate:

The Criminalization of Fat: Have We Gone Too Far?

Although prejudice of all kinds still exists, our society espouses values of tolerance and compassion toward all people, despite their disease state, religious beliefs, sexual orientation, or racial and ethnic background. However, there seems to be one group of people against whom prejudice is still acceptable, and that is obese people. They remain the punch line of many jokes, are socially ostracized, and experience widespread harassment and embarrassment at work and in most avenues of life. The recent efforts of airlines to deny flights to individuals who are too large to fit in standard airline seats are only one example of how our society deals with obesity. Although this effort by the airlines may appear to make perfect sense to many people, it is perceived by others as demeaning, punitive, and overtly prejudicial.

Most people do not understand that obesity is a disease, just as heart disease and diabetes are diseases. Contrary to this fact, society generally views obesity as a condition that results from being lazy and having no willpower. As you have learned in this chapter, obesity is a complex, multifactorial disease that is not caused solely by overeating or doing too little exercise. As we continue to struggle with how best to prevent and treat obesity, our society must take measures to reduce the social stigma of living with this disease. Such measures might include using more overweight men and women in print and television advertisements and increasing public awareness of regulations prohibiting job and housing discrimination based on weight.

Recently, some compelling arguments have been put forth that we should stop our obsession with weight. Although more than $30 billion is spent every year on weight loss efforts, the average weight loss is only about 10% of body weight. Even more discouraging is that most of the weight lost is regained within five years. As most diets are not effective over the long term, many nutrition and exercise professionals are proposing that we encourage a healthful lifestyle defined by eating a balanced diet and staying physically active on a regular basis and stop defining a person's health by his or her body weight.

Dr. Glen Gaesser (1999) and others have challenged long-held assumptions that increased body weight is associated with increased mortality. According to these researchers, there is no clear-cut evidence to define the "best" body weight to increase our life span. In contrast, evidence does support the contention that

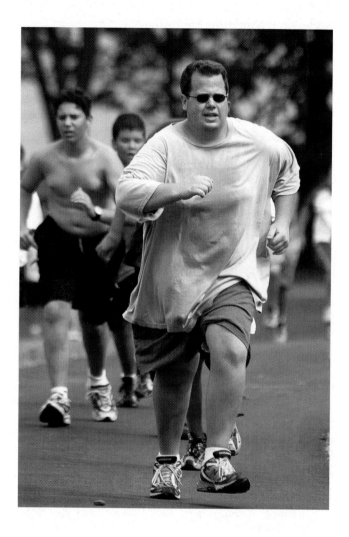

regular physical activity leads to significant improvements in health without weight loss. For instance, increasing aerobic fitness helps reduce mortality rates, whether or not the person performing the aerobic activity also loses weight. Thus, experts question whether it makes sense to spend limited healthcare resources encouraging individuals who are moderately overweight, particularly those with no significant disease risk factors, to meet a predefined "ideal" weight.

This topic will most likely remain controversial for many years. However, some professional organizations are beginning to embrace a new way of thinking about the definition of ideal body weight and the negative effects of dieting. For instance, "About Face" is a media literacy organization focused on the impact that mass media has on the mental, emotional, and physical well-being of girls. "Bullying" is a Web site written by students on the topic of bullying and weight prejudice among youth. The U.S. Department of Health and Human Services sponsors a Web site called "Girl Power!", which is a national education campaign aimed to encourage and motivate 9- to 14-year-old girls to make most of their lives using targeted health messages. The Society for Nutrition Education has formed a division called "Nutrition and Weight Realities" to assist dietitians, nutrition educators, and the general public about coping with unrealistic body image expectations and an unhealthy pursuit of thinness. Refer to the Web site at http://www.sne.org/weightrealitiesdivision.htm

to gain access to these Web links and other resources related to positive attitudes about body image and healthful alternatives to dieting.

Earlier, we identified a few measures for reducing the social stigma of obesity. What other measures can you think of? How can we deal with practical concerns such as small airline seats, movie theater seats, and narrow department store aisles? Can you think of ways we can be more compassionate toward obese family members, friends, and acquaintances, and support them in their quest for health? As the obesity epidemic continues to grow, our need to answer these questions becomes more critical.

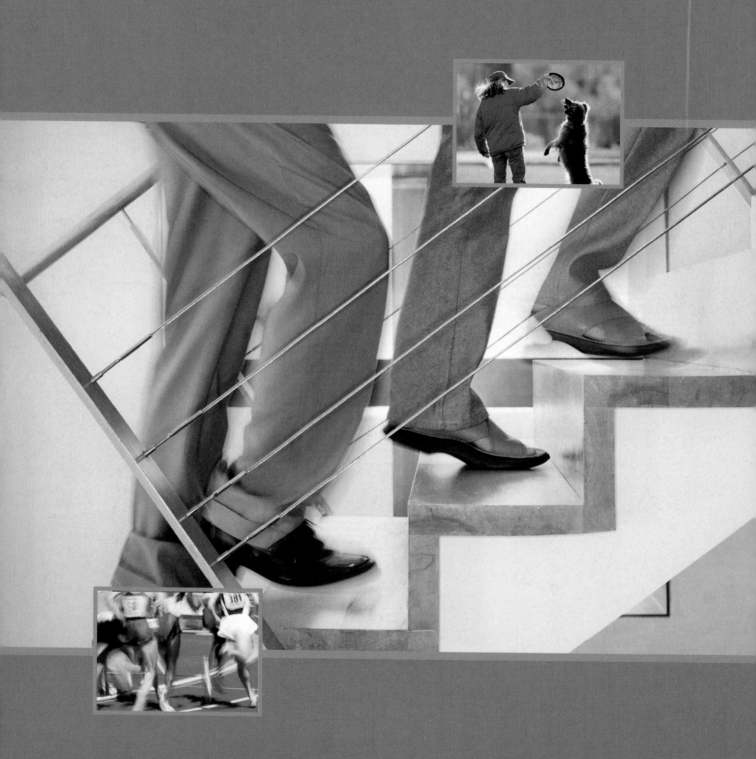

Chapter 12

Nutrition and Physical Activity: Keys to Good Health

Chapter Objectives

After reading this chapter you will be able to:

1. Compare and contrast the concepts of physical activity, leisure-time physical activity, exercise, and physical fitness, pp. 420–421.

2. List at least four health benefits of being physically active on a regular basis, pp. 421–423.

3. Define the four components of fitness, pp. 420–421.

4. Describe the FIT principle and calculate your maximal and training heart rate range, pp. 425–429.

5. List and describe at least three processes we use to break down fuels to support physical activity, pp. 430–436.

6. Discuss at least three changes in nutrient needs that can occur in response to an increase in physical activity or vigorous exercise training, pp. 436–448.

7. Define the heat illnesses, including heat syncope, heat cramps, heat exhaustion, and heatstroke, pp. 445–446.

8. Define the term *ergogenic aids* and discuss the potential benefits and risks of at least four ergogenic aids that are currently on the market, pp. 449–453.

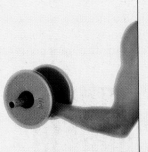
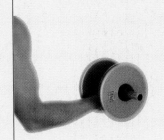

Test Yourself True or False

1. *Physical activity* and *exercise* mean basically the same thing and are terms that can be used interchangeably. T or F

2. Despite the multitude of health benefits of participating in regular physical activity, almost half of all Americans report being inactive. T or F

3. To achieve fitness, a person needs to exercise at least one hour each day. T or F

4. Lactic acid is not a major contributor to muscle soreness. T or F

5. Most ergogenic aids are not effective, and many can be dangerous or cause serious health consequences. T or F

Test Yourself answers can be found at the end of the chapter.

In June, 2003, Harold Hoffman of North Carolina won several gold medals in track and field at the National Senior Olympics. He clocked 38.36 seconds in the 100-meter dash to beat the listed American record of 38.66. He also won the 200-meter dash (in 1:37.46), the 5K (in 38.3 minutes), and the long jump. If Hoffman's performance times don't amaze you, perhaps they will when you consider his age: at the time he gave these winning performances, he was 95 years old!

There's no doubt about it: regular physical activity dramatically improves our strength, stamina, health, and longevity. But what qualifies as "regular physical activity"? In other words, how much do we need to do to reap the benefits? And if we do become more active, does our diet have to change, too?

Healthy eating practices and regular physical activity are like two sides of the same coin, interacting in a variety of ways to improve our strength and stamina and to increase our resistance to many chronic diseases and acute illnesses. In fact, the nutrition and physical activity recommendations for reducing your risk of heart disease also reduce your risk of high blood pressure, type 2 diabetes, obesity, and some forms of cancer! In this chapter, we define physical activity, identify its many benefits, and discuss the nutrients needed to maintain an active life.

Physical Activity, Exercise, and Physical Fitness: What's the Difference?

Do the terms *physical activity, exercise,* and *physical fitness* mean the same thing? They are used interchangeably in many situations, but they actually represent quite different concepts. **Physical activity** describes any movement produced by muscles that increases energy expenditure. Different categories of physical activity include occupational, household, leisure-time, and transportation (U.S. Department of Health and Human Services 1996). **Leisure-time physical activity** is any activity not related to a person's occupation and includes competitive sports, planned exercise training, and recreational activities such as hiking, walking, and bicycling. **Exercise** is therefore considered a subcategory of leisure-time physical activity and refers to activity that is purposeful, planned, and structured (Caspersen, Powell, and Christensen 1985).

Physical fitness is a state of being that arises largely from the interaction between nutrition and physical activity. It is defined as the ability to carry out daily tasks with vigor and alertness, without undue fatigue, and with ample energy to enjoy leisure-time pursuits and meet unforeseen emergencies (U.S. Department of Health and Human Services 1996). Physical fitness has many components

physical activity Any movement produced by muscles that increases energy expenditure; includes occupational, household, leisure-time, and transportation activities.

leisure-time physical activity Any activity not related to a person's occupation; includes competitive sports, recreational activities, and planned exercise training.

exercise A subcategory of leisure-time physical activity; any activity that is purposeful, planned, and structured.

physical fitness The ability to carry out daily tasks with vigor and alertness, without undue fatigue, and with ample energy to enjoy leisure-time pursuits and meet unforeseen emergencies.

Hiking is a leisure-time physical activity that can contribute to your physical fitness.

Table 12.1 The Components of Fitness

Fitness Component	Examples of Activities One Can Do to Achieve Fitness in Each Component
Cardiorespiratory	Aerobic-type activities such as walking, running, swimming, cross-country skiing
Musculoskeletal fitness:	Resistance training, weightlifting, calisthenics, sit-ups, push-ups
Muscular strength	Weightlifting or related activities using heavier weights with few repetitions
Muscular endurance	Weightlifting or related activities using lighter weights with greater number of repetitions
Flexibility	Stretching exercises, yoga
Body composition	Aerobic exercise and resistance training can help optimize body composition

(Table 12.1) (Heyward 1998). These include **cardiorespiratory fitness**, which is defined as the ability of the heart, lungs, and circulatory system to efficiently supply oxygen and nutrients to working muscles. **Musculoskeletal fitness** involves fitness of both the muscles and bones and includes *muscular strength* and *muscular endurance*. **Muscular strength** is the maximal force or tension level that can be produced by a muscle group, and **muscular endurance** is the ability of a muscle to maintain submaximal force levels for extended periods of time. **Flexibility** is the ability to move a joint fluidly through the complete range of motion, and **body composition** is the amount of bone, muscle, and fat tissue in the body. Although many people are interested in improving their physical fitness, some are more interested in maintaining general fitness, while others are interested in achieving higher levels of fitness to optimize their athletic performance.

> **Recap:** Physical activity is any movement produced by muscles that increases energy expenditure. Leisure-time physical activity is any activity not related to a person's occupation. Exercise is a subcategory of leisure-time physical activity and is purposeful, planned, and structured. Physical fitness is the ability to carry out daily tasks with vigor and alertness, without undue fatigue, and with ample energy to enjoy leisure-time pursuits and meet unforeseen emergencies. The components of physical fitness include cardiorespiratory fitness, musculoskeletal fitness, flexibility, and body composition.

cardiorespiratory fitness Fitness of the heart and lungs; achieved through regular participation in aerobic-type activities.

musculoskeletal fitness Fitness of the muscles and bones.

muscular strength A subcomponent of musculoskeletal fitness defined as the maximal force or tension level that can be produced by a muscle group.

muscular endurance A subcomponent of musculoskeletal fitness defined as the ability of a muscle to maintain submaximal force levels for extended periods of time.

flexibility The ability to move a joint through its full range of motion.

body composition The amount of bone, muscle, and fat tissue in the body.

Why Engage in Physical Activity?

A lot of people are looking for a "magic pill" that will help them maintain weight loss, reduce their risk of diseases, make them feel better, and improve their quality of sleep. Although many people are not aware of it, regular physical activity is this magic pill. Some of the many benefits of regular physical activity include:

- *Reduces our risks for, and complications of, heart disease, stroke, and high blood pressure:* Regular physical activity increases high-density lipoprotein cholesterol (HDL, the "good" cholesterol) and lowers triglycerides in the blood; improves the strength of the heart; helps maintain healthy blood pressure; and limits the progression of atherosclerosis (or hardening of the arteries).

- *Reduces our risk for obesity:* Regular physical activity maintains lean body mass and promotes more healthful levels of body fat; may help in appetite control; increases energy expenditure and the use of fat as an energy source.

- *Reduces our risk for type 2 diabetes:* Regular physical activity enhances the action of insulin, which improves the cells' uptake of glucose from the blood; can improve blood glucose control in people with diabetes, which in turn reduces the risk for, or delays the onset of, diabetes-related complications.

- *Potential reduction in our risk for colon cancer:* Although the exact role that physical activity may play in reducing colon cancer risk is still unknown, we do know that regular physical activity enhances gastric motility, which reduces transit time of potential cancer-causing agents through the gut.

- *Reduces our risk for osteoporosis:* Regular physical activity strengthens bones and enhances muscular strength and flexibility, thereby reducing the likelihood of falls and the incidence of fractures and other injuries when falls occur.

Regular physical activity is also known to improve our sleep patterns, reduce our risk for upper respiratory infections by improving immune function, and reduce anxiety and mental stress. It also can be effective in treating mild and moderate depression. In women receiving chemotherapy treatment for breast cancer, regular physical activity may reduce fatigue (Schwartz et al. 2001). During pregnancy, regular physical activity helps maintain the mother's fitness and muscle tone and helps control weight gain. It is also associated with lower fetal distress during labor, shorter labor, lower risk of cesarean birth, and improved recovery for the mother after the birth (Olds et al. 2003).

Despite the plethora of benefits derived from regular physical activity, most people find that this magic pill is not easy to swallow. In fact, most people in the United States are physically inactive. The Centers for Disease Control and Prevention (2003) report that over half of all U.S. adults do not do enough physical activity to meet national health recommendations, and 26% of adults in the United States admit to doing no leisure-time physical activity at all (Figure 12.1). These statistics mirror the reported increases in obesity, heart disease, and type 2 diabetes in industrialized countries.

This trend toward inadequate physical activity levels is also occurring in young people. Only 17% of middle and junior high schools and only 2% of senior high schools require daily physical activity for all students (U.S. Department of Health and Human Services 2000). Low rates of voluntary participation in physical education (PE) compound this problem, as less than 30% of high school students participate in daily PE. Since our habits related to eating and physical activity are formed early in

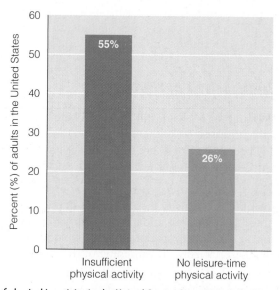

Figure 12.1   Rates of physical inactivity in the United States. Over 50% of the U.S. population do not do enough physical activity to meet national health recommendations, and about 26% report doing no leisure-time physical activity. (Centers for Disease Control and Prevention (CDC), Prevalence of physical activity, including lifestyle activities among adults—United States, 2000–2001, *Morbidity and Mortality Weekly* 52(32)[2003]: 764–769.)

life, it is imperative that we provide opportunities for children and adolescents to engage in regular, enjoyable physical activity. An active lifestyle during childhood increases the likelihood of a healthier life as an adult.

Recap: Physical activity provides a multitude of health benefits, including reducing our risks for obesity and many chronic diseases and relieving anxiety and stress. Despite the many health benefits of physical activity, most people in the United States, including many children, are inactive.

What Is a Sound Fitness Program?

There are several widely-recognized qualities of a sound fitness program, as well as guidelines to help you design one that is right for you. These are explored here.

A Sound Fitness Program Meets Your Personal Goals

A fitness program may be ideal for someone else, but that doesn't necessarily mean it is right for you. Before you design or evaluate any program, you need to know what you intend to get from it; in other words, you need to define your personal fitness goals. Do you want to prevent osteoporosis, diabetes, or another chronic disease that runs in your family? Do you simply want to increase your energy and stamina? Or do you intend to compete in athletic events? Each of these scenarios would require a very different fitness program.

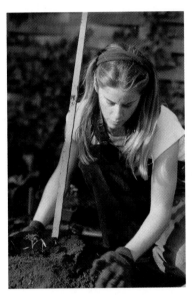

Moderate physical activity, such as gardening, helps maintain overall health.

For example, if you want to train for athletic competition, a traditional approach that includes planned, purposive exercise sessions under the guidance of a trainer or coach would probably be most beneficial. Similarly, if you want to achieve cardiorespiratory fitness, you would likely be advised to participate in an aerobics class at least three times per week, or jog for at least 20 minutes three times per week.

In contrast, if your goal were to maintain your overall health, you might do better to follow the 1996 report of the Surgeon General on achieving health through regular physical activity (U.S. Department of Health and Human Services 1996). This report emphasizes that significant health benefits, including reducing your risk for chronic diseases (such as heart disease, osteoporosis, and type 2 diabetes), can be achieved by participating in a moderate amount of physical activity (such as 30 minutes of gardening, 15 minutes of jogging, or 45 minutes of basketball) on most, if not all, days of the week. These health benefits occur even when the time spent performing the physical activities is cumulative (for example, brisk walking for 10 minutes three times per day). While these guidelines are appropriate for achieving health benefits, they are not necessarily of sufficient intensity and duration to improve physical fitness.

Recently, the Institute of Medicine published guidelines that state that the minimum amount of physical activity that should be done each day to maintain health and fitness is 60 minutes, not 30 minutes as published in the Surgeon General's report (Institute of Medicine 2002; U.S. Department of Health and Human Services 1996). This discrepancy in fitness guidelines has caused some confusion among consumers. Refer to the Nutrition Debate at the end of this chapter to learn more about this controversy.

A Sound Fitness Program Is Fun

One of the most important goals for everyone is fun; unless you enjoy being active, you will find it very difficult to maintain your physical fitness. What activities do you consider fun? If you enjoy the outdoors, hiking, camping, fishing, and rock climbing are potential activities for you. If you would rather exercise with friends on your lunch break, walking, climbing stairs, and bicycle riding may be more appropriate. Or you may find it more enjoyable to stay indoors and use the programs and equipment at your local fitness club. . . or purchase your own treadmill and free weights.

A Sound Fitness Program Includes Variety and Consistency

Variety is critical to maintaining your fitness. While some people enjoy doing similar activities day after day, most of us get bored with the same fitness routine. Incorporating a variety of activities into your fitness program will help maintain your interest and increase your enjoyment while you are active. Variety can be achieved by: combining indoor and outdoor activities throughout the week; taking a different route when you walk each day; watching a movie or reading a book while you ride a stationary bicycle or walk on a treadmill; or participating in different activities each week such as walking, bicycling, swimming, taking the stairs, hiking, and gardening. This smorgasbord of activities can increase your activity level without leading to monotony and boredom.

Fortunately, a fun and useful tool has been developed to help you increase the variety of your physical activity choices (Figure 12.2). Like the Food Guide Pyramid, the **Physical Activity Pyramid** makes recommendations for the type and amount of activity that should be done weekly to increase your physical activity level. The bottom of the pyramid describes activities that should be done every day, including walking more, taking the stairs instead of the elevator, and working in your garden. Aerobic types of exercises (such as bicycling and brisk walking) and recreational activities (such as soccer, tennis, and basketball) should be done three to five times each week, for at least 20 or 30 minutes. Flexibility, strength, and

Physical Activity Pyramid   A pyramid similar to the Food Guide Pyramid that makes recommendations for the type and amount of activity that should be done weekly to increase physical activity levels.

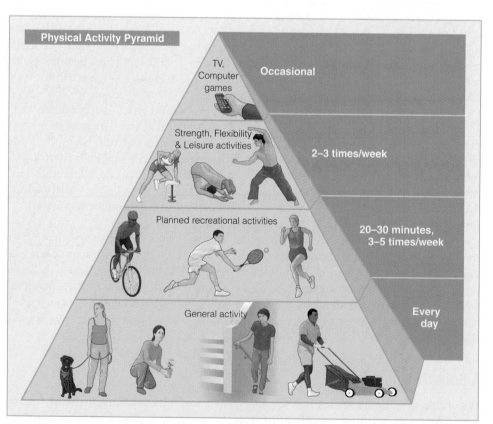

Figure 12.2   You can use this Physical Activity Pyramid as a guide to increase your level of physical activity. (From Corbin, C. B. and R. D. Pangrazi. Physical Activity Pyramid rebuffs peak experience. *ACSM's Health and Fitness Journal* 2(1) 1998. Copyright © 1998. Used with permission.)

leisure activities should be done two to three times each week. The top of the pyramid emphasizes things we should do less of, including watching TV, playing computer games, or sitting for more than 30 minutes at one time.

It is important to understand you cannot do just one activity to achieve overall fitness. Refer back to Table 12.1, and notice that different activities are listed as examples to achieve the various components of fitness. There is simply not one activity that we can do to achieve overall fitness because physical fitness is specific to each component. For instance, participating in aerobic-type activities will improve our cardiorespiratory fitness but will do little to improve muscular strength. To achieve that goal, we must participate in some form of **resistance training,** or exercises in which our muscles work against resistance. Flexibility is achieved by participating in stretching activities. By following the recommendations put forth in the Physical Activity Pyramid, physical fitness can be achieved in all components.

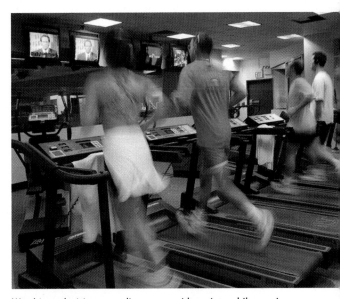

Watching television or reading can provide variety while running on a treadmill.

> **Recap:** A sound fitness program has many components. First, it must meet your personal fitness goals, such as reducing your risks for disease or preparing for competition in athletic events. Second, a fitness program should be fun and include activities you enjoy. Third, it should include variety and consistency to help you maintain interest and reap the benefits of regular physical activity. Physical fitness is specific to each of the components of fitness.

resistance training   Exercises in which our muscles act against resistance.

A Sound Fitness Program Appropriately Overloads the Body

In order to improve your fitness level, you must place an extra physical demand on your body. This is referred to as the **overload principle.** A word of caution is in order here: *the overload principle does not advocate subjecting your body to inappropriately high stress* because this can lead to exhaustion and injuries. In contrast, an appropriate overload on various body systems will result in healthy improvements in fitness.

To achieve an appropriate overload, you should consider three factors, collectively known as the **FIT principle:** frequency, intensity, and time of activity. You can use the FIT principle to design either a general physical fitness program or a performance-based exercise program. Table 12.2 shows how the FIT principle can be applied to a cardiorespiratory and muscular fitness program.

Let's consider each of the FIT principle's three factors in more detail.

overload principle   Placing an extra physical demand on your body in order to improve your fitness level.

FIT principle   The principle used to achieve an appropriate overload for physical training. Stands for frequency, intensity, and time of activity.

Frequency

Frequency refers to the number of activity sessions per week. Depending upon your goals for fitness, the frequency of your activities will vary. To achieve cardiorespiratory fitness, training should be more than two days per week. On the other hand, training more than five days per week does not cause significant gains in fitness but can substantially increase your risk for injury. Training three to five days per week appears optimal to achieve and maintain cardiorespiratory fitness. In contrast, only two to three days are needed to achieve muscular fitness.

Think about Theo's goals for fitness during the off-season and the frequency needed to achieve these goals. He is interested in maintaining his general physical fitness so he can continue to play basketball, and he also wants to significantly improve muscular strength and size. Using the Physical Activity Pyramid as a guide, Theo should do the activities as suggested for every day and those prescribed three to five times a week. To further improve muscular strength and size,

frequency   Refers to the number of activity sessions per week you perform.

Table 12.2   Using the FIT Principle to Achieve Cardiorespiratory and Muscular Fitness

	Cardiorespiratory Fitness	**Muscular Fitness**
Frequency:	3–5 days per week	2–3 days per week
Intensity:	55 to 90% of maximal heart rate Or an RPE[1] of 12–15 (Somewhat Hard to Hard)	70 to 85% of maximal weight you can lift Or an RPE[1] of 13–16 (Somewhat Hard to Very Hard)
Time:	At least 20 consecutive minutes	1–3 sets of 8–12 lifts[2] for each set

[1] RPE stands for *rating of perceived exertion,* defined in the text.
[2] A minimum of 8 to 10 exercises involving the major muscle groups such as arms, shoulders, chest, abdomen, back, hips, and legs is recommended.
Source: Adapted from American College of Sports Medicine Position Stand. The recommended quantity and quality of exercise for developing and maintaining cardiorespiratory and muscular fitness, and flexibility in healthy adults. *Med. Sci. Sports Exerc.* 30 (1998): 975–991. Used with permission.

intensity Refers to the amount of effort expended during the activity, or how difficult the activity is to perform.

low intensity activities Activities that cause very mild increases in breathing, sweating, and heart rate.

moderate intensity activities Activities that cause moderate increases in breathing, sweating, and heart rate.

vigorous intensity activities Activities that produce significant increases in breathing, sweating, and heart rate; talking is difficult when exercising at a vigorous intensity.

Theo should perform weight lifting at least two to three days each week. With this type of program, Theo will be able to reach his goals. Theo should also regularly participate in flexibility activities to enhance his quality of training and to prevent potential injuries.

Intensity

Intensity refers to the amount of effort expended or, to put it another way, how difficult the activity is to perform. In general, **low intensity activities** are those that cause very mild increases in breathing, sweating, and heart rate, while **moderate intensity activities** cause moderate increases in these responses. **Vigorous intensity activities** produce significant increases in breathing, sweating, and heart rate so that talking is difficult when exercising at a vigorous intensity.

Traditionally, heart rate has been used to indicate level of intensity during aerobic activities. Figure 12.3 shows an example of a heart rate training chart. You can

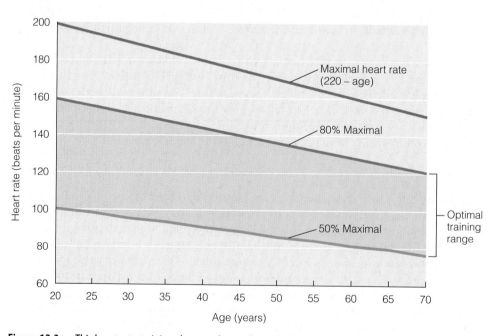

Figure 12.3   This heart rate training chart can be used to estimate your aerobic exercise intensity. The top line indicates the predicted maximal heart rate value for a person's age (220 − age). The shaded area represents the heart rate values that fall between 50% and 80% of maximal heart rate, which is the range generally recommended to achieve aerobic fitness.

Calculating Your Maximal and Training Heart Rate Range

Prior to getting pregnant, Nadia became interested in starting an exercise program. Her brother has type 1 diabetes, her mother had recently been diagnosed with type 2 diabetes, and Nadia was like the rest of her family, always struggling with being moderately overweight. She is interested in participating in a regular exercise program that will improve her cardiorespiratory fitness and help her maintain a more healthful weight. As she enjoys walking and bike riding, Nadia plans to begin by either riding the stationary bicycle or walking on the treadmill at the gym three times per week for 30 minutes each time. She now needs to determine the aerobic exercise training intensity that will help her improve her cardiorespiratory fitness. Nadia is 28 years of age and healthy, and she does a lot of light walking and lifting in her work in the retail business. Based on this information, Nadia should set her training heart rate range between 50 and 80% of her maximal heart rate.

Let's work with Nadia while she calculates these values:

- Maximal heart rate: 220 − age = 220 − 28 = 192 beats per minute (bpm)
- Lower end of intensity range: 50% of 192 bpm = 0.50 × 192 bpm = 96 bpm
- Higher end of intensity range: 80% of 192 bpm = 0.80 × 192 bpm = 154 bpm

When Nadia rides the bicycle or walks on the treadmill, her heart rate (when counted for an entire minute) should be between 96 and 154 bpm; this puts her in her aerobic training zone and will allow her to achieve cardiorespiratory fitness. Although Nadia does some walking at work, she is not accustomed to exercising for 30 minutes without stopping, and it is very likely that she will be unable to complete the entire 30 minutes of exercise when she first begins her program. It is important that she start at a level that she can achieve (for example, an intensity that allows her to exercise for 15 to 20 minutes) and that she slowly increase her exercise time and intensity until she meets her fitness goal. ●

---

calculate the range of exercise intensity that is appropriate for you by estimating your **maximal heart rate,** which is the rate at which your heart beats during maximal intensity exercise (see the You Do the Math box, above). Maximal heart rate is estimated by subtracting your age from 220 and is described in more detail below. For achieving and maintaining physical fitness, the intensity range typically recommended is 50 to 80% of your estimated maximal heart rate. People who are older or who have been inactive for a long time may want to exercise at the lower end of the range. Those who are more physically fit or are striving for a more rapid improvement in fitness may want to exercise at the higher end of the range. Competitive athletes generally train at a higher intensity, around 80 to 95% of their maximum heart rate.

Although the calculation *220 − age* has been used extensively for years to predict maximal heart rate, it was never intended to accurately represent everyone's true maximal heart rate or to be used as the standard of aerobic training intensity. There are limitations to using the calculation, and it has recently been challenged (Tanaka, Monahan, and Seals 2001). The most accurate way to determine your own maximal heart rate is to complete a maximal exercise test in a fitness laboratory; however, this test is not commonly conducted with the general public and can be very expensive. Although not completely accurate, the estimated maximal heart rate method can still be used to give you a general idea of your aerobic training range.

An alternative way to estimate intensity during activity is to use the Borg Scale of Perceived Exertion, also called the **rating of perceived exertion** (or **RPE**) (Figure 12.4; Ettinger, Mitchell, and Blair 1996). This scale helps you to assess how difficult any activity is for you. For example, a very light exertion at level 8

maximal heart rate The rate at which your heart beats during maximal intensity exercise.

rating of perceived exertion (RPE) A scale that defines the difficulty level of any activity; this scale can be used to estimate intensity during exercise.

Rating of Perceived Exertion (RPE)

Scale	Perceived Exertion	Physical Signs
6 7	Very, very light	No perceptible sign
8 9	Very light	No perceptible sign
10 11	Fairly light	Feeling of motion
12 13	Somewhat hard	Warmth on cold day, slight sweat on warm days
14 15	Hard	Sweating but can still talk without difficulty
16 17	Very hard	Heavy sweating, difficulty talking
18 19 20	Very, very hard	Feeling of near exhaustion

Figure 12.4   Rating of perceived exertion (RPE) scale to estimate exercise intensity. An intensity of 12 to 15, or somewhat hard to hard, is recommended to achieve physical fitness. (From G. V. Borg, 1982, *Medicine and Science in Sports and Exercise* 14: 377–387. Copyright © 1982. Used with permission.)

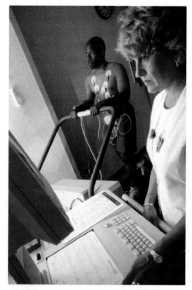

Testing in a fitness lab is the most accurate way to determine maximal heart rate.

time of activity How long each exercise session lasts.

would produce no perceptible physical signs, whereas a very hard exertion at level 16 would be indicated by heavy sweating and difficulty talking. An intensity of 12 to 15, or somewhat hard to hard, is recommended to achieve physical fitness. At this suggested intensity, you should breathe more rapidly, feel warm, and even sweat, but still be able to talk.

Time of Activity

Time of activity refers to how long each session lasts. To achieve general health, you can do multiple short bouts of activity that add up to 30 minutes each day. However, to achieve higher levels of fitness, it is important that the activities be done for at least 20 to 30 consecutive minutes.

For example, let's say you want to compete in triathlons. To be successful during the running segment of the triathlon, you will need to be able to run quickly for at least 5 miles. Thus, it is appropriate for you to train so that you can complete 5 miles during one session and still have enough energy to swim and bicycle during the race. Running for two or three 10-minute sessions each day would not be a sufficient overload to prepare you for this competition. You will need to consistently train at a distance of 5 miles; you will also benefit from running longer distances. In contrast, bicycling for 10 minutes two or three times each day would be appropriate for someone like Nadia to achieve her health-related cardiorespiratory fitness goal.

Table 12.3 compares the guidelines for achieving health to those for achieving physical fitness. The guidelines you follow will depend on your personal goals. These recommendations apply to people of all ages, and following either set will allow you to improve and maintain your health. For people with established disease, these guidelines may help postpone complications and reduce their reliance on medications. People with heart disease, high blood pressure, diabetes, osteoporosis, or arthritis should get approval to exercise from their health care practitioner prior to starting a fitness program. In addition, a medical evaluation should be conducted before starting an exercise program for an apparently healthy but currently inactive man 40 years or older or woman 50 years or older.

Table 12.3   Physical Activity Guidelines for Achieving Health versus Physical Fitness

	Health	Physical Fitness
Frequency:	Daily	2 – 5 days per week (3 – 5 days for cardiorespiratory fitness, 2 – 3 days for muscular fitness and flexibility)
Intensity:	Any level	50 – 80% of maximal heart rate or an RPE[1] of 12 – 16
Time:	Accumulation of a minimum of 30 minutes each day	20 – 60 minutes of continuous or intermittent activity
Type:	Any activity	Aerobic-type activities, resistance exercises to enhance muscular strength and endurance, and flexibility exercises

[1]RPE is rating of perceived exertion

Source: Adapted from American College of Sports Medicine Position Stand, The recommended quantity and quality of exercise for developing and maintaining cardiorespiratory and muscular fitness, and flexibility in healthy adults, *Med. Sci. Sports Exerc.* 30 (1998):975–991. U.S. Department of Health and Human Services, *Physical Activity and Health: A Report of the Surgeon General.* (Atlanta, GA: U.S. Department of Health and Human Services, Centers for Disease Control and Prevention, National Center for Chronic Disease Prevention and Health Promotion, 1996).

Recap: To improve fitness, you must place an extra physical demand, or an overload, on your body. To achieve appropriate overload, the FIT principle should be followed; FIT stands for frequency, intensity, and time of activity. Frequency refers to the number of activity sessions per week. Intensity refers to how difficult the activity is to perform. Time refers to how long each activity session lasts.

A Sound Fitness Plan Includes a Warm-Up and a Cool-Down Period

To properly prepare for and recover from an exercise session, warm-up and cool-down activities should be performed. **Warm-up,** also called preliminary exercise, includes general activities (such as stretching and calisthenics) and specific activities that prepare you for the actual activity (such as jogging or swinging a golf club). Your warm-up should be brief (5 to 10 minutes), gradual, and sufficient to increase muscle and body temperature but should not cause fatigue or deplete energy stores.

Warming up prior to exercise is important, as it properly prepares the muscles for exertion by increasing blood flow and temperature. It may also help to prepare a person psychologically for the exercise session or athletic event.

Cool-down activities are done after the exercise session is completed. Similar to the warm-up, the cool-down should be gradual and allow your body to slowly recover. Your cool-down should include some of the same activities you performed during the exercise session but done at a low intensity, and you should allow ample time for stretching. Cooling down after exercise assists in the prevention of injury and may help reduce muscle soreness.

warm-up   Also called preliminary exercise; includes activities that prepare you for an exercise bout, including stretching, calisthenics, and movements specific to the exercise bout.

cool-down   Activities done after an exercise session is completed. Should be gradual and allow your body to slowly recover from exercise.

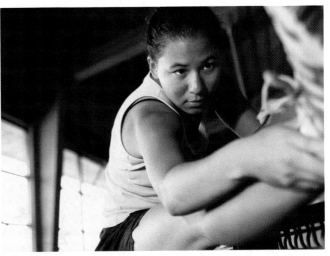

Stretching should be included in the warm-up and the cool-down for exercise.

Recap: Warm-up, or preliminary exercise, is important to get prepared for exercise. Warm-up exercises prepare the muscles for exertion by increasing blood flow and temperature. Cool-down activities are done after an exercise session is complete. Cool-down activities should be done at a low intensity, and cooling down after activity assists in the prevention of injury and may help reduce muscle soreness.

Nadia   *Nutri-Case:*

"I've been working out on the exercise bike for thirty minutes every other day for six weeks now, and I feel so great, I decided to increase the resistance on the bike! Yesterday, I went up two levels, and I made it, all thirty minutes at the new level! I was sweating so much I soaked my T-shirt through and felt sort of shaky for a few minutes afterward, but I was really proud of myself, too! If I can keep this up, my baby is going to have a strong mama!"

Imagine that you were a trainer at the gym where Nadia exercises, and she told you about her new workout routine. How would you respond? Before you answer, think about both positive and negative aspects of the information she has shared with you. Why would it be especially important to begin your response with encouragement and praise, and which aspects of her new routine would you identify as potentially harmful? Think of at least two additional questions you might want to ask her about her practices before, during, and/or after her workouts.

What Fuels Our Activities?

In order to perform exercise, or muscular work, we must be able to generate energy. The common currency of energy for virtually all cells in the body is **ATP,** or **adenosine triphosphate.** As you might guess from its name, a molecule of ATP includes an organic compound called adenosine and three phosphate groups (Figure 12.5). When one of the phosphates is cleaved, or broken away, from ATP, energy is released. The products remaining after this reaction are adenosine diphosphate (ADP) and an independent inorganic phosphate group (P_i). In a mirror image of this reaction, the body regenerates ATP by adding a phosphate group back to ADP. In this way, we continually provide energy to our cells.

The amount of ATP stored in a muscle cell is very limited; it can keep the muscle active for only about 1 to 3 seconds. Thus, we need to generate ATP from other sources to fuel activities for longer periods of time. Fortunately, we are able to generate ATP from the breakdown of carbohydrate, fat, and protein, providing our cells with a variety of sources from which to receive energy. The primary energy systems we rely upon to provide energy for physical activities are the adenosine triphosphate –

adenosine triphosphate (ATP) The common currency of energy for virtually all cells of the body.

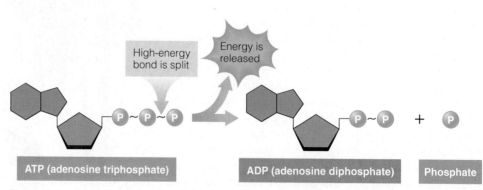

Figure 12.5 Structure of adenosine triphosphate (ATP). Energy is produced when ATP is split into adenosine diphosphate (ADP) and inorganic phosphate (P_i).

creatine phosphate (ATP-CP) energy system and the anaerobic and aerobic break-down of carbohydrates. Our bodies also generate energy from the breakdown of fats. As you will see, the type, intensity, and duration of the activities we perform determine the amount of ATP we need and therefore the energy system we use.

The ATP-CP Energy System Uses Creatine Phosphate to Regenerate ATP

As we said, muscle cells store only enough ATP to maintain activity for 1 to 3 seconds. When more energy is needed, a high-energy compound called **creatine phosphate (CP)** (also called **phosphocreatine, or PCr**) can be broken down to support the regeneration of ATP (Figure 12.6). Because this reaction can occur in the absence of oxygen, it is referred to as an **anaerobic** reaction (meaning "without oxygen").

Muscle tissue contains about four to six times as much CP as ATP, but there is still not enough CP available to fuel activities longer than two minutes. We tend to use CP the most during very intense, short bouts of activity such as lifting, jumping, and sprinting (Figure 12.7). Together, our stores of ATP and CP can only support a *maximal* physical effort for about 3 to 15 seconds. We must rely on other energy sources, such as carbohydrate and fat, to support activities of longer duration.

> **Recap:** Adenosine triphosphate, or ATP, is the common energy source for all cells of the body. When one of the phosphate groups is cleaved from the ATP molecule, energy is released. The amount of ATP stored in a muscle cell is limited and can only keep a muscle active for about 1 to 3 seconds. For maximal-physical-effort activities lasting about 3 to 15 seconds, creatine phosphate can be broken down in an anaerobic reaction to provide energy and support the regeneration of ATP. To support activities that last longer than 2 minutes, we must derive energy from the breakdown of carbohydrates, fats, and protein.

The Breakdown of Carbohydrates Provides Energy for Brief and Long-Term Exercise

During activities lasting about 30 seconds to 3 minutes, we cannot generate enough ATP from the breakdown of CP to fully support our efforts. Thus, we need an energy source that we can use quickly to produce ATP. The breakdown of carbohydrates,

creatine phosphate (CP) A high-energy compound that can be broken down for energy and used to regenerate ATP.

anaerobic Means "without oxygen." Term used to refer to metabolic reactions that occur in the absence of oxygen.

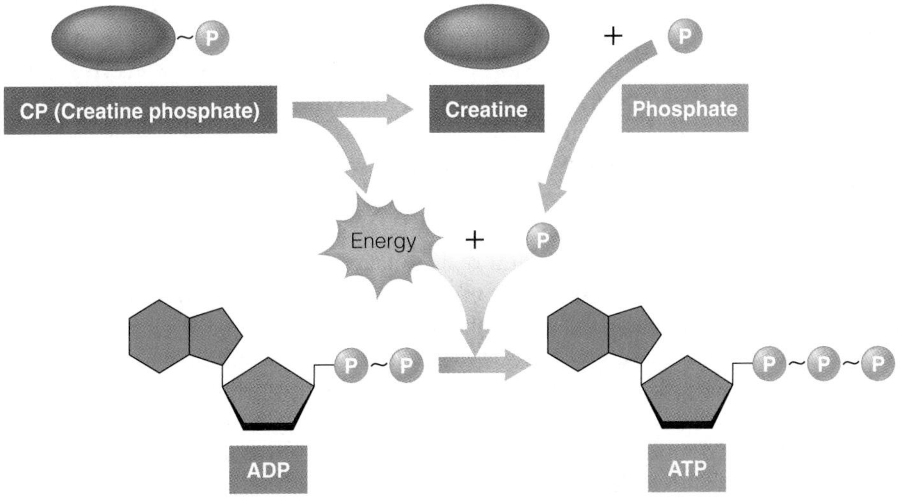

Figure 12.6 When the compound creatine phosphate (CP) is broken down into a molecule of creatine and an independent phosphate molecule, energy is released. This energy, along with the independent phosphate molecule, can then be used to regenerate ATP.

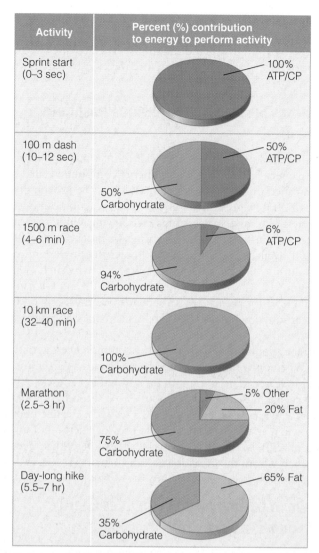

Figure 12.7 The relative contribution of ATP-CP, carbohydrate, and fat to activities of various durations and intensities.

glycolysis The breakdown of glucose; yields two ATP molecules and two pyruvic acid molecules for each molecule of glucose.

pyruvic acid The primary end product of glycolysis.

lactic acid A compound that results when pyruvic acid is metabolized in the presence of insufficient oxygen.

specifically glucose, provides this quick energy in a process called **glycolysis.** The most common source of glucose during exercise comes from glycogen stored in the muscles and glucose found in the blood. As shown in Figure 12.8, for every glucose molecule that goes through glycolysis, two ATP molecules are produced. The primary end product of glycolysis is **pyruvic acid.**

When oxygen availability is limited in the cell, pyruvic acid is converted to **lactic acid.** For years it was assumed that lactic acid was a useless, even potentially toxic, by-product of high-intensity exercise. We now know that lactic acid is an important intermediate of glucose breakdown and that it plays a critical role in supplying fuel for working muscles, the heart, and resting tissues (see the Nutrition Myth or Fact: Lactic Acid Causes Muscle Fatigue and Soreness box, page 434).

The major advantage of glycolysis is that it is the fastest way that we can regenerate ATP for exercise, other than the ATP-CP system. However, this high rate of ATP production can be sustained only for a brief period of time, generally less than 3 minutes. To perform exercise that lasts longer than 3 minutes, we must rely on the aerobic energy system to provide adequate ATP.

To generate even more ATP molecules, pyruvic acid can go through additional metabolic pathways in the presence of oxygen (see Figure 12.8). Although this

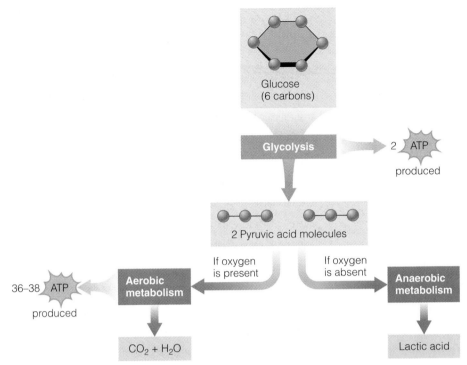

Figure 12.8   The breakdown of one molecule of glucose, or the process of glycolysis, yields two molecules of pyruvic acid and two ATP molecules. The further metabolism of pyruvic acid in the presence of insufficient oxygen (anaerobic process) results in the production of lactic acid. The metabolism of pyruvic acid in the presence of adequate oxygen (aerobic process) yields 36 to 38 molecules of ATP.

process is slower than glycolysis occurring under anaerobic conditions, the breakdown of one glucose molecule going through aerobic metabolism yields 36 to 38 ATP molecules for energy, while the anaerobic process yields only 2 ATP molecules. Thus, this aerobic process supplies 18 times more energy! Another advantage of the aerobic process is that it does not result in the significant production of acids and other compounds that contribute to muscle fatigue, which means that a low-intensity activity can be performed for hours. Aerobic metabolism of glucose is the primary source of fuel for our muscles during activities lasting from 3 minutes to 4 hours (see Figure 12.7).

As you learned in Chapter 4, we can store only a limited amount of glycogen in our bodies. An average, well-nourished man who weighs about 154 pounds (70 kg) can store about 200 to 500 g of muscle glycogen, which is equal to 800 to 2000 kcal of energy. Although trained athletes can store more muscle glycogen than the average person, there is still not enough glycogen stored in our bodies to provide an unlimited energy supply for long-term activities. Thus, we also need a fuel source that is very abundant and can be broken down under aerobic conditions so that it can support activities of lower intensity and longer duration. This fuel source is fat.

Recap: To support activities that last from 30 seconds to 2 minutes, energy is produced from the breakdown of glucose, called glycolysis. Two ATP molecules are produced for every glucose molecule broken down, and pyruvic acid is the primary end product of this reaction. Lactic acid is formed when pyruvic acid is metabolized under anaerobic conditions. To support activities that last from 3 minutes to 4 hours, energy is produced from the aerobic metabolism of pyruvic acid. During this process, pyruvic acid is broken down in the presence of oxygen, and each molecule can yield 36 to 38 ATP molecules.

Lactic Acid Causes Muscle Fatigue and Soreness

Lactic acid is a by-product of glycolysis. For many years it was believed that lactic acid caused both muscle fatigue and soreness. Does recent scientific evidence support this belief?

The exact causes of muscle fatigue are not known, and there appear to be many contributing factors. Recent evidence suggests that fatigue may be due not only to the accumulation of acids and other metabolic by-products, but also to the depletion of creatine phosphate and changes in calcium in the cells that affect muscle contraction. Depletion of muscle glycogen, liver glycogen, and blood glucose, as well as psychological factors, can all contribute to fatigue (Brooks et al. 2000). Thus, lactic acid contributes to fatigue but does not appear to cause fatigue independently.

So what factors cause muscle soreness? As with fatigue, there are probably many contributors. It is hypothesized that soreness usually results from microscopic tears in the muscle fibers as a result of strenuous exercise. This damage triggers an inflammatory reaction that causes an influx of fluid and various chemicals to the damaged area. These substances work to remove damaged tissue and initiate tissue repair, but they may also stimulate pain (Brooks et al. 2000). However, it appears highly unlikely that lactic acid is an independent cause of muscle soreness.

Recent studies indicate that lactic acid is produced even under aerobic conditions! This means it is produced at rest as well as during any intensity of exercise. The reasons for this constant production of lactic acid are still being studied. What we do know is that lactic acid is an important fuel for resting tissues and for working cardiac and skeletal muscles. That's right—skeletal muscles not only *produce* lactic acid, but they also *use* it for energy, both directly and after it is converted into glucose and glycogen in the liver (Brooks 2000; Gladden 2000). We also know that endurance training improves the muscle's ability to use lactic acid for energy. Thus, contrary to being a waste product of glucose metabolism, lactic acid is actually an important energy source for muscle cells during rest and exercise. ●

Aerobic Breakdown of Fats Supports Exercise of Low Intensity and Long Duration

When we refer to fat as a fuel source, we mean the triglyceride molecule, which is the primary storage form of fat in our cells. As you learned in Chapter 5, a triglyceride molecule is comprised of a glycerol backbone attached to three fatty acid molecules (see Figure 5.1, page 159). It is these fatty acid molecules that provide much of the energy we need to support long-term activity. Fatty acids are classified by their length; that is, by the number of carbons they contain. The longer the fatty acid, the more ATP that can be generated from its breakdown. For instance, palmitic acid is a fatty acid with sixteen carbons. If palmitic acid is broken down completely, it yields 129 ATP molecules! Obviously, far more energy is produced from this one fatty acid molecule than from the aerobic breakdown of a glucose molecule.

There are two major advantages of using fat as a fuel. First, fat is a very abundant energy source, even in lean people. For example, a man who weighs 154 pounds (70 kg) who has a body fat level of 10% has approximately 15 pounds of body fat, which is equivalent to over 50,000 kcal of energy! This is significantly more energy than can be provided by his stored muscle glycogen (800 to 2000 kcal). Second, fat provides 9 kcal of energy per gram, while carbohydrate provides only 4 kcal of energy per gram, which means that fat supplies more than twice as much energy per gram as carbohydrate. The primary disadvantage of using fat as a fuel is that the breakdown process is relatively slow; thus fat is used predominantly as a fuel source during activities of lower intensity and longer duration. Fat is also our primary energy source during rest, sitting, and standing in place.

What specific activities are primarily fueled by fat? Walking long distances uses fat stores, as do other low to moderate intensity forms of exercise. Fat is also an important fuel source during endurance events such as marathons (26.2 miles) and ultra-

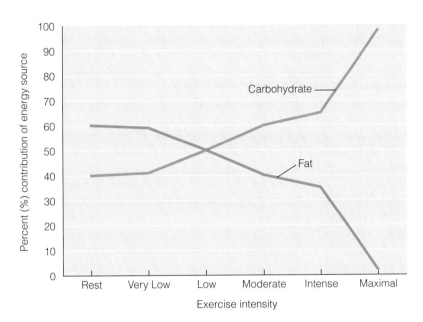

Figure 12.9   For most daily activities, including exercise, we use a mixture of carbohydrate and fat for energy. At lower exercise intensities, we rely more on fat as a fuel source. As exercise intensity increases, we rely more on carbohydrate for energy. (Adapted from M. Manore and J. Thompson, *Sports Nutrition for Health and Performance* [Champaign, IL: Human Kinetics Publishers, 2000].)

marathon races (49.9 miles). Endurance exercise training improves our ability to use fat for energy, which may be one reason that people who exercise regularly tend to have lower body fat levels than people who do not exercise.

It is important to remember that we are almost always using some combination of carbohydrate and fat for energy. At rest, we use very little carbohydrate, relying mostly on fat. During maximal exercise (at 100% effort), we are using mostly carbohydrate and very little fat. However, most activities we do each day involve some use of both fuels (Figure 12.9).

When it comes to eating properly to support regular physical activity or exercise training, the nutrient to focus on is carbohydrate. This is because most people store more than enough fat to support exercise, whereas our storage of carbohydrate is limited. It is especially important that we maintain adequate stores of glycogen for moderate to intense exercise. Dietary recommendations for fat, carbohydrate, and protein are reviewed later in this chapter (pages 436–444).

> **Recap:** Fat can be broken down aerobically to support activities of low intensity and long duration. Each fatty acid from a triglyceride molecule is broken down for energy, and the amount of energy derived depends upon the length of the fatty acid chain. The two major advantages of using fat as a fuel is that it is an abundant energy source and it provides more than twice the energy per gram as compared to carbohydrate. The primary disadvantage of using fat as a fuel is that the breakdown process is relatively slow so it cannot support quick, high intensity activities.

Amino Acids Are Not Major Sources of Fuel During Exercise

Proteins, or more specifically amino acids, are not major energy sources during exercise. As discussed in Chapter 6, amino acids can be used directly for energy if necessary, but they are more often used to make glucose to maintain our blood glucose levels during exercise. Amino acids also help build and repair tissues after exercise. Depending upon the intensity and duration of the activity, amino acids may contribute about 3 to 6% of the energy needed (Tarnolpolsky 2000).

Given this, why is it that so many people are concerned about their protein intakes? As you learned in Chapter 6, our muscles are not stimulated to grow when we eat extra dietary protein. Only appropriate physical training can stimulate our muscles to grow and strengthen. Thus, while we need enough dietary protein to support activity and recovery, consuming very high amounts does not provide an added benefit. The protein needs of athletes are only slightly higher than the needs of non-athletes, and most of us eat more than enough protein to support even the highest requirements for competitive athletes! Thus, there is generally no need for recreationally active people or even competitive athletes to consume protein or amino acid supplements.

> **Recap:** Amino acids may contribute from 3 to 6% of the energy needed during exercise, depending upon the intensity and duration of the activity. Amino acids help build and repair tissues after exercise. We generally consume more than enough protein in our diets to support regular exercise, and there is typically no need for protein or amino acid supplementation even for competitive athletes.

What Kind of Diet Supports Physical Activity?

Lots of people wonder, "Do my nutrient needs change if I become more physically active?" The answer to this question depends upon the type, intensity, and duration of activity in which you participate. It is not necessarily true that our requirement for every nutrient is greater if we are physically active.

People who are performing moderate-intensity daily activities for health can follow the general guidelines put forth in the Food Guide Pyramid. For smaller or less active people, the lower end of the range of recommendations for each food group may be appropriate. For larger or more active people, the higher end of the range is suggested. Modifications may need to be made for people who exercise vigorously every day, and particularly for athletes training for competition. Table 12.4 provides an overview of the nutrients that can be affected by regular, vigorous exercise training. Each of these nutrients is described in more detail below (American College of Sports Medicine et al., 2000).

grazing Consistently eating small meals throughout the day; done by many athletes to meet their high energy demands.

Vigorous Exercise Increases Energy Needs

Athletes generally have higher energy needs than moderately physically active or sedentary people. The amount of extra energy needed to support regular training is determined by the type, intensity, and duration of the activity. In addition, the energy needs of male athletes are higher than those of female athletes because male athletes weigh more, have more muscle mass, and will expend more energy during activity than women. This is relative, of course: a large woman who trains three to five hours each day will probably need more energy than a small man who trains one hour each day. The energy needs of athletes can range from only 1500 to 1800 kcal per day for a small female gymnast to over 7500 kcal per day for a male cyclist competing in the Tour de France cross-country cycling race!

Figure 12.10 shows a sample of meals that total 1500 kcal per day and 4000 kcal per day, with the carbohydrate content of these meals meeting more than 60% of total energy intake. As you can see, athletes who need more than 4000 kcal per day need to consume very large quantities of food. However, the heavy demands of daily physical training, work, school, and family responsibilities often leaves these athletes with little time to eat adequately. Thus, many athletes meet their energy demands by planning regular meals and snacks and **grazing** (eating small meals throughout the day) consistently. They may also take advantage of the energy-dense snack foods and meal replacements specifically designed for athletes participating in vigorous training. These steps help athletes to maintain their blood glucose and energy stores.

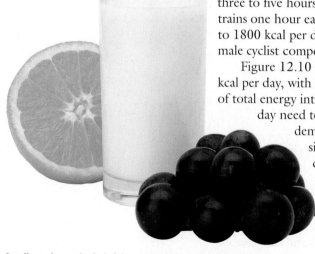

Small snacks can be helpful to meet daily energy demands.

Table 12.4   Suggested Intakes of Nutrients to Support Vigorous Exercise

Nutrient	Functions	Suggested Intake
Energy	Supports exercise, activities of daily living, and basic body functions	Depends upon body size and the type, intensity, and duration of activity. For many female athletes: 1800 to 3500 kcal/day For many male athletes: 2500 to 7500 kcal/day
Carbohydrate	Provides energy, maintains adequate muscle glycogen and blood glucose; high complex carbohydrate foods provide vitamins and minerals	At least 60% of total energy intake Depending upon sport and gender, should consume 6–10 grams of carbohydrate per kg body weight per day
Fat	Provides energy, fat-soluble vitamins, and essential fatty acids; supports production of hormones and transport of nutrients	15–25% of total energy intake
Protein	Helps build and maintain muscle; provides building material for glucose; energy source during endurance exercise; aids recovery from exercise	12–20% of total energy intake Endurance athletes: 1.4–1.6 grams per kg body weight Strength athletes: 1.0–1.7 grams per kg body weight
Water	Maintains temperature regulation (adequate cooling); maintains blood volume and blood pressure; supports all cell functions	Consume fluid before, during, and after exercise Consume enough to maintain body weight Consume at least 8 cups (or 64 fl. oz.) of water daily to maintain regular health and activity Athletes may need up to 10 liters (or 170 fl. oz.) every day; more is required if exercising in a hot environment
B vitamins	Critical for energy production from carbohydrate, fat, and protein	May need slightly more (1–2 times the RDA) for thiamin, riboflavin, and vitamin B_6
Calcium	Builds and maintains bone mass; assists with nervous system function, muscle contraction, hormone function, and transport of nutrients across cell membrane	Meet the current AI: 14–18 yrs: 1300 mg/day 19–50 yrs: 1000 mg/day 51 and older: 1200 mg/day
Iron	Primarily responsible for the transport of oxygen in blood to cells; assists with energy production	Consume at least the RDA: Males: 14–18 yrs: 11 mg/day 19 and older: 8 mg/day Females: 14–18 yrs: 15 mg/day 19–50 yrs: 18 mg/day 51 and older: 8 mg/day

If an athlete is losing body weight, then his or her energy intake is inadequate. Conversely, weight gain may indicate that energy intake is too high. Weight maintenance is generally recommended to maximize performance. If weight loss is warranted, food intake should be lowered no more than 200 to 500 kcal per day, and athletes should try to lose weight prior to the competitive season if at all possible. Weight gain may be

1500 kcal/day Diet	4000 kcal/day Diet
1 1/2 cup Cheerios 4 oz. skim milk 1 medium banana 8 fl. oz. orange juice	3 cups Cheerios 8 fl. oz. skim milk 1 medium banana 2 slices whole wheat toast 1 tbsp. butter 8 fl. oz. orange juice

Turkey sandwich with:
  2 slices whole wheat bread
  3 oz. turkey lunch meat
  1 ounce Swiss cheese slice
  1 leaf iceberg lettuce
  2 slices tomato
  1 cup tomato soup
    (made with water)
	Two Turkey sandwiches with:
	  2 slices whole wheat bread
	  3 oz. turkey lunch meat
	  1 ounce Swiss cheese slice
	  1 leaf iceberg lettuce
	  2 slices tomato
	  2 cups tomato soup
	    (made with water)
	Two 8-oz. containers of
	  low-fat fruit yogurt
	24 fl. oz. of Gatorade

3 oz. grilled skinless
  chicken breast
1 1/2 cup mixed salad greens
1 tbsp. French salad dressing
1 cup steamed broccoli
1/2 cup cooked brown rice
8 fl. oz. skim milk
	6 oz. grilled skinless
	  chicken breast
	3 cups mixed salad greens
	3 tbsp. French salad dressing
	2 cups cooked
	  spaghetti noodles
	1 cup spaghetti sauce
	  with meat
	16 fl. oz. skim milk

Figure 12.10   High carbohydrate (approximately 60% of total energy) meals that contain approximately 1500 kcal per day (on left) and 4000 kcal per day (on right). Athletes must plan their meals carefully to meet energy demands, particularly those with very high energy needs.

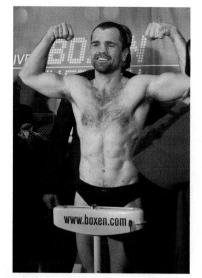

Some athletes may diet to meet a pre-defined weight category.

necessary for some athletes and can usually be accomplished by consuming 500 to 700 kcal per day more than needed for weight maintenance. The extra energy should come from a healthy balance of carbohydrate (55 to 60% of total energy intake), fat (25 to 30% of total energy intake), and protein (10 to 20% of total energy intake).

Many athletes are concerned about their weight for reasons of performance or physical appearance. Jockeys, boxers, wrestlers, judo athletes, and others are required to "make weight," or meet a predefined weight category. Others, such as distance runners, gymnasts, figure skaters, and dancers, are required to maintain a very lean figure for performance and aesthetic reasons. These athletes tend to eat less energy than they need to support vigorous training, which puts them at risk for inadequate intakes of all nutrients. These athletes are at a higher risk of suffering from health consequences resulting from poor energy and nutrient intake, including eating disorders, osteoporosis, menstrual disturbances, dehydration, heat and physical injuries, and even death. Refer to the Highlight box, "When Sports Nutrition Becomes a Matter of Life or Death" to learn more about the consequences of risky nutritional practices among athletes.

Recap: The type, intensity, and duration of activities you participate in will determine your nutrient needs. Vigorous intensity exercise requires extra energy, and male athletes typically need more energy than female athletes because of their higher muscle mass and larger body weight. Weight maintenance is recommended to maximize athletic performance. Some athletes who are concerned with making a competitive weight or with the aesthetic demands of their sport may be at risk for poor energy and nutrient intakes.

When Sports Nutrition Becomes a Matter of Life or Death

Athletes are generally strong and very physically fit. However, some athletes push their bodies to the extreme, placing themselves in danger of illness and even death. The two examples described below illustrate how poor nutrition and excessive exercise can lead to serious, life-threatening consequences.

In 1997, three previously healthy collegiate wrestlers died of cardiac arrest. These wrestlers were competing in three different university programs. All of them were attempting to compete in weight classes that were 25 to 33 pounds lower than their preseason body weight (Remick et al. 1998) and were using dehydration strategies to lose weight. They restricted fluid and food intake, exercised excessively in hot environments, and wore heavy sweat suits that pre-

vented evaporative cooling. These athletes lost 4 to 9 pounds within 2 to 4 hours; they continued to exercise until they collapsed of heart failure.

Christy Henrich was an Olympic-caliber gymnast. In 1988, she missed the Olympic team by 0.0188 of a point. During an international competition that same year, a judge made an off-handed comment to her that she needed to watch her weight. At the time, she was 4′ 11″ tall and weighed only 98 pounds. This comment triggered something inside of Christy, and she resorted to anorexia and bulimia in order to reduce her body weight. At one point her weight dropped to only 47 pounds. She withdrew from gymnastics in 1991. After years of battling these two eating disorders, Christy died of multiple organ failure in 1994 at the age of 22 (Thompson 2001). ●

Carbohydrate Needs Increase for Many Active People

As you know, carbohydrate (in the form of glucose) is one of the primary sources of energy needed to support exercise. Both endurance athletes and strength athletes require adequate carbohydrate to maintain their glycogen stores and provide quick energy.

How Much of an Athlete's Diet Should Be Carbohydrates?

You may recall from Chapter 4 that the AMDR for carbohydrates is 45 to 65% of total energy intake. Athletes should consume at least 60% of their total energy intake as carbohydrates, which falls within this recommended range. Athletes who are participating in strength-type activities, sprinting, or other explosive-type events, or are not training for more than one hour each day may find that consuming 55% of their total energy intake as carbohydrate is sufficient.

To illustrate how inadequate carbohydrate affects glycogen stores, let's see what happens to Theo when he participates in a study designed to determine how carbohydrate intake affects glycogen stores during a period of heavy training. Theo was asked to come to the exercise laboratory at the university and ride a stationary bicycle for 2 hours a day for three consecutive days at 75% of his maximal heart rate. Before and after each ride, samples of muscle tissue were taken from his thighs to determine the amount of glycogen stored in the working muscles. Theo performed these rides on two different occasions — once when he had eaten a high carbohydrate diet (80% of total energy intake) and again when he had eaten a moderate carbohydrate diet (40% of total energy intake). As you can see in Figure 12.11, Theo's muscle glycogen levels decreased dramatically after each training session. More importantly, his

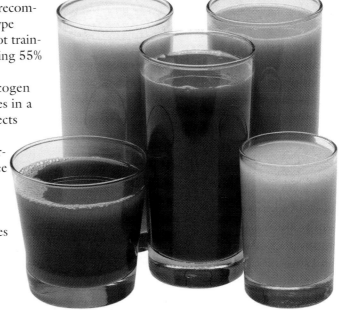

Fruit and vegetable juices can be a good source of carbohydrates.

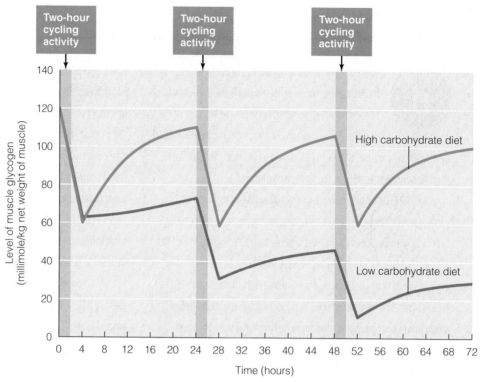

Figure 12.11 The effects of a low carbohydrate diet on muscle glycogen stores. When a low carbohydrate diet is consumed, glycogen stores cannot be restored during a period of regular vigorous training. (Adapted from D. L. Costill and J. M. Miller, Nutrition for endurance sport: CHO and fluid balance. *Int. J. Sports Med.* 1 (1980): 2–14. Copyright © 1980 Georg Thieme Verlag. Used with permission.)

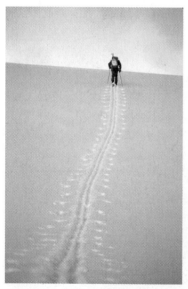

Carbohydrate loading may benefit endurance athletes, such as cross-country skiers.

muscle glycogen levels did not recover to baseline levels over the three days when Theo ate the lower carbohydrate diet. He was able to maintain his muscle glycogen levels only when he was eating the higher carbohydrate diet. Theo also told the researchers that completing the 2-hour rides was much more difficult when he had eaten the moderate carbohydrate diet as compared to when he ate the diet that was higher in carbohydrate.

When Should Carbohydrates Be Consumed?

It is important for athletes not only to consume enough carbohydrate to maintain glycogen stores, but also to time their intake optimally. Our bodies store glycogen very rapidly during the first 24 hours of recovery from exercise, with the highest storage rates occurring during the first few hours (Burke 2000). If an athlete has to perform or participate in training bouts that are scheduled less than 8 hours apart, then he or she should try to consume enough carbohydrate in the few hours following training to allow for ample glycogen storage. However, with a longer recovery time (generally 12 hours or more) the athlete can eat when he or she chooses, and glycogen levels should be restored as long as the total carbohydrate eaten is sufficient.

What Food Sources of Carbohydrates Are Good for Athletes?

What are good carbohydrate sources to support vigorous training? In general, complex, less-processed carbohydrate foods such as whole grains and cereals, fruits, vegetables, and juices are excellent sources that also supply fiber, vitamins, and minerals. Guidelines for intake of simple sugars is less than 10% of total energy intake, but some athletes who need very large energy intakes to support training may need to consume more. There are also many beverages and snack bars designed to assist athletes with increasing carbohydrate intake. Simple, inexpensive foods that contain 50 to 100 grams of carbohydrate are listed in Table 12.5, as are some snack bars designed for athletes.

Table 12.5   Nutrient Composition of Various Foods and Sport Bars

Food	Amount	Carbohydrate (grams)	Energy from Carbohydrate (%)	Protein (grams)	Fat (grams)	Total Energy (kcal)
Sweetened applesauce	1 cup	50	97	0.5	0.5	207
Large apple	1 each	50	82	3	4	248
Saltine crackers	8 each					
Whole wheat bread	1 oz. slice	50	71	16	2	282
Jelly	4 tsp					
Skim milk	12 fl. oz.					
Spaghetti noodles (cooked)	1 cup	50	75	8	4	268
Tomato sauce	¼ cup					
Brown rice (cooked)	1 cup	100	88	8	2	450
Mixed vegetables	½ cup					
Apple juice	12 fl. oz.					
Large bagel	1 each (3.5 oz.)	100	81	19	2	494
Jelly	8 tsp					
Skim milk	8 fl. oz.					
Grape Nuts cereal	½ cup	100	84	16	1	473
Raisins	⅜ cup					
Skim milk	8 fl. oz.					
Balance food bar	1.76 oz.	22	44	14	6	200
Clif Bar (chocolate chip)	2.4 oz.	45	72	10	4	250
Kellogg's Nutri-grain Bar (raspberry)	1.3 oz.	27	77	2	3	140
Meta-Rx (fudge brownie)	3.53 oz.	48	60	27	2.5	320
Nature Valley Granola Bar	1.5 oz.	29	64	5	6	180
Power Bar (chocolate)	2.25 oz.	42	75	10	2	225
PR Bar Ironman	2 oz.	24	42	17	7	230

Source: Adapted from M. Manore and J. Thompson. *Sport Nutrition for Health and Performance.* (Champaign, IL: Human Kinetics Publishers, 2000), 42, 49.

When Does Carbohydrate Loading Make Sense?

As you know, carbohydrate is a critical energy source to support exercise, particularly endurance-type activities. Because of the importance of carbohydrates as an exercise fuel and our limited capacity to store them, discovering ways to maximize our storage of carbohydrates has been at the forefront of sports nutrition research for many years. The practice of **carbohydrate loading,** also called *glycogen loading,* involves altering both exercise duration and carbohydrate intake such that it maximizes the amount of muscle glycogen. Table 12.6 reviews a schedule for carbohydrate loading for an endurance athlete. Athletes who may benefit from maximizing muscle glycogen stores are those competing in marathons, ultramarathons, long-distance swimming, cross-country skiing, and triathlons. Athletes who compete in baseball, American football, 10-kilometer runs, walking, hiking, weightlifting, and most swimming events will not gain any performance benefits from this practice, nor will people who regularly participate in moderately intense physical activities to maintain fitness.

carbohydrate loading   Also known as glycogen loading. A process that involves altering training and carbohydrate intake so that muscle glycogen storage is maximized.

Table 12.6 Recommended Carbohydrate Loading Procedure for Endurance Athletes

Days Prior to Event	Exercise Duration (minutes)	Carbohydrate Content of Diet (grams per kg of body weight)
6	90	5
5	40	5
4	40	5
3	20	10
2	20	10
1	None (rest day)	10
Day of Race	Competition	Precompetition food and fluid

Source: Coleman, E. 2000. Carbohydrate and exercise, in: C. A. Rosenbloom, Editor. *Sports Nutrition,* 3d ed. Chicago, IL: The American Dietetic Association. Used with permission.

It is important to emphasize that carbohydrate loading does not always improve performance. There are many adverse side effects of this practice, including extreme gastrointestinal distress, particularly diarrhea. We store water along with the extra glycogen in our muscles, which leaves many athletes feeling heavy and sluggish. Athletes who want to try carbohydrate loading should experiment prior to competition to determine if it is an acceptable and beneficial approach for them (Manore and Thompson 2000).

Recap: Carbohydrate needs increase for active people. In general, athletes should consume 55 to 60% of their total energy as carbohydrate. Consuming carbohydrate sources within the first few hours of recovery can maximize carbohydrate storage rates. Good food sources of carbohydrates for active people include whole grains and cereals, fruits, vegetables, and juices. Carbohydrate loading involves altering physical training and the diet such that the storage of muscle glycogen is maximized in an attempt to enhance endurance performance.

Moderate Fat Consumption Is Enough to Support Most Activities

As you have learned, fat is an important energy source for both moderate physical activity and vigorous endurance training. When athletes reach a physically trained state, they are able to use more fat for energy; in other words, they become better "fat burners." This can also occur in people who are not athletes but who regularly participate in aerobic-type fitness activities. This training effect occurs for a number of reasons including an increase in the number and activity of various enzymes involved in fat metabolism, improved ability of the muscle to store fat, and improved ability to extract fat from the blood for use during exercise. By using fat as a fuel, athletes can spare carbohydrate so they can use it during prolonged, intense training or competition.

Many athletes concerned with body weight and physical appearance believe they should eat less than 15% of their total energy intake as fat, but this is inadequate for vigorous activity. Instead, a fat intake of 15 to 25% of total energy intake is generally recommended for most athletes, with less than 10% of total energy intake as saturated fat. These same recommendations can also be followed by people who are not competitive athletes. Recall from Chapter 5 that fat provides not only energy, but also fat-soluble vitamins and essential fatty acids that are critical to maintaining general health. If fat consumption is too low, inadequate levels of these can eventually prove detrimental to training and performance. Athletes who have chronic disease risk factors such as high blood lipids, high blood pressure, or unhealthful blood glucose levels should work with their physician to adjust their intake of fat and carbohydrate according to their health risks.

> **Recap:** Athletes and physically active people use more fat than carbohydrates for energy because they experience an increase in the number and activity of the enzymes involved in fat metabolism, and they have an improved ability to store fat and extract it from the blood for use during exercise. A dietary fat intake of 15 to 25% is generally recommended for athletes, with less than 10% of total energy intake as saturated fat.

Active People Need More Protein Than Do Inactive People, but Many Already Eat Enough

The protein intakes suggested for competitive athletes and moderately active people are in Table 12.7. Competitive male and female endurance athletes are those individuals who train five to seven days per week for more than an hour each day; many of these individuals may train for 3 to 6 hours per day. These athletes need protein in amounts similar to strength athletes, while the needs of moderate-intensity endurance athletes are slightly higher than the current RDA of 0.8 grams of protein per kg body weight. Moderate-intensity endurance athletes are people exercising four to five times per week for 45 to 60 minutes each time; these individuals may compete in community races and other activities. Recreational endurance athletes are people who exercise four to five times per week for 30 minutes at less than 60% of their maximal effort. These individuals have a protein need that is equal to, or slightly higher than the needs of sedentary people. Strength athletes who are already trained need less protein than those who are initiating training. Studies do not support the contention that consuming more than 2 grams of protein per kg body weight improves protein synthesis, muscle strength, or performance (Tarnopolsky 2000).

As we mentioned earlier, most inactive people and many athletes in the United States consume more than enough protein to support their needs (Manore and Thompson 2000). However, some athletes do not consume enough protein; these typically include individuals with very low energy intakes, vegetarians or vegans who do not consume high-protein food sources, and young athletes who are growing and are not aware of their higher protein needs.

In 1995, Dr. Barry Sears published *The Zone: A Dietary Road Map*, a book that claims numerous benefits of a high-protein, low-carbohydrate diet for athletes (Sears 1995). As we discussed in Chapter 6, low-carbohydrate, high-protein diets have

Table 12.7 Estimated Protein Requirements for Athletes

Group	Protein Requirements (grams per kg body weight)
Competitive male and female athletes	1.4 – 1.6
Moderate-intensity endurance athletes	1.2
Recreational endurance athletes	0.8 – 1.0
Football, power sports	1.4 – 1.7
Resistance athletes, weightlifters (early training)	1.5 – 1.7
Resistance athletes, weightlifters (steady-state training)	1.0 – 1.2

Source: Adapted from M. Tarnopolsky, Protein and amino acid needs for training and bulking up, in *Clinical Sports Nutrition*, edited by L. Burke and V. Deakin (Sydney, AUS: The McGraw-Hill Companies, Inc., 2000), 109.

become quite popular, especially among people who want to lose weight (see Nutrition Debate in Chapter 6, page 228). Unlike many of these diets, the Zone Diet was developed and marketed specifically for competitive athletes. It recommends that athletes eat a 40–30–30 diet, or one comprised of 40% carbohydrate, 30% fat, and 30% protein. Dr. Sears claims that high-carbohydrate diets impair athletic performance because of unhealthy effects of insulin. These claims have never been supported by research — in fact, many of Dr. Sears' claims are not consistent with human physiology. The primary problems with the Zone Diet for athletes are:

- A low-carbohydrate diet is recommended. Years of research have shown that the only way to store sufficient glycogen for athletic performance is to consume a diet relatively high in carbohydrate. For most serious athletes, the Zone Diet is too low in carbohydrate to support training and performance.

- A high-protein diet is recommended, in levels much higher than can ever be used by the body. Some athletes have reported feeling better when eating the Zone Diet. It may be that their protein intake prior to trying the Zone Diet was inadequate so their overall nutrient intake may have improved by following this diet.

- A diet containing 30% of total energy intake from fat is recommended. We know that eating less than 30% of total energy intake from fat helps reduce the risk of chronic diseases for all individuals, including athletes, and eating a higher fat diet is not recommended for health reasons.

- The Zone Diet, if followed as recommended, is a low-energy diet. This diet only provides 1200 to 1300 kcal per day, which is not enough energy for any athlete or even for a recreationally active person.

- It is difficult for the average person to really know if they are eating a 40–30–30 diet. Estimating diet composition involves meticulous counting and recording of calories and grams of fat, carbohydrate, and protein. Many people do not have the time, energy, desire, or expertise to make this determination.

As described in Chapter 6, high-quality protein sources include lean meats, poultry, fish, eggs and egg whites, low-fat dairy products, legumes, and soy products. By following the Food Guide Pyramid and meeting energy needs, people of all fitness levels can consume more than enough protein without the use of supplements or specially formulated foods.

> **Recap:** Protein needs can be higher for athletes and active people. However, most people in the United States already consume more than twice their daily needs for protein. Athletes at risk for low protein intakes include those with low-energy intakes, vegetarians or vegans who do not consume high-protein food sources, and young athletes who are growing and not aware of their higher protein needs. Although low-carbohydrate, high-protein diets have been marketed to athletes, these diets are generally too low in carbohydrate and energy to support regular training and competition.

Regular Exercise Increases Our Need for Fluids

A detailed discussion of fluid and electrolyte balance is provided in Chapter 7. In this chapter, we will briefly review some of the basic functions of water and its role during exercise.

Functions of Water

Water serves many important functions in the body. It is:

- A lubricant that bathes the tissues and cells
- A transport medium for nutrients, hormones, and waste products
- An important component of many chemical reactions, particularly those related to energy production

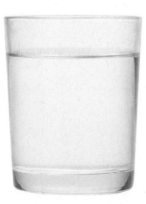

Water is essential for maintaining fluid balance and preventing dehydration.

- A structural part of body tissues such as proteins and glycogen
- A vital component in temperature regulation; without adequate water, we cannot cool our bodies properly through sweating and thereby can cause severe heat illness and even death.

Cooling Mechanisms

When you exercise, your body generates heat. In fact, heat production can increase 15 to 20 times during heavy exercise! The primary way in which we dissipate this heat is through sweating, which is also called **evaporative cooling.** When body temperature rises, more blood (which contains water) flows to the surface of the skin. Heat is carried in this way from the core of our bodies to the surface of our skin. By sweating, the water (and body heat) leaves our bodies and the air around us picks up the evaporating water from our skin, cooling our bodies.

Dehydration and Heat-Related Illnesses

Exercising in extreme heat and humidity is very dangerous for two reasons: the extreme heat dramatically raises body temperature, and the high humidity prohibits evaporative cooling. During periods of high humidity, the environmental air is so saturated with water that it is unable to pull the water from the surface of our skin. Under these conditions, we are unable to cool ourselves adequately, and heat illnesses are likely to occur. It is important to remember that dehydration significantly increases our risk for heat illnesses. General signs of dehydration for adults and children were introduced in Chapter 3, and are listed in Table 3.1 (see page 107). In Table 12.8, specific signs of dehydration during heavy exercise are listed.

Heat illnesses include heat syncope, heat cramps, heat exhaustion, and heatstroke. **Heat syncope** is dizziness that occurs when people stand for too long in the heat, and the blood pools in their lower extremities rather than fully supplying their brains. It can also occur when people stop suddenly after a race or stand suddenly from a lying position. **Heat cramps** are muscle spasms that occur several hours after strenuous exercise. They occur during times when sweat losses and fluid intakes are high, urine volume is low, and sodium intake was inadequate to replace losses. These cramps generally are felt in the legs, arms, or abdomen after a person cools down from exercise.

Heat exhaustion and **heatstroke** occur on a continuum, with unchecked heat exhaustion leading to heatstroke. Early signs of heat exhaustion include excessive sweating, weakness, nausea, dizziness, headache, and difficulty concentrating. As this condition progresses, consciousness becomes impaired. Signs that a person is progressing to heatstroke are hot, dry skin, rapid heart rate, vomiting, diarrhea, an increase in body temperature greater than or equal to 104°F, hallucinations, and coma. It is critical that a person gets proper medical care, or death can result. These illnesses occur because during exercise in the heat, our muscles and skin are constantly competing for blood flow. When there is no longer enough blood flow to simultaneously provide adequate blood to our muscles and to our skin, muscle blood flow takes priority over the skin, which prevents us from cooling ourselves. Body temperature during these conditions becomes dangerously high, and the dehydration that occurs during this situation worsens this overheating condition. Heat cramps and heat exhaustion are highly likely to occur, and

evaporative cooling Another term for sweating, which is the primary way in which we dissipate heat.

heat syncope Dizziness that occurs when people stand for too long in the heat or when they stop suddenly after a race or stand suddenly from a lying position; results from blood pooling in the lower extremities.

heat cramps Muscle spasms that occur several hours after strenuous exercise; most often occur when sweat losses and fluid intakes are high, urine volume is low, and sodium intake is inadequate.

heat exhaustion A heat illness that is characterized by excessive sweating, weakness, nausea, dizziness, headache, and difficulty concentrating. Unchecked heat exhaustion can lead to heatstroke.

heatstroke A potentially fatal heat illness that is characterized by hot, dry skin, rapid heart rate, vomiting, diarrhea, an increase in body temperature greater than or equal to 104°F, hallucinations, and coma.

Table 12.8 Signs of Dehydration During Heavy Exercise

Decreases In:	Increases In:
Exercise performance	Heart rate at a given exercise intensity
Urine output (and urine is dark yellow or brown in color)	Rating of perceived exertion (RPE) during exercise
Appetite	Fatigue and weakness

heatstroke is possible with prolonged exposure or exercise in environmental temperatures between 90 to 130°F; heatstroke is highly likely in temperatures of at least 130°F (National Weather Service 1998).

Guidelines for Proper Fluid Replacement

How can we prevent dehydration and heat illnesses? Obviously, adequate fluid intake is critical before, during, and after exercise. Unfortunately, our thirst mechanism cannot be relied upon to signal when we need to drink. If we rely only on our feelings of thirst, we will not consume enough fluid to support exercise.

General fluid replacement recommendations are based on maintaining body weight. As introduced in Chapter 7, athletes who are training and competing in hot environments should weigh themselves before and after the training session or event and should regain the weight lost over the subsequent 24-hour period. They should avoid losing more than 2 to 3% of body weight during exercise, as performance can be impaired with fluid losses as small as 1% of body weight.

Table 12.9 reviews guidelines for proper fluid replacement. For activities lasting less than one hour, plain water is generally adequate to replace fluid losses. However, for training and competition lasting longer than one hour in any weather, sport beverages containing carbohydrates and electrolytes are recommended. These beverages are also recommended for people who will not drink enough water because they don't like the taste. If drinking these beverages will guarantee adequate hydration, they are appropriate to use. For more specific information about sport beverages, refer to pages 260–261.

> **Recap:** Regular exercise increases our fluid needs. Fluid is critical to cool our internal body temperature and prevent heat illnesses. Dehydration is a serious threat during exercise in extreme heat and high humidity. Heat illnesses include heat syncope, heat cramps, heat exhaustion, and heatstroke. Adequate fluid intake before, during, and after exercise is critical to prevent heat illnesses.

Inadequate Intakes of Some Vitamins and Minerals Can Diminish Health and Performance

When individuals train vigorously for athletic events, their requirements for certain vitamins and minerals may be altered. Many highly active people do not eat enough food or a variety of foods that allows them to consume enough of these nutrients, yet it is imperative that active people do their very best to eat an adequate, varied, and balanced diet to try and meet the increased needs associated with vigorous training.

B Vitamins

The B-complex vitamins are directly involved in energy metabolism (see pages 350–353). There is reliable evidence that the requirements of active people for thiamin, riboflavin, and vitamin B_6 may be slightly higher than the current RDA (Manore and Thompson 2000). However, these increased needs are easily met by consuming adequate energy and a lot of complex carbohydrates, fruits, and vegetables. Athletes and physically active people at risk for poor B-complex vitamin status are those who consume inadequate energy or who consume mostly refined carbohydrate foods such as soda pop and sugary snacks. Vegan athletes and active individuals may be at risk for inadequate intake of vitamin B_{12}; food sources enriched with this nutrient include soy and cereal products.

Calcium and the Female Athlete Triad

Calcium supports proper muscle contraction and ensures bone health (see pages 315–322). Calcium intakes are inadequate for most women in the United States, including both sedentary and active women. This is most likely due to the failure to consume

Table 12.9 Guidelines for Fluid Replacement

Activity Level	Environment	Fluid Requirements (liters per day)
Sedentary	Cool	2 – 3
Active	Cool	3 – 6
Sedentary	Warm	3 – 5
Active	Warm	5 – 10 +

Before Exercise or Competition:

- Drink adequate fluids during 24 hours before event; should be able to maintain body weight

- Drink about 2 – 3 cups (17 – 20 fl. oz.) of water or a sports drink 2 – 3 hours prior to exercise or event to allow time for excretion of excess fluid prior to event

- Drink 1 – 1.5 cups (7 – 10 fl. oz.) of water or a sports drink 10 – 20 minutes prior to event

During Exercise or Competition:

- Drink early and regularly throughout event to sufficiently replace all water lost through sweating, or consume the maximal amount of fluid that can be tolerated; generally 1 – 1.5 cups (7 – 10 fl. oz.) every 10 to 20 minutes is adequate

- Fluids should be cooler than the environmental temperature and flavored to enhance taste and promote fluid replacement

During Exercise or Competition That Lasts More than One Hour:

- Fluid replacement beverage should contain 4 – 8% carbohydrate to maintain blood glucose levels; sodium and other electrolytes should be included in the beverage in amounts of 0.5 – 0.7 grams of sodium per liter of water to replace the sodium lost by sweating.

Following Exercise or Competition:

- Consume at least 2 cups of fluid for each pound of body weight lost

- Fluids after exercise should contain water to restore hydration status, carbohydrates to replenish glycogen stores, and electrolytes (for example, sodium and potassium) to speed rehydration

- Consume enough fluid to permit regular urination and to ensure the urine color is very light or light yellow in color; drinking about 125 to 150% of fluid loss is usually sufficient to ensure complete rehydration

In General:

- Products that contain fructose should be limited, as these may cause gastrointestinal distress

- Caffeine and alcohol should be avoided, as these products increase urine output and reduce fluid retention

- Carbonated beverages should be avoided as they reduce the desire for fluid intake due to stomach fullness

Source: Adapted from R. Murray, Drink more! Advice from a world class expert, *ACSM's Health and Fitness Journal* 1 (1997):19–23. American College of Sports Medicine Position Stand, Exercise and fluid replacement, *Med. Sci. Sports Exerc.* 28 (1996): i–vii. D. J. Casa, L. E. Armstrong, S. K. Hillman, S. J. Montain, R. V. Reiff, B. S. E. Rich, W. O. Roberts, and J. A. Stone, National Athletic Trainers' Association position statement: fluid replacement for athletes, *J. Athletic Training* 35 (2000): 212–224.

foods that are high in calcium, particularly dairy products. While vigorous training does not appear to increase our need for calcium, we need to consume enough calcium to support bone health. If we do not, stress fractures and severe loss of bone can result.

Some female athletes suffer from what is referred to as the Female Athlete Triad (see pages 480–483 for more details). The triad includes three syndromes: eating disorders, osteoporosis, and **amenorrhea** (lack of menstruation for at least three consecutive months in the absence of pregnancy). In this triad, nutritional inadequacies from disordered eating cause irregularities in the menstrual cycle; these in turn cause hormonal disturbances which lead to a significant loss of bone mass. Reduction in bone

amenorrhea Lack of menstruation for at least three consecutive months in the absence of pregnancy.

mass may cause *osteoporosis*, a disease in which the bones become porous and break easily (see page 333). Consuming the recommended amounts of calcium can help prevent osteoporosis. For female athletes who are physically small and consume lower energy intakes, supplementation may be needed to meet current recommendations.

Iron

Iron is a part of the hemoglobin molecule and is critical for the transport of oxygen in our blood to our cells and working muscles. Iron also is involved in energy production. Research has shown that active individuals lose more iron in the sweat, feces, and urine than do inactive individuals and that endurance runners lose iron when their red blood cells break down in their feet due to the high impact of running (Weaver and Rajaram 1992). Female athletes and non-athletes lose more iron than male athletes because of menstrual blood losses, and females in general tend to eat less iron in their diet. Vegetarian athletes and active people may also consume less iron. Thus, many athletes and active people are at higher risk of iron deficiency. Depending upon its severity, poor iron status can impair athletic performance and our ability to maintain regular physical activity.

Not all athletes suffer from iron deficiency. A phenomenon known as *sports anemia* was identified in the 1960s. Sports anemia is not true anemia, but a transient decrease in iron stores that occurs at the start of an exercise program for some people, and it is also seen in athletes who increase their training intensity. Exercise training increases the amount of water in our blood (called *plasma volume*); however, the amount of hemoglobin does not increase until later into the training period. Thus, the iron content in the blood appears to be low but instead is falsely depressed due to increases in plasma volume. Sports anemia, since it is not true anemia, does not affect performance.

The stages of iron deficiency are described in pages 367–368. In general, it appears that physically active females are at relatively high risk of suffering from the first stage of iron depletion, in which iron stores are low (Haymes 1998; Haymes and Clarkson 1998). Because of this it is suggested that blood tests of iron stores and monitoring dietary iron intakes be routinely done for active females (Manore and Thompson 2000). In some cases, iron needs cannot be met through the diet, and supplementation is necessary. Iron supplementation should be done with a physician's approval and proper medical supervision.

> **Recap:** Some athletes may have a greater need for certain vitamins and minerals. Active people may need more thiamin, riboflavin, and vitamin B_6 than inactive people. Exercise itself does not increase our calcium needs, but most women, including active women, do not consume enough calcium. Some female athletes suffer from the female athlete triad, a condition that involves the interaction of disordered eating, osteoporosis, and amenorrhea. Many active individuals require more iron, particularly female athletes and vegetarian athletes.

Theo   *Nutri-Case*

"Ever since I did that cycling test in the fitness lab, I've been watching my carbohydrates. Lately, I've been topping 500 grams of carbs a day. But now I'm beginning to wonder, am I getting enough protein? I'm starting to feel really wiped out, especially after games. We've won four out of the last five games, and I'm giving it everything I've got, but today I was really dragging myself through practice. I'm eating about 150 grams of protein a day, but I think I'm going to try one of those protein powders they sell at my gym. I guess I just feel like, when I'm competing, I need some added insurance."

Theo's weight averages about 170 pounds during practice season. Given what you've learned about the role of the energy nutrients in vigorous physical activity, what do you think might be causing Theo to feel "wiped out"? Would you recommend that Theo try the protein supplement? What other strategies might be helpful for him to consider?

Are Ergogenic Aids Necessary for Active People?

Many competitive athletes and even some recreationally active people continually search for that something extra that will enhance their performance. **Ergogenic aids** are substances used to improve exercise and athletic performance. For example, nutrition supplements can be classified as ergogenic aids, as can anabolic steroids and other pharmaceuticals. Interestingly, people report using ergogenic aids not only to enhance athletic performance, but also to improve their physical appearance, prevent or treat injuries, treat diseases, and help them cope with stress. Some people even report using them because of peer pressure!

As you have learned in this chapter, adequate nutrition is critical to athletic performance and to regular physical activity, and products such as sport bars and beverages can assist athletes with maintaining their competitive edge. However, as we will explore shortly, many of these products are not effective, some are dangerous, and most are very expensive. For the average consumer, it is virtually impossible to track the latest research findings for these products. In addition, many have not been adequately studied, and unsubstantiated false claims surrounding them are rampant. How can you become a more educated consumer about ergogenic aids?

Lightsey and Attaway (1992) describe the most common deceptive practices used to sell ergogenic aids; these are identified in the Highlight box, "Nine Deceptive Practices Used to Market Ergogenic Aids" (page 450). You should also know that, in many cases, research done on a product is misrepresented or is conducted by an inexperienced investigator. It is important that independent laboratories conduct some of the research, as they are more likely to be unbiased. Many companies claim that research is being conducted but state that the findings cannot be shared with the public. This is a warning sign, as there is no need to hide research findings. The use of a celebrity spokesperson is also very common, as celebrity testimonials help to sell products. However, many times this spokesperson is simply being paid to endorse the product and does not actually use it. Finally, it is critical that consumers realize that a patent on a product does not guarantee the effectiveness or safety of that product. Patents are granted solely to distinguish differences among products; indeed, they can be granted on a product that has never been scientifically tested for effectiveness or safety.

New ergogenic aids are available virtually every month, and keeping track of these substances is a daunting task. It is therefore not possible to discuss every available product in this chapter. However, a brief review of a number of currently popular ergogenic aids is provided.

Recap: Ergogenic aids are substances used to improve exercise and athletic performance. Some people also use these substances to improve physical appearance, prevent or treat injuries, treat diseases, or to help them cope with stress. Many ergogenic aids are not effective, some are dangerous, and most are expensive.

Anabolic Products Are Touted as Muscle and Strength Enhancers

Many ergogenic aids are said to be **anabolic,** meaning that they build muscle and increase strength. Most anabolic substances promise to increase testosterone, which is the hormone associated with male sex characteristics and increases muscle size and strength. Although some anabolic substances are effective, they are generally associated with harmful side effects.

Anabolic Steroids

Anabolic steroids are testosterone-based drugs that have been used extensively by strength and power athletes. Anabolic steroids are known to be effective in increasing muscle size, strength, power, and speed. These products are illegal in the United States, and their use is banned by all major collegiate and professional sports organizations, in

ergogenic aids Substances used to improve exercise and athletic performance.

anabolic Refers to a substance that builds muscle and increases strength.

Nine Deceptive Practices Used to Market Ergogenic Aids

1. **General misrepresentation of research:**

   - Published research is taken out of context or findings are applied in an unproven manner.

   - Claims that the product is university-tested may be true, but the investigator may be inexperienced or the manufacturer may control all aspects of the study.

   - Research may not have been done, but company falsely claims it has been conducted.

2. **Company claims that research is currently being done:** Although many companies claim they are doing properly controlled research, most are unable to provide specific information about this research.

3. **Company claims that research is not available for public review:** Consumers have a right to obtain proof about performance claims, and there is no rationale to support hiding research findings.

4. **Testimonials:** Celebrities who endorse a product may only be doing so for the money. Testimonials can be faked, bought, and exaggerated. If the product does work for that person, it may be due to the placebo effect. The **placebo effect** means that even though a product has been proven to have no physiologic benefits, a person believes so strongly in the product that his or her performance improves. It is estimated that there is a 40% chance that any substance will enhance mental or physical performance through the placebo effect.

5. **Patents:** These are granted to indicate distinguishable differences among products. Patents do not indicate effectiveness or safety of a product and can be given without any research being done on a product.

6. **Inappropriately referenced research:**

   - References may include poorly designed and inadequately controlled studies.

   - The company may refer to research that was published in another country and is not accessible in the United States or may base claims on unsubstantiated rumors or unconfirmed reports.

   - The company may cite outdated research that has been proven wrong or fail to quote studies that do not support their claims.

7. **Media approaches:** Advertising modes include infomercials and mass-media marketing videos. While the Federal Trade Commission (FTC) regulates false claims in advertising, products are generally investigated only if they pose significant danger to the public.

8. **Mail-order fitness evaluations:** Used to attract consumers to their products. Most of these evaluations are not specific enough to be useful to the consumer, and their accuracy is highly questionable.

9. **Anabolic measurements:** Some companies perform in-house tests of hair and blood to give consumers information on protein balance. Many times these tests are used inappropriately and only to sell their ergogenic products. The test results may be inaccurate or may indicate nutritional deficiencies that can be remedied with proper nutrition.

Source: All information adapted from D. M. Lightsey and J. R. Attaway. Deceptive tactics used in marketing purported ergogenic aids. *Natl. Strength Cond. Assoc. J.* 14(2) (1992): 26–31. Reprinted by permission of Alliance Communications Group, a division of Allen Press, Inc. ●

---

placebo effect The belief that a product improves performance although it has been proven to have no physiologic benefits.

addition to both the U.S. and the International Olympic Committees. They cause dangerous side effects, including premature closure of growth plates in bones, which can stunt the growth of young athletes who use them. Other side effects include liver cysts, liver dysfunction, increased heart disease risk, high blood pressure, and reproductive dysfunction. Some of the irreversible side effects experienced by women include increased growth of body and facial hair and an enlarged clitoris. Men may grow breast tissue that must be surgically removed. Anabolic steroids also cause mood disturbances, increased aggressiveness, and sleep disturbances.

Androstenedione and Dehydroepiandrosterone

Androstenedione and dehydroepiandrosterone (DHEA) are precursors of testosterone. Manufacturers of these products claim that taking them will increase testosterone levels and muscle strength. Recent studies have found that these products do not increase testosterone levels, and androstenedione has been shown to increase the risk of heart disease in men aged 35 to 65 years (Broeder et al. 2000). There are no studies that support the products' claims of improving strength or increasing muscle mass.

Gamma-Hydroxybutyric Acid

Gamma-hydroxybutyric acid, or GHB, has been promoted as an alternative to anabolic steroids for building muscle. The production and sale of GHB has never been approved in the United States; however, it was illegally produced and sold on the black market. For many users, GHB caused only dizziness, tremors, or vomiting, but others experienced severe side effects, including seizures. Many people were hospitalized and some died.

After GHB was banned, a similar product (gamma-butyrolactone, or GBL) was marketed in its place. This product was also found to be dangerous and was removed from the market. Recently, another replacement product called BD, or 1,4-butanediol was banned because it has caused at least 71 deaths, with 40 more under investigation. BD is an industrial solvent and is listed on ingredient labels as tetramethylene glycol, butylene glycol, or sucol-B. Side effects include wild, aggressive behavior, nausea, incontinence, and sudden loss of consciousness.

Creatine

Creatine is a supplement that has become wildly popular with strength and power athletes. Creatine, or creatine phosphate, is found in meat and fish and stored in our muscles. As described earlier in this chapter, we use creatine phosphate (or CP) to regenerate ATP. By taking creatine supplements, it is hypothesized that more CP is available to replenish ATP, which will prolong a person's ability to train and perform in short-term, explosive activities such as weightlifting and sprinting. Between 1994 and 2004, over 700 research articles related to creatine and exercise in humans were published. Creatine does not seem to enhance performance in aerobic-type events, but this product has been shown to enhance sprint performance in swimming, running, and cycling (Balsom et al. 1995; Grindstaff et al. 1997; Kreider, 1998; Tarnopolsky and MacLennan 2000). Other studies have shown that creatine increases the work performed and the amount of strength gained during resistance exercise (Kreider et al., 1998; Kreider et al. 1999; Volek et al., 1999).

In January 2001, the *New York Times* reported that the French government claimed that creatine use could lead to cancer (Reuters 2001). The news spread quickly across national and international news organizations and over the Internet. These claims were found to be false, as there are absolutely no studies in humans that suggest an increased risk of cancer with creatine use. In fact, there are numerous studies that show an anticancer effect of creatine (Jeong 2000; Ara et al. 1998). Although side effects such as dehydration, muscle cramps, and gastrointestinal disturbances have been reported with creatine use, we have very little information on how long-term use of creatine impacts health. A recent study by Schilling and colleagues (2001) found that the incidence of muscle cramps, injuries, or other side effects were similar for athletes who had never used creatine as compared to those using creatine up to four years. Further research is needed to determine the effectiveness and safety of creatine use over prolonged periods of time.

Recap: Anabolic products are marketed to build muscle and increase strength. Anabolic steroids are effective in increasing muscle size, power, and strength, but they are illegal and can cause serious health consequences. Androstenedione and dehydroepiandrosterone are precursors of testosterone; neither of these products have been shown to effectively increase testosterone levels or to increase strength or muscle mass. Gamma-hydroxybutyric acid was marketed as an alternative to steroids but was banned due to severe and sometimes fatal side effects. Creatine supplements are popular and can enhance sprint performance in swimming, running, and cycling. Little is known about the long-term use of creatine.

Some Products Are Said to Optimize Fuel Use During Exercise

Certain ergogenic aids are touted as increasing energy levels and improving athletic performance by optimizing our use of fat, carbohydrate, and protein. The products reviewed here include caffeine, ephedrine, carnitine, chromium, and ribose.

Caffeine

Caffeine is a stimulant that makes us feel more alert and energetic, decreasing feelings of fatigue during exercise. Caffeine has been shown to increase the use of fat as a fuel during endurance exercise, which spares muscle glycogen and improves performance (Anderson et al. 2000; Spriet and Howlett 2000). It should be recognized that caffeine is a controlled or restricted drug in the athletic world, and athletes can be banned from Olympic competition if urine levels are too high. However, the amount of caffeine that is banned is quite high, and athletes would need to consume caffeine in pill form to reach this level. Side effects of caffeine use include increased blood pressure, increased heart rate, dizziness, insomnia, headache, and gastrointestinal distress.

Ephedrine

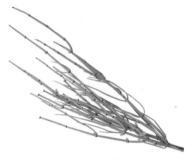

Ephedrine is made from the herb *Ephedra sinica* (Chinese ephedra).

Ephedrine, also known as ephedra, Chinese ephedra, or ma huang, is a strong stimulant marketed as a weight loss supplement and energy enhancer. In reality, many products sold as Chinese ephedra (or herbal ephedra) contain ephedrine from the laboratory and other stimulants such as caffeine. The use of ephedra supplements does not appear to enhance performance, but supplements containing both caffeine and ephedra have been shown to prolong the amount of exercise that can be done until exhaustion is reached (Bucci 2000). Ephedra is known to reduce body weight and body fat in sedentary women, but its impact on weight loss and body fat levels in athletes is unknown. Side effects of ephedra use include headaches, nausea, nervousness, anxiety, irregular heart rate, and high blood pressure, and at least 17 deaths have been attributed to its use (Williams 1998). Ephedra has been banned by the International Olympic Committee for many years, and the U.S. FDA banned the manufacture and sale of ephedra in the United States in 2004 due to its potentially fatal side effects.

Carnitine

Carnitine is a compound made from amino acids that is found in the mitochondrial membrane of our cells. Carnitine helps shuttle fatty acids into the mitochondria so they can be used for energy. In theory, it has been proposed that exercise training depletes our cells of carnitine and that supplementation should increase the amount of carnitine in our cell membranes. By increasing cellular levels of carnitine, we should be able to improve the use of fat as a fuel source. Thus, carnitine is marketed not only as a performance-enhancing substance, but also as a "fat burner." Research studies of carnitine supplementation do not support these claims (Heinonen 1996), as exercise does not appear to reduce the amounts of carnitine in our cells. Use of carnitine supplements has not been associated with significant side effects.

Chromium

Chromium is a trace mineral that enhances insulin's action of increasing the transport of amino acids into the cell (see Chapter 10). It is found in whole grain foods, cheese, nuts, mushrooms, and asparagus. It is theorized that many people are chromium deficient and that supplementation will enhance the uptake of amino acids into muscle cells, which will increase muscle growth and strength. Like carnitine, chromium is marketed as a fat burner, as it is speculated that its effect on insulin stimulates the brain to decrease food intake (Williams 1998). Chromium supplements are available as chromium picolinate and chromium nicotinate. Early studies of chromium supplementation showed promise, but more recent, better-designed studies do not support any benefit of chromium supplementation on muscle mass, muscle strength, body fat, or exercise performance.

Ribose

Ribose is a five-carbon sugar that is critical to the production of ATP. Ribose supplementation is claimed to improve athletic performance by increasing work output and by promoting a faster recovery time from vigorous training. While ribose has been shown to improve exercise tolerance in patients with heart disease (Pliml et al. 1992), no published studies have examined its impact on athletic performance (Coleman 2000).

From this review of ergogenic aids, you can see that most of these products are not effective in enhancing athletic performance or in optimizing muscle strength or body composition. It is important to be a savvy consumer when examining these products to make sure you are not wasting your money or putting your health at risk by using them.

> **Recap:** Caffeine is a stimulant that increases the use of fat during exercise; caffeine is a banned substance in the athletic world due to its potential impact on performance. Ephedrine is a stimulant that has been banned from the United States due to its potentially fatal side effects. Carnitine helps shuttle fatty acids into our mitochondria so they can be used for energy. Carnitine supplements do not enhance fat utilization during exercise or improve athletic performance. Chromium is a trace mineral that is marketed as a fat burner, but chromium supplements do not appear to enhance body composition or athletic performance. Ribose supplementation is claimed to increase work output and promote faster recovery time from training, but no studies have yet been done in athletes to support these claims.

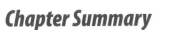

Chapter Summary

- Physical activity is any movement produced by muscles that increases energy expenditure and includes occupational, household, leisure-time, and transportation.

- Leisure-time physical activity is any activity not related to a person's occupation and includes competitive sports and recreational activities. Exercise is a subcategory of leisure-time physical activity and is purposeful, planned, and structured.

- Physical fitness has many components and is defined as the ability to carry out daily tasks with vigor and alertness, without undue fatigue, and with ample energy to enjoy leisure-time pursuits and meet unforeseen emergencies.

- Physical activity provides a multitude of health benefits, including reducing our risks for heart disease, stroke, high blood pressure, obesity, type 2 diabetes, and osteoporosis. Despite these benefits, most Americans are inactive.

- The components of fitness include cardiorespiratory fitness, musculoskeletal fitness (which includes muscular strength and endurance), flexibility, and body composition. Physical fitness is specific to each one of these components.

- To achieve the appropriate overload for fitness, the FIT principle should be followed (frequency, intensity, and time of activity). Frequency refers to the number of activity sessions per week. Intensity refers to how difficult the activity is to perform. Time refers to how long each activity session lasts.

- Warm-up, or preliminary exercise, is important to get prepared for exercise. Warm-up exercises prepare the muscles for exertion by increasing blood flow and temperature.

- Cool-down activities are done after an exercise session is complete. Cool-down activities assist in the prevention of injury and may help reduce muscle soreness.

- Adenosine triphosphate, or ATP, is the common energy source for all cells of the body. The amount of ATP stored in a muscle cell is limited and can only keep a muscle active for about 1 to 3 seconds.

- For maximal activities lasting about 3 to 15 seconds, creatine phosphate can be broken down in an anaerobic reaction to provide energy and support the regeneration of ATP.

- To support activities that last from 30 seconds to 2 minutes, energy is produced from glycolysis. Glycolysis produces 2 ATP molecules for every glucose molecule broken down. Pyruvic acid is the final end product of glycolysis.

- The further metabolism of pyruvic acid in the presence of adequate oxygen provides energy for activities that last from 3 minutes to 4 hours. During this aerobic process, each molecule of glucose can yield 36 to 38 ATP molecules.

- Fat can be broken down aerobically to support activities of low intensity and long duration. Fat is an abundant energy source and it provides more than twice the energy per gram as compared to carbohydrate, but its breakdown process is relatively slow, and it cannot support quick, high intensity activities.

- Amino acids can be used to make glucose to maintain our blood glucose levels during exercise and can contribute from 3 to 6% of the energy needed during exercise. Amino acids also help build and repair tissues after exercise.

- Vigorous intensity exercise requires extra energy, and male athletes typically need more energy than female athletes because of their higher muscle mass and larger body weight. Athletes who are concerned with making a competitive weight or with the aesthetic demands of their sport may be at risk for poor energy and nutrient intakes.

- It is generally recommended that athletes should consume 55 to 60% of their total energy as carbohydrate.

- Carbohydrate loading involves altering physical training and the diet such that the storage of muscle glycogen is maximized in an attempt to enhance endurance performance.

- A dietary fat intake of 15 to 25% is generally recommended for athletes, with less than 10% of total energy intake as saturated fat.

- Protein needs can be higher for athletes and regularly active people, but most people in the United States already consume more than twice their daily needs for protein.

- Athletes at risk for low protein intakes include those with low energy intakes, vegetarians or vegans who do not consume high-protein food sources, and young athletes who are growing and not aware of their higher protein needs.

- Regular exercise increases our fluid needs to help cool our internal body temperature and prevent heat illnesses. Heat illnesses include heat syncope, heat cramps, heat exhaustion, and heatstroke. Adequate fluid intake before, during, and after exercise will help prevent heat illnesses.

- Active people may need more thiamin, riboflavin, and vitamin B_6 than inactive people. Most women, including active women, do not consume enough calcium. Many active individuals also require more iron, particularly female athletes and vegetarian athletes.

- Ergogenic aids are substances used to improve exercise and athletic performance, to improve physical appearance, prevent or treat injuries, treat diseases, or to cope with stress. Many ergogenic aids are not effective, some are dangerous, and most are expensive.

Review Questions

1. For achieving and maintaining cardiorespiratory fitness, the intensity range typically recommended is
   a. 25 to 50% of your estimated maximal heart rate.
   b. 35 to 75% of your estimated maximal heart rate.
   c. 50 to 80% of your estimated maximal heart rate.
   d. 75 to 95% of your estimated maximal heart rate.

2. The amount of ATP stored in a muscle cell can keep a muscle active for about
   a. 1 to 3 seconds.
   b. 10 to 30 seconds.
   c. 1 to 3 minutes.
   d. 1 to 3 hours.

3. To support a long afternoon of gardening, the body predominantly uses which nutrient for energy?
   a. carbohydrate
   b. fat
   c. amino acids
   d. lactic acid

4. Creatine
   a. seems to enhance performance in aerobic-type events.
   b. appears to increase an individual's risk for bladder cancer.
   c. seems to increase strength gained in resistance exercise.
   d. is stored in our liver.

5. Which of the following statements about the rating of perceived exertion (RPE) is true?
   a. An intensity of 12 to 15, or somewhat hard to hard, is recommended to achieve physical fitness.
   b. An intensity of 6 to 9 produces warmth on a cold day and a slight sweat on a warm day.
   c. An intensity of 10 to 11, fairly light, is all that is necessary to achieve cardiovascular fitness.
   d. An intensity of 16 to 19, very hard, should be achieved for at least a few minutes during each exercise session to achieve health-related benefits.

6. **True or false?** A sound fitness program overloads the body.

7. **True or false?** A dietary fat intake of 15 to 25% is generally recommended for athletes.

8. **True or false?** Carbohydrate loading involves altering duration and intensity of exercise and intake of carbohydrate such that the storage of fat is minimized.

9. **True or false?** Sports anemia is a chronic decrease in iron stores that occurs in some athletes who have been training intensely for several months to years.

10. **True or false?** FIT stands for frequency, intensity, and time.

11. Write a plan for a weekly activity/exercise routine that does the following:
    - meets your personal fitness goals
    - is fun for you to do
    - includes variety and consistency
    - uses all components of the FIT principle
    - includes a warm-up and cool-down period

12. Determine how many grams of carbohydrate, protein, and fat you need to consume daily to support the activity/exercise routine you described in the previous question.

13. You decide to start training for your school's annual marathon. After studying this chapter, which of the following preparation strategies would you pursue, and why?
    - use of B vitamin supplements
    - use of creatine supplements
    - use of sports beverages
    - carbohydrate loading

14. Given what you have learned about Gustavo in the Nutri-Cases in previous chapters, would you advise him to begin a planned exercise program of low to moderate intensity? Why or why not? If so, what steps should he take before starting an exercise program?

15. Marisa and Conrad are students at the same city college. Marisa walks to and from school each morning from her home seven blocks away. Conrad lives in a suburb twelve miles away and drives to school. Marisa, an early childhood education major, covers the lunch shift, two hours a day, at the college's day care center, cleaning up the lunchroom and supervising the children in the playground. Conrad, an accounting major, works in his department office two hours a day, entering data into computer spreadsheets. On weekends, Marisa and her sister walk downtown and go shopping. Conrad goes to the movies with his friends. Neither Marisa nor Conrad participate in sports or scheduled exercise sessions. Marisa has maintained a normal, healthful weight throughout the school year, but in the same period of time, Conrad has gained several pounds. Identify at least two factors that might play a role in Marisa's and Conrad's current weight.

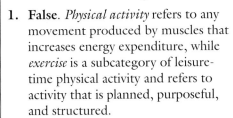

Test Yourself Answers

1. **False**. *Physical activity* refers to any movement produced by muscles that increases energy expenditure, while *exercise* is a subcategory of leisure-time physical activity and refers to activity that is planned, purposeful, and structured.

2. **True**. Up to 40% of Americans report doing no leisure-time physical activity, and another 23% report doing no activity at all, not even on the job.

3. **False**. Each person has to design a fitness program based on his or her own interests and needs. Depending upon a person's fitness goals, being active 20 to 30 minutes each day could be enough for a given individual.

4. **True**. Although lactic acid is one of many contributors to muscle fatigue, recent research has shown that it is not a primary cause of muscle soreness.

5. **True**. Most ergogenic aids are ineffective or do not produce the results that are advertised. Many ergogenic aids, such as anabolic steroids and ephedrine, can actually cause serious health consequences and can even cause death in some instances.

Web Links

www.americanheart.org
American Heart Association
The Healthy Lifestyle section of this site has sections on health tools, exercise and fitness, healthy diet, managing your lifestyle and more.

www.acsm.org
American College of Sports Medicine
Look under Health and Fitness Information for guidelines on healthy aerobic activity, calculating your exercise heart rate range, and the ACSM's Fit Society Page newsletter.

www.webmd.com
WebMD Health
Visit this site to learn about a variety of lifestyle topics, including fitness and exercise.

www.hss.gov
U.S. Department of Health and Human Services
Review this site for multiple statistics on health, exercise,

and weight as well as information on supplements, wellness, and more.

www.niddk.nih.gov/health/nutrit/pubs/physact.
htm
Physical Activity and Weight Control
Find out more about healthy fitness programs.

http://dietary-supplements.info.nih.gov/
NIH Office of Dietary Supplements
Look on this National Institutes of Health site to learn more about the health effects of specific nutritional supplements.

www.nal.usda.gov/fnic/etext/ds_ergogenic.html
Food and Nutrition Information Center
Visit this site for links to detailed information about ergogenic aids and sports nutrition.

http://ag.arizona.edu/nsc/new/sn/publications.htm
Nutrition Exercise Wellness
Check this University of Arizona site for information for athletes on nutrition, fluid intake, and ergogenic aids.

References

American College of Sports Medicine, American Dietetic Association, and Dietitians of Canada. 2000. Nutrition and athletic performance. Joint position statement. *Med. Sci. Sports Exerc.* 32: 2130–2145.

Anderson, M. E., C. R. Bruce, S. F. Fraser, N. K. Stepto, R. Klein, W. G. Hopkins, and J. A. Hawley. 2000. Improved 2000-meter rowing performance in competitive oarswomen after caffeine ingestion. *Int. J. Sport Nutr. Exerc. Metab.* 10: 464–475.

Ara, G., L. M. Gravelin, R. Kaddurah-Daouk, and B. A. Teicher. 1998. Antitumor activity of creatine analogs produced by alterations in pancreatic hormones and glucose metabolism. *In Vivo* 12: 223–231.

Balsom, P. D., K. Söderlund, B. Sjödin, and B. Ekblom. 1995. Skeletal muscle metabolism during short duration high-intensity exercise: influence of creatine supplementation. *Acta Physiol. Scand.* 1154: 303–310.

Blair, S. N., H. W. Kohl III, C. E. Barlow, R. S. Paffenbarger Jr., L. W. Gibbons, and C. A. Macera. 1995. Changes in physical fitness and all-cause mortality: a prospective study of healthy and unhealthy men. *JAMA* 273: 1093–1098.

Broeder, C. E., J. Quindry, K. Brittingham, L. Panton, J. Thomson, S. Appakondu, K. Breuel, R. Byrd, J. Douglas, C. Earnest, C. Mitchell, M. Olson, T. Roy, and C. Yarlagadda. 2000. The Andro Project: physiological and hormonal influences of androstenedione supplementation in men 35 to 65 years old participating in a high-intensity resistance training program. *Arch. Intern. Med.* 160: 3093–3104.

Brooks, G. A. 2000. Intra- and extra-cellular lactate shuttles. *Med. Sci. Sports Exerc.* 32: 790–799.

Brooks, G. A, T. D. Fahey, T. P. White, and K. M. Baldwin. 2000. *Exercise Physiology. Human Bioenergetics*

and Its Applications. Mountain View, CA: Mayfield Publishing Company.

Bucci, L. 2000. Selected herbals and human exercise performance. *Am. J. Clin. Nutr.* 72: 624S–636S.

Burke, L. 2000. Nutrition for recovery after competition and training. In *Clinical Sports Nutrition*, 2d ed., edited by L. Burke and V. Deakin, 396–427.

Caspersen, C. J., K. E. Powell, and G. M. Christensen. 1985. Physical activity, exercise, and physical fitness: definitions and distinctions for heath-related research. *Public Health Reports* 100: 126–131.

Centers for Disease Control and Prevention (CDC). 2003. Prevalence of physical activity, including lifestyle activities among adults — United States, 2000–2001. *Morbid. Mortal. Wkly. Rep.* 52(32): 764–769.

Coleman, E. 2000. Ribose — an ergogenic aid? *Sports Med. Digest* 22: 54.

Gladden, L. B. 2000. Muscle as a consumer of lactate. *Med. Sci. Sports Exerc.* 32: 764–771.

Grindstaff, P. D., R. Kreider, R. Bishop, M. Wilson, L. Wood, C. Alexander, and A. Almada. 1997. Effects of creatine supplementation on repetitive sprint performance and body composition in competitive swimmers. *Int. J. Sport Nutr.* 7: 330–346.

Haymes, E. M. 1998. Trace minerals and exercise. In *Nutrition and Exercise and Sport*, edited by I. Wolinsky. Boca Raton, FL: CRC Press, 1997–2218.

Haymes, E. M., and P. M. Clarkson. 1998. Minerals and trace minerals. In *Nutrition and Sport and Exercise*, edited by J. R. Berning and S. N. Steen. Gaithersburg, MD: Aspen Publishers, 77–107.

Heinonen, O. J. 1996. Carnitine and physical exercise. *Sports Med.* 22: 109–132.

Helmrich, S. P., D. R. Ragland, R. W. Leung, and R. S. Paffenbarger Jr. 1991. Physical activity and reduced occurrence of non-insulin-dependent diabetes mellitus. *N. Engl. J. Med.* 325: 147–152.

Heyward, V. H. 1998. *Advanced Fitness Assessment and Exercise Prescription*, 3d ed. Champaign, IL: Human Kinetics Publishers.

Institute of Medicine, Food and Nutrition Board. 2002. *Dietary Reference Intakes for Energy, Carbohydrates, Fiber, Fat, Protein and Amino Acids (Macronutrients)*. Washington, DC: The National Academy of Sciences.

Jeong, K. S., S. J. Park, C. S. Lee, T. W. Kim, S. H. Kim, S. Y. Ryu, B. H. Williams, R. L. Veech, and Y. S. Lee. 2000. Effects of cyclocreatine in rat hepatocarcinogenesis model. *Anticancer Res.* 20(3A): 1627–1633.

King, A. C., W. L. Haskell, C. B. Taylor, H. C. Kraemer, and R. F. DeBusk. 1991. Group- vs home-based exercise training in healthy older men and women: a community-based clinical trial. *JAMA* 266: 1535–1542.

Kohrt, W. M., M. T. Malley, A. R. Coggan, R. J. Spina, T. Ogawa, A. A. Ehsani, R. E. Bourey, W. H. Martin

3rd, and J. O. Holloszy. 1991. Effects of gender, age, and fitness level on response of Vo$_{2max}$ to training in 60–71 yr olds. *J. Appl. Physiol.* 71: 2004–2011.

Kreider, R. B., M. Ferreira, M. Wilson, P. Grindstaff, S. Plisk, J. Reinardy, E. Cantler, and A. L. Almada. 1998. Effects of creatine supplementation on body composition, strength, and sprint performance. *Med. Sci. Sports Exerc.* 30: 73–82.

Kreider R., M. Ferreira, M. Wilson, and A. L. Almada. 1999. Effects of calcium beta-hydroxy-beta methylbu-tyrate (HMB) supplementation during resistance-training on markers of catabolism, body composition and strength. *Int. J. Sports Med.* 20(8): 503–509.

LaCroix, A. Z., S. G. Leveille, J. A. Hecht, L. C. Grothaus, and E. H. Wagner. 1996. Does walking decrease the risk of cardiovascular disease hospitaliza-tions and death in older adults? *J. Am. Geriatr. Soc.* 44: 113–120.

Leon, A. S., J. Connett, D. R. Jacobs Jr., and R. Raura-maa. 1987. Leisure-time physical activity levels and risk of coronary heart disease and death: the Multiple Risk Factor Intervention Trial. *JAMA* 258: 2388–2395.

Lightsey, D. M., and J. R. Attaway. 1992. Deceptive tac-tics used in marketing purported ergogenic aids. *Natl. Strength Cond. Assoc. J.* 14: 26–31.

Manore, M., and J. Thompson. 2000. *Sports Nutrition for Health and Performance.* Champaign, IL: Human Kinetics Publishers.

National Weather Service, National Oceanic and Atmo-spheric Administration, Department of Commerce. December, 2003 Heat Index Chart. www.crh. noaa.gov/pub/heat.htm (Accessed April 2004).

Olds, S. B., M. L. London, P. W. Ladewig, and M. R. Davidson. 2003. *Maternal-Newborn Nursing and Women's Health Care,* 7th ed. Upper Saddle River, NJ: Prentice Hall Health, 373–374.

Paffenbarger, R. S. Jr., R. T. Hyde, A. L. Wing, and C.-C. Hsieh. 1986. Physical activity, all-cause mortality, and longevity of college alumni. *N. Engl. J. Med.* 314: 605–613.

Pliml, W., T. von Arnim, A. Stablein, H. Hofmann, H. G. Zimmer, and E. Erdmann. 1992. Effects of ribose on exercise-induced ischaemia in stable coronary artery disease. *Lancet* 340(8818): 507–510.

Remick, D., K. Chancellor, J. Pederson, E. J. Zambraski, M. N. Sawka, and C. D. Wenger. 1998. Hyperther-mia and dehydration-related deaths associated with intentional rapid weight loss in three collegiate wrestlers — North Carolina, Wisconsin, and Michi-gan, November – December, 1997. *Morbid. and Mor-tal. Wkly. Rep.* 47: 105–108.

Reuters. 2001. Creatine use could lead to cancer, French government reports. *New York Times,* January 25.

Schilling, B. K., M. H. Stone, A. Utter, J. T. Kearney, M. Johnson, R. Coglianese, L. Smith, H. S. O'Bryant, A. C. Fry, M. Starks, R. Keith, and M. E. Stone. 2001. Creatine supplementation and health variable: a retro-spective study. *Med. Sci. Sports Exerc.* 33: 183–188.

Schwartz, A. L., M. Mori, R. Gao, L. M. Nail, and M. E. King. 2001. Exercise reduces daily fatigue in women with breast cancer receiving chemotherapy. *Med. Sci. Sports Exerc.* 33: 718–723.

Sears, B. 1995. *The Zone: A Dietary Road Map.* New York: HarperCollins Publishers.

Spriet, L. L., and R. A. Howlett. 2000. Caffeine. In *Nutrition in Sport,* edited by R. J. Maughan. Oxford: Blackwell Science, 379–392.

Slattery, M. L., D. R. Jacobs Jr., and M. Z. Nichaman. 1989. Leisure-time physical activity and coronary heart disease death: the U.S. Railroad Study. *Circu-lation* 79: 304–311.

Tanaka, H., K. D. Monahan, and D. R. Seals. 2001. Age-predicted maximal heart rate revisited. *J. Am. Coll. Cardiol.* 37: 153–156.

Tarnopolsky, M. 2000. Protein and amino acid needs for training and bulking up. In *Clinical Sports Nutrition,* edited by L. Burke and V. Deakin, Sydney, AUS: The McGraw-Hill Companies, Inc.

Tarnopolsky, M. A., and D. P. MacLennan. 2000. Crea-tine monohydrate supplementation enhances high-intensity exercise performance in males and females. *Int. J. Sport Nutr. Exerc. Metab.* 10: 452–463.

Thompson, C. 2001. Athletes and eating disorders. http://www.mirror-mirror.org/athlete.htm (Accessed April 2004.)

U.S. Department of Health and Human Services. 1996. *Physical Activity and Health: A Report of the Surgeon General.* Atlanta, GA: U.S. Department of Health and Human Services, Centers for Disease Control and Prevention, National Centers for Chronic Disease Prevention and Health Promotion.

U.S. Department of Health and Human Services. 2000, January. *Healthy People 2010* (Conference Edition, in Two Volumes). Washington, DC.

Volek, J. S., N. D. Duncan, S. A. Mazzetti, R. S. Staron, M. Putukian, A. L. Gomez, D. R. Pearson, W. J. Fink, and W. J. Kraemer. 1999. Performance and muscle fiber adaptations to creatine supplementation and heavy resist-ance training. *Med. Sci. Sports Exerc.* 31: 1147–1156.

Weaver, C. M., and S. Rajaram. 1992. Exercise and iron status. *J. Nutr.* 122: 782–787.

Williams, M. H. 1998. *The Ergogenics Edge.* Champaign, IL: Human Kinetics Publishers.

Nutrition Debate:

How Much Physical Activity Is Enough?

Your aerobics instructor tells you to work out at your target heart rate for twenty minutes a day, whereas your doctor tells you to walk for half an hour three or four times a week. A magazine article exhorts you to work out to the point of exhaustion, while a new weight-loss book claims that you can be perfectly healthy without ever breaking a sweat. And as if these mixed messages about what constitutes "regular physical activity" weren't enough, a recent report from the Institute of Medicine (2002) has inadvertently added to the confusion. In this report, it is recommended that Americans should be active 60 minutes per day to optimize health. This message appears contradictory to the Surgeon General's report published in 1996 (U.S. Department of Health and Human Services 1996), in which it was recommended that Americans need to accumulate 30 minutes of physical activity on most, if not all, days of the week to optimize health.

The publication of the report by the Institute of Medicine resulted in an immediate firestorm of responses from various health organizations condemning the recommendations. The primary concern of these organizations was that consumers would be confused about how much physical activity was enough and that this confusion would result in frustration and lead to people giving up on participating in any physical activity. Another concern was that 60 minutes of physical activity each day is too much to ask a population in which over half are already insufficiently active.

So how much activity is really enough? To try to answer this question, let's take a closer look at how the reports of the Surgeon General and Institute of Medicine differ. The Surgeon General's report considers a combination of what we have learned from exercise training studies and from population-based epidemiological studies. *Exercise training studies* involve taking individuals, putting them through a clearly defined training program, and assessing fitness and health outcomes. These studies consistently show that less fit and older individuals can significantly improve their cardiorespiratory fitness and reduce their risk for chronic diseases by participating in moderate levels of physical activity (King et al. 1991; Kohrt et al. 1991). In contrast, *population-based epidemiological studies* compare self-reports of physical activity and/or fitness to rates of illness and mortality (LaCroix et al., 1996; Blair et al., 1995). In other words, the direct effect of exercise training is not being assessed in these studies; instead, they assess only the relationship between level of physical activity/fitness and rates of disease and premature death. These studies show that unfit, sedentary people suffer from the highest rates of disease and premature mortality and that increased physical activity significantly correlates to decreased risks for chronic diseases and premature mortality.

One challenge highlighted in the Surgeon General's report was how to determine the exact dose of exercise needed to improve physical fitness and health. The authors of this report clearly state that using epidemiological studies to determine this dose is problematic. However, some studies indicate that expending an average of 150 kcal per day, which is equivalent to about 30

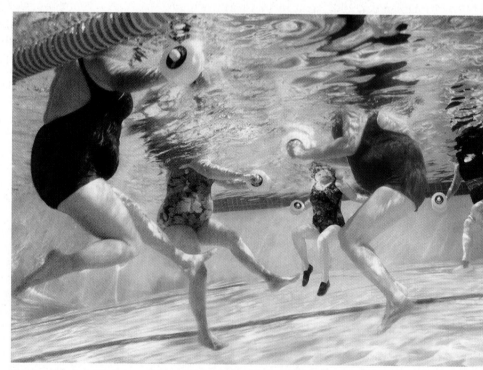

Older and less fit individuals can improve their health and physical fitness with moderate daily activity.

minutes of moderate physical activity per day, is associated with significant reductions in disease risk and premature mortality (Paffenbarger et al. 1986; Leon et al. 1987; Slattery, Jacobs, and Nichaman 1989; Helmrich et al. 1991). This information was used to shape the recommendations put forth in the Surgeon General's report. It is important to emphasize that these recommendations are intended for individuals who are currently inactive. They are not intended to apply to individuals who are already physically active and doing more activity that results in moderate to high fitness levels. In fact, the Surgeon General's report emphasizes that additional health and fitness benefits will result by adding in more time doing moderate-intensity physical activity or by substituting vigorous physical activities for those that are moderate in intensity.

In contrast, the Institute of Medicine based their physical activity recommendations on the assumption of a healthful energy balance, in which energy intake should be equal to the energy expenditure associated with maintaining a healthful body weight. Thus, this group of experts examined studies that measured the amount of energy people expend to maintain a BMI of 18.5 to 25 kg/m^2. After reviewing a large number of studies that assessed energy expenditure and BMI, the Institute of Medicine concluded that participating in about 60 minutes of moderately intense physical activity per day will move people from a very sedentary to an active lifestyle and will allow them to maintain a healthful body weight.

Although this recommendation appears to be very different from that from the Surgeon General's report, and may seem unrealistic, the Institute of Medicine emphasizes that this recommendation includes all activities a person does above resting levels, including gardening, dog-walking, light housekeeping, and shopping.

So are these two recommendations really that different? Probably not. The Surgeon General's recommendation is based on associations among self-reported physical activity levels, physical fitness levels, and disease and mortality rates. Its report clearly states that 30 minutes per day, most days of the week, is the minimum amount of physical activity recommended to improve physical fitness and optimize health. The Institute of Medicine's recommendation is based on studies that precisely determined an energy expenditure associated with a healthful body weight. Its report more clearly defines how much physical activity is needed to maintain a healthful weight and does not focus specifically on disease risk or premature mortality. It is commonly recognized by nutrition and exercise experts and other health professionals that weight loss and healthful weight maintenance is easier to achieve in people who do more physical activity each day, not less.

So how much physical activity is enough for you? To answer this question, you must determine what your fitness goals are and how you can best achieve them. For weight loss, maintenance of weight loss, and to train for athletic competition, you will need to be active for at least 60 minutes each day to achieve your goals. To move from a sedentary to a relatively fit person and to improve your health status, doing at least 30 minutes of moderate physical activity each day will be sufficient. Thus, there is no one right answer to this question for everyone. By considering your health status, current fitness level, personal interests, the time you have available, and your fitness goals, you can determine the right amount of physical activity to meet your goals.

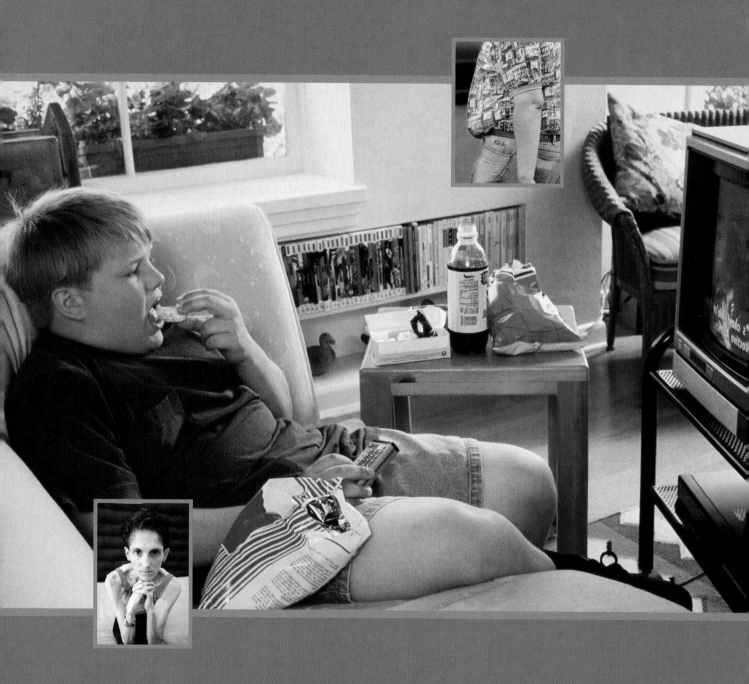

Chapter 13
Disordered Eating

Chapter Objectives

After reading this chapter you will be able to:

1. Explain what is meant by the statement that eating behaviors occur along a continuum, pp. 462–463.

2. Compare and contrast disordered eating behaviors and true clinical eating disorders, pp. 463–464.

3. Identify at least four factors that may contribute to the development of an eating disorder, pp. 464–468.

4. Create a table listing the symptoms and health risks of anorexia nervosa, bulimia nervosa, binge-eating disorder, and chronic dieting, pp. 468–479.

5. Discuss the steps you can use when discussing an eating disorder with a friend or family member, p. 471.

6. List the three components of the female athlete triad and explain how they are interconnected, pp. 479–482.

7. Describe the various treatment options available for people with anorexia nervosa or bulimia nervosa, pp. 482–485.

8. Discuss ways of preventing the development of eating disorders and disordered eating, pp. 485–486.

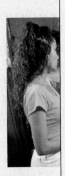

Test Yourself True or False?

1. Only females get eating disorders. T or F

2. No one ever recovers from an eating disorder. T or F

3. Anorexia nervosa has one primary cause. T or F

4. Disordered eating behaviors may lead to the development of a true eating disorder. T or F

5. Obesity can be associated with an eating disorder. T or F

Test Yourself answers can be found at the end of the chapter.

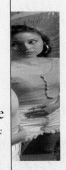

In 1988, at age 16, gymnast Christy Henrich bragged to her coach that she could exist on three apples a day. In 1994, she was dead. A national champion, Henrich failed to make the 1988 Olympic team. During a critique session, a United States judge told her that, at 4'11" tall and 98 pounds, she was too fat. Following that remark, she began restricting her food intake and exercising obsessively. Laxative abuse and forced vomiting soon followed. Her weight fell so dramatically that, a year later, her coach insisted she begin counseling with a psychotherapist and nutritionist. When she stopped attending the sessions, he removed her from the team. Her weight then plummeted to a low of 47 pounds, despite repeated hospital stays of several months and the loving concern of her fiancé, parents, coaches, and friends. In July of 1994, she suffered multiple organ failure, slipped into a coma, and died. When she heard of Henrich's death, Olympic gymnast Kathy Rigby, who twice suffered heart attacks during her own twelve-year battle with eating disorders, burst into tears. Rigby called gymnastics "fertile ground" for eating disorders, which the American College of Sports Medicine confirms afflict a majority of young women in the sport.

Everybody knows that food is essential for life, so why would anyone stop eating? When does normal dieting cross the line into disordered eating? Are there any early warning signs that would tip you off that a friend was crossing that line? If you noticed the signs in one of your friends or teammates, would you confront him or her? If so, what would you say?

This chapter will discuss the continuum of eating behaviors and the negative consequences of moving from more normal to disordered to abnormal eating behaviors. First, we describe eating behaviors and body image as a continuum. We then discuss specific eating disorders and disordered eating behaviors that commonly occur in adolescents and adults. We will also discuss the female athlete triad. Finally, we provide the various treatment options available to those with an eating disorder.

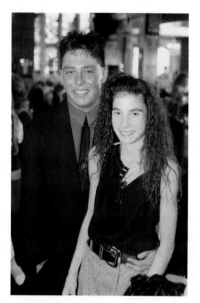

Former gymnast Christy Henrich and her fiancé, a year before she died.

Eating Behaviors Occur on a Continuum

Over the last twenty years, food availability and lifestyle choices have changed dramatically, making it more difficult to describe "normal eating behaviors." The days of a nuclear family sitting down to a home-cooked meal together every evening at 6:00 P.M. seem part of our culture's distant past. Nowadays, our schedules are crammed with classes, jobs, and activities, and our meals are often packaged or eaten out. Skipping meals, eating at odd times, and trying a variety of fad diets are all behaviors commonly accepted as normal. So when does normal eating in a disorderly life cross over into disordered eating or a medically diagnosed eating disorder?

This question is tricky to answer because eating behaviors occur on a *continuum*, a spectrum that can't be divided neatly into parts. An example is a rainbow—where exactly does the red end and the orange begin? Thinking about eating behaviors as a continuum makes it easier to understand how a person could progress from relatively normal eating behaviors to a pattern that is disordered. For instance, let's say that for several years you've skipped breakfast in favor of a midmorning snack, but now you find yourself avoiding the cafeteria until early afternoon. Is this normal? To answer that question, you'd need to consider your feelings about food and your **body image**—the way you perceive your body.

Take a moment to study the Eating Issues and Body Image Continuum in Figure 13.1. Which of the five columns best describes your feelings about food and your body? If you find yourself identifying with the statements on the left side of the continuum, you probably have few issues with food or body image. Most likely you accept your body size and view food as a normal part of maintaining your health and fueling your daily physical activity. As you progress to the right side of the continuum, food and body image become bigger issues, with food restriction becoming the norm. If you identify with the statements on the far right, you are probably afraid of eating and dislike your body. If so, what can you do to begin to move

body image A person's perception of his or her body's appearance and functioning.

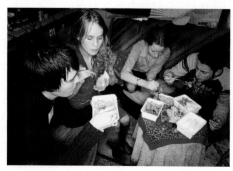

Hectic schedules often force us to grab a quick meal "on the go."

• I am not concerned about what others think regarding what and how much I eat. • When I am upset or depressed I eat whatever I am hungry for without any guilt or shame. • I feel no guilt or shame no matter how much I eat or what I eat. • Food is an important part of my life but only occupies a small part of my time. • I trust my body to tell me what and how much to eat.	• I pay attention to what I eat in order to maintain a healthy body. • I may weigh more than what I like, but I enjoy eating and balance my pleasure with eating with my concern for a healthy body. • I am moderate and flexible in goals for eating well. • I try to follow Dietary Guidelines for healthy eating.	• I think about food a lot. • I feel I don't eat well most of the time. • It's hard for me to enjoy eating with others. • I feel ashamed when I eat more than others or more than what I feel I should be eating. • I am afraid of getting fat. • I wish I could change how much I want to eat and what I am hungry for.	• I have tried diet pills, laxatives, vomiting or extra time exercising in order to lose or maintain my weight. • I have fasted or avoided eating for long periods of time in order to lose or maintain my weight. • I feel strong when I can restrict how much I eat. • Eating more than I wanted to makes me feel out of control.	• I regularly stuff myself and then exercise, vomit, use diet pills or laxatives to get rid of the food or calories. • My friends/family tell me I am too thin. • I am terrified of eating fat. • When I let myself eat, I have a hard time controlling the amount of food I eat. • I am afraid to eat in front of others.
FOOD IS NOT AN ISSUE	**CONCERNED WELL**	**FOOD PREOCCUPIED/ OBSESSED**	**DISRUPTIVE EATING PATTERNS**	**EATING DISORDERED**
BODY OWNERSHIP	**BODY ACCEPTANCE**	**BODY PREOCCUPIED/ OBSESSED**	**DISTORTED BODY IMAGE**	**BODY HATE/ DISASSOCIATION**
• Body image is not an issue for me. • My body is beautiful to me. • My feelings about my body are not influenced by society's concept of an ideal body shape. • I know that the significant others in my life will always find me attractive. • I trust my body to find the weight it needs to be at so I can move and feel confident of my physical body.	• I base my body image equally on social norms and my own self-concept. • I pay attention to my body and my appearance because it is important to me, but it only occupies a small part of my day. • I nourish my body so it has the strength and energy to achieve my physical goals. • I am able to assert myself and maintain a healthy body without losing my self-esteem.	• I spend a significant time viewing my body in the mirror. • I spend a significant time comparing my body to others. • I have days when I feel fat. • I am preoccupied with my body. • I accept society's ideal body shape and size as the best body shape and size. • I'd be more attractive if I was thinner, more muscular, etc...	• I spend a significant amount of time exercising and dieting to change my body. • My body shape and size keeps me from dating or finding someone who will treat me the way I want to be treated. • I have considered changing or have changed my body shape and size through surgical means so I can accept myself. • I wish I could change the way I look in the mirror.	• I often feel separated and distant from my body—as if it belongs to someone else. • I hate my body and I often isolate myself from others. • I don't see anything positive or even neutral about my body shape and size. • I don't believe others when they tell me I look OK. • I hate the way I look in the mirror.

Figure 13.1   The Eating Issues and Body Image Continuum. The progression from normal eating to eating disorders occurs on a continuum. People whose responses fall to the far left of the continuum have normal eating patterns and do not suffer from an eating disorder. People whose responses fall to the far right of the continuum most likely suffer from an eating disorder such as anorexia nervosa or bulimia nervosa. (Smiley/King/Avoy: Campus Health Service. Original Continuum, C. Shlaalak: Preventive Medicine and Public Health. Copyright © 1997 Arizona Board of Regents. Used with permission.)

toward the left side of the continuum? How can you begin to develop a more healthful approach to food selection and to view your body in a more positive light? Before you can begin to find solutions, you need to understand the many complex factors that contribute to eating disorders and disordered eating and the differences between these terms.

What Is the Difference between an Eating Disorder and Disordered Eating?

The media, consumers, and health professionals frequently use the terms *eating disorder* and *disordered eating* interchangeably. Do they mean the same thing? The answer is no! An **eating disorder** is a psychiatric condition that must be diagnosed by a physician and involves extreme body dissatisfaction and long-term eating patterns that

eating disorder   An eating disorder is a psychiatric disorder that must be clinically diagnosed by a physician and is characterized by severe disturbances in body image and eating behaviors. Anorexia nervosa and bulimia nervosa are two examples of eating disorders for which specific diagnostic criteria must be present for diagnosis.

negatively affect body functioning. The behaviors of someone with an eating disorder typically include severe food restriction, obsessive exercising, self-induced vomiting, and/or laxative abuse. Before a physician can diagnose an eating disorder, the patient's condition and behavior must meet specific diagnostic criteria outlined by the American Psychiatric Association's (APA) *Diagnostic and Statistical Manual of Mental Disorders (DSM-IV)* (1994).

The two more commonly diagnosed eating disorders are anorexia nervosa and bulimia nervosa. *Anorexia nervosa* is a potentially life-threatening eating disorder that is characterized by self-starvation, which eventually leads to severe nutrient deficiencies. In contrast, *bulimia nervosa* is characterized by recurrent episodes of extreme overeating and compensatory behaviors to prevent weight gain, such as self-induced vomiting, misuse of laxatives, fasting, or excessive exercise. Both disorders will be discussed in detail later in the chapter.

In contrast, **disordered eating** is a general term used to describe a variety of abnormal or atypical eating behaviors that people use to achieve or maintain a lower body weight. These behaviors may be as simple as going on and off diets or as extreme as refusing to eat any fat. Such behaviors don't usually continue for long enough to make the person seriously ill, nor do they significantly disrupt the person's normal routine. In fact, most people who engage in disordered eating behaviors from time to time don't consider what they're doing as abnormal. However, sometimes such behaviors disturb people enough to cause them to seek medical care. The American Psychiatric Association's *DSM–IV* diagnosis that would apply to these individuals is "Eating Disorders Not Otherwise Specified" (EDNOS) (Walsh and Garner 1997; APA 1994). It is estimated that one-third of all people treated for eating disorders receive a diagnosis of EDNOS (Patrick 2002). As we have said, not all atypical eating behaviors qualify as EDNOS; thus, we use the more inclusive term *disordered eating* throughout the remainder of this chapter.

> **Recap:** Eating behaviors occur along a continuum from normal to somewhat abnormal to disordered. Our feelings about food and our body images influence our eating behaviors. True eating disorders are psychiatric conditions characterized by long-term behavior patterns that negatively affect body functioning, whereas disordered eating is a more general term applicable to any of a variety of abnormal or atypical eating behaviors that may not seriously impair health or functioning.

What Factors Contribute to the Development of Eating Disorders?

The factors that result in the development of an eating disorder are very complex, but research indicates that a number of psychological, interpersonal, social, and genetic and biological factors may contribute in any particular individual (Table 13.1).

Family Environment

Most of us recognize that family conditioning influences our eating behaviors. During childhood, our parents and other family members provided most of the food we ate, limiting our choices and influencing our developing concept of how much food to eat, when, how often, and so forth. As we grew, our families developed unique mealtime rituals. For example, perhaps your family never sat down together at a meal, and you were responsible for getting your own meals. Or perhaps your family insisted on a shared mealtime, and one family member was responsible for preparing the meal for the whole family. We also had experiences that caused us to associate food with particular family members or shared activities. Maybe you really like hot oatmeal with brown sugar and raisins on winter days because your grandmother prepared this for

disordered eating Disordered eating is a general term used to describe a variety of abnormal or atypical eating behaviors that are used to keep or maintain a lower body weight. Individuals with disordered eating behaviors do not have severe enough eating disturbances to be medically diagnosed with an eating disorder such as anorexia nervosa or bulimia nervosa. The designation of "Eating Disorders Not Otherwise Specified" is the medical term used to describe these individuals.

Table 13.1   Risk Factors that May Contribute to the Development of an Eating Disorder

Psychological Factors	Interpersonal Factors	Social Factors	Genetic and Biological Factors*
Low self-esteem Feelings of inadequacy or lack of control over life Depression, anxiety, anger, or loneliness	Troubled family and personal relationships Difficulty expressing emotions and feelings History of being teased or ridiculed based on size or weight History of physical or sexual abuse	Cultural pressures to be "thin" and the high value placed on a "perfect body" Narrow definitions of beauty that include only women and men of a certain body size Cultural norms that value people on the basis of physical appearances and not inner qualities and strengths	Chemical imbalances that control hunger, appetite, and digestion Possible gene or set of genes that predisposes individual

*These factors are still under investigation.

Source: Adapted from National Eating Disorders Association (NEDA), © 2002. Causes of Eating Disorders. Used with permission. http://www.nationaleatingdisorders.org/p.asp?WebPage_ID5322&Profile_ID541144 Accessed April 2004.

you when you visited for the holidays. Because of such family patterns, rituals, and associations, our response to food and our eating behaviors are to some extent conditioned. Thus, it is not difficult to believe that the family eating environment might contribute to the development of an eating disorder.

Researchers have examined a number of family-related factors to determine whether or not they contribute to the development of eating disorders. Currently, there are no data to suggest that family size or birth order is influential. Research on siblings, however, does show a greater likelihood of developing an eating disorder if a sibling also has an eating disorder. The precise reason for this is unclear. Family structure and patterns of interaction have also been implicated. Based on observational studies, compared to "normal" families, families with an anorexic member show more rigidity in their family structure, less clear interpersonal boundaries, and a tendency to avoid open discussions on topics of disagreement. Conversely, families with a member diagnosed with bulimia nervosa have a less stable family organization, are less nurturing, and more angry and disruptive than "normal" families (Vandereycken 2002). In addition, childhood physical or sexual abuse can increase the risk of an eating disorder developing in a child (Patrick 2002). In short, family conditioning, structure, and patterns of interaction, including abuse, can influence the development of an eating disorder.

Unrealistic Media Images

As media saturation has increased over the last century, so has the incidence of eating disorders among white women (Striegel-Moore and Smolak 2002). Every day, we are confronted with advertisements in which computer-enhanced images of lean, beautiful women promote everything from beer to cars (Figure 13.2). Most adult men and women understand that these images are unrealistic, but adolescents, who are still developing a sense of their identity and body image, lack the same ability to distance themselves from what they see (Steinberg 2002). Adolescent girls are likely to compare themselves unfavorably to these "perfect" female bodies and to develop a negative body image as a result. Since body image influences eating behaviors, it is not unlikely that the barrage of media models may be contributing to an increase in eating disorders. Unfortunately, scientific evidence demonstrating whether the media is *causing* increased eating disorders is difficult to obtain.

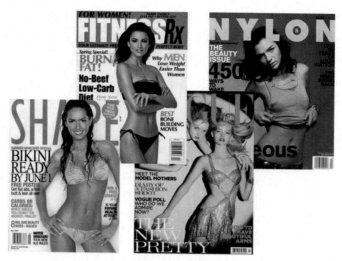

Figure 13.2 Photos of celebrities or models are often airbrushed or altered to "enhance" physical appearance. Unfortunately, many people believe that these are accurate images and strive to reach this unrealistic image of physical beauty.

Sociocultural Values

Evidence suggesting that Western sociocultural values contribute to eating disorders is also hard to deny. For instance, consider the fact that eating disorders are significantly more common in white females in Western societies than in other women worldwide. This may be due in part to our culture's valuing of slenderness, not only for aesthetic reasons, but because Westerners tend to consider it as an indication that the person is self-disciplined, a generally valued characteristic. Westerners also associate slenderness with health and often with wealth. In contrast, until quite recently, the prevailing view in developing societies has been that excess body fat is desirable as a sign of material abundance.

Recent research among Native American children illustrates that body dissatisfaction and desire for thinness is more common in this population than previously assumed. Rural (Davis and Lambert 2000; Stevens et al. 1999) and urban (Rinderknecht and Smith 2002) Native American children were asked to rate their own satisfaction with their bodies using the images shown in Figure 13.3. In all of these studies, girls reported higher rates of body dissatisfaction than boys, and overweight children more often chose a thinner body size as more desirable. Surprisingly, 38 to 61% of fourth and fifth grade children reported already trying to lose weight at this young age.

Only limited research has examined the prevalence of eating disorders in nonwhite populations and in non-Western cultures; thus, we have a lot to learn about how culture affects the development of eating disorders. However, as cross-cultural interactions increase, some researchers hypothesize that non-Western cultures will adapt Western norms for beauty, and this may increase the development of eating disorders in those cultures.

The members of society with whom we most often interact—our family members, friends, teachers, and coworkers—also influence the way we see ourselves. Their comments related to our body weight or shape can be particularly hurtful—enough so to cause some people to start down the path of disordered eating. For example, individuals with bulimia nervosa report that they perceived greater pressure from their peers to be thin than controls, while research shows that peer teasing about weight increases body dissatisfaction and eating disturbances (Stice 2002). Thus, our comments to others regarding their weight do count.

Girls

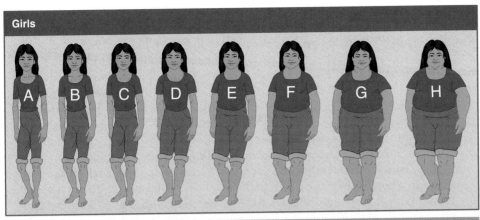

Boys

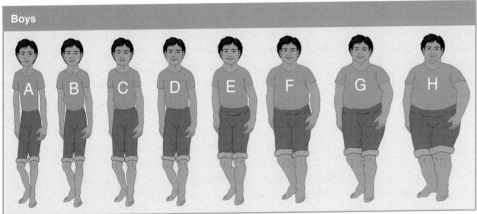

Figure 13.3   These line drawings were used in studies of Native American schoolchildren to assess levels of body dissatisfaction in this population. (J. Stevens, M. Story, A. Becenti, S. A. French, J. Gittelsohn, S. B. Going, Juhaeri, S. Levin, and D. M. Murray. Weight-related attitudes and behaviors in fourth grade American Indian children. *Obes. Res.* 7 (1999): 34–42.)

Personality Traits

Researchers have long been interested in the question of whether certain personalities predispose one to the development of an eating disorder. The reverse question has also been asked: Does an eating disorder modify personality traits, making changes in personality a consequence of the disorder instead of a cause?

A number of studies suggest that people with anorexia nervosa exhibit increased rates of obsessive-compulsive behaviors and perfectionism. They also tend to be socially inhibited, compliant, and emotionally restrained (Wonderlich 2002). Unfortunately, many studies observe these behaviors only in individuals who are very ill and in a state of starvation, which may affect personality. Thus, it is difficult to determine if personality is the cause or effect of the disorder. For example, research shows that perfectionism is high in malnourished individuals and takes a long time to change after recovery (Wonderlich 2002).

In contrast to individuals with anorexia nervosa, individuals with bulimia nervosa tend to be more impulsive, have low self-esteem, and demonstrate an extroverted erratic personality style that seeks attention and admiration. For example, a comparison of diaries kept by individuals with bulimia nervosa and healthy controls indicated that those with bulimia nervosa showed greater self-criticism and deterioration in mood following a stressful interpersonal interaction (Steiger, Lehoux, and Gauvin 1999). In individuals with bulimia nervosa, negative moods are more likely to cause overeating than food restriction (Wonderlich 2002). Finally, individuals with bulimia nervosa are more likely to practice substance abuse and suffer from anxiety disorders.

Genetic and Biological Factors

Overall, the diagnosis of anorexia nervosa and bulimia nervosa is several times more common in biological relatives who also have the diagnosis than in the general population (Strober and Bulik 2002). This observation would imply that existence of some mechanism of transmission of the disease occurs within families; however, it is difficult to separate the impact of genetic and environmental components in many studies. One way to address this issue is to look at the incidence of eating disorders in twins. The heritability of bulimia nervosa was examined in this way in a series of studies from the Virginia Twin Registry (Kendler et al. 1991). They found that heritability and specific environmental influences each accounted for approximately 50% of the variability in who was diagnosed with bulimia nervosa. Although researchers are looking for a specific gene or sets of genes that may be a factor in eating disorders, there are no candidate genes identified at this time.

In addition, biological factors may play a role, although this contention is also under investigation. Currently, researchers are looking at imbalances in the chemicals that control hunger, appetite, and digestion. Among these are hormones produced in our central nervous system, such as serotonin, dopamine, and cholecystokinin, and ghrelin, a polypeptide released from our stomach and small intestine (Bailor and Kaye 2003; Tanaka et al. 2003).

> **Recap:** A number of factors are thought to influence the development of eating disorders. These include our family environment, the media, society, and culture, as well as our personalities and our genetic make-up. However, the combination of factors triggering the development of an eating disorder in any individual is probably unique.

What Does an Eating Disorder Look Like?

An eating disorder can be defined as a "persistent disturbance of eating behavior which significantly impairs physical health or psychosocial functioning" (Fairburn and Walsh 2002, p. 171). As we will discuss below, anorexia nervosa and bulimia nervosa fit this description.

Anorexia Nervosa Is a Potentially Deadly Eating Disorder

anorexia nervosa A serious, potentially life-threatening eating disorder that is characterized by self-starvation, which eventually leads to a deficiency in energy and essential nutrients that are required by the body to function normally. For an individual to be considered to have anorexia nervosa, he/she must be medically diagnosed by a physician and meet specific diagnostic criteria.

Anorexia nervosa is a medical disorder in which an individual uses a number of unhealthful practices to maintain a body weight less than 85% of expected, as based on height and weight. According to the American Psychiatric Association (1994), 90 to 95% of individuals with anorexia nervosa are young girls or women. Approximately 0.5 to 1% of U.S. females develop anorexia, and between 5 and 20% of these will die from complications of the disorder within ten years of initial diagnosis (Patrick 2002). These statistics make anorexia nervosa the most common and deadly psychiatric disorder diagnosed in women and the leading cause of death in females between the ages of 15 and 24 years (Patrick 2002). Anorexia nervosa also occurs in males, but the prevalence is much lower than in females (Robb and Dadson 2002).

Symptoms of Anorexia Nervosa

amenorrhea Amenorrhea is the absence of a menstrual period. Primary amenorrhea is the absence of menstruation by the age of sixteen years in a girl who has secondary sex characteristics, while secondary amenorrhea is the absence of the menstrual period for three or more months after menarche. The presence of amenorrhea is a criterion for the diagnosis of anorexia nervosa.

For people who develop anorexia nervosa, the trigger factors that initiated the disorder may differ widely, but the results are the same: extremely restrictive eating practices that lead to self-starvation (Figure 13.4). These individuals have such an intense drive for thinness and need for weight loss that they may fast completely, restrict energy intake to only a few calories per day, or eliminate all but one or two food groups from their diet. They also have an intense fear of weight gain or becoming fat, even though they are underweight. In anorexic individuals, small amounts of weight gain (e.g., one or two pounds) trigger high stress and anxiety. Finally, **amenorrhea** (no menstrual periods for at least three months) is a feature of anorexia nervosa in females. *Primary amenorrhea* occurs when a girl has not yet begun to menstruate by age 16, even though she has secondary sex characteristics; *secondary amenorrhea* is the absence of a menstrual peroid for three or more months after menarche. It occurs when a young woman consumes insufficient calories to maintain normal body functions.

The *DSM-IV* (APA, 1994) identifies the following conditions of anorexia nervosa:

- Refusal to maintain body weight at or above a minimally normal weight for age and height
- Intense fear of gaining weight or becoming fat, even though considered underweight by all medical criteria
- Disturbance in the way in which one's body weight or shape is experienced, undue influence of body weight or shape on self-evaluation, or denial of the seriousness of the current low body weight
- Amenorrhea in females who are past puberty. Amenorrhea is defined as the absence of at least three consecutive menstrual cycles. A woman is considered to have amenorrhea if her periods occur only when given hormones, such as estrogen or oral contraceptives.

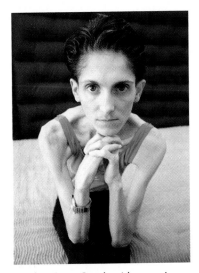

Figure 13.4 People with anorexia experience an extreme drive for thinness, resulting in potentially fatal weight loss.

Do you know anyone who might have anorexia nervosa? How can you determine if they have this eating disorder? Table 13.2 lists behavioral, emotional, mental, and physical signs of anorexia nervosa that you might look for in someone you suspect may have this disorder. Remember, one person may not display all of these characteristics, but you may observe one or two characteristics in each category.

Health Risks of Anorexia Nervosa

Left untreated, anorexia nervosa eventually leads to a deficiency in energy and other nutrients that are required by the body to function normally. During this period of self-imposed starvation, the body will use stored fat and lean tissue (e.g., organ and muscle tissue) as energy sources to maintain brain tissue and vital body functions. The body will also shut down or reduce nonvital body functions to conserve energy. For example, the menstrual cycle will stop, thus conserving the energy required for normal periods and eliminating the chance of pregnancy during a period when there are inadequate nutrients to support a growing fetus. In children and adolescents, growth slows or stops because the body does not have enough energy to support the formation of new tissue.

In addition, people with anorexia nervosa may have many of the following health problems. The severity of these problems will depend on the length of time they have had the disorder and the degree of weight loss that has occurred.

- Electrolyte imbalances—These imbalances can lead to irregular heartbeats, heart failure, and death. The role of electrolytes in our health is discussed in detail in Chapter 7.
- Cardiovascular problems—Rapid heart rate, low blood pressure, dizziness, and fainting can all occur as a result of starvation.
- Gastrointestinal problems—The gastrointestinal tract can become weak and lose its ability to function. These changes result in irritable bowel syndrome, constipation, loss of peristalsis, and delayed emptying of food from the intestines. People with anorexia nervosa frequently complain of stomach pain.
- Bone problems—The malnutrition that accompanies starvation can deprive the body of bone-building nutrients such as calcium. The amenorrhea that occurs is associated with a decrease in estrogen production, which causes poor bone health and can lead to osteoporosis (see Chapter 9).

Because the best chances for recovery occur when an individual receives intensive treatment early, it is important to recognize the early warning signs of anorexia nervosa. Use these warning signs as a guide to help identify those at risk for anorexia

Table 13.2   Behavioral, Emotional, Mental, and Physical Signs of Anorexia Nervosa

Behavioral Signs	Emotional and Mental Signs	Physical Signs
Difficulty eating with others, lying about eating	Depression and social isolation (e.g., withdrawal from usual friends and avoiding any social situations where food is being served)	Low body weight (15% or more below what is expected for age, height, activity level)
Frequently weighing self; measuring food portions, caloric intake, and/or fat grams	Strong need to be in control; rigid and inflexible	Lack of energy, fatigue, muscle weakness due to low energy intakes and malnutrition
Development of food rituals such as eating foods in a certain order, excessive chewing, and/or rearranging food on the plate	Decreased interest in sex or fears around sex	Decreased balance and unsteady gait due to loss of muscle tissue and bone density
Refusal to eat certain foods, such as carbohydrates, fats, and/or foods of a particular color	Low sense of self worth — uses weight as a measure of worth	Lowered body temperature, blood pressure, and pulse rate and irregular heartbeat due to malnutrition, poor maintenance of blood electrolytes and loss of body fat and lean tissue
Avoidance of meal times or other situations involving food	Difficulty expressing feelings; afraid to discuss their food and body issues with others	Tingling in hands and feet due to poor circulation
Excessive, rigid exercise regimen	Perfectionistic — strives to be the neatest, thinnest, or smartest person in the group	Thinning hair or hair loss, lanugo (downy growth of body hair due to poor nutrition)
Frequent comments revealing disgust with body size or shape and focusing on parts of the body that are not perfect (e.g., buttocks, thighs, stomach)	Difficulty thinking clearly or concentrating due to malnutrition and poor energy intake	
Distortion of body size (e.g., feels fat even though others tell them they are too thin)	Irritability, denial — believes others are overreacting to their low weight or energy restriction	
Denial of hunger	Insomnia	

nervosa and to encourage them to seek help. Discussing a friend's eating disorder can be difficult. It is important to choose an appropriate time and place to raise your concerns, and that you listen closely and with great sensitivity to their feelings. The accompanying Highlight box, Discussing an Eating Disorder with a Friend or Family Member: What Do You Say?, outlines an approach you might use in confronting a friend or family member who might have an eating disorder.

> **Recap:** Anorexia nervosa is a severe, life-threatening disorder in which the person refuses to maintain a minimally normal body weight, is intensely afraid of gaining weight, and exhibits a significant distortion in the perception of body size and shape. Knowing the early warning signs of anorexia nervosa can help you identify friends and family members at risk for this disorder.

Bulimia Nervosa Is Characterized by Binging and Purging

bulimia nervosa A serious eating disorder characterized by recurrent episodes of binge eating and recurrent inappropriate compensatory behaviors (such as self-induced vomiting; misuse of laxatives, diuretics, enemas, or other medications; fasting or excessive exercise) in order to prevent weight gain.

binge eating Consumption of a large amount of food in a short period of time, usually accompanied by a feeling of loss of self-control.

purging An attempt to rid the body of unwanted food by vomiting or other compensatory means, such as excessive exercise, fasting, or laxative abuse.

Bulimia nervosa is an eating disorder characterized by repeated episodes of **binge eating,** followed by some form of **purging.** While binge eating, the person feels a loss of self-control (Garfinkel 2002), including an inability to end the binge once it has started. At the same time, the person feels a sense of euphoria not unlike a drug-induced high. For practical purposes, a binge is usually determined on an individual basis, but generally it is a quantity of food that would be large for the individual, compared to what other people eat, and for the time period and social occasion (Garfinkel 2002). For example, a person may eat a dozen brownies with two quarts of ice cream in thirty minutes. Binge episodes occur an average of twice a week or more (APA 1994). An individual with bulimia nervosa typically purges after most episodes,

Discussing an Eating Disorder with a Friend or Family Member: What Do You Say?

Background: Before approaching a friend or family member you suspect to have an eating disorder, learn as much as possible as you can about the eating disorder. Make sure you know the difference between the facts and myths about eating disorders. Locate a health professional specializing in eating disorders to whom you can refer your friend, and be ready to go with your friend if he or she does not want to go alone. If you are at a university or college, check with your local health center to see if they have an eating disorder team or can recommend someone to you. Set the stage for your discussion by finding a relaxed and private setting.

Steps to use in your discussion:

• Schedule a time to talk. Set aside a time and place for a private discussion where you can share your concerns openly and honestly in a caring and supportive way. Make sure the setting is quiet and away from other distractions.

• Communicate your concerns. Share your memories and knowledge of specific times when you felt concerned about your friend's eating or exercise behaviors. Explain that you think these things may indicate that there could be a problem that needs professional attention.

• Ask your friend to explore these concerns with a counselor, doctor, nutritionist, or other health professional who is knowledgeable about eating issues.

• Avoid conflicts or a "battle of the wills" with your friend. If your friend refuses to acknowledge that there is a problem, restate your feelings and the reasons for them and leave yourself open and available as a supportive listener.

• Avoid placing shame, blame, or guilt on your friend regarding their actions or attitudes. Do not use accusatory "you" statements such as, "You just need to eat" or "You are acting irresponsibly." Instead use "I" statements such as, "I am concerned about you because you refuse to eat breakfast and lunch" or "It makes me afraid when I hear you vomit."

• Avoid giving simple solutions. For example, "If you would just stop, everything would be fine."

• Express your continued support. Remind your friend that you care and want your friend to be healthy and happy.

Source: Adapted from National Eating Disorders Association. 2002. Communication: What Should I Say? http://www.nationaleatingdisorders.org/p.asp?WebPage_ID=322&Profile_ID=41174 Accessed April 2004. Used with permission. ●

---

but not necessarily on every occasion, and weight gain as a result of binge eating can be significant.

The prevalence of bulimia nervosa is higher than anorexia nervosa and estimated to affect 1 to 4% of women. Like anorexia nervosa, bulimia nervosa is found predominately in women, with the male-female prevalence ratio ranging from 1:6 to 1:10 (APA 2000). This means that for every one male diagnosed with bulimia nervosa, six to ten females are diagnosed with this disorder. The mortality rate is much lower than for anorexia nervosa, with 1% of patients dying within 10 years of diagnosis (Patrick 2002). Statistics on bulimia nervosa are somewhat misleading, because about half of anorexic individuals will also be diagnosed with bulimia at some point. Thus, many of the women who die of anorexia nervosa may also have bulimia.

Although the prevalence of bulimia nervosa is much higher in women than men (Robb and Dadson 2002), rates for men are higher in some predominately thin-build male sports in which participants are encouraged to maintain a low body weight (e.g., horse racing, wrestling, crew, and gymnastics). Individuals in these sports typically do not have all the characteristics of bulimia nervosa, however, and the purging behaviors they practice typically stop once the sport is discontinued.

The binge-purge pattern of disordered eating may begin as an infrequent occurrence in which a person attempts to deal with unwanted food in a social situation. For example, friends are having a pizza party and the person wants to join in but feels

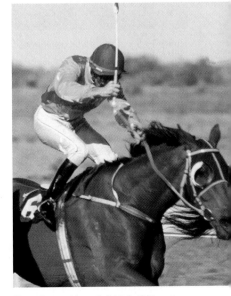

Men who participate in "thin build" sports, such as jockeys, have a higher risk for bulimia nervosa than men who do not.

guilty about eating so much food. So upon returning home, the person induces vomiting, takes laxatives, or stays up late exercising to burn off the extra calories. What may begin as an isolated incident can develop into a daily event, with purging occurring even after the person has eaten only a small amount of food. Binging and purging behaviors can also be triggered by periods of dieting: depriving oneself of adequate food and energy for a long period of time requires tremendous self-control, and when the control fails, such as if the person "cheats" even once, he or she can quickly lose any ability to deal with food rationally.

Many people with bulimia engage in vomiting as a way of purging unwanted foods. Other methods of purging are laxative or diuretic abuse, enemas, or excessive exercise. For example, after a binge a runner may increase her daily mileage to equal the "calculated" energy content of the binge. Some people with bulimia fast for a day or two until they feel they have compensated for the extra calories from the binge (Garfinkel 2002).

Symptoms of Bulimia Nervosa

As with anorexia nervosa, the *DMV-IV* has identified conditions of bulimia nervosa (APA 1994):

- Recurrent episodes of binge eating (e.g., eating a large amount of food in a short period of time, such as within two hours) (Figure 13.5)
- Recurrent inappropriate compensatory behavior in order to prevent weight gain, such as self-induced vomiting, misuse of laxatives, diuretics, enemas, or other medications, fasting, or excessive exercise
- Binge eating occurs on average at least twice a week for three months
- Body shape and weight unduly influence self-evaluation
- The disturbance does not occur exclusively during episodes of anorexia nervosa. Some individuals will have periods of binge eating and then periods of starvation, which makes classification of their disorder difficult.

How can you tell if a family member or friend has bulimia nervosa? The National Eating Disorders Association identifies the following early warning signs:

- Disappearance of large amounts of food in a short period of time, or the existence of wrappers or containers indicating the consumption of large amounts of food
- Frequent trips to the bathroom after a meal, signs or smells of vomiting, presence of wrappers or packages of laxatives or diuretics
- Excessive exercising
- Visual signs such as unusual swelling of the cheeks or jaw area, calluses on the back of the hands and knuckles, and/or discoloration of the teeth
- Withdrawal from usual friends and family
- Statements and behaviors indicating that weight loss, dieting, and control of food are becoming primary concerns

To learn more about the realities of having bulimia nervosa, refer to the Highlight box, A Day in the Life of a Bulimic.

Health Risks of Bulimia Nervosa

The destructive behaviors of bulimia nervosa can lead to illness and even death. The most common health consequences associated with bulimia nervosa are:

- Electrolyte imbalance — This can lead to irregular heartbeat and even heart failure and death. The electrolyte imbalance seen in bulimia nervosa is caused by dehydration and the loss of potassium and sodium from the body with frequent vomiting.

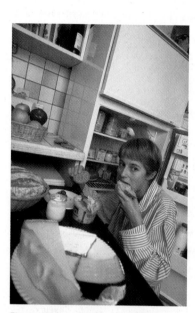

Figure 13.5   People who suffer from bulimia nervosa can consume relatively large amounts of food in brief periods of time.

A Day in the Life of a Bulimic

Hi, my name is Katie.* Through high school and my first two years of college, I suffered from bulimia nervosa and used exercise as a method of purging. Initially, I was able to keep it a secret because people saw me eat meals, and I looked normal because I had learned to purge my calories through exercise. After a few years, I knew I had a problem and so did people around me. My excessive exercise is what clued in my friends and family. Below, I give you an example of what a typical day was like for me during my first two years of college.

5:30 A.M.

Alarm goes off. I ate too much yesterday. I was the only one to finish my plate of food at dinner. I must get up and go running. If I can run this morning and eat only a small bowl of cereal at breakfast then everything that happened last night won't matter.

6:10 A.M.

Two miles in 15:45 minutes. That's horrible. What is my problem? OK, if I won't run fast enough, I'll just have to increase my miles. Instead of running three miles, I'm going to run five. Why are my legs so heavy? I've got to run faster than this.

8:30 A.M.

The run was pathetic. It wasn't even worth going out. If I just skip going to the cafeteria, then I won't eat breakfast. That's what I should do. No breakfast today. Just get to class and then you'll be OK until lunch.

9:00 A.M.

Oh no, there's Julie. I know she's going to ask me to go into the cafeteria with her. I can't. Katie, do not let yourself go in to the cafeteria, no matter what Julie says or does. Just wait three more hours until lunch. Don't go.

9:25 A.M.

I can't believe I went to the cafeteria with Julie. Of course, they were serving my favorite scones and I ate two! They are huge — there must be 400 calories in each of them. I'm so utterly disgusting. Julie does not even understand how hard that is for me. I'm so mad at myself. After class, I'll go to the gym. Katie, do not worry about the scones. You can get rid of them by taking the kickboxing class after your workout.

1:00 P.M.

If I can walk straight past the cafeteria and not eat lunch, I can get home faster, and get to the gym sooner.

1:15 P.M.

I did it — I walked past the cafeteria. Not eating lunch is going to make my workout feel so much better. I'll drink a diet coke first and then I'll go.

2:30 P.M.

Three hundred calories burned on the treadmill and 400 burned on the elliptical machine. That's 700 calories! If I go to the kickboxing class, then I can stop thinking about the scones I ate for breakfast and I'll be able to eat a normal dinner with my roommates.

4:00 P.M.

I'm exhausted. I've got to lie down.

4:15 P.M.

I can't lie down. You don't burn calories while you're sleeping. Get up!

5:00 P.M.

I'm so dizzy. I hate that feeling, but I love it at the same time. It's good to know that I was strong enough to deny myself food long enough to feel dizzy. I get such a sense of strength from feeling so weak, it's strange. I'm safe to go to dinner now as long as I don't eat any dessert afterwards.

7:00 P.M.

It's amazing how normal I can act when I eat dinner. Even my roommates don't have any idea how hard it is for me to just enjoy a meal with them. I ate my complete dinner and took seconds — I couldn't believe I kept eating. I will add a couple of miles to my run in the morning to make up for the extra 300 calories. I'm too tired to think about it now.

8:30 P.M.

I've got to go to bed. I can't move my body. I can't concentrate on my homework. I don't know when I'm ever going to get caught up in my classes. I'll have to read some after I run in the morning. I have to do better tomorrow — more exercise and less food.

*Not her real name. This true story was submitted by a student of one of the authors. ●

- Gastrointestinal problems — Inflammation, ulceration, and possible rupture of the esophagus and stomach from frequent binging and vomiting. Chronic irregular bowel movements and constipation may result in people with bulimia who regularly abuse laxatives.
- Dental problems — Tooth decay and staining and mouth sores from stomach acids released during frequent vomiting.
- Calluses on the back of the hands and knuckles from self-induced vomiting
- Swelling of the cheeks or jaw area from recurrent vomiting.

As with anorexia nervosa, the chance of recovery from bulimia nervosa increases, and the negative effects on health decrease, if the disorder is detected at an early stage. Familiarity with the warning signs of bulimia nervosa can help you identify friends and family members who might be at risk.

> **Recap:** Bulimia nervosa is a severe, life-threatening disorder characterized by recurrent episodes of binge eating followed by self-induced vomiting or another method of purging (e.g., laxatives, diuretics, excessive exercise, fasting) in an attempt to avoid weight gain. Knowing the early warning signs of bulimia nervosa can help you identify friends and family members who may be at risk.

What Does Disordered Eating Look Like?

As we discussed earlier, a variety of unhealthful behaviors constitute disordered eating. Chronic overeating and chronic dieting are the milder and more common forms and fall in the middle of the eating issues continuum (see Figure 13.1, page 463). As one progresses to the right of the continuum, a more severe pattern of disordered eating called binge-eating disorder can develop. It is estimated that 3 to 6% of middle-school–aged females and 2 to 24% of high-school–aged females have some type of disordered eating behavior, with the incidence in college-aged athletes and active women being much higher (Patrick 2002).

Binge-Eating Disorder Can Cause Significant Weight Gain

When was the last time a friend or relative confessed to you about "going on an eating binge?" Most likely, they explained that the behavior followed some sort of stressful event, such as a problem at work, the break-up of a relationship, or a poor grade on an exam. As we noted earlier, binge-eating is defined as the consumption of a large amount of food *in a short period of time*. This time factor distinguishes binge-eating from "continual snacking" or "grazing." Many people have one or two binge episodes every year or so, in response to stress. But when the behavior occurs an average of twice a week or more, the person is categorized in the *DSM-IV* as having a **binge-eating disorder** (APA 1994).

binge-eating disorder A disorder characterized by binge eating an average of twice a week or more.

The prevalence of binge-eating disorder is estimated to be 2 to 3% of the adult population and 8% of the obese population; however, some obesity treatment programs report that 20 to 40% of their patients suffer from this disorder (Grilo 2002). In contrast to anorexia nervosa and bulimia nervosa, binge-eating disorder is also common in men (an approximate ratio of 1.5 female to 1 male) and minority groups.

Symptoms of Binge-Eating Disorder

Not surprisingly, people with binge-eating disorder are often overweight. This is not only because of the amount of food they eat, but also because they do not end the binge by purging themselves of the food. In the absence of purging, the increased energy intake that occurs with each binge can significantly increase the person's overall energy intake and contribute to weight gain. Some evidence suggests that a large proportion of people who suffer from binge-eating disorder (35 to 55%) experienced their first binge-eating episode prior to beginning a diet (Grilo 2002). As in bulimia nervosa, an individual suffering from binge-eating disorder has a sense of lack of control during the binge episode and cannot will themselves to stop eating. The *DSM-IV* (*APA* 1994) associates the binge-eating episode with three or more of the following experiences: eating much more rapidly than normal; eating until feeling uncomfortably full; eating large amounts of food when you are not feeling hungry; eating alone because you are embarrassed by how much you are eating; or feeling disgusted with yourself, depressed, or guilty about overeating.

In addition, individuals who suffer from binge-eating disorder generally have chaotic eating behaviors, low levels of dietary restraint (e.g., when food is available they cannot resist), and may suffer from more chronic overeating behaviors (e.g., regularly overeating but without losing control). As you would expect, our current food environment, which offers an abundance of good-tasting, cheap food any time of the day, makes it difficult for people with binge-eating disorder to avoid food triggers.

People with binge-eating disorder frequently suffer from negative self-esteem, are distressed over their eating behaviors and body size, and have dysfunctional attitudes about their weight and shape (Grilo 2002). Depression is reported in 50 to 60% of people with binge-eating disorder. Substance abuse and anxiety disorders are also common.

Health Risks of Binge-Eating Disorder

As you would expect, the destructive overeating behaviors of people suffering from binge-eating disorder can have long-term health consequences. First, the increased caloric intake associated with each binge significantly increases a person's risk of being overweight or obese. As discussed in detail in Chapter 11, obesity significantly increases the risk of other health problems such as heart disease, high blood pressure, stroke, diabetes, and arthritis. Second, the types of foods individuals typically consume during a binge episode are high in fat and sugar, which can increase blood lipids. Third, the stress associated with binge eating can have psychological consequences, such as low self-esteem, avoidance of social contact, depression, and negative thoughts related to body size. Constantly battling the negative thought processes that occur following each binge can be overwhelming and increase stress levels. In general, there is a high level of psychological distress associated with this disorder.

> **Recap:** Binge-eating disorder is a severe, life-threatening disorder characterized by recurrent episodes of compulsive overeating or binge eating. The binge occurs on average two times a week but is not associated with the regular use of inappropriate compensatory behaviors (including vomiting, fasting, excessive exercise) seen in bulimia nervosa. Many people suffering from binge-eating disorder are overweight and have depression.

Chronic Dieting Is a Common Pattern of Disordered Eating

Do you find yourself dieting every January to make up for holiday eating or dieting every spring in preparation for beach season? If so, you're not alone. Many people diet occasionally to lose those three or four extra pounds, and their behavior certainly doesn't qualify as disordered eating. But at some point for some people, those occasional weight-loss diets become habitual, and a cycle of chronic dieting begins. **Chronic dieting** is usually defined as consistently and successfully restricting energy intake to maintain an average or below average body weight (Manore 1996). The chronic dieter is often referred to as a "restrained eater" in the research literature and may be at risk for poor health and nutrition.

chronic dieting Consistently and successfully restricting energy intake to maintain an average or below average body weight.

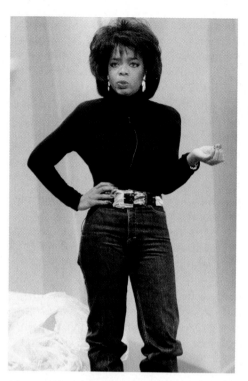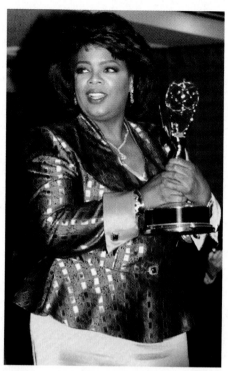

After several attempts at dieting and regaining weight, Oprah Winfrey has stated that she is now comfortable with her weight. Here are two extreme examples of her weight cycling. At left, Oprah in 1988, after losing 67 pounds. At right, in 1992, having regained the weight.

weight cycling   The condition of successfully dieting to lose weight, regaining the weight, and repeating the cycle again.

Conversely, **weight cycling** or "yo-yo" dieting occurs when a person who is normal weight or overweight successfully diets to lose weight, then regains the lost weight, and then repeats the cycle all over again (Manore 1996). One reason why weight cyclers are thought to be unsuccessful at maintaining long-term weight loss is their failure to make permanent lifestyle changes in their eating and exercise behaviors.

Although energy restriction during the dieting phase can be severe, weight cycling is unlikely to cause serious illness unless the diet is long and unmonitored by a physician. This is because the person overeats during the non-dieting phase, restoring the body's nutritional status. The long-term health consequences associated with this type of dieting, such as increased risk of heart disease, remain controversial. However, everyone agrees that there is a great deal of physiological stress associated with losing and then regaining weight.

Symptoms of Chronic Dieting

How can you tell if someone is a chronic dieter? What characteristics would you look for? Remember the eating continuum (see Figure 13.1, page 463)? Notice that as you move from column 3 to column 4, the comments related to dieting and body image become more extreme. That means that someone who chronically diets is very aware of what they are eating and may constantly have negative thoughts related to food. If they allow themselves to eat foods they feel are "bad," they become upset with themselves for having so little self-control. Understandably, chronic dieters experience a lot of stress related to eating, and research has shown that their production of the stress hormone cortisol is higher. Some of the symptoms you may observe in a friend or family member who is chronically dieting are related to this increased stress. Below are listed some of the signs of chronic dieting behavior:

Dietary Patterns/Eating Behaviors

- Preoccupation with food, calories, and/or weight
- Strict dieting
- Classifies foods as "good" or "bad"

Exercise/Training Patterns

- Relentless, excessive exercise to help burn off calories
- Chronically fatigued and finds it hard to exercise

Psychological Functioning

- Loss of concentration
- Mood swings
- Overly concerned with comparing themselves with others (body shape, training regime)
- Increased criticism of body size or shape

Health Risks of Chronic Dieting

For most of us, going on a diet for a short time presents few nutritional or long-term health problems. However, serious health problems may arise for individuals who chronically restrict their energy intake, especially if they are expending high amounts of energy in exercise. In fact, the female athlete triad (discussed on page 479) is one example of a serious health consequence that can arise from chronic energy restriction in active females. Some other health risks associated with chronic dieting include (Manore 1998, 2002):

- Poor nutrient and energy intakes—If you restrict energy intake to less than 1600 to 1800 kcal/day, it is almost impossible to get adequate nutrients (protein, carbohydrates, vitamins, and minerals), even if you are inactive. In general, inactive women need at least 1600 kcal/day to maintain weight. Recreationally active females (females who exercise 6 to 10 hours a week) typically need 2200 to 2500 kcal/day for weight maintenance, while active males may need 2800 to 3500 kcal/day. For the competitive athlete who exercises 10 to 20 hours or more per week, energy requirements are at least 2500 to 2800 kcal/day for females and 3500 to 4000 kcal/day for males to maintain body weight. Both inactive and active individuals who restrict energy intake in order to lose weight will frequently have poor vitamin and mineral intakes, especially calcium, magnesium, iron, zinc, B-complex vitamins, and antioxidants. Individuals who diet need to carefully select the foods they eat to make sure their micronutrient needs are met. They may also need to consider taking a multivitamin-mineral supplement.
- Decreased total daily energy expenditure—It is well documented that as you severely restrict energy intake, your resting or basal metabolic rate (BMR) decreases at a greater rate than your change in body size. As you know, your BMR represents the amount of energy required just to keep your body functioning at rest—your heart beating, brain functioning, and organs working. This represents about 60 to 75% of the energy you need each day. Thus, reductions in this energy expenditure result in your needing an even greater caloric restriction to bring about the weight loss you want. A more reasonable approach to weight loss is to increase energy expenditure (by about 300 to 500 kcal/day on four to five days per week) using both endurance and strength training, while making only moderate decreases in energy intake (no more than 300 to 500 kcal/day). This decrease can usually be achieved by altering food choices and serving size, without counting calories. When this more moderate approach to weight loss is used, more fat tissue is lost, while decreases in lean tissue and BMR are minimized. See the Highlight box, How Does Severe Dieting Alter Basal Metabolic Rate (BMR)? (page 478).
- Decreased ability to exercise—Remember that in order to maintain body weight, one must consume enough energy (calories) to cover the energy costs of basic metabolism, the building and repair of muscle tissue, activities of daily

How Does Severe Dieting Alter Basal Metabolic Rate (BMR)?

Researchers at the University of Nebraska-Kearney (Donnelly et al. 1994) looked at the effect of severe dieting (520 kcal/day) and exercise on changes in BMR and lean tissue in obese females. This classic study is especially interesting because they studied both aerobic and weight-training types of exercise. The researchers recruited 115 sedentary female subjects, who were then randomly assigned to one of six exercise groups for a 12-week period. Each of the six exercise groups was fed the same low energy diet (520 kcal/day), and the researchers monitored all exercise. The exercise consisted of no exercise, aerobic exercise, strength-training exercise, or a combination of aerobic and strength-training exercise administered in different ways.

The researchers found that all groups lost weight, as you would expect on such a low calorie diet, but total weight loss did not differ between the groups and ranged from 16.7 to 22.3% of their initial body weight. All individuals also lost similar amounts of body fat, ranging from 6.9 to 9.3%. As expected, BMR decreased as a result of the diet and exercise. Interestingly, the greatest decrease in BMR (240 kcal/day decrease; 13.5% decrease) was seen in the dieters who did both aerobic and strength-training exercise (Figure 13.6). However, the amount of lean tissue lost in this group was similar to that lost in the other five groups (approximately 4 kg, or 9 pounds). This study shows that severe energy restriction reduces BMR and that exercise does not slow the decrease of lean tissue or BMR compared to dieting without exercise. The exercise group had the highest energy expenditure and had the greatest decrease in BMR during the 12-week dieting period because they had the greatest energy deficit. Thus, the body decreases BMR to conserve energy when our energy intake is low and our energy expenditure is high. ●

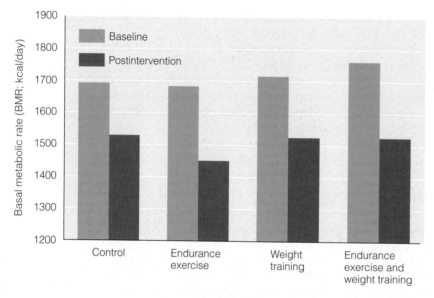

Figure 13.6   Obese women who combined severe dieting with exercise experienced a significant decrease in basal metabolic rate. This decrease in basal metabolic rate can inhibit weight loss over the long term. (J. E. Donnelly, D. J. Jacobsen, J. M. Jakicic, and J. E. Whatley. Very low calorie diet with concurrent versus delayed and sequential exercise. *Int. J. Obesity* 18 [1994]: 469–475.)

living, and exercise. Females of reproductive age must also cover the energy costs of menstruation, while children and adolescents must cover the energy costs of growth. If, in addition, you are trying to maintain an exercise or training program or are competing regularly in sports or dance, the energy costs are much greater. Therefore, among athletes and dancers, chronic dieting not only reduces the level of nutrients available to cover these energy costs, but also dramatically increases risk of injury and the time it takes to recover from injury, decreases the ability to concentrate, and reduces exercise performance (Beals and Manore 1998). In addition, a number of psychological stresses are reported with severe dieting in athletes, such as increased depression, obsession with food and body weight, increased incidence of binge-purge eating behaviors, increased stress of constantly trying to "make weight" or maintain an unrealistic body weight, and increased risk of developing an eating disorder (Beals and Manore 1998; 2002).

- Increased risk of developing a psychiatric eating disorder—One fact that eating-disorder specialists agree on is that constant dieting can lead to more severe forms of disordered eating, including anorexia nervosa. As individuals become more and more restrictive in their dieting behaviors they move further to the right on the eating continuum and their perception of what constitutes normal eating behaviors becomes more distorted.

Recap: An individual who consistently and successfully restricts energy intake to maintain an average or below average body weight is considered a chronic dieter. Because this type of behavior can last for years, the long-term health consequences may be poor nutrient status, loss of lean tissue, poor bone health, fatigue, and decreased ability to exercise. Chronic dieters are also at risk for developing a more severe eating disorder such as anorexia nervosa or bulimia nervosa.

Hannah *Nutri-Case*

"This morning, my mom and I each had half a grapefruit for breakfast. I asked her for my Cocoa Puffs, but she said we need to lose some weight, so she was trying this new grapefruit diet. "Oh great," I think, "here we go again!" She's always trying some stupid diet, and they never work. Then she gets all depressed and eats chips and cookies and stuff. The worst thing is, when she goes on a diet, she makes Dad and me do it, too. And now here it is not even close to lunch time, and I'm starving!"

If you could counsel Hannah's mother about her eating behaviors, what would you say? Specifically, what information might persuade her to change her pattern of disordered eating? What weight-loss strategies might you suggest instead of chronic dieting? Why would it be especially important to try to persuade her not to involve Hannah in her chronic dieting?

What Is the Female Athlete Triad?

The **female athlete triad** is a term used to describe a serious syndrome that consists of three medical disorders frequently seen in female athletes: disordered eating, menstrual dysfunction, and osteoporosis (Figure 13.7). To emphasize the seriousness of this syndrome, the American College of Sports Medicine issued a position stand on the female athlete triad in 1997 (Otis et al. 1997), which outlined the seriousness of this syndrome in active women and girls and delineated its three components. These components are described in more detail on the following page.

female athlete triad A serious syndrome that consists of three medical disorders frequently seen in female athletes: disordered eating, amenorrhea, and osteoporosis.

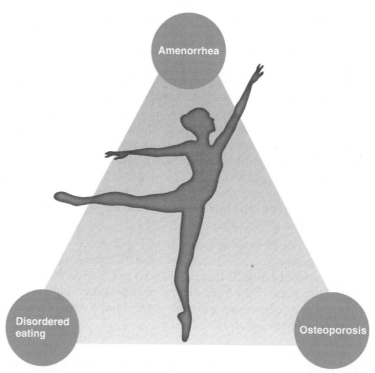

Figure 13.7   The female athlete triad is a syndrome comprised of three coexisting disorders: disordered eating, amenorrhea, and osteoporosis.

Sports that Emphasize Leanness Increase the Risk for the Female Athlete Triad

Sports that emphasize leanness or a thin body build may place a young girl or a woman at risk for the female athlete triad. The American College of Sports Medicine has identified these sports and activities as follows (Otis et al. 1997):

- Sports that have subjective performance scoring, such as dance, skating, diving, and gymnastics
- Endurance sports that emphasize a lean build and/or a low body weight, such as long-distance running, cycling, and cross-country skiing
- Sports that require the athlete to wear body-contouring or body-revealing clothing, such as gymnastics, swimming, volleyball, aerobics, track, and dance
- Sports that require athletes to weigh in or that use weight-specific categories for participation, such as horse racing, martial arts, and rowing
- Sports that emphasize a preadolescent body build for success, such as gymnastics, figure skating, and diving

Three Disorders Characterize the Female Athlete Triad

Active females, like most women in our society, are often preoccupied with their body weight and shape. They feel pressure to conform to certain ideal body shapes and sizes; however, their source of pressure is two-fold. These women experience the general social and cultural demands placed on women to be thin, but also experience pressure from their coach, teammates, judges, and/or spectators to meet weight standards or body-size expectations for their sport. Failure to meet these standards can result in severe consequences such as being cut from the team, losing an athletic scholarship, decreased participation with the team, or elimination from competition.

As the pressure to be thin mounts, active women may engage in disordered eating behaviors. This in turn may disrupt the menstrual cycle and result in amenorrhea. Without a normal menstrual cycle and adequate reproductive hormones, which play an important role in bone health, osteoporosis can result. Thus, for many female athletes, disordered eating is the event that leads to absence of menstruation (amenorrhea) and premature bone loss (osteoporosis). In the following sections we describe each of the components of the female athlete triad.

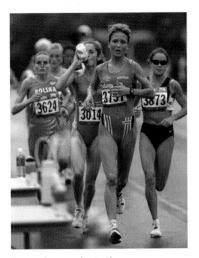

Sports that emphasize leanness or require the athlete to wear body-contouring clothing increase the risk for the female athlete triad.

Disordered Eating

The first component of the female athlete triad is disordered eating. The way that severe energy restriction in active individuals can increase the incidence of disordered eating was illustrated in a study of military personnel who were required to maintain low body weight in order to keep their jobs (Peterson et al. 1995). This study found that individuals in the military weight-management group engaged in bulimic weight-loss behaviors two to five times more often than volunteers in a civilian weight-management group. Thus, under pressures to lose weight or face possible discharge, these soldiers resorted to excessive and unhealthful weight-loss measures. This study can easily be applied to the female athlete who is required to lose weight to make the team or to please a coach or parent. When the pressure and stakes are high for weight loss to occur, female athletes will frequently turn to harmful dieting practices to achieve their goal.

A number of factors may predispose active women to disordered eating, including a prolonged period of dieting, an increase in exercise, a stressful event, or the pressure to maintain a low body weight (Peterson et al. 1995; Sundgot-Borgen 1994). In addition, active women frequently avoid animal products and strictly limit their fat intake (Beals and Manore 1998), and these factors can increase their risk even further. Table 13.2 (page 470) lists some of the signs and symptoms that an active individual, either male or female, may not be eating enough.

Menstrual Dysfunction

The second component of the female athlete triad is menstrual dysfunction, such as irregular periods, amenorrhea, or failure to ovulate. As we discussed earlier, energy restriction combined with high levels of physical activity can disrupt the menstrual cycle. Research suggests that the menstrual dysfunction may be due in part to periods of negative energy balance, where there is a high level of exercise and psychological or physical stress combined with inadequate intakes of energy (Dueck, Manore, and Matt 1996; Manore 2002). The prevalence of exercise-induced menstrual dysfunction may be as high as 50% in female athletes (Dueck, Manore, and Matt 1996; Beals and Manore 1998).

Osteoporosis

The final component of the female athlete triad is osteoporosis, which was defined in Chapter 9 as loss of bone mineral density. Female athletes with menstrual dysfunction typically display reduced levels of the reproductive hormones estrogen and progesterone. When estrogen levels in the body are low, it is difficult for bone to retain calcium, and gradual loss of bone mass occurs. Research shows that in the lumbar region of the spine, bone mineral density is reduced by about 14% in amenorrheic athletes compared to athletes with regular menstrual cycles, and by as much as 27% compared to normally menstruating sedentary women (Dueck, Manore, and Matt 1996). Loss of bone mineral density also increases the risk of muscle and bone injuries, such as stress fractures. Thus, despite the positive stimulus of exercise on bone, the hormonal changes associated with menstrual dysfunction compromise bone mineral density and increase the risk for fracture.

Liz *Nutri-Case*

"I used to dance with a really cool modern company, where everybody looked sort of healthy and "real." No waifs! When they folded after Christmas, I was really bummed, but this spring, I'm planning to audition for the City Ballet. My best friend dances with them, and she told me that they won't even look at anybody over a hundred pounds. That means I have three months to lose eight pounds. With morning and afternoon dance classes, teaching, and school performances, I've got the exercise part down, but I've had to put myself on a pretty strict diet, too. Most days, I come in under 1,200 calories, though some days I cheat and then I feel so out of control. Last week, my dance teacher stopped me after class and asked me whether or not I was menstruating. I thought that was a pretty weird question, so I just said sure, but then when I thought about it, I realized that I haven't had my period for a couple of months now. And I do feel tired a lot. But the audition is only a week away, and after that I can relax a little. I still have one pound to go, but I'm going to try a juice fast this weekend. I've just got to make it into the City Ballet!"

What factors increase Liz's risk for the female athlete triad? If you were to explain to her about osteoporosis, stress fractures, and increased injuries, do you think that this might change her disordered eating behaviors? Why or why not? What, if anything, do you think Liz's dance teacher should do? Why is intervention even necessary, since the audition is only a week away?

Recognizing and Treating the Female Athlete Triad Can Be Challenging

Recognition of an athlete with one or more of the components of the female athlete triad can be difficult, especially if the athlete is reluctant to be honest when questioned about the symptoms. For this reason, familiarity with the early warning signs is critical. These include excessive dieting and/or weight loss, excessive exercise, stress fractures, and self-esteem that appears to be dictated by body weight and shape. You may not know whether a female friend or teammate is experiencing irregular periods, but you might overhear her commenting negatively on her body or see her head off to the gym after eating only a lettuce salad for lunch.

Treating an athlete requires a multidisciplinary approach. This means that the sports medicine team, nutritionist, exercise physiologist, psychologist, coach, trainer, parents, friends of the athlete, and the athlete all must work together. As with any health problem, prevention is the best treatment. Thus, recognition of the risk factors by the sports medicine team and education of athletes, coaches, and parents is imperative. If the athlete is having trouble with weight and body shape issues, care should be taken to deal with these issues before they develop into something more serious.

Recap: The female athlete triad is a syndrome consisting of three distinct disorders: disordered eating, menstrual dysfunction, and osteoporosis. It is initiated when energy intake is reduced to the point of disrupting the menstrual cycle. When menstrual cycles become irregular or cease, there is a significant decrease in estrogen, a reproductive hormone that improves calcium absorption and the maintenance of healthy bones. Eventually, osteoporosis develops.

What Therapies Work for People with an Eating Disorder?

Recognition and treatment of someone with an eating disorder can be difficult, especially if the person is reluctant to answer questions about the symptoms and does not want treatment. Since eating disorders can be triggered by any number of factors (discussed earlier), multiple issues may need to be addressed in treatment.

Most treatment programs use a multidisciplinary team-management approach that incorporates medical and nutritional management, psychological treatment, and a number of other therapies, depending on the individual problems and issues that need to be addressed.

A team-management approach to treating an individual suffering from an eating disorder will begin with a physical examination, diagnosis, and identification of underlying causes or trigger factors. The team will meet and decide on the approach each will use in working with the patient (Joy et al. 1997). At this time the team may choose to develop a contract for treatment that is then signed by the patient. Team members meet individually with the patient and on a regular basis as a team to determine the progress being made and the next steps in the treatment process. Team members may also meet with family and friends of the patient and involve them in the treatment plan; this is especially true if the patient is still living at home. Discussed below are the various steps and options that are available for the treatment of eating disorders.

Choosing a Treatment Approach for an Eating Disorder

There are a variety of services available to treat eating disorders, ranging from intensive hospitalization to varied levels of outpatient care (Figure 13.8). For example, an individual who is severely underweight, displaying signs of malnutrition, is medically unstable (e.g., has elevated pulse rate, low blood pressure, inability to maintain core body temperature, abnormal blood electrolytes), or is suicidal may require immediate hospitalization to stabilize his or her condition and initiate refeeding. Patients may be hospitalized for several days until stabilized, and then transferred to a residential care facility specifically designed to treat people with eating disorders.

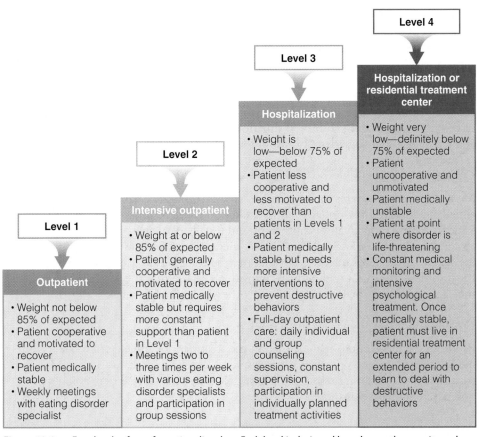

Figure 13.8   Four levels of care for eating disorders. Each level is designed based upon the severity and type of eating disorder. (Adapted from American Psychiatric Association. *Practice Guidelines for the Treatment of Patients with Eating Disorders.* [Washington, DC: American Psychiatric Association, 2000]. Reprinted with permission of the American Psychiatric Association.)

Conversely, patients who are underweight but are still medically stable may enter an outpatient program designed to meet their specific needs. For example, some outpatient programs are extremely intensive, requiring patients to come in each day for treatment, while others are less rigorous, requiring only weekly visits for meetings with a psychiatrist or eating disorder specialist. The type of program an individual selects will be determined by their medical condition, options available, personal preference of the individual and family members involved, and affordability.

Treatment Options for Patients With Anorexia Nervosa

The goals of treatment for patients with anorexia nervosa are to restore the patient to a healthy weight, treat any physical complications that may be present, motivate the patient to restore healthful eating habits and lifestyle patterns, correct any dysfunctional feelings related to their eating disorder, treat associated psychiatric conditions, enlist the aid of family and friends to support the patient's healing, and prevent relapse. Nutritional rehabilitation, psychosocial interventions, and medications are the therapies most commonly used to reach these goals.

Nutritional Therapies Are Critical in Anorexia Nervosa Treatment

The goals of nutritional therapies are to restore the individual to a healthy body weight and resolve the nutrition-related eating issues. For hospitalized patients, the expected weight gain per week ranges from 1 to 3 pounds. For outpatient settings, the expected weight gain is much lower (0.5 to 1pound/week). During the weight-gain phase of a treatment program, energy intake goals may be set at 1000 to 1600 kcal/day, depending on body size, severity of the disease, and achievable levels of intake. Patients frequently try a variety of methods to avoid consuming the food presented to them. They may discard the food, vomit, exercise excessively, or engage in a high level of non-exercise motor activity to eliminate the calories they just consumed. In addition to increasing amounts of food, patients may be given vitamin and mineral supplements to assure adequate micronutrients are consumed.

Nutrition counseling is an important aspect of the treatment to deal with the body image issues that occur as weight is regained. Once the patient reaches an acceptable body weight, nutrition counseling will address issues such as acceptability of certain foods, dealing with food situations such as family gatherings and eating out, and learning to put together a healthful food plan for weight maintenance.

Psychosocial Interventions Are Important

Most treatment programs for anorexia nervosa incorporate a variety of treatments aimed at addressing the underlying psychological issues related to the disorder. Patients receive individual psychotherapy and usually participate in both family therapy and group counseling sessions. Family therapy is useful in identifying and alleviating family dynamics or relationships that may be contributing to the maintenance of the disorder. Group counseling helps individuals realize that they are not alone in their struggles with the disorder and that others have similar issues.

Psychotropic Medications May Be Helpful

Psychotropic medications may be used in the treatment of anorexia nervosa. These medications are aimed primarily at preventing relapse in patients who have undergone treatment and in treating associated psychiatric disorders, such as depression or obsessive-compulsive disorder.

Treatment Options for Patients With Bulimia Nervosa

The primary goals of treatment for patients with bulimia nervosa are the identification and modification of events, behaviors, or environments that trigger binging and purging behaviors. As with anorexia nervosa, a variety of approaches are used to reach these goals. The most common include nutritional rehabilitation, psychosocial interventions, and medications.

Nutritional Therapies Are Critical in Bulimia Nervosa Treatment

Most individuals with bulimia nervosa are of normal weight or overweight, so restoring body weight is generally not the focus of treatment as it is with anorexia nervosa. Instead, nutrition counseling generally focuses on identifying and dealing with events and feelings that trigger binging, reducing purging, and establishing eating behaviors that can maintain a healthful body weight. In addition, nutrition counseling will address negative feelings about foods and the fear associated with uncontrolled binge eating of foods.

Psychosocial Interventions Are Important

Cognitive therapy that helps patients monitor and alter their thought patterns related to eating issues and body image has been shown to be the most effective form of treatment for bulimia nervosa. Behavior modification can help patients stop a binge episode from occurring or interrupt one in progress. As with anorexia nervosa, both group and family therapy are important. These approaches help identify food issues, body image concerns, interpersonal conflicts, difficulties with anger and aggression management, family dysfunctions, and coping styles that contribute to the disorder.

Antidepressant Medications May Be Helpful

The treatment of bulimia nervosa frequently involves the use of antidepressant medications in conjunction with nutritional and psychotherapy. Antidepressants are prescribed to alleviate the symptoms of depression, anxiety, obsessions, and overriding impulses that trigger a binge-and-purge event.

Recap: Treatments for patients with an eating disorder may combine a variety of therapies, including nutrition counseling, individual psychotherapy, family counseling, support groups, and medications. Individuals may progress through various levels of treatment (e.g., hospitalization to weekly outpatient counseling) over a period of months or years. Some individuals need ongoing counseling and medications to help prevent a recurrence of their eating disorder.

How Can We Prevent Eating Disorders and Disordered Eating?

We have suggested throughout this book that, rather than trying to achieve an unrealistic body weight, you try to achieve a weight that is healthful for you and one that can be maintained for life. This process requires you to think about your genetics, current body size and shape, environment, social life, exercise habits, and psychological factors. A healthful weight is one that can be realistically maintained, allows for involvement in physical activity, and reduces risk factors for chronic disease. It is not realistic to pick a body weight that you cannot maintain except by constant dieting or resorting to disordered eating behaviors. See the Highlight box on page 402 for practical advice on identifying and maintaining a healthful body weight. In addition, at the end of this chapter is a list of Web links to additional resources related to dieting and eating disorders.

As we noted earlier, it is difficult to delineate precisely what factors precipitate the development of eating disorders. Nevertheless, research does suggest that the following techniques may be useful in prevention (Piran 2002).

- Reducing peer and family weight-related criticism and teasing; educating parents and teachers about the destructiveness of such behavior
- Teaching children and adolescents that changes of body shape and size are a natural part of human development

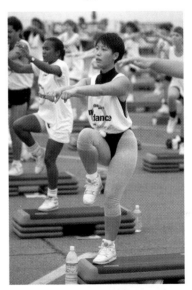

It is most healthful to maintain a body weight that is appropriate for your body type, that allows you to be involved in physical activity, and that reduces risk factors for chronic disease.

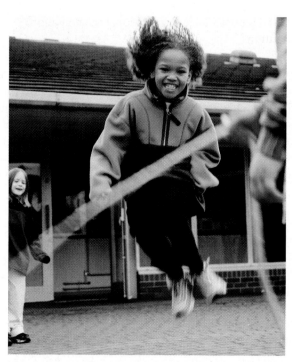

Encouraging an active lifestyle early on helps to prevent excessive weight gain and eating disorders.

- Improving media literacy skills and helping children and adolescents identify unrealistic body images and subliminal messages
- Establishing public policies related to media messages about body weight and size aimed at children and adolescents
- Identifying body weight and image concerns among children and adolescents early in the developmental years
- Encouraging participation in physical activity and sports early in life to help prevent excessive weight gain
- Establishing healthy eating behaviors within the home, school, and social environments, both for adults and children. Making positive changes in the food environment to reduce unlimited access to high-fat, high-sugar foods in large portions. Finding alternative rewards for successful behaviors to replace the use of food (e.g., snacks, candy, sweets, fast-food) and sedentary behavior (e.g., more time at the computer or in front of the television) as rewards.
- Establishing opportunities for activity throughout the day, at work, school, and during periods of leisure time. Encouraging the development of walking programs that allow children and adolescents to walk safely to school and within their neighborhoods.
- Modeling of healthy diet and exercise habits by parents
- Commenting positively on attributes of children's and adolescents' bodies that are not related to appearance, such as strength, flexibility, endurance, and gross and fine motor skills.

Recap: The prevention of eating disorders is a relatively young field in which researchers are still developing models for prevention. The current goals of eating disorder prevention programs are to identify precipitating factors in the home, school, and social environment, and to implement strategies to reduce or eliminate these factors.

Chapter Summary

- Eating behaviors occur along a continuum from normal to somewhat abnormal to disordered. Our feelings about food and our body images influence our eating behaviors.

- An eating disorder is a psychiatric disorder characterized by extreme body dissatisfaction and long-term eating patterns that negatively affect body functioning.

- Disordered eating is a general term used to describe a variety of abnormal or atypical eating behaviors that are used to achieve or maintain a lower body weight.

- The two most common clinically diagnosed eating disorders in the United States are anorexia nervosa and bulimia nervosa.

- A number of factors are thought to contribute to the development of eating disorders, including family environment, the media, social and cultural factors, personality traits, and genetics.

- Anorexia nervosa is a medical disorder in which an individual uses severe food restriction and other practices to maintain a body weight that is less than 85% of expected.

- Health risks associated with anorexia nervosa include electrolyte imbalance, cardiovascular and gastrointestinal problems, malnutrition, and poor bone health. Between 5 and 20% of people with anorexia will die from complications of the disorder within ten years of initial diagnosis.

- Bulimia nervosa is an eating disorder characterized by recurrent episodes of binge eating, followed by some form of purging.

- The health consequences associated with bulimia nervosa include electrolyte imbalance, dental decay and mouth sores, gastrointestinal ulcerations from binging and vomiting, and constipation. Bulimia nervosa results in death in 1% of patients within ten years of diagnosis.

- Binge-eating disorder is the consumption of a large amount of food in a short period of time (such as within two hours) without compensatory behaviors.

- Increased rates of obesity, cardiovascular disease, diabetes, hypertension, cancer, and depression are associated with binge-eating disorder.

- Chronic dieting is defined as consistently and successfully restricting energy intake to maintain an average or below average body weight.

- Some of the health consequences of chronic dieting may include the following: poor energy and nutrient intakes, poor nutritional status, decreased metabolic rate and total daily energy expenditure, increased psychological stress, increased risk of developing a clinical eating disorder, and increased risk of exercise-induced menstrual dysfunction.

- The female athlete triad is a syndrome characterized by the presence of three coexisting disorders: disordered eating, amenorrhea, and osteoporosis.

- Treatment of a clinical eating disorder typically involves a team approach that includes nutritional management, psychological treatment, medications, and other treatment options as necessary.

- Patients with life-threatening symptoms are hospitalized until their vital signs become stable. They are then typically transferred to an inpatient facility specializing in the treatment of patients with eating disorders. Patients with less severe symptoms typically receive outpatient care that may range from intensive daily appointments to weekly sessions.

- Strategies for preventing eating disorders include strategies to promote children's and adolescents' self-esteem and to help them develop and maintain healthful eating behaviors and exercise habits throughout life.

Review Questions

1. Damage to the esophagus, dental decay, and electrolyte imbalances are health risks of what disorder?
   a. binge-eating disorder
   b. bulimia nervosa
   c. chronic dieting
   d. anorexia nervosa

2. Chronic dieting
   a. increases your risk of developing a psychiatric eating disorder.
   b. increases your basal metabolic rate.
   c. is a psychiatric eating disorder.
   d. is a characteristic of bulimia nervosa.

3. The components of the female athlete triad are
   a. disordered eating, amenorrhea, and osteoarthritis.
   b. anorexia nervosa, menstrual dysfunction, and increased injuries.
   c. anorexia nervosa, irregular periods, and osteoporosis.
   d. disordered eating, menstrual dysfunction, and osteoporosis.

4. One recommended strategy for maintaining a healthful body image is to
   a. exercise regularly.
   b. read sports magazines.

    c. reduce your fat intake to no more than 10% of your daily energy consumption.

    d. reduce your intake of sweets to no more than one "treat" a day.

5. Which of the following statements reflects a distorted body image?

    a. I am afraid that if I eat whenever I am hungry I will get fat.

    b. I wish I could change the way I look in the mirror.

    c. I felt devastated yesterday when my best friend told me I was getting fat.

    d. I think about food a lot.

6. True or false? People with binge-eating disorder typically purge to compensate for the binge.

7. True or false? Media images of idealized female bodies are known to cause eating disorders in some adolescent girls.

8. True or false? People with eating disorders typically fear eating in front of others.

9. True or false? People with anorexia typically claim to be ravenously hungry, but then fail to eat.

10. True or false? Chronic overeating is the common name for binge-eating disorder.

11. Explain why there is some truth to the saying that the more you diet, the harder it is to lose weight.

12. Create a flow chart showing how restricted energy intake in female athletes can eventually lead to loss of bone mineral density.

13. Compare and contrast anorexia nervosa and bulimia nervosa. In what ways are they similar? In what ways are they different?

14. You start a new aerobics class and make friends with another student named Kashi. Although Kashi wears oversized clothes in class, you notice right away that she is extremely thin. After class, you go out for coffee and are surprised when Kashi eats two large pastries with her skim-milk latte. Propose at least two theories as to what might be going on with Kashi.

15. You've noticed that your friend Carlo, who is on your crew team, has been losing a lot of weight over the last few months. Today you sit next to him in class and notice that his cheeks look swollen and the knuckles on the back of his right hand are scabbed. After class, you ask him if he is feeling okay and he frowns. "Never felt better!" he says—and abruptly walks away. What might you do next?

Test Yourself Answers

1. False. Males also are diagnosed with eating disorders, but the incidence is much lower than for females.

2. False. People can and do recover from medically diagnosed eating disorders, with the best outcomes occurring in those who seek and get treatment early in their illness.

3. False. There are a number of factors that may play a role in the development of anorexia nervosa in any one individual.

4. True. As eating behaviors become more and more atypical, there is an increased risk of a clinical eating disorder developing.

5. True. Individuals who suffer from bulimia nervosa and binge-eating disorder may be obese. This is especially true of individuals who suffer from binge-eating disorder because they do not purge the extra energy consumed during the binge-eating episode. Overall, 8% of obese people have a problem with binge-eating, and some clinics report the incidence to be as high as 20 to 40% of their obese clients.

Web Links

www.hedc.org
Harvard Eating Disorders Center
This site provides information about current eating disorder research, as well as sections on understanding eating disorders and resources for those with eating disorders.

www.nimh.nih.gov
National Institute of Mental Health (NIMH)
Search this site for "disordered eating" or "eating disorders" to find numerous articles on the subject.

www.anad.org
National Association of Anorexia Nervosa and Associated Disorders
Visit this site for information and resources about eating disorders to the public and professional eating disorder specialists.

www.nationaleatingdisorders.org
National Eating Disorders Association
This site is dedicated to expanding public understanding of eating disorders and promoting access to treatment for those affected and support for their families.

www.menstuff.org/issues/byissue/
eatingdisorders.html
Menstuff Eating Disorders
A resource for men about eating disorders. Contains information about male anorexia and eating disorders in general, self-assessments, disordered eating statistics, and prevention information.

www.somethingfishy.org/
Something Fishy Website on Eating Disorders
A comprehensive Web site about the dangers of eating disorders, eating disorder treatment, and signs of symptoms of disorders. This site includes first-hand survivors' stories and online chats.

www.eatright.org
American Dietetic Association
Visit this site to learn about healthy eating habits.

References

American Psychiatric Association (APA). 1994. *Diagnostic and Statistical Manual of Mental Disorders (DSM-IV)*, 4th ed. Washington, DC: American Psychiatric Association.

American Psychiatric Association. 2000. *Practice Guidelines for the Treatment of Patients with Eating Disorders*. Washington, DC: American Psychiatric Association.

Andersen, A. E. 1992. Eating disorders in male athletes: A special case? In *Eating, Body Weight and Performance in Athletes: Disorders of Modern Society*, edited by K. D. Brownell, J. Rodin, and J. H. Wilmore. Philadelphia, PA: Lea and Fegiger, 172–188.

Andersen, A. E. 2001, Spring. Eating disorders in males: Gender divergence management. *Currents*. Volume 2, Number 2. University of Iowa Health Care. http://www.uihealthcare.com/news/currents/vol2issue2/eatingdisordersinmen.html Accessed February 2004.

Andersen, R. E., S. J. Bartlett, G. D. Morgan, and K. D. Brownell. 1995. Weight loss, psychological and nutritional patterns in competitive male body builders. *Int. J. Eating Disord*. 18: 49–57.

Anorexia Nervosa and Related Eating Disorders, Inc. (ANRED). 2002. Males with eating disorders. http://www.anred.com/males.html Accessed February 2004.

Bailor, U. F., and W. H. Kaye. 2003. A review of neuropeptide and neuroendocrine dysregulation in anorexia and bulimia nervosa. *Curr. Drug Target CNS Neurol. Disord*. 2: 53–59.

Beals, K. A. 2003. Mirror, Mirror on the Wall, who is the most muscular one of all? Disordered eating and body image disturbances in male athletes. *ACSM Health and Fitness J*. 7(2): 6–11.

Beals, K. A. 2004. *Disordered Eating in Athletes: A Comprehensive Guide for Health Professionals*. Champaign, IL: Human Kinetics Publishers.

Beals, K. A., and M. M. Manore. 1998. Nutritional status of female athletes with subclinical eating disorders. *J. Am. Diet. Assoc*. 98: 419–425.

Beals, K. A., and M. M. Manore. 2002. Disordered eating and menstrual dysfunction in female collegiate athletes. *Int. J. Sport Nutr. Exerc. Metabolism*. 12: 281–293.

Carlat, D. J., C. A. Camargo, and D. B. Herzog. 1997. Eating disorders in males: A report on 135 patients. *Am. J. Psychiatry* 154(8): 1127–1132.

Davis, S. M., and L. C. Lambert. 2000. Body image and weight concerns among Southwestern American Indian preadolescent schoolchildren. *Ethn. Dis*. 10: 184–194.

Donnelly, J. E., D. J. Jacobsen, J. M. Jakicic, and J. E. Whatley. 1994. Very low calorie diet with concurrent versus delayed and sequential exercise. *Int. J. Obesity* 18: 469–475.

Dueck, C. A., M. M. Manore, and K. S. Matt. 1996. Role of energy balance in athletic menstrual dysfunction. *Int. J. Sport Nutr*. 6: 90–116.

Fairburn, C. G., and T. B. Walsh. 2002. Atypcial eating disorders. In *Eating Disorders and Obesity: A Comprehensive Handbook*, 2nd ed., edited by D. G. Fairburn and K. D. Brownell. New York: Guilford Press, 171–177.

Garfinkel, P. E. 2002. Classification and diagnosis of eating disorders. In *Eating Disorders and Obesity: A Comprehensive Handbook*. 2nd ed., edited by D. G. Fairburn and K. D. Brownell. New York: Guilford Press, 155–161.

Grilo, C. M. 2002. Binge eating disorder. In *Eating Disorders and Obesity: A Comprehensive Handbook*. 2nd ed., edited by D. G. Fairburn and K. D. Brownell. New York: Guilford Press, 178–182.

Joy, E., N. Clark, M. L. Ireland, J. Martie, A. Nattiv, and S. Varechok. 1997. Team management of the female athlete triad. Part 2: Optimal treatment and prevention tactics. *Physician Sports Med*. 25(4): 55–69.

Kendler, K. S., C. MacLean, M. Neal, R. Kessler, A. Heath, and L. Eaves. 1991. The genetic epidemiology of bulimia nervosa. *Am. J. Psychiatry* 148: 1627–1637.

Mangweth, B., H. G. Pope, G. Kemmler, C. Ebenbichler, A. Hausmann, C. DeCol, B. Kreutner, J. Kinzl, and W. Biebl. 2001. Body image and psychopathology in male bodybuilders. *Psychother. Psychosom*. 70: 38–43.

Manore, M. M. 1996. Chronic dieting in active women: What are the health consequences? *Women's Health Issues* 6(6): 332–341.

Manore, M. M. 1998. Running on Empty: Health consequences of chronic dieting in active women. *ACMS Health Fitness J*. 2(2): 24–31.

Manore, M. M. 2002. Dietary recommendations and athletic menstrual dysfunction. *Sports Med*. 32(14): 887–901.

Nemeroff, C. J., R. I. Stein, N. S. Diehl, and K. M. Smilack. 1994. From the Cleavers to the Clintons: Role choices and body orientation as reflected in magazine article content. *Int. J. Eating Disord.* 16: 167–176.

Otis, C. L., B. Drinkwater, M. Johnson, A. Loucks, and J. Wilmore. 1997. American College of Sports Medicine Position Stand: The female athlete triad. *Med. Sci. Sports Exerc.* 29: i-ix.

Patrick, L. 2002. Eating disorders: a review of the literature with emphasis on medical complication and clinical nutrition. *Altern. Med. Rev.* 7(3): 184–202.

Peterson, A. L., W. Talcott, W. J. Kelleher, and S. D. Smith. 1995. Bulimic weight-loss behaviors in military versus civilian weight-management programs. *Military Med.* 160: 616–620.

Piran, N. 2002. Prevention of eating disorders. In *Eating Disorders and Obesity: A Comprehensive Handbook.* 2nd ed., edited by D. G. Fairburn and K. D. Brownell. New York: Guilford Press, 367–371.

Pope, H. G., and D. L. Katz. 1994. Psychiatric and medical effects of anabolic-androgenic steroid use: a controlled study of 160 athletes. *Arch. Gen. Psychiatry* 51: 375–382.

Pope, H. G., K. A. Phillips, and R. Olivardia. 2000. *The Adonis Complex: The Secret Crisis of Male Body Obsession.* New York: The Free Press.

Rinderknecht, K., and C. Smith. 2002. Body-image perceptions among urban Native American youth. *Obes. Res.* 10: 315–327.

Robb, A. S., and M. J. Dadson. 2002. Eating disorders in males. *Child Adolesc. Psychiatr. Clin. N. Am.* 11: 399–418.

Steiger, H., P. M. Lehoux, and L. Gauvin. 1999. Impulsivity, dietary control and the urge to binge in bulimic syndromes. *Inter. J. Eating Disord.* 26: 261–274.

Steinberg, L. 2002. *Adolescence,* 6th ed. New York: McGraw-Hill.

Stevens, J., M. Story, A. Becenti, S. A. French, J. Gittelsohn, S. B. Going, Juhaeri, S. Levin, and D. M. Murray. 1999. Weight-related attitudes and behaviors in fourth grade American Indian children. *Obes. Res.* 7: 34–42.

Stice, E. 2002. Sociocultural influences on body image and eating disturbances. In *Eating Disorders and Obesity: A Comprehensive Handbook,* 2nd ed., edited by D. G. Fairburn and K. D. Brownell. New York: Guilford Press, 103–107.

Striegel-Moore, R. H., and L. Smolak. 2002. Gender, ethnicity, and eating disorders. In *Eating Disorders and Obesity: A Comprehensive Handbook,* 2nd ed., edited by D. G. Fairburn and K. D. Brownell. New York: Guilford Press, 251–255.

Strober, M., and C. M. Bulik. 2002. Genetic epidemiology of eating disorders. In *Eating Disorders and Obesity: A Comprehensive Handbook,* 2nd ed., edited by D. G. Fairburn and K. D. Brownell. New York: Guilford Press, 238–242.

Sundgot-Borgen, J. 1994. Risk and trigger factors for the development of eating disorders in female elite athletes. *Med. Sci. Sport Exerc.* 26: 414–419.

Tanaka, M., T. Naruo, N. Nagai, N. Kuroki, T. Shiiya, M. Nakazato, S. Matsukura, and S. Nozoe. 2003. Habitual binge/purge behavior influences circulating ghrelin levels in eating disorders. *J. Psychiat. Res.* 37: 17–22.

Vandereycken, W. 2002. Families of patients with eating disorders. In *Eating Disorders and Obesity: A Comprehensive Handbook,* 2nd ed., edited by D. G. Fairburn and K. D. Brownell. New York: Guilford Press, 215–220.

Walsh, B. T., and D. M. Garner. 1997. *Diagnostic Issues. Handbook of Treatment for Eating Disorders,* 2nd ed. New York: Guilford Press.

Wonderlich, S. A. 2002. Personality and eating disorders. In *Eating Disorders and Obesity: A Comprehensive Handbook,* 2nd ed., edited by D. G. Fairburn and K. D. Brownell. New York: Guilford Press, 204–209.

Woodside, D. B., P. E. Garfinkel, E. Lin, P. Goering, A. S. Kaplan, D. S. Goldbloom, and S. H. Kennedy. 2001. Comparisons of men with full or partial eating disorders, men without eating disorders, and women with eating disorders in the community. *Am. J. Psychiatry* 158(4): 570–574.

Nutrition Debate:

Eating Disorders in Men: Are They Different?

David was tired of being called "fat boy." But the real motivation behind his weight loss was his coach's end-of-season threat: if he didn't lose at least twenty pounds, he wouldn't make the soccer team again next year. David couldn't imagine his life without soccer, so he started cutting back on his snacks and running a couple of mornings a week at the gym. He lost two pounds, but it took him four weeks. Discouraged by the slow pace, he eliminated all snacking, put less on his plate at mealtimes, and ran every day, first two miles, then three, then five. The weight started dropping more dramatically, and he loved the high he got from "running on empty." Four months into his program, he'd lost all twenty pounds, and he kept on going. By the time the soccer season started, he'd lost thirty-two pounds, and his coach rewarded him with more time on the field. He knew he should slack off on the dieting and running now that he was in practice every day, but something made him keep at it. Every time he got on the scale and saw he weighed another pound less, he felt better, stronger, more in control.

Like many people, you might find it hard to believe that "real men" like David develop eating disorders . . . or if they do, their disorders must be somehow different, right? To explore this question, let's take a look at what research has revealed about similarities and differences between men and women with eating disorders.

Comparing Men and Women with Eating Disorders

Until about a decade ago, little research was conducted on eating disorders in males (Beals 2003, 2004). Recently, however, eating disorder experts have begun to examine the gender-differences debate in detail and have discovered that "men with eating disorders are very similar to women with eating disorders on most variables" (Woodside et al. 2001). Or, to put it more simply, no current evidence suggests that eating disorders in males are atypical or somehow different from the eating disorders experienced by females (Anorexia Nervosa and Related Eating Disorders, Inc. [ANRED] 2002). Following is a list of what *is* currently known regarding the similarities and differences between males and females with eating disorders.

Predisposing Factors, Personality Traits, and Dieting History Are Similar

Many of the factors that appear to predispose an individual to an eating disorder are similar for males and females. For example, both have a high probability of coming from families with mental illness and/or have a personal history of mental illness (Carlat, Camargo, and Herzog 1997; Andersen 1992; Beals 2003, 2004). Both males and females are also frequently connected with some type of social group, such as a family, peer group, or sports team, where leanness is encouraged (Andersen et al. 1995). In addition, media studies suggest that males are increasingly becoming the target of articles and ads promoting dieting and an ideal of lean muscularity that is difficult to achieve (Nemeroff et al. 1994).

Both males and females with eating disorders, especially anorexia nervosa, tend to be perfectionists, goal-oriented, and introverted (Wonderlich 2002; Beals 2004). However, as with women, the extent to which these personality traits are effects of the illness rather than risk factors is not clear (Woodside et al. 2001).

Finally, dieting is one of the most powerful eating disorder triggers for both males and females (ANRED 2002). Eating disorders in both males and females typically develop after a period of dieting that becomes increasingly stringent (in anorexia nervosa) or increasingly erratic (in bulimia nervosa).

History of Overweight, Triggers for Dieting, and Methods of Weight Loss Are Different

We discussed in this chapter the fact that females with eating disorders say they *feel* fat even though they typically are normal weight or even underweight before they develop the disorder. In contrast, males who develop eating disorders are more likely to have actually *been* overweight or even obese (Robb and Dadson 2002; Beals 2004). Thus, the male's fear of "getting fat again" is based on reality. In addition, males with disordered eating are less concerned with actual body weight (scale weight) than females but are more concerned with body composition (percentage of muscle mass compared to fat mass). For example, Mangweth and colleagues (2001) found that male bodybuilders obsessed with eating and exercising focused on gaining muscle mass, as opposed to losing fat or weight, and were preoccupied with body image.

Whereas dieting itself is a common trigger for eating disorders in both males and females, research suggests that the factors *initiating* the dieting behavior are different (Anderson 1992). There appear to be four reasons why males diet: to improve athletic performance, to avoid being teased for being fat, to avoid obesity-related illnesses observed in male family members, and to improve a homosexual relationship (Andersen 2001). Similar factors are rarely reported by women.

The methods that men and women use to achieve weight loss also appear to differ. Males are more likely to use excessive exercise as a means of weight control, while females use more passive methods such as severe energy restriction, vomiting, and laxative abuse. These weight control differences may stem from the societal biases surrounding dieting and male behavior; that is, dieting is considered to be more acceptable for women, whereas the overwhelming sociocultural belief is that "real men don't diet" (Beals 2004).

Reverse Anorexia Nervosa: The New Male Eating Disorder?

Is there an eating disorder unique to men? Recently, some eating disorder experts who work with men have suggested that there is. Observing men who are distressed by the idea that they are not sufficiently lean and muscular, who spend long hours lifting weights, and who follow an extremely restrictive diet, they have defined a disorder called *reverse anorexia nervosa*. (The disorder is also called *muscle dysphoria* or *muscle dysmorphia*.) Men with reverse anorexia nervosa perceive themselves as small and frail even though they are actually quite large and muscular. Thus, like men with true anorexia nervosa, they suffer from a body image distortion, but it is reversed. No matter how "buff" or "chiseled" he becomes, his biology cannot match his idealized body size and shape (Andersen 2001).

There are other "reversals" in these men compared to men with anorexia and other eating disorders. For instance, men with reverse anorexia nervosa frequently abuse performance-enhancing drugs: in one study, approximately half of the participants reported using anabolic steroids (Pope, Phillips, and Olivardia

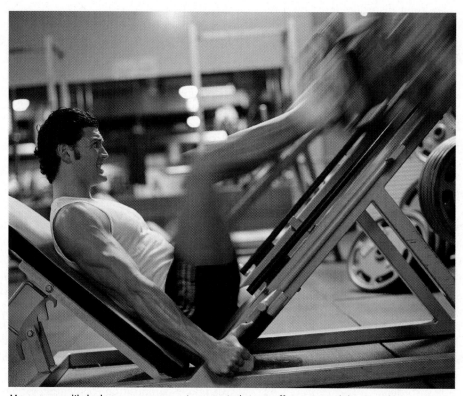

Men are more likely than women to exercise excessively in an effort to control their weight.

2000). Additionally, whereas people with anorexia eat little of anything, men with reverse anorexia tend to consume excessive high-protein foods and dietary supplements, especially products like protein powders that promise increased muscle mass and weight gain (Pope and Katz 1994).

On the other hand, men with reverse anorexia share some characteristics with men and women with other eating disorders. For instance, they too report "feeling fat" and engage in the same behaviors indicating an obsession with appearance (such as looking in the mirror). They also express significant discomfort with the idea of having to expose their body to others (e.g., taking off their clothes in the locker room) and have increased rates of mental illness (Pope, Phillips, and Olivardia 2000).

Do you know anyone who might have reverse anorexia nervosa? If you do, maybe you're wondering how you can tell whether your friend's concern about his body size is extreme or a simple enthusiasm for weightlifting. The warning signs listed in the accompanying box may help. If you think they apply to your friend, talk to him about it. Whereas reverse anorexia nervosa isn't typically life-threatening, it can certainly cause distress and despair, and therapy—especially participation in an all-male support group—can help.

Warning Signs of Reverse Anorexia Nervosa

These are some of the outward indications that someone may be struggling with reverse anorexia nervosa. Not all of them apply to all men with the disorder. If you notice any of these behaviors in a friend or relative, talk about it with him and let him know that help is available.

- Rigid and excessive schedule of weight training.

- Strict adherence to a high-protein, muscle-enhancing diet.

- Use of anabolic steroids, protein powders, or other muscle-enhancing drugs or supplements.

- Poor attendance at work, school, or sports activities because of interference with rigid weight-training schedule.

- Avoidance of social engagements where the person will not be able to follow his strict diet.

- Avoidance of situations in which the person would have to expose his body to others.

- Frequent and critical self-evaluation of body composition.

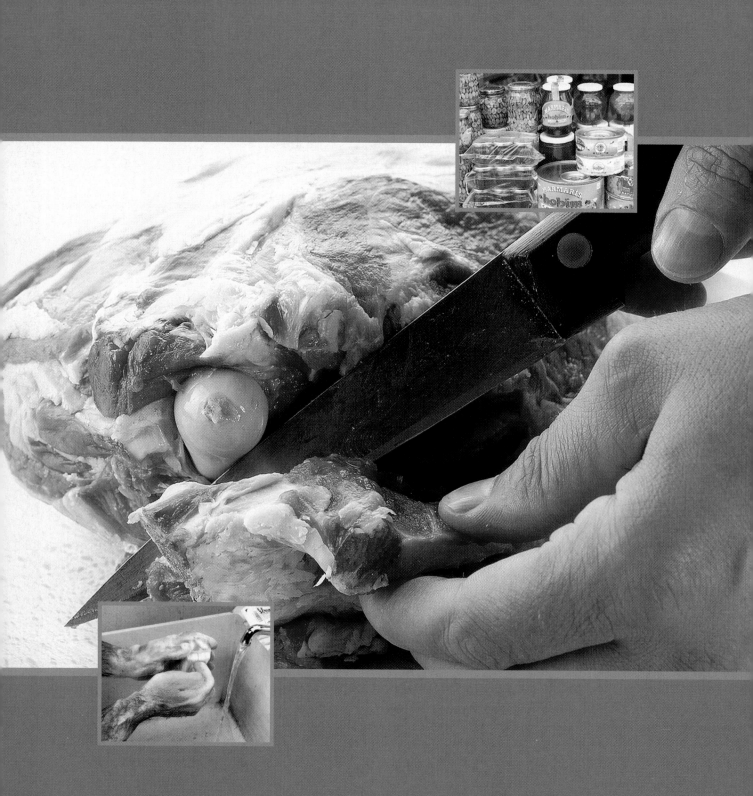

Chapter 14
Food Safety and Technology: Impact on Consumers

Chapter Objectives

After reading this chapter you will be able to:

1. Discuss four reasons why food safety is an important concern, pp. 496–498.

2. Identify the types of microorganisms involved in food-borne illness, pp. 498–505.

3. Describe strategies for preventing food-borne illness at home, while eating out, and when traveling to other countries, pp. 505–512.

4. Explain the advantages and disadvantages of canning, pasteurization, use of preservatives, aseptic packaging, and irradiation to preserve foods, pp. 512–518.

5. Identify at least five categories of food additives and explain why they are used, pp. 518–520.

6. Debate the safety of food additives, including the role of the GRAS list, pp. 520–521.

7. Discuss the benefits and safety concerns related to pesticides, pp. 522–524.

8. Explain the current system of labeling for organic foods, pp. 525–528.

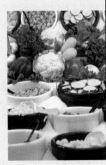

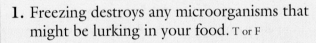

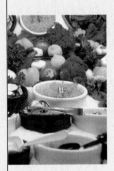

Test Yourself True or False?

1. Freezing destroys any microorganisms that might be lurking in your food. T or F

2. Some canned foods have been proven safe to eat more than forty years after canning. T or F

3. Mold is the most common cause of food poisoning. T or F

4. Research has failed to show any nutritional advantage of organic foods. T or F

5. Every food additive approved for use by food companies in the United States has been tested and proven safe. T or F

Test Yourself answers can be found at the end of the chapter.

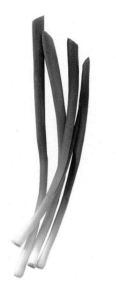

Contaminated scallions in salsa were the cause of a deadly hepatitis A outbreak.

Next time you go out with friends to your favorite Mexican restaurant, you might consider skipping the salsa. Why? In October and November of 2003, over six hundred people became ill with hepatitis A, a viral infection, and three died after eating raw green onions (scallions), primarily in salsa, at a Mexican restaurant in Pennsylvania. Officials from the Food and Drug Administration later confirmed that earlier hepatitis outbreaks in Tennessee and Georgia were also caused by contaminated scallions. When FDA investigators inspected the four farms in Mexico that had produced the scallions, they found poor sanitation, worker health, and hygiene, including inadequate handwashing, as well as concerns about water quality.

What is food poisoning? How common is it, and what causes it? Would scallions produced in the United States have caused the same reaction? What about organic scallions? Are there any guarantees that our food is safe? If not, what can we do to reduce our risk of food-borne illness?

In this chapter, you'll discover how contaminants enter our food supply, and learn some simple ways to protect yourself from getting sick. You will also learn about techniques for food preservation, food additives and residues, and the difference between organic and non-organic farming. But whether your food comes from South America, a corporate farm, an organic grower, or your own backyard, you'll see that safeguards must be in place at every step from field to table, to ensure food safety.

Why Is Food Safety Important?

Modern science and technology have given us a wide array of techniques to produce and preserve food. With these advances, there are also risks. Food safety is a major global public health issue, as foods are produced further and further away from the regions in which they are consumed, and contamination can occur at any point from farm to table. Concerns about food safety typically focus on food-borne illness, food spoilage, and technologic manipulation of food. We introduce these topics briefly here.

Food-Borne Illness Affects Seventy-Six Million Americans Each Year

food-borne illness An illness transmitted through food or water; either by an infectious agent, a poisonous substance, or a protein that causes an immune reaction.

Food-borne illness is a term used to encompass any symptom or illness that arises from ingesting food or water that contains an infectious agent, poisonous substance, or protein that causes an immune reaction. Food-borne illness is commonly called *food poisoning*. Some researchers also consider *food allergy*, a topic we introduced in Chapter 3, a type of food-borne illness.

According to the Centers for Disease Control and Prevention approximately seventy-six million Americans report experiencing food-borne illness each year. It is estimated that over half the population of the United States have had symptoms of food-borne illness without ever knowing or reporting it. Of those afflicted by food-borne illness, 300,000 are hospitalized and 5,000 die each year (CDC 2003b).

Spoilage Affects a Food's Appeal and Safety

The majority of our food is derived from living plants and animals. Because living cells gradually die and decompose after being separated from their nutrient source, it makes sense that foods start to spoil over time. The breakdown of food is due to both enzymes naturally found in the food and microorganisms that colonize the food.

Spoilage alters food in several ways. Slice an apple and leave it exposed to air for a few minutes and you'll notice how it changes in appearance. Both fruits and meats turn brown, vegetables wilt, and milk starts to curdle and sometimes takes on a yellow tinge. The texture of foods also changes as components that give food their fibrous structure begin to break down. Think of the difference between a perfectly ripe tomato and one that has turned to "mush." Taste and smell also change as a food spoils. The taste and smell of soured milk or an apple that is mealy is very distinct to anyone who has the misfortune of consuming them. Most importantly, spoiled food is no longer safe to eat: since decomposition of foods is accomplished in part by microbes, if you eat a food that has spoiled, you risk developing a food-borne illness.

Food spoilage is certainly a concern for fresh foods such as meats, fruits, and vegetables, but if you're like most Westerners, a large part of your daily diet consists of processed foods. Do they spoil, too? **Processed foods** are created by mechanical or chemical manipulation of whole foods. For example, milk is manipulated to produce cheese, which is further manipulated to become the topping for your favorite frozen pizza. Although they are often very different in appearance from their original ingredients, many processed foods actually have the same potential for spoiling as unprocessed foods. They may not change in color as they age, but their flavor, texture, and smell typically degrade, and they begin to support microbial growth. Of course, some processed foods, such as dry pasta or canned soups, resist spoilage.

Oxygen, heat, and light are the three factors most often responsible for spoilage of foods. That is why proper packaging and storage are so important in keeping foods safe to eat and enjoy. Techniques for food preservation are discussed later in this chapter.

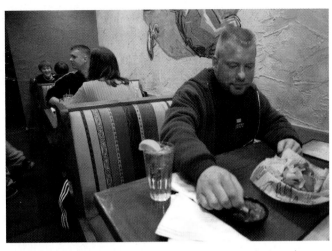

A customer samples salsa at the Pennsylvania restaurant that was the source of a hepatitis A outbreak. The restaurant no longer uses scallions in its salsa or other dishes.

processed foods Foods that are manipulated mechanically or chemically during their production or packaging. Processed foods may or may not resemble the original ingredients in their final form.

Technologic Manipulation of Food Raises Safety Concerns

Technologic manipulation of food also raises concerns related to food safety. Food producers manipulate their products by adding chemicals, using drugs and other substances that can remain in food as residues, and employing techniques such as irradiation and genetic modification that cause some food safety experts concern.

Food additives are not foods in themselves, but are chemicals added to foods to enhance them in some way. For instance, the food dye yellow #6 makes a processed cheese spread look more like real cheese, corn syrup makes processed peanut butters taste sweet, and calcium increases the nutrient value of orange juice. One category of food additives are **food preservatives,** chemicals added to foods to help maintain their freshness and appearance.

Pesticides are a family of chemicals used in both the field and storage areas to destroy plant, fungal, and animal pests. Other residues, such as organic and industrial pollutants or growth hormones used in livestock, can also remain in foods. High levels of such residues can be harmful to human health. The use of food additives, pesticides, and other chemicals and processes for food production and preservation are discussed in more detail later in this chapter.

food additives A substance or mixture of substances intentionally put into food to enhance its appearance, palatability, and quality.

food preservatives Chemicals that help prevent microbial spoilage and enzymatic deterioration.

pesticides Chemicals used either in the field or in storage to destroy plant, fungal, and animal pests.

Government Regulations Control Food Safety

Many government agencies such as the United States Department of Agriculture (USDA), the U.S. Food and Drug Administration (FDA), the Centers for Disease Control and Prevention (CDC), and the Environmental Protection Agency (EPA) monitor and regulate food production and preservation, and help to set standards to ensure food safety. Information about these agencies and how to access them is in Table 14.1.

Table 14.1   Government Agencies That Regulate Food Safety

Name of Agency	Year Established	Role in Food Regulations	Web Site
U.S. Department of Agriculture (USDA)	1785	Oversees safety of meat, poultry, and eggs sold across state lines. Also regulates which drugs can be used to treat sick cattle and poultry.	www.usda.gov
Centers for Disease Control and Prevention (CDC)	1946	Works with public health officials to promote and educate the public about health and safety. Able to track information needed in identifying food-borne illness outbreaks.	www.cdc.gov
Environmental Protection Agency (EPA)	1970	Regulates use of pesticides and which crops they can be applied to. Establishes standards for water quality.	www.epa.gov
U.S. Food and Drug Administration (FDA)	1862	Regulates food standards of all food products (except meat, poultry, and eggs) and bottled water. Regulates food labeling and enforces pesticide use as established by EPA.	www.fda.gov

Recap: Concerns about food safety center on three areas: food-borne illness, food spoilage, and technologic manipulation of food. Food-borne illness arises from ingesting food or water that contains harmful microorganisms or their products. Food spoilage affects a food's appearance, texture, taste, smell, and safety. Oxygen, heat, and light are the three factors most often responsible for spoilage of foods. The food industry uses additives, pesticides, and other chemicals and techniques in food production and preservation that concern some food safety experts. A variety of government agencies monitor and regulate food production and preservation and help to set standards to ensure food safety.

What Causes Food-Borne Illness?

Microbes or their toxic by-products cause most cases of food-borne illness. However, as we will discuss later in the chapter (page 521), chemical residues in foods can also cause illness.

Food-Borne Illness Is Caused by Microorganisms and Their Toxins

Two types of food-borne illness are common: *food infections* result from the consumption of food containing living microorganisms, whereas *food intoxications* result from consuming food in which microbes have secreted poisonous substances called *toxins* (Bauman 2004).

Several Types of Microbes Poison Foods

The microbes that most commonly cause food infections are bacteria and viruses; however, helminths, fungi, and prions also poison foods.

According to the CDC (2003b), the majority of food infections are caused by **bacteria** (Table 14.2). Bacteria are microorganisms that lack a true nucleus and have a chemical called peptidoglycan in their cell walls. Of the several species involved, *Campylobacter jejuni* is thought to be the most common culprit, causing more than two million cases each year in the United States (Figure 14.1). Most cases result from eating foods or drinking milk or water contaminated with infected animal feces. The bacteria cause fever, pain, and bloody and frequent diarrhea (Bauman 2004).

bacteria Microorganisms that lack a true nucleus and have a chemical called peptidoglycan in their cell walls.

Table 14.2   Common Bacterial Causes of Food-Borne Illness

Bacteria	Incubation Period	Duration	Symptoms	Foods Most Commonly Affected	Usual Source of Contamination	Steps for Prevention
Campylobacter jejuni	1–7 days	7–10 days	Fever Headache and muscle pain followed by diarrhea (sometimes bloody) Nausea Abdominal cramps	Raw and undercooked meat, poultry or shellfish Raw eggs Cake icing Untreated water Unpasteurized milk	Intestinal tracts of animals and birds Raw milk Untreated water and sewage sludge	Only drink pasteurized milk Cook foods properly Avoid cross contamination
Salmonella (over 2,300 types)	12–24 hours	4–7 days	Diarrhea Abdominal pain Chills Fever Vomiting Dehydration	Raw or undercooked eggs Undercooked poultry and meat Raw milk and dairy products Seafood Fruits and vegetables	Intestinal tract and feces of poultry *Salmonella enteritidis* in raw shell eggs	Cook thoroughly Avoid cross contamination Use sanitary practices
Escherichia coli (O157:H7 and other strains that can cause human illness)	2–4 days	5–10 days	Diarrhea (may be bloody) Abdominal cramps Nausea Can lead to kidney and blood complications	Contaminated water Raw milk Raw or rare ground beef, sausages Unpasteurized apple juice or cider Uncooked fruits and vegetables	Intestinal tracts of cattle Raw milk Unchlorinated water	Thoroughly cook meat Avoid cross contamination
Clostridium botulinum	12–36 hours	1–8 days	Nausea Vomiting Diarrhea Fatigue Headache Dry mouth Double vision Muscle paralysis (droopy eyelids) Difficulty speaking and swallowing Difficulty breathing	Improperly canned or vacuum-packed food Meats Sausage Fish Garlic in oil Honey	Widely distributed in nature Soil, water, on plants and intestinal tracts of animals and fish Grows only in little or no oxygen	Properly can foods following recommended procedures Cook foods properly Children under 16 months should not consume raw honey

continued

Table 14.2   *Continued*

Bacteria	Incubation Period	Duration	Symptoms	Foods Most Commonly Affected	Usual Source of Contamination	Steps for Prevention
Staphylococcus	1–6 hours	2–3 days	Severe nausea and vomiting Abdominal cramps Diarrhea	Custard-or-cream filled baked goods Ham Poultry Dressing Gravy Eggs Mayonnaise based salads and sandwiches Cream sauces	Human skin Infected cuts Pimples Noses and throats	Refrigerate foods Use sanitary practices
Shigella (over 30 types)	12–50 hours	2 days– 2 weeks	Bloody and mucus-containing diarrhea Fever Abdominal cramps Chills Vomiting	Contaminated water Salads Milk and dairy products	Human intestinal tract Rarely found in other animals	Use sanitary practices
Listeria monocytogenes	2 days– 3 weeks	None reported	Fever Muscle aches Nausea Diarrhea Headache, stiff neck, confusion, loss of balance, or convulsions can occur if infection spreads to nervous system Infections during pregnancy can lead to miscarriage or stillbirth, premature delivery, or infection of newborn	Uncooked meats and vegetables Soft cheeses Lunch meats and hot dogs Unpasteurized milk	Intestinal tract and feces of animals Soil and manure used as fertilizer Raw milk	Thoroughly cook all meats Wash raw vegetables before eating Keep uncooked meats separate from vegetables and cooked foods Avoid unpasteurized milk or foods made from unpasteurized milk People at high risk should: not eat hot dogs or lunch meats unless they are reheated until steaming hot avoid getting fluid from hot dog packages on foods, utensils, and surfaces wash hands after handling hot dogs or lunch meats avoid eating soft cheeses such as feta, Brie, and Camembert avoid eating refrigerated smoked seafood unless it is cooked

Source: Iowa State University Extension, Food safety and quality project 2000, Safe food: It's your job too! (www.extension.iastate.edu/foodsafety/Lesson/L1.html, accessed July 2003). U.S. Food and Drug Administration (FDA), How can I prevent foodborne illness? (www.cfsan.fda.gov/~dms/qa-fdb1.html, accessed June 2003). Centers for Disease Control and Prevention (CDC), Division of Bacterial and Mycotic Diseases, Disease information, Foodborne illness (http://www.cdc.gov/ncidod/dbmd/diseaseinfo/foodborneinfections_g.htm, accessed April 2004).

Salmonella is the second most common bacterial culprit in food infections. As with *Campylobacter,* most *Salmonella* infections result from eating food contaminated with animal feces, and poultry and eggs are commonly implicated. Salmonellosis causes diarrhea, nausea, and vomiting, and cells of some strains of the bacteria can perforate the intestines and infect the blood. The accompanying Highlight box discusses a particular strain of *Salmonella* that causes a food-borne disease called *typhoid fever* and its most famous host.

Although bacteria are the primary cause of food infections, some food-borne **viruses** also cause disease. Viruses are infectious agents that are much smaller than bacteria, lack independent metabolism, and are incapable of growth or reproduction apart from living cells. As we discussed at the beginning of the chapter, the hepatitis A virus can contaminate raw produce and cause liver damage. Hepatitis E also damages the liver and is fatal in about 20% of pregnant women. In terms of sheer numbers, the rotaviruses are among the most serious: in the United States, they cause about 50,000 cases of severe diarrhea in children each year, and, in developing nations, they are responsible for about one million childhood deaths. The Norwalk virus, which was identified after an epidemic in Norwalk, Ohio, can contaminate water supplies to cause diarrhea, nausea, and vomiting.

Helminths are commonly called worms, and include tapeworms, flukes, and roundworms (Figure 14.2). These microbes release their eggs into the environment, such as in vegetation or water. Animals, most commonly cattle, pigs, or fish then consume the contaminated matter. The eggs hatch inside their host, and larvae develop in the host's tissue. The larvae can survive in the flesh long after the host is killed for food. Cooking beef, pork, or fish thoroughly destroys the larvae. In contrast, if you eat the contaminated meat or fish either raw or undercooked, you consume living larvae, which then mature into adult worms in your small intestine. Some worms cause mild symptoms such as nausea and diarrhea, but others can grow large enough to cause intestinal obstruction. Some spread beyond the gastrointestinal tract to damage other organs, such as the liver, bladder, or lungs. Some can cause death.

A parasite known as *Giardia intestinalis* (or *Giardia lamblia*) causes a diarrheal illness called **giardiasis.** *Giardia* lives in the intestines of animals and humans, and it is passed in the stool of infected people and animals. It is one of the most common causes of waterborne disease in humans in the United States. You can consume *Giardia* by putting something in your mouth or by swallowing something that has come into contact with the stool of an infected person or animal, by drinking contaminated water (this includes water in lakes, streams, rivers, swimming pools, hot tubs, or fountains), or by eating uncooked food contaminated with *Giardia.* Symptoms include diarrhea, loose or watery stools, stomach cramps, and upset stomach, but some people show no symptoms. The symptoms usually begin within one to two weeks of being infected, and generally last two to six weeks. Symptoms may last longer in some people.

Fungi are plantlike spore forming organisms that can grow either as single cells or multi-cellular colonies. Two types of fungi are: yeasts, which are globular, and molds, which are long and thin. Growths of these microbes on foods rarely cause food infection. This is due in part to the fact that very few species of fungi cause serious disease in people with healthy immune systems (Bauman 2004). In addition, unlike bacterial growth, which is invisible and often tasteless, fungal growth typically makes food look and taste so unappealing that we quickly discard it (Figure 14.3).

A food-borne illness that has had front-page exposure in recent years is mad cow disease, or *bovine spongiform encephalopathy (BSE).* Cattle contract this disease from eating feed contaminated with tissue and blood from other infected animals.

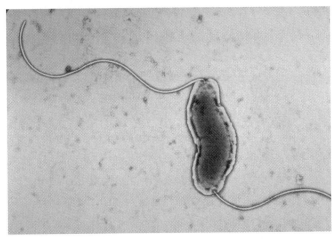

Figure 14.1 The bacteria called *Campylobacter jejuni* causes more than two million cases of food infection each year in the United States.

viruses A group of infectious agents that are much smaller than bacteria, lack independent metabolism, and are incapable of growth or reproduction apart from living cells.

helminth Multicellular microscopic worm.

giardiasis A diarrheal illness caused by the intestinal parasite *Giardia intestinalis* (or *Giardia lamblia*).

fungi Plantlike spore forming organisms that can grow either as single cells or multi-cellular colonies.

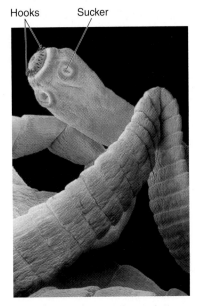

Hooks   Sucker

Figure 14.2 Tapeworms have long, worm-like bodies and hooks and suckers, which help them to attach to human tissues.

How Typhoid Mary Earned Her Place in History

"Typhoid Mary" is a name commonly given to someone who has a contagious disease, but not many people know much about the real Typhoid Mary, an Irish immigrant named Mary Mallon. In 1868, Mallon came to the United States and found work as a cook. She first came to the attention of health officials after working for the Warren family at their summer home on Oyster Bay, Long Island. Soon after settling in for a summer vacation, one of the children became ill with typhoid fever, followed by her mother, a sister, and three of the hired help.

Typhoid fever's symptoms include a high fever (104°F) and continuous headaches, followed by diarrhea. It is caused by *Salmonella typhi* and is passed through food and water contaminated by an infected person's feces. An examination of the Warren family's outbreaks caused the health investigator to stumble across Mary Mallon's employment history, which revealed that she had worked at seven previous jobs in which twenty-two people had contracted typhoid fever, with one death, after Mary began cooking for them (Leavitt 1996). When first approached as a suspect, Mary grew defensive and refused to submit blood and fecal samples, which are necessary to confirm infection. The persistent health investigator returned to Mary's place of employment with additional New York City Health Department personnel, police, and an ambulance. Mary was apprehended after a struggle and taken to a local hospital where it was confirmed that she was indeed a carrier. She had no symptoms; and so she became the United States' first "healthy carrier," a designation she refused to believe. A healthy carrier is someone who seems healthy but carries a contagious form of a disease that can infect others.

Mary was then sent to North Brother Island, part of the Riverside Hospital's facilities, in the East River to live in isolation. Mary believed she was unfairly persecuted and sued the health department. The judgment was found in favor of the health department, and Mary stayed on North Brother Island for another year, until a new health commissioner decided to release Mary on the condition that she never work as a cook again. Unfortunately, no one ever explained to Mary how she could be a "healthy carrier," as some people can have a weak

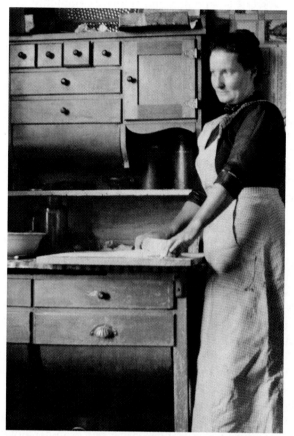

Working as a cook, Mary Mallon, also known as Typhoid Mary, caused over 50 outbreaks of typhoid.

case of typhoid fever that resembles the common flu and never know they were infected.

Now using the pseudonym Mrs. Brown, Mary again found employment as a cook, and five years after her release from North Brother Island, caused another outbreak of typhoid fever at the Sloan Maternity Hospital in Manhattan. This time, twenty-five people became ill, two of whom died. When it was discovered that Mrs. Brown was really Mary Mallon, she was immediately sent back to confinement where she lived out the remainder of her life. In all, it is believed that Typhoid Mary was the cause of fifty-three outbreaks, including the 1903 Ithaca, New York, epidemic in which 1,400 people were infected, including three deaths. (Cunningham 2002) ●

First discovered in the early 1980s in Britain, this neurological disorder is caused by a **prion,** a proteinaceous infectious particle that is self-replicating. The first reported case in the United States was in December of 2003 in Washington state, when an animal tested positive for the disease after it was slaughtered. Prions are not destroyed with cooking and are only found in the tissue of the central nervous system, retina, and lower intestines—not in the milk or muscle meats. BSE can be passed to humans who consume contaminated meat or tissue that has been ground into items such as sausages or burger. For more information on mad cow disease, check out the Highlight box, Mad Cow Disease: What's the Beef?, on page 216.

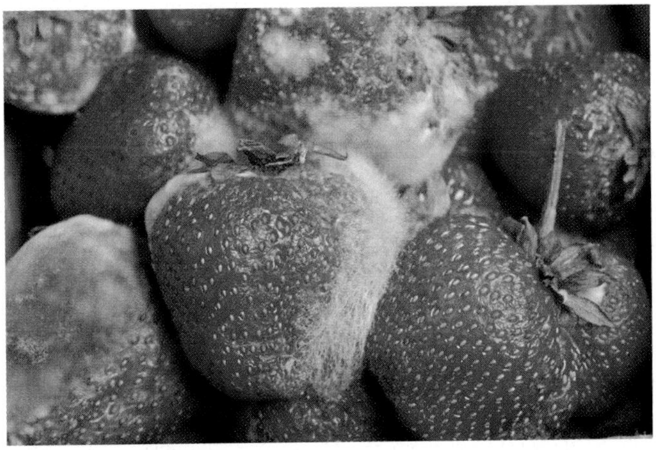

Figure 14.3 Molds rarely cause human illness, in part because they look so unappealing that we throw the food away.

Some Microbes Release Toxins

The microbes just discussed cause illness by directly infecting and destroying body cells. In contrast, other bacteria and fungi secrete chemicals called **toxins** that are responsible for serious and even life-threatening illnesses. These toxins bind to body cells and can cause a variety of symptoms such as diarrhea, vomiting, organ damage, convulsions, and paralysis.

One of the most common and deadly toxins is produced by the bacteria *Clostridium botulinum.* The botulism toxin blocks nerve transmission to muscle cells and causes paralysis, including of the muscles required for breathing.

Some fungi produce poisonous chemicals called *mycotoxins.* (The prefix *myco-* means "fungus.") These toxins are typically found in grains stored in moist environments. In some instances, moist conditions in the field encourage fungi to reproduce and release their toxins on the surface of growing crops. Long-term consumption of mycotoxins can cause organ damage or cancer, and they can be fatal if consumed in large doses. A mycotoxin called *aflatoxin* is produced by the mold *Aspergillus flavus.* Aflatoxin has been associated with peanuts and other crops and, if ingested, can cause illness in livestock and humans.

A highly visible fungus that causes food intoxication is the poisonous mushroom. Most mushrooms are not toxic, but a few, such as the deathcap mushroom (*Amanita phalloides*), can be fatal. Some poisonous mushrooms are quite colorful (Figure 14.4), a fact which helps to explain why the victims of mushroom poisoning are often children (Bauman 2004).

Toxins can be categorized depending on the type of cell they bind to; the two primary types of toxins associated with food-borne illness are **neurotoxins** and **enterotoxins.** Neurotoxins damage the nervous system, usually causing paralysis, while enterotoxins target the gastrointestinal system and generally cause severe diarrhea and vomiting.

Our Bodies Respond to Food-Borne Microbes and Toxins with Acute Illness

Many food-borne microbes are killed in the mouth by antimicrobial enzymes in saliva or in the stomach by hydrochloric acid. Any microbe that survives these chemical assaults will usually trigger vomiting and/or diarrhea as the gastrointestinal tract attempts to expel the offender. Simultaneously, the white blood cells of the immune system will be activated, and a generalized inflammatory response will cause the person to experience nausea, fatigue, fever, and muscle cramps. Refer back to Table 14.2 (page 499) to identify many possible symptoms resulting from food infection with various bacteria.

People most affected by food-borne illnesses are those with compromised immune systems, such as people with HIV or undergoing chemotherapy, the elderly,

prion An infectious, self-replicating protein.

toxin Any harmful substance; specifically, a chemical produced by a microorganism that harms tissues or causes harmful immune responses.

neurotoxins A type of exotoxin that targets the nervous system cells.

enterotoxins A type of exotoxin that targets the gastrointestinal tract cells.

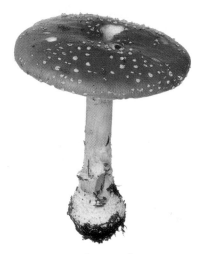

Figure 14.4 Some mushrooms, such as this fly agaric, contain toxins that can cause illness or even death.

children under the age of ten, and pregnant women. However, food-borne illness can affect anyone. Depending on our state of health, the precise microbe involved, and the number of microbes ingested, the symptoms can range from mild to severe, including double vision, loss of muscle control, and excessive or bloody diarrhea. As noted earlier, some cases, if left untreated, can result in death.

To diagnose a food-borne illness, a specimen must be obtained and cultured. This means the specimen is analyzed in a laboratory setting in which the offending microorganisms are grown in a specific chemical medium. Stool (fecal) cultures are usually analyzed, especially if diarrhea is a symptom. Blood is cultured if the patient has a high fever. A physician who suspects that a patient is suffering from a food-borne illness will take a detailed history including a 24-hour dietary recall. Treatment usually involves keeping the person hydrated and comfortable, as most food-borne illness tends to be self-limiting; the person's vomiting and/or diarrhea, though unpleasant, serve to rid the body of the offending microbe. In severe illnesses such as botulism, the patient's intestinal tract will be repeatedly treated to remove the microbe, and antibodies will be injected to neutralize its deadly toxin.

In the United States, all confirmed cases of food-borne illness must be reported to the state health department, which in turn reports these illnesses to the CDC in Atlanta, Georgia. The CDC monitors its reports for indications of epidemics of food-borne illness and assists local and state agencies in controlling such outbreaks.

Certain Environmental Conditions Help Microbes Multiply in Foods

Given the correct conditions, microbes can thrive and multiply in many types of food. These growth-favoring conditions include a precise range of temperature, humidity, acidity, and oxygen content. For example, many bacteria are destroyed by normal heating, and many cannot reproduce in a food that is refrigerated or frozen. Many microbes require a high level of moisture, and thus foods like boxed dried pasta do not make suitable microbial homes, though cooked pasta left at room temperature might prove hospitable.

As just noted, many microbes cannot tolerate acidic foods. For example, *Clostridium botulinum* cannot grow or produce its toxin in an acidic environment, so the risk of botulism is decreased in citrus fruits, pickles, and tomato-based foods. In contrast, more alkaline foods such as eggs are a magnet for *C. botulinum*.

In addition, microbes need an entryway into a food. Just as our skin protects our bodies from microbial invasion, the peels, rinds, and shells of many foods seal off access to microbes. Eggshells are a good example of a barrier that keeps almost all bacteria from entering the nutrient-rich environment within. Once such a barrier is removed, however, the food loses its primary defense against contamination.

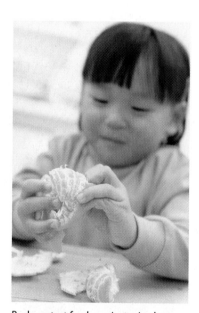

Peels protect foods against microbes.

Recap: Food infections result from the consumption of food containing living microorganisms, such as bacteria, whereas food intoxications result from consuming food in which microbes have secreted toxins. Food infections can be caused by bacteria, viruses, fungi, helminths, and prions. The body has several defense mechanisms, such as saliva, stomach acid, vomiting, diarrhea, and the inflammatory response, which help rid us of offending microorganisms or their toxins. In order to reproduce in foods, microbes require a precise range of temperature, humidity, acidity, and oxygen content.

Food Allergies Also Cause Illness

The ancient saying, "one man's meat is another man's poison" has a good deal of truth behind it. As discussed in Chapter 3, some people experience allergic reactions to foods. These can vary from delayed-onset reactions such as rashes, headaches, or bowel disturbances hours or days after the offending food was eaten, to immediate-onset reactions, such as life-threatening anaphylactic shock. The foods that most commonly cause allergic reactions include cow's milk and milk products, eggs, nuts, citrus fruit, seafood, wheat, corn, and soy. Although people can have food allergies to starches or additives, 90% of all food allergies are related to proteins that make up the foods themselves (Emsley and Fell 2002).

Children's delayed reactions to food allergens are often different from those of adults. Some common symptoms in children include chronic ear infections, bedwetting, dark circles under the eyes, irritability, and eczema. Interestingly enough, many young children outgrow their allergies. Over 50% of children under the age of three who were diagnosed with a food allergy to eggs or milk became tolerant of these foods when their gastrointestinal tracts matured (Emsley and Fell 2002).

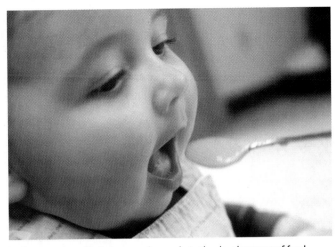

Earlier weaning of infants may play a role in the development of food allergies, especially if infants are introduced to highly-allergenic foods early on.

Food allergies can either be fixed or cyclic. A fixed food reaction occurs whenever an offending food is eaten. People with fixed food allergies need to avoid foods that cause a reaction. A cyclic allergic response, which accounts for 85% of food allergies, develops slowly over time. If the offending food is avoided for at least three to six months, then it can be reintroduced into the diet in small, infrequent amounts without any reactions (Braly 2000).

It is estimated that one out of five Americans experiences some symptoms related to their diet (Emsley and Fell 2002). Although most people do not have immediate-onset food allergies, with repeated exposure to the same food components, many people develop delayed-onset reactions. Some theories as to why we react to food or its components are:

- Increased stresses on the immune system from chemicals in the environment, such as water or air pollution.
- Earlier weaning and introduction of solid food to infants, especially foods that are highly allergenic, such as dairy, eggs, wheat, citrus, nuts, soy, and chocolate.
- Genetic manipulation of plants and animals (known as GMOs, or genetically modified organisms) results in food components which contain proteins that are not normally in that organism, but cause an antibody response in that individual.
- Frequent exposure to the same food in various forms, many times not intentionally. For example, you can purchase frozen French fries that have milk protein listed as an ingredient and rice chips that have corn in them—who would have guessed!

Regardless of the reasons why people develop food allergies, it is important to eat a variety of foods so potential irritants are not repeatedly exposed to our systems. It is also prudent to eat less processed and more organically grown foods to minimize the amount of added chemicals in your diet, especially if you have relatives who suffer from food allergies.

Recap: Allergic reactions to foods can be immediate or delayed by several hours or days. To prevent the development of delayed-onset food allergies, it is important to eat a variety of foods so that your immune system is not repeatedly exposed to the same potential irritants.

How Can You Prevent Food-Borne Illness?

Foods of animal origin are most commonly associated with food-borne illness. These include not only raw meat, poultry, and fish, but also eggs, shellfish, and unpasteurized milk. Foods that may be the product of several animals (such as ground beef) can

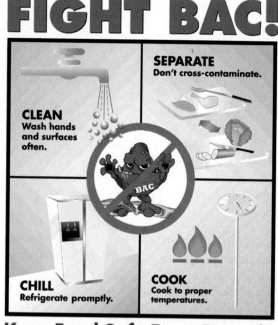

Figure 14.5   The FightBAC! logo is the food safety logo of the United States Department of Agriculture.

be especially hazardous. In addition, a bacteria or virus present in one animal has the potential to contaminate the entire herd.

Fruits and vegetables can also cause problems when they are consumed unwashed and raw. Washing decreases, but cannot eliminate, all contaminants, and the quality of the water used in washing is sometimes a factor. Unpasteurized fruit or vegetable juices may also be contaminated if the produce used to make these juices contained pathogens (CDC 2003b).

When Preparing Foods at Home

When you prepare foods at home, you can prevent food-borne illness by following four basic rules (Figure 14.5):

1. Wash your hands and kitchen surfaces often.
2. Separate foods to prevent **cross contamination;** that is, the spread of bacteria or other microbes from one food to another. This commonly occurs when raw, unwashed foods are cut on the same cutting board or served together on the same plate.
3. Cook foods to their proper temperatures (discussed on pages 509–511).
4. Chill foods to prevent microbes from growing.

Wash Your Hands

One of the easiest and most effective ways to prevent food-borne illness is to wash your hands both before and after preparing food. Scrub for at least twenty seconds with gentle soap under warm running water (sing "Happy Birthday" or say the ABC's to time yourself). Hot water is too harsh: it causes the surface layer of the skin to break down, increasing the risk that microbes will be able to penetrate your skin. Pay special attention to the areas underneath your fingernails and between your fingers. Also, it's a good idea to remove rings while cooking, as they can harbor bacteria. To prevent cross contamination, always wash your hands after working with each raw food and before progressing to the next one.

cross contamination Contamination of one food by another via the unintended transfer of microbes through physical contact.

Wash Kitchen Utensils and Surfaces

A clean area and tools are also essential in reducing cross contamination. Wash utensils, containers, and cutting boards in the dishwasher or with hot soapy water before and after contact with food; this is especially critical with raw and cooked meat, poultry, and seafood (Food Marketing Institute 2003). It's also important to wash counter tops and utensils with hot soapy water after preparing each food type to reduce the chance of cross contamination. Use a non-porous, smooth plastic or stone cutting board because porous wood and scratched plastic can hold juices and harbor bacteria.

Dishtowels, cloths and aprons should be washed in hot water often. It's a good idea to wash sponges in the dishwasher each time you run it and to replace them regularly. If you don't have a dishwasher, put sponges in boiling water for three minutes to sterilize them on a routine basis.

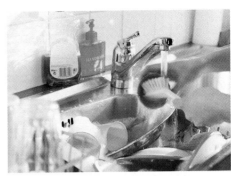

Washing dishes, utensils, and cutting boards with hot soapy water reduces the chances for food contamination.

Isolate Raw Foods

Raw meat, poultry, and seafood harbor an array of microbes and can easily contaminate other foods through direct contact, as well as by the juices they leave behind on surfaces (including hands) that are not cleaned after each food's preparation. Contact between food that won't be cooked, like salad ingredients, with these foods or their juices can result in food-borne illness. Also be careful not to place cooked food on a plate that previously held raw meat, seafood, or poultry. When preparing meals with a marinade, make sure you reserve some of the marinade in a clean container before adding raw ingredients if you will need some noncontaminated marinade to use later in the cooking process. Remember to always marinate raw food in the refrigerator.

Store Foods in the Refrigerator or Freezer

Different microbes thrive in different environmental temperatures. The majority of bacteria that cause food-borne illness prefer temperatures between 60 and 130°F, (15 to 50°C), with the majority growing best in temperatures between 80 and 100°F (25 to 40°C) (Tortora, Funke, and Case 2003). Because of this, refrigeration (storage between 32 and 40°F) and freezing (storage below 32°F) are two of the most reliable methods of diminishing bacteria's ability to cause illness. Not all bacteria in cool environments are killed, but the rate at which they reproduce is drastically reduced. Also, naturally occurring enzymes that cause food decomposition are stopped at freezing temperatures.

Shopping Tips   When shopping for food, purchase refrigerated and frozen foods last. Many grocery stores are actually designed so that these foods are in the last aisles. When you are buying meats, poultry, seafood, and dairy products, look for the "sell by" or "use by" date on their packaging. The "sell by" date indicates the last day a product can be sold and still maintain its quality during normal home storage and consumption. It is generally best to try to purchase foods prior to this date. The "use by" date tells you how long a product will maintain optimum quality before eating (Food Marketing Institute 2003). It is best to avoid buying foods past the "use by" date, even though they are generally still safe to eat. For nonperishable foods such as cereal and baking mixes, the "best if used by (or before)" dates indicate the shelf-life of the product or the date at which the product is no longer at peak flavor, texture, and appearance. These foods can be safely eaten past the listed date if they have been stored properly, but they may not taste as good or be as nutritious as they were before this date. Proper storage for nonperishable items includes storage in a dry, clean, cool (less than 85°F) cabinet or pantry.

After you purchase perishable foods, get them home and into the refrigerator or freezer within one hour. If your trip home will be longer than an hour, bring along a cooler to transport them in.

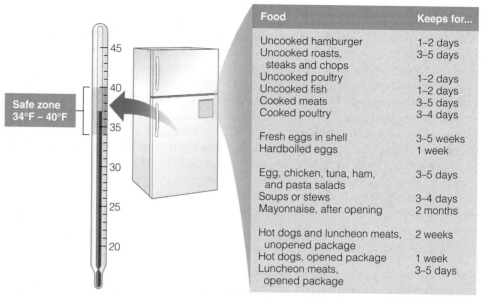

Food	Keeps for...
Uncooked hamburger	1–2 days
Uncooked roasts, steaks and chops	3–5 days
Uncooked poultry	1–2 days
Uncooked fish	1–2 days
Cooked meats	3–5 days
Cooked poultry	3–4 days
Fresh eggs in shell	3–5 weeks
Hardboiled eggs	1 week
Egg, chicken, tuna, ham, and pasta salads	3–5 days
Soups or stews	3–4 days
Mayonnaise, after opening	2 months
Hot dogs and luncheon meats, unopened package	2 weeks
Hot dogs, opened package	1 week
Luncheon meats, opened package	3–5 days

Safe zone 34°F – 40°F

Figure 14.6   While it's important to keep a well-stocked refrigerator, it's also important to know how long foods will keep. (U.S. Department of Agriculture, Food Safety and Inspection Service, January 1999, Consumer Education and Information. Refrigeration and Food Safety, www.fsis.usda.gov/OA/pubs/focus_ref.htm Accessed April 2004.)

Refrigerating Foods   Once you get home, meat, poultry, and seafood should be put in the coldest part of the refrigerator. They should also be properly wrapped so their juices do not drip onto any other foods. If you are not going to use meat, poultry, or seafood within forty-eight hours of purchase, store them in the freezer (Food Marketing Institute 2003). Remember that eggs are also perishable and should be kept refrigerated. Avoid overstocking your refrigerator or freezer, as air needs to circulate around food to cool it quickly and discourage microbial growth.

After a meal, leftovers should be promptly refrigerated—even if still hot—to discourage microbial growth. The standard rule for storing leftovers is: *2 hours/2 inches/4 days*. Food should be refrigerated *within 2 hours* of serving. If the temperature is 90°F or higher, such as at a picnic, then foods should be refrigerated within one hour (USDA 2003). Because a larger quantity of food takes longer to cool and will allow more microbes to thrive, food should be stored at a depth of no greater than *2 inches*. The interior of deeper containers of foods can remain warm long enough to allow bacteria to multiply rapidly even when the surface of the food has cooled. Leftovers should only be refrigerated for *up to 4 days*. If you don't plan on using the food within four days, freeze it. A guide for storing foods in your refrigerator is provided in Figure 14.6.

Freezing and Thawing Foods   The temperature in your freezer should not exceed 32°F (0°C). Use a thermometer to check it periodically to make sure this temperature is being maintained. If your electricity goes out, avoid opening the freezer until the power is restored. When the power does come back on, check to make sure the temperature is at least 23°F (−5°C) on the top shelf. If it is warmer, you should inspect your freezer's contents and discard any items that are not firmly frozen, thus lessening chances of an overgrowth of bacteria.

When freezing items, remember that smaller packages will freeze more quickly. So rather than attempting to freeze an entire casserole or a whole batch of homemade spaghetti sauce, divide the food into multiple portions in freezer-safe containers, then freeze.

Sufficient thawing will ensure adequate cooking throughout, which is essential to preventing food-borne illness. Raw poultry is a good example of a food item that

Table 14.3 A Guide to Thawing Poultry

Method Needed	Size of Poultry	Approximate Length of Time
Refrigerator	1–3 pounds, small chickens, pieces	1 day
	3–6 pounds, large chickens, ducks, small turkeys	2 days
	6–12 pounds, large turkeys	3 days
	12–16 pounds, whole turkey	3–4 days
	16–20 pounds, whole turkey	4–5 days
Microwave (read instructions)	1–3 pounds, small chickens, pieces	8–15 minutes* (standing time 10 minutes)
	3–6 pounds, large chickens, ducks, small turkeys	15–30 minutes* (standing time 20 minutes)

*Approximate, read microwave's instructions
Note: Turkeys purchased stuffed and frozen with the USDA or state mark of inspection on the packaging are safe because they have been processed under controlled conditions. These turkeys *should not* be thawed before cooking. Follow package directions for handling.
Sources: R. W. Lacey, *Hard to Swallow: A brief history of food* (Cambridge: Cambridge University Press, 1994), 85–187. U.S. Department of Agriculture, Food Safety and Inspection Service, 2000, Turkey basics: Safe thawing (www.fsis.usda.gov/oa/pubs/tbthaw.htm, accessed July 2003).

needs to be carefully contained as it thaws, so its juices don't contaminate other foods. The perfect place to thaw poultry is on the bottom shelf of the refrigerator and in a large bowl to catch any of its juices. Table 14.3 shows recommended poultry thawing times based on weight. Never thaw frozen meat, poultry, or seafood on a kitchen counter or in a basin of warm water. Room temperatures allow growth of bacteria on the surface of food, although the inside may still be frozen (Food Marketing Institute 2003). A microwave is also useful for thawing, but be sure to read your microwave's instructions carefully first. Thawing with a microwave is generally recommended only if the food is to be cooked immediately afterwards.

Molds in Refrigerated Foods   Have you ever taken cheese out of the refrigerator and noticed that it had a fuzzy blue growth on it? This is mold, one of the two types of fungus. Interestingly, cool temperatures do not slow the growth of some molds; in fact, some prefer refrigeration. For instance, when acidic foods such as applesauce, leftover coffee, and spaghetti sauce are refrigerated, they readily support the growth of mold. So how did the mold get into the sealed, refrigerated package? Mold spores are common in the atmosphere, and they randomly land on food either in the processing plant or in open containers at your home. If the temperature and acidity of the food is hospitable, they will grow.

Most people throw away moldy foods because they are so unappealing, but as we noted earlier, food-borne illnesses aren't commonly caused by fungi. If a small portion of a solid food such as cheese becomes moldy, it is generally safe to cut off that section and eat the unspoiled portion.

Some fungi are actually used in the food industry to create popular foods and beverages. The distinct flavor of Roquefort and blue cheeses can be attributed to the molds used in their ripening process. Yeast, the globular form of fungi, gives a distinct flavor to fermented foods such as sourdough bread, miso, soy sauce, beer, wine, and distilled spirits. Even the production of chocolate requires the help of yeasts, which ferment the cacao seeds, causing them to lose their bitter taste.

Cook Foods Thoroughly

Remember those intestinal worms we discussed earlier? Thoroughly cooking food is a sure way to kill these and other microbes. The appropriate temperatures for cooking raw meat, poultry, seafood, and eggs vary, as shown in Figure 14.7.

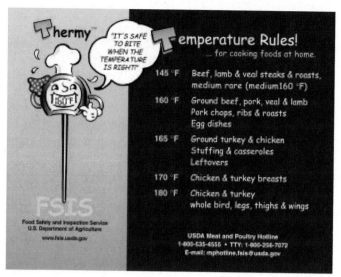

Figure 14.7   The United States Department of Agriculture's "Thermy" provides temperature rules for safely cooking foods at home.

The color of cooked meat can be deceiving. Grilled meat and poultry often brown very quickly on the outside but may not be thoroughly cooked on the inside. The only way to be sure meat is thoroughly cooked is with a food thermometer. Test your food in several places to be sure it's cooked evenly, and remember to wash the thermometer after each use. If you don't have a thermometer available, do not eat hamburger that is still pink inside, as the CDC links eating undercooked, pink hamburger with a higher risk of food-borne illness (USDA 2003).

Microwave cooking is convenient, but you need to be sure your food is thoroughly cooked, and there are no cold spots in the food where bacteria can thrive. For best results when microwaving, remember to cover food, stir often, and rotate for even cooking (USDA 2003). If you are microwaving meat or poultry, use a thermometer to check internal temperatures in several spots, since temperatures vary in different parts of food more in microwave cooking than in conventional ovens (Food Marketing Institute 2003).

Raw fish delicacies such as sushi are tempting, but their safety cannot be guaranteed. Always cook fish thoroughly. When done, fish should be opaque and flake easily with a fork.

You may have memories of licking the cake batter off a spoon when you were a kid, but such practices are no longer safe. That's because cake batter contains raw eggs, and an estimated one-third of chicken eggs in the United States is contaminated with *Salmonella*. For this reason, the USDA now recommends that you cook eggs until the yolk and whites are firm. Scrambled eggs should not be runny. If you are using eggs in a casserole or custard, make sure that the internal temperature reaches at least 160°F (Center for Science in the Public Interest [CSPI] 2004b).

Killing microorganisms with heat is an important step in keeping food safe, but it won't protect you against their toxins. That's because toxins are unaffected by heat and are capable of causing severe illness even when the microbes that produced them have been destroyed. For example, let's say you prepare a casserole for a team picnic. Too bad you forget to wash your hands before serving it to your teammates because you contaminate the casserole with the bacteria *Staphylococcus aureus*. You and your friends go off and play soccer, leaving the food in the sun, and a few hours later, you take the rest of the casserole home. At supper, you heat the leftovers thoroughly, thinking as you do so that this will kill any bacteria that might have multiplied while it was left out. That night you wake up with nausea, vomiting, diarrhea, and abdominal pain. What happened? While your food was left out, the bacteria from your hands multiplied and produced their toxin (Figure 14.8). When you reheated the food, you

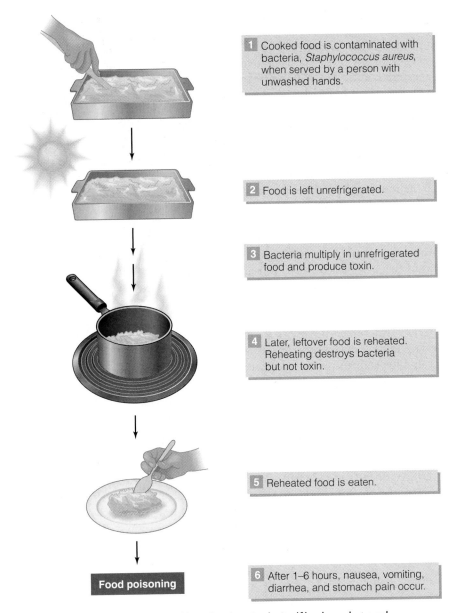

1. Cooked food is contaminated with bacteria, *Staphylococcus aureus*, when served by a person with unwashed hands.

2. Food is left unrefrigerated.

3. Bacteria multiply in unrefrigerated food and produce toxin.

4. Later, leftover food is reheated. Reheating destroys bacteria but not toxin.

5. Reheated food is eaten.

Food poisoning

6. After 1–6 hours, nausea, vomiting, diarrhea, and stomach pain occur.

Figure 14.8 Food intoxication can occur long after the microbe itself has been destroyed.

killed the microorganisms, but their toxin was unaffected by the heat. When you then ate the food, the toxin made you sick. Fortunately, in the case of *S. aureus,* symptoms typically resolve on their own in about 24 hours.

When Eating Out

When choosing a place to eat out, avoid restaurants that don't look clean. Grimy tabletops and dirty restrooms indicate indifference to hygiene. On the other hand, cleanliness of areas used by the public doesn't guarantee that the kitchen is clean. That is why health inspections are important. Public health inspectors randomly visit and inspect the food preparation areas of all businesses that serve food, whether eaten in or taken out. You can usually find the results of these inspections in the local newspaper or by contacting your local health department.

Another way to protect yourself when dining out is by ordering foods to be cooked thoroughly. If you order a hamburger that arrives pink in the middle, send it back and ask for it to be cooked longer. If you order scrambled eggs that arrive runny, send them back or order something else.

When Traveling to Other Countries

When planning your trip, tell your physician your travel plans and ask about vaccinations needed or any medications that you should take along in case you get sick. Also pack a waterless antibacterial hand cleanser, and use it frequently during your trip. When dining, select foods and beverages carefully. All raw food has the potential for contamination, especially in areas where hygiene and sanitation are inadequate. All travelers are cautioned to avoid salads, uncooked fruits and vegetables, and unpasteurized dairy products. Fruits and vegetables are safe to eat if you first wash them thoroughly in bottled water or water that has been boiled for one minute and then allowed to cool. Peeling washed fruits and vegetables also reduces the likelihood of contamination. If fish is a local delicacy, be aware that many tropical species from the insular areas of the Caribbean and the Pacific and Indian Oceans can contain poisonous **biotoxins,** even when well cooked (CDC 2003a). Biotoxins are naturally occurring poisonous chemicals.

biotoxins Naturally occurring poisonous chemicals.

Water is seldom a safe option, even if chlorinated, as chlorine doesn't kill all organisms that can cause disease. In regions where hygiene and sanitation are suspect, only consume the following: canned or bottled carbonated beverages such as bottled water and soft drinks, beverages made with boiled water such as tea, and fermented drinks such as beer and wine, as their processing will neutralize any potential pathogens. Also, remember to ask for drinks without ice, as freezing contaminated water does not kill microbes and parasites. If you think the water may be contaminated, don't even brush your teeth with it: use bottled water or boil the water for one minute, then allow the water to return to room temperature before brushing. You can find more information about food and water safety when traveling by visiting the CDC's Web site (www.cdc.gov.travel.food-drink-risks.htm) or by contacting your local health department.

> **Recap:** You can prevent food-borne illness at home by following these tips: wash your hands and kitchen surfaces often; separate foods to prevent cross contamination; cook foods to their proper temperatures; store foods in the refrigerator or freezer; thaw frozen foods in the refrigerator; and heat foods long enough and at proper temperatures to ensure proper cooking. When traveling, avoid all raw foods unless thoroughly washed in bottled or boiled water, and choose beverages that are boiled, bottled, or canned, without ice.

Theo   *Nutri-Case*

"I got really sick yesterday after eating lunch in the cafeteria. I had a turkey sandwich, potato salad, and a cola. Halfway through my afternoon class, I had to leave. I barely made it to the bathroom in time. I spent the rest of the day in my dorm room in bed. This morning I feel okay, just sort of weak. I asked some of my friends who ate in the caf yesterday if they got sick, and none of them did, but I still think it was the food. I'm going off-campus for lunch today!"

Do you think that Theo's illness was food-borne? If so, what food(s) do you most suspect? What do you think of his plan to go off-campus for lunch today? And what other actions might you advise Theo to take?

How Is Food Spoilage Prevented?

Any food that has been harvested and that people aren't ready to eat must be preserved in some way or, before long, it will degrade chemically and become home to a variety of microorganisms. Here, we look at some techniques that people have used for centuries to preserve food, as well as more modern techniques used in the food industry.

Tried and True—Preserving Foods through Natural Techniques

Some methods of preserving foods have been used for thousands of years and employ naturally derived substances such as salt, sugars, and smoke or techniques such as drying and cooling.

Salting and Sugaring

Both salt and sugar preserve food by drawing the water out of the plant or animal cells by *osmosis,* as discussed in Chapter 7 (see Figure 7.4, page 237). Salting or sugaring essentially dehydrates the food, making it inhospitable to microbes, especially bacteria. Dehydration also dramatically slows the action of enzymes that would otherwise degrade the food. A good way to see how effectively salt draws water from food, and to understand osmosis, is to rub salt on cucumber slices, then let them sit for an hour. When the hour has passed, the surface of the cucumber will be covered with water that has "sweated" out of the cucumber.

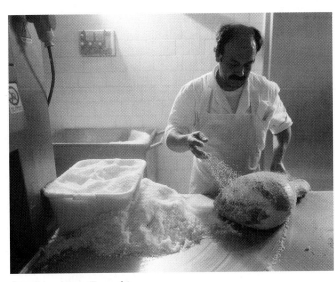

A worker salting a Parma ham.

Salt, one of the oldest and most effective preservatives, is especially good at drawing water from food. The amount of salt required to be effective as a preservative is much higher than what is normally used for seasoning. Traditionally, salt was the primary preservative used in all meats and seafood, but because of current concerns about sodium intake and hypertension, this method is not used as much as it was in the past. Some kinds of meat jerky still rely on salting, but few other products do.

Salt has been traditionally used for curing pork products. Many countries have specialty hams that rely on regional customs to produce a unique and quality meat. A good example is the Parma ham from Italy, which is dry-salted with sea salt during the winter for about a month, then wiped clean and hung in huge curing rooms in long rows where plenty of fresh air can circulate around them. The curers must constantly adjust windows to accommodate changing winds. It takes almost nine months for a Parma ham to mature (Shephard 2000).

Sugar has a remarkable ability to preserve foods while retaining much of their shape, color, and texture because some of the sugar is absorbed into the cells, replacing the water drawn out. The downside to using sugar is that fungi tend to flourish in sweet, acidic environments, such as jams. Sugar also adds calories and can contribute to dental caries (cavities).

Honey, a natural sweetener, is also an effective preserver. Thousands of years ago, long before the processing of white or cane sugar, honey was used to preserve meats and fruits (Shephard 2000). Hams are often covered in honey to create an antibacterial coating to protect them during storage.

Drying

Drying is an ancient method of preserving food, used by many cultures in a variety of climates. There is evidence that the Egyptians dried fish and poultry in the hot desert sun as early as 12,000 BC (Shephard 2000). Beans, peas, and fruits are also commonly preserved by drying.

Drying works by the same principle as osmosis: by removing water, it makes a food inhospitable to bacteria, fungi, and other microorganisms and slows its chemical deterioration. However, depending on the method used, the food's color, texture, and flavor may change, and the vitamin content can be decreased.

Another method of drying food is called *freeze-drying;* this is a rapid and complete drying of food. The food is first flash-frozen: any water is rapidly converted to fine ice crystals, which are evaporated in a vacuum. The product is then immediately packaged and sealed to ensure no penetration of moisture occurs. Freeze-drying preserves flavor, color, and texture, and allows a shelf life of several years as long as the seal is not broken. Food manufacturers use freeze-drying for products such as coffee, tea, dried milk, gravy, and soup powders. This method is also used to make freeze-dried backpacker's food.

Smoking

Smoking has been used for centuries for preservation of meats, poultry, and fish. If food was not drying well, it would be hung near the campfire or chimney so the smoke of the fire would permeate the food, further drying it.

For short-term preservation, food can be *cold-smoked* at a temperature no higher then 85°F (29°C). The smoke will give a mild, smoky flavor to the food as it dries but will not actually cook the food. This method is good for meat or fish but will only preserve them for a limited time before they start to spoil. Cold-smoking is commonly used for foods that are eaten raw such as beef fillets or smoked salmon.

Hot-smoking uses temperatures above 130°F (55°C). It not only dries, but also partially cooks the food. This process is used for foods such as venison, poultry, smoked trout, pork, lamb and beef. Originally heavy salting was used in conjunction with hot-smoking, but now modern hot-smoked food uses much less salt.

The type of wood used to smoke foods contributes to the food's flavor. Birch, hickory, apple, juniper, mesquite and willow are woods that have distinctive flavors. Smoked foods still need to be covered and stored in areas where air, heat, and insects cannot have easy access to them.

Cooling

As mentioned earlier, bacterial metabolism works best at temperatures at or above 60°F. As the temperature of a food is lowered, the bacteria's metabolism is slowed, and it becomes less able to reproduce or give off toxic by-products. So what did people use to cool and store foods before they had electric refrigerators?

For thousands of years, people have stored foods in underground cellars, caves, running streams, and even "cold pantries," rooms of the house that were kept dark and unheated and often were stocked with ice. The use of icehouses to store food is discussed in records from second century China. Thirteenth and fourteenth century Egyptian royalty were also storing food in icehouses, stocked with ice brought from the mountains of Lebanon (Shephard 2000). The transport of freshly caught fish using ice is also first attributed to the Chinese, and European merchants fascinated with the idea soon perfected the use of cold to design and build refrigerated vessels to transport all types of foods. Ice therefore became an important commodity. A Massachusetts company developed the forerunner of our refrigerator, the miniature icehouse, in the early 1800s, and in cities and towns, the local iceman would make rounds delivering ice to homes.

> **Recap:** Natural food preservation techniques include salting, sugaring, drying, and smoking, all of which draw water out of foods, making them inhospitable to microbes. Storage in ice houses, cold pantries, cellars, running streams, and other cold areas has been used for centuries to preserve food.

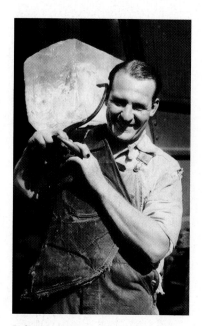

Before the modern refrigerator, an "iceman" would deliver ice to homes and businesses.

Better Living through Chemistry—Synthetic Preservative Techniques Improve Food Safety

To be successful, food producers have had to find ways to preserve the integrity of their products during the days, weeks, or months between harvesting and consumption. Until the latter part of the twentieth century, industrial techniques for food preservation were limited to drying, canning, pasteurization, and the addition of certain preservative chemicals. However, in the last few decades, the modern techniques of aseptic packaging, irradiation, and genetic modification have greatly expanded our food choices.

Industrial Canning

The French inventor Nicolas-François Appert first developed the canning process in the late 1700s, and modern techniques have contributed to the retention of flavor, texture, and nutrients in canned foods. In the United States, twenty million canned foods are consumed per day (Shephard 2000).

Producers of canned foods are required by law to ensure that all endospores of *Clostridium botulinum* be eliminated from their goods. As you recall, if the spores of this bacteria were to germinate inside a can of food, the food would soon become saturated with the deadly botulism toxin. The same process that destroys *C. botulinum* endospores also kills other microorganisms that have food-poisoning potential. This process involves several steps:

1. The food to be canned is sorted, and any spoiled food is removed.
2. The food is washed.
3. The food is blanched. Blanching involves the use of hot water or steam to parboil or scald the food, thereby stopping enzymatic processes and killing microorganisms on the food's surface. It can also be used to help remove skins from certain fruits and vegetables.
4. Cans are filled and heated, air is siphoned out, and they are sealed.
5. The sealed cans are heated to a very high temperature by steam under pressure and then cooled in a water bath.

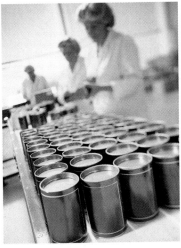

Canning food involves several steps to ensure all microorganisms in the food are killed.

Canned food has an average shelf life of at least two years from the date of purchase. It is recommended that all canned food be stored in moderate temperatures (75°F and below).

The U.S. Army has found that canned meats, vegetables and jam have been in "excellent states of preservation" after 46 years. However, long storage of canned foods is not recommended. For high quality (versus safety), the broadest guideline given by the USDA is to use high-acid canned food (fruits, tomatoes and pickled products) in 18 to 24 months and low-acid (meats and vegetables) in two to five years.

Pasteurization

Pasteurization was developed in 1864 by Louis Pasteur to destroy microorganisms that spoiled wine. Its quick use of heat to eliminate pathogens without altering the taste or quality of the food product makes it a particularly useful and important process in the dairy and juice industry. Heating to 162°F (72°C) for fifteen seconds pasteurizes milk, while ice cream, which is higher in fat, requires pasteurization at 180°F (82°C) for twenty seconds. Pasteurization does not eliminate all microbes but significantly decreases the numbers of heat-sensitive microorganisms, which tend to be the most harmful.

pasteurization   A form of sterilization using high temperatures for short periods of time.

Addition of Preservatives

Food preservatives are substances added to a variety of foods to prevent or slow food spoilage. There are many natural and synthetically derived preservatives used in our food supply. One of the most commonly used natural preservatives is vitamin C. This nutrient is a powerful antioxidant and helps protect foods from damage due to oxygen exposure. EDTA (ethylenediaminetetraacetic acid) is a commonly used synthetic preservative. It is used to trap trace amounts of metal impurities that can get into foods from containers and processing machinery.

Preservatives help extend the shelf life of many foods, decreasing costs and allowing consumers to buy items in bulk. Some preservatives such as vitamin C also enhance the nutrient quality of foods. However, a small segment of the population is sensitive to certain preservatives. These people can experience asthma, headaches, or other symptoms after eating food containing preservatives.

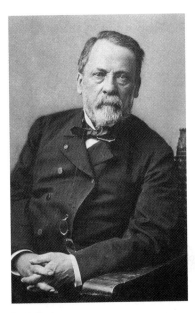

Louis Pasteur.

Table 14.4   Common Food Preservatives

Preservative	Foods Found In
Alpha-tocopheral (vitamin E)	Vegetable oils
Ascorbic acid (vitamin C)	Breakfast cereal, cured meat, fruit drinks
BHA	Breakfast cereal, chewing gum, oil, potato chips
BHT	Breakfast cereal, chewing gum, oil, potato chips
Calcium proprionate / Sodium proprionate	Breads, cakes, pies, rolls
EDTA	Canned shellfish, margarine, mayonnaise, processed fruits and vegetables, salad dressings, sandwich spreads, soft drinks
Propyl gallate	Mayonnaise, chewing gum, chicken soup base, vegetable oil, meat products, potato sticks, mashed potato flakes, fruits, ice cream
Sodium benzoate	Carbonated drinks, fruit juice, pickles, preserves
Sodium chloride (salt)	Most processed foods
Sodium nitrate/sodium nitrite	Bacon, corned beef, ham, luncheon meat, hot dogs, smoked fish
Sorbic acid/potassium sorbate	Cakes, cheese, dried fruit, jelly, syrup, wine
Sulfites (Sodium bisulfite, Sulfur dioxide)	Dried fruit, processed potatoes, wine

Most processed foods contain preservatives, unless the package touts that it is "preservative free." All preservatives must be listed in the ingredients, but you must know a wide array of chemical names to know and understand which ingredients are preservatives. Table 14.4 lists some common preservatives and the types of foods you might expect to find them in. We discuss a few of these in more detail here.

BHA/BHT   **BHT (butylated hydroxytoluene)** and **BHA (butylated hydroxyanisole)** are two commonly used antioxidants in foods. BHT and BHA are found in a wide variety of products and are used to keep oils and fats from going rancid. BHT is frequently added to many breakfast cereal packages to decrease spoilage. BHA is stable at high temperatures and is often used in products such as soup bases, ice cream, potato flakes, gelatin desserts, dry mixes for desserts, unsmoked dry sausage, and chewing gum.

Propyl gallate, another antioxidant, works synergistically with both BHA and BHT to enhance their effectiveness. Propyl gallate is used in products such as mayonnaise, mashed potato flakes, fruits, chewing gum, ice cream, baked goods, and gelatin desserts.

Propionic Acid   The bread you bought, left on the counter, and finally got around to eating a week later would start to mold if it hadn't been treated with mold inhibitors such as propionic acid, calcium propionate, or sodium propionate. *Propionic acid* occurs naturally in apples, strawberries, and tea and is used to prevent mold growth in baked goods and processed cheese. *Sodium propionate* and *calcium propionate* are salts synthesized from propionic acid and are used as mold inhibitors in a variety of foods.

Sulfites   **Sulfites** such as sodium bisulfite and sulfur dioxide are effective preservatives, antioxidants, and antibrowning agents. Sulfites have antibacterial properties and are used as a bleaching agent for flour. They are also used in the beer and wine industry to inhibit mold growth as well as in dehydrated foods, maraschino cherries, and processed potatoes. Sulfites are not used in enriched grain products because of their capacity to bind with thiamin (vitamin B$_1$), making it unavailable for absorption.

Sulfur dioxide is used to control mold growth on fresh fruits and vegetables. For example, it has become standard commercial practice to fumigate stored grapes every

BHT (butylated hydroxytoluene) An antioxidant used primarily to stop rancidity in fats and oils.

BHA (butylated hydroxyanisole) An antioxidant used primarily to stop rancidity in fats and oils.

sulfites Agents that are effective as preservatives, antioxidants, and prevent browning. Sulfites also have antibacterial properties, are used to bleach flour, and inhibit mold growth in grapes, wine, and other foods.

ten days with this chemical. Because of such procedures, it's important to remember to wash all fresh fruit and vegetables before eating.

The FDA has banned the use of sulfites as a preservative in salad bars because some people have had adverse asthmatic reactions. All foods that contain added sulfites must be labeled to warn those with sensitivities.

Nitrates and Nitrites   **Nitrates** and **nitrites** have been used in the processed meat industry for many years as antibacterial agents and color enhancers. They give ham, hot dogs, and bologna their familiar pink color. They also inhibit microbial growth and rancidity. However, nitrites can easily be converted to *nitrosamines* during the cooking process. Nitrosamines have been found to be carcinogenic in animals, so the FDA has required all foods with nitrites to contain additional antioxidants to decrease the formation of nitrosamines.

Aseptic Packaging   Many different packaging techniques have arisen over the past several decades. The newest and most environmentally sound one is **aseptic packaging** (Figure 14.9). You probably know it best as "juice boxes." Widely used in Europe and Asia, aseptic packaging was first introduced in the United States in the 1980s. Food and beverages that are packaged in aseptic containers are first sterilized in a flash-heating and cooling process, then placed in the sterile container. Nutrient quality, as well as overall food quality, remain high without the need for preservatives or refrigeration as long as the package seals are not broken. The process uses less energy than traditional canning.

Aseptic packaging material consists of six layers: several outer polyethylene layers make the package liquid-tight. An inner paper layer gives strength and shape, while an ultrathin inner aluminum layer eliminates the need for refrigeration and preservatives by forming a barrier against light and oxygen (Aseptic Packaging Council 2003).

Although the six layers sounds like a lot of packaging, there is actually less packaging material used than in any other comparable container. A typical single serving aseptic package provides a product-to-package ratio that is 96% product to only 4% packaging by weight. Aseptic cartons also use less energy to manufacture, fill, ship, and store, and they are recyclable. By eliminating the need for refrigeration or preservatives, aseptic packaging reduces subsequent energy use and its potential environmental burden (Aseptic Packaging Council 2003).

Irradiation

Irradiation is an effective process for eliminating harmful bacteria often found in foods, such as *Trichinella spiralis* and *Salmonella* in meats and poultry, and inhibits spoilage by fungus. It involves the use of X rays, beams of high-energy electrons produced by electron accelerators, or gamma rays from cobalt 60 or cesium 137. In the United States, gamma rays are typically used for irradiation. Energy from gamma rays penetrates food and its packaging. Most of this energy simply passes through the food, similar to microwaves, leaving no residue (Magnuson 1997). While the food remains relatively unchanged, bacteria and fungi are killed or left unable to reproduce, thus decreasing their ability to spoil food or cause food-borne illness.

In the United States, many foods are preserved using irradiation; among them spices, grains, fruits, pork products, beef, and poultry. The National Aeronautics and Space Administration (NASA) uses irradiated foods for space flights (Loaharanu 2003). Although irradiation rids foods of most pathogenic microbes, frozen foods remain frozen and raw foods stay raw through the process. While many foods can be safely irradiated without any noticeable changes, dairy products cannot. The flavor of milk and dairy products becomes unpalatable after irradiation, making them inappropriate for this process. A recent consumer report on irradiated meat did note that the flavor of both beef and chicken had a subtle off-taste and smell, but one that many consumers might not necessarily notice (Consumer

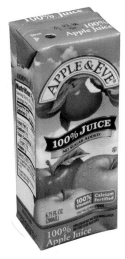

Figure 14.9   Aseptic packaging allows foods to be stored unrefrigerated for several months without spoilage.

nitrates   Chemicals used in meat curing to develop and stabilize the pink color associated with cured meat; also function as antibacterial agents.

nitrites   Chemicals used in meat curing to develop and stabilize the pink color associated with cured meat; also function as antibacterial agents.

aseptic packaging   Sterile packaging that does not require refrigeration or preservatives while seal is maintained.

irradiation   A sterilization process utilizing gamma rays or other forms of radiation, but which does not impart any radiation to the food being treated.

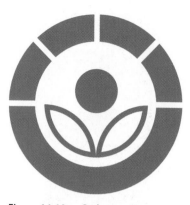

Figure 14.10   Radura—the international symbol of irradiated food—is required by the Food and Drug Administration to be displayed on all irradiated food sold in the United States.

genetic modification Changing an organism by manipulating its genetic material.

Reports 2003). Only a few nutrients, including vitamins A, E, K, and thiamin seem to be affected by irradiation. Losses of these nutrients are comparable to what would be lost in conventional processing and preparation.

Although irradiated food has been shown to be safe, the FDA requires that all irradiated foods be labeled with a "radura" symbol, and the words "treated by irradiation, do not irradiate again" or "treated with radiation, do not irradiate again" must accompany the symbol (Figure 14.10). Irradiated food can be re-infected by inadequate handling and preparation practices, so consumers still need to be diligent in their storage and preparation practices. Irradiation has been approved for use by fifty countries and endorsed by the World Health Organization (WHO), the Food and Agricultural Organization of the United Nations (FAO) and the International Atomic Energy Agency (IAEA).

Genetic Modification

In **genetic modification,** the DNA of an organism is altered to bring about specific changes in its seeds or offspring, for instance making tomatoes plumper, juicier, and more pest-resistant or making beef cattle that produce a higher quality of meat. The relative benefits and harm of genetic modification have been debated worldwide. For instance, some environmentalists have raised the concern that seeds from genetically modified crops disrupt other crops through cross-pollination, even those many miles from where the altered ones are growing. Another concern is the long-term effect of genetically modified crops on the plants, insects, and animals that consume them or use them for their habitat. For more information on genetic modification, see the Nutrition Debate box at the end of this chapter.

> **Recap:** The canning process was developed in the late eighteenth century. Pasteurization has been in use for over a hundred years to destroy microbes using high heat for short durations on liquids such as milk and juice. Preservatives such as vitamin C, sulfites, and nitrates are often added to keep foods fresher longer. Aseptic packaging is a relatively new form of packaging in which sterilized foods can be stored for long periods of time without refrigeration. In the United States, irradiation typically involves the use of gamma rays to destroy the microbes in foods. The DNA of plants and animals can be genetically modified to enhance certain qualities of the food, such as its ability to resist pests.

What Are Food Additives, and Are They Safe?

Have you ever picked up a loaf of bread and started reading its ingredients? You'd expect to see flour, yeast, water, and some sugar, but what are all those other items? And why does it feel as if you have to have a degree in chemistry to understand what they are? They are collectively called food additives, and they are in almost every processed food. Without additives, that loaf of bread would go stale within a day or two.

Although their use is regulated by the FDA, food additives have been a source of controversy for the past fifty years. Nevertheless, their use has steadily increased, allowing food producers to offer consumers a greater variety of foods at lower costs.

Additives Can Enhance a Food's Taste, Appearance, Safety, or Nutrition

It's estimated that over three thousand different additives are currently used in the United States. By becoming familiar with some of the most common, you'll gain a better understanding of what's in your food.

Additives Can Be Natural or Synthetic

Many of the additives used by the food industry come from natural sources. Beet juice, a natural food coloring, salt, and citric acid are common, naturally derived food additives, but in cases when supply or cost would prohibit using naturally derived additives, additives are synthesized. For instance, vanillin, the main flavoring substance in vanilla beans, is synthesized at a cost considerably lower than the cost of extracting it from the natural beans. Even if the costs were comparable, it is doubtful that natural sources of vanillin could meet consumer demands.

Flavorings

Roughly half of all additives are flavorings used to replace the natural flavor lost during food processing (Winter 1994). **Flavoring agents** can be obtained from natural or synthetic sources. Essential oils, extracts, and spices supply most of the naturally derived flavorings. Flavorings are typically found in soft drinks, baked goods, and frozen confections.

flavoring agents Obtained from either natural or synthetic sources; allow manufacturers to maintain a consistent flavor from batch to batch.

Flavor enhancers are also widely used. These additives have little or no flavor of their own but accentuate the natural flavor of foods. They are often added when very little of a natural ingredient is used (CSPI 2004a). The most common flavor enhancers used are maltol and MSG (monosodium glutamate). MSG is the sodium salt of glutamic acid, one of the nonessential amino acids, which also serves as a neurotransmitter. Originally derived from sea kelp by the Japanese and introduced to Americans during World War II, MSG is found in many processed foods. However, in some people, MSG causes symptoms such as headaches, difficulty breathing, and heart palpitations. It has been demonstrated that the glutamate portion of MSG can cross the blood-brain barrier and cause over-stimulation of neurons, especially in the young. Because of this research, Congress mandated in the 1960s that MSG be removed from baby food (Blaylock 1996).

Colorings

Food colorings, derived from both natural and synthetic sources, are used extensively in processed foods. In the past, many food colorings were made from **coaltar,** a thick or semisolid tar derived from bituminous coal. Derivatives of coaltar have been found to cause cancer in animals, and most have been banned by the FDA from use in foods. Natural colorings such as beet juice (which gives a red color), beta-carotene (which gives a yellow color), and caramel (which adds brown color), are now used instead and do not need to be tested for safety. The coloring tartrazine (FD&C yellow #5) causes an allergic reaction in some people, and its use must be indicated on the product packaging.

coaltar A food additive made from thick or semisolid tar derived from bituminous coal, the by-products of which have been found to cause cancer in animals.

Vitamins and Other Nutrients

Vitamin E is usually added to fat-based products to keep them from going rancid, and ascorbic acid is commonly added to food such as frozen fruit, dry milk, apple juice, soft drinks, candy, and meat products containing sodium nitrates. Sodium ascorbate, a form of vitamin C with sodium added to produce a salt, is used as an antioxidant in foods such as concentrated milk products, cereals, and cured meats.

Iodine and vitamin D are purely nutritive additives. Their function in foods is to reduce the occurrence of a deficiency disease. Iodine was originally added to table salt to help decrease the incidence of goiter, a condition that causes the thyroid gland to enlarge. Vitamin D is added to milk because in northern latitudes during the late fall and winter it is not possible to produce adequate vitamin D from sun exposure. As you learned in Chapter 9, vitamin D is necessary for calcium metabolism and has been found to be important in preventing osteoporosis in adults and rickets in infants and children.

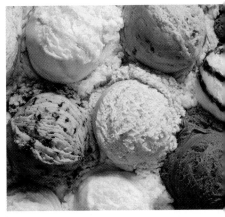

Many foods, such as ice cream, contain colorings.

Texturizers, Stabilizers, and Emulsifiers

Texturizers such as calcium chloride are added to foods to improve their texture. For instance, they are added to canned tomatoes and potatoes so they don't fall apart. **Stabilizers** are added to products to give them "body" and help them maintain a desired texture or color. **Thickening agents** are used to absorb water and keep the complex mixtures of oils, water, acids, and solids in foods balanced (CSPI 2004a). Natural thickeners include pectin, alginate, and carrageenan. **Emulsifiers,** like thickening agents and stabilizers, help to keep fats evenly dispersed within foods. Texturizers, stabilizers, thickening agents, and emulsifiers have no known adverse effect on humans when used according to regulations.

Humectants and Desiccants

Moisture content is a critical component to food, and **humectants** and **desiccants** are added to maintain the correct moisture levels. Humectants keep foods like marshmallows, chewing gum, and shredded coconut soft and stretchy. Common humectants are glycerin, sorbitol, and propylene glycol. Waxes used on produce also help maintain moisture content. The best way to remove wax is to peel the outerlayer off or scrub it with hot, soapy water and rinse well. Desiccants prevent moisture absorption from the air; for example, they are used to prevent table salt from forming clumps.

Bleaching Agents

Bleaching agents are used primarily in baked goods. Fresh ground flour is pale yellow, and when stored it slowly becomes white. Processors have added bleaching agents to flour to speed this process and decrease the possibility of spoilage or insect infestation. Benzoyl peroxide is commonly used to bleach flour as well as blue and Gorgonzola cheeses (Winter 1994).

Some Additives Get into Our Food Unintentionally

Trace amounts of substances (such as insects, fragments of packaging materials, pesticides, and hormones or antibiotics given to livestock) can get into our food during harvesting, processing, storage, or packaging. These are called *unintentional* or *incidental additives* and do not have to be included on the label. This small amount of incidental food additives present in food has not been shown to cause any problems with quality or safety.

The GRAS List Identifies Food Additives

It is estimated that by 1958 the food industry in the United States was using over six hundred natural and synthetic additives. Federal legislation was passed to regulate food additives, and the **Generally Recognized as Safe (GRAS) list** was established. A substance was accorded GRAS status if it was generally recognized by experts as having been adequately shown through scientific procedures or experience based on common use in food to be safe under the conditions of its intended use. The Delaney Clause, also enacted in 1958, states that "No additive may be permitted in any amount if tests show that it produces cancer when fed to man or animals or by other appropriate tests."

In 1985, the FDA established the Adverse Reaction Monitoring System (ARMS). Under this system, the FDA investigates complaints from consumers, physicians, or food companies. Many of the complaints are about artificial sweeteners and sulfite preservatives causing headaches, asthmatic reactions, and in some cases anaphylactic shock. Because of these complaints and the investigations that followed, the FDA has banned the use of sulfites on raw fruit and vegetables, with the exception of potatoes, while continuing to monitor sulfite use on other foods.

---

texturizers A chemical used to improve the texture of various foods.

stabilizers Help maintain smooth texture and uniform color and flavor in some foods.

thickening agents Natural or chemically modified carbohydrates that absorb some of the water present in food, making the food thicker while keeping food components balanced.

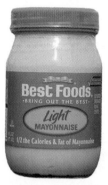

Mayonnaise contains emulsifiers to prevent separation of fats.

emulsifiers Chemicals that improve texture and smoothness in foods; stabilizes oil-water mixtures.

humectants Chemicals that help retain moisture in foods, keeping them soft and pliable.

desiccants Chemicals that prevents foods from absorbing moisture from the air.

bleaching agents Chemicals used to speed the natural process of ground flour changing from pale yellow to white.

Generally Recognized as Safe (GRAS) list Established by Congress to identify and regulate food additives.

Are Food Additives Safe?

Although there is much controversy over food additives, those on the GRAS list have been tested and found to be safe. These additives have allowed our food supply to increase and diversify, providing consumers more variety at lower costs. Without additives such as flavorings, strawberry ice cream would only be available for a short time and only in limited quantities during the early summer. If you are interested in reducing the amount of food additives in your diet, you should start by comparing food labels of different brands of the same foods. Some brands use fewer additives than others, and some brands are additive-free.

Recap: Food additives are chemicals intentionally added to foods to enhance their color, flavor, texture, nutrient density, moisture level, or shelf life. Unintentional additives are trace amounts of substances that get into our food during harvesting, processing, storage, or packaging. Although there is continuing controversy over food additives, those on the GRAS list have been tested and found to be safe.

Do Residues Harm Our Food Supply?

Food **residues** are chemicals that remain in the foods we eat despite cleaning and processing. Two residues of global concern are pollutants and pesticides.

residues Chemicals that remain in the foods we eat despite cleaning and processing.

Persistent Organic Pollutants Can Cause Illness

Many different organic chemicals are released into the atmosphere as a result of industry, agriculture, automobile emissions, and improper waste disposal. These chemicals, collectively referred to as **persistent organic pollutants (POPs),** eventually enter the food supply through the soil or water. If a pollutant gets into the soil, a plant can absorb the chemical into its structure and can pass it on as part of the food chain. Animals can also absorb the pollutants into their tissues or can consume them when feeding on plants growing in the polluted soil. Fat-soluble pollutants are especially problematic, as they tend to accumulate in the animal's body tissues and are then absorbed by humans when the animal is used as a food source.

persistent organic pollutants (POPs) Chemicals released into the environment as a result of industry, agriculture, or improper waste disposal; automobile emissions also are considered POPs.

POP residues have been found in virtually all categories of foods, including baked goods, fruit, vegetables, meat, poultry, and dairy products. The chemicals can travel long distance in trade winds and water currents, moving from tropical and temperate regions to concentrate in the northern latitudes. It is believed that all living organisms on Earth carry a measurable level of POPs in their tissues (Schafer and Kegley 2002).

Mercury and Lead Are Nerve Toxins Found in the Environment

Mercury, a naturally occurring element, is found in soil and rocks, lakes, streams, and oceans. It is also released into the environment by pulp and paper processing and the burning of garbage and fossil fuels. As mercury is released into the environment, it falls from the air, eventually finding its way to streams, lakes, and the ocean, where it accumulates. Fish absorb mercury as they feed on aquatic organisms. This mercury is passed on to us when we consume the fish. As mercury accumulates in the body, it has a toxic effect on the nervous system.

Large predatory fish, such as swordfish, shark, king mackerel, and tilefish tend to contain the highest levels of mercury (FDA 2003). Because mercury is especially toxic to the developing nervous system of fetuses and growing children, pregnant and breastfeeding women and young children are advised to avoid eating these types of fish. Canned tuna, salmon, cod, pollock, sole, shrimp, mussels and scallops do not contain high levels of mercury and are safe to consume; however, the FDA advises against eating any one

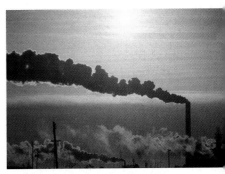

One of the ways mercury is released into the environment is by pulp mills.

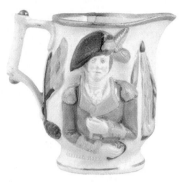

Antique porcelain is often coated with lead-based glaze.

polychlorinated biphenyls (PCBs) An industrial pollutant most commonly attributed to discarded transformers.

dioxins An industrial pollutant most commonly attributed to waste incineration.

type of fish more often than once a week (FDA 2003). Freshwater fish caught in local lakes and rivers have variable levels of mercury; thus, local and state governments routinely monitor mercury levels and post advisories when levels are too high. To learn more about the risks of mercury in seafood, visit the FDA's food safety Web site (www.cfsan.fda.gov) or call their 24-hour information line (at 1[888] SAFEFOOD).

Lead, another naturally occurring element, can be found in the soil, water, and even the air. It also occurs as industrial waste from leaded gasolines, lead-based paints, and lead-soldered cans, now outlawed but decomposing in landfills. Some ceramic mugs and other dishes are fired with lead-based glaze. Thus, residues can build up in foods. Excessive lead exposure can cause learning and behavioral impediments in children and cardiovascular and kidney disease in adults. It is impossible to avoid lead residues completely, but because of its health implications, everyone should try to limit their exposure.

Industrial Pollutants Also Create Residues

Polychlorinated biphenyls (PCBs) and **dioxins** are two industrial pollutants that have been found in food worldwide. Dioxins (byproducts of waste incineration) and PCBs (from discarded transformers) enter the soil and can persist in the environment for years, easily accumulating in fatty tissues. Many studies done in Belgium show that chicken, pork, and eggs have been found to have concentrations of these chemicals in excess of international standards (Larenbeke et al. 2002). PCBs and dioxins, along with other POPs, have been linked to cancer, learning disorders, impaired immune function, and infertility (Schafer and Kegley 2002).

Reducing POPs Is a Global Concern

International agreements sponsored by the United Nations seek to ban or restrict POPs. For example, the Stockholm Convention, originally drafted in May 2001, is intended to enable the international community to collaborate on an agreeable solution to reducing and eventually phasing out the use of POPs. Its mandate also includes the development of alternatives and the safe and environmentally sound disposal of POPs. If you're interested in reading the full text of the Stockholm Convention, go to http://www.pops.int.

Recap: Persistent organic pollutants (POPs) have been found in virtually all categories of foods. Mercury contaminates certain fish, and lead contaminates many foods. Both are toxic to the nervous system. Polychlorinated biphenyls (PCBs) and dioxins are two industrial pollutants that have been found in food worldwide. International agreements sponsored by the United Nations seek to ban or restrict POPs.

Pesticides Protect Against Crop Losses

Pesticides are used to help protect crop losses due to weeds, insects, fungi, and other organisms, including birds and mammals. Rodents, for example, in addition to consuming food, also contaminate large quantities of food with their excreta. Pesticides also help reduce the potential of disease by decreasing the number of microorganisms on crops. They increase overall crop yield and crop diversity. The three most common types of pesticides used in food production are insecticides, herbicides, and fungicides. Insecticides are used to control insects that can infest crops; herbicides are used to control weeds and other unwanted plant growth; and fungicides are used to control plant-destroying fungal growth. It is estimated that 65% of all pesticides produced in the United States are herbicides.

Pesticides Can Be Natural or Synthetic

Many plants naturally produce pesticides to help protect themselves from predators and disease. Man has found a way to use naturally derived or synthetic analogs of this protective mechanism for agricultural use. Despite the negative connotations associated with pesticides, many pesticides used today are naturally derived, and/or have a low impact on the environment. Gardeners and farmers are starting to use **biopesticides,** which are primarily insecticides. Biopesticides are less toxic to humans and the environment. They are species-specific and work to suppress a pest's population, not eliminate it. Biopesticides do not leave residues on crops—most degrade rapidly and are easily washed away with water.

biopesticides Primarily insecticides, these chemicals use natural methods to reduce damage to crops.

There are two types of biopesticides: biochemical and microbial. Pheromones are a type of biochemical pesticide. In nature, insects use pheromones to attract mates. Man-made pheromones are used to disrupt insect mating by attracting males into traps. Microbial pesticides are derived from naturally occurring or genetically altered microorganisms like bacteria, viruses, or fungi. A widely used microbial biopesticide is *Bacillus thuringiensis,* or *Bt.* This is a common soil bacterium that is genetically altered to be toxic to several species of insects.

Aside from biopesticides, many common products such as boric acid or diatomaceous earth are used as pesticides. A Pacific Northwestern remedy for decreasing the damage to gardens by slugs is to sprinkle table salt around the perimeter of the garden, which deters slugs from entering. The salt dehydrates the slug, slowly killing it. However, salt can also change a soil's pH and interfere with roots' ability to absorb water and nutrients.

Pesticides can also be synthetically derived. Many are made from petroleum-based products. Examples of commonly used synthetic pesticides include thiabendazole (a fungicide used on potatoes) and fungicides commonly used to prevent apple diseases (such as dithane, manzate, and polyram).

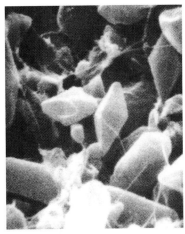

Bt bacteria produces crystals, shown here, that are a widely used microbial biopesticide.

Pesticides Are Potential Toxins

Years of studies show that chemicals, whether natural or synthetic, can remain on food and affect immune system function in people whose systems are already compromised. The liver is responsible for detoxifying the chemicals that enter our bodies; but if diseases such as cancer or toxins such as alcohol already stress it, then the liver cannot effectively remove pesticide residues. When pesticide residues are not effectively removed, they can damage body tissues. Some are fat-soluble and can be deposited in adipose tissues, which may later be metabolized for energy—and the residues then may be released into the body and cause damage. Others target nervous system and endocrine system cells. Thus, although originally intended for other organisms, pesticides do have the potential to cause problems in humans.

Children may be more susceptible to pesticide residues as they consume more food and water per unit of body weight than adults and may have a limited ability to detoxify these substances. Because of the potential risks from chemicals to a developing child, pregnant and breastfeeding women should peel fruit and vegetable rinds to decrease their exposure to residues. This is also a sensible precaution when preparing fruit or vegetables for small children, though removing the rinds may also reduce the nutritional content of the food (Heaton 2003).

In short, although pesticides are a necessary component of agricultural practice, they are potential toxins. It is therefore essential to wash all produce carefully.

Government Regulations Control the Use of Pesticides

The Environmental Protection Agency is the government agency responsible for regulating the labeling, sale, distribution, use, and disposal of all pesticides in the United States. The EPA also sets a tolerance level, which is the maximum residue level of a pesticide permitted in or on food or feed grown in the United States or imported into the United States from other countries (EPA 2003). The EPA reviews every registered pesticide on a fifteen-year cycle (EPA 2003).

Before a pesticide can be accepted by the EPA for use, it must be determined that it performs its intended function with minimal impact to the environment. Once the EPA has certified a pesticide, states may set their own regulations for its use. Canadian regulation of pesticides closely resembles U.S. laws, with provinces and territories given free range to limit pesticide use.

Recap: Pesticides are chemicals used to prevent or reduce food crop losses due to weeds, insects, fungi, and other organisms, including birds and mammals. Biopesticides may be biochemical or microbial. Many synthetic pesticides are petroleum-based products. Pesticides are potential toxins; therefore, it is essential to wash all produce carefully. Pregnant and breastfeeding women and young children should eat produce without the peel. The Environmental Protection Agency (EPA) regulates the labeling, sale, distribution, use, and disposal of all pesticides in the United States.

Gustavo · *Nutri-Case*

"All of a sudden, a feisty bunch of newcomers to town are complaining about vineyards around here using too many pesticides. They're worried that somehow the pesticides we use are going to hurt them, but that's not possible because winemaking destroys all those bad chemicals before you drink it. I've been working with pesticides for fifty years, and they haven't hurt me!"

What do you think of Gustavo's claim that the pesticides are not harmful? Before you answer, think not only about their effect on the grapes used to make wine, but also about other potential forms of contamination.

Growth Hormones Are Injected into Cows to Increase Production of Meat and Milk

recombinant bovine growth hormone (rBGH) A genetically engineered hormone injected into dairy cows to enhance their milk output.

Introduced in the United States food supply in 1994, **recombinant bovine growth hormone (rBGH),** also known as *recombinant bovine somatotropin (rBST)*, is a genetically engineered growth hormone. It is used in beef herds to induce animals to grow more muscle tissue and less fat. It is also injected into a third of U.S. dairy cows and increases milk output by as much as 20 to 30%. The meat and milk products from these animals are then shipped throughout the country and internationally. Currently, there are no labeling requirements for products containing rBGH.

Although the FDA has allowed the use of rBGH in the United States, Canada and the European Union have banned its use because of studies showing that there is an increased risk of mastitis (inflamed udders), infertility, and lameness in dairy cows (LeSage 1999). However, according to Health Canada (LeSage 1999), there is no strong evidence to support increased risk to humans who ingest products from animals who have been injected with rBGH. Some individuals are still concerned with consuming products of animals injected with rBGH, as the milk of cows receiving this hormone has higher levels of insulin-like growth factor (IGF-1). IGF-1 is a protein that can pass into the bloodstream of humans who drink milk from cows who receive rBGH, and some studies have shown that an elevated level of IGF-1 in humans may increase the risk of breast and prostate cancers (Montague 1998). However, there are no studies directly linking increased risk of these cancers with eating products from animals injected with rBGH.

While the risks of rBGH to humans are still being studied, dairy cows subject to this chemical are known to have an increased tendency to develop mastitis (udder swelling), which requires medical treatment and administration of antibiotics. These antibiotics commonly find their way into the milk supply and into the consumer, possibly fostering the development of antibiotic-resistant strains of bacteria.

Advocates of rBGH say that its use allows farmers to use less feed for the same yield, reducing resource use by each ranch or farm. In addition, they argue that approximately 90% of the hormone in milk is destroyed during pasteurization and that the remaining percentage is destroyed during digestion in the human gastrointestinal tract.

Recap: Recombinant bovine growth hormone (rBGH) is a genetically engineered growth hormone injected into meat and dairy cows to increase meat production and milk output. Concerns about rBGH include possible immune system impairment, increased risk of prostate and breast cancers, and increased administration of antibiotics to dairy cows receiving the hormone.

Are Organic Foods More Healthful?

The term *organic* is commonly used to describe foods that are grown without the use of synthetic pesticides. The thought of organic food used to conjure up images of hippies and bean sprouts. Now organic food has become part of the mainstream food supply. Organic food sales in the United States have more than quadrupled in the past two decades, with sales estimated to reach $3.6 billion in 2003 (Kortbech-Olesen 2002). Many small organic companies have been acquired by large corporations, resulting in many processed and snack foods carrying an organic label.

To Be Labeled Organic, Foods Must Meet Federal Standards

The National Organic Program (NOP) of the USDA came into law in October of 2002. The organic industry itself had asked for national standards on organic labeling, as different U.S. states had different requirements for organic food labels and some had no rules at all. The European Union enforced a common standard for organic plant produce in 1991. Without a national standard, it was feared that European countries might seek to exclude U.S. organic exports.

The new Organic Standards established uniform definitions for all organic products. Any label or product claiming to be organic must comply with the following definitions:

- *100% organic:* Products containing only organically produced ingredients, excluding water and salt.
- *Organic:* Products containing 95% organically produced ingredients by weight, excluding water and salt; with the remaining ingredients consisting of those products not commercially available in organic form.
- *Made with organic ingredients:* A product containing more than 70% organic ingredients.

If a processed product contains less than 70% organically produced ingredients, then those products cannot use the term *organic* in the principal display panel, but ingredients that are organically produced can be specified on the ingredients statement on the information panel.

Products that are "100% organic" and "organic" may display the USDA seal (Figure 14.11) or mark of certifying agents. Any product that is labeled as organic must identify each organically produced item in the ingredient statement of the label. The name and address of the certifying agency must also be on the label.

The USDA Regulates Organic Farming

The USDA regulates organic farming standards, and farms must be certified as organic by a government-approved certifier who inspects the farm and verifies that the farmer is following all USDA organic standards. Companies that handle or process organic food before it arrives at your local supermarket or restaurant must also be certified (Aiyana 2002). Organic farming methods are strict and require farmers to find natural alternatives to many common problems, such as weeds and insects. Contrary to common belief, organic farmers can use pesticides as a final option for pest control when all other methods have failed or are known to be ineffective, but they are restricted to a limited number that have been approved for use based on their origin, environmental impact, and potential to persist as residues (Heaton 2003). Organic farmers emphasize the use of renewable resources and the conservation of soil and water to enhance environmental and nutritional quality. Once a crop is harvested, a winter crop (usually of a legume origin) is planted to help fix nitrogen in the soil and decrease erosion, which also lessens the need for fertilizers.

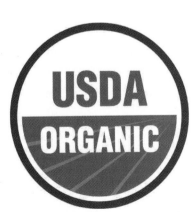

Figure 14.11   The USDA organic seal identifies foods that are at least 95% organic.

Deciphering the Ingredients

Figure 14.12 shows labels for two breakfast cereals. The cereal on the left is a typical national brand of processed breakfast cereal for children, and the one on the right is one of the new organic, whole-grain brands with a minimum of processing. Their prices are relatively close: the national brand is a 12-ounce box for $3.79 (32 cents/oz.) while the less-familiar brand is a 10-ounce box for $3.99 (40 cents/oz.).

A quick glance reveals that the label on the left has about three times as many ingredients as the other. What are all those ingredients, and are they really necessary? The product on the right lists organic grains, sweeteners, oils, and natural colorings and flavorings. Because the cereal on the right is certified as organic, we know that it contains 95% organically produced ingredients by weight, excluding water and salt, and the remaining ingredients consist of products not commercially available in organic form. In addition, either no pesticides were used or pesticide use was limited. With the cereal on the left, we cannot determine whether pesticides were used or if the grains were derived from genetically engineered crops.

The 8th and 9th ingredients on the left label are guar gum and gum arabic, water-soluble fibers derived from plants and used as thickeners and texturizers to help foods maintain consistency. The label on the right does not contain any texturizers or thickeners. However, these water-soluble fibers are considered safe to consume. The cereal on the left also contains calcium carbonate, which is added to products to boost their calcium content. Although this is an additive, it does result in the cereal on the left being a better source of calcium than the organic cereal on the right. Other ingredients contained in the cereal on the left are dicalcium phosphate and trisodium phosphate; these are anticaking agents that also help boost phosphorous and calcium levels.

Both labels list coloring agents. The label on the left lists Red 40, Yellow 6, Blue 1, and other color added. Based on this label, we do not know if all of these colors are artificially derived. The label on the right lists natural colors derived from vegetable extracts and annatto, the latter of which is a vegetable dye from a tropical tree.

Flavors are listed on the left label as natural and artificial flavor, wording which does not provide a lot of information. Sodium citrate, citric acid, and malic acid are added as acidifiers, and they also affect flavor, as they give foods tartness. Malic acid is derived from apples, and citric acid is obtained from lemons and oranges. The label on the right lists only natural flavor, and also contains citric acid. Incidentally, a small taste-test panel of 5th graders rated the two cereals as very similar. When not able to see the cereal, they could not tell the difference by taste alone.

The very last ingredient listed in the national brand is BHT, which is an antioxidant used to help stop rancidity in fats and oils.

Probably the most striking difference in the labels is the higher vitamin and mineral content in the national brand. Clearly the manufacturer added these nutrients to enrich the grains. Nutrient food additives were not used in the other product. Thus, depending upon your preferences, you may consider the cereal on the left to be more nutritious, as it contains more vitamins and minerals than the cereal on the right. Or, you may feel that foods are more nutritious if they contain less additives; in this case, you would most likely prefer to eat the cereal on the right.

Knowing what the ingredients are, would you purchase either of these cereals for yourself? Why or why not? Before you answer, check out the sugars, sodium content, oils, and grains. How do these influence your choice? Which cereal would you choose if you worked at a day-care center and wanted something to serve toddlers? ●

Organic meat, poultry, eggs, and dairy products come from animals fed only organic feed, and if the animals become ill, they are removed from the others until well again. None of these animals are given growth hormones to increase their size or ability to produce milk. Irradiation is also prohibited in organic production.

Organic Foods Can Be More Nutritious

Recent studies at the University of California, Davis, and other institutions indicate that organic foods are 2.5 times more nutritious than their non-organic counterparts and that organic plants are lower in toxic metals (Grinder-Pedersen et al., 2003). For example,

Non-organic breakfast cereal

Nutrition Facts

Serving Size 1 cup (30g)
Servings Per Container 11

Amount Per Serving

	Cereal	With 1/2 Cup Skim Milk
Calories	120	160
Calories from Fat	10	15

	% Daily Value**	
Total Fat 1g*	2%	2%
Saturated Fat 0g	0%	0%
Polyunsaturated Fat 0g		
Monounsaturated Fat 0.5g		
Cholesterol 0mg	0%	1%
Sodium 200mg	8%	11%
Potassium 20mg	1%	6%
Total Carbohydrate 27g	9%	11%
Dietary Fiber 1g	4%	4%
Sugars 13g		
Other Carbohydrate 13g		
Protein 1g		
Vitamin A	10%	15%
Vitamin C	10%	10%
Calcium	10%	25%
Iron	25%	25%
Vitamin D	10%	25%
Thiamin	25%	30%
Riboflavin	25%	35%
Niacin	25%	25%
Vitamin B$_6$	25%	25%
Folic Acid	25%	25%
Vitamin B$_{12}$	25%	35%
Phosphorus	2%	15%
Magnesium	0%	4%
Zinc	25%	30%

* Amount in cereal. A serving of cereal plus skim milk provides 1.5g total fat, less than 5mg cholesterol, 260mg sodium, 220mg potassium, 33g total carbohydrate (19g sugars) and 5g protein.

** Percent Daily Values are based on a 2,000 calorie diet. Your daily values may be higher or lower depending on your calorie needs:

Calories		2,000	2,500
Total Fat	Less than	65g	80g
Sat. Fat	Less than	20g	25g
Cholesterol	Less than	300mg	300mg
Sodium	Less than	2,400mg	2,400mg
Potassium		3,500mg	3,500mg
Total Carbohydrate		300g	375g
Dietary fiber		25g	30g

INGREDIENTS: Corn (Meal, Flour), Sugar, Corn Syrup, Partially Hydrogenated Soybean Oil, Modified Corn Starch, Corn Starch, Salt, Guar Gum, Gum Arabic, High Fructose Corn Syrup, Calcium Carbonate, Dicalcium Phosphate, Tridsodium Phosphate, Red 40, Yellow 6, Blue 1, and Other Color Added, Baking Soda, Sodium Citrate, Natural & Artificial Flavor, Citric Acid, Malic Acid, Zinc and Iron (Mineral Nutrients), Vitamin C (Sodium Ascorbate), A B Vitamin (Niacinamide), Vitamin B$_6$ (Pyridoxine Hydrochloride), Vitamin B$_2$ (Riboflavin), Vitamin B$_1$ (Thiamin Mononitrate), Vitamin A (Palmitate), A B Vitamin (Folic Acid), Vitamin B$_{12}$, Vitamin D, Wheat Starch. Freshness preserved by BHT.

Organic breakfast cereal

Nutrition Facts

Serving Size 3/4 cup (30g)
Servings Per Package: About 9

Amount Per Serving

Calories 120	Calories from Fat 5

	% Daily Value**
Total Fat 0.5g*	1%
Saturated Fat 0g	0%
Cholesterol 0mg	0%
Sodium 58mg	2%
Potassium 23mg	1%
Total Carbohydrate 26g	9%
Dietary Fiber 0g	1%
Sugars 9g	
Protein 2g	

Vitamin A	0%	•	Vitamin C	0%
Calcium	0%	•	Iron	0%

* Amount in cereal. 1/2 cup skim milk contributes an additional 40 calories, 65mg sodium, 190mg potassium, 6g total carbohydrate (6g sugars), and 4g protein.

** Percent Daily Values are based on a 2,000 calorie diet. Your daily values may be higher or lower depending on your calorie needs:

Calories		2,000	2,500
Total Fat	Less than	65g	80g
Sat. Fat	Less than	20g	25g
Cholesterol	Less than	300mg	300mg
Sodium	Less than	2,400mg	2,400mg
Potassium		3,500mg	3,500mg
Total Carbohydrate		300g	375g
Dietary fiber		25g	30g

Calories per gram:
Fat 9 • Carbohydrate 4 • Protein 4

INGREDIENTS: Organic Yellow Corn, Organic Dehydrated Cane Juice, Organic Whole Oat Flour, Organic Expeller Pressed Canola and/or Sunflower Oil, Natural Colors (Vegetable Extracts and Annatto), Natural Flavor, Sea Salt, Citric Acid.

Certified Oganic by Quality Assurance International.

Figure 14.12 These labels for a non-organic breakfast cereal (left) and an organic breakfast cereal (right) illustrate the differences in additives between these two products. Determining which cereal is more nutritions depends on your personal preferences.

organic plants are generally 29% lower in lead, 25% lower in mercury, and 40% lower in land aluminum than plants not grown organically (Spectrum 1995). On average, vitamin C content in many organically grown crops is found in higher concentrations than in similar non-organically grown crops. Differences range from an increase of 6 to 100%, depending on the type of plant (potatoes versus carrots) (Heaton 2003). Higher mineral content has also been found in organically grown crops. The accompanying Nutrition Label Activity can help you evaluate the quality of comparable nonorganic and organic foods.

Recap: Organic Standards established in 2002 established uniform definitions for all organic products sold in the United States. The USDA regulates organic farming standards and inspects and certifies farms that follow all USDA organic standards. Recent studies indicate that organic foods can be more nutritious and lower in toxic metals than non-organic foods.

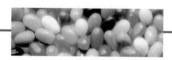

Chapter Summary

- Concerns about food safety typically focus on food-borne illness, food spoilage, and technologic manipulation of food.

- Approximately seventy-six million Americans report experiencing food-borne illness each year.

- Food infections result from the consumption of food containing living microorganisms, such as bacteria, whereas food intoxications result from consuming food in which microbes have secreted toxins.

- Food infections can be caused by bacteria, viruses, fungi, helminths, and prions.

- The body has several defense mechanisms, such as saliva, stomach acid, vomiting, diarrhea, and the inflammatory response, which help rid us of offending microorganisms and toxins.

- In order to reproduce in foods, microbes require a precise range of temperature, humidity, acidity, and oxygen content.

- It is estimated that one-fifth of Americans experience some type of reaction to foods in their diet. Allergic reactions to foods can be immediate or delayed by several hours or days.

- To prevent the development of delayed-onset food allergies, it is important to eat a variety of foods so that your immune system is not repeatedly exposed to the same potential irritants.

- You can prevent food-borne illness at home by following these tips: Wash your hands and kitchen surfaces often. Separate foods to prevent cross contamination. Cook foods to their proper temperatures. Store foods in the refrigerator or freezer. Thaw frozen foods in the refrigerator, and heat them long enough and at the required temperature to ensure proper cooking.

- When traveling, avoid all raw foods unless thoroughly washed in bottled or boiled water, and choose beverages that are boiled, bottled, or canned, without ice.

- Food spoilage affects a food's appearance, texture, taste, smell, and safety. Both fresh and processed foods are vulnerable to spoilage.

- Some natural techniques for food preservation include salting and sugaring, drying, smoking, and cooling.

- Synthetic food preservation techniques include canning, pasteurization, addition of preservatives, aseptic packaging, irradiation, and genetic modification.

- Food additives are natural or synthetic ingredients added to foods during processing to enhance them in some way. They include flavorings, colorings, nutrients, texturizers, and other additives.

- The GRAS list identifies the several hundred food additives approved for use by United States food manufacturers.

- Persistent organic pollutants (POPs) are chemicals released into the atmosphere as a result of industry, agriculture, automobile emissions, and improper waste disposal. Plants, animals, and fish absorb the chemicals from contaminated soil or water and pass them on as part of the food chain.

- Large predatory fish, such as swordfish, shark, king mackerel, and tilefish tend to contain high levels of mercury, which is especially toxic to the developing nervous system.

- Although pesticides prevent or reduce crop losses, they are potential toxins; thus, their use is regulated by the Environmental Protection Agency.

- All produce should be washed carefully before eating. Produce prepared for pregnant women, breastfeeding women, and young children should be peeled whenever possible.
- Recombinant bovine growth hormone (rBGH) is injected into beef and dairy cows to increase their yield. Although the hormone is largely destroyed by pasteurization of milk and by human digestion, concerns remain about residues.
- Cows injected with rBGH have a higher rate of antibiotic use: the residue from these antibiotics may be contributing to the increased development of antibiotic-resistant strains of microorganisms.
- Organic Standards established in 2002 established uniform definitions for all organic products sold in the United States.
- The USDA regulates organic farming standards and inspects and certifies farms that follow all USDA organic standards.
- Recent studies indicate that organic foods can be more nutritious and lower in toxic metals than non-organic foods.

Review Questions

1. The three factors most often responsible for spoilage of foods are
   a. oxygen, heat, and light.
   b. moisture, heat, and light.
   c. moisture, heat, and cold.
   d. oxygen, light, and cold.

2. Yeasts are
   a. a type of mold used to make bread rise.
   b. a type of bacteria that can cause food intoxication.
   c. a type of fungus used to ferment foods.
   d. a type of mold inhibitor used as a food preservative.

3. Monosodium glutamate (MSG) is
   a. a thickening agent used in baby foods.
   b. a flavor enhancer used in a variety of foods.
   c. a mold inhibitor used on grapes and other foods.
   d. an amino acid added as a nutrient to some foods.

4. Foods that are labeled *100% organic*
   a. contain only organically produced ingredients, excluding water and salt.
   b. may display the EPA's organic seal.
   c. were produced without the use of pesticides.
   d. contain no discernible level of toxic metals.

5. Beginning with the most ancient method, what is the correct chronological order for the following techniques for food preservation?
   a. freezing, drying, pasteurization, aseptic packaging
   b. freeze-drying, smoking, irradiation, pasteurization
   c. freezing, pasteurization, canning, aseptic packaging
   d. cooling, canning, pasteurization, irradiation

6. **True or false?** Heating foods to at least 160°F guarantees that a food will not cause food-borne illness.

7. **True or false?** The Centers for Disease Control and Prevention (CDC) has established an Adverse Reaction Monitoring System (ARMS) to investigate complaints of adverse reactions to food additives.

8. **True or false?** In the United States, farms certified as organic are allowed to use pesticides under certain conditions.

9. **True or false?** Recombinant bovine growth hormone (rBGH) is used to increase the amount and quality of meat in beef herds and milk production in dairy cows.

10. **True or false?** Some colorings used as food additives do not need to be tested for safety.

11. A box of macaroni and cheese has the words *Certified Organic* on the front and the following ingredients listed on the side: "Organic durum semolina pasta (organic durum semolina, water), organic cheddar cheese (organic cultured pasteurized milk, salt, enzymes), whey, salt." Is this food 100% organic? Why or why not? Does it contain any food additives? If so, identify them.

12. Steven and Dante go to a convenience store after a tennis match looking for something to quench their thirst. Steven chooses a national brand of orange juice, and Dante chooses a bottle of locally produced, organic, unpasteurized apple juice. Steven points out to Dante that his juice is not pasteurized, but he shrugs and says, "I'm more afraid of the pesticides they used on the oranges in your juice than I am about microorganisms in mine!" Which juice would *you* choose, and why?

13. Pickling is a food-preservation technique that involves soaking foods such as cucumbers in a solution containing vinegar (acetic acid). Why would pickling be effective in preventing food spoilage?

14. In the 1950s and 1960s in Minamata, Japan, over one hundred cases of a similar illness were recorded: patients, many of whom were infants or young children, suffered irreversible damage to the nervous system. A total of 46 people died. Adults with the disease and mothers of afflicted young children had one thing in common: they had frequently eaten fish caught in Minamata Bay. What do you think might have been the cause of this disease? Using key words from this description, research the event on the Internet and identify the culprit(s).

15. Your sister Joy, who attends a culinary arts school, is visiting you for dinner. You want to impress her, so

you've decided to make chicken marsala. You begin that afternoon by removing two chicken breasts from the freezer and putting them in a bowl in the refrigerator to thaw. Then you go shopping for fresh salad ingredients. When you get home from the market, you wash your hands in cold water, then take the chicken breasts from the refrigerator and wash them thoroughly. You set them aside on a clean cutting board. You then take the lettuce, red pepper, and scallions you just bought, put them in a colander, and rinse them. Next, you slice them with a clean knife on your marble countertop and toss them together in a salad. You put the chicken breasts in a frying pan and cook them until they lose their pink color. In a separate pan, you prepare the sauce, using a new carton of cream and the marsala. Finally, using a clean knife, you slice some freshly-baked bread on the counter top. You then wash the knives and the cutting board you used for the chicken. Joy arrives and admires your skill in cooking. Later that night, you both wake up vomiting. Identify *at least two* aspects of your food preparation that might have contributed to your illness.

Test Yourself Answers

1. **False.** Freezing inhibits the ability of microbes to reproduce, but when the food is thawed, reproduction resumes.

2. **True.** The U.S. Army has found that canned meats, vegetables and jam have been in "excellent states of preservation" after 46 years. Nevertheless, the USDA recommends consuming low-acid canned goods within five years and high-acid canned goods within two years.

3. **False.** Bacteria cause the vast majority of cases of food-borne illness.

4. **False.** Recent studies at U. C. Davis indicate that organic foods are up to 2.5 times more nutritious than their non-organic counterparts as well as being lower in toxic metals than in non-organic foods of similar type.

5. **True.** The Generally Recognized as Safe (GRAS) list identifies all additives that have been tested, found to be safe, and approved for use in the food industry. The Delaney Clause, enacted in 1958, states that "No additive may be permitted in any amount if tests show that it produces cancer when fed to man or animals or by other appropriate tests."

Web Links

www.foodsafety.gov/
Foodsafety.gov
Use this Web site as a gateway to government food safety information; it contains news and safety alerts, an area to report illnesses and product complaints, information on food-borne pathogens, and much more.

www.fsis.usda.gov
The USDA Food Safety and Inspection Service
A comprehensive site providing information on all aspects of food safety. Click on Publications for links to the informative publications about food preparation, storage, handling, and other specific safety issues.

www.cspinet.org/foodsafety/index.html
Center for Science in the Public Interest: Food Safety
Visit this Web site for summaries of food additives and their safety, alerts and other information, and interactive quizzes.

www.consumerreports.org
Consumer Reports: Food
Click on Food at the top right or use the search index on top left to find topics such as irradiated meat, produce washes, poultry safety, and mad cow disease.

www.cfsan.fda.gov
The USDA Center for Food Safety and Applied Nutrition
This site contains thorough information on topics such as national food safety programs, recent news, and food labeling. It also contains links to special program areas, such as regulation of mercury levels in fish, food colorings, and biotechnology.

www.extension.iastate.edu/foodsafety/
Food Safety Project
The Food Safety Projects compiles educational materials about food safety for consumer use. Provided on the site are links for food safety from farm to table.

www.epa.gov/pesticides
The U.S. Environmental Protection Agency: Pesticides
This site provides information about agricultural and home-use pesticides, pesticide health and safety issues, environmental effects, and the government regulation.

www.ams.usda.gov
The USDA National Organic Program
Click on National Organic Program to find the Web site describing the NOP's standards and labeling program, consumer information, and publications.

References

Aiyana, J. 2002. What consumers should know about the new USDA organic labeling standard. The pulse of oriental medicine. www.pulsemed.org/usdaorganic. htm (Accessed April 2004.)

Aseptic Packaging Council. 2003. The award-winning, Earth smart packaging for a healthy lifestyle. http://www.aseptic.org/main.shtml (Accessed April 2004.)

Bauman, R. W. 2004. *Microbiology*. San Francisco: Pearson Benjamin Cummings.

Blaylock, R. L. 1996. *Excitoxins: The Taste That Kills*. Santa Fe, NM: Health Press.

Braly, J. 2000. *Food Allergy Relief*. Los Angeles: Keats Publishing.

Centers for Disease Control and Prevention (CDC). 2003a, July. National Center for Infectious Diseases. Traveler's health. Risks from food and drink. http://www.cdc.gov/travel/food-drink-risks.htm (Accessed April 2004.)

Centers for Disease Control and Prevention (CDC). 2003b, September. Division of Bacterial and Mycotic Diseases. Disease information. Foodborne illness. http://www.cdc.gov/ncidod/dbmd/diseaseinfo/foodborneinfections_g.htm (Accessed April 2004.)

Center for Science in the Public Interest (CSPI). 2004a (accessed). Food safety. Chemical cuisine. CSPI's guide to food additives. http://www.cspinet.org/reports/chemcuisine.htm (Accessed April 2004.)

Center for Science in the Public Interest (CSPI). 2004b (accessed). Tips to prevent food poisoning: CSPI's "eggspert" egg advice. http://www.cspinet.org/foodsafety/eggspert_advice.html (Accessed April 2004.)

Consumer Reports. 2003, August. The truth about irradiated meat. http://www.consumerreports.org/main/detailv2.jsp?CONTENT%3C%3Ecnt_id=322725&FOLDER%3C%3Efolder_id=162689 (Accessed September 2003.)

Cunningham, A. (ed.) 2000, *Guiness World Records 2002*. Guiness World Records, Ltd. New York: Bantam.

Emsley, J., and P. Fell. 2002. *Was it Something You Ate? Food Intolerance: What Causes It and How to Avoid It*. Oxford: Oxford University Press.

Environmental Protection Agency (EPA). 2003. *About Pesticides*. http://www.epa.gov/pesticides/about/index.htm Accessed September 2003.

Food Marketing Institute. 2003. *A Consumer Guide to Food Quality and Safe Handling: Meat, Poultry, Seafood, Eggs*. [pamphlet]

Grinder-Pedersen L., S. E. Rasmussen, S. Bügel, L. O. Jørgensen, D. Vagn Gundersen, and B. Sandström. 2003. Effect of diets based on foods from conventional versus organic production on intake and excretion of flavonoids and markers of antioxidative defense in humans. *Agric. Food Chem.* 51(19): 5671–5676.

Heaton, S. 2003. *Organic Farming, Food Quality and Human Health: A Review of the Evidence*. Soil Association. Bristol: Briston House.

Kortbech-Olesen, R. 2002. The United States Market for Organic Food and Beverages. International Trade Center, United Nations Conference on Trade and Development 2002. http://www.intracen.org/mds/sectors/organic/foodbev.pdf (Accessed October 2003.)

Larenbeke, N. Van, A. Covaci, P. Schepens, and L. Hens. 2002. Food contamination with polychlorinated biphenyls and dioxins in Belgium, Effects of the body burden. *Epidemiol. Community Health* 56 (11): 828–830.

Leavitt, J. W. 1996. *Typhoid Mary: Captive to the Public's Health*. Boston: Beacon Press.

LeSage L. January 14, 1999. News Release. Health Canada rejects bovine growth hormone in Canada. Health Canada Online. http://www.hc-sc.gc.ca/english/media/releases/1999/99_03e.htm Accessed April 2004.

Loaharanu, P. 2003. *Irradiated Foods*. New York: American Council on Science & Health Booklets.

Magnuson, B. 1997. Extoxnet. Safety of irradiated food page. The food irradiation process: How is food irradiation done? ace.orst.edu/info/extoxnet/faqs/irradiat/howdone.htm (Accessed September 2003.)

McHughen, A. 2000. *Pandora's Picnic Basket: The potential and hazards of genetically modified foods*. Oxford: Oxford University Press, pgs 17–45.

Montague, P. 1998. Organic Consumers Association. Breast cancer, rBGH and milk. http://www.organicconsumers.org/rBGH/rach598.htm (Accessed January 2004.)

Schafer, K. S., and S. E. Kegley. 2002. Persistent toxic chemicals in the US food supply. *J. Epidemiol. Community Health* 56: 813–817.

Shephard, S. 2000. *Pickled, Potted and Canned: The Story of Food Preserving*. London: Headline Publishing.

Tortora, G. J., B. R. Funke, and C. L. Case. 2003. *Microbiology: An Introduction*, 8th ed. San Francisco: Pearson Benjamin Cummings.

U.S. Department of Agriculture (USDA), 2003, July 2. News Release: For an enjoyable Fourth, consumers should practice food safety. www.usda.gov/news/releases/2003/07/0239.htm (Accessed July 2003.)

U.S. Food and Drug Administration (FDA). 2003. Draft advice for women who are pregnant, or who might become pregnant, and nursing mothers, about avoiding harm to your baby or young child from mercury in fish and shellfish. www.fda.gov/oc/opacom/mehgadvisory 1208.html (Accessed February 2004.)

Whitman, D. B. April 2000. Cambridge Scientific Abstracts: Hot Topics Series: *Genetically Modified Foods: Harmful or Helpful?* http://www.csa.com/hottopics/gmfood/oview.html Accessed September 2003.

Windsor, R. G. 1995, September/October. *Spectrum: The Wholistic News Magazine*. Organically Grown Really Is Better Issue 44: p. 5.

Winter, R. 1994. *A Consumer's Dictionary of Food Additives*. New York: Three Rivers Press.

Nutrition Debate:

Genetically Modified Organisms: A Blessing or a Curse?

Current advances in biotechnology have opened the door to one of the most controversial topics in food science, genetically modified organisms (GMOs). GMOs are organisms that are created through genetic engineering, the standard U.S. term for a process in which foreign genes are spliced into a nonrelated species, creating an entirely new (transgenic) organism. Biotech foods, gene foods, bioengineered food, gene-altered foods, and transgenic foods are other terms used to describe foods that have been created through genetic engineering.

Any plant, animal, or living organism (such as bacteria or yeast) that has had its DNA altered in a laboratory to enhance or change certain characteristics is considered genetically engineered. For example, *Bacillus thuringiensis* is a genetically engineered bacterium that is used as a pesticide. Research labs at University of California, Berkeley, and Stanford University led the process of genetic engineering in the early 1970s.

Developing GMOs is a lengthy, tedious, and costly process requiring years of research and testing. After carefully selecting cultivated cells, genes are removed and scientists are able to identify individual genes that code for specific functions. Using bacteria to transfer these genes, scientists incorporate them into new cells where the introduced genes trigger chosen functions. By using bacteria as the selected medium, DNA can be easily and efficiently produced and incorporated into any cell. Several important medical therapeutics have been developed using this process including human insulin, human growth factor, and factor VIII (a protein needed for blood clotting in hemophiliacs).

Genetically engineered plants and animals may have the potential to solve many food production problems encountered worldwide by improving nutrient content, increasing yield, decreasing the need for pesticides, and allowing plants to grow in inhospitable soils. Animals, in addition to plants, have also been genetically modified to grow quicker and bigger. In 1994, the FlavrSavr tomato became the first commercially sold GMO. Developing this tomato involved identifying the gene that codes for an enzyme called polygalacturonase, which causes ripening in the tomato. This gene was removed and inserted back in reverse orientation. As a result, polygalacturonase was not synthesized, and ripening slowed dramatically—making the tomato appear "fresh" longer and enabling it to maintain a longer shelf life (McHughen 2000).

Since 1994, hundreds of plants and animals have been genetically modified and incorporated into our current food market. In the United States, soy, corn, canola, and cotton crops make up nearly all the genetically modified crop acreage (Whitman 2000). In 2000, approximately 54% of all soybeans and 25% of all the corn grown in the United States were GMOs (Whitman 2000).

Many proponents of genetic modification argue that genetic engineering is an extension of plant and animal breeding methods, producing a superior organism by only transferring the desired traits. Indeed, in traditional farming practices, plants have been selected for desired traits such as higher yield, better taste, size, and color by saving seeds. Sometimes one plant is crossed with another plant in a process called *hybridization*. In this process, a plant or animal is paired with another of a similar species—such as tangelos, which are a hybrid of grapefruit and tangerines, or nectarines, which are modified peaches.

Many animals have been targeted by genetic engineering, leading to the development of cattle, sheep, pigs, and poultry that grow quicker and with a higher

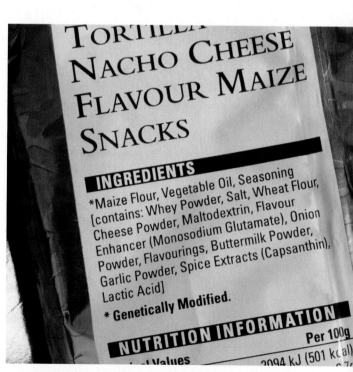

In the United States, companies are not required to list whether ingredients are genetically modified. This label from England indicates the genetically modified content of the food.

disease resistance and lower fat levels. Fish, such as salmon, have also been genetically modified. Transgenic salmon are significantly larger than their wild relatives, producing a higher yield of meat. They are also manipulated for other traits, including disease resistance.

Opponents to genetic engineering argue that hybridization is a safer and a more natural way of manipulating plants and animals. Their concerns regarding GMOs include environmental hazards, human health risks, and economic concerns. Gene transfer to nontarget species is a concern, especially if plants that are engineered for herbicide tolerance are crossbred with non-altered plants. One result could be a "super weed"—a plant tolerant to herbicides and thereby requiring that newer and stronger chemicals be produced to control it.

The risk of allergens being introduced or created by GMOs is another legitimate concern. Introducing a gene into a plant may create a new allergen or cause an allergic reaction in a susceptible individual (Whitman 2000). In the United States, legislation was passed in 1992 that requires all new GMOs to be tested and labeled for allergy sensitivity if the DNA introduced is from any food containing a common allergen. It is estimated that it will take several generations before the full impact of genetically modified organisms will be known.

Genetically modified organisms are welcomed in some countries and outlawed in others. In the United States, many processed foods already contain GMOs and do not require labeling to indicate their presence. The regulation of GMOs in the United States is shared by several governmental agencies including the National Institutes of Health (NIH), USDA, FDA and EPA. Many U.S. consumer groups are pressuring the government to require labeling for all foods containing GMOs.

There are many potential benefits to GMOs, but there are also many potential risks to their development and use. Only time will tell if they are a blessing or a curse.

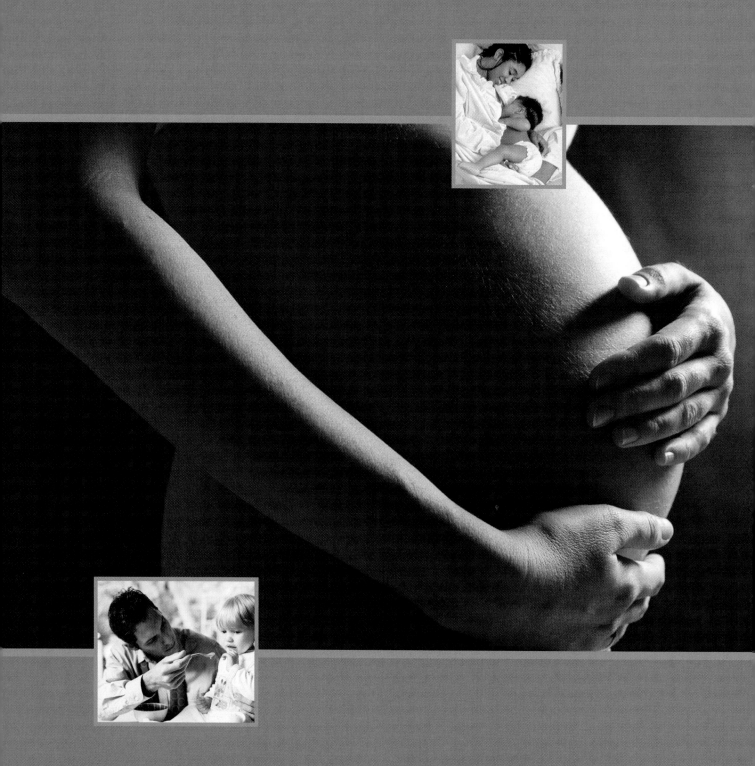

Chapter 15

Nutrition Through the Lifecycle: Pregnancy and the First Year of Life

Chapter Objectives

After reading this chapter you will be able to:

1. Explain why maintaining a nutritious diet is important for prospective parents even before conception, pp. 536–537.

2. Explore the relationship between fetal development, changes in the mother, and increasing nutrient requirements during the course of a pregnancy, pp. 537–540.

3. Identify the range of optimal weight gain for a pregnant woman in the first, second, and third trimesters, pp. 541–542.

4. Describe the physiologic events that lead to lactation, pp. 553–555.

5. Compare and contrast the nutrient requirements of pregnant and lactating women, pp. 542–547 and 555–556.

6. Identify the primary advantages and most common challenges of breastfeeding, pp. 557–561.

7. Relate the growth and activity patterns of infants to their nutrient needs, pp. 562–566.

8. Discuss some common nutrition-related concerns for infants, pp. 566–568.

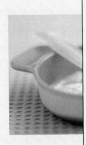

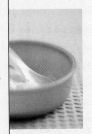

Test Yourself True or False?

1. The amount of weight a woman gains during pregnancy has little influence on the outcome of the pregnancy. T or F

2. Despite popular belief, very few pregnant women actually experience morning sickness, food cravings, or food aversions. T or F

3. Breast-fed infants tend to have fewer infections and allergies than formula-fed infants. T or F

4. Physical growth is the best way to assess whether an infant is adequately nourished. T or F

5. Most infants begin to require solid foods by about three months (12 weeks) of age. T or F

Test Yourself answers can be found at the end of the chapter.

Pregnancy shouldn't be a death sentence . . . but for a malnourished woman, it often is. A report in the *Journal of the Indian Medical Association* found that maternal nutritional deficiency was one of the most important factors contributing to death during pregnancy or childbirth (Mitra and Chowdhury 2002). Statistics from the United Nations Children's Fund indicate that over 100,000 women worldwide die each year during pregnancy or childbirth as a result of iron-deficiency anemia alone (UNICEF 2004). Deficiencies of iodine, folate, vitamin A, zinc, and protein also dramatically increase the risk of the mother and/or her newborn dying. Perhaps maternal malnutrition partly explains the traditional Filipino saying quoted in the UNICEF report: "A woman giving birth has one foot in the grave."

Is maternal malnutrition a problem only in developing nations? What role, if any, does nutrition play in maternal-newborn illness and death in the industrialized countries such as the United States and Canada? Why is inadequate iron especially dangerous to a pregnant woman and her fetus? What role do protein, folate, and other nutrients play in maternal health and fetal development? In this chapter, we discuss how adequate nutrition supports fetal development, maintains the pregnant woman's health, and contributes to lactation. We then explore the nutrient needs of breastfeeding and formula-feeding infants.

Starting Out Right: Healthful Nutrition in Pregnancy

At no stage of life is nutrition more crucial than during fetal development and infancy. Especially from conception through the end of the first year of life, adequate nutrition is essential for tissue formation, neurological development, and bone growth, modeling, and remodeling. Your ability to reach your peak physical and intellectual potential in adult life is in part determined by the nutrition you received during the earliest years of your development.

Is Nutrition Important before Conception?

Several factors make adequate nutrition important even before **conception,** the point at which a woman's ovum (egg) is fertilized with a man's sperm. First, some deficiency-related problems develop extremely early in the pregnancy, typically before the mother even realizes she is pregnant. An adequate and varied preconception diet reduces the risk of such problems, providing "insurance" during those first few weeks of life. For example, failure of the spinal cord to close results in *neural tube defects;* these defects are closely related to inadequate levels of folate during the first few weeks following conception. For this reason, all sexually active women of childbearing age are encouraged to consume 400 μg of folic acid daily, whether or not they plan to become pregnant.

Second, adopting a healthful diet prior to conception includes the avoidance of alcohol, illegal drugs, and other known **teratogens** (substances that cause birth defects). Women should also consult their healthcare provider about their consumption of caffeine, medications, herbs, and supplements, and if they smoke, they should attempt to quit. Finally, maintaining a balanced and nourishing diet before conception reduces a woman's risk of developing a nutrition-related disorder during her pregnancy. These disorders, which we discuss later in the chapter, include gestational diabetes and *preeclampsia,* a form of hypertension specific to pregnant women. Although genetic and metabolic abnormalities are beyond the woman's control, following a healthful diet prior to conception is something a woman can do to help her fetus develop into a healthy baby.

The man's nutrition prior to pregnancy is important as well, since malnutrition contributes to abnormalities in sperm (Olds et al. 2003). Both sperm number and motility (ability to move) are reduced by alcohol consumption, as well as the use of

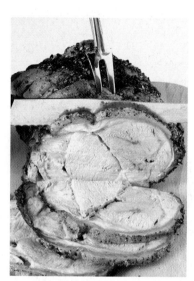

Meats, like pork roast, provide protein and heme iron that are important for maternal and fetal nutrition.

conception   (also called *fertilization*) The uniting of an ovum (egg) and sperm to create a fertilized egg, or zygote.

teratogen   Any substance that can cause a birth defect.

certain prescription and illegal drugs. Finally, infections accompanied by a high fever can destroy sperm; so, to the extent that adequate nutrition keeps the immune system strong, it also promotes a man's fertility.

Why Is Nutrition Important during Pregnancy?

A plentiful, nourishing diet is important throughout pregnancy to provide the nutrients needed to support fetal development without depriving the mother of nutrients she needs to maintain her own health.

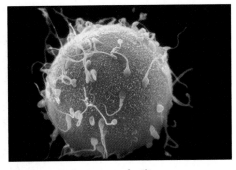

During conception a sperm fertilizes an egg, creating a zygote.

The First Trimester

In clinical practice, the calculation of weeks in a pregnancy begins with the date of the first day of a woman's last menstrual period. A full term pregnancy lasts 38 to 42 weeks and is divided into three **trimesters,** with each trimester lasting about 13 to 14 weeks. The first trimester begins when the ovum and sperm unite to form a single, fertilized cell called a **zygote.** As the zygote travels through the uterine (fallopian) tube, it further divides into a ball of 12 to 16 cells which, at about day four, arrives in the uterus (Figure 15.1). By day 10, the inner portion of the zygote, called the *blastocyst,* implants into the uterine lining. The outer portion becomes part of the placenta, which is discussed shortly.

Further cell growth and multiplication occurs, and the blastocyst differentiates into distinct layers of cells. At this stage, approximately day 15, the mass is called an **embryo.** Over the next six weeks, embryonic tissues differentiate and fold into a primitive tubelike structure with limb buds, organs, and facial features recognizable as human (Figure 15.2). It isn't surprising, then, that the embryo is most vulnerable to teratogens during this time. Not only alcohol and illegal drugs, but also prescription and over-the-counter medications, megadoses of supplements such as vitamin A, certain herbs, viruses, cigarette smoking, and radiation can interfere with embryonic

trimester Any one of three stages of pregnancy, each lasting 13 to 14 weeks.

zygote A fertilized egg (ovum) consisting of a single cell.

embryo Human growth and developmental stage lasting from the third week to the end of the eighth week after fertilization.

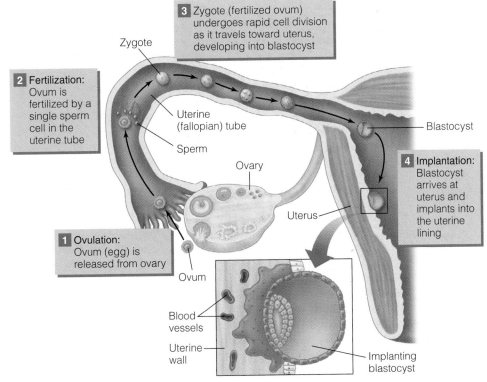

Figure 15.1 Ovulation, conception, and implantation.

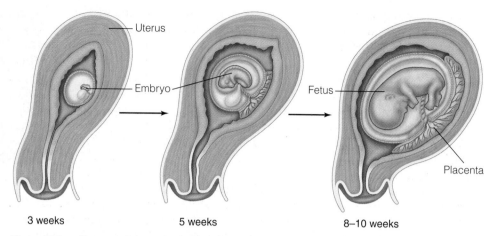

Figure 15.2   Human embryonic development during the first ten weeks. Organ systems are most vulnerable to teratogens during this time, when cells are dividing and differentiating.

spontaneous abortion (also called *miscarriage*)   Natural termination of a pregnancy and expulsion of pregnancy tissues because of a genetic, developmental, or physiological abnormality that is so severe that the pregnancy cannot be maintained.

placenta   A pregnancy-specific organ formed from both maternal and embryonic tissues. It is responsible for oxygen, nutrient, and waste exchange between mother and fetus.

development and cause birth defects (Olds et al. 2003). In some cases, the damage is so severe that the pregnancy is naturally terminated in a **spontaneous abortion** (*miscarriage*), most of which occur in the first trimester.

During the first weeks of pregnancy, the embryo obtains its nutrients from cells lining the uterus. But by the fourth week, a primitive **placenta** has formed in the uterus from both embryonic and maternal tissue. Within a few more weeks, the placenta will be a fully functioning organ through which the mother will provide nutrients and remove fetal wastes (Figure 15.3).

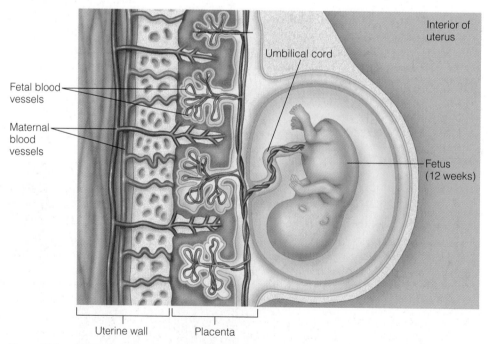

Figure 15.3   Placental development. The placenta is formed from both embryonic and maternal tissues. When the placenta is fully functional, fetal blood vessels and maternal blood vessels are intimately intertwined, allowing the exchange of nutrients and wastes between the two. The mother transfers nutrients and oxygen to the fetus, and the fetus transfers wastes to the mother for disposal.

By the end of the embryonic stage, about eight weeks postconception, the embryo's tissues and organs have differentiated dramatically: a primitive skeleton, including fingers and toes, has formed. Since muscles have begun to develop in the trunk, limbs, and head, some movement is now possible. A primitive heart has also formed and begun to beat, and the digestive system is differentiating into distinct organs (stomach, liver, etc.). The brain and cranial nerves have differentiated, and the head has a mouth, eyespots with eyelids, and primitive ears (Olds et al. 2003).

The third month of pregnancy marks the transition from embryo to **fetus.** The fetus requires abundant nutrients from the mother's body to support its dramatic growth during this period. The placenta is now a mature organ that can provide these nutrients. It is connected to the fetal circulatory system via the **umbilical cord,** an extension of fetal blood vessels emerging from the fetus's navel (called the *umbilicus*). Blood rich in oxygen and nutrients flows through the placenta and into the umbilical vein (see Figure 15.3). Once inside the fetus's body, the blood travels to the fetal liver and heart. Wastes are excreted in blood returning from the fetus to the placenta via the umbilical arteries.

fetus Human growth and developmental stage lasting from the beginning of the ninth week after conception to birth.

umbilical cord The cord containing arteries and veins that connect the baby (from the navel) to the mother via the placenta.

The Second Trimester

During the second trimester (weeks 14 to 27 of pregnancy), the fetus continues to grow and mature. The torso begins to elongate, bones are getting harder and stronger, and the arms and legs are moving. Organ systems also continue to develop and mature. During this period, the fetus can suck its thumb, its ears begin to hear and distinguish sounds, and its eyes can open and close and react to light. The placenta is now fully functional.

At the beginning of the second trimester, the fetus is about 3 inches long and weighs about 1½ pounds. By the end of the second trimester, the fetus is generally over a foot long and weighs over 2 pounds. Some babies born prematurely in the last weeks of the second trimester survive with intensive **neonatal** care.

neonatal Referring to a newborn.

The Third Trimester

The third trimester (weeks 28 to 40) is a time of remarkable growth for the fetus. During three short months, the fetus gains nearly half its body length and three-quarters of its body weight! At the time of birth, an average baby will be approximately 18 to 22 inches long and about 7.5 pounds in weight (Figure 15.4). Brain growth (which continues to be rapid for the first two years of life) is also quite remarkable, and the lungs become fully mature. The fetus acquires eyebrows, eyelashes, and hair on the head. Because of the intense growth and maturation of the fetus during the third trimester, it is critical that the mother eat an adequate and balanced diet.

Impact of Nutrition on Maturity and Birth Weight

An adequate, nourishing diet is one of the most important modifiable variables increasing the chances for birth of a mature newborn (at 38 to 42 weeks of **gestation**). If a baby is mature, sufficient fetal development, particularly of the lungs, will usually have occurred to ensure survival. Proper nutrition also increases the likelihood that the newborn's weight will be appropriate for his or her gestational age. Generally, a birth weight of at least 5.5 pounds is considered a marker of a successful pregnancy.

An undernourished mother is likely to give birth to a **low-birth-weight** baby (UNICEF 2004). Any infant weighing less than 5.5 pounds at birth is considered to be of low birth weight and is at increased risk of infection, learning disabilities, impaired physical development, and death in the first year of life (Figure 15.5). Many low-birth-weight babies are born **preterm;** that is, before 38 weeks gestation. Others are born at term but weigh less than would be expected for their gestational age. While nutrition is not the only factor contributing to maturity and birth weight, its role cannot be overstated.

gestation The period of intrauterine development from conception to birth.

low-birth weight A weight of less than 5.5 pounds at birth.

preterm Birth of a baby prior to 38 weeks gestation.

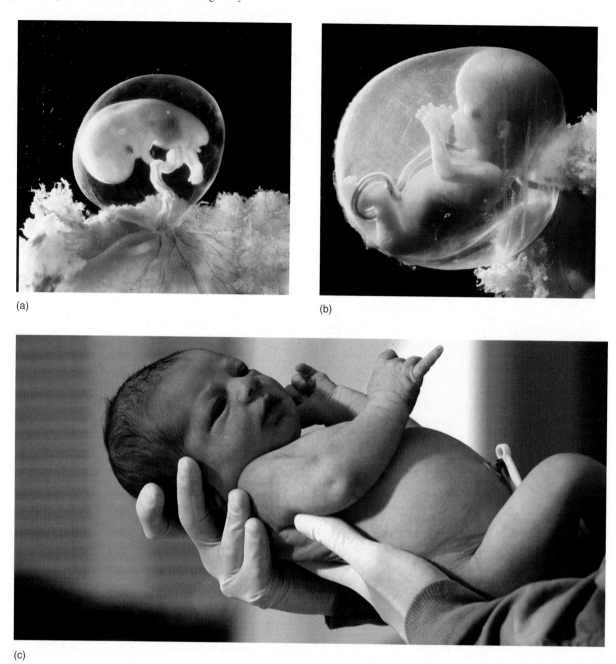

(a)

(b)

(c)

Figure 15.4 Stages of fetal development. **(a)** A fetus at 8 weeks. **(b)** A fetus at 16 weeks. **(c)** A full-term baby at birth.

Recap: A full term pregnancy lasts from 38 to 42 weeks and is traditionally divided into trimesters lasting 13 to 14 weeks. During the first trimester, cells differentiate and divide rapidly to form the various tissues of the human body. The fetus is especially susceptible to teratogens during this time. The second trimester is characterized by continued growth and maturation of organ systems and body structures. The third trimester is a time of profound growth and maturation, especially of the fetal lungs and brain. Nutrition is important before and throughout pregnancy to support fetal development without depleting the mother's reserves. An adequate, nourishing diet increases the chance that a baby will be born after 37 weeks and weighing at least 5.5 pounds.

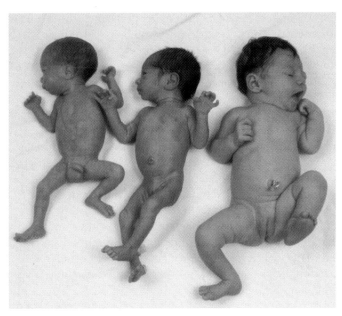

Figure 15.5 A healthy 2-day-old infant (right) compared with two low-birth-weight infants.

How Much Weight Should a Pregnant Woman Gain?

Recommendations for weight gain vary according to a woman's weight *before* she became pregnant (Table 15.1). As you can see in this table, the average recommended weight gain for women of normal pre-pregnancy weight is 25 to 35 pounds; underweight women should gain a little more than this amount, and overweight and obese women should gain less.

As stated earlier, women who gain too little weight increase their risk of having a preterm or low-birth-weight baby and of dangerously depleting their own nutrient reserves, but gaining *too* much weight is also risky. Excessive weight gain increases the risk that the fetus will be large for his or her gestational age, increasing the likelihood of trauma during vaginal delivery and of cesarean birth. In addition, the more weight gained during pregnancy, the more difficult it is to return to pre-pregnancy weight; therefore, women who gain excessive weight have an increased risk of permanent weight gain that can become especially problematic if the woman has two or more children.

In addition to amount of weight, the *pattern* of weight gain is important. During the first trimester, a woman of normal weight should gain no more than 3 to 5 pounds. During the second and third trimester, about one pound a week is considered healthful. If weight gain is excessive in a single week, month, or trimester, the woman should not attempt to lose weight. Dieting during pregnancy jeopardizes the health of both mother and fetus by depriving both of critical nutrients and energy. Instead, the woman should merely attempt to slow the rate of weight gain. On the other hand, if a woman has not

Table 15.1 Recommended Weight Gain for Women During Pregnancy

Pre-Pregnancy Weight Status	Body Mass Index (kg/m²)	Recommended Weight Gain (lbs)
Normal	18.5 – 25	25 – 35
Underweight	<18.5	28 – 40
Overweight	25.1 – 29.9	15 – 25
Obese	≥ 30	No more than 15

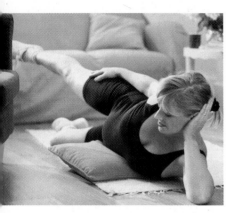

Figure 15.6   Following a physician-approved exercise program helps pregnant women maintain a positive body image and prevent excess weight gain.

gained sufficient weight in the early months of her pregnancy, she should gradually increase her nutrient intake but not attempt to "catch up" all at once. In short, weight gain throughout pregnancy should be slow and steady.

In a society obsessed with thinness, it is easy for pregnant women to worry about weight gain. Focusing on the quality of food consumed, rather than the quantity, can help women feel more in control. In addition, following a physician-approved exercise program helps women maintain a positive body image and prevent excessive weight gain (Figure 15.6).

A pregnant woman may also feel less anxious about her weight gain if she understands how that weight is distributed. Of the total weight gained in pregnancy, 10 to 12 pounds are accounted for by the fetus itself, the amniotic fluid, and the placenta (Figure 15.7). Since these are delivered at birth, a woman can expect to be about 10 to 12 pounds lighter immediately afterward. In addition, within about two weeks, another 5 to 8 pounds of fluid (from increased blood volume and extracellular fluid) is lost. After that, losing the remainder of pregnancy weight depends on more energy being expended than is taken in. Since production of breast milk requires significant energy, breastfeeding helps many new mothers lose the remaining weight. We discuss breastfeeding on pages 553–561.

What Are a Pregnant Woman's Nutrient Needs?

The requirement for nearly all nutrients increases during pregnancy to accommodate the growth and development of the fetus without depriving the mother of the nutrients she needs to maintain her own health.

Macronutrient Needs of Pregnant Women

In pregnancy, macronutrients provide necessary energy for building tissue. They are also the building blocks for the physical form and structure of the fetus, as well as for other pregnancy-associated tissues.

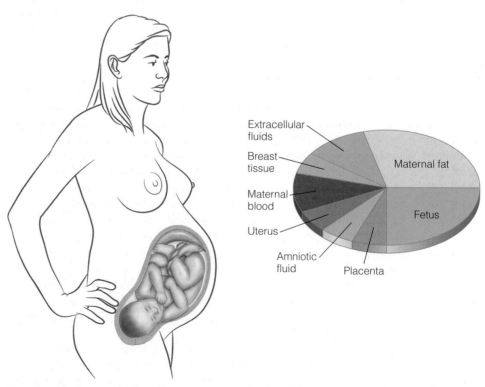

Figure 15.7   The weight gained during pregnancy is distributed between the mother's own tissues and the pregnancy-specific tissues.

Energy   Given what you've just learned about pregnancy weight gain, you've probably figured out that energy requirements increase only modestly during pregnancy. In fact, during the first trimester, a woman should consume approximately the same number of calories daily as during her non-pregnant days. Instead of eating more, she should attempt to maximize the nutrient density of what she eats. For example, drinking low-fat milk is preferable to drinking soft drinks. Low-fat milk provides valuable protein, vitamins, and minerals to feed the fetus's rapidly dividing cells, while soft drinks provide nutritionally empty calories.

During the last two trimesters of pregnancy, caloric needs increase by about 350 to 450 kcal/day. For a woman normally consuming 2000 kcal/day, an extra 400 kcal represents only a 20% increase in calorie intake, a goal that can be met more easily than many pregnant women realize. For example, one cup of low-fat yogurt and a graham cracker with jam is about 400 kilocalories. At the same time, some vitamin and mineral needs increase by as much as 50%, so again, the key for getting adequate micronutrients while not consuming too many extra calories is choosing nutrient-dense foods.

Protein and Carbohydrate   During pregnancy, protein needs increase to 1.1 grams of protein per day per kg body weight over the entire nine-month period. This is an increase of 25 grams of protein per day over the needs for nonpregnant, adult women. Keep in mind that many women already eat this much protein each day, especially in the United States. Dairy products, meats, eggs, and soy products are all rich sources of protein, as are legumes, whole grains, nuts, and seeds.

Carbohydrate intake should be at least 130 grams/day to prevent ketosis (discussed on page 131). Additional carbohydrate is also needed to support daily physical activity. This recommendation is easily met by consuming a sensible diet but should be verified in each individual case. The majority of carbohydrate intake should come from whole foods, such as whole-grain breads and cereals, brown rice, fruits, vegetables, and legumes. Not only are these carbohydrates good sources of micronutrients such as the B vitamins, but they also contain a lot of fiber, which can help prevent constipation. They are fairly filling and can be a boon to women who need to be careful not to gain too much weight. Refined carbohydrates in crackers, cakes, cookies, etc., are both calorie-dense and nutrient-poor. While there's nothing wrong with an occasional treat, it is more healthful for a pregnant woman to satisfy her "sweet tooth" with fresh or dried fruits, which contain vitamins, fiber, and phytochemicals.

Fat   The percentage of daily calories that comes from fat does not change during pregnancy. Pregnant women should be aware that, because new tissues and cells are being built, some fat in the diet is essential. In addition, the fetus stores fat during the third trimester that is a critical source of fuel in the newborn period. Without adequate fat stores, for example, newborns cannot effectively regulate their body temperature.

Moderation and eating the right kinds of fats is important. Like anyone else, pregnant women should limit saturated fat and avoid trans fats because of their negative impact on cardiovascular health (as discussed in Chapter 5). Poly- and monounsaturated fats should be chosen whenever possible. Particularly, an omega-3 polyunsaturated fatty acid known as *docosahexaenoic acid (DHA)* has been found to be critical for both brain growth and eye development. Since the fetal brain grows dramatically during the third trimester, DHA is especially important in the maternal diet then (and also after birth, for those who breast-feed, because of the rapid brain growth that occurs during the first three months of life outside the womb). Good sources of DHA are the oily fish: anchovies, mackerel, salmon, and sardines. It is also found in lesser amounts in tuna, chicken, and eggs (some eggs are DHA-enhanced by feeding hens a DHA-rich diet).

Pregnant women who eat fish should be aware of the potential for mercury contamination, as even a limited intake of mercury during pregnancy can impair a fetus's developing nervous system. While pregnant women should avoid large fish like swordfish, shark, tile fish, and king mackerel, they can safely consume up to 12 ounces of most other types of fish per week, as long as it is cooked. Canned tuna is considered safer than fresh tuna, and commercially caught and farm-raised fish are considered safer than wild fish caught recreationally.

Micronutrient Needs of Pregnant Women

During pregnancy, expansion of the mother's blood supply and growth of the uterus, placenta, breasts, body fat levels, and the fetus itself all contribute to an increased need for micronutrients. In addition, the increased need for energy during pregnancy correlates with an increased need for micronutrients involved in the metabolism of macronutrients and ATP production. Discussions of the micronutrients most critical during pregnancy follow. Refer to Table 15.2 for an overview of the changes in micronutrient needs with pregnancy.

Folate Since folate, or folic acid, is necessary for cell division, it follows that during a time when both maternal and fetal cells are dividing rapidly, the requirement for this vitamin would be increased. Adequate folate is especially critical during the first twenty-eight days after conception, when it is required for the formation and closure of the **neural tube,** an embryonic structure that eventually becomes the brain and spinal cord. Folate deficiency is associated with neural tube defects such as **anencephaly,** a fatal defect in which there is partial absence of brain tissue most likely caused by failure of the neural tube to close (Institute of Medicine 1998). Adequate folate intake does not guarantee normal neural tube development, as the precise cause of neural tube defects is unknown, and there is a genetic component in some cases. Still, it is estimated that 70% of all neural tube defects could be prevented by simply consuming enough folate (CDC 2003).

To reduce the risk of a neural tube defect, all sexually active women of childbearing age are encouraged to consume 400 μg of folate per day. Of course, folate remains very important even after the neural tube has closed. The RDA for folate for pregnant women is therefore 600 μg/day, a full 50% increase over the RDA for a nonpregnant female (Institute of Medicine 1998). A deficiency of folate during pregnancy can result in macrocytic anemia (a condition in which blood cells do not mature properly) and has been associated with low birth weight, preterm delivery, and failure of the fetus to grow properly. Types and sources of folate are discussed on page 354 and include fortified cereals and grains, spinach, and lentils.

Vitamin B₁₂ Vitamin B₁₂ (cobalamin) is vital during pregnancy because it regenerates the active form of folate. Not surprisingly, deficiencies of vitamin B₁₂ can also result in macrocytic anemia. Yet the RDA for vitamin B₁₂ for pregnant women is

neural tube Embryonic tissue that forms a tube, which eventually becomes the brain and spinal cord.

anencephaly A fatal neural tube defect in which there is partial absence of brain tissue most likely caused by failure of the neural tube to close.

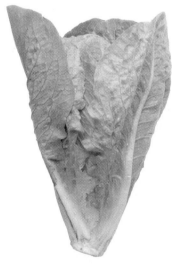

Romaine lettuce is a good source of folate.

Table 15.2 Changes in Nutrient Recommendations With Pregnancy for Adult Women

Micronutrient	Pre-Pregnancy	Pregnancy	% Increase
Folate	400 μg/day	600 μg/day	50
Vitamin B₁₂	2.4 μg/day	2.6 μg/day	8
Vitamin C	75 mg/day	85 mg/day	13
Vitamin A	700 μg/day	770 μg/day	10
Vitamin D	5 μg/day	5 μg/day	0
Calcium	1000 mg/day	1000 mg/day	0
Iron	18 mg/day	27 mg/day	50
Zinc	8 mg/day	11 mg/day	38
Sodium	1500 mg/day	1500 mg/day	0
Iodine	150 μg/day	220 μg/day	47

only 2.6 µg/day, a mere 8% increase over the RDA of 2.4 µg/day for nonpregnant women. How can this be? One reason is that during pregnancy, absorption of vitamin B_{12} is more efficient. The required amount of vitamin B_{12} can easily be obtained from animal food sources. However, deficiencies have been observed in women who follow a vegan diet. Fortified foods or supplementation provide these women with the requisite B_{12}.

Vitamin C   Vitamin C is necessary for the synthesis of collagen, a component of connective tissue (including skin, blood vessels, and tendons) and part of the organic matrix of bones. Because blood plasma volume increases during pregnancy, and because vitamin C is being transferred to the fetus, the concentration of vitamin C in maternal blood decreases. In order to make up the vitamin C deficit, the RDA for vitamin C during pregnancy is increased by a little more than 10% over the RDA for nonpregnant women (from 75 mg to 85 mg per day). A deficiency of vitamin C during pregnancy increases the risk for infections, preterm birth, and other problems. As described on page 273, vitamin C is found abundantly in many food sources, such as citrus fruits, citrus juices, and numerous other fruits and vegetables.

Vitamin A   Vitamin A needs increase during pregnancy by about 10%, to 770 µg per day. However, excess preformed vitamin A can cause fetal abnormalities, particularly in the kidneys and nervous system, even when it is not consumed in extremely high quantities. Since an adequate diet supplies sufficient vitamin A, supplementation is not recommended. Note that provitamin A, in the form of beta carotene (which is converted to vitamin A in the body) has not been associated with birth defects.

Vitamin D   Despite the role of vitamin D in calcium absorption, the AI for this nutrient does not increase during pregnancy. According to the Institute of Medicine (1997), the amount of vitamin D transferred from the mother to the fetus is relatively small and does not appear to affect overall vitamin D status. Pregnant women who receive adequate exposure to sunlight do not need vitamin D supplements. However, pregnant women with limited sun exposure who do not regularly drink milk will benefit from vitamin D supplementation. Most prenatal vitamin supplements contain 10 µg/day of vitamin D, which is considered safe and acceptable (Institute of Medicine 1997). Pregnant women should be cautious and avoid consuming excessive vitamin D from supplements, as this can cause developmental disability in the newborn.

Calcium   Growth of the fetal skeleton requires a significant amount of calcium. However, the AI for adult pregnant women is the same as that for nonpregnant adult women, 1000 mg/day, for two reasons. First, pregnant women absorb calcium from the diet more efficiently than do nonpregnant women. This increased absorption may be due to the fact that they have higher levels of the active form of vitamin D (Cross et al. 1995) and high levels of estrogen in their blood, both of which enhance calcium absorption. Second, the extra demand for calcium has not been found to cause demineralization of the mother's bones or to increase fracture risk (Institute of Medicine, 1997). Sources of calcium are discussed on pages 315–322.

Iron   Recall from Chapter 10 the importance of iron in the formation of red blood cells, which transport oxygen throughout the body so that cells can produce ATP. During pregnancy, the demand for red blood cells increases to accommodate the needs of the growing uterus, placenta, and the fetus itself. Thus, more iron is needed. Fetal demand for iron increases even further during the last trimester, when the fetus stores iron in the liver for use during the first few months of life. This iron storage is protective because breast milk is low in iron.

Severely inadequate iron intake certainly has the potential to harm the fetus, resulting in an increased rate of low birth weight, preterm birth, stillbirth, and death of the newborn in the first weeks after birth. However, in most cases the fetus in a

iron-deficiency anemia A reduction in the number of red blood cells or hemoglobin or both, resulting in pallor and fatigue. Caused by a lack of the mineral iron, in this case.

low-iron state builds adequate stores by "robbing" maternal iron, prompting **iron-deficiency anemia** in the mother. During pregnancy, maternal iron deficiency causes pallor and exhaustion, but at birth, it endangers her life: anemic women are more likely to die during or shortly following childbirth because they are less able to tolerate blood loss and fight infection.

The RDA for iron for pregnant women is 27 mg per day, compared with 18 mg per day for nonpregnant women. This represents a 50% increase, despite the fact that iron loss is minimized during pregnancy because menstruation ceases. Typically, women of childbearing age have poor iron stores, and the demands of pregnancy are likely to produce deficiency. To ensure adequate iron stores during pregnancy, an iron supplement (as part of, or distinct from, a total prenatal supplement) is routinely prescribed during the last two trimesters. Vitamin C enhances iron absorption, as do dietary sources of heme iron, whereas substances in coffee, tea, milk, bran, and oxalates decrease absorption. Therefore, many healthcare providers recommend taking iron supplements with foods high in vitamin C and/or heme iron. Sources of iron are discussed on pages 364–368.

Zinc   The RDA for zinc for adult pregnant women increases by about 38% over the RDA for nonpregnant adult women, from 8 mg per day to 11 mg per day. Since zinc has critical roles in DNA synthesis, RNA synthesis, and protein synthesis, it is imperative that adequate zinc status be maintained during pregnancy to facilitate proper growth and development of both maternal and fetal tissues. Inadequate zinc can lead to malformations in the fetus, premature delivery, and extended labor. It should be noted that the absorption of zinc is inhibited by iron when these two minerals are taken with water. However, when iron and zinc are consumed together in a meal, absorption of zinc is not affected (Whittaker 1998; Davidsson et al. 1995). In addition, the heme form of iron does not appear to inhibit zinc absorption. When iron supplements are prescribed during pregnancy, it is good practice to consume these supplements with food and with a good vitamin C source to enhance the absorption of both zinc and iron.

Sodium and Iodine   During pregnancy, the AI for sodium is the same for a nonpregnant adult woman, or 1500 mg (1.5 g) per day (Institute of Medicine 2004). Although too much sodium is associated with fluid retention and bloating, as well as high blood pressure, increased fluids are a normal and necessary part of pregnancy, so some sodium is necessary to maintain fluid balance.

Iodine needs increase significantly during pregnancy, but the RDA of 220 μg per day is easy to achieve by using a modest amount of iodized salt (sodium chloride) during cooking. Sprinkling salt onto food at the table is unnecessary.

Do Pregnant Women Need Supplements?

Prenatal multivitamin and mineral supplements are not strictly necessary during pregnancy, but most healthcare providers recommend them. Meeting all the nutrient needs would otherwise take careful and somewhat complex dietary planning. Prenatal supplements are especially good insurance for special populations such as vegans, adolescents, and others whose diet might normally be low in one or more micronutrients. It is important that pregnant women understand, however, that supplements are to be taken *in addition to,* not as a substitute for, a nutrient-rich diet.

Fluid Needs of Pregnant Women

Fluid plays many vital roles during pregnancy. It allows for the necessary increase in the mother's blood volume, acts as a lubricant, aids in regulating body temperature, and is necessary for many metabolic reactions. Fluid that the mother consumes also helps maintain the **amniotic fluid** that surrounds, cushions, and protects the fetus in the uterus. The AI for total fluid intake, which includes drinking water, beverages,

amniotic fluid The watery fluid contained within the innermost membrane of the sac containing the fetus. It cushions and protects the growing fetus.

and food, is 3 liters per day (or about 12.7 cups). This recommendation includes approximately 2.3 liters (10 cups) of fluid as total beverages, including drinking water (Institute of Medicine 2004).

Drinking adequate fluid also helps combat fluid retention and constipation, two common discomforts of pregnancy. Drinking lots of fluids (and going to the bathroom as soon as the need is felt) will also help prevent **urinary tract infections,** which are very common in pregnancy. Urinary tract infections are bacterial infections of the urethra, which is the tube that leads from the bladder to the exterior of the body. Fluids also combat dehydration, which can develop if a woman with morning sickness has frequent bouts of vomiting. For these women, any nondiuretic fluid can help prevent dehydration, including soups, juices, and sport beverages.

urinary tract infection A bacterial infection of the urethra, the tube leading from the bladder to the body exterior.

> **Recap:** Sufficient calories should be consumed so that a pregnant woman gains an appropriate amount of weight, typically 25 to 35 pounds, to ensure adequate growth of the fetus. The calories consumed during pregnancy should be nutrient-dense so that both the mother and the fetus obtain the nutrients they need from food. Protein, carbohydrates, and fats provide the building blocks for fetal growth. Folate deficiency has been associated with neural tube defects. Most healthcare providers recommend prenatal supplements for pregnant women to ensure that sufficient micronutrients are consumed. Fluid provides for increased maternal blood volume and amniotic fluid.

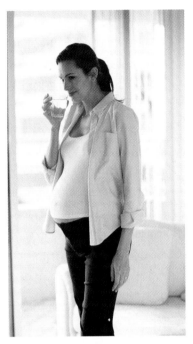

It is important that pregnant women drink about 10 cups of fluid a day.

Nutrition-Related Concerns for Pregnant Women

Pregnancy-related conditions involving a particular nutrient, such as iron-deficiency anemia, have already been discussed. The following sections describe some of the most common discomforts and disorders of pregnant women that are related to their general nutrition.

Morning Sickness

morning sickness Varying degrees of nausea and vomiting associated with pregnancy, most commonly in the first trimester.

Morning sickness, or *nausea and vomiting of pregnancy (NVP)*, is increasingly gaining recognition as a legitimate and potentially serious medical condition worthy of study and treatment (von Dadelszen 2000). The symptoms vary in severity, from occasional mild queasiness to constant nausea with bouts of vomiting. In truth, "morning sickness" is not an appropriate name because the nausea and vomiting can begin at any time of the day, and about 80% of pregnant women report that it lasts all day. More than half of all pregnant women experience morning sickness, and some have it with one pregnancy but not with another. It usually begins shortly after the first missed period and abates by week 12 to 16, but a minority of women experience it throughout the pregnancy. Except in severe cases, the mother and fetus do not suffer lasting harm. However, some women experience such frequent vomiting that they are unable to nourish or hydrate themselves or their fetus adequately, and thus they require hospitalization.

Rising levels of two pregnancy-related hormones are thought to be at least partly responsible for morning sickness. Metabolic and emotional factors may also play some role.

There is no cure for morning sickness. However, here are some practical tips for reducing the severity:

- Eat lightly throughout the day. An empty stomach can actually trigger nausea so eating small, frequent meals and snacks is usually helpful. Many women experiencing queasiness find that once they start eating, they begin to feel better. Protein and complex carbohydrates are especially useful in combating nausea.

- Some women find it helpful to keep snacks at their bedside to ease nighttime queasiness. A small snack before rising in the morning helps some women, as does rising from bed slowly.

The Danger of Nonfood Cravings

For most of her life, Darcy had thoroughly enjoyed good food. Her husband even bragged about her being a "gourmet cook." But a few weeks after learning she was pregnant, her appetite seemed to disappear. She would wander through the aisles of the grocery store with an empty cart, knowing she should be choosing nutritious foods for her growing baby but feeling unable to find a single food that appealed to her. Eventually, she'd return home with a few things for her husband . . . and a large bag of ice. On weekends, she'd keep a cupful of ice with her almost constantly. She brought ice to work in a cold pack and ate it throughout the day, and she even kept a glass of ice by her bed at night. At her prenatal healthcare visits, her physician became concerned because she wasn't gaining weight. "I try to eat right," she confessed, "but nothing appeals to me." She was too embarrassed to admit to anyone, even her husband, that the only thing she really wanted to eat was ice.

Some people contend that a pregnant woman with unusual food cravings is intuitively seeking needed nutrients. Arguing against this claim is the phenomenon of *pica*—the craving and consumption of nonfood material during pregnancy. A woman with pica may crave ice, freezer frost, clay, dirt, chalk, coffee grounds, baking soda, laundry starch, and many other substances. The cause of these nonfood cravings is not known, though cultural factors, socioeconomic status, emotional support, and family tendencies seem to contribute to the incidence. No matter the cause, pica is dangerous. Consuming ice cubes or freezer frost can lead to inadequate weight gain if the substance substitutes for food. Ingestion of clay, starch, and other substances can cause deficiency of iron and other nutrients, as well as constipation, intestinal blockage, and even excessive weight gain.

Some women find it helpful to substitute food items for the craved nonfood. For instance, frozen juice bars can be substituted for ice, and nonfat powdered milk can replace starch (Olds et al. 2003). ●

- Taking a prenatal supplement ensures that at least some vitamins and minerals are being absorbed. Obviously, the supplement should be taken at a time of day when vomiting is not likely.
- Women should also drink plenty of fluids to prevent dehydration from vomiting.
- Women should avoid sights, sounds, smells, and tastes that bring on or exacerbate queasiness.
- For some women, alternative therapies such as acupuncture, acupressure wrist bands, biofeedback, meditation, and hypnosis help. Raspberry tea soothes nausea in some women. Ginger tea may also be helpful but should be consumed in moderation. Women should check with their healthcare provider regarding alternative therapies to ensure that the therapy they are using is safe and does not interact with other medications, supplements, or health considerations.
- Decrease stress and get some rest and relaxation time, if possible.

Cravings and Aversions

It seems like nothing is more stereotypical about pregnancy than the image of a frazzled husband getting up in the middle of the night to run to the convenience store to get his pregnant wife some pickles and ice cream. This image, although humorous, is far from reality for most women. Although some women have specific cravings, most crave a particular type (such as "something sweet" or "something salty") rather than a particular food.

Why do pregnant women crave certain tastes? Does a desire for salty foods mean that the woman is experiencing a sodium deficit? While there may be some truth to the assertion that we crave what we need, scientific evidence for this claim is lacking. More likely, it is thought that cravings during pregnancy are due to hormonal fluctuations or physiological changes or have familial or cultural roots. In some cases, when a

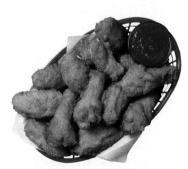

Deep-fried foods are often unappealing to pregnant women.

woman improves her diet after learning she is pregnant, she simply misses the "forbidden" foods that she used to eat.

Most cravings are, of course, for edible substances. But a surprising number of pregnant women crave nonfoods like freezer frost and clay. This craving, called **pica,** is the subject of the Highlight box on the previous page.

pica   An abnormal craving to eat something not fit for food, such as clay, paint, etc.

Food aversions are also common during pregnancy but are by no means universal. Many women experience an aversion to coffee during the early months, for example. Does this mean a woman's body somehow "knows" she should avoid caffeine? Again, probably not, although this happens to be a fortuitous, convenient aversion if you're a habitual coffee drinker! It is also fairly common for deep-fried foods to elicit a gag response. Most likely food aversions have similar roots as food cravings.

Heartburn

Heartburn, along with indigestion, is common during pregnancy. Heartburn occurs when the sphincter between the esophagus and the stomach relaxes, allowing acid and partially digested food from the stomach to well up and irritate the tissues of the esophagus. Because hormones released during pregnancy relax smooth muscle, heartburn incidence increases at this time. During the last two trimesters, enlargement of the uterus pushes up on the stomach, compounding the problem. Practical tips for minimizing the distress associated with heartburn and indigestion during pregnancy include the following:

- Avoid excessive weight gain.
- Eat small frequent meals and chew food slowly.
- Don't wear tight clothing.
- Avoid foods that seem to trigger the problem.
- Wait for at least one hour after eating before lying down.
- Sleep with your head elevated.
- Ask your doctor and/or midwife for an antacid that is safe for use during pregnancy.

Foods high in fiber, such as dried fruits, reduce the chances of constipation.

Constipation and Hemorrhoids

Hormone production during pregnancy causes the smooth muscles to relax, including the muscles of the large intestine. This causes movement of material through the colon to be sluggish. In addition, pressure exerted by the growing uterus on the colon can slow movement even further, making elimination difficult. **Hemorrhoids**—swollen varicose veins in the rectum—are caused by constipation or exacerbated by it. They are usually painful and may itch and bleed. Practical hints to avoid constipation include the following:

hemorrhoids   Swollen varicose veins in the rectum.

- Include 25 to 35 grams of fiber in the daily diet, concentrating on fresh fruits and vegetables, legumes, and whole grains. Dried fruits are fiber-rich and very portable snacks.
- Keep fluid intake high. Drink plenty of water, and eat water-rich fruits and vegetables to keep stools soft and moving, thus making them easier to eliminate.
- Exercise, as it helps increase motility of the large intestine.
- Don't hold bowel movements in. Go to the bathroom as soon as you feel the need.

Gestational Diabetes

Gestational diabetes is generally a temporary condition in which a pregnant woman is unable to produce sufficient insulin or becomes insulin resistant. Either of these conditions results in elevated levels of blood glucose. Fortunately, gestational diabetes has no ill effects on either the mother or the fetus if blood glucose levels are strictly

gestational diabetes   Insufficient insulin production or insulin resistance that results in consistently high blood glucose levels, specifically during pregnancy; condition typically resolves after birth occurs.

controlled through diet, exercise, and/or medication. Screening for gestational diabetes is routine for almost all healthcare practitioners and is necessary because the symptoms, which include frequent urination, fatigue, and an increase in thirst and appetite, among others, can be indistinguishable from normal pregnancy symptoms. If uncontrolled, gestational diabetes can result in *preeclampsia*, which is discussed in greater detail below. It can also result in a baby that is too large as a result of receiving too much glucose across the placenta during fetal life. Babies that are overly large are at risk for early delivery, trauma during birth, and other problems and may need to be born by cesarean section. There is also evidence that exposing a fetus to diabetes while in the womb significantly increases the risk for type 2 diabetes during adolescence and adulthood (Benyshek, Martin, and Johnston 2001; Dabelea et al. 1998). Women who are obese have a greater risk of developing gestational diabetes, and any woman who develops gestational diabetes remains at greater risk of developing type 2 diabetes later in life—particularly if she is obese to begin with or fails to maintain normal body weight after pregnancy. As with type 2 diabetes, attention to diet, weight control, and exercise reduce the risk of gestational diabetes.

Nadia *Nutri-Case*

"After talking to the clinic's registered dietitian, I found out that I don't have to give myself insulin shots right now, and I probably won't have to as long as I can keep the diabetes under control on my own. However, I do need to watch what I eat. This is distressing for me because I feel like I'm hungry all the time, but I can't have the foods I crave the most! I don't know how I'm going to endure it for the entire pregnancy. I am still concerned about the possible lifelong effects of gestational diabetes, both for me and my baby."

Review what you learned about diabetes in Chapter 4. What foods do you think the dietitian might have advised Nadia to limit or avoid? What strategies could you suggest to help her cope with her constant hunger and carbohydrate cravings? Besides diet, what other measures can Nadia take to help control her gestational diabetes? Assuming Nadia's condition is controlled, need she be afraid for her baby's health? Will she need to maintain her restricted diet for the rest of her life?

Preeclampsia

preeclampsia High blood pressure that is pregnancy-specific and accompanied by protein in the urine, edema and unexpected weight gain.

Preeclampsia (also called *pregnancy-induced hypertension*) is characterized by sudden, high maternal blood pressure, swelling, excessive and rapid weight gain unrelated to food intake, and protein in the urine. If left untreated, it can result in death for both the mother and fetus.

No one knows exactly what causes preeclampsia, but there appears to be a genetic link as well as a nutritional connection. Deficiencies in vitamin C, vitamin E, and magnesium seem to increase the risk. High levels of blood triglycerides (associated with high-sugar diets) have been correlated with preeclampsia. Also at higher risk than the general population are women who are over the age of forty, women who already have chronic high blood pressure, women with diabetes (gestational or otherwise), women carrying multiple fetuses, and African American women (Mostello et al. 2002).

Management of preeclampsia focuses mainly on blood pressure control. Typical treatment includes bed rest. Ultimately, the only thing that will cure the condition is childbirth. Depending on the severity of the symptoms and the gestational age of the fetus, delivery may be a viable treatment, either by inducing labor or by cesarean section. If the symptoms are mild and the onset is before the fetus would likely survive outside the womb, conservative treatment and bed rest are the usual course of action so that the fetus has the opportunity to mature further. Unfortunately, sometimes severe preeclampsia occurs early in the pregnancy, and labor must be induced even though there is little chance of survival for the fetus. Today, with good prenatal care, preeclampsia is nearly always detected early and can be appropriately managed, and prospects for both mother and fetus are usually very good. In nearly all women without prior chronic high blood pressure, blood pressure returns to normal within about a day after the birth.

> **Recap:** About half of all pregnant women experience nausea and/or vomiting during pregnancy, called morning sickness, and many crave or feel aversions to specific types of foods. Pica is a craving for nonfood items experienced by some pregnant women. Heartburn and constipation in pregnancy are related to the relaxation of smooth muscle caused by certain pregnancy-related hormones. Gestational diabetes and preeclampsia are nutrition-related disorders that can seriously affect maternal and fetal health.

Adolescent Pregnancy

Adolescents who become pregnant are subject to greater nutritional risks than adult women. Throughout the adolescent years, a woman's body is still changing and growing. Peak bone mass has not yet been reached. Full physical stature may not have been attained, and teens are more likely to be underweight than are young adult women. This demand for tissue growth keeps nutrient needs during adolescence very high. In addition, many adolescents have not established healthful nutritional patterns; thus, the added burden of a pregnancy on an adolescent body creates a nutrient demand that can be very difficult to meet. Hence, adolescent mothers are more likely to have preterm births, low-birth-weight babies, and other complications related to nutritional deficiencies than are more mature women. With adequate and thorough prenatal care and close attention to proper nutrition and other healthful behaviors, the likelihood of a positive outcome for both the adolescent mother and infant is greatly increased (Barnet, Duggan, and Devoe 2003).

Vegetarianism

Vegetarian women who consume dairy products and/or eggs (lacto-ovo-vegetarians) have no nutritional concerns beyond those encountered by every pregnant woman. In contrast, women who are totally vegetarian (vegan) need to be more vigilant than usual about their intake of nutrients that are derived primarily or wholly from animal products. These include vitamin D (unless exposed to sunlight), vitamin B_6, vitamin B_{12}, calcium, iron, and zinc. Supplements containing these nutrients are usually necessary. A regular prenatal supplement will fully meet the vitamin and iron needs of a vegan woman but does not fulfill calcium needs, so a separate calcium supplement, or consumption of calcium-fortified soy milk or orange juice, might be required.

Dieting

Dieting to lose weight is not advisable during pregnancy. When calories are restricted, neither the woman nor the fetus obtains the nutrients necessary to grow and develop appropriately. Similarly, fad diets that are unbalanced in macronutrients (for example, high protein/low carbohydrate, or vice versa) are also unbalanced in micronutrients. Both total fasting and abstaining from carbohydrates are especially dangerous practices during pregnancy: recall from Chapter 4 that ketones are released when the body must rely on stored fats for fuel. These ketones are readily taken up and metabolized by the fetal brain, which could be detrimental to proper brain growth and development. Lack of glucose (carbohydrates) in the mother's diet also has been shown to result in reduced fetal growth (Harding 2001). The best strategy during pregnancy to ensure health of mother and baby is a healthful balance of all nutrients.

Consumption of Caffeine

Caffeine is a stimulant found in several foods, including coffee, tea, soft drinks, and chocolate. Caffeine crosses the placenta and thus reaches the fetus, but at what dose and to what extent it causes harm is still a subject of controversy and study. Current

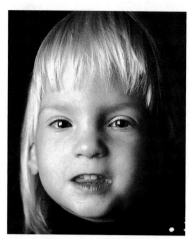

Figure 15.8   A child with fetal alcohol syndrome (FAS). The facial features characteristic of children with FAS include a short nose with a low, wide bridge, drooping eyes with an extra skinfold, and a flat, thin upper lip. Behavioral problems and learning disorders are also characteristic. The effects of FAS are irreversible.

fetal alcohol syndrome (FAS)   A set of serious, irreversible alcohol-related birth defects characterized by certain physical and mental abnormalities.

fetal alcohol effects (FAE)   A milder set of alcohol-related birth defects characterized by behavioral problems such as hyperactivity, attention deficit disorder, poor judgment, sleep disorders and delayed learning.

thinking holds that women who consume less than about 200 mg of caffeine per day (the equivalent of one to two cups of coffee) are very likely doing no harm to the fetus. Evidence suggests that consuming higher daily doses of caffeine (the higher the dose, the more compelling the evidence) may slightly increase the risk of miscarriage and low birth weight. It is sensible, then, for pregnant women to limit daily caffeine intake to no more than the equivalent of two cups of coffee (March of Dimes 2003a). In addition to its possible harm to the fetus, keep in mind that caffeine is a diuretic and will thus exacerbate maternal fluid loss and cause even more frequent trips to the bathroom. Because coffee and colas are devoid of nutritional value, drinking them can be especially detrimental during pregnancy because they can make one feel full and provide considerable calories (if sweetened) without contributing any nutrients at a time when nutrient intake is critical.

Consumption of Alcohol

Alcohol is a known teratogen that readily crosses the placenta and accumulates in the fetal bloodstream. The immature fetal liver cannot readily metabolize alcohol, and its presence in the fetal tissues is associated with a variety of birth defects. These effects are dose-dependent: the more the mother drinks, the greater the potential harm to the fetus.

Heavy drinking (greater than three to four drinks per day) throughout pregnancy can result in a condition called **fetal alcohol syndrome (FAS)** (Figure 15.8). Babies born with FAS have characteristic malformations, particularly of the face, limbs, heart, and nervous system. They have a high mortality rate, and those who survive typically have emotional, behavioral, social, learning, and developmental problems throughout life.

Moderate drinking (two drinks per day) or occasional binge drinking during pregnancy increases the risk for miscarriage as well as serious complications during delivery, preterm birth, developmental delays, and **fetal alcohol effects (FAE).** Also caused by alcohol consumption during pregnancy, FAE is a milder set of alcohol-related birth defects manifested in the child as developmental and behavioral problems (for example, hyperactivity and attention deficit disorder) and possibly physical abnormalities. Although some women do have the occasional alcoholic drink with no apparent ill effects, there is no amount of alcohol that is known to be safe. The best advice regarding alcohol during pregnancy is to abstain, if not from before conception, then as soon as pregnancy is suspected (March of Dimes 2003b).

Exercise

Physical activity during pregnancy can be of tremendous benefit to a mother-to-be and is recommended for women experiencing normal pregnancies and who are otherwise in good health (Lumbers 2002). Exercise can help keep a woman physically fit during pregnancy, an important asset when enduring the physical stress of labor and delivery. In addition, exercise is a great mood booster, helping women feel more in control of their changing bodies. Expending additional energy through exercise will also allow intake of compensatory energy when a ravenous appetite kicks in. Moreover, regular moderate exercise will help keep blood pressure down and confer all the cardiovascular benefits that it does for nonpregnant individuals. Regular exercise can reduce the risks for preeclampsia (Yeo and Davidge 2001). Finally, a woman who keeps fit during pregnancy will have an easier time resuming a fitness routine and losing weight after pregnancy.

If a woman was not active prior to pregnancy, then she should begin an exercise program slowly and progress gradually under the guidance of her healthcare provider. If a woman was physically active before pregnancy, she can continue to be physically active during pregnancy, within comfort and reason. The exercise should be comfortable for the woman. Low- or no-impact exercises are excellent choices for most women, although women who have been avid runners before pregnancy can often continue to run, as long as they feel comfortable. However, they should probably limit the distance and intensity of their runs.

All pregnant women should be careful not to unduly raise their heart rate or body temperature. They should avoid sports where there is potential for falling or jarring physical contact. Special care should also be taken when exercising in hot weather; careful attention should be given to fluid replenishment. Exercise while laying on one's back should be avoided after the fourth month, since the growing weight of the uterus can compress important blood vessels. Generally, it is recommended that exercise gradually taper off during the last trimester, especially during the ninth month. Any exercise program should meet with the approval of the woman's healthcare provider, as some conditions encountered during pregnancy explicitly contraindicate exercise.

> **Recap:** As adolescents' bodies are still growing and developing, their nutrient needs during pregnancy become so high that adequate nourishment for the mother and baby becomes difficult. Women who follow a vegan diet usually need to consume multivitamin and mineral supplements, plus supplemental calcium, during pregnancy. Dieting during pregnancy is not advised, as it leads to inadequate nutrition for mother and fetus. Caffeine intake should not exceed two cups of coffee per day throughout pregnancy. Alcohol is a teratogen and should not be consumed in any amount during pregnancy. Exercise (provided the mother has no contraindications) can enhance the health of a pregnant woman.

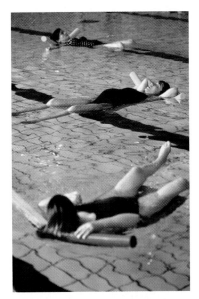

During pregnancy, women should adjust their physical activity to comfortable low-impact exercises.

Breastfeeding

Throughout most of human history, infants have thrived on only one food: breast milk. But during the first half of the twentieth century, commercially prepared infant formulas slowly began to replace breast milk as the mother's preferred feeding method. Aggressive marketing campaigns promoting formula as more nutritious than breast milk convinced many families, even in developing nations, to switch. Soon formula-feeding had become a status symbol, proof of the family's wealth and modern thinking. In the 1970s, this trend began to reverse as the "back-to-the-land" movement led to a renewed appreciation for the natural simplicity of breastfeeding and a distaste for corporate involvement in infant feeding. At the same time, several international organizations, including the World Health Organization, UNICEF, and La Leche League, began to promote the nutritional, immunologic, financial, and emotional advantages of breastfeeding and developed programs to encourage and support breastfeeding worldwide. These efforts have paid off: in 2002, U. S. breastfeeding rates reached an all-time high with just over 70% of new mothers now initiating breastfeeding in the hospital and over 33% of mothers still breastfeeding their babies at six months of age (Abbott Laboratories 2003). Worldwide, slightly more than half of all women breastfeed exclusively for at least six months (UNICEF 2003); however, this value is significantly lower in the United States where only 10% of children are breastfed exclusively at six months of age (Li et al. 2002).

How, exactly, does breastfeeding occur? What nutrients are important for breastfeeding mothers? Is breastfeeding painful and difficult? And what exactly are the advantages that everyone is talking about? The answers to these questions are presented in the following sections.

How Does Lactation Occur?

Lactation, the production of breast milk, is a process that is set in motion during pregnancy in response to several hormones. Once established, lactation can be sustained as long as the mammary glands continue to receive the proper stimuli.

lactation   The production of breast milk.

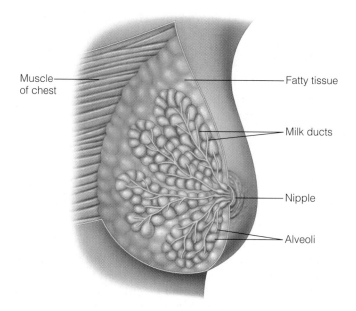

Figure 15.9 Anatomy of the breast. During pregnancy, estrogen and progesterone secreted by the placenta foster the preparation of breast tissue for lactation. This process includes breast enlargement and development of the milk-producing glands, or alveoli.

The Body Prepares During Pregnancy

Throughout pregnancy, the placenta produces estrogen and progesterone. In addition to performing various functions to maintain the pregnancy, these hormones prepare the breasts physically for lactation. The breasts increase in size, and milk-producing glands (alveoli) and milk ducts are formed (Figure 15.9). Toward the end of pregnancy, the hormone *prolactin* increases. Prolactin is released by the anterior pituitary gland and is responsible for milk synthesis. However, estrogen and progesterone suppress the effects of prolactin during pregnancy.

What Happens After Childbirth

By the time a pregnancy has come to full term, the level of prolactin is about ten times higher than it was at the beginning of pregnancy. At birth, the suppressive effect of estrogen and progesterone ends, and prolactin is free to stimulate milk production. The first substance to be released from the breasts and to be ingested by a suckling infant is **colostrum,** sometimes called pre-milk or first milk. It is thick, yellowish in color, and rich in protein, and includes antibodies that help protect the newborn from infection. It is also relatively high in vitamin and mineral content, compared to the mature milk that comes later. Colostrum also contains a factor that fosters the growth of a particular species of bacteria in the infant GI tract. These bacteria in turn prevent the growth of other bacteria that could potentially be harmful. Finally, colostrum has a laxative effect in infants, helping the infant to expel *meconium,* the sticky "first stool."

Within two to four days in most women, colostrum is fully replaced by mature milk. Mature breast milk contains protein, fat, and carbohydrate (in the form of the sugar lactose). Much of the protein and fat are synthesized in the breast, while the rest enter the milk from the mother's bloodstream.

Mother-Infant Interaction Maintains Milk Production

Continued, sustained breast milk production depends entirely on infant suckling (or a similar stimulus like a mechanical pump). Infant suckling stimulates the continued production of prolactin, which in turn stimulates more milk production. The longer

colostrum The first fluid made and secreted by the breasts from late in pregnancy to about a week after birth. It is rich in immune factors and protein.

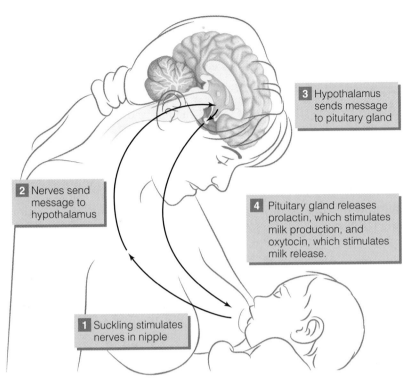

3 Hypothalamus sends message to pituitary gland

2 Nerves send message to hypothalamus

4 Pituitary gland releases prolactin, which stimulates milk production, and oxytocin, which stimulates milk release.

1 Suckling stimulates nerves in nipple

Figure 15.10 Sustained milk production depends on the mother-child interaction during breastfeeding, specifically the suckling of the infant. Suckling stimulates the continued production of prolactin, which is responsible for milk production, and also oxytocin, which is responsible for the let-down response.

and more vigorous the feeding, the more milk will be produced. Thus even twins can be successfully breastfed.

Prolactin allows for milk to be produced, but that milk has to move through the milk ducts to the nipple in order to reach the baby's mouth. The hormone responsible for this "let down" of milk is *oxytocin*. Like prolactin, oxytocin is produced by the pituitary gland and its production is dependent on the suckling stimulus at the beginning of a feeding (Figure 15.10). This response usually occurs within 10 to 30 seconds but can be significantly inhibited by stress, resulting in frustration on the part of both mother and baby. Finding a relaxed environment in which to breastfeed is therefore important. On the other hand, many women experience let down in response to other cues, such as breast fullness, hearing a baby cry, or even thinking about their infant.

What Are a Breastfeeding Woman's Nutrient Needs?

You might be surprised to learn that breastfeeding requires even more energy than pregnancy! This is because breast milk has to supply an adequate amount of all of the nutrients an infant needs to grow and develop.

Nutrient Recommendations for Breastfeeding Women

It is estimated that milk production requires about 700 to 800 kcal/day. It is generally recommended that lactating women consume 500 kcal/day above their prepregnancy energy needs. This additional energy is sufficient to support adequate milk production. The resulting energy deficit of 200 to 300 kcal/day will assist in the gradual loss of excess fat and body weight gained during pregnancy. It is critical that lactating women avoid severe energy restriction, as this practice can result in decreased milk production.

The weight loss that occurs during breastfeeding should be gradual, approximately one to four pounds per month. Both breastfeeding and participating in regular physical activity can assist with weight loss. Interestingly, some active women may lose too much weight during breastfeeding and must either increase their energy intake or reduce their activity level to maintain health.

Of the macronutrients, only protein needs are different from pregnancy requirements. An increase of 15 to 20 grams/day above pre-pregnancy requirements is recommended during lactation.

For the micronutrients, the needs of several vitamins and minerals increase over the requirements of pregnancy. These include vitamins A, C, E, riboflavin, vitamin B_{12}, biotin, and choline, and the minerals copper, chromium, manganese, iodine, selenium, and zinc. The requirement for folate during lactation is 500 µg/day, which is decreased from the 600 µg/day required during pregnancy; but this requirement is higher than pre-pregnancy needs (400 µg/day).

Requirements for iron decrease significantly during lactation. For lactating women, iron needs are a mere 9 mg/day compared with pregnant women at 27 mg/day and non-pregnant, non-lactating women at about 18 mg/day. This is because iron is not a significant component of breast milk, and in addition, breastfeeding usually suppresses menstruation for at least a few months, defraying iron losses.

Calcium is a significant component of breast milk; but, as in pregnancy, calcium absorption is enhanced during lactation, and urinary loss of calcium is decreased. In addition, some calcium appears to come from the demineralization of the mother's bones, and increased dietary calcium does not prevent this. Thus, the recommended intake for calcium for a lactating woman is unchanged from pregnancy; that is, 1,000 mg/day. Because of their own continuing growth, however, teen mothers who are breastfeeding should continue to consume 1300 mg/day. Typically, a woman's bone density returns to normal after lactation ends.

Do Breastfeeding Women Need Supplements?

If a breastfeeding woman increases her energy intake by 500 kcal/day above pre-pregnancy levels, and does so with nutrient-dense foods, her nutrient needs can usually be met without supplements. However, there is nothing wrong with taking a basic multivitamin for insurance, as long as it is not considered a substitute for proper nutrition. Lactating women should consume omega-3 fatty acids either in fish or supplements to support the infant's developing nervous system, and women who don't consume dairy products should monitor their calcium intake carefully.

Fluid Recommendations for Breastfeeding Women

Since extra fluid is expended with every feeding, lactating women need to consume about an extra quart (about one liter) of fluid per day. This extra fluid facilitates milk production and staves off dehydration. Many women report that, within a minute or two of beginning to nurse their baby, they become intensely thirsty. To prevent this thirst and achieve the recommended fluid intake, women are encouraged to drink a nutritious beverage (water, juice, milk, etc.) each time they nurse their baby. However, it is not good practice to drink hot beverages while nursing because accidental spills could burn the infant.

Recap: Lactation is the result of the coordinated effort of several hormones, including estrogen, progesterone, prolactin, and oxytocin. Breasts are prepared for lactation during pregnancy, and infant suckling provides the stimulus that sustains the production of prolactin and oxytocin needed to maintain the milk supply. It is recommended that lactating women consume an extra 500 kcal/day above pre-pregnancy energy intake, including increased protein, certain vitamins and minerals, and fluids. The requirements for folate and iron decrease from pregnancy levels, while the requirement for calcium remains the same.

Getting Real About Breastfeeding: Pros and Cons

Breastfeeding is the perfect way to provide the best food for a baby's first six months of life (UNICEF 2003). However, the technique does require patience and practice on the part of both mother and infant, and being taught by an experienced mother is important. For some women, illness, medication use, or other factors may make breastfeeding a difficult choice. The decision to breastfeed or use formula must be made independently by each family after careful consideration of all the factors that apply to their particular situation.

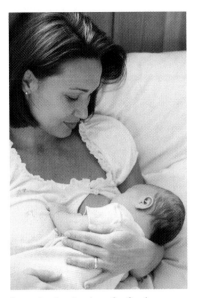

Breastfeeding has benefits for the mother and infant.

Advantages of Breastfeeding

As adept as formula manufacturers have been at simulating components of breast milk, an exact replica has never been produced. In addition, there are other benefits that mother and baby can access only through breastfeeding.

Nutritional Quality of Breast Milk   The main protein in breast milk, lactalbumin, is broken down easily in infants' immature GI tracts, and the whey-to-casein protein ratio in breast milk is more easily digested and absorbed than that of formula. Other proteins in breast milk bind iron and prevent the growth of harmful bacteria that require iron. Antibodies from the mother are additional proteins that help prevent infection while the infant's immune system is still immature. Cow's milk contains far too much protein for infant consumption.

The carbohydrate in milk is lactose, a disaccharide composed of glucose and galactose. The galactose component is important in nervous system development. Lactose provides energy and prevents ketosis in the infant, as well as promotes the growth of beneficial bacteria. It also aids in the absorption of calcium.

The fats in breast milk, especially DHA and arachidonic acid (ARA), have been shown to be essential for growth and development of the infant's nervous system and for development of the retina of the eyes. Until 2002, these fatty acids were omitted from commercial infant formulas in the United States, although they have been available in formulas in other parts of the world for the better part of a decade. Interestingly, the concentration of DHA in breast milk varies considerably, is sensitive to maternal diet, and is highest in women who consume large quantities of fish (Brenna 2003).

The fat content of breast milk changes according to the gestational age of the infant, providing a ratio of fatty acid types unique to the infant's needs. The fat content also changes during the course of every feeding: The milk that is initially released is watery and low in fat, somewhat like skim milk. This milk is thought to satisfy the infant's initial thirst. As the feeding progresses, the milk acquires more fat and becomes more like whole milk. Finally, the very last 5% or so of the milk produced during a feeding (called the *hindmilk*) is very high in fat, similar to cream. This milk is thought to satiate the infant. It is important to let infants suckle for at least twenty minutes at each feeding so that they get this hindmilk.

Another important aspect of breastfeeding (or any type of feeding) is the fluid it provides the infant. Because of their small size, infants are at risk of dehydration, which is one reason why feedings must be consistent and frequent. This topic will be discussed at greater length in the section on infant nutrition.

In terms of micronutrients, breast milk is a good source of calcium and magnesium. It is low in iron, but the iron it does contain is easily absorbed (recall that infants store iron in preparation for the first few months of life).

Breast milk composition continues to change as the infant grows and develops. Because of this ability to change as the baby changes, breast milk alone is entirely sufficient to sustain infant growth for the first six months of life. Throughout the next six months of infancy, as solid foods are gradually introduced, breast milk remains the baby's primary source of superior-quality nutrition. The World Health Organization

(1995) recommends continuing breastfeeding until at least age two, to maintain optimal nutrition of the growing toddler.

Protection from Infections and Allergies

Immune factors from the mother, including antibodies and immune cells, are passed directly from the mother to the newborn through breast milk. These factors provide important disease protection for the infant while its immune system is still immature. It has been shown that breastfed infants have a lower incidence of respiratory tract, GI tract, and urinary tract infections than formula-fed infants. Even a few weeks of breastfeeding is beneficial, but the longer a child is breastfed, the greater the level of passive immunity from the mother. A report from the United Nations Children's Fund estimates that, in part because of this immunologic protection, if every baby were exclusively breastfed from birth for six months, 1.3 million lives would be saved (UNICEF 2003).

In addition, breast milk is non-allergenic, and breastfeeding is associated with a reduced risk of allergies during childhood and adulthood. Breastfed babies also have fewer ear infections, die less frequently from **sudden infant death syndrome (SIDS),** and have a decreased chance of developing diabetes and chronic digestive disorders. SIDs refers to the sudden death of a previously healthy infant.

Physiologic Benefits for Mother

Breastfeeding causes uterine contractions that quicken the return of the uterus to pre-pregnancy size and reduce bleeding. Many women also find that breastfeeding helps them lose the weight they gained during pregnancy, particularly if it continues for more than six months. In addition, breastfeeding appears to be associated with a decreased risk for breast cancer (Salih and Fentiman 2001). The relationship between breastfeeding and osteoporosis is still unclear, and more research on this topic is needed (Grimes and Wimalawansa 2003).

Breastfeeding also suppresses **ovulation,** lengthening the time between pregnancies and giving a mother's body the chance to recover before she conceives again. This benefit can be life-saving for malnourished women living in countries that discourage or outlaw the use of contraceptives. Ovulation may not cease completely, however, so it is still possible to become pregnant while breastfeeding. Healthcare providers typically recommend use of additional birth control methods while breastfeeding to avoid another conception occurring too soon to allow a mother's body to recover from the earlier pregnancy. See the accompanying Highlight box to learn more about encouraging breastfeeding in developing nations.

Mother-Infant Bonding

Breastfeeding is among the most intimate of human interactions. Ideally, it is a quiet time away from distractions when mother and baby begin to develop an enduring bond of affection known as *attachment*. Breastfeeding enhances attachment by providing the opportunity for frequent, direct skin-to-skin contact, which stimulates the baby's sense of touch and is a primary means of communication (Olds et al. 2003). The cuddling and intense watching that occur during breastfeeding begin to teach the mother and baby about the other's behavioral cues. Breastfeeding also reassures the mother that she is providing the best possible nutrition for her baby.

Undoubtedly, bottle-feeding does not preclude parent-infant attachment! As long as attention is paid to closeness, cuddling, and skin contact, bottle-feeding can foster bonding as well.

Convenience and Cost

Breast milk is always ready, clean, at the right temperature, and available on demand, whenever and wherever it's needed. In the middle of the night, when the baby wakes up hungry, a breastfeeding mother can respond almost instantaneously, and both are soon back to sleep. In contrast, formula-feeding is a time-consuming process: parents have to continually wash and sterilize bottles, and each batch of formula must be mixed and heated to the proper temperature.

Global Nutrition: Encouraging Breastfeeding in the Developing World

In the United States and other industrialized nations, the benefits of breastfeeding include its precise correspondence to the infant's nutritional needs, protection of the infant from infections and allergies, promotion of mother-infant bonding, low cost, and convenience. In developing countries, however, breastfeeding may also save the newborn's or mother's life. Here are some reasons why.

It is estimated that a quarter of the earth's population may lack sanitary drinking water. breastfeeding protects newborns from contaminated water supplies. The least expensive form of infant formula is a packaged powder that must be carefully measured and mixed with a precise quantity of sterilized water. If the water is not sterilized and is contaminated with disease-causing organisms, the baby will become ill. A baby who is fed formula instead of breast milk receives none of the mother's beneficial antibodies; this means that when formula-fed infants do contract an infection, whether from contaminated water or another source, they are not as well-prepared to fight it off as breastfed infants would be. Many studies indicate that, for these reasons, a nonbreastfed child living in disease-ridden and unhygienic conditions is between 6 and 25 times more likely to die of diarrhea and 4 times more likely to die of pneumonia than breastfed infants living in the same region (UNICEF 2003).

In addition, in an attempt to make their supply of formula last longer, many impoverished parents add more water than the amount specified by the manufacturer. In this case, even when the water is sterilized, the child is at risk of malnutrition because the nutrients in the formula are being diluted (Elliot 2003; Reuters 2000).

These factors explain why breastfeeding is protective of the infant, but why does it help the mother? First, breastfeeding stimulates the uterus to contract vigorously after childbirth. This reduces the woman's risk of prolonged or excessive postpartum bleeding, a common cause of death in developing nations. Second, breastfeeding reduces a woman's risk of developing ovarian and breast cancer. Third, as mentioned earlier, breastfeeding is a natural form of birth control. While her infant is exclusively breastfeeding, a mother is rarely fertile because frequent breastfeeding suppresses ovulation. In regions where access to contraceptives may be lacking, breastfeeding can help women to space births, giving their bodies a chance to fully recover from the physical and metabolic changes of pregnancy, and to nourish their baby adequately without also having to support the development of a growing fetus.

The human immunodeficiency virus (HIV), which causes AIDS, can be transmitted from mother to child via breast milk. For this reason, in areas with sanitary water supplies, women with HIV or AIDS are routinely counseled against breastfeeding. In contrast, in regions where the risk of infant death from infectious disease is high, mothers are counseled about the risks, benefits, and costs of all infant-feeding options. They are then encouraged to make an informed but independent feeding choice (Jackson et al. 2003; UNICEF 2003).

For these reasons, international organizations like the World Health Organization and UNICEF encourage all HIV-negative women to breastfeed exclusively until their baby is six months of age and to continue supplemented breastfeeding until at least the age of two. ●

In addition, breastfeeding costs nothing other than the price of a modest amount of additional food for the mother. In contrast, formula can be relatively expensive, and there are the additional costs of bottles and other supplies, as well as the cost of energy used for washing and sterilization.

A hidden cost of formula-feeding is its effect on the environment. Consider the energy used and waste produced during formula manufacturing, marketing, shipping and distribution, preparation, and disposal of used packaging. In contrast, breastfeeding is environmentally responsible, using no external energy and producing no external wastes.

Difficulties Encountered with Breastfeeding

For some women and infants, breastfeeding is easy from the very first day. Others experience some initial difficulty due to mechanical factors, such as incorrect positioning or poor sucking technique, either of which can cause soreness or cracked nipples. With teaching from an experienced nurse, lactation consultant, or volunteer mother from La Leche League, these women are usually able to correct such problems, and the experience becomes mutually pleasurable. In contrast, some families encounter difficulties that make formula-feeding their best choice. This section discusses some roadblocks that may impede the success of breastfeeding.

Effects of Drugs and Other Substances on Breast Milk   Many substances make their way into breast milk. Among them are illegal and prescription drugs, over-the-counter drugs, and even substances from foods the mother eats. All illegal drugs should be assumed to pass into breast milk and should be avoided by breastfeeding mothers. Prescription drugs vary in the degree to which they pass into breast milk. Breastfeeding mothers should inform their physician that they are breastfeeding. Many drugs can be taken safely while lactating. If a safe and effective form of the necessary medication cannot be found, however, the mother will have to avoid breastfeeding while she is taking the drug. During this time, she can pump and discard her breast milk so that her milk supply will be adequate when she resumes breastfeeding. Similarly, a physician should be consulted before taking any over-the-counter medications.

Caffeine and alcohol do enter breast milk. Caffeine can make the baby agitated and fussy, whereas alcohol can make the baby sleepy, depress the central nervous system, and slow motor development, in addition to inhibiting the mother's milk supply. During the initial stages when breastfeeding takes place nearly around the clock, intake of either caffeine or alcohol is not recommended. When feedings become less frequent, an occasional cup of coffee or glass of wine is considered safe, as long as there is sufficient time before the next feeding to allow the substance to clear from the breast milk.

Nicotine also passes into breast milk; therefore, it is best for the woman to quit smoking altogether. A recent study showed that smoking can impair fetal growth and impair bioavailability of various nutrients (Berlanga et al. 2002).

Foods that pass into the breast milk may seem innocuous; however, some substances that the mother eats, such as garlic, onions, peppers, broccoli, and cabbage, are distasteful enough to the infant to prevent proper feeding. Many babies have allergic reactions to things the mother ate, such as wheat, cow's milk, eggs, or citrus, and suffer GI upset, diaper rash, or another reaction. The offending foods must then be identified and avoided.

Maternal HIV Infection   HIV, which causes AIDS, can be transmitted from mother to baby through breast milk. Thus, HIV-positive women in the United States and Canada are encouraged to feed their infants formula (Jackson et al. 2003). This recommendation does not apply to all women worldwide, as is discussed in the Highlight box on page 559.

Conflict Between Breastfeeding and the Mother's Employment   Breast milk is absorbed more readily than formula, making more frequent feedings necessary. Newborns commonly require breastfeedings every one to three hours versus every two to four hours for formula feedings. After the first month, the infant's digestive system matures and the feedings become slightly less frequent. Nevertheless, mothers who are exclusively breastfeeding and return to work within the first six months after the baby's birth must leave several bottles of pumped breast milk for others to use in their absence each day. This means that, to keep up their milk supply, working women have to pump their breasts to express the breast milk during the work day. This can be a challenge in companies that do not provide the time, space, and privacy required. In addition, many in society do not feel it is appropriate for women to breastfeed in public places. Societal pressures against breastfeeding have led many community leaders and politicians who understand the importance of breastfeeding to introduce worksite policies and legislation that supports breastfeeding in public and to support working mothers who are breastfeeding. Refer to the Nutrition Debate at the end of this chapter to learn more about breastfeeding legislation.

In addition, night feedings become unnecessary for formula-fed infants several weeks or even months before breastfed infants sleep through the night. This means that working mothers get less rest than formula-feeding mothers, and sleep deprivation—if severe and ongoing—may impair their performance at work.

Work travel is also a concern: if the mother needs to be away from home for longer than 24 to 48 hours, she can typically pump and freeze enough breast milk for others to give the baby in her absence. When longer business trips are required, some mothers bring the baby with them and arrange for childcare at their destination. Others resort to pumping, freezing, and shipping breast milk home via overnight mail. Understandably, many women cite returning to work as the reason they switch to formula-feeding (Adams et al. 2001).

Some working women successfully combine breastfeeding with commercial formula. For example, a woman might breastfeed in the morning before she leaves for work, as soon as she returns home, and once again before retiring at night. The remainder of the feedings are formula given by the infant's father or a childcare provider. Women who choose supplemental formula feedings usually find that their bodies adapt quickly to the change and produce ample milk for the remaining breastfeedings.

Social Concerns   In North America, women have been conditioned to keep their breasts covered in public even when feeding an infant. For some women, this conditioning can be a significant barrier to breastfeeding. However, public places are beginning to be more accommodating for nursing mothers. For example, separate nursing rooms can often be found adjacent to public restrooms. Some states have passed legislation preserving a woman's right to breastfeed in public (see the Nutrition Debate at the end of this chapter). Special nursing clothing or judicious placement of a scarf or shawl allows women to breastfeed discreetly. When women feel free to breastfeed in public, the baby's feeding schedule becomes much less confining.

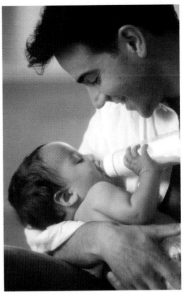

Fathers and siblings can bond with infants through bottle-feeding.

What About Bonding for Fathers and Siblings?

With all the attention given to attachment between a breastfeeding mother and infant, it is easy for fathers and siblings to feel left out. One option that allows other family members to participate in infant feeding is to supplement breastfeedings with bottle-feedings of stored breast milk or formula. If a family decides to share infant feeding in this manner, bottle-feedings can begin as soon as breastfeeding has become well established. That way, the mother's milk supply will be established, and the infant will not become confused by the artificial nipple. A final option that works well for some families is to breastfeed for the first few months, and then switch entirely to formula. There are many formulas from which to choose, including formulas based on modified cow's milk, formulas based on soy, formulas that are lactose-free, and others.

> **Recap:** Breastfeeding provides many benefits to both mother and newborn, including superior nutrition, heightened immunity, mother-infant bonding, convenience, and cost. However, breastfeeding may not be the best option for every family. The mother may need to use a medication that enters the breast milk and makes it unsafe for consumption. She may be HIV-positive. Or her job may interfere with the baby's requirement for frequent feedings. The infant's father and siblings can participate in feedings using a bottle filled with either pumped breast milk or formula.

Theo   *Nutri-Case*

"I'm only 19, but my mom is already after me and my girlfriend, Tina, to get married and have babies. In Nigeria, where my folks grew up, people marry a lot younger than here, and they have kids right away. Tina and I talk about it, but we both want to finish school first. Besides, we like to stay out late at the clubs, and who'd be home watching the kids?"

Considering what you've learned so far in this chapter, do you think there is any ideal age at which to have children? If so, what would that age be, and why? What practical information could you suggest Theo offer his mom to justify his decision to wait a few years before starting a family?

Infant Nutrition: From Birth to One Year

Most first-time parents are amazed at how rapidly their infant grows. Optimal nutrition is extremely important during the first year, as the baby's organs and nervous system continue to develop and mature and as the baby grows physically and acquires new skills. In fact, physicians use length and weight measurements as the main tools for assessing an infant's nutritional status. These measurements are plotted on growth charts (there are separate charts for boys and girls), which track an infant's growth over time (Figure 15.11). Although every infant is unique, in general, physicians look for a correlation between length and weight. In other words, an infant who is in the sixtieth percentile for length is usually in about the fiftieth to seventieth percentile for

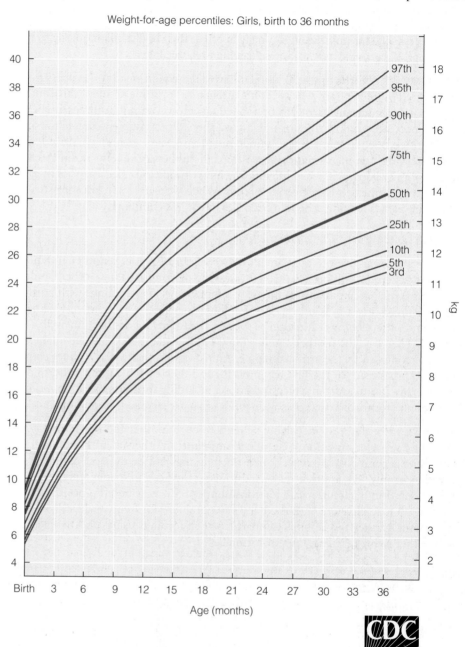

Weight-for-age percentiles: Girls, birth to 36 months

Figure 15.11   This weight-for-age growth chart is a much smaller version of charts used by health care practitioners to monitor and assess the growth of an infant/toddler from birth to 36 months. This example shows the growth curves of girls over time, each at different percentiles. (Developed by the National Center for Health Statistics in collaboration with the National Center for Chronic Disease Prevention and Health Promotion [2000].)

weight. An infant who is in the ninetieth percentile for weight but is in the twentieth percentile for length might be overfed. Consistency over time is also a consideration: for example, an infant who suddenly drops well below her established profile for weight might be underfed or ill.

Typical Infant Growth and Activity Patterns

Babies' basal metabolic rates are high, in part because their body surface area is large compared to their body size. Still, their limited physical activity keeps total energy expenditure relatively low. For the first few months of life, an infant's activities consist mainly of eating and sleeping. As the first year progresses, the repertoire of activity gradually expands to include rolling over, sitting up, crawling, standing, and finally taking the first few wobbly steps. Nevertheless, relatively few calories are expended in movement, and the primary use of energy during the first year of life is to support growth.

In the first year of life, an infant generally grows about 10 inches in length and triples in weight—a growth rate more rapid than will ever occur again. Not surprisingly, energy needs per unit body weight are also the highest they will ever be in order to support this phenomenal growth and metabolism.

Part of the rapid growth of an infant involves the brain, the growth of which is more rapid during the first year than at any other time. To accommodate such a large increase in brain size, infants' heads are typically quite large in proportion to the rest of their bodies. Pediatricians use head circumference as an additional tool for the assessment of growth and nutritional status. After around eighteen months of age, the rate of brain growth slows, and gradually the body "catches up" to head size.

An infant's physical activity will progress beyond crawling before the first year of life is over.

Nutrient Needs for Infants

Three characteristics of infants combine to make their nutritional needs unique. These are: 1) their high energy needs per unit body weight to support rapid growth; 2) their immature digestive tracts and kidneys; and 3) their small size.

Macronutrient Needs of Infants

An infant needs to consume about 50 kcal/pound of body weight per day. This amounts to about 700 kcal/day at around 6 months of age. Given infants' immature digestive tracts and kidneys, as well as their high fluid needs, providing this much energy may seem difficult. Fortunately, breast milk and commercial formulas are energy-dense, contributing about 650 kcal/quart of fluid. When solid foods are introduced after about four to six months of age, they provide even more energy in addition to the breast milk or formula.

Infants are not merely small versions of adults. The proportions of macronutrients they require differ from adult proportions, as do the types of food they can tolerate. It is generally agreed that about 40 to 50% of an infant's diet should come from fat during the first year of life and that fat intake below this level can be harmful before the age of two. Given the high energy needs of infants just discussed, it makes sense to take advantage of the energy density of fat (9 kcal/gram) to help meet these requirements. Breast milk and commercial formulas are both high in fat (about 50% of total energy). In addition to being a dense source of energy, fats are essential for the rapid brain growth and nervous system development that happens in the first one to two years of life.

No more than 20% of an infant's daily energy requirement should come from protein. This is plenty to accommodate an infant's rapid growth. Immature infant kidneys are not able to process and excrete the excess amine groups from higher-protein diets. Breast milk and commercial formulas both provide adequate overall protein and appropriate essential amino acids to support growth and development.

Micronutrient Needs of Infants

An infant's micronutrient needs are also high to accommodate their rapid growth and development. Micronutrients of particular note include iron, vitamin D, zinc, and iodide. Fortunately, breast milk and commercial formulas provide most of the micronutrients needed for infant growth and development, with some special considerations discussed later in this chapter.

In addition, all infants are routinely given an injection of vitamin K shortly after birth. This provides vitamin K until the infant's intestine can develop its own healthful bacteria, which provide vitamin K thereafter.

Do Infants Need Supplements?

Breast milk and commercial formulas provide most of the vitamins and minerals infants need. However, there are several micronutrients that may warrant supplementation. For breastfed infants, a supplement containing vitamin D is commonly prescribed from birth to around six months of age. Breastfed infants also require additional iron beginning no later than six months of age because the infant's iron stores become depleted and breast milk is a poor source of iron. Iron is extremely important for cognitive development and prevention of iron-deficiency anemia. Starting solid foods (baby cereal) fortified with iron at four to six months of age can also serve as an additional iron source. Fluoride is important for strong tooth development, but fluoride supplementation is not recommended during the first six months of life.

For formula-fed infants, supplementation depends on the formula composition and the water supply used to make the formula. Many formulas are already fortified with iron, for example, and some municipal water supplies contain fluoride. If this is the case, and the baby is getting adequate vitamin D either in the formula or via sun exposure, then an extra supplement may not be necessary.

There are also special conditions in which additional supplements may be wise. For example, if a woman is a vegan, her breast milk may be low in vitamin B_{12}, and a supplement of this vitamin should be given to the baby. Vitamin D supplements may also be necessary for babies who do not get adequate sun exposure.

If a supplement is given, careful consideration should be given to dose. The supplement should be formulated specifically for infants, and the daily dose should not be exceeded. High doses of micronutrients can be dangerous. Too much iron can be fatal, as accidental iron poisoning is the leading cause of death in children under 6 years of age in the U.S. (FDA 1997).

Fluid Recommendations for Infants

Fluid is critical for everyone, but for infants the balance is more delicate for two reasons. First, because infants are so small, they proportionally lose more water through evaporation than adults. Second, their kidneys are immature and unable to concentrate urine. Hence, they are at even greater risk of dehydration. An infant needs about 2 ounces of fluid per pound of body weight, and either breast milk or formula is usually enough to provide this amount. However, there are certain conditions, such as diarrhea, vomiting, fever, or hot weather, which can exacerbate fluid loss. In these instances, supplemental fluid may be warranted. However, too much fluid can also be particularly dangerous for an infant. Thus, supplemental fluids (whether water or an infant electrolyte formula) should be given judiciously and under the advice of a physician. Generally, it is advised that supplemental fluids not exceed 4 ounces per day. A guide for parents to determine whether fluid intake is appropriate is to look for six to eight wet diapers per day.

What Types of Formula Are Available?

We discussed the advantages of breastfeeding earlier in this chapter, and indeed both national and international healthcare organizations consider breastfeeding the best choice for infant nutrition, when possible. However, if breastfeeding is not feasible, several types of commercial formulas provide nutritious alternatives.

Most formulas are based on altered cow's milk proteins, casein and whey, which have been heated to denature them. The sugars lactose and sucrose, alone or in combination, provide carbohydrates, and vegetable oils or microbiologically produced fatty acids provide the fat component (Uauy and Mena 1999).

Soy-based formulas are a viable alternative for infants who are lactose intolerant (although this is rare in infants) or cannot tolerate the proteins in cow's milk-based formulas. Soy formulas may also satisfy the requirements of families who are strict vegans. However, soy-based formulas are not without controversy. Because soy contains isoflavones, or plant forms of estrogens, there is some concern over the effects these compounds have on growing infants. Currently it is believed that soy formulas are safe, but they should only be used when breast milk or cow's milk-based formulas are contraindicated. Babies can also have allergic reactions to soy based formulas (American Academy of Pediatrics 2000). Soy-based formulas are not the same as soy milk, which is not suitable for infant feeding.

Finally, there are specialized formula preparations for specific conditions. Some contain proteins that have been predigested, for example, or have compositions designed to accommodate certain medical conditions. Some have been specially formulated for older infants and toddlers. The final choice of formula depends on cost, infant tolerance, stage of infant development, and the advice of the infant's pediatrician.

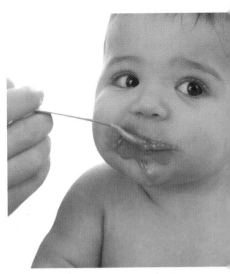

The suckling reflex will push solid food out of an infant's mouth.

When Do Infants Begin to Need Solid Foods?

Infants begin to need solid foods at around four to six months of age. Before this age, most infants are not physically able to consume solid food. The suckling response depends on a particular movement of the tongue that draws liquid out of breast or bottle. In response to solid foods introduced with a spoon, this tongue movement merely results in pushing most of the food back out of the mouth. Not only must the tongue's extrusion reflex begin to abate, but the infant must have gained muscular control of the head and neck and must be able to sit up (with or without support).

Another part of being ready for solid foods is sufficient maturity of the digestive system, so that it can digest and absorb nutrients from solid food. If an infant is fed solid foods too soon, nutrient molecules (particularly proteins) can be absorbed intact and undigested, setting the stage for allergies. In addition, the kidneys must have matured so that they are better able to process proteins and concentrate urine.

Finally, the nutritional need for foods besides breast milk or formula becomes evident at about six months of age, when infant iron stores become depleted. Typically the first foods introduced are iron-fortified infant cereals, starting with rice, which rarely provokes an allergic response and is easy to digest. Once a child reaches six months of age, other grains, strained vegetables, fruits, and protein sources can gradually be incorporated into the diet.

Infant foods should be introduced one at a time, with no other new foods for a week, so that allergies can be watched for. Gradually, a repertoire including a variety of foods should be built by the end of the first year. Throughout the first year, solid foods should only be a supplement to, not a substitute for, breast milk or formula. Infants still need the nutrient density and energy that breast milk and formula provide. Notice that it is not safe for infants to consume regular cow's milk.

What *Not* to Feed an Infant

The following foods should never be offered to an infant:

- *Foods that could cause choking.* Foods such as grapes, hot dogs, nuts, popcorn, raw carrots, raisins, and hard candies cannot be chewed adequately by infants and can cause choking.
- *Corn syrup and honey.* These may contain spores of the bacterium *Clostridium botulinum.* These spores can germinate and grow into viable bacteria in the immature digestive tracts of infants, whereupon they produce a potent toxin that can be fatal. Children older than one year can safely consume these substances because their digestive tracts are mature enough to kill any *C. botulinum* bacteria.

- *Goat's milk.* Goat's milk is notoriously low in many nutrients that infants need, such as folate, vitamin C, vitamin D, and iron.

- *Cow's milk.* For children under one year, cow's milk is too concentrated in minerals and protein and contains too few carbohydrates to meet infant energy needs. Infants can begin to consume whole cow's milk after the age of one year. Infants and toddlers should not be given reduced-fat cow's milk before the age of two, as it does not contain enough fat and is too high in mineral content for the kidneys to handle effectively. Infants should not be given evaporated milk or sweetened condensed milk.

- *Large quantities of fruit juices.* Fruit juices are poorly absorbed in the infant digestive tract, causing diarrhea if consumed in excess. Large quantities of fruit juice can make an infant feel full and reject breast milk or formula at feeding time, thus causing him or her to miss out on essential nutrients. It is considered safe for infants older than 6 months to consume 4 to 8 ounces of pure fruit juice (no sweeteners added) per day, with no more than 2 to 4 ounces given at a time; however, plain water will quench an infant's thirst. Diluting fruit juice with water is another option.

- *Too much salt and sugar.* Infant foods should not be seasoned with salt or other seasonings. Naturally-occurring sugars such as those found in fruits can provide needed energy. Cookies, cakes, and other excessively sweet, processed foods should be avoided.

- *Too much breast milk or formula.* As nutritious as breast milk and/or formula are, once infants reach the age of six months, solid foods should be introduced gradually. Six months of age is a critical time, as it is when a baby's iron stores begin to be depleted and must be replenished with iron from enriched rice cereal. In addition, infants are physically and psychologically ready to incorporate solid foods at this time, and solid foods can help appease their increasing appetites. Between six months and the time of weaning (from breast or bottle), solid foods should gradually make up an increasing proportion of the infant's diet.

Nutrition-Related Concerns for Infants

Nutrition is one of the biggest concerns of new parents. Infants cannot speak, and their cries are sometimes indecipherable. Feeding time can be very frustrating for parents, especially if the child is not eating, not growing appropriately, or has problems like diarrhea, vomiting, or persistent skin rashes. Below are some nutrition-related concerns for infants.

Allergies

Many foods have the potential to stimulate an allergic reaction (see pages 104–105). Breastfeeding helps deter allergy development, as does delaying introduction of solid foods until the age of six months. One of the most common allergies in infants is to the proteins in cow's milk-based formulas. Some of these proteins are denatured with heat during the production process, but others remain intact. Symptoms include those of gastrointestinal distress such as diarrhea, constipation, bloating, blood in the stool, and vomiting. In such cases, an alternative such as soy-based formula or a formula with predigested proteins may be used (the potential to develop allergies to the proteins in soy also exists, however).

As stated above, every food should be introduced in isolation, so that any allergic reaction can be spotted and attributed to a particular food which can then be avoided.

Dehydration

Whether the cause is diarrhea, vomiting, or inadequate fluid intake, dehydration is extremely dangerous to infants, and if left untreated can quickly result in death. The factors behind infants' increased risk of dehydration were discussed on pages 239–241.

Treatment includes providing fluids, a task that is difficult if vomiting is occurring. In some cases, the physician may recommend that a pediatric electrolyte solution be administered on a temporary basis. In more severe cases, hospitalization may be necessary. If possible, breastfeeding should continue throughout an illness. A physician should be consulted concerning formula feeding and solid foods.

Colic

Perhaps nothing is more frustrating to new parents than the relentless crying spells of some infants, typically referred to as **colic.** In this condition, newborns and young infants who appear happy, healthy, and well-nourished suddenly begin to cry or even shriek, and continue no matter what their caregiver does to console them. The spells tend to occur at the same time of day, typically late in the afternoon or early in the evening, and often occur daily for a period of several weeks. Crying lasts for hours at a time. Overstimulation of the nervous system, feeding too rapidly, swallowing of air, and intestinal gas pain are considered possible culprits, but the precise cause is unknown.

As with allergies, if a colicky infant is breastfed, breastfeeding should be continued, but the mother should try to determine whether eating certain foods seems to prompt crying and, if so, eliminate the offending food(s) from her diet. Avoidance of spicy or other strongly flavored foods may also help. Formula-fed infants may benefit from a change in type of formula. In the worst cases of colic, a physician may prescribe medication. Fortunately, most cases disappear spontaneously, possibly because of maturity of the GI tract, around three months of age.

Anemia

As stated earlier, infants are born with sufficient iron stores to last for approximately the first six months of life. In older infants and toddlers, however, iron is the mineral most likely to be deficient. Iron-deficiency anemia causes pallor, lethargy, and impaired growth. Iron-fortified formula is a good source for formula-fed infants. Some pediatricians prescribe a supplement containing iron especially formulated for infants. Iron for older infants is typically supplied by iron-fortified rice cereal.

Nursing Bottle Syndrome

Infants should never be left alone with a bottle, whether lying down or sitting up. As infants manipulate the nipple of the bottle in their mouths, the high-carbohydrate fluid (whether breast milk, formula, or fruit juice) drips out, coming into prolonged contact with the developing teeth. This high-carbohydrate fluid provides an optimal food source for bacteria that are the underlying cause of **dental caries** (cavities), which are defined as dental erosion and decay caused by acid-secreting bacteria in the mouth and on the teeth. Severe tooth decay can result (Figure 15.12). Encouraging the use of a cup around the age of eight months helps prevent nursing bottle syndrome, along with weaning the baby from a bottle entirely by the age of eighteen months.

Preterm Infants

What a preterm infant is fed depends on his or her gestational age, weight, and state of health. Sometimes a preterm infant can be fed breast milk, but often the milk must be pumped first and fed to the infant through a tube. Sometimes, depending on the condition of the infant, breast milk can be fortified with vitamins, minerals, or protein to meet the growth needs of the infant. Sometimes the immaturity of the infant's GI tract precludes breast milk or formula-feeding entirely and nutrition via an intravenous tube is necessary.

Lead Poisoning

Lead is especially toxic to infants and children because their brains and central nervous systems are still developing. Lead poisoning can result in decreased mental

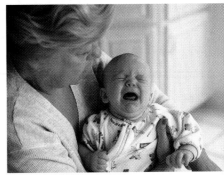

Colicky babies will begin crying for no apparent reason even if they otherwise appear well-nourished and happy.

colic Inconsolable infant crying that lasts for hours at a time.

dental caries Dental erosion and decay caused by acid-secreting bacteria in the mouth and on the teeth. The acid produced is a by-product of bacterial metabolism of carbohydrates deposited on the teeth.

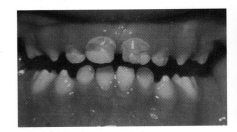

Figure 15.12 Leaving a baby alone with a bottle can result in the tooth decay of nursing bottle syndrome.

capacity, behavioral problems, impaired growth, impaired hearing, and other problems. Laws have been passed in recent decades to decrease lead exposure for everyone, including introducing unleaded gasoline, eliminating lead solder, and outlawing the use of lead-based paint. Unfortunately, lead in old pipes can still leach into a home's water supply, and lead paint can still be found in older homes and buildings. If the paint in an older home is flaking and peeling, an infant or toddler may easily pop these flakes into their mouths (as they do everything else). Measures to reduce lead exposure include:

- Allowing tap water to run for a minute or so before use, to clear the pipes of any lead-contaminated water that may have leached from solder.
- Using only cold tap water for drinking and cooking, as hot tap water is more likely to leach lead.
- Professionally removing lead-based paint, painting it over with latex paint, or at least removing paint flakes and dust.

Recap: Infancy is characterized by the most rapid growth a human being will ever experience. Infants need large amounts of energy per unit body weight to keep up with growth, but because they cannot consume large amounts of food, nutrient levels per kilocalorie must be high. Breast milk or formula provides necessary nutrients for the first 4 to 6 months of life. Solid foods can gradually be introduced into an infant's diet thereafter. A supplement containing iron and fluoride may be prescribed after age six months. Infants must be monitored for allergies, dehydration, and other signs of distress. Growth is the most reliable longitudinal assessment of infant nutrition.

Chapter Summary

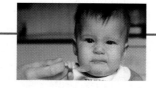

- Nutrition is important before conception because critical stages of cell division, tissue differentiation, and organ development occur in the early weeks of pregnancy, often before a woman even knows she is pregnant.
- A plentiful, nourishing diet is important throughout pregnancy to provide the nutrients needed to support fetal development without depriving the mother of nutrients she needs to maintain her own health.
- A normal pregnancy progresses over the course of 38 to 42 weeks. This time is divided into three trimesters of 13 to 14 weeks. Each trimester is associated with particular developmental phases of the embryo/fetus.
- Pregnant women of normal weight should consume adequate energy to gain 25 to 35 lbs. during pregnancy. Women who are underweight should gain slightly more, and women who are overweight or obese should gain less.
- Pregnant women need to be especially careful to consume adequate amounts of folate, vitamin B_{12}, vitamin C, vitamin D, calcium, iron, and zinc. A supplement is often prescribed to ensure adequate intake of these nutrients.
- A majority of pregnant women experience nausea and/or vomiting during pregnancy, called morning sickness, and many crave or feel aversions to specific types of foods and nonfood substances.
- Heartburn and constipation in pregnancy are related to the relaxation of smooth muscle caused by certain pregnancy-related hormones.
- Gestational diabetes and preeclampsia are nutrition-related disorders that can seriously affect maternal and fetal health.
- Adolescents' bodies are still growing and developing; thus, their nutrient needs during pregnancy are higher than those of older pregnant women.
- Dieting during pregnancy leads to inadequate nutrition for mother and fetus.
- Alcohol is a teratogen and should not be consumed in any amount during pregnancy.
- Successful breastfeeding requires the coordination of several hormones, including estrogen, progesterone, prolactin, and oxytocin. These hormones govern the preparation of the breasts, as well as actual milk production and the let down response.
- Breastfeeding women require more energy than during pregnancy. Protein needs increase, and an overall nutritious diet with plentiful fluids is important in maintaining milk quality and quantity, as well as preserving the mother's health.

- The advantages of breastfeeding include nutritional superiority of breast milk, protection from infections and allergies, promotion of attachment, convenience, and lower cost.

- Breastfeeding exclusively for at least the first 4 to 6 months of a baby's life is recommended by both North American and international healthcare organizations.

- Difficulties that might be encountered with breastfeeding include effect of medications on breast milk, concerns related to transmission of HIV to a breastfeeding infant, scheduling conflicts for mothers who return to work, and social concerns.

- Infants are characterized by their extremely rapid growth and brain development.

- Physicians use length and weight measurements as the main tools for assessing an infant's nutritional status.

- An infant needs to consume about 50 kcal/pound of body weight/day.

- Since infant stores of iron become depleted after about six months, a supplement is sometimes prescribed for breastfeeding infants.

- Breast milk or formula is entirely sufficient for the first 4 to 6 months of life. After that, solid foods can be introduced (rice cereal fortified with iron at first) and expanded gradually, with breast milk or formula remaining very important throughout the first year.

- Infants need to be monitored carefully for appropriate growth and appropriate number of wet diapers every day to assess adequate nutrient intake and hydration.

- Nutrition-related concerns for infants include the potential for allergies, dehydration, colic, nursing bottle syndrome, and ingestion of lead.

Review Questions

1. Folate deficiency in the first weeks after conception has been linked with which of the following problems in the newborn?
   a. anemia
   b. neural tube defects
   c. low birth weight
   d. preterm delivery

2. Which of the following hormones is responsible for the let down response?
   a. progesterone
   b. estrogen
   c. oxytocin
   d. prolactin

3. Which of the following nutrients is essential to ensure in every newborn's diet?
   a. fiber
   b. fat
   c. iron
   d. vitamin D

4. A pregnancy weight gain of 28 to 40 pounds is recommended for

a. all women.
b. women who begin their pregnancy underweight.
c. women who begin their pregnancy overweight.
d. women who begin their pregnancy at a normal weight.

5. The best solid food to introduce first to infants is
   a. cream of wheat cereal.
   b. applesauce.
   c. teething biscuits.
   d. iron-fortified rice cereal.

6. **True or false?** Major developmental errors and birth defects are most likely to occur in the third trimester of pregnancy.

7. **True or false?** Infant suckling is a critical component of successful and continued lactation.

8. **True or false?** Growth is a key indicator of adequate infant nutrition.

9. **True or false?** Fetal alcohol effects can occur in children born to mothers who drink only two alcoholic beverages per day during pregnancy.

10. **True or false?** Most infants have a physiologic need for solid food by about four months of age.

11. Explain the relationship between the increased need for iron and the increased need for fluid in a pregnant woman.

12. Identify five advantages and five disadvantages of breastfeeding. Can you think of others?

13. Your cousin, who is pregnant with her first child, tells you that her physician prescribed supplemental iron tablets for her but that she decided not to take them. "You know me," she says, "I'm a natural food nut! I'm absolutely certain that my careful diet is providing all the nutrients my baby needs!" Is it possible that your cousin is partly right and partly wrong? Explain.

14. You visit your neighbors one afternoon to congratulate them on the birth of their new daughter, Katie. While you are there, two-week-old Katie suddenly starts crying as if she is in terrible pain. "Oh, no," Katie's dad says to his wife. "Here we go again!" He turns to you and explains, "She's been like this every afternoon for the past week, and it goes on until sunset. I just wish we could figure out what we're doing wrong." What would you say?

15. You are on a picnic with your sister at a park, who drapes a shawl over her shoulders and breastfeeds her fourteen-month-old son. A woman walking by stops and says, "Isn't that child getting too old for that?" What information could you share with her in response to her question?

Test Yourself Answers

1. **False.** Gaining too much weight might result in a large baby and difficult delivery, as well as difficulty in losing the weight after pregnancy. Gaining too little weight can result in a low-birth-weight baby, which increases the risk of various complications that can be life-threatening.

2. **False.** More than half of all pregnant women experience morning sickness, and food cravings or aversions are also common.

3. **True.** Breast milk contains various immune factors (antibodies and immune system cells) from the mother that protect the infant against infection. The nutrients in breast milk are structured to be easily digested by an infant, resulting in fewer symptoms of gastrointestinal distress and fewer allergies.

4. **True.** Physical growth, including length, weight, and head circumference, is the best indicator for assessing an infant's nutrition status.

5. **False.** Most infants do not have a physiologic need for solid food until about six months of age.

Web Links

http://aappolicy.aappublications.org
American Academy of Pediatrics
Visit this Web site for information on infants' and children's health. Searches can be performed for topics such as "neural tube defects" or "infant formulas."

www.nal.usda.gov/fnic
Food Nutrition Information Center
Click on Topics A–Z and then Child Nutrition and Health for a list of infant nutrition topics and a listing of child nutrition programs, links, and resources.

www.emedicine.com/ped
eMedicine: Pediatrics
Select "Toxicology" and then "Toxicity, Iron" to learn about accidental iron poisoning and its signs in children and infants.

www.marchofdimes.com/pnhec/pnhec.asp
March of Dimes
Click on Pregnancy & Newborn to find links on nutrition during pregnancy, breastfeeding, and baby care.

www.diabetes.org
American Diabetes Association
Search for "gestational diabetes" to find information about diabetes that develops during pregnancy.

www.lalecheleague.org
La Leche League
Search this site to find multiple articles on the health effects of breastfeeding for mother and infant.

www.obgyn.net
OBGYN.net
Visit this site to learn about pregnancy health and nutrition, as well as breastfeeding and infant nutrition.

www.nofas.org
National Organization on Fetal Alcohol Syndrome
This site provides news and information relating to fetal alcohol syndrome.

References

Abbott Laboratories. 2003. New data show US breastfeeding rates at all-time recorded high. www.obgyn.net/ newsheadlines/womens-health-Breastfeeding-20031225-11.asp (Accessed January 2004.)

Adams, C., R. Berger, P. Conning, L. Cruikshank, and K. Dore. 2001. Breastfeeding trends at a community breastfeeding center: An evaluative survey. *Journal of Obstetric, Gynecologic, and Neonatal Nursing* 30(4): 392–400.

American Academy of Pediatrics, Policy Statement, Committee on Nutrition. 2000. Hypoallergenic Infant Formulas (RE0005).
http://www.aap.org/policy/re0005.html

Baldwin, E. N., and K. A. Friedman. 2004. A current summary of breastfeeding legislation in the U.S. La Leche League International. http://www.lalecheleague. org/Law/Bills4.html (Accessed April 2004.)

Barnet, B., A. K. Duggan, and M. Devoe. 2003. Reduced low birth weight for teenagers receiving prenatal care at a school-based health center: effect of access and comprehensive care. *J. Adolesc. Health* 33(5): 349–358.

Benyshek, D. C., J. F. Martin, and C. S. Johnston. 2001. A reconsideration of the origins of type 2 diabetes epidemic among Native Americans and the implications for intervention policy. *Med. Anthropol.* 20(1): 25–64.

Berlanga, M. R., G. Salazar, C. Garcia, and J. Hernandez. 2002. Maternal smoking effects on infant growth. *Food & Nutrition Bulletin* 23(3 Suppl): 142–145.

Brenna, J. T. 2003. Cornell Cooperative Extension, Ask the Nutrition Expert. Infant Formulas Containing DHA and ARA. http://cce.cornell.edu/food/ expfiles/topics/brenna/brennaoverview.html

Centers for Disease Control and Prevention (CDC). 2003. Folic Acid: Topic Home. http://www.cdc.gov. node.do/id/0900f3ec80010af 9 (Accessed April 2004.)

Cohen, R., M. B. Mrtek, and R. G. Mrtek. 1995. Comparison of maternal absenteeism and infant illness rates among breastfeeding and formula-feeding women in two corporations. *Am. J. Health Promotion* 10(2): 148–153.

Cross, N. A., L. S. Hillman, S. H. Allen, G. F. Krause, and N. E. Vieira. 1995. Calcium homeostasis and bone metabolism during pregnancy, lactation, and postweaning: A longitudinal study. *Am. J. Clin. Nutr.* 61: 514–523.

Dabelea, D., R. L. Hanson, P. H. Bennett, J. Roumain, W. C. Knowler, and D. J. Pettitt. 1998. Increasing prevalence of type 2 diabetes in American Indian children. *Diabetologia* 41: 904–910.

Davidsson, L., A. Almgren, B. Sandstrom, and R. F. Hurrell. 1995. Zinc absorption in adult humans. The effect of iron fortification. *Br. J. Nutr.* 74: 417–425.

Elliot, J. 2003. Breastfeeding could save lives. BBC News, http://news.bbc.co.uk/1/hi/health/2973845.stm

Grimes, J. P., and S. J. Wimalawansa. 2003. Breastfeeding and postmenopausal osteoporosis. *Current Women's Health Reports* 3(3): 193–198.

Harding, J. E. 2001. The nutritional basis of the fetal origins of adult disease. *Int. J. Epidemiol.* 30: 15–23.

Institute of Medicine, Food and Nutrition Board. 1997. *Dietary Reference Intakes for Calcium, Phosphorus, Magnesium, Vitamin D, and Fluoride.* Washington, DC: National Academy Press.

Institute of Medicine, Food and Nutrition Board. 1998. *Dietary Reference Intakes for Thiamin, Riboflavin, Niacin, Vitamin B_6, Folate, Vitamin B_{12}, Pantothenic Acid, Biotin, and Choline.* Washington, DC: National Academy Press.

Institute of Medicine, Food and Nutrition Board. 2004. *Dietary Reference for Water, Potassium, Sodium, Chloride, and Sulfate.* Washington, DC: National Academy Press.

Jackson, D. J., M. Chopra, C. Witten, and M. J. Sengwana. 2003. HIV and infant feeding: Issues in developed and developing countries. *Journal of Obstetric, Gynecologic, and Neonatal Nursing* 32(1): 117–127.

Li, R., C. Ogden, C. Ballew, C. Gillespie, and L. Grummer-Strawn. 2002. Prevalence of exclusive breastfeeding among US infants: The Third National Health and Nutrition Examination Survey (Phase II, 1991–1994). *Am. J. Public Health* 92(7): 1107–1110.

Lumbers, E. R. 2002. Exercise in pregnancy: physiological basis of exercise prescription for the pregnant woman. *J. Sci. Med. Sport* 5(1): 20–31.

March of Dimes. 2003a. Caffeine in Pregnancy. http://modimes.org/professionals/681_1148.asp (Accessed April 2004.)

March of Dimes. 2003b. Drinking Alcohol During Pregnancy. http://www.modimes.org/professionals/681_1170.asp (Accessed April 2004.)

Mitra, K., and M. K. Chowdhury. 2002. Maternal malnutrition, perinatal mortality and fetal pathology: A clinico-pathological study. *Journal of the Indian Medical Association,* February, 2002. http://www.jimaonline.org/Feb2002/report04.html (Accessed January 2004.)

Mostello, D., T. K. Catlin, L. Roman, W. L. Holcomb Jr., and T. Leet. 2002. Preeclampsia in the parous woman: Who is at risk? *Am. J. Obstet. Gynecol.* 187(2): 425–429.

Olds, S. B., M. L. London, P. W. Ladewig, and M. R. Davidson. 2003. *Maternal-Newborn Nursing and Women's Health Care,* 7th ed. Upper Saddle River, NJ: Prentice Hall Health.

Porter, D. V. 2003. breastfeeding: Impact on health, employment, and society. CRS Report for Congress. Congressional Research Service. The Library of Congress. http://www.breastfeeding.org/law/CRS1.pdf (Accessed April 2004.)

Reuters. 2000. Peers encourage third world women to breastfeed. http://www.durhamobgyn.com/viewArticle?ID=22184

Salih, A. K., and I. S. Fentiman. 2001. Breast cancer prevention: present and future. *Cancer Treatment Rev.* 27(5): 261–273.

Uauy, R., and P. Mena. 1999. Requirements for long-chain polyunsaturated fatty acids in the preterm infant. *Curr. Opin. Pediatr.* 11(2): 115–120.

UNICEF. 2003. Protecting, promoting and supporting breastfeeding. http://www.unicef.org/nutrition/index_breastfeeding.html (Accessed January 2004.)

UNICEF (United Nations Childrens' Fund). 2004. Maternal nutrition and low birth weight. http://www.unicef.org/nutrition/index_lowbirthweight.html (Accessed January 2004.)

U.S. Food and Drug Administration (FDA). 1997. Preventing Iron Poisoning in Children. FDA Backgrounder. http://www.fda.gov/opacom/backgrounders/ironbg.html (Accessed January 2004.)

von Dadelszen, P. 2000. The Etiology of Nausea and Vomiting in Pregnancy. In: First International Congress on NVP. http://www.nvp-volumes.org/index.htm (Accessed April 2004.)

Weimer, D. R. 2003. Summary of state breastfeeding laws. CRS Report for Congress. Congressional Research Service. The Library of Congress. http://www.breastfeeding.org/law/CRS2.pdf

Whittaker, P. 1998. Iron and zinc interactions in humans. *Am. J. Clin. Nutr.* 68: 442S–446S.

World Health Organization (WHO). 1995. The World Health Organization's infant-feeding recommendation. *Wkly. Epidemiol. Rec.* 70: 119–120.

Yeo, S., and S. T. Davidge. 2001. Possible beneficial effect of exercise, by reducing oxidative stress, on the incidence of preeclampsia. *J. Women's Health Gender-Based Med.* 10(10): 983–989.

Nutrition Debate:

Should Breastfeeding Be Allowed in Public and in the Workplace?

A woman sitting at the food court at the mall is openly breastfeeding. A colleague excuses herself from an important meeting to pump her breast milk in the restroom. How do you feel about these two scenarios? Do they make you uncomfortable? How do you feel about a woman being excused from jury duty because she is breastfeeding or a guard removing a woman from a public legislative session because she was breastfeeding her infant during the proceedings? Should maternity leave benefits be extended for women who are exclusively breastfeeding? Should a working woman be allowed paid break time to breastfeed or should this time away from her work be unpaid? What rights do you feel a breastfeeding mother should have?

The benefits of breastfeeding for infant health are well established. Leading national and international healthcare organizations such as the American Academy of Pediatrics, UNICEF, and the World Health Organization advocate breastfeeding exclusively for the first six months and breastfeeding with supplemental foods until age two to optimize the nutrition, growth, and overall health of the world's children. Despite these endorsements, many people in the United States support social and workplace restrictions on breastfeeding.

For example, some Americans feel that breastfeeding in public is indecent. In fact, only thirteen states have legislation that specifically exempts breastfeeding from being classified as indecent exposure. Thus, although breastfeeding in public is more common than it was twenty years ago, there is still a great deal of pressure for mothers to breastfeed only in private settings. Unfortunately, because breastfed babies require far more frequent feedings than formula-fed babies, and many breastfed babies refuse artificial nipples, this pressure to breastfeed in private can severely restrict the lives of these mothers.

What about jury duty? Although it doesn't at first seem fair that breastfeeding women should "get out of it," consider the consequences if women who are exclusively breastfeeding were forced to serve. Bringing the baby to court for what may end up being several hours, days, or even weeks would inevitably cause disruptions whenever the baby fussed, cried, needed diaper changes, etc. In fact, many courtrooms have policies banning children outright. Leaving the baby behind would be equally unacceptable, as babies who are exclusively breastfed are unlikely to suddenly accept an artificial nipple and thus would go without food and hydration.

As you have learned in this chapter, breastfeeding mothers who work outside the home face additional challenges, including lack of privacy and time to pump breast milk at the worksite. Some of this lack of support for breastfeeding at worksites most likely stems from the historical facts that, throughout much of the twentieth century, most women stayed home and cared for children and worksite environments were designed for men. Although millions of women are now working outside of the home, the social norms are relatively slow to change. Think of how challenging it must be for a female police officer to find the time and opportunity to pump breast milk. Most of her colleagues are males, and the work environment is typically fast-paced and demanding. Women returning to work in these types of environments are more likely to give up breastfeeding.

Numerous incidences of outright harassment of working women who breastfeed include:

- Not allowing women to pump breast milk during lunch or other sanctioned work breaks.
- Withholding pay to women who use work time to pump breast milk.

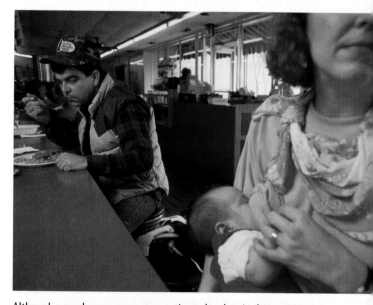

Although a much more common practice today than in the past, many people still consider it inappropriate to breastfeed in public.

- Assigning women to less desirable work shifts as punishment for breastfeeding.
- Laying off or firing women who request time to express milk during standard working hours.

Ironically, working women who continue to breastfeed despite such harassment actually have less absenteeism due to infant-related illnesses as compared to working mothers who do not breastfeed (Cohen, Mrtek, and Mrtek 1995).

Because of these instances of social and worksite harassment, breastfeeding legislation has been enacted in over half of the states in the United States. It is important to emphasize that breastfeeding is not illegal, and legislation is not necessary to legalize this natural act. The primary purpose of legislation is to clarify that women have a right to breastfeed in public, and they should not be harassed or shunned if they do so (Baldwin and Friedman 2004). Porter (2003) reports that as of 2002, thirty-two states had enacted legislation related to breastfeeding. Many states have legislation stating that breastfeeding in public is not illegal, and seventeen states permit women to breastfeed in any public or private location where children and mothers are authorized to be. Five states exempt women from jury duty if they are breastfeeding, and Connecticut, Hawaii, Illinois, and Minnesota have laws that require employers to accommodate breastfeeding mothers who return to work (Weimer 2003). U.S. Congresswoman Carolyn Maloney (NY) has drafted a federal bill that goes much further in supporting breastfeeding mothers who go back to work (Baldwin and Friedman 2004). If passed, this bill would:

- Provide a tax credit to employers who set up a lactation location, purchase or rent lactation equipment, hire a health professional, or take other actions to promote a lactation-friendly environment.
- Ensure that breastfeeding is protected under civil rights law.
- Require the FDA to develop minimum quality standards for breast pumps

What do you think of this legislation? Is it necessary? Does it go far enough? Does it go too far? What rights do you feel breastfeeding women should have? And what about infants—do they have a right to breastfeed? This debate will likely continue as both national and international healthcare organizations continue to urge policy makers, healthcare providers, and business leaders to support breastfeeding.

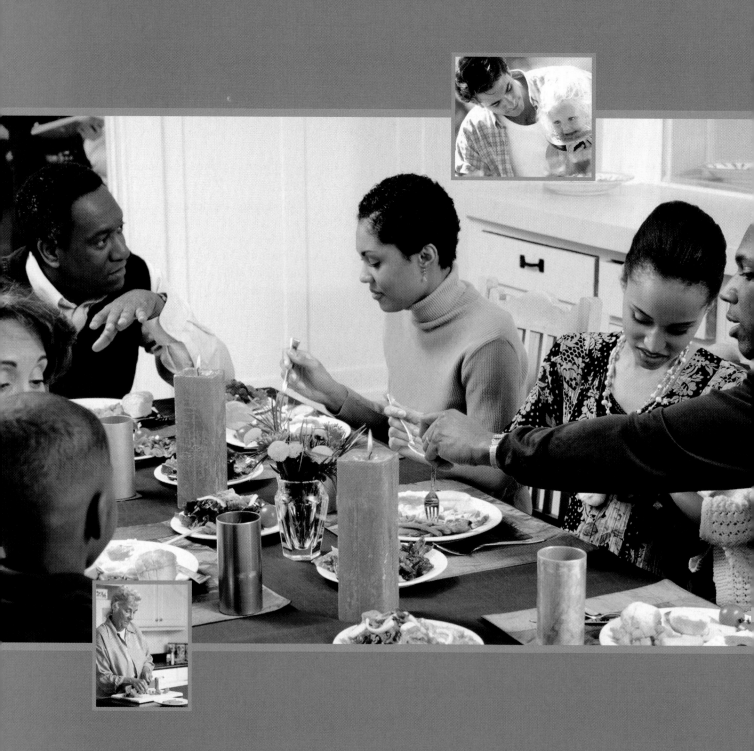

Chapter 16
Nutrition Through the Lifecycle: Childhood to Late Adulthood

Chapter Objectives

After reading this chapter you should be able to:

1. Compare and contrast the growth and activity patterns of toddlers and preschoolers, pp. 576 and 583.

2. List at least three nutrients of concern when feeding a vegan diet to young children, pp. 581–582.

3. Describe how micronutrient needs change as a child matures from school-aged years to adolescence, pp. 588–589 and 595–596.

4. List at least two factors that can result in obesity during childhood and adolescence, pp. 585–587 and 597.

5. Define puberty and describe how it influences changes in body composition, p. 594.

6. Identify at least three physiological changes that occur with aging and describe how these changes affect nutrient needs of older adults, pp. 599–602.

7. Give two reasons why older adults may avoid drinking adequate amounts of fluid, p. 602.

8. Discuss how changes in oral health can affect nutrient intake in older adults, p. 603.

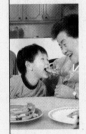

Test Yourself True or False?

1. Toddlers should be fed nonfat milk products to reduce their risk for obesity. T or F

2. The average girl reaches almost full height by the onset of menstruation. T or F

3. The move toward consuming a heart-healthy diet should begin around two years of age. T or F

4. Participating in regular physical activity can delay or reduce some of the loss of muscle mass that occurs with aging. T or F

5. Older adults should take supplements whenever possible because they cannot consistently meet their nutritional needs by eating a healthful diet. T or F

Test Yourself answers can be found at the end of the chapter.

At age 16 and 350 pounds, José Jímenez underwent bariatric surgery (also called gastric bypass or "stomach stapling" surgery) in a drastic attempt to lose weight. In the year following his surgery, he lost 100 pounds (Cable News Network [CNN] 2003). At age 19, Irene Orr weighed 363 pounds and chose the same surgery. Two years later, she had lost more than half her body weight (Talanian 2003). José and Irene are not alone: as the rate of morbid obesity has skyrocketed in the past decade, more and more adults, teens, and even some preteens are resorting to weight-loss surgery. In 1995, just 20,000 weight-loss operations were performed in the United States. In 2003, there were 103,000 (Grady 2004).

The procedure is far from a miracle cure: afterwards, patients can never eat more than one cup of food at one time. Ironically, because the pouch stretches over time, the majority of patients gain the weight back within about twenty years (Grady, 2004). The procedure also carries significant risks, including persistent diarrhea, wound infection, hernias, bowel obstruction, liver disease, severe vitamin and mineral deficiencies, and death. In fact, the death rate from the surgery is estimated at about 2%, and is thought to be much higher in patients over age 65 and those whose surgeons are not highly experienced in the difficult procedure.

So why are patients—and their physicians—willing to take such risks? Many say they turned to surgery because they could no longer bear the social problems that accompanied their obesity, such as job discrimination or the intense teasing that led Irene Orr to drop out of school. Their physicians tend to cite the severe health consequences of morbid obesity, such as increased risk for type 2 diabetes, hypertension, heart disease, cancer, asthma, sleep apnea, and joint problems. The most serious risk of obesity is premature death: the American Obesity Association reports that each year, obesity causes at least 300,000 unnecessary deaths in the United States alone (American Obesity Association 2004). Researchers expect obesity to soon overtake smoking as the primary cause of preventable death. As one obesity expert put it, for obese patients with heart and lung disease, a 2% mortality rate from bariatric surgery might be a reasonable risk (Grady 2004).

Obesity is a serious concern across the lifespan: more than 15% of American children and adolescents (age 6 to 19) and more than 30% of American adults are now obese (American Obesity Association 2004). Since obesity is now so prevalent, chances are you know someone who struggles with this problem. Why have obesity rates skyrocketed in the past ten years, and what can be done to promote weight management across the lifespan? How do our nutrient needs change as we grow and age, and what other nutrition-related concerns develop in each life stage? This chapter will help you answer these questions.

Nutrition for Toddlers, Age 1–3 Years

As babies begin to walk and explore, they transition out of infancy and into the active world of toddlers.

Toddler Growth and Activity Patterns

The rapid growth rate of infancy begins to slow during toddlerhood. During the second and third years of life, a toddler will grow a total of about 5.5 to 7.5 inches and gain an average of 9 to 11 pounds. Toddlers expend more energy to fuel increasing levels of activity as they explore their ever-expanding world and develop new skills (Figure 16.1). They progress from taking a few wobbly steps to running, jumping, and climbing with confidence, and they begin to dress, feed, and toilet themselves. Thus, their diet should provide an appropriate quantity and quality of nutrients to fuel their growth and activity.

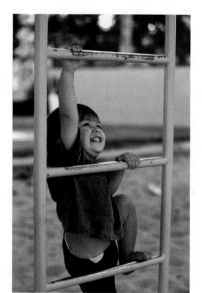

Figure 16.1   Toddlers expend significant amounts of energy actively exploring their world.

What Are a Toddler's Nutrient Needs?

Nutrient needs increase as a child progresses from infancy to toddlerhood. Refer to Table 16.1 on page 584 for a review of specific nutrient recommendations.

Energy and Macronutrient Recommendations for Toddlers

Although the energy requirement per kilogram of body weight for toddlers is just slightly less than for infants, *total* energy requirements are higher because toddlers are larger and much more active than infants. The **estimated energy requirements (EER),** or the total energy needed per day, varies according to the toddler's age, body weight, and level of activity. The equation to calculate EER for toddlers is (Institute of Medicine 2002):

estimated energy requirements (EER)
The total amount of energy needed per day for any age group.

$$\text{kcal/day} = (89 \times \text{weight (kg)} - 100) + 20$$

Toddlers need more fat than adults. However, studies show that there does not appear to be a significant effect of fat intake on growth and development, assuming fat intake is at least 21% of total energy intake and that energy intake is adequate (Lagström et al., 1999; Obarzanek et al., 1997; Niinikoski et al., 1997). We know that fat provides a concentrated source of energy in a relatively small amount of food, and this is important for toddlers, especially those who are fussy eaters or have little appetite. Fat is also necessary during the toddler years to support the continuously developing nervous system. Although at the present time there is insufficient evidence available to set a DRI for fat for toddlers, it is recommended that toddlers consume 30 to 40% of their total daily energy intake as fat (Institute of Medicine 2002).

Toddlers' protein needs increase modestly because they weigh more than infants and are still growing rapidly. The RDA for protein for toddlers is 1.10 grams/kg body weight per day, or approximately 13 grams of protein daily (Institute of Medicine 2002).

The RDA for carbohydrate for toddlers is 130 grams/day, and carbohydrate intake should be about 45 to 65% of total energy intake (Institute of Medicine 2002). As is the case for older children and adults, most of the carbohydrates eaten should be complex, and refined carbohydrates from snack foods should be kept to a minimum. Fruits and fruit juices are nutritious sources of simple carbohydrates that can also be included. Keep in mind, however, that too much fruit juice can displace other foods and nutrients and can cause diarrhea.

Adequate fiber is important for toddlers to maintain regularity and prevent constipation. The AI is 14 grams of fiber per 1,000 kcal of energy, or 19 grams/day (Institute of Medicine 2002). Too much fiber can inhibit essential nutrient absorption, harm toddler's small digestive tracts, and cause them to feel too full to consume adequate nutrients.

Determining the macronutrient requirements of toddlers can be challenging. See the You Do the Math box on p. 578 for analysis of the macronutrient levels in one toddler's daily diet.

Micronutrient Recommendations for Toddlers

As toddlers grow, their micronutrient needs increase. Of particular concern with toddlers are adequate intakes of the micronutrients associated with fruits and vegetables, such as vitamins A, C and E, as well as the minerals calcium, iron, and zinc (Table 16.1).

Calcium is necessary for children to promote optimal bone mass, which continues to accumulate until early adulthood. For toddlers, the AI for calcium is 500 mg/day (Institute of Medicine 1997). Dairy products are excellent sources of calcium. When a child reaches the age of one year, whole cow's milk can be given; however, reduced-fat milk (2%) should *not* be given until age two. If dairy products are not feasible, fortified orange juice or soy milk can supply calcium, or children's calcium supplements can be given. Toddlers generally cannot consume enough food to depend on alternate calcium sources such as dark green vegetables.

Iron-deficiency anemia is the most common nutrient deficiency in young children in the United States and around the world. Iron-deficiency anemia can affect a child's energy level, attention span, and mood. The RDA for iron for toddlers is 7 mg/day (Institute of Medicine 2001). Good sources of iron include lean meats, eggs, and

Is This Menu Good for a Toddler?

A dedicated mother and father want to provide the best nutrition for their young son, Ethan, who is now 1½ years old and has just been completely weaned from breast milk. Ethan weighs about 26 pounds (or 11.8 kg). Below is a typical day's menu for Ethan. Grams of protein, fat, and carbohydrate, respectively, are given after each food in parentheses. The day's total energy intake is 1,168 kcal. Calculate the percent of Ethan's calories that come from protein, fat, and carbohydrate (numbers may not add up to exactly 100% because of rounding). Where are Ethan's parents doing well, and where could they use some advice for improvement?

Note: This activity focuses on the macronutrients. It does not ask you to consider Ethan's intake of micronutrients or fluids.

Meal	Foods	Protein (grams)	Fat (grams)	Carbo-hydrate (grams)
Breakfast	Oatmeal (½ cup, cooked)	2.5	1.5	13.5
	Brown sugar (1 tsp.)	0	0	4
	Milk (1%, 4 fl. oz.)	4	1.25	5.5
	Grape juice (4 fl. oz.)	0	0	20
Mid-morning Snack	Banana slices (1 small banana)	0	0	16
	Yogurt (nonfat fruit flavored, 3 fl. oz.)	5.5	0	15.5
	Orange juice (4 fl. oz.)	1	0	13
Lunch	Whole-wheat bread (1 slice)	1.5	0.5	10
	Peanut butter (1 tbsp.)	4	8	3.5
	Strawberry jam (1 tbsp.)	0	0	13
	Carrots (cooked, ⅛ cup)	0	0	2
	Applesauce (sweetened, ¼ cup)	0	0	12
	Milk (1%, 4 fl. oz.)	4	1.25	5.5
Afternoon Snack	Bagel (½)	3	1	20
	American cheese product (1 slice)	3	5	1
	Water	0	0	0
Dinner	Scrambled egg (1)	11	5	1
	Baby food spinach (3 oz.)	2	0.5	5.5
	Whole-wheat toast (1 slice)	1.5	0.5	10
	Mandarin orange slices (¼ cup)	0.5	0	10
	Milk (1%, 4 fl. oz.)	4	1.25	5.5

Calculations:
There is a total of 47.5 grams protein in Ethan's menu.

47.5 grams × 4 kcal/gram = 190 kcal
190 kcal protein/1,168 total kcal × 100 = 16% protein

There is a total of 25.75 grams fat in Ethan's menu.

25.75 grams × 9 kcal/gram = 232 kcal
232 kcal fat/1,168 total kcal × 100 = 20% fat

There is a total of 186.5 grams carbohydrate in Ethan's menu.

186.5 grams × 4 cal/gram = 746 kcal
746 kcal carbohydrate/1,168 total kcal × 100 = 64% carbohydrate

Analysis: Ethan's parents are doing very well at offering a wide variety of foods from various food groups; they are especially doing well with fruits and vegetables. Also, according to his estimated energy requirement, Ethan requires about 970 kcal/day, and he is consuming 1,168 kcal/day, thus meeting his energy needs.

Ethan's total carbohydrate intake for the day is 186.5 grams, which is higher than the RDA of 130 grams per day; however, this value falls within the recommended 45 to 65% of total energy intake that should come from carbohydrates. Thus, high carbohydrate intake is adequate to meet his energy needs.

However, Ethan is being offered far more than enough protein. The DRI for protein for toddlers is about 13 grams per day, and Ethan is being offered more than three times that much!

It is also readily apparent that Ethan is being offered too little fat for his age. Toddlers need at least 30 to 40% of their total energy intake from fat, and Ethan is only consuming about 20% of his calories from fat. He should be drinking whole milk, not 1% milk. He should occasionally be offered higher fat foods like cheese for his snacks or macaroni and cheese for a meal. Yogurt is fine, but it shouldn't be nonfat at Ethan's age.

In conclusion, Ethan's parents should be commended for offering a variety of nutritious foods but should be counseled that a little more fat is critical for toddlers' growth and development. Some of the energy currently being consumed as protein and carbohydrate should be shifted to fat. ●

fortified foods such as breakfast cereals. If a toddler is willing to accept a non-heme source of iron, such as beans or greens, remember that consuming a source of vitamin C at the same meal will enhance the absorption of iron from these sources.

Fluid Recommendations for Toddlers

Toddlers lose less fluid from evaporation than infants, and their more mature kidneys are able to concentrate urine, thereby sparing fluid. However, as toddlers become active, they start to lose significant fluid through sweat, especially in hot weather. Toddlers and young children sometimes become so busy playing that they ignore or fail to recognize the thirst sensation, so parents need to make sure an active toddler is drinking adequately. The recommended fluid intake for toddlers is 1.3 liters per day (or 5.5 cups per day), which includes about 0.9 liters (or 4 cups) as total beverages, including drinking water (Institute of Medicine 2004). Parents can also monitor the number and heaviness of wet diapers to make sure the child is urinating appropriately. Suggested beverages include plain water, milk and soy milk, diluted fruit juice, and foods high in water content, such as vegetables and fruits.

Do Toddlers Need Nutritional Supplements?

Toddlers can be well nourished by consuming a balanced, varied diet. But given their typically erratic eating habits, the child's physician may recommend a multivitamin and mineral supplement as a precaution against deficiencies. The toddler's physician or dentist may also prescribe a fluoride supplement, if the community water supply is not fluoridated. Supplements should always be considered for any child at risk for deficiency of one or more nutrients. These may include children in vegan families, children from families who are financially limited, children with certain medical conditions or dietary restrictions, or very picky or erratic eaters.

As always, if a supplement is given, it should be formulated especially for toddlers and the recommended dose should not be exceeded. A supplement should not contain more than 100% of the Daily Value of any nutrient per dose.

Recap: Growth during toddlerhood is slower than during infancy; however, toddlers are highly active and need to consume enough energy to fuel growth and activity. Energy, fat, and protein requirements are higher for toddlers than for infants. Many toddlers will not eat vegetables, so micronutrients of concern include vitamins A, C, and E. Until age two, toddlers should drink whole milk rather than reduced-fat (2%) milk to meet calcium requirements. Iron deficiency is a concern in the toddler years and can be avoided by feeding toddlers lean meats, eggs, and iron-fortified foods.

Encouraging Nutritious Food Choices with Toddlers

Parents and pediatricians have long recognized that toddlers tend to be choosy about what they eat. Some avoid entire food groups, such as all meats or vegetables. Others will abruptly refuse all but one or two favorite foods (such as peanut butter on crackers) for several days or longer. Still others eat in extremely small amounts, seemingly satisfied by a single slice of apple or two bites of toast. These behaviors frustrate and worry many parents, but in fact, studies have consistently shown that, as long as food is abundant and choices varied, toddlers have an innate ability to match their intake with their needs. It is the whole nutrition profile over time that matters most, and the toddler will most likely make up for it later. Parents who offer only foods of high nutritional quality can feel confident that their children are getting the nutrition they need even if their choices seem odd or erratic on any particular day. Food should never be "forced" on a child, as doing so sets the stage for eating and control issues later in life.

To encourage nutritious food choices in toddlers, it's important to recognize that their stomachs are still very small and they cannot consume all of the calories they

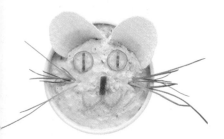

Figure 16.2 Most toddlers are delighted by food prepared in a fun way.

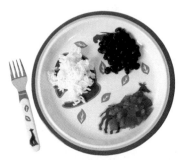

Figure 16.3 Portion sizes for preschoolers are much smaller than for older children. Use the following guideline: one tablespoon of the food for each year of age equals one serving. For example, the meal shown here—two tablespoons of rice, two tablespoons of black beans, and two tablespoons of chopped tomatoes—is appropriate for a two-year-old toddler.

need in three meals. They need small meals, interspersed with nutritious snacks, every two to three hours, and should not be forced to sit still until they finish every bite. A successful snack-time technique used by many experienced parents is to create a snack tray filled with small portions of nutritious food choices, such as one-third of a banana, two pieces of cheese, and three whole-grain pretzels, and leave it within reach of the child's play area. The child can then "graze" on these healthful foods while he or she plays. A snack tray plus a spill-proof cup of milk or water is particularly useful on car trips.

Foods prepared for toddlers should be developmentally appropriate. Firm, raw foods such as nuts, carrots, grapes, raisins, and cherry tomatoes are difficult for a toddler to chew and pose a choking hazard. Foods should be soft and sliced into strips or wedges that are easy for children to grasp. As the child develops more teeth and becomes more coordinated, the food repertoire can become more varied.

Foods prepared for toddlers should also be fun (Figure 16.2). Parents can use cookie-cutters to turn a peanut-butter sandwich into a pumpkin face, or arrange cooked peas or carrot slices to look like a smiling face on top of mashed potatoes. Juice and low-fat yogurt can be frozen into "popsicles" or blended into "milkshakes."

A positive mealtime environment helps toddlers develop good mealtime habits as well. Parents should seat the toddler in the same place at the table consistently and make sure that the child is served first. Television and other distractions should be turned off, and pleasant conversation should include the toddler, even if the toddler is preverbal.

Even at mealtime, portion sizes should be small. One tablespoon of a food for each year of age constitutes a serving throughout the preschool years (Figure 16.3). Realistic portion sizes can give toddlers a sense of accomplishment when they "eat it all up" and allay parents' fears that their child is not eating enough.

Introduce new foods gradually. Most toddlers are leery of new foods, spicy foods, hot (temperature) foods, mixed foods such as casseroles, and foods with strange textures. A helpful rule is to require the child to eat at least one bite of a new food: if the child does not want the rest, nothing negative should be said and the child should be praised just for the willingness to try. The food should be reintroduced a few weeks later. Eventually, the child might accept the food; however, some foods won't be accepted until well into adulthood as tastes expand and develop. One tactic that parents should not resort to is bribing; for example, promising dessert if the child finishes her squash. Bribing teaches children that food can be used to reward and manipulate. Instead, try to positively reinforce good behaviors; for example, "Wow! You ate every bite of your squash! That's going to help you grow big and strong!"

Role modeling is important when teaching toddlers how to make nutritious food choices. Toddlers emulate older children and adults: if they see their parents eating a variety of healthful foods, they will be likely to do so as well.

Providing limited healthful alternatives early on will also help toddlers to make nutritious food choices. For example, parents might say, "It's snack time! Would you like apples and cheese or bananas and yogurt?" Toddlers can also help select from a limited range of nutritious foods at the grocery store. Finally, toddlers are more likely to eat food they help prepare: encourage them to assist in the preparation of simple foods, such as helping pour a bowl of cereal or helping to arrange the raw vegetables on a plate.

Nutrition-Related Concerns for Toddlers

Just as toddlers have their own specific nutrient needs, they also have toddler-specific nutrition concerns. Some continue from infancy, while others are new.

Continued Allergy Watch

As during infancy, new foods should be presented one at a time, and the toddler should be monitored for allergic reactions for a week before introducing additional new foods. To prevent the development of food allergies, even foods that are established in the diet should be rotated, rather than served every day.

Obesity: A Concern Now?

Believe it or not, early signs indicating a tendency toward overweight can occur as early as the toddler years. Toddlers should *not* be denied nutritious food; however, they should not be force-fed nor should they be encouraged to eat when they are full. In the toddler years, a child who is above the 80th percentile for weight (that is, who weighs more than 80% of children of the same age and height) should be monitored. These children should be encouraged and supported in increasing their physical activity, and as for all children, foods with low nutrient density should be limited.

Vegetarian Families

For toddlers, a vegetarian diet in which eggs and dairy foods are included can be as wholesome as a diet including meats and fish. However, since red meat is an excellent source of heme iron, the most bioavailable form, families who do not serve red meat must be careful to include enough iron from other sources in their child's diet.

In contrast, a vegan diet, in which no foods of animal origin are consumed, poses several potential nutritional risks for toddlers:

- Protein—Vegan diets can be too low in protein for toddlers, who need protein for growth and increasing activity. Few toddlers can consume enough legumes and whole grains to provide sufficient protein.
- Iron, calcium, and zinc—Iron is an even greater concern in vegan diets than in vegetarian diets that include eggs. Calcium is a concern because of the avoidance of milk, yogurt, and cheese. As with protein, few children can consume enough calcium from plant sources to meet their daily requirement, and supplementation is advised. Zinc is also commonly low in vegan diets.
- Vitamins D and B_{12}—Both vitamins are typically lower in strict vegan diets. Vitamin B_{12} is not available in any amount from plant foods and must be supplemented.
- Fiber—Vegan diets often contain a higher percentage of fiber than is recommended for toddlers.

Although adults have the ability to choose alternative foods and/or supplements to meet the demands for these nutrients, toddlers must depend on their parents to make appropriate food choices for them. If parents are very dedicated to maintaining a vegan diet for their toddler, choices such as fortified juices, soy milk, and other soy products, along with judicious supplement use should be employed to ensure adequate nutrition.

The practice of feeding a vegan diet to infants and young children is highly controversial. See the Nutrition Myth or Fact box on p. 582 for more information about this controversy.

> **Recap:** Toddlers require small, frequent, nutritious meals and snacks, and food should be cut in small pieces so it is easy to handle, mash, and swallow. Because toddlers are becoming more independent and can self-feed, parents need to be alert for choking and should watch for allergies and monitor weight gain. Role modeling by parents and access to ample healthful foods can help toddlers make nutritious choices for snacks and meals. Feeding vegan diets to toddlers is controversial and poses potential deficiencies for iron, calcium, zinc, vitamin D, and vitamin B_{12}.

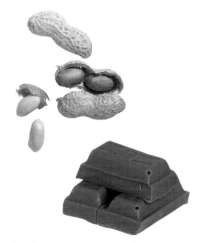

Foods that may cause allergies, such as peanuts and chocolate, should be introduced to toddlers one at a time.

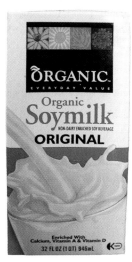

Soy milk can be a part of a healthy vegan diet for toddlers.

Vegan Diets Are Not Appropriate for Young Children

It only takes a look at the headlines to realize that feeding a vegan diet to young children is a controversial issue. Strong proponents of veganism state that any consumption of animal products is wrong and that feeding animal products to children is forcing them into a life of obesity, clogged arteries, and chronic diet-related diseases. In addition, many people who consume a vegan diet feel that consumption of animal products wastes natural resources and contributes to environmental damage and is therefore morally wrong. In contrast, strong antagonists of veganism emphasize that feeding a vegan diet to young children deprives them of essential nutrients that can only be found in animal products. Some people even suggest that veganism for young children is, in essence, a form of child abuse.

As with many controversies, there are truths on both sides. For example, there have been documented cases of children failing to thrive, and even dying, on extreme vegan diets (Bailey 2001; CDC 2001; Second Opinions 2002). Cases have been cited of vitamin B_{12}, and probable calcium, zinc, and vitamin D deficiencies in vegan children. These nutrients are found primarily or almost exclusively in animal products, and deficiencies can have serious and lifelong consequences. For example, not all of the neurologic impairments caused by vitamin B_{12} deficiency can be reversed by timely B_{12} supplement intervention. In addition, inadequate zinc, calcium, and vitamin D can result in impaired bone growth and strength, failure to reach peak bone mass, and retarded growth in general.

However, close inspection of the cases of nutrition-related illness in children that cite veganism as the culprit reveals that lack of education, fanaticism, and/or extremism is usually at the root of the problem. Informed parents following responsible vegan diets are rarely involved. On the other hand, such cases do point out that veganism is not a lifestyle one can safely undertake without thorough education regarding the necessity of supplementation of those nutrients not available in plant products. Parents also need to understand that typical vegan diets are high in fiber and low in fat, a combination that can be dangerous for very young children (Mangels 2001). Moreover, certain staples of the vegan diet, such as wheat, soy, and nuts, commonly provoke allergic reactions in children; when this happens, finding a plant-based substitute that contains adequate nutrients can be challenging.

On the other hand, both the American Dietetic Association and the American Academy of Pediatrics have stated that a vegan diet can promote normal growth and development—*provided* that adequate supplements and/or fortified foods are consumed to account for the nutrients that are normally found in animal products. However, most healthcare organizations stop short of outright endorsement of a vegan diet for young children. Instead, many advocate a more moderate approach during the early childhood years. Reasons for this level of caution include acknowledgement of several factors:

- Some vegan parents are not adequately educated on the planning of meals, the balancing of foods, and the inclusion of supplements to ensure adequate levels of all nutrients.

- Most young children are picky eaters and are hesitant to eat certain food groups, particularly vegetables, a staple in the vegan diet.

- The high fiber content of vegan diets may not be appropriate for very young children.

- Young children have small stomachs, and they are not able to consume enough plant-based foods to ensure adequate intakes of all nutrients and energy.

Because of these concerns, most nutrition experts advise parents to take a more moderate dietary approach, one that emphasizes plant foods but also includes some animal based foods, such as fish, dairy, and/or eggs.

Once children reach school age, the low fat, abundant fiber, antioxidants, and many micronutrients in a vegan diet will promote their health as they progress into adulthood. However, those who consume animal products can also live a healthful life and reduce their risk for chronic diseases by choosing low-fat, nutrient-dense foods such as lean meats, nonfat dairy products, whole grains, and fruits and vegetables. Since animal products are consumed, there are fewer worries about consuming adequate amounts of micronutrients such as vitamin B_{12}, calcium, vitamin D, iron, and zinc. ●

Nutrition for Preschoolers, Age 4–5 Years

Distinct developmental markers such as increased language fluency, decision-making skills, and physical coordination and dexterity are characteristic of the preschool years. Here, we discuss preschooler growth and activity, nutrient requirements, and nutrition issues that reflect these changes.

Preschooler Growth and Activity Patterns

During the preschool years, growth rate continues to slow. Preschoolers experience an average growth of 3 to 4 inches per year, accompanied by an annual weight gain of 5 to 6 pounds. Because of the slowed growth, the appetite of preschoolers is often noticeably diminished.

Activity levels in preschool children generally increase as they become more skillful and confident in running, jumping, and climbing. Most preschoolers can kick, throw, catch, and hit balls. Many ride their bikes, skate, swim, or perform other vigorous activities nearly every day. Sometimes it is hard to get preschoolers to stop for snacks and meals because they are so involved in their play and so intent on exerting their independence.

Preschool children have acquired all of their baby teeth so they can chew most foods adequately enough to prevent choking. They can also use a cup, spoon, and fork with relative ease.

Recap: Preschoolers have a slower growth rate than toddlers and may have a reduced appetite. Preschoolers are more physically active than toddlers, and playing can sometimes interfere with eating adequate food.

What Are a Preschooler's Nutrient Needs?

By age three, children exposed to a wide variety of foods typically have developed a varied diet. Nevertheless, since they are still small, they cannot be expected to consume the required amounts of nutrients in three main meals. Thus, nutrient-dense snacks continue to be important.

Energy and Macronutrient Recommendations for Preschoolers

Fat remains a key macronutrient in the preschool years. During this time, the total fat in a child's diet should gradually be reduced to a level closer to that of an adult, to around 25 to 35% of total energy (Institute of Medicine 2002). One easy way to start reducing dietary fat is to gradually introduce preschoolers to lower-fat dairy products such as 2% milk.

Total needs for protein and energy increase for preschoolers because of their larger size, even though their growth rate has slowed. For preschoolers, the RDA for protein is 0.95 grams/kg body weight per day, or approximately 19 grams of protein per day (Institute of Medicine 2002).

The RDA for carbohydrate for preschoolers is 130 grams/day. By the end of the preschool years, carbohydrate intake should resemble the pattern of the recommended adult diet. That is, carbohydrates should make up about 45 to 65% of total daily energy intake, and carbohydrates should be mostly complex in nature. Simple sugars should come from fruits and fruit juices, with refined-sugar items such as cakes, cookies, and candies saved for occasional indulgences. The AI for fiber for children of preschool age is 14 grams of fiber per 1,000 kcal of energy consumed, or 25 grams/day (Institute of Medicine 2002). As was the case with toddlers, too much fiber can be detrimental because it can make a child feel full and interfere with food intake and nutrient absorption.

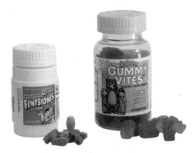

Children's multivitamins often appear in shapes or bright colors.

Micronutrient Recommendations for Preschoolers

Children who fail to consume the recommended five servings of fruits and vegetables each day may become deficient in vitamins A, C, and E. Minerals of concern continue to be calcium, iron, and zinc, which come primarily from animal-based foods. For preschoolers, the AI for calcium is increased to 800 mg/day (Institute of Medicine 1997). The RDAs for iron and zinc increase slightly to 10 mg/day and 5 mg/day, respectively (Institute of Medicine 2001). Refer to Table 16.1 for a review of the nutrient needs of preschoolers.

A multivitamin and mineral supplement for preschoolers, though not strictly necessary, may help to make up for those times when the preschooler's appetite is low or when particular food groups are not being consumed with regularity. As is always the case with children, vitamin and mineral supplements for preschoolers should be specific for their age, and the recommended dose (not more than 100% DV) should not be exceeded.

Fluid Recommendations for Preschoolers

The fluid recommendation for preschoolers is 1.7 liters (or about 7 cups) of total water per day, which includes approximately 1.2 liters (or about 5 cups) as total beverages, including drinking water (Institute of Medicine 2004). The exact amount of

Table 16.1 Nutrient Recommendations for Children and Adolescents

Nutrient	Toddlers (1–3 years)	Preschoolers (4–5 years)	School-Aged Children (6–8 years)	School-Aged Children (9–13 years)	Adolescents (14–18 years)
Fat	No DRI	No DRI	No DRI	No DRI	No DRI
Protein	1.10 grams/kg body weight per day	0.95 grams/kg body weight per day	0.95 grams/kg body weight per day	0.95 grams/kg body weight per day	0.85 grams/kg body weight per day
Carbohydrate	130 g/day	130 g/day	130 g/day	130 g/day	130 g/day
Vitamin A	300 µg/day	400 µg/day	400 µg/day	600 µg/day	Boys = 900 µg/day Girls = 700 µg/day
Vitamin C	15 mg/day	25 mg/day	25 mg/day	45 mg/day	Boys = 75 mg/day Girls = 65 mg/day
Vitamin E	6 mg/day	7 mg/day	7 mg/day	11 mg/day	15 mg/day
Calcium	500 mg/day	800 mg/day	800 mg/day	1,300 mg/day	1,300 mg/day
Iron	7 mg/day	10 mg/day	10 mg/day	8 mg/day	Boys = 11 mg/day Girls = 15 mg/day
Zinc	3 mg/day	5 mg/day	5 mg/day	8 mg/day	Boys = 11 mg/day Girls = 9 mg/day
Fluid	1.3 liters/day	1.7 liters/day	1.7 liters/day	Boys = 2.4 liters/day Girls = 2.1 liters/day	Boys = 3.3 liters/day Girls = 2.3 liters/day

fluid a preschooler needs varies according to level of physical activity and weather conditions. Preschoolers can use the bathroom on their own, but parents should keep an eye on number of trips to the bathroom and occasionally check the child's urine to make sure it is pale. Preschoolers can easily become dehydrated because they get so involved in their play that they ignore or fail to recognize the sensation of thirst. Offer fluid breaks to preschoolers during prolonged periods of play, especially if the weather is hot (Figure 16.4).

> **Recap:** Preschoolers have teeth and can better chew their food, and they also can use dishes and eating utensils. Preschoolers need less fat than toddlers but slightly more than adults. Protein and energy needs are higher for preschoolers due to their larger size and higher activity levels. Calcium, iron, and zinc requirements are slightly higher for preschoolers than toddlers. Preschoolers can become easily dehydrated because they fail to recognize or ignore their thirst.

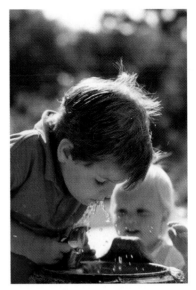

Figure 16.4   Fluid intake is important for preschoolers, who may become so involved in their play that they ignore the sensation of thirst.

Encouraging Nutritious Food Choices with Preschoolers

Preschoolers can understand that some foods will "give them energy" and "help them grow up healthy and strong," and that other foods should be used only for treats. Thus, parents can now teach their children, using age-appropriate language and concepts, what makes some foods better choices than others. Most preschoolers want to grow as quickly as possible, so parents can capitalize on this natural desire when they encourage foods high in protein, for example, and micronutrients.

A Food Guide Pyramid designed for preschoolers is shown in Figure 16.5. Parents can introduce preschoolers to the pyramid and guide them in using it to make food choices on their own.

Nutrition-Related Concerns for Preschoolers

In addition to potential nutrient deficiencies that have already been discussed, new concerns arise during the preschool years.

Obesity Watch: Encouraging an Active Lifestyle

The preschool years are an important time for parents to be watchful of potential overweight and obesity. This is the time when most children are becoming seriously active in their play. In addition, most preschoolers are prone to a decreased appetite. Combined, these two factors should work to combat obesity and overweight. If a preschooler is overweight, energy balance is disrupted at some level.

Childhood overweight is defined as having a BMI at or above the 85th percentile; that is, the child's body mass is heavier than that of 85% of U.S. children of the same age and height. A child is considered obese if his or her BMI is above the 95th percentile.

childhood overweight   Having a body mass index (BMI) at or above the 85th percentile.

Overweight children are at higher risk of becoming overweight adults than are normal weight children, so preventing childhood overweight is important for the long-term health and happiness of the child. It is also important for the child's current health and happiness: even in early childhood, significant overweight can exacerbate asthma, cause sleep apnea, impair the child's mobility, and lead to intense teasing, low self-esteem, and social isolation.

The preschool years are formative; thus, establishing healthful eating and physical activity practices is very important during this time. One important guideline is to limit television watching to no more than two hours per day. Studies have linked higher rates of television watching to higher rates of obesity in children (Torgan 2002). Too much television can also interfere with the acquisition of physical skills and can hinder preschoolers' use of their own imagination, dampening creativity. Moreover, an abundance of television commercials during children's programs advertise less healthful

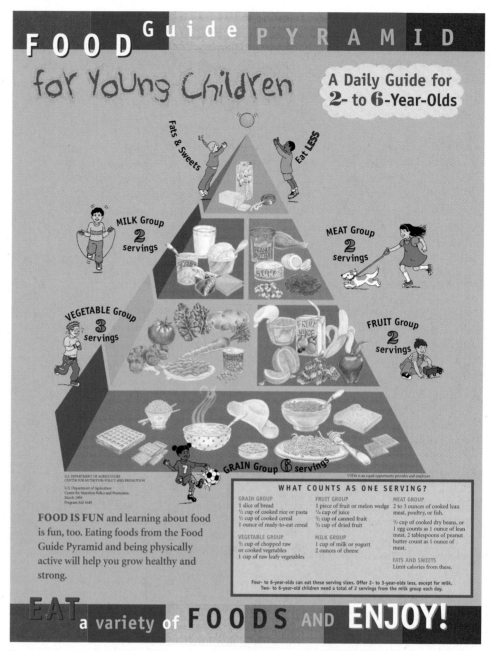

Figure 16.5   Food Guide Pyramid for Children. This version of the USDA Food Guide Pyramid is designed to be fun for young children. In addition to eating healthful foods, this pyramid emphasizes active play.

foods, such as sweetened breakfast cereals made with refined grains, high-sugar yogurt products, candies, pastries, and high-fat snacks. Even parents who limit television watching should sit with their children during several commercials and explain to them, in age-appropriate language, that these foods are made to look appealing to kids and are not healthful choices.

Because of the high nutrient needs of preschoolers, restrictive diets are not advised even when the child is diagnosed as overweight. Rather, parents should strive to consistently provide more nutritious food choices, sitting down together to a shared family meal each evening. The television should be off throughout dinner to encourage slow eating and true enjoyment of the food. To encourage activity throughout the day, parents should limit their own and their children's television watching, computer games, and other sedentary activities and instead encourage increased physical activity, especially shared activities such as ball games, hikes, etc. When parents and children are active together, healthful activity patterns are established early. Over time, overweight children who are offered nutritious foods and encouraged to be active can "catch up" to their weight as they grow taller without restricting food (and thus nutrient) intake. Increased activity also helps young children acquire motor skills and muscle strength and develop self-esteem as they feel themselves becoming faster, stronger, and more skilled.

Dental Caries

As discussed in Chapter 4, *dental caries,* or cavities, occur when bacteria in the mouth feed on carbohydrates deposited on teeth. As a result of metabolizing the carbohydrates, the bacteria then secrete acid that begins to erode tooth enamel, leading to tooth decay. The occurrence of dental caries can be minimized by limiting sugary sweets, especially those that stick to teeth, like jelly beans. Frequent brushing helps to eliminate the sugars on teeth, as well as the bacteria that feed on them.

During the preschool years, children begin learning to brush their own teeth. Because preschoolers' fine-motor skills are not yet mature, parents should help, or at least supervise, to make sure that brushing is effective and thorough. Fluoride, either through a municipal water supply or through supplements, will also help deter the development of dental caries. Even though the teeth of a preschooler will be replaced by permanent teeth in several years, it is critical to keep them healthy and strong. This is because they make room for and guide the permanent teeth into position. Children should start having regular dental visits at the age of three.

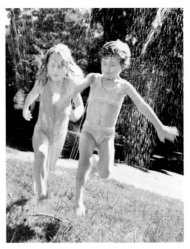

Active, healthy weight children are less likely to become overweight adults.

> **Recap:** Parents can communicate effectively with preschoolers to encourage healthful eating and can act as role models in regard to food choices, preparation, and level of physical activity. Overweight and obesity are potential concerns for preschoolers and can be prevented with a healthful diet and regular physical activity. An additional concern with preschoolers is dental caries, and they should be taught to brush their teeth regularly, limit sweets, and visit the dentist regularly beginning at age three.

Nutrition for School-Aged Children, Age 6–13 Years

The beginning of school marks the first time for many children to make some of their own food choices. The impact these decisions can make on the health of children can be profound and habit forming, so the education and training of school-aged children to make nutritious food choices is critical.

School Age Growth and Activity Patterns

School-aged children can be expected to grow an average of 2 to 3 inches per year at a slow and steady pace. In fact, these years are sometimes referred to as the "calm before the storm" of adolescence, when growth rates again become very rapid. Activity levels among school-aged children vary dramatically—some love sports and physical activity, while others prefer quieter activities like reading and drawing. All children can be encouraged to enjoy walking, to appreciate nature and exploration, and to have fun using their minds and their muscles in various ways that suit their interests.

> **Recap:** School-aged children are more independent and can make more of their own food choices. Their physical growth is slow and steady, and physical activity levels can vary dramatically between children.

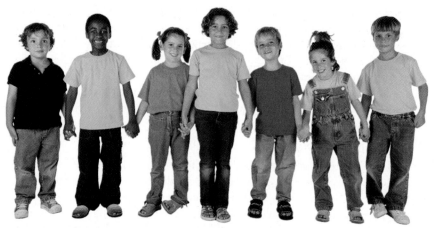

School-aged children grow an average of 2 to 3 inches per year.

What Are a School-Aged Child's Nutrient Needs?

The beginning of sexual maturation is an important phenomenon that has a dramatic impact on the nutrient needs of children. Boys' and girls' bodies develop differently in response to gender-specific hormones. These changes in sexual maturation can begin subtly between the ages of 8 and 9 years; because of this, the DRI values for the macronutrients, fiber, and micronutrients are grouped together for children aged 1 to 3 years and 4 to 8 years, and are redefined for boys and girls between the ages of 9 to 13 years (Institute of Medicine 2002). Table 16.1 (page 584) identifies the nutrient needs of school-aged children and adolescents.

Energy and Macronutrient Recommendations for School-Aged Children

Children of school age should ideally consume a variety of foods from each major food group. Children should be guided to eat a diet that contains about 25 to 35% of total energy from fat. A diet lower in fat is not recommended for children of school age, as they are still growing, developing, and maturing. Foods such as meats and dairy products should not be withheld solely because of their fat content since they otherwise have important nutrient value. Indeed, too much emphasis should not be placed on fat at this age. Impressionable and peer-influenced school-age kids can easily be led to categorize foods as "good" or "bad"; this can lead to skewed views of food, eating, and body image, and ultimately even eating disorders.

As you can see in Table 16.1, the protein recommendation for school-aged boys and girls is 0.95 grams/kg body weight per day. Although the recommended protein intake per kg body weight for children aged 4 to 13 years is lower than that of toddlers, the total protein intake of school-aged is higher due to their higher body weight.

The RDA for carbohydrate for school-aged children is the same as for toddlers through adults: 130 grams/day. Carbohydrate intake should be about 45 to 65% of total daily energy intake. As always, most carbohydrates eaten should be complex. The recommended fiber intake for school-aged children is 14 grams per 1000 kcal.

Micronutrient Recommendations for School-Aged Children

The need for most micronutrients increases slightly for school-aged children up to 8 years old because of their increasing size. A sharper increase in micronutrient needs occurs during the transition into full adolescence; this increase is due to the beginning of sexual maturation and in preparation for the impending adolescent growth spurt. Of continued interest during the school age years are the minerals calcium and iron. The AI for calcium increases from 800 mg/day for children aged 4 to 8 years to 1,300 mg/day for children aged 9 to 13 years (Institute of Medicine 1997). The RDA for iron for children aged 4 to 8 years is 10 mg/day, and this value drops to 8 mg/day for boys and girls aged 9 to 13 years. These recommendations are based on the assumption that most girls do not begin menstruation until after age 13 (Institute of Medicine 2001).

If there is any doubt that a child's nutrient needs are not being met for any reason (for instance, breakfasts are skipped, lunches are traded, parents lack money for nourishing food, etc.) a vitamin/mineral supplement that provides no more than 100% of the daily value for the micronutrients may help to correct any existing deficit.

Fluid Recommendations for School-Aged Children

The AI for school-aged children aged 4 to 8 years is 1.7 liters per day (or about 7 cups) of total water, with about 1.2 liters (or 5 cups) as total beverages, including drinking water. The AI for fluid for school-aged boys aged 9 to 13 years is 2.4 liters per day (or about 10 cups) of total water, with about 1.8 liters (or 8 cups) as total beverages, including drinking water. The AI for fluid for school-aged girls aged 9 to 13 years is 2.1 liters per day (or about 9 cups) of total water, with about 1.6 liters (or 7 cups) as total beverages, including drinking water (Institute of Medicine 2004).

At this point in life, children are mostly in control of their own fluid intake. However, as they engage in physical activity classes at school and in extracurricular sporting activities and general play, reminders to drink when they are thirsty are important to assist them in staying properly hydrated.

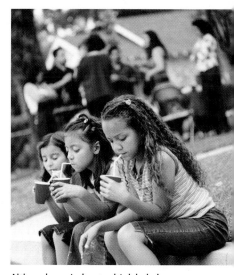

Although reminders to drink help keep school-aged children hydrated, they mostly control their own fluid intake.

> **Recap:** Sexual maturation begins during the school-age years. The DRI values reflect these changes by differentiating between nutrient needs for children 4 to 8 years and 9 to 13 years. School-aged children should eat 25 to 35% of their total energy as fat and 45 to 65% of their total energy as carbohydrate. Micronutrient needs increase because of growth and maturation. Calcium needs increase as children mature, while iron needs decrease slightly.

Encouraging Nutritious Food Choices with School-Aged Children

Peer pressure can be extremely difficult for both parents and their children to deal with during this life stage. Most children want to feel as if they "belong," and they admire and like to emulate children they believe to be popular. If the popular children at school are eating chips and drinking sugared soft drinks, it may be hard for a child to eat her tuna-on-whole wheat, apple, and milk without embarrassment.

Parents and children can work together to find compromises they can both live with by regularly communicating about healthful nutrition. One strategy that parents might consider is to introduce to their kids "cool" role models such as star athletes who follow nutritious diets. Emphasize that in order to perform at elite levels, athletes must pay close attention to their nutrition. Elite athletic performance cannot be sustained on chips and sugared soft drinks! However, the common practice of athletes endorsing fast-food restaurants can be confusing for some children. One way to help deal with this confusion is to explain that even an occasional fast-food meal can be part of a healthful diet, but it is not the type of food that star athletes eat every day.

Continuing to involve children in food choices for the family and in meal preparation is also a good idea. If they have input into what is going into their bodies, they may be more likely to take an active role in their health. In addition, parents should continue to act as healthful role models throughout this time to maintain consistent messages and images that children can rely upon when establishing their own eating and physical activity patterns.

What Is the Effect of School Attendance on Nutrition?

School attendance can affect a child's nutrition in several ways. First, in the hectic time between waking and getting out the door, many children minimize or skip breakfast completely. School children who don't eat breakfast may not get a chance to eat until lunch. If the entire morning is spent in a state of hunger, they are more likely to do poorly on schoolwork, have decreased attention spans, and have more behavioral problems than their peers who do eat breakfast (USDA Food and Nutrition Service 2003; USDA/ARS Children's Nutrition Research Center at Baylor College of Medicine 1999). For this reason, public schools now offer low-cost school breakfasts that are free of charge to low-income families. These breakfasts help children to optimize their nutrient intake and avoid the behavioral and learning problems associated with hunger in the classroom.

Another consequence of attending school is that, with no one monitoring what they eat, children do not always consume adequate amounts of food. They may spend their lunch time conversing or playing with friends rather than eating. If a school lunch is purchased, they might not like the foods being served, or their peers might influence them to skip certain foods with comments such as, "This broccoli is yucky!" Even homemade lunches that contain nutritious foods may be left uneaten or traded for less nutritious fare.

Finally, many schools have become places where soft drink and snack food companies advertise and sell their products to children in exchange for providing important revenues to maintain necessary school programs (see the Nutrition Debate in Chapter 2, p. 76, for more information on this topic). Many schools provide vending machines filled with snacks that are high in energy, sugar, and fat. Eating too many of these foods, either in place of or in addition to lunch, can lead to overweight and potential nutrient deficiencies.

The first years of school are an exciting time for learning, meeting new friends, and exerting a new degree of independence. However, it can also be a time of stress, the first real exposure to peer pressure, and the first real awareness of "who" and "what" are popular or acceptable to peers. Peer pressure and popularity influence food choices as much as they do friends, fashion, and other lifestyle choices.

Are School Lunches Nutritious?

On the surface, the answer to this question is "yes." All school lunches must meet certain nutrition requirements set forth by federal guidelines. Every lunch must provide one third of the 1989 Recommended Dietary Allowances for protein, vitamin A, vitamin C, iron, calcium, and energy (Food and Nutrition Board 1989). No more than 10% and 30% of the total energy in a meal should come from saturated fat and total fat, respectively.

However, when we delve into this question a little bit deeper, we find that the answer is not so clear. This is because the actual proportion of nutrients a student *gets* depends on what the student actually *eats* (Figure 16.6). School lunch programs do not have to meet the federal guidelines every day, but only over the course of a week's meals (USDA Food and Nutrition Service 2003; Armstrong 2001). Thus, the school lunches that students actually eat (not necessarily those planned on the menu) tend to be higher in fat than 30% of total energy because students choose to eat the foods they like the best, such as the higher fat entrées like pizza, hamburgers, and hot dogs. Children prefer to eat French fries instead of the other vegetables offered, such as green beans or carrots. Keep in mind that children in many schools can buy high-fat and high-sugar snacks and beverages from vending machines, and some schools actually have fast-food restaurants selling their food in competition with the school lunch program! Thus, even though school lunches are considered a healthful choice, children may not be getting the benefit of these meals due to selective eating and consumption of competitive foods.

The good news is that many schools are working to ensure a more healthful food environment. This change in environment is due to the efforts of school administrators, school lunch program personnel, parents, and student groups. Attention to nutrition is resulting in the offering of healthful alternatives such as salad bars and is changing how foods are bought and prepared by food service staff. A recent school-based obesity prevention study in Native American schools found that by educating food service staff about healthful food purchasing and preparation, the fat content of

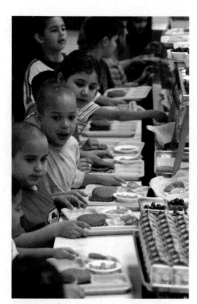

Figure 16.6   School-aged children may receive a standard school lunch, but many young people choose to eat less healthful foods when given the opportunity.

school breakfasts and lunches could be reduced without sacrificing nutritional quality (Cunningham-Sabo et al. 2003; Himes et al. 2003).

> **Recap:** Peer pressure has a strong influence on nutritional choices in school-aged children. Involving children in food purchasing and meal planning and preparation can help them make more healthful food choices. Attending school can interfere with eating breakfast, and children may not always choose healthful foods during school lunch. Peer pressure and popularity are strong influences on food choices. School lunches are nutritious and must meet federal guidelines, but the foods that children choose to eat at school, both during and outside of the lunch break, can be high in fat, sugar, and energy and low in nutrients.

Nutrition-Related Concerns for School-Aged Children

The nutrition-related concerns for school-aged children revolve around weight concerns and body image issues. These concerns are discussed below.

Obesity Watch: Keeping Active for Life

Obesity in school-aged children is now epidemic in the United States (Torgan 2002). In the past decade, the skyrocketing rate of childhood obesity has become a concern of nutritionists, physicians, educators, policy makers, and parents across the United States. Experts agree that the main culprits are the same as those involved in adult obesity: eating too much and moving too little (Torgan 2002). Rather than placing school-aged children on restrictive diets, however, experts advise encouraging physical activity.

In the past, children played freely outdoors and were relatively active indoors in times of bad weather or during the evening hours. In recent years, however, several factors have prompted childhood activities to become increasingly sedentary. One such factor is simply the availability of entertainment technologies, including television, video games, and computer games. Another factor is that the number of households in which no adult is home after school has risen in recent decades, either because of single-parent families or because both parents have to work to support their families. Safety concerns cause working parents to forbid their children when they are home alone after school to venture out of the house. Given these circumstances and limited options for indoor physical activities at home, the television or the computer are quite logical choices. Children often eat snack foods while they watch television or play video games, and they don't have sufficient parental guidance to curb overeating or encourage physical play when they are home alone.

What are some strategies for encouraging daily physical activity in children of working parents? Many communities and even public school districts offer after-school programs that include team sports, running, swimming, and other physical activities. If these are not available, working parents can form partnerships with classmates' families in which a parent is home after school and agrees to encourage after-school physical activity. If children must return from school to an empty house, a phone call from mom or dad can encourage them to complete their homework and promise them an hour of quality time "shooting hoops" or bike-riding as soon as the parents return from work. Children can also be paid an allowance to complete a list of active chores such as vacuuming while they are waiting for their parents to come home.

The Dietary Guidelines for Americans (U.S. Department of Agriculture 2000) recommend that children be very active for at least an hour each day. For younger children, this can be divided into two or three shorter sessions,

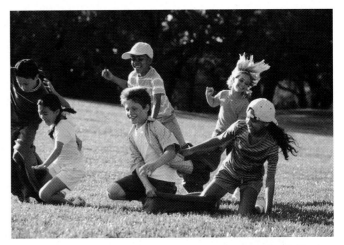

Encouraging physical play with friends is a good way to combat childhood obesity.

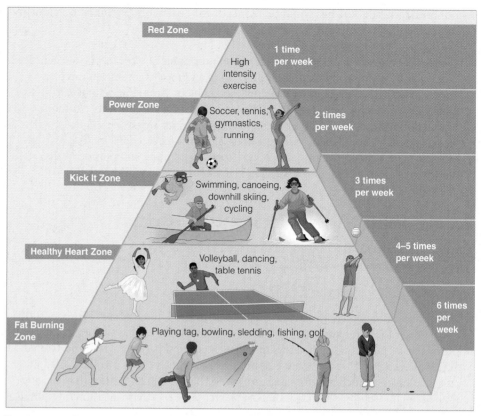

Figure 16.7 The American Dietetic Association's Fitness Pyramid for Kids gives guidelines for the duration, intensity, and frequency of various types of activities that are appropriate for children aged 2 to 11 years.

allowing them to regroup, recoup, and refocus in between activity sessions. Older children may be able to be active for an hour without stopping. Children should be exposed to a variety of activities so that they move different muscles, play at various intensities, avoid boredom, and find out what they like and don't like to do. The American Dietetic Association has designed a Fitness Pyramid for Kids to help guide children towards a physically active lifestyle (Figure 16.7).

The ACTIVATE/Kidnetic.com Program is another approach aimed at encouraging children and their families to communicate and work together to be more physically active and to eat a more healthful diet. This is done through an interactive computer-based program. This program was developed through a partnership of many organizations that are committed to improving the nutritional status and physical activity levels of children and families, including the International Food Information Council, the American Academy of Family Physicians, and the American College of Sports Medicine. The interactive computer-based program can be found at http://www.kidnetic.com (Figure 16.8).

Project VERB™ "It's What You Do" is a youth media campaign targeting "tweens", or school-aged children between the ages of 9 and 13 years. It is coordinated by the Centers for Disease Control and the Department of Health and Human Services. This campaign is a national, multicultural, social marketing campaign to encourage these children to be more active and to stay active, done through paid advertising, marketing strategies, and partnership efforts. More information about Project VERB™ can be found at the Centers for Disease Control and Prevention home page at www.cdc.gov.

Body-Image Concerns

As children, particularly females, approach puberty, appearance and body image play increasingly important roles in food choice. Concerns about appearance and body image are not necessarily detrimental to health, particularly if they result in children making more healthful food choices, such as eating more whole grains, fruits, and vegetables. However, it is important for children to understand that being thin does not guarantee health, popularity, or happiness and that a healthy body image includes accepting our own individual body type and recognizing that we can be physically fit and healthy at a variety of weights, shapes, and sizes. Excessive concern with thinness can lead children to experiment with fad diets, food restriction, and other behaviors that can result in undernutrition and perhaps even trigger a clinical eating disorder. (Refer to Chapter 13 to learn more about disordered eating and eating disorders and how they can be prevented and treated.)

Inadequate Calcium Intake

Another nutrition-related concern for school-aged children is an inadequate intake of calcium. Adequate calcium is necessary to achieve peak bone mass, as well as for numerous other critical body and cell functions. As you learned in Chapter 9, we achieve peak bone mass in our late teens or early twenties, and childhood and adolescence are critical times to ensure adequate deposition of bone tissue. Inadequate calcium intake during childhood and adolescence leads to poor bone health and potential osteoporosis in our later years.

Dairy products are the most common source of calcium for children in the U.S. (Institute of Medicine 1997). During the infant, toddler, and preschool years, milk consumption can largely be monitored by parents or caregivers. However, once children begin to attend school, they may choose to spend the money intended for milk on soft drinks, if available. This "milk displacement" is a recognized factor in low calcium intake and poor bone health (Heaney and Rafferty 2001). Diets that are low in calcium also tend to be low in other nutrients, so attention to calcium intake can help ensure a more healthful overall diet for children.

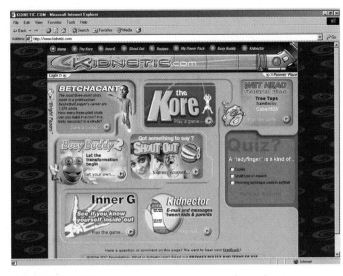

Figure 16.8   Kidnetic.com is an on-line program focused on increasing physical activity levels and promoting healthful eating among children and their families.

> **Recap:** Obesity is an important concern for school-aged children. All children should be active at least one hour every day. Programs and campaigns aimed at increasing the physical activity levels of children and their families include the Fitness Pyramid for Kids, the ACTIVATE/Kidnetic.com Program, and Project VERB™ "It's What You Do." Appearance and body image play increasingly important roles in this age group, and disordered eating and eating disorders can result from these concerns. Consuming adequate calcium to support the development of peak bone mass is also a primary concern for school-aged children.

Hannah   *Nutri-Case*

"Today at school I got picked last for kickball, and I heard some boys on the other team laughing at me. Our phys. ed. teacher keeps telling me I should eat less, so this morning I didn't eat any breakfast at all, and I didn't eat all of my hamburger and French fries at lunch. I'm still sad though, because nobody wants to be my friend, except for Julia. She's chubby too, and we're going to try to help each other lose weight. We're going to watch TV together after school today, and we promised each other we're only going to drink the diet soda my mom has in the fridge."

Given what you know about Hannah, her family, and the nutrient needs for school age children, what would you say about the overall quality of Hannah's diet? What about her activity level? How might you use Hannah's interest in science to help her achieve a more healthful body weight? What advice would you give to her parents?

Nutrition for Adolescents, Age 14–18 Years

puberty The period in life in which secondary sexual characteristics develop and people are biologically capable of reproducing.

The adolescent years begin with the onset of **puberty**, the period in life in which secondary sexual characteristics develop and we become capable of reproducing. This is a physically and emotionally tumultuous time for adolescents and their families. The nutritional needs of adolescents are influenced by their rapid growth in height, increased weight, changes in body composition, and their individual levels of physical activity.

Adolescent Growth and Activity Patterns

Growth during adolescence is primarily driven by hormonal changes, including increased levels of testosterone for boys and estrogen for girls. Both boys and girls experience *growth spurts*, or periods of accelerated growth, during later childhood and adolescence. Growth spurts for girls tend to begin around 10 to 11 years of age, while growth spurts for boys begin around 12 to 13 years of age. These growth periods last about two years.

menarche The beginning of menstruation, or the menstrual period.

Adolescents experience an average 20 to 25% increase in height during the pubertal years. On average, girls tend to grow 2 to 8 inches and boys tend to grow 4 to 12 inches (Polan and Taylor 2003). The average girl reaches almost full height by the onset of menstruation (called **menarche**). Boys typically experience continual growth throughout adolescence, and some may even grow slightly taller during early adulthood.

epiphyseal plates Plates of cartilage located toward the end of long bones that provide for growth in the length of long bones.

Skeletal growth ceases once closure of the *epiphyseal plates* occurs (Figure 16.9). The **epiphyseal plates** are plates of cartilage located toward the end of the long bones that provide for growth in length of the long bones. In some circumstances the epiphyseal plates can close early in adolescents and result in a failure to reach full stature. The most common causes of this failure are malnourishment during childhood and adolescence or use of anabolic steroids during this critical growth period.

Weight and body composition also change dramatically during adolescence. Weight gain is extremely variable during this time and reflects the adolescent's energy intake, physical activity level, and genetics. The average weight gained by girls and boys during this time is 35 and 45 pounds, respectively. The weight gained by girls and boys is dramatically different in terms of its composition. Girls tend to gain significantly more body fat than boys, with this fat accumulating around the buttocks, hips, breasts, thighs, and upper arms. Although many girls are uncomfortable or embarrassed by these changes, they are a natural result of maturation. Boys gain significantly more muscle mass than girls, and they experience an increase in muscle definition. Both girls and boys experience significant growth of their internal organs, including the liver, kidneys, heart, lungs, and sexual organs. Other changes that occur with sexual maturation include a deepening of the voice in boys and growth of pubic hair in both boys and girls.

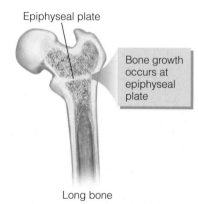

Epiphyseal plate

Bone growth occurs at epiphyseal plate

Long bone

Figure 16.9 Skeletal growth ceases once closure of the epiphyseal plates occurs.

The physical activity levels of adolescents are highly variable. Many are physically active in sports or other organized physical activities, whereas others become less interested in sports and more interested in intellectual or artistic pursuits. This variability in activity levels of adolescents results in highly individual energy needs. Although the rapid growth and sexual maturation that occur during puberty requires a significant amount of energy, adolescence is often a time in which overweight begins. The following section discusses the unique nutrient needs of adolescents.

Recap: Adolescence is predominated by puberty, or the period in life in which secondary sexual characteristics develop and the physical ability to reproduce begins. Adolescents experience rapid increases in height, weight, and lean body mass and fat mass. Physical activity levels of adolescents are highly variable, and overweight may begin during this period.

What Are an Adolescent's Nutrient Needs?

The nutrient needs of adolescents are influenced by rapid growth, weight gain, and sexual maturation, in addition to the demands of physical activity.

Energy and Macronutrient Recommendations for Adolescents

Adequate energy intake is necessary to maintain adolescents' health, support their dramatic growth and maturation, and fuel their physical activity. Because of these competing demands, the energy needs of adolescents can be quite high. The EER for adolescents can be calculated by using one of the equations presented in Table 16.2. To calculate the EER for this life stage, you must know the person's age, physical activity level, weight, and height.

As with the younger age groups, there is no DRI for fat for adolescents. However, adolescents are at risk for the same chronic diseases as adults, including type 2 diabetes, obesity, coronary heart disease, and various cancers. Thus, it is prudent for adolescents to consume 25 to 35% of total energy from fat and to consume no more than 10% of total energy from saturated fat sources.

The RDA for carbohydrate for adolescents is 130 grams/day. As with adults, this amount of carbohydrate covers what is needed to supply adequate glucose to the brain, but it does not cover the amount of carbohydrate needed to support daily activities. Thus, it is recommended that adolescents consume more than the RDA, or about 45 to 65% of their total energy as carbohydrate, and most carbohydrate should come from complex carbohydrate sources. The AI for fiber for adolescents is 26 grams/day, which is similar to adult values.

The RDA for protein for adolescents is similar to that of adults at 0.85 grams of protein per kg body weight per day. This value was selected because data are not available to determine protein maintenance requirements for this age group, and the amount of nitrogen needed to maintain protein balance in children is similar to that of adults (Institute of Medicine 2002). This amount is assumed to be sufficient to support health and to cover the additional needs of growth and development during the adolescent stage.

Micronutrient Recommendations for Adolescents

Micronutrients of particular concern for adolescents include calcium, iron, and vitamin A. Adequate calcium intake is critical to achieve peak bone density, and the AI for calcium for adolescents is 1,300 mg/day. This amount of calcium can be difficult to consume for many adolescents because the quality of foods they select is often less than optimal to meet their nutrient needs. This level of calcium intake can be achieved by eating at least three servings of dairy foods or calcium-fortified products daily.

Table 16.2 Equations Used to Calculate the Estimated Energy Requirements (EER) of Children and Adolescents Ages 9 to 18 years

Gender	EER Equation	Physical Activity (PA) Values
Males	EER (kcal/day) = 88.5 − (61.9 × Age [yrs]) + {Physical Activity × [(26.7 × Weight [kg]) + (903 × Height [m])]} + 25	PA = 1.00 if physical activity level is sedentary PA = 1.13 if physical activity level is low active PA = 1.26 if physical activity level is active PA = 1.42 if physical activity level is very active
Females	EER (kcal/day) = 135.3 − (30.8 × Age [yrs]) + {Physical Activity × [(10.0 × Weight [kg]) + (934 × Height [m])]} + 25	PA = 1.00 if physical activity level is sedentary PA = 1.16 if physical activity level is low active PA = 1.31 if physical activity level is active PA = 1.56 if physical activity level is very active

Source: Institute of Medicine, Food and Nutrition Board, *Dietary Reference Intakes for Energy, Carbohydrates, Fiber, Fat, Protein and Amino Acids (Macronutrients)* (Washington, DC: The National Academy of Sciences, 2002), 5–55 and 5–56.

The iron needs of adolescents are relatively high; this is because iron is needed to replace the blood lost during menstruation in girls and to support the growth of muscle mass in boys. The RDA for iron for boys is 11 mg/day, while the RDA for girls is 15 mg/day. If energy intake is adequate and adolescents consume heme-iron food sources such as animal products each day, they should be able to meet the RDA for iron. However, many young people adopt a vegetarian lifestyle during this life stage, or they consume foods that have limited nutrient density. Both of these situations can prevent adolescents from meeting the RDA for iron.

Vitamin A is critical to support the rapid growth and development that occurs during adolescence. The RDA for vitamin A is 900 µg per day for boys and 700 µg per day for girls. These individuals can meet this RDA by consuming at least 5 servings of fruits and vegetables each day. As with iron and calcium, meeting the RDA for vitamin A can be a challenging goal in this age group due to their potential to make less healthful food choices.

If an adolescent is unable or unwilling to eat adequate amounts of nutrient-dense foods, then a multivitamin and mineral supplement that provides no more than 100% of the Daily Value for the micronutrients could be very beneficial as a safety net. As with younger children and adults, a supplement should not be considered a substitute for a balanced, healthful diet.

Fluid Recommendations for Adolescents

The fluid needs of adolescents are higher than those for children due to their higher physical activity levels and to the extensive growth and development that occurs during this phase of life. The AI for total fluid for adolescent boys is 3.3 liters per day (or 14 cups), which includes about 2.6 liters (or 11 cups) as total beverages, including drinking water. The AI for total fluid for adolescent girls is 2.3 liters per day (or 10 cups), which includes about 1.8 liters (or 8 cups) as total beverages, including drinking water. Boys are generally more active than girls and have more lean tissue, thus they require a higher fluid intake to maintain fluid balance. Highly active adolescents who are exercising in the heat may have higher fluid needs than the AI, and these individuals should be encouraged to drink often to quench their thirst and avoid dehydration.

> **Recap:** Energy needs for adolescents can be very high, and adequate energy is needed to support growth, maturation, and physical activity. Fat intake should be 25 to 35% of total energy, and carbohydrate intake should be 45 to 65% of total energy intake. Because many adolescents fail to eat a variety of nutrient-dense foods, intakes of many nutrients such as calcium, iron, and vitamin A may be deficient. Calcium is needed to optimize bone growth and to achieve peak bone density, and iron needs are increased due to increased muscle mass in boys and to menstruation in girls.

Encouraging Nutritious Food Choices with Adolescents

At this point in their lives, adolescents are making most of their own food choices, and many are also buying and preparing a significant amount of the foods they consume. Although parents can still be effective role models, adolescents are generally strongly influenced by their peers, their preferences, and their own developing sense of what foods comprise a healthful and adequate diet.

One particular area of concern in the adolescent diet is a lack of vegetables, fruits, and whole grains. Many teens eat on the run, skip meals, and select fast foods and convenience foods because they are inexpensive, accessible, and taste good. Parents, caretakers, and school food-service programs can capitalize on adolescents' preferences for pizza, burgers, spaghetti, and sandwiches by providing more healthful meat and cheese alternatives, whole-grain breads, and plenty of appealing vegetable-based sides or additions to these foods. In addition, keeping healthful snacks such as fruits

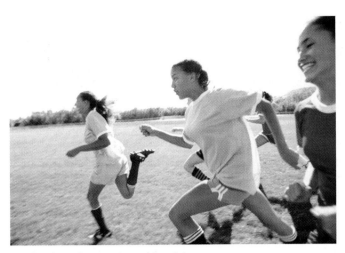

Regular physical activity is good for adolescents.

and vegetables that are already cleaned and prepared in easy-to-eat pieces may encourage adolescents to consume more of these foods as between-meal snacks. Teens should also be encouraged to consume adequate milk and other calcium-enriched beverages.

Nutrition-Related Concerns for Adolescents

Nutrition-related concerns for adolescents continue to include weight concerns and body-image issues. Additional concerns include cigarette smoking and the use of alcohol and illegal drugs.

Obesity Watch: Balancing Food and Physical Activity to Encourage Healthful Weight Gain

Although expected and desirable, weight gain during adolescence can become excessive if increased energy intake is not balanced with adequate physical activity. Overweight and obesity is on the rise for children and adults of all ages, and it is estimated that about 15% of all youth are overweight (Nutrition and Physical Activity Work Group 2002). Many overweight and obese adolescents already have at least one risk factor for heart disease such as high blood pressure, elevated blood cholesterol, or type 2 diabetes.

As with younger children, a reduction in regular physical activity is a significant factor in adolescent obesity. Nearly half of all youths ages 12 to 21 years in the United States are not vigorously active on a regular basis, and about 14% of young people report doing no physical activity; physical inactivity is more common in females (14%) than in males (7%) (CDC 1999). By offering daily physical education in school and by providing more opportunities and encouragement for adolescents to participate in regular physical activity outside of school, the prevalence of overweight and obesity among adolescents can be reduced.

Disordered Eating and Eating Disorders

An initially healthful concern about body image and weight can turn into a dangerous obsession during this emotionally challenging life stage. Clinical eating disorders frequently begin during adolescence and can occur in boys as well as girls. Parents, teachers, and friends should be aware of the warning signs, which include rapid and excessive weight loss, a preoccupation with weight and body image, going to the bathroom regularly after meals, and signs of frequent vomiting or laxative use. Refer to Chapter 13 for a full discussion of eating disorders.

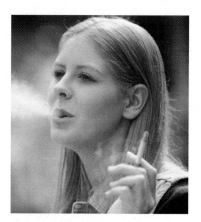

Cigarette smoking may interfere with nutrient absorption.

Other Nutrition-Related Concerns

Cigarette smoking and alcohol and illegal drug use are additional nutritional concerns that face adolescents. Adolescents are naturally curious and most are open to experimenting with tobacco, illegal drugs, and alcohol. Cigarette smoking diminishes appetite and can interfere with nutrient absorption. Indeed, it is frequently used by adolescent girls to maintain a low body weight. The short-term effects of smoking include damage to the lungs and respiratory system, addiction to nicotine, and increased incidence of participation in other risky behaviors such as alcohol and drug abuse, fighting, and engaging in unprotected sex. Most people who begin smoking during adolescence continue to smoke throughout adulthood, increasing their risks for lung cancer, heart disease, osteoporosis, and emphysema. Other consequences of cigarette smoking for adolescents include (CDC 2000):

- Reduced physical fitness and poor exercise endurance
- Inhibition of normal lung growth and maximal lung function
- Increased incidence of respiratory illnesses
- Increased risk of addiction to nicotine
- Poor overall health

Alcohol and drug use can start at early ages, even in school-aged children. The primary cause of death among high-school aged youth is a motor vehicle accident; the risk of being involved in an accident is greatly increased by using alcohol and illegal drugs. Alcohol can also interfere with proper nutrient absorption and metabolism, and it can take the place of foods in an adolescent's diet; these adverse effects of alcohol put adolescents at risk for various nutrient deficiencies. Alcohol and marijuana use are also associated with getting "the munchies," a feeling of food craving which usually results in people eating large quantities of high-fat, high-sugar, nutrient-poor foods. This behavior can result in overweight or obesity, and also increases the risk of nutrient deficiencies. Teens who use drugs and alcohol are typically in poor condition, are either underweight or overweight, have poor appetites, and perform poorly in school.

> **Recap:** Adolescents' food choices are influenced by peer pressure, personal preferences, and their own developing sense of what foods are healthful. Adolescents are at risk for skipping meals and selecting fast foods and snack foods in place of whole grains, fruits, and vegetables. Milk is commonly replaced with sugared soft drinks. Obesity can occur during adolescence because of increased appetite and food intake and decreased physical activity. Disordered eating behaviors, eating disorders, cigarette smoking, and use of alcohol and illegal drugs are also concerns for this age group.

Nutrition for Young and Middle Adults, Age 19–64 Years

The majority of information in this text is directed toward nutrition for young and middle-aged adults. Thus, here we provide simply a brief summary for this age group.

Adult Growth and Activity Patterns

The young adult and middle-aged years are primarily concerned with maintenance of health and our body tissues. Maximal height has been attained, and our goal is to maintain a healthful body weight. Peak bone mass is generally achieved by some time in our twenties, and bone mass starts to decline in our mid- to late-thirties. Thus, our goal in relation to bone is to build as much as we can during our childhood and adolescence and to maintain as much as we can during young- and middle-adulthood so we can decrease our risk for osteoporosis as we age. We can accomplish this by being physically active on a regular basis, getting enough sun or taking a supplement to maintain a healthful vitamin D status, and by eating a balanced diet that contains adequate energy, calcium, phosphorus, and magnesium.

Young- and middle-adulthood is also a time where we become more concerned with our risk for chronic diseases such as heart disease, type 2 diabetes, and various cancers. This is a critical time to establish and maintain a physically active lifestyle and to pay particularly close attention to consuming adequate amounts of fruits, vegetables, whole grains, and lower fat foods.

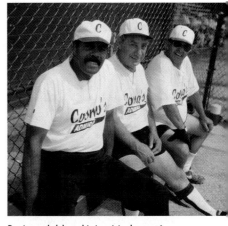

During adulthood it is critical to maintain an active lifestyle; a sports team is one way to stay active.

What Are an Adult's Nutrient Needs?

The nutrient needs for young- and middle-aged adults are covered in detail throughout this text. Refer to the appropriate chapter to review needs related to specific nutrients and illnesses. In addition, the DRIs for all life stages can be found inside the back cover of this text.

Nutrition-Related Concerns for Adults

The primary nutrition-related concerns of young and middle-aged adults are maintaining a balanced, healthful diet and a physically active lifestyle that can help reduce our risks for chronic diseases and the disabilities and premature death that can accompany them. This age group also needs to consume a diet that supports optimal functioning of the immune system and the maintenance and repair of body tissues.

> **Recap:** The majority of this text is directed toward the nutritional needs of young and middle-aged adults. The young adult and middle-aged years are primarily concerned with the maintenance of health and body tissues. Nutritional concerns include bone loss and increased risk for osteoporosis, obesity, and chronic diseases such as heart disease, type 2 diabetes, and various cancers. Eating a healthful diet, maintaining a healthful body weight, and being physically active on a regular basis reduces the risks for these diseases.

Nutrition for Older Adults, Age 65 Years and Older

The U.S. population is getting older each year. It is estimated that by the year 2030, about 20% of Americans will be 65 years of age and older (CDC 2004). In 2001, average life expectancy reached 77.2 years (CDC 2004). These statistics have important implications for people of all ages, since a nutritious diet and regular physical activity can help prevent chronic diseases and keep us happy and productive in our later years. Let's now explore the unique nutritional needs and concerns of older adults.

Older Adult Growth and Activity Patterns

Older adulthood is a time in which growth is complete and our body systems begin to slow and degenerate. While aging of our body tissues is inevitable, eating a healthful diet and living a physically active lifestyle can help slow this process.

Some of the physiological changes that occur with aging include:

- Decreased muscle mass and lean tissue
- Increased fat mass
- Decreased bone density
- Decreased immune function
- Impaired ability to absorb or metabolize various nutrients

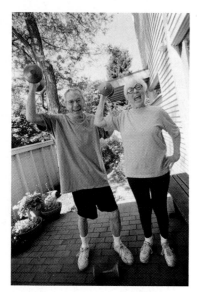

Older adults should participate in strengthening exercises to reduce the risks for low bone mass and muscle weakness.

If these changes disturb you, remember that they are at least partly within your control. For instance, some of the decrease seen in muscle mass, bone mass, and muscle strength is due to low physical activity levels. Older adults who regularly participate in strengthening exercises and aerobic-type activities have reduced risks for low bone mass and muscle atrophy and weakness, which in turn reduces their risk for falls and the fractures related to falls that commonly occur in this population.

Recap: Older adults have the greatest risk for chronic diseases and related disabilities. Growth is complete, and body systems begin to degenerate with aging. The physiological changes that occur with aging include loss of muscle mass and lean tissue, increased fat mass, decreased bone density, decreased immune function, and impaired ability to absorb and metabolize various nutrients. These changes influence the nutritional needs of older adults.

What Are an Older Adult's Nutrient Needs?

The requirements for many nutrients are the same for older adults as for young and middle-aged adults. A few nutrient requirements increase, and a few are actually lower. Table 16.3 identifies nutrient recommendations that do change, as well as the physiologic reason behind these changes.

Energy and Macronutrient Recommendations for Older Adults

The energy needs of older adults are lower than those of younger adults. This decrease is due to loss of muscle mass and lean tissue, a reduction in thyroid hormones, and a less physically active lifestyle. It is estimated that total daily energy expenditure decreases approximately 10 kcal each year for men and 7 kcal each year for women ages 19 and older (Institute of Medicine 2002). This means that a woman who needs 2,000 kcal at age 20 needs just 1,650 at age 70. Some of this decrease in energy expenditure is an inevitable response to aging, but some of the decrease can be delayed or minimized by staying physically active. Because their total daily energy needs are lower, older adults need to pay particularly close attention to consuming a diet high in nutrient-dense foods but not too high in energy in order to avoid weight gain. Refer to the Nutrition Debate at the end of this chapter to learn more about how energy-restricted diets may significantly prolong our lives.

Table 16.3   Nutrient Recommendations That Change with Increased Age

Changes in Nutrient Recommendations	Rationale for Changes
Increased need for vitamin D from 5 µg/day for young adults to 10 µg/day for adults 51 to 70 years and to 15 µg/day for adults over age 70 years.	• Decreased bone density • Decreased ability to convert vitamin D to its active form in our skin • Decreased absorption of dietary calcium
Increased need for calcium from 1,000 mg/day for young adults to 1,200 mg/day for adults 51 years of age and older.	• Decreased bone density • Decreased absorption of dietary calcium
Decreased need for fiber from 38 grams/day for young men to 30 grams/day for men 51 years and older. Decreases for women are from 25 grams/day for young women to 21 grams/day for women 51 years and older.	• Decreased energy intake
Increased need for vitamins B$_6$ and B$_{12}$	• Lower levels of stomach acid • Decreased absorption from gastrointestinal tract • Increased need to reduce homocysteine levels and to optimize immune function

Because there is no evidence suggesting a minimal amount of dietary fat needed to maintain health, there is no DRI for total fat intake for older adults. However, to reduce their risk for heart disease and other chronic diseases, it is recommended that total fat intake remain within 20 to 35% of total daily energy intake, with no more than 10% of total energy intake coming from saturated fat.

The RDA for carbohydrate for older adults is 130 grams/day. As with all other age groups, this level of carbohydrate is sufficient to support brain glucose utilization. There is no evidence to indicate what percentage of carbohydrate should come from sugars or starches. However, it is recommended that older individuals consume a diet that contains no more than 30% of total energy intake as sugars (Institute of Medicine 2002). The fiber recommendations are slightly lower for older adults than for younger adults because older adults eat less energy. After age 50, 30 grams of fiber per day for men and 21 for women is assumed sufficient to reduce the risks for constipation and diverticular disease, maintain healthful blood levels of glucose and lipids, and provide good sources of nutrient-dense, low-energy foods.

The recommendation for protein is the same for adults of all ages: 0.80 grams/protein per body weight per day. Protein is critically needed to help reduce the loss of muscle and lean tissue, and it is also critical to help prevent excessive loss of bone. Many protein foods are also important sources of vitamins and minerals that are typically low in the diets of older adults; thus, protein is an important nutrient for this age group.

Micronutrient Recommendations for Older Adults

The vitamins and minerals of particular concern for older adults are identified in Table 16.3 (page 600). Preventing or minimizing the consequences of osteoporosis is a top priority for older adults. The requirements for both calcium and vitamin D are higher because of a reduced absorption of calcium from the gut, along with reduced production of the active form of vitamin D in our skin as a result of aging. Many older adults are at risk for vitamin D deficiency because they are institutionalized and are not exposed to adequate amounts of sunlight. It is critical that older adults consume foods that are high in calcium and vitamin D, and in many cases supplements are necessary.

Iron needs decrease with aging. This decrease is primarily due to reduced muscle and lean tissue in both men and women and the cessation of menstruation in women. The decreased need for iron in older men is not significant enough to change the recommendations for iron intake in this group, thus the RDA for iron is the same for older men as for younger, 8 mg/day. However, the RDA for iron in older women is 8 mg/day, which is 10 mg/day lower than the RDA for younger women. Although zinc recommendations are the same for all adults, it is important to emphasize that zinc is a critical nutrient for optimizing immune function and wound healing in older adults. Intakes of both zinc and iron can be inadequate in older adults because they may eat less of the food sources that supply these nutrients, such as red meats, poultry, and fish. These foods are relatively expensive and many older adults on a limited income cannot afford to eat them regularly. Also, older adults may have a difficult time chewing meats due to loss of teeth and/or use of dentures.

Although it is speculated that older adults have increased oxidative stress, the recommendations for vitamin C and vitamin E are the same as for younger adults because there is insufficient evidence that consuming amounts higher than the current RDA for these nutrients has any additional health benefits (Institute of Medicine 2000).

Older adults need to pay close attention to consuming adequate amounts of the B-complex vitamins, specifically vitamin B_{12}, vitamin B_6, and folate. As discussed in detail on pages 353–355, inadequate intakes of these nutrients increases the levels of the amino acid homocysteine in the blood, and elevated homocysteine levels are associated with an increased risk for cardiovascular, cerebrovascular, and peripheral vascular diseases (Beresford and Boushey 1997). These diseases are common among older adults. The RDA for vitamin B_{12} is the same for younger and older adults, but up to 30% of older adults cannot absorb enough vitamin B_{12} from foods due to atrophic gastritis (see page 354). It is recommended that older adults consume foods that are fortified with vitamin B_{12} or supplements because the vitamin B_{12} in these sources is absorbed more readily. Vitamin B_6 recommendations are slightly higher for older adults, as these higher levels appear necessary to reduce homocysteine levels and optimize immune function in this population (Institute of Medicine 1998).

Vitamin A requirements are the same for adults of all ages; however, older adults should be careful not to consume more than the RDA, as absorption of vitamin A is actually greater in older adults. Thus, this group is at greater risk for vitamin A toxicity, which can cause liver damage and neurological problems. However, consuming foods high in beta-carotene or other carotenoids is safe and does not lead to vitamin A toxicity in this age group.

A variety of factors may limit an older adult's ability to eat healthfully. These include limited financial resources that prevent some older people from buying nutrient-dense foods on a regular basis, reduced appetite, social isolation, inability to prepare foods, and illnesses and physiological changes that limit the absorption and metabolism of many nutrients. Thus, some older adults may benefit from taking a multivitamin and mineral supplement that contains no more than the RDA for all nutrients contained in the supplement. Additional supplementation may be necessary for nutrients such as calcium, vitamin D, and vitamin B_{12}. However, supplementation with individual nutrients should only be done under the supervision of the individual's primary healthcare provider, as the risk of nutrient toxicity is high in this population.

Gustavo *Nutri-Case*

"I don't believe in taking vitamins. If you eat good food, you get everything you need and it's the way nature intended it. My daughter kept nagging at my wife and me to start taking B vitamins. She said when people get to be our age they have problems with their nerves if they don't. I didn't fall for it, but my wife did, and then her doctor told her she needed calcium pills and vitamin D, too. The kitchen counter is starting to look like a medicine chest! You know what I think? I think this whole vitamin thing is just a hoax to get you to empty your wallet."

Would you support Gustavo's decision to avoid taking B vitamin supplements? Given what you have learned in previous Nutri-Cases about Gustavo's wife, would you support or oppose her taking a vitamin B, calcium, or vitamin D supplement? Explain your choices.

Fluid Recommendations for Older Adults

The AI for fluid is the same for older and younger adults. Men should consume 3.7 liters (about 15.5 cups) of total water per day, which includes 3.0 liters (about 13 cups) as total beverages, including drinking water. Women should consume 2.7 liters (about 12.7 cups) of total water per day, which includes 2.2 liters (about 9 cups) as total beverages, including drinking water. It is important to emphasize that kidney function changes as we age, and the thirst mechanism of older people can be impaired. These changes can result in chronic dehydration and hypernatremia (elevated blood sodium levels) in this population. Some older adults will intentionally limit their beverage intake because they have urinary incontinence. This practice can endanger their health, so it is important for these individuals to seek treatment for the incontinence and continue to drink plenty of fluids.

Recap: Older adults have lower energy needs due to their loss of lean tissue and lower physical activity levels. Older adults should consume 20 to 35% of total energy as fat and 45 to 65% of their energy as carbohydrate. Protein recommendations are the same as for younger adults. Micronutrients of concern for older adults include calcium, vitamin D, iron, zinc, vitamin B_{12}, vitamin B_6, and folate. Older adults need to carefully select nutrient-dense foods to meet their micronutrient needs, and supplementation may be necessary. Older adults are at risk for chronic dehydration and hypernatremia, so ample fluid intake should be encouraged.

Nutrition-Related Concerns for Older Adults

Older adults have a number of unique nutritional concerns. In addition to body weight issues, they commonly experience changes in taste and appetite. They may also face dental problems, potential interactions between nutrients and medications, and diseases that affect their memory. Each of these concerns is discussed briefly in the following sections.

Overweight and Underweight: A Delicate Balancing Act

Not surprisingly, overweight and obesity are also a concern for older adults. This population has a high risk for heart disease, hypertension, type 2 diabetes, and cancer, and these diseases are more prevalent in people who are overweight or obese. In contrast, overweight can be protective against osteoporosis and fall-related fractures in older adults.

Underweight is also risky for older adults. Many older adults lose weight as a result of illness, disability, poor nutritional status, alcoholism, or smoking. Many lose the ability to smell and taste, and the loss of these senses is associated with lower appetite and reduced food and nutrient intakes (Kim et al. 2003). Limited income, mobility or transportation problems, or concerns about neighborhood safety may make food shopping difficult for elders. Other significant risk factors for underweight in older adults are depression and social isolation, which can develop following the death of family members and friends, or when adult children move out of the area. Depression and isolation can cause older adults to lose the desire to prepare nourishing meals for themselves. Any of these factors can result in underweight and frailty, significantly increasing the person's risk of serious illnesses and injuries. Community food-service programs can thus be life-saving. These include:

- Seniors' Farmers Market Nutrition Program, which is sponsored by the U.S. Department of Agriculture, provides coupons to low-income seniors so they can buy eligible foods at farmers' markets, roadside stands, and community-supported agricultural programs
- food stamps and commodity foods, which are available to low-income seniors through the state departments of health
- food pantries, which typically offer canned goods and other nonperishable items free of charge
- soup kitchens, which offer lunches and other meals at a community location such as a church hall
- Meals on Wheels, a nonprofit organization that delivers fully prepared meals to homebound ill and elderly clients (Figure 16.10).

In summary, maintaining a healthful weight and a physically and socially active lifestyle helps elders live stronger, healthier, and more satisfying lives.

Dental Health Issues

Many older adults have lost their teeth, suffer from gum disease, or have poorly fitting dentures. These conditions cause considerable mouth pain and make chewing difficult and sometimes embarrassing. Because of these dental health challenges, older adults may avoid eating foods such as meats and firm fruits and vegetables. Avoidance of these foods leads to nutrient deficiencies and an increased risk for illness and infection. Gum disease and other infections in the mouth can also increase the risk for heart disease. Maintaining good oral health and having regular dental checkups are thus critical to an older adult's nutrition and overall health.

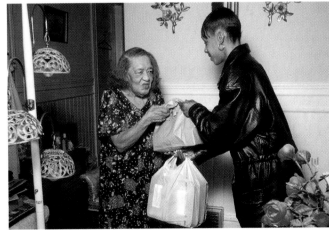

Figure 16.10   For homebound disabled and older adults, community programs such as Meals on Wheels provide nourishing, balanced meals as well as vital social contact.

Other Nutrition-Related Concerns

Many older adults take multiple medications daily. Some of these medications can alter nutrient absorption and metabolism, and many affect appetite. For example, people taking the blood-thinning drug Coumadin should avoid consuming excess vitamin E, as vitamin E magnifies the effects of this drug. Both ibuprofen (Motrin) and acetaminophen (Tylenol) are commonly prescribed for muscle, joint, and headache pain, but taking these drugs with alcohol increases the risk for liver damage and bleeding, so alcohol should not be consumed with these medications.

Older adults are also at higher risk for Alzheimer's disease and other forms of dementia. These illnesses affect memory and movement, interfering and potentially preventing older adults from being able to choose, prepare, and consume a healthful diet. Interestingly, recent studies show that eating a balanced, wholesome diet that includes ample folate, vitamin B_{12} and macronutrients can improve memory and decrease the risk for Alzheimer's disease and other forms of dementia in older adults (Kaplan et al. 2001; Barberger-Gateau et al. 2002; Morris et al. 2003). These studies emphasize the critical importance to older adults of consuming a balanced, healthful diet and supplementing as needed.

Recap: Overweight and obesity are an important concern for older adults, as they increase the risk for chronic diseases. Underweight and frailty are also concerns, as these conditions can lead to increased illness and injury. Older adults may lose their sense of smell and taste, and dental problems can limit intake of meats, fruits, and vegetables; this can lead to nutrient deficiencies. Medications and certain nutrients can have adverse interactions. Alzheimer's disease and other forms of dementia affect memory and mobility and interfere with food preparation and consumption. Nutrient-rich diets have been shown to improve memory and reduce the risk of Alzheimer's disease and other forms of dementia in older adults.

Chapter Summary

- Toddlers grow more slowly than infants but are far more active. They require small, frequent, nutritious snacks and meals, and food should be cut in small pieces so it is easy to handle and swallow.

- For toddlers and preschoolers, a serving of food equals one tablespoon for each year of age. For example, four tablespoons of yogurt is a full serving for a four-year-old child.

- Energy, fat, and protein requirements are higher for toddlers than for infants. Many toddlers will not eat vegetables, so micronutrients of concern include vitamins A, C, and E.

- Until age two, toddlers should drink whole milk rather than reduced-fat milk to meet calcium requirements. Iron deficiency is a concern in the toddler years and can be minimized by the consumption of foods naturally high in iron and iron-fortified foods.

- Toddlers are still at risk for choking, and parents should watch for allergies and monitor weight gain.

- Feeding vegan diets to toddlers is controversial and poses potential deficiencies for protein, iron, calcium, zinc, vitamin D, and vitamin B_{12}.

- Preschoolers have a slower growth rate than toddlers and may have a reduced appetite. Preschoolers are more physically active than toddlers, and playing can sometimes interfere with eating adequate food.

- Preschoolers need less fat than toddlers but slightly more than adults. Protein and energy needs are higher for preschoolers due to their larger size and higher activity levels. Calcium, iron, and zinc requirements are slightly higher for preschoolers than toddlers. Preschoolers can become easily dehydrated because they ignore or fail to recognize their thirst.

- Overweight and obesity are concerns for preschoolers and can be avoided by regular physical activity and eating a healthful diet. Dental caries are also of concern,

- and preschoolers should brush their teeth regularly, limit sweets, and visit the dentist regularly beginning at age three.

- School-aged children are more independent and can make more of their own food choices. Physical activity levels can vary dramatically.

- Sexual maturation begins during the early school-age years. School-aged children should eat 25 to 35% of their total energy as fat and 45 to 65% of their total energy as carbohydrate. Calcium needs increase as children mature, while iron needs decrease slightly.

- Many school-aged children skip breakfast and do not choose healthful foods during school lunch. Peer pressure and popularity are strong influences on food choices. School lunches are nutritious and meet federal guidelines, but the foods that children choose to eat at school, both during and outside of the lunch break, can be high in fat, sugar, and energy and low in nutrients.

- Obesity is an increasing concern for school-aged children. Children should be physically active at least one hour every day. Disordered eating behaviors and eating disorders can result from concerns about body image. Consuming adequate calcium to support the development of peak bone mass is a primary concern for school-aged children.

- Puberty is the period in life in which secondary sexual characteristics develop and the physical capability to reproduce begins. Puberty results in rapid increases in height, weight, and lean body mass and fat mass.

- Energy needs for adolescents are variable and can be quite high, and adequate energy is needed to support growth, maturation, and physical activity. Fat intake should be 25 to 35% of total energy, and carbohydrate intake should be 45 to 65% of total energy intake.

- Many adolescents replace whole grains, fruits, and vegetables with fast foods and snack foods, placing them at risk for deficiencies for calcium, iron, and vitamin A. Calcium is needed to optimize bone growth and to achieve peak bone density, and iron needs are increased because of increased muscle mass in boys and menstruation in girls.

- Obesity can occur during adolescence if food intake increases and physical activity decreases. Disordered eating behaviors, eating disorders, cigarette smoking, and use of alcohol and illegal drugs are also concerns for this age group.

- The young adult and middle-aged years are primarily concerned with the maintenance of health and body tissues. Nutritional concerns include bone loss and increased risk for osteoporosis, obesity, and chronic diseases such as heart disease, type 2 diabetes, and various cancers.

- Growth is complete in older adults, and their body systems begin to degenerate as part of the normal aging process. Some of the physiological changes that occur with aging include loss of muscle mass and lean tissue, increased fat mass, decreased bone density, decreased immune function, and impaired ability to absorb and metabolize various nutrients. A nutritious diet and regular physical activity can reduce the rate of some of these changes.

- Older adults have lower energy needs due to their loss of lean tissue and lower physical activity levels. Older adults should consume 20 to 35% of total energy as fat and 45 to 65% of their energy as carbohydrate. Protein recommendations are the same as for younger adults.

- Micronutrients of concern for older adults include calcium, vitamin D, iron, zinc, vitamin B_{12}, vitamin B_6, and folate. Older adults need to carefully select nutrient-dense foods to meet their micronutrient needs, and supplementation may be necessary. Older adults are at risk for chronic dehydration and hypernatremia, so ample fluid intake should be encouraged.

- Overweight and obesity are important concerns for older adults, as they increase the risk for chronic diseases. A variety of factors also increase the older adult's risk for underweight.

- Medications can interfere with nutrient absorption and metabolism, and nutrients can also interfere with the actions of medications.

- Alzheimer's disease and other forms of dementia affect memory and movement and interfere with food preparation and consumption. Varied, nutritious diets have been shown to improve memory and reduce the risk of Alzheimer's disease and other forms of dementia in older adults.

Review Questions

1. Which of the following nutrients is needed in increased amounts in older adulthood?
   a. fiber
   b. vitamin D
   c. protein
   d. vitamin A

2. Carbohydrate should make up what percentage of total energy for school-aged children?
   a. 25 to 40%
   b. 35 to 50%
   c. 45 to 60%
   d. 45 to 70%

3. Which of the following is a major nutrition-related concern for preschoolers?
    a. choking
    b. skipping breakfast
    c. botulism
    d. dental caries

4. Which of the following breakfasts would be most appropriate to serve a twenty-month-old child?
    a. ½ cup of iron-fortified cooked oat cereal, two tablespoons of mashed pineapple, and one cup of whole milk
    b. two tablespoons of nonfat yogurt, two tablespoons of applesauce, one slice of melba toast spread with strawberry preserve, and one cup of calcium-fortified orange juice
    c. ½ cup of iron-fortified cooked oat cereal, ¼ cup of cubed pineapple, and one cup of low-fat milk
    d. two small link sausages cut in 1-inch pieces, two tablespoons of scrambled egg, one slice of whole-wheat toast, four cherry tomatoes, two tablespoons of applesauce, and one cup of whole milk.

5. Which of the following statements about cigarette smoking is true?
    a. Cigarette smoking can interfere with the absorption of nutrients.
    b. Cigarette smoking commonly causes food cravings such as "getting the munchies."
    c. Cigarette smoking is the number-one cause of death in adolescents.
    d. All of the above statements are true.

6. True or False? Preschool children are too young to understand and be influenced by their parents' examples.

7. True or False? The food choice patterns of school-aged children are heavily influenced by circumstances at school.

8. True or false? Among adolescents, the prevalence of clinical eating disorders exceeds that of obesity.

9. True or false? The DRI for fat for toddlers is 40 grams/day.

10. True or false? Older adults who regularly participate in strengthening and aerobic exercises have a reduced risk for fractures.

11. Identify some advantages and disadvantages of modern technology (such as television and computers) in terms of their impact on lifestyle and nutrition.

12. Explain why a toddler in a vegan family might be at risk for protein deficiency.

13. Imagine that you are taking care of four five-year-old children for an afternoon. Design a menu for the children's lunch that is nutritious and that will be fun for them to eat.

14. Imagine that you manage a college cafeteria. Design a menu with three lunch choices that are nutritious and that are likely to be popular with 18 to 21-year-old students.

15. You and your parents live in Dallas, where you attend college and your parents are employed as architects. A year ago, your maternal grandmother, who lives in Boston, stayed with you for several weeks following the death of your grandfather. She seemed fit at the time, going for walks with you and your dog, and cooking large meals for your family and special treats for you throughout her stay. Last night your mother received a phone call from a Boston hospital saying that her mother had been admitted following a hip fracture suffered in a fall at home and was battling significant dehydration and moderate dementia as well. Identify several factors that might have contributed to your grandmother's condition.

Test Yourself Answers

1. **False**. Toddlers have a higher need for fat than do older children or adults so they should consume foods that are higher in fat.

2. **True**. Girls may only grow a few more inches after menstruation begins, while boys continue to grow throughout adolescence and even into early adulthood.

3. **True**. Although toddlers and preschoolers need slightly more fat than adults, these children should be encouraged to consume whole grain foods, fruits, and vegetables.

4. **True**. Although a reduction of muscle mass and lean tissue is inevitable with aging, some of this loss can be attenuated with regular physical activity.

5. **False**. Older adults may need to supplement certain nutrients such as calcium and vitamin B$_{12}$, but people in this age group are at increased risk for vitamin toxicity. In addition, certain nutrients and medications can interact to cause significant health problems, so supplementation with individual nutrients should occur only with the supervision of a trained healthcare professional.

Web Links

www.kidnetic.com

Kidnetic.com

A fun Web site developed to help children and families get active, providing instructions and ideas for physical games and challenges, recipes for kids to make, and information about nutrition and the body.

www.kidsnutrition.org

USDA/ARS Children's Nutrition Research Center at Baylor College of Medicine

This site provides information about current research projects, nutrition Web links, and consumer and nutrition news.

www.keepkidshealthy.com

Keep Kids Healthy.com

Find information about nutrition and health for toddlers, children, and adolescents on this Web site.

www.cdc.gov

The Centers for Disease Control

Click on Health Promotion, then you can select topics such as Adolescent Health, Project VERB_{TM}, Aging & Elderly Health, Men's Health, or Women's Health, plus many others.

www.vrg.org

The Vegetarian Resource Group

Visit this Web site to learn more about vegetarianism for all ages. Included on the site are special sections for teens and kids, as well as recipes and guides for vegetarian and vegan eating in all kinds of situations.

www.health.gov/dietaryguidelines

Dietary Guidelines for Americans

Visit this site to read the current edition of Dietary Guidelines for Americans and to learn about their development.

www.fns.usda.gov

USDA Food & Nutrition Services

Read about governmental programs to provide food to all ages, including school meals programs; the Child and Adult Care Food Program; and the Women, Infants, and Children Program.

www.nlm.nih.gov/medlineplus/dentalhealth.html

Medline Plus Dental Health

Contained on this site are links to articles about dental health for all ages.

www.eatright.org

American Dietetic Association

Visit this Web site to learn about healthy eating habits for all stages of life.

www.healthandage.com

Health and Age

This site lists comprehensive information about nutrition, exercise, and preventative medicine with relation to aging. Features include a section for caregivers and a newsletter.

References

American Obesity Association. 2004. Obesity in the U.S. http://www.obesity.org/fastfacts/obesity_US.shtml (Accessed 30 April 2004).

Anderson, R. M., M. Latorre-Esteves, A. R. Neves, S. Lavu, O. Medvedik, C. Taylor, K. T. Howitz, H. Santos, and D. A. Sinclair. 2003. Yeast life-span extension by calorie restriction is independent of NAD fluctuation. *Science* 302(5653):2124–2126.

Armstrong, C. 2001. Discoveryhealth.com. Nutrition. School Lunch Program. http://health.discovery.com/diseasesandcond/encyclopedias/1936.html (Accessed April 2004).

Bailey, I. 2001. *National Post.* Daughters, 9 and 5, Starving on a Vegan Diet, Father Claims. http://fact.on.ca/news/news0103/np010305.htm (Accessed April 2004).

Barberger-Gateau P., L. Letenneur, V. Deschamps, K. Peres, J.-F. Dartigues, and S. Renaud. 2002. Fish, meat, and risk of dementia: cohort study. *Br. Med. J.* 325:932–934.

Barrows, C. H., and G. C. Kokkonen. 1982. Dietary restriction and life extension, biological mechanisms. In *Nutritional Approaches to Aging Research*, edited by G. B. Moment. Boca Raton, FL: CRC Press, Inc.

Beresford, S. A., and C. J. Boushey. 1997. Homocysteine, folic acid, and cardiovascular disease risk. In *Preventive Nutrition: The Comprehensive Guide for Health Professionals*, edited by A. Bendich and R. J. Deckelbaum. Totowa, NJ: Humana Press.

Cable News Network (CNN). (2003, June 23). Some obese teens turn to surgery. http://www.cnn.com/2003/HEALTH/diet.fitne . . . /teen.obesity.surgery (Accessed 30 April 2004).

Centers for Disease Control and Prevention (CDC). 1999. National Center for Chronic Disease Prevention and Health Promotion. Physical Activity and Health. A Report of the Surgeon General. Adolescents and Young Adults. http://www.cdc.gov/nccdphp/sgr/adoles.htm (Accessed April 2004).

Centers for Disease Control and Prevention. 2000. National Center for Chronic Disease Prevention and Health Promotion. Tobacco Information and Prevention Source (TIPS). Facts on Youth Smoking, Health, and Performance. http://www.cdc.gov/tobacco/research_data/youth/ythsprt.htm (Accessed April 2004).

Centers for Disease Control and Prevention. 2001. Neurologic impairment in children associated with maternal dietary deficiency of cobalamin. *Morbid. Mortal. Wkly. Rep.* 52(04):61–64.

Centers for Disease Control and Prevention. 2004. National Center for Chronic Disease Prevention and Health Promotion. Healthy Aging. Healthy Aging for Older Adults. http://www.cdc.gov/aging/ (Accessed April 2004).

Cunningham-Sabo, L., M. P. Snyder, J. Anliker, J. Thompson, J. L. Weber, O. Thomas, K. Ring,

D. Stewart, H. Platero, and L. Nielsen. 2003. Impact of the Pathways food service intervention on breakfast served in American-Indian schools. *Preventive Medicine* 37:S46–S54.

Dhahbi, J. M., H.-J. Kim, P. L. Mote, R. J. Beaver, and S. R. Spindler. 2004. Temporal linkage between the phenotypic and genomic responses to caloric restriction. *Proceedings of the National Academy of Sciences* 101(15):5524–5529.

Food and Nutrition Board. Institute of Medicine. 1989. *Recommended Dietary Allowances*, 10th ed. Washington, DC: National Academy Press.

Grady, D. 2004. Operation for obesity leaves some in misery. *New York Times* Science Times Supplement May 4:1, 6.

Heaney, R. P., and K. Rafferty. 2001. Carbonated beverages and urinary calcium excretion. *Am. J. Clin. Nutr.* 74:343–347.

Heilbronn, L. K., and E. Ravussin. 2003. Calorie restriction and aging: review of the literature and implications for studies in humans. *Am. J. Clin. Nutr.* 78(3):361–369.

Himes, J. H., K. Ring, J. Gittelsohn, L. Cunningham-Sabo, J. Weber, J. Thompson, L. Harnack, and C. Suchinidran. 2003. Impact of the Pathways intervention on the dietary intakes of American Indian schoolchildren. *Preventive Medicine* 37:S55–S61.

Institute of Medicine, Food and Nutrition Board. 1997. *Dietary Reference Intakes for Calcium, Phosphorus, Magnesium, Vitamin D, and Fluoride.* Washington, DC: National Academy Press.

Institute of Medicine, Food and Nutrition Board. 1998. *Dietary Reference Intakes for Thiamin, Riboflavin, Niacin, Vitamin B$_6$, Folate, Vitamin B$_{12}$, Pantothenic Acid, Biotin, and Choline.* Washington, DC: National Academy Press.

Institute of Medicine, Food and Nutrition Board. 2000. *Dietary Reference Intakes for Vitamin C, Vitamin E, Selenium, and Carotenoids.* Washington, DC: National Academy Press.

Institute of Medicine, Food and Nutrition Board. 2001. *Dietary Reference Intakes for Vitamin A, Vitamin K, Arsenic, Boron, Chromium, Copper, Iodine, Iron, Manganese, Molybdenum, Nickel, Silicon, Vanadium, and Zinc.* Washington, DC: National Academy Press.

Institute of Medicine, Food and Nutrition Board. 2002. *Dietary Reference Intakes for Energy, Carbohydrates, Fiber, Fat, Protein and Amino Acids (Macronutrients).* Washington, DC: The National Academy of Sciences.

Institute of Medicine, Food and Nutrition Board. 2004. *Dietary Reference Intakes for Water, Potassium, Sodium, Chloride, and Sulfate.* Washington, DC: National Academy Press.

Kaplan, R. J., C. E. Greenwood, G. Winocur, and T. M. S. Wolever. 2001. Dietary protein, carbohydrate, and fat enhance memory performance in the healthy elderly. *Am. J. Clin. Nutr.* 74:687–693.

Kim, W. Y., M. Hur, M. S. Cho, and H. S. Lee. 2003. Effect of olfactory function on nutritional status of Korean elderly women. *Nutr. Res.* 23:723–734.

Kostoff, R. N. 2001. Energy restriction. *Am. J. Clin. Nutr.* 74(4):556–557.

Lagström H., R. Seppänen, E. Jokinen, H. Niinikoski, T. Rönnemaa, J. Viikari, and O. Simell. 1999. Influence of dietary fat on the nutrient intake and growth of children from 1 to 5 years of age: The Special Turku Coronary Risk Factor Intervention Project. *Am. J. Clin. Nutr.* 69:516–523.

Mangels, R. 2001. The Vegetarian Resource Group. Vegetarianism in a Nutshell. Feeding Vegan Kids. http://www.vrg.org/nutshell/kids.htm (Accessed April 2004).

Morris, M. C., D. A. Evans, J. L. Bienias, C. C. Tangney, D. A. Bennett, R. S. Wilson, N. Aggarwal, and J. Schneider. 2003. Consumption of fish and n-3 fatty acids and risk of incident Alzheimer disease. *Arch. Neurol.* 60:940–946.

Niinikoski, H., J. Viikari, T. Rönnemaa, H. Helenius, E. Jokinen, H. Lapinleimu, T. Routi, H. Lagström, R. Seppänen, I. Välimäki, and O. Simell. 1997. Regulation of growth of 7- to 36-month-old children by energy and fat intake in the prospective, randomized STRIP baby trial. *Pediatrics* 100:810–816.

Nutrition and Physical Activity Work Group. 2002. *Guidelines for Comprehensive Programs to Promote Healthy Eating and Physical Activity.* Champaign, IL: Human Kinetics Publishers.

Obarzanek, E., S. A. Hunsberger, L. Van Horn, V. V. Hartmuller, B. A. Barton, V. J. Stevens, P. O. Kwiterovich, F. A. Franklin, S. Y. S. Kimm, N. L. Lasser, D. G. Simons-Morton, and R. M. Lauer. 1997. Safety of a fat-reduced diet: The Dietary Intervention Study in Children (DISC). *Pediatrics* 100:51–59.

Polan, E. U., and D. R. Taylor. 2003. *Journey Across the Lifespan*, 2nd ed. Philadelphia: F. A. Davis.

Roth, G. S., D. K. Ingram, A. Black, and M. A. Lane. 2000. Effects of reduced energy intake on the biology of aging: the primate model. *Eur. J. Clin. Nutr.* 54(Suppl 3):S15–S20.

Second Opinions. 2002. Vegan Child Abuse. http://www.second-opinions.co.uk/child_abuse.html (Accessed April 2004).

Talanian, D. 2003. Young people opt for bariatric surgery. *The Orange County Register.* March 3, http://www.charleston.net/stories/030303/Sci_03 bari.shtml (Accessed April 2004).

Torgan, C. 2002, June. Childhood Obesity on the Rise. The NIH Word on Health. http://www.nih.gov/news/WordonHealth/jun2002/childhoodobesity.htm (Accessed April 30, 2004).

USDA/ARS Children's Nutrition Research Center at Baylor College of Medicine. 1999. Consumer News—Facts and Answers. Hunger Hinders School Performance. http://www.kidsnutrition.org/

consumer/archives/breakfast-fuel.htm (Accessed April 2004).

U.S. Department of Agriculture (USDA) and U.S. Department of Health and Human Services (USDHHS). 2000. Dietary Guidelines for Americans, 2000. 5th ed., Home and Garden Bulletin, No. 232. (Available at http://www.health.gov/dietaryguidelines/dga2000/document/frontcover.htm Accessed March 2004).

USDA. Food and Nutrition Service. 2003. National School Lunch Program. http://www.fns.usda.gov/cnd/Lunch/AboutLunch/NSLPFactSheet.htm (Accessed April 2004).

USDA. Food and Nutrition Service. 2003. School Breakfast Program. Healthy Eating Helps You Make the Grade. http://www.fns.usda.gov/cnd/Breakfast/SchoolBfastCampaign/theresearch.html (Accessed April 2004).

Wang, C., R. Weindruch, J. R. Fernández, C. S. Coffey, P. Patel, and D. B. Allison. 2004. Caloric restriction and body weight independently affect longevity in Wistar rats. *Int. J. Obesity* 28(3):357–362.

Weindruch, R., and R. L. Walford. 1988. *The Retardation of Aging and Disease by Dietary Restriction*. Springfield, IL: Charles C. Thomas Publisher.

Nutrition Debate:

Can We Live Longer by Eating a Low-Energy Diet?

How old do you want to live to be—80 years, 100 years, 120 years? If you were to discover that you could live to be 150 years of age by eating a little more than half of your current energy intake and still be healthy as you age, would you do it? Believe it or not, many people are already doing this in response to studies indicating that low-energy diets can significantly increase the lifespan of animals.

Existing research shows that consuming low-energy diets, also referred to as *caloric restriction*, can significantly extend the lifespan of small species; most of this research has been done in rats, mice, fish, flies, and yeast cells (Barrows and Kokkonen 1982; Weindruch and Walford 1988; Dhahbi et al. 2004; Wang et al. 2004; Anderson et al. 2003). Until recently, we did not know if this same effect would be seen in nonhuman primates and in humans. Roth and colleagues (2000) have summarized the results of ongoing studies of caloric restriction in nonhuman primates, and these results show promise that caloric restriction can improve the health and significantly extend the lifespan of mammals that are very similar to humans.

How can caloric restriction prolong our lifespan? We do not yet know the answer to this question, but it is speculated that the reduction in metabolic rate that occurs with restricting energy intake results in a much lower production of free radicals, which in turn significantly reduces oxidative damage and can prolong life. Caloric restriction also causes marked improvements in insulin sensitivity and results in hormonal changes that result in a lower incidence of chronic diseases such as heart disease and diabetes. In fact, caloric restriction can alter gene expression, which can reduce the effects of aging and prevent diseases such as cancer (Dhahbi et al. 2004). Some of the effects of prolonged caloric restriction in rodents include (Heilbronn and Ravussin 2003):

- Decreased insulin levels and improved insulin sensitivity
- Decreased body temperature
- Decreased energy expenditure
- Decreased oxidative stress
- Decreased fat mass and lean body mass
- Increased levels of voluntary physical activity

It is important to emphasize that species that live longer due to caloric restriction are still fed nutritious diets. Unhealthful energy-restriction situations such as starvation, wasting caused by diseases such as cancer, and eating disorders such as anorexia nervosa do not result in prolonged life. In fact, these situations are associated with increased risks for illness and premature death (Kostoff 2001).

Although caloric restriction is successful in extending the lives of some animal species, there is no direct evidence that this same effect will occur in humans. Studies that can answer this question in humans might never be conducted because of ethical and logistical concerns. Finding enough people to participate in any research study over their entire lifetime would be extremely difficult. In addition, most people find it challenging to follow a caloric-restricted diet for just a few

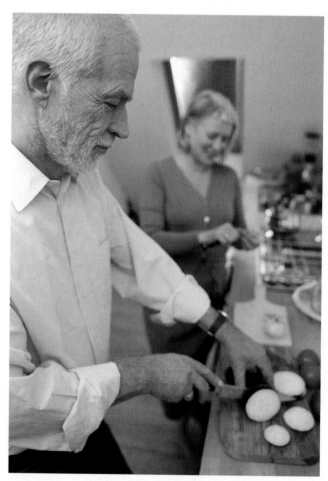

Maintaining a calorically-restricted diet that is also highly nutritious requires significant planning and preparing most of your own meals.

months; compliance to this type of diet over 80 years or more could be almost impossible. Institutional committees that review research studies are hesitant to approve caloric-restriction research in humans not only because of these logistical problems, but also because of the potential risks of malnutrition that could occur.

You may be wondering how much less energy you would have to consume to meet the caloric-restriction levels studied in animals. Most studies have found a significant extension of life span when animals are fed 30 to 40% less energy than control animals. If you are a woman who normally eats about 2,000 kcal/day, this level of reduction would result in an energy intake of about 1,200 to 1,400 kcal per day. While this amount of energy reduction does not seem excessive, it is very difficult to achieve this reduction every day over a lifetime —particularly if you live to be 130 years of age! You must also keep in mind that this diet must be of very high nutritional quality,

which presents a plethora of challenges, including meticulous planning of meals, preparation of most, if not all, of your own foods, limited options for eating meals outside of the home, and the challenge of working the demands of your special diet around the eating behaviors of family members and friends.

Considering the potential benefits of caloric restriction, do you think it is worth following this type of diet? Are you willing to make the sacrifices necessary to try to significantly prolong your life, even though we are unsure if this practice can prolong the lives of humans? If we do find that caloric restriction substantially improves the health of humans and in turn can prolong their lives, should caloric restriction be recommended for all people? This debate will continue as more research is conducted. In the meantime, many people are already consuming diets that are low in energy in the hope that they will live much longer, healthier lives.

Appendices

Appendix A *Nutrient Values of Foods*

The following table of nutrient values is taken from the EvaluEat diet analysis software that is included with every new copy of this text. The foods in the table are just a fraction of the foods provided in the software. When using the software you can quickly find foods shown here by entering the EvaluEat code in the search field. Values are obtained from the USDA Nutrient Database for Standard Reference, Release 16. A "0" indicates that nutrient value is determined to be zero; a blank space indicates that nutrient information is not available.

Amt = serving amount; **Wt** = weight; **Ener** = energy; **Prot** = protein; **Carb** = carbohydrate; **Fiber** = dietary fiber; **Fat** = total fat; **Mono** = mono-unsaturated fat; **Poly** = poly-unsaturated fat; **Sat** = saturated fat; **Chol** = cholesterol; **Calc** = calcium; **Iron** = iron; **Mag** = magnesium; **Phos** = phosphate; **Sodi** = sodium; **Zinc** = zinc; **Vit A** = vitamin A; **Vit C** = vitamin C; **Thia** = thiamin; **Ribo** = riboflavin; **Niac** = niacin; **Vit B$_6$** = vitamin B$_6$; **Vit B$_{12}$**-vitamin B$_{12}$; **Vit E** = Vitamin E; **Fol** = folate; **Alc** = alcohol.

EvaluEat Code	Food Name	Amt	Wt (g)	Energy (kcal)	Prot (g)	Carb (g)	Fiber (g)	Fat (g)	Mono (g)	Poly (g)	Sat (g)
2047	Salt, table (sodium chloride)	1 tsp	6	0	0	0	0	0	0	0	0
4609	Animal fat, bacon grease	1 tbsp	12.8	114.8	0	0	0	12.736	5.744	1.426	4.993
4542	Animal fat, chicken	1 cup	205	1845	0	0	0	204.59	91.635	42.845	61.09
43388	Apple cider-flavored drink, powder, low calorie, with vitamin C, prepared	1 fl. oz.	29.8	0.298	0	0.089	0	0	0	0	0
9357	Apricots, canned, heavy syrup, drained	1 fruit	122	101.26	0.781	25.998	3.294	0.134	0.055	0.026	0.009
7921	Bacon and beef sticks	1 oz	28	145.6	8.148	0.224	0	12.376	6.132	1.204	4.48
43212	Bacon bits, meatless	1 cup	186	885.36	59.52	53.196	18.972	48.174	11.578	25.199	7.542
16104	Bacon, vegetarian, meatless	1 strip	5	15.5	0.534	0.316	0.13	1.476	0.355	0.772	0.231
18005	Bagel, cinnamon-raisin	1 bagel (4" dia)	89	243.86	8.722	49.128	2.047	1.513	0.156	0.597	0.244
18003	Bagel, egg	1 large bagel (4-1/2" dia)	131	364.18	13.886	69.43	3.013	2.751	0.55	0.841	0.552
18504	Bagel, Lender's Bagel Shop Blueberry	1 bagel (4" dia)	102	264.18	10.71	53.377	1.734	1.53	0.408	0.51	0.306
18007	Bagel, oatbran	1 bagel (4" dia)	89	226.95	9.523	47.437	3.204	1.068	0.222	0.433	0.17
18001	Bagel, plain/onion/poppy/sesame, enriched	1 bagel (4" dia)	89	244.75	9.345	47.526	2.047	1.424	0.117	0.619	0.196
43449	Baked beans, canned, no salt added	1 fl. oz.	29.8	31.29	1.43	6.142	1.639	0.119	0.01	0.051	0.031
42182	Bean beverage	1 oz	28.34	9.636	0.794	1.644	0	0	0	0	0
16115	Bean flour, soy, fullfat, raw	1 cup, stirred	84	366.24	29.014	29.56	8.064	17.346	3.831	9.792	2.509
16119	Bean meal, soy, defatted, raw	1 cup	122	413.58	54.839	48.971		2.916	0.499	1.275	0.327
16112	Bean sauce, fermented soy product, Miso	1 cup	275	566.5	32.478	76.89	14.85	16.693	3.688	9.427	2.414
16113	Bean sauce, fermented soy product, Natto	1 cup	175	371	31.01	25.13	9.45	19.25	4.253	10.868	2.784
16114	Bean sauce, fermented soy product, Tempeh	1 cup	166	320.38	30.776	15.587		17.928	4.98	6.353	3.685
16424	Bean sauce, soy & wheat (Shoyu) low sodium	1 tbsp	18	9.54	0.931	1.532	0.144	0.014	0.002	0.006	0.002
16124	Bean sauce, soy (Tamari)	1 tsp	6	3.6	0.631	0.334	0.048	0.006	0.001	0.003	0.001
16375	Beans, baby lima, mature seed, boiled w/salt	1 cup	182	229.32	14.633	42.424	14.014	0.692	0.062	0.308	0.16
16008	Beans, baked w/franks, canned	1 cup	259	367.78	17.483	39.86	17.871	17.016	7.33	2.165	6.092
16006	Beans, baked, plain or vegetarian, canned	1 cup	254	236.22	12.167	52.121	12.7	1.143	0.099	0.493	0.295
16015	Beans, black, mature seeds, boiled w/o salt	1 cup	172	227.04	15.239	40.781	14.964	0.929	0.081	0.397	0.239
16353	Beans, broadbeans (Fava) mature seed, boiled w/salt	1 cup	170	187	12.92	33.405	9.18	0.68	0.134	0.279	0.112
43112	Beans, chili, barbeque, ranch style, cooked	1 cup	186	180.42	9.3	31.527	7.812	1.86	0.143	1.032	0.27

Chol (g)	Calc (mg)	Iron (mg)	Mag (mg)	Phos (mg)	Pota (mg)	Sodi (mg)	Zinc (mg)	Vit A (RAE)	Vit C (mg)	Thia (mg)	Ribo (mg)	Niac (mg)	Vit B$_6$ (mg)	Vit B$_{12}$ (µg)	Vit E (mg)	Fol (µg)	Alc (g)
0	1.44	0.02	0.06	0	0.48	2325.48	0.006	0	0	0	0	0	0	0	0	0	0
12.16	0	0	0	0	0	19.2	0.014	0	0	0	0	0	0	0	0.077	0	0
174.25	0	0	0	0	0	0	0	0	0	0	0	0	0	0	5.535	0	0
0	3.278	0.009	0.298	3.576	0		0.009	0		0	0	0	0	0	0	0	0
0	12.2	0.366	8.54	15.86	174.46	4.88	0.134	178.1	3.782	0.026	0.029	0.459	0.067	0	1.086	2.44	0
28.56	3.92	0.521	4.76	39.76	107.8	397.6	0.904	0	0	0.168	0.08	1.363	0.14	0.532	0.078	0.56	0
0	187.86	1.339	176.7	403.62	269.7	3292.2	3.478	0	3.534	1.116	0.13	2.976	0.149	2.232	12.834	236.2	0
0	1.15	0.121	0.95	3.5	8.5	73.25	0.021	0.2	0	0.22	0.024	0.378	0.024	0	0.345	2.1	0
0	16.91	3.382	24.92	89	131.72	286.58	1.006	18.69	0.623	0.342	0.247	2.741	0.055	0	0.276	98.79	0
31.44	17.03	5.214	32.75	110.04	89.08	661.55	1.009	43.23	0.786	0.702	0.308	4.51	0.114	0.21		115.3	0
0	57.12	1.836			158.1	427.38			0	0.265	0.204	4.08	0.061	0		75.48	
0	10.68	2.741	27.59	97.9	102.35	451.23	0.801	0.89	0.178	0.295	0.301	2.634	0.038	0	0.294	87.22	0
0	65.86	3.168	25.81	85.44	89.89	475.26	0.783	0	0	0.479	0.28	4.06	0.045	0	0.258	94.34	0
0	14.9	0.086	9.536	30.992	88.208	0.298	0.417	1.49	0.924	0.045	0.018	0.128	0.039	0	0.158	7.152	0
0	4.818	0.354	13.603	26.073	95.506	0.567	0.105	0	0	0.043	0.028	0.176	0.028	0	0.068	17	0
0	173.04	5.351	360.36	414.96	2112.6	10.92	3.293	5.04	0	0.488	0.974	3.629	0.387	0	1.638	289.8	0
0	297.68	16.714	373.32	855.22	3037.8	3.66	6.173	2.44	0	0.843	0.306	3.156	0.694	0		369.67	0
0	181.5	7.535	115.5	420.75	451	10029.23	9.13	11	0	0.267	0.688	2.365	0.591	0	0.027	90.75	0
0	379.75	15.05	201.25	304.5	1275.75	12.25	5.302	0	22.75	0.28	0.332	0	0.227	0	0.018	14	0
0	184.26	4.482	134.46	441.56	683.92	14.94	1.892	0	0	0.129	0.594	4.382	0.357	0.133		39.84	0
0	3.06	0.364	6.12	19.8	32.4	599.94	0.067	0	0	0.009	0.023	0.605	0.031	0	0	2.88	0
0	1.2	0.143	2.4	7.8	12.72	335.16	0.026	0	0	0.004	0.009	0.237	0.012	0	0	1.08	0
0	52.78	4.368	96.46	231.14	729.82	434.98	1.875	0	0	0.293	0.1	1.201	0.142	0		273	0
15.54	124.32	4.481	72.52	269.36	608.65	1113.7	4.843	10.36	5.957	0.15	0.145	2.334	0.119	0	1.191	77.7	0
0	127	0.737	81.28	264.16	751.84	1008.38	3.556	12.7	7.874	0.389	0.152	1.087	0.34	0	1.346	60.96	0
0	46.44	3.612	120.4	240.8	610.6	1.72	1.926	0	0	0.42	0.101	0.869	0.119	0		256.3	0
0	61.2	2.55	73.1	212.5	455.6	409.7	1.717	1.7	0.51	0.165	0.151	1.209	0.122	0	0.034	176.8	0
0	57.66	3.46	83.7	286.44	837	1348.5	3.72	1.86	3.162	0.074	0.279	0.67	0.502	0.019	0.391	48.36	

EvaluEat Code	Food Name	Amt	Wt (g)	Energy (kcal)	Prot (g)	Carb (g)	Fiber (g)	Fat (g)	Mono (g)	Poly (g)	Sat (g)
16137	Beans, hummus, garbanzo or chickpea spread, homemade	1 tbsp	15	26.55	0.729	3.018	0.6	1.289	0.737	0.312	0.168
16029	Beans, kidney, mature seeds, canned	1 cup	256	207.36	13.312	38.093	8.96	0.794	0.061	0.44	0.115
16033	Beans, kidney, red, mature seeds, boiled w/o salt	1 cup	177	224.79	15.346	40.356	13.098	0.885	0.069	0.487	0.127
16072	Beans, large lima, mature seeds, boiled w/o salt	1 cup	188	216.2	14.664	39.254	13.16	0.714	0.064	0.321	0.167
16073	Beans, large lima, mature seeds, canned	1 cup	241	190.39	11.881	35.933	11.568	0.41	0.036	0.178	0.094
16070	Beans, lentils, mature seeds, boiled w/o salt	1 cup	198	229.68	17.86	39.857	15.642	0.752	0.127	0.347	0.105
16081	Beans, mung, mature seeds, boiled w/o salt	1 cup	202	212.1	14.18	38.683	15.352	0.768	0.109	0.259	0.234
16080	Beans, mung, mature seeds, raw	1 tbsp	13	45.11	3.102	8.141	2.119	0.149	0.021	0.05	0.045
16038	Beans, navy, mature seeds, boiled w/o salt	1 cup	182	258.44	15.834	47.884	11.648	1.037	0.091	0.448	0.269
16039	Beans, navy, mature seeds, canned	1 cup	262	296.06	19.729	53.579	13.362	1.127	0.1	0.487	0.293
16044	Beans, pinto, mature seeds, canned	1 cup	240	206.4	11.664	36.6	11.04	1.944	0.389	0.694	0.401
16109	Beans, soy, mature seeds, boiled w/o salt	1 cup	172	297.56	28.621	17.08	10.32	15.428	3.407	8.71	2.231
16108	Beans, soy, mature seeds, raw	1 cup	186	773.76	67.871	56.098	17.298	37.088	8.191	20.934	5.364
16110	Beans, soy, mature seeds, roasted w/salt	1 cup	172	810.12	60.578	57.706	30.444	43.688	9.649	24.663	6.319
16162	Beans, soy, tofu, Mori-Nu, silken, firm	1 slice	84	52.08	5.796	2.016	0.084	2.268	0.453	1.247	0.341
16164	Beans, soy, tofu, Mori-Nu, silken, lite firm	1 slice	84	31.08	5.292	0.924	0	0.672	0.114	0.377	0.112
16161	Beans, soy, tofu, Mori-Nu, silken, soft	1 slice	84	46.2	4.032	2.436	0.084	2.268	0.438	1.302	0.3
16129	Beans, soy, tofu, nigari, fried	1 oz	28.35	76.829	4.873	2.974	1.106	5.721	1.263	3.229	0.827
16050	Beans, white, mature seeds, boiled w/o salt	1 cup	179	248.81	17.417	44.911	11.277	0.626	0.055	0.272	0.163
16051	Beans, white, mature seeds, canned	1 cup	262	306.54	19.021	57.483	12.576	0.76	0.065	0.322	0.194
16048	Beans, yellow, mature seeds, boiled w/o salt	1 cup	177	254.88	16.213	44.728	18.408	1.912	0.166	0.825	0.494
51696	Beef & onion patty, flame broiled, Lean Magic product #9676	1 piece	74	138.38	17.094	1.939	1.036	6.727	2.857	0.276	2.633
51738	Beef & turkey, flame broiled patty w/teriyaki sauce, Lean Magic 30 product #9128	1 piece	20	28.2	3.892	1.672	0.26	0.72	0.306	0.099	0.248
51737	Beef & turkey, flame broiled rib-B-Q w/BBQ sauce, Rib-B-Q lean magic 30	1 piece	85	115.6	14.348	8.024	1.36	3.094	1.301	0.42	1.008
13168	Beef bottom round, all grades, lean (1/4" trim) braised	3 oz	85	177.65	26.852	0	0	6.97	3.052	0.264	2.355
13160	Beef bottom round, all grades, lean & fat (1/4" trim) braised	3 oz	85	233.75	24.361	0	0	14.365	6.247	0.544	5.415
13319	Beef brain, pan fried	3 oz	85	166.6	10.684	0	0	13.456	3.383	1.964	3.179
13022	Beef brisket, whole, all grades, lean & fat (1/4" trim) braised	3 oz	85	327.25	19.975	0	0	26.826	11.815	0.961	10.523
13345	Beef cured breakfast strip, cooked	3 slices	34	152.66	10.642	0.476	0	11.696	5.729	0.537	4.879
13322	Beef heart, simmered	3 oz	85	133.45	24.208	0.128	0	4.021	0.859	0.837	1.193
13324	Beef kidney, simmered	3 oz	85	128.35	23.18	0	0	3.953	0.604	0.703	0.906
13327	Beef liver, pan fried	1 slice (yield from 112 g raw liver)	81	141.75	21.481	4.18	0	3.791	0.529	0.471	1.209
22529	Beef pot pie, frozen	1 package	198	449.46	13.266	44.154	2.178	24.354	9.682	2.673	8.514
7956	Beef sausage, fresh, cooked	1 hot dog	52	172.64	9.469	0.182	0	14.55	6.572	0.345	5.671
7954	Beef sausage, pre-cooked	1 hot dog	52	210.6	8.06	0.016	0	19.536	8.521	0.457	7.851
13458	Beef short loin, porterhouse steak, all grades, lean & fat (1/4" trim) broiled	3 oz	85	279.65	19.134	0	0	21.964	9.822	0.849	8.642
13472	Beef short loin, T-bone steak, all grades, lean & fat (1/4" trim) broiled	3 oz	85	260.1	19.949	0	0	19.363	8.63	0.701	7.582
13270	Beef short loin, top loin, all grades, lean (1/4" trim) broiled	3 oz	85	175.95	24.327	0	0	7.99	3.213	0.264	3.052

Chol (g)	Calc (mg)	Iron (mg)	Mag (mg)	Phos (mg)	Pota (mg)	Sodi (mg)	Zinc (mg)	Vit A (RAE)	Vit C (mg)	Thia (mg)	Ribo (mg)	Niac (mg)	Vit B_6 (mg)	Vit B_{12} (µg)	Vit E (mg)	Fol (µg)	Alc (g)
0	7.35	0.236	4.35	16.5	25.95	36.3	0.164	0	1.185	0.013	0.008	0.06	0.06	0	0.113	8.85	0
0	69.12	3.149	79.36	268.8	657.92	888.32	1.408	0	3.072	0.279	0.184	1.285	0.177	0		125.4	0
0	49.56	5.204	79.65	251.34	713.31	3.54	1.894	0	2.124	0.283	0.103	1.023	0.212	0	1.54	230.1	0
0	31.96	4.493	80.84	208.68	955.04	3.76	1.786	0	0	0.303	0.103	0.791	0.303	0	0.338	156	0
0	50.61	4.362	93.99	178.34	530.2	809.76	1.566	0	0	0.133	0.082	0.629	0.219	0		120.5	0
0	37.62	6.593	71.28	356.4	730.62	3.96	2.515	0	2.97	0.335	0.145	2.099	0.352	0	0.218	358.4	0
0	54.54	2.828	96.96	199.98	537.32	4.04	1.697	2.02	2.02	0.331	0.123	1.166	0.135	0	0.303	321.2	0
0	17.16	0.876	24.57	47.71	161.98	1.95	0.348	0.78	0.624	0.081	0.03	0.293	0.05	0	0.066	81.25	0
0	127.4	4.514	107.38	285.74	669.76	1.82	1.929	0	1.638	0.368	0.111	0.966	0.298	0		254.8	0
0	123.14	4.847	123.14	351.08	754.56	1173.76	2.017	0	1.834	0.369	0.144	1.276	0.27	0	2.044	162.4	0
0	103.2	3.504	64.8	220.8	583.2	705.6	1.656	0	2.16	0.242	0.151	0.701	0.178	0	1.416	144	0
0	175.44	8.841	147.92	421.4	885.8	1.72	1.978	0	2.924	0.267	0.49	0.686	0.402	0	0.602	92.88	0
0	515.22	29.202	520.8	1309.44	3342.42	3.72	9.095	0	11.16	1.626	1.618	3.019	0.701	0	1.581	697.5	0
0	237.36	6.708	249.4	624.36	2528.4	280.36	5.401	17.2	3.784	0.172	0.249	2.425	0.358	0	1.565	362.9	0
0	26.88	0.865	22.68	75.6	162.96	30.24	0.512	0	0	0.085	0.034	0.207	0.009	0	0.16		0
0	30.24	0.63	8.4	68.04	52.92	71.4	0.277	0	0	0.034	0.017	0.092	0	0	0.05		0
0	26.04	0.689	24.36	52.08	151.2	4.2	0.437	0	0	0.084	0.034	0.252	0.009	0	0.168		0
0	105.462	1.381	17.01	81.365	41.391	4.536	0.564	0.284	0	0.048	0.014	0.028	0.028	0	0.011	7.655	0
0	161.1	6.623	112.77	202.27	1004.19	10.74	2.47	0	0	0.211	0.082	0.251	0.166	0	1.736	145	0
0	191.26	7.834	133.62	238.42	1189.48	13.1	2.934	0	0	0.252	0.097	0.296	0.197	0		170.3	0
0	109.74	4.39	130.98	323.91	575.25	8.85	1.876	0	3.186	0.331	0.182	1.253	0.228	0		143.4	0
42.18	23.68	2.153	28.86	240.5	283.42	313.02	5.025		0.518	0.139	0.152	2.917	0.278	1.643	0.068	5.18	0
8.2	6.2	0.43	6.6	45.8	59.2	127.4	0.878		0	0.034	0.023	0.561	0.058	0.264	0.005	0.4	0
28.9	33.15	1.87	26.35	202.3	244.8	560.15	3.179		1.275	0.144	0.086	2.356	0.264	1.403	0.046	1.7	0
81.6	4.25	2.941	21.25	231.2	261.8	43.35	4.658	0	0	0.06	0.221	3.468	0.306	2.1	0.119	9.35	0
81.6	5.1	2.652	18.7	208.25	239.7	42.5	4.174	0	0	0.06	0.204	3.171	0.281	1.997	0.162	8.5	0
1695.75	7.65	1.887	12.75	328.1	300.9	134.3	1.148	0	2.805	0.111	0.221	3.213	0.331	12.92		5.1	0
79.9	6.8	1.904	15.3	158.95	196.35	51.85	4.335	0	0	0.051	0.153	2.55	0.204	1.938	0.204	5.1	0
40.46	3.06	1.068	9.18	80.24	140.08	766.02	2.166	0	0	0.031	0.088	2.2	0.105	1.173	0.099	2.72	0
180.2	4.25	5.423	17.85	215.9	186.15	50.15	2.439	0	0	0.086	1.029	5.678	0.208	9.18	0.247	4.25	0
608.6	16.15	4.93	10.2	258.4	114.75	79.9	2.414	0	0	0.136	2.525	3.332	0.332	21.165	0.068	70.55	0
308.61	4.86	4.998	17.82	392.85	284.31	62.37	4.236	6273	0.567	0.143	2.774	14.155	0.832	67.335	0.373	210.6	0
37.62						736.56											
42.64	5.72	0.816	7.28	73.32	134.16	339.04	2.278	6.76	0	0.025	0.078	1.872	0.163	1.045	0.125	1.56	0
43.16	7.8	0.796	6.76	96.2	121.68	473.2	1.518	13	0.364	0.015	0.061	1.669	0.1	1.056	0.255	2.6	0
61.2	6.8	2.278	17	150.45	216.75	52.7	3.511	0	0	0.077	0.178	3.272	0.284	1.793	0.187	5.95	0
55.25	5.95	2.626	18.7	157.25	239.7	56.95	3.655	0	0	0.079	0.183	3.367	0.286	1.811	0.178	5.95	0
64.6	6.8	2.1	22.95	185.3	336.6	57.8	4.437	0	0	0.077	0.17	4.539	0.357	1.7	0.119	6.8	0

EvaluEat Code	Food Name	Amt	Wt (g)	Energy (kcal)	Prot (g)	Carb (g)	Fiber (g)	Fat (g)	Mono (g)	Poly (g)	Sat (g)
13262	Beef short loin, top loin, all grades, lean & fat (1/4" trim) broiled	3 oz	85	243.95	21.726	0	0	16.796	7.064	0.604	6.647
13340	Beef tongue, simmered	3 oz	85	236.3	16.397	0	0	18.955	8.587	0.557	6.906
13341	Beef tripe, raw	1 oz	28.35	23.247	3.422	0	0	1.046	0.435	0.051	0.366
13012	Beef, all cuts, all grades, lean (1/4"trim) cooked	3 oz	85	183.6	25.143	0	0	8.424	3.545	0.289	3.222
13004	Beef, all cuts, all grades, lean & fat (1/4"trim) cooked	3 oz	85	259.25	22.049	0	0	18.309	7.837	0.663	7.259
43384	Beef, bologna, reduced sodium	1 fl. oz.	29.8	93.274	3.487	0.596	0	8.463	3.963	0.313	3.479
13870	Beef, bottom round, all grades, lean & fat (1/8" trim) roasted	1 piece, cooked, (yield from 1 lb raw meat)	338	736.84	89.266	0	0	39.343	16.778	1.518	14.933
13953	Beef, bottom sirloin, tri-tip roast, separable lean and fat, 0"trim, all grades, cooked, roasted	3 oz (1 serving)	85	176.8	22.142	0	0	9.41	4.659	0.309	3.46
13055	Beef, brisket, flat half, separable lean and fat, 1/8"trim, select, cooked, braised	3 oz	85	238	24.625	0	0	14.765	6.359	0.546	5.855
13034	Beef, chuck, arm pot roast, all grades, lean & fat (1/4"trim) braised	3 oz	85	282.2	23.316	0	0	20.239	8.679	0.774	7.973
13050	Beef, chuck, blade roast, all grades, lean & fat (1/4"trim) braised	3 oz	85	293.25	22.585	0	0	21.837	9.435	0.782	8.695
23553	Beef, chuck, clod roast, separable lean and fat, trimmed to 1/4"fat, all grades, cooked, roasted	3 oz (1 serving)	85	205.7	20.587	0	0	13.107	5.952	0.521	4.877
23555	Beef, chuck, clod steak, separable lean and fat, trimmed to 1/4"fat, all grades, cooked, braised	3 oz (1 serving)	85	231.2	22.262	0	0	15.071	6.809	0.599	5.694
23547	Beef, chuck, tender steak, separable lean and fat, trimmed to 0"fat, all grades, cooked, broiled	3 oz (1 serving)	85	136	21.99	0	0	4.692	2.256	0.329	1.59
23523	Beef, chuck, top blade, separable lean and fat, trimmed to 0"fat, USDA Choice, cooked, broiled	3 oz (1 serving)	85	192.95	21.905	0	0	10.991	5.329	0.39	3.538
22698	Beef, corned beef hash, canned entree/Hormel	1 cup	236	387.04	20.603	21.877	2.596	24.166	12.414	0.708	10.195
22908	Beef, corned beef hash, canned, with potato	100 grams	100	164	8.73	9.27	1.1	10.24	5.26	0.3	4.32
51658	Beef, country fried finger/Pierre product #3813	1 piece	26	82.16	4.334	4.009	0.364	5.486	1.704	1.897	1.372
51613	Beef, country fried nugget/Pierre product #1935	1 piece	14.2	48.706	2.424	2.256	0.185	3.385	1.113	1.078	0.9
51605	Beef, country fried patty/Pierre product #1840	1 piece	108	356.4	17.55	16.459	1.512	24.786	7.951	7.957	6.515
51602	Beef, country fried steak/Pierre product #1610	1 piece	108	356.4	16.859	14.083	0.432	25.607	9.168	6.324	7.897
13358	Beef, cured, smoked, chopped	1 slice (1 oz)	28	37.24	5.653	0.521	0	1.238	0.512	0.064	0.507
13360	Beef, cured, thin sliced	10 slices	28	42.84	8.708	0.773	0	0.543	0.235	0.02	0.266
13350	Beef, dried, cured	10 slices	28	42.84	8.708	0.773	0	0.543	0.235	0.02	0.267
13176	Beef, eye of round, all grades, lean & fat (1/4"trim) roasted	3 oz	85	194.65	22.772	0	0	10.838	4.658	0.391	4.233
13682	Beef, eye of round, Prime, lean & fat (1/2"trim) roasted	3 oz	85	212.5	22.958	0	0	12.708	5.67	0.459	5.117
13096	Beef, eye/small end ribs (10–12 ribs), Choice, lean & fat (1/4"trim) broiled	1 steak	236	625.4	62.729	0	0	39.554	16.197	1.468	15.354
51718	Beef, flame broiled fajita/Lean Magic Wonderbites Dipper product #9974	1 piece	18	32.58	3.897	1.089	0.27	1.483	0.626	0.062	0.576
51663	Beef, flame broiled meatloaf/Lean Magic product #3825	1 piece	74	148	16.643	4.151	0.814	7.2	3.092	0.362	2.793
51677	Beef, flame broiled patty/Pierre product #3871	1 piece	69	158.01	16.187	1.546	1.035	9.536	4.082	0.386	3.782

Chol (g)	Calc (mg)	Iron (mg)	Mag (mg)	Phos (mg)	Pota (mg)	Sodi (mg)	Zinc (mg)	Vit A (RAE)	Vit C (mg)	Thia (mg)	Ribo (mg)	Niac (mg)	Vit B_6 (mg)	Vit B_{12} (µg)	Vit E (mg)	Fol (µg)	Alc (g)
67.15	7.65	1.896	19.55	164.9	296.65	53.55	3.885	0	0	0.068	0.153	3.995	0.315	1.649	0.017	5.95	0
112.2	4.25	2.218	12.75	123.25	156.4	55.25	34.77	0	1.105	0.019	0.25	2.967	0.132	2.661	0.255	5.95	0
34.587	19.562	0.167	3.686	18.144	18.995	27.5	0.403	0	0	0	0.018	0.25	0.004	0.394	0.026	1.418	0
73.1	7.65	2.542	22.1	198.05	306	56.95	5.891	0	0	0.085	0.204	3.511	0.315	2.244	0.119	6.8	0
74.8	8.5	2.227	18.7	172.55	266.05	52.7	4.972	0	0	0.068	0.178	3.094	0.281	2.074	0.17	5.95	0
16.688	3.576	0.417	2.98	24.436	46.19	203.236	0.596	0	0	0.018	0.039	0.784	0.054	0.42	0.057	1.49	0
253.5	20.28	7.301	57.46	554.32	723.32	118.3	14.97	0	0	0.206	0.477	15.602	1.173	4.969	1.386	27.04	0
71.4	16.15	1.411	18.7	170.85	274.55	45.05	3.97	0	0	0.06	0.107	5.893	0.463	1.301	0.34	6.8	0
60.35	14.45	2.04	16.15	153	201.45	41.65	5.882	0	0	0.054	0.134	3.549	0.242	1.632	0.425	7.65	0
84.15	8.5	2.644	16.15	187	209.1	51	5.814	0	0	0.06	0.204	2.703	0.238	2.508	0.187	7.65	0
88.4	11.05	2.635	16.15	170	196.35	54.4	7.072	0	0	0.06	0.204	2.057	0.221	1.938	0.17	4.25	0
63.75	6.8	2.388	17	166.6	286.45	56.95	4.854	0	0	0.069	0.192	2.726	0.217	2.405	0.119	7.65	0
79.9	7.65	2.831	16.15	175.95	220.15	48.45	5.772	0	0	0.057	0.192	2.428	0.205	2.329	0.094	6.8	0
53.55	6.8	2.491	19.55	192.95	249.05	60.35	6.647	0	0	0.094	0.196	3.087	0.273	2.882	0.136	6.8	0
49.3	5.95	2.355	20.4	182.75	255	57.8	7.446	0	0	0.094	0.195	3.076	0.272	2.873	0.153	6.8	0
75.52	44.84	2.36	30.68		405.92	1003	3.304	2.124									0
32	19	1	13	56	172	425	1.4	0	0.9	0.069	0.05	1.572	0.231	0.41	0.04	7	0
9.88	8.32	0.783	7.02	60.06	71.76	125.58	1.191		0	0.08	0.064	1.083	0.066	0.387	0.548	9.36	0
5.254	5.538	0.454	3.834	34.932	39.192	71.284	0.626		0	0.044	0.039	0.563	0.036	0.25	0.298	6.106	0
42.12	34.56	3.208	29.16	246.24	293.76	519.48	4.828		0	0.329	0.261	4.441	0.27	1.588	2.272	38.88	0
51.84	15.12	2.657	12.96	177.12	217.08	376.92	3.402		0	0.211	0.233	3.776	0.159	1.512	1.859	37.8	0
12.88	2.24	0.798	5.88	50.68	105.56	352.24	1.1	0	0	0.023	0.049	1.282	0.098	0.484		2.24	0
22.12	1.68	0.781	5.6	61.04	69.16	781.2	1.229	0	0	0.016	0.059	0.914	0.081	0.554	0.031	2.52	0
22.12	1.4	0.812	6.16	54.88	81.48	781.2	1.112	0	0	0.017	0.062	0.927	0.069	0.661	0	2.24	0
61.2	5.1	1.564	20.4	176.8	307.7	50.15	3.689	0	0	0.068	0.136	2.967	0.298	1.785	0.153	5.95	0
61.2	5.1	1.573	21.25	178.5	311.1	50.15	3.723	0	0	0.068	0.138	2.986	0.298	1.793		5.95	0
297.36	42.48	4.248	51.92	474.36	769.36	125.08	11.3	0	0	0.156	0.276	17.013	1.251	4.13	1.109	18.88	0
9.36	6.3	0.531	7.2	57.24	67.68	85.86	1.195		0.054	0.035	0.036	0.689	0.065	0.38	0.012	0.9	0
41.44	25.9	2.079	23.68	142.08	244.94	399.6	4.359		2.072	0.109	0.155	2.53	0.242	1.643	0.073	7.4	0
41.4	24.15	2.105	29.67	228.39	276	291.18	4.975		0	0.149	0.146	2.904	0.275	1.615	0.042	3.45	0

EvaluEat Code	Food Name	Amt	Wt (g)	Energy (kcal)	Prot (g)	Carb (g)	Fiber (g)	Fat (g)	Mono (g)	Poly (g)	Sat (g)
51683	Beef, flame broiled steak/Pierre product #9010	1 piece	74	248.64	17.856	0.326	0	18.944	8.161	0.712	7.586
13067	Beef, flank, choice, lean & fat (0″ trim) broiled	1 steak	387	781.74	106.62	0	0	36.03	14.516	1.409	14.861
23580	Beef, ground, 75% lean meat/25% fat, crumbles, cooked, pan-browned	3 oz	85	235.45	22.338	0	0	15.478	7.131	0.386	6.027
23575	Beef, ground, 80% lean meat/20% fat, crumbles, cooked, pan-browned	3 oz	85	231.2	22.95	0	0	14.756	6.542	0.428	5.586
23570	Beef, ground, 85% lean meat/15% fat, crumbles, cooked, pan-browned	3 oz	85	217.6	23.57	0	0	13.005	5.605	0.406	4.925
23565	Beef, ground, 90% lean meat/10% fat, crumbles, cooked, pan-browned	3 oz	85	195.5	24.183	0	0	10.234	4.316	0.315	4.053
23560	Beef, ground, 95% lean meat/5% fat, crumbles, cooked, pan-browned	3 oz	85	164.05	24.795	0	0	6.443	2.825	0.328	3.022
13299	Beef, ground, extra lean, broiled, well done	3 oz	85	225.25	24.293	0	0	13.43	5.882	0.502	5.279
13306	Beef, ground, lean, broiled, well done	3 oz	85	238	23.97	0	0	14.994	6.562	0.561	5.891
13313	Beef, ground, regular, broiled, well done	3 oz	85	248.2	23.12	0	0	16.541	7.242	0.621	6.503
13113	Beef, large end ribs (6–9 ribs) all grades, lean (1/4″ trim) roasted	yield from 1 lb raw meat	210	497.7	57.813	0	0	27.72	11.592	0.798	11.067
13101	Beef, large end ribs (6–9 ribs) all grades, lean & fat (1/4″ trim) roasted	yield from 1 lb raw meat	293	1069.5	66.335	0	0	87.226	37.358	3.047	35.189
23545	Beef, loin, bottom sirloin butt, tri-tip steak, separable lean and fat (0″ trim) all grades	3 oz	85	225.25	25.475	0	0	12.903	6.599	0.457	4.851
23540	Beef, plate, inside skirt steak, separable lean and fat, trimmed to 0″ fat, all grades, broiled	3 oz	85	187	22.211	0	0	10.243	5.147	0.371	3.966
13979	Beef, plate, outside skirt steak, separable lean only, trimmed to 0″ fat, all grades, broiled	3 oz	85	198.05	20.553	0	0	12.215	6.273	0.51	5.075
13952	Beef, rib eye, small end (ribs 10–12), separable lean and fat, 0″ trim, all grades, cooked, broiled	3 oz	85	209.95	23.18	0	0	12.529	5.129	0.465	4.862
23626	Beef, rib, small end ribs (ribs 10–12), separable lean only, 1/8″ trim, Choice, cooked, broiled	3 oz	85	171.7	24.047	0	0	7.693	3.07	0.275	2.928
22721	Beef, roast beef hash, canned entree/Hormel	3 oz	236	384.68	21.311	22.916	3.54	23.647	11.281	0.637	9.912
23592	Beef, round, top round, separable lean only, 1/8″ trim, select, cooked, broiled	3 oz	85	150.45	26.869	0	0	3.953	1.652	0.16	1.362
23002	Beef, short loin, porterhouse steak, all grades, lean & fat (1/8″ trim) broiled	3 oz	85	252.45	19.984	0	0	18.556	8.152	0.697	7.157
23006	Beef, short loin, T-bone steak, all grades, lean & fat (1/8″ trim) broiled	3 oz	85	238	20.681	0	0	16.549	7.259	0.595	6.426
23630	Beef, short loin, top loin, separable lean only, 1/8″ trim, Choice, cooked, broiled	3 oz	85	170.85	24.786	0	0	7.182	2.867	0.257	2.734
13148	Beef, short ribs, Choice, lean & fat, braised	3 oz	85	400.35	18.334	0	0	35.683	16.048	1.301	15.13
13124	Beef, small end ribs (10–12 ribs) all grades, lean & fat (1/4″ trim) broiled	3 oz	85	285.6	20.137	0	0	22.083	9.486	0.765	8.942
13238	Beef, tenderloin, all grades, lean & fat (1/4″ trim) broiled	3 oz	85	247.35	21.471	0	0	17.221	7.064	0.655	6.758
13192	Beef, tip round, all grades, lean & fat (1/4″ trim) roasted	3 oz	85	198.9	22.874	0	0	11.254	4.684	0.433	4.267
13427	Beef, top round, all grades, lean & fat (1/4″ trim) braised	3 oz	85	210.8	28.756	0	0	9.716	4.012	0.4	3.672
13278	Beef, top sirloin, all grades, lean & fat (1/4″ trim) broiled	3 oz	85	219.3	23.639	0	0	13.099	5.636	0.502	5.219

Chol (g)	Calc (mg)	Iron (mg)	Mag (mg)	Phos (mg)	Pota (mg)	Sodi (mg)	Zinc (mg)	Vit A (RAE)	Vit C (mg)	Thia (mg)	Ribo (mg)	Niac (mg)	Vit B$_6$ (mg)	Vit B$_{12}$ (µg)	Vit E (mg)	Fol (µg)	Alc (g)
64.38	7.4	1.791	14.8	229.4	208.68	284.9	3.826		0	0.053	0.144	2.398	0.211	1.717	0.057	4.44	0
197.37	69.66	6.966	85.14	777.87	1261.62	205.11	18.54	0	0	0.267	0.468	28.913	2.125	7.043	1.509	34.83	0
75.65	28.9	2.236	18.7	181.9	300.9	79.05	5.245	0	0	0.039	0.159	4.543	0.365	2.499	0.408	10.2	0
75.65	23.8	2.363	19.55	192.1	323	77.35	5.44	0	0	0.038	0.161	4.956	0.364	2.431	0.408	9.35	0
76.5	18.7	2.491	21.25	202.3	345.95	75.65	5.627	0	0	0.037	0.162	5.37	0.364	2.372	0.4	8.5	0
75.65	13.6	2.618	22.95	212.5	368.05	73.95	5.814	0	0	0.037	0.164	5.783	0.364	2.304	0.374	6.8	0
75.65	7.65	2.746	23.8	223.55	390.15	72.25	6.001	0	0	0.036	0.166	6.197	0.364	2.244	0.34	5.95	0
84.15	7.65	2.355	21.25	161.5	313.65	69.7	5.465		0	0.06	0.272	4.972	0.272	2.176	0.153	9.35	0
85.85	10.2	2.082	20.4	154.7	296.65	75.65	5.27		0	0.051	0.204	5.075	0.255	2.312	0.173	9.35	0
85.85	10.2	2.329	18.7	162.35	277.95	79.05	4.938		0	0.034	0.178	5.499	0.255	2.788	0.196	8.5	0
170.1	16.8	5.922	52.5	438.9	749.7	153.3	15.67	0	0	0.189	0.462	9.345	0.546	5.481	0.294	18.9	0
249.05	29.3	6.768	55.67	498.1	843.84	187.52	16.7	0	0	0.205	0.527	10.577	0.674	6.798	0.674	20.51	0
57.8	10.2	3.094	22.1	225.25	371.45	61.2	5.993	0	0	0.109	0.243	3.591	0.377	2.405	0.145	8.5	0
51	9.35	2.355	20.4	195.5	245.65	63.75	6.146	0	0	0.077	0.162	3.183	0.273	3.162	0.085	5.95	0
49.3	8.5	2.261	21.25	187.85	334.05	79.9	4.862	0	0	0.101	0.166	3.681	0.421	3.655	0.094	6.8	0
94.35	17	1.488	19.55	180.2	289	47.6	4.19	0	0	0.063	0.111	6.168	0.485	1.36	0.382	6.8	0
72.25	13.6	1.632	20.4	186.15	299.2	49.3	4.514	0	0	0.064	0.123	7.095	0.501	1.505	0.357	7.65	0
73.16	42.48	2.36	33.04		431.88	792.96	3.304	1.888									0
51.85	5.95	2.261	18.7	175.95	229.5	36.55	4.735	0	0	0.065	0.145	4.621	0.354	1.377	0.289	9.35	0
60.35	6.8	2.329	19.55	158.95	272.85	54.4	3.893	0	0	0.085	0.187	3.46	0.298	1.828	0.17	5.95	0
52.7	6.8	2.405	20.4	164.05	285.6	56.1	3.978	0	0	0.085	0.187	3.519	0.298	1.845	0.162	5.95	0
67.15	13.6	1.675	21.25	192.1	307.7	51	4.649	0	0	0.065	0.127	7.313	0.516	1.547	0.349	8.5	0
79.9	10.2	1.964	12.75	137.7	190.4	42.5	4.148	0	0	0.043	0.128	2.084	0.187	2.227	0.247	4.25	0
71.4	11.05	1.862	18.7	148.75	276.25	52.7	4.752	0	0	0.077	0.153	3.391	0.281	2.457	0.187	5.95	0
73.1	6.8	2.678	22.1	178.5	312.8	50.15	4.148	0	0	0.094	0.221	2.992	0.331	2.049	0.162	5.1	0
69.7	5.1	2.338	21.25	191.25	305.15	53.55	5.525	0	0	0.077	0.213	2.992	0.315	2.346	0.145	5.95	0
76.5	4.25	2.652	20.4	180.2	267.75	38.25	3.638	0	0	0.06	0.204	3.069	0.23	2.21	0.145	7.65	0
76.5	9.35	2.601	24.65	188.7	311.1	53.55	4.972	0	0	0.094	0.23	3.341	0.349	2.287	0.153	7.65	0

EvaluEat Code	Food Name	Amt	Wt (g)	Energy (kcal)	Prot (g)	Carb (g)	Fiber (g)	Fat (g)	Mono (g)	Poly (g)	Sat (g)
13073	Beef, whole ribs (6–12 ribs) all grades, lean & fat (1/4"trim) roasted	3 oz	85	304.3	19.125	0	0	24.659	10.6	0.876	9.945
14169	Beverage mix, carob flavor, dry, prep w/milk	1 cup (8 fl. oz.)	256	192	8.09	22.221	1.024	7.962	1.989	0.484	4.554
14177	Beverage mix, chocolate flavor, dry mix, prep w/milk	1 cup (8 fl. oz.)	266	226.1	8.592	31.681	1.064	8.618	2.205	0.495	4.948
14318	Beverage mix, chocolate malted milk powder, no added nutrients, prep w/milk	1 cup (8 fl. oz.)	265	225.25	8.931	29.68	1.325	8.719	2.192	0.551	4.99
14312	Beverage mix, natural malt powder, no added nutrients, prep w/milk	1 cup (8 fl. oz.)	265	233.2	10.229	27.109	0.265	9.593	2.393	0.731	5.403
14351	Beverage mix, strawberry flavor, dry, prep w/milk	1 cup (8 fl. oz.)	266	234.08	7.98	32.718	0	8.246	2.357	0.303	5.081
14006	Beverage, alcoholic, beer, light	1 can or bottle (12 fl. oz.)	354	99.12	0.708	4.602	0	0	0	0	0
14003	Beverage, alcoholic, beer, regular	1 can	356	117.48	1.068	5.732	0.356	0.214	0	0	0
14534	Beverage, alcoholic, coffee liqueur 63 proof	1 jigger (1.5 fl. oz.)	52	160.16	0.052	16.744	0	0.156	0.011	0.055	0.055
14415	Beverage, alcoholic, coffee w/cream liqueur, 34 proof	1 jigger (1.5 fl. oz.)	47	153.69	1.316	9.823	0	7.379	2.095	0.314	4.542
14034	Beverage, alcoholic, creme de menthe, 72 proof	1 jigger (1.5 fl. oz.)	50	185.5	0	20.8	0	0.15	0.007	0.083	0.007
14010	Beverage, alcoholic, daiquiri, prep from recipe	1 cocktail (2 fl. oz.)	60	111.6	0.036	4.164	0.06	0.036	0.004	0.01	0.004
14049	Beverage, alcoholic, distilled spirits, gin 90 proof	1 jigger (1.5 fl. oz.)	42	110.46	0	0	0	0	0	0	0
14050	Beverage, alcoholic, distilled spirits, rum 80 proof	1 jigger (1.5 fl. oz.)	42	97.02	0	0	0	0	0	0	0
14051	Beverage, alcoholic, distilled spirits, vodka 80 proof	1 jigger (1.5 fl. oz.)	42	97.02	0	0	0	0	0	0	0
14052	Beverage, alcoholic, distilled spirits, whiskey 86 proof	1 jigger	42	105	0	0.042	0	0	0	0	0
14014	Beverage, alcoholic, martini, prepared from recipe	1 cocktail (2 fl. oz.)	60	145.8	0.024	1.224	0	0	0	0	0
14017	Beverage, alcoholic, pina colada, prep from recipe	1 cocktail (4.5 fl. oz.)	141	245.34	0.592	31.951	0.423	2.651	0.116	0.047	2.307
43479	Beverage, alcoholic, rice (sake)	1 oz	28.34	37.976	0.142	1.417	0	0	0	0	0
14084	Beverage, alcoholic, wine (all table)	1 glass (3.5 fl. oz.)	103	79.31	0.206	3.296	0	0	0	0	0
43154	Beverage, alcoholic, wine, cooking	1 cup	186	93	0.93	11.718	0	0	0	0	0
14536	Beverage, alcoholic, wine, dry dessert	1 glass (3.5 fl. oz.)	103	156.56	0.206	12.02	0	0	0	0	0
14096	Beverage, alcoholic, wine, red	1 glass (3.5 fl. oz.)	103	74.16	0.206	1.751	0	0	0	0	0
14104	Beverage, alcoholic, wine, rose	1 glass (3.5 fl. oz.)	103	73.13	0.206	1.442	0	0	0	0	0
14057	Beverage, alcoholic, wine, sweet dessert	1 glass (3.5 fl. oz.)	103	164.8	0.206	14.101	0	0	0	0	0
14106	Beverage, alcoholic, wine, white	1 glass (3.5 fl. oz.)	103	70.04	0.103	0.824	0	0	0	0	0
14182	Beverage, chocolate syrup w/o added nutrients, prep w/milk	1 cup (8 fl. oz.)	282	253.8	8.657	36.04	0.846	8.347	2.087	0.485	4.74
14390	Beverage, cocoa mix w/aspartame, dry, low kcal, prep w/H₂O	1 packet dry mix with 6 fl. oz. water	192	55.68	2.419	10.445	0.96	0.442	0.146	0.013	0
14194	Beverage, cocoa mix, dry, w/o added nutrients, prep w/H₂O	1 oz packet with 6 fl. oz. water	206	113.3	1.669	23.978	1.03	1.133	0.375	0.035	0.672
14195	Beverage, cocoa, hot cocoa mix w/marshmallows/Carnation	1 envelope	28	111.72	1.347	24.254	0.504	1.025	0.307	0.376	0.412
14418	Beverage, coffee mix w/sugar (cappuccino) dry, prep w/H₂O	6 fl. oz. H₂O & 2 rounded tsp mix	192	61.44	0.384	10.752	0	2.112	0.123	0.038	1.83
14419	Beverage, coffee mix w/sugar (French) dry, prep w/H₂O	6 fl. oz. H₂O & 2 rounded tsp mix	189	56.7	0.567	6.615	0	3.402	0.198	0.062	2.947
14420	Beverage, coffee mix w/sugar (mocha) dry, prep w/H₂O	6 fl. oz. & 2 round tsp mix	188	50.76	0.564	8.46	0.188	1.88	0.109	0.034	1.609
14232	Beverage, coffee mix, Kraft Intl Sugar-Free Fat-Free Low-Calorie French Vanilla	1 NLEA serving	7	25.41	0.217	5.32	0.343	0.343			0.056
14209	Beverage, coffee, brewed	1 cup (8 fl. oz.)	237	9.48	0.332	0	0	1.801	0	0	0

Chol (g)	Calc (mg)	Iron (mg)	Mag (mg)	Phos (mg)	Pota (mg)	Sodi (mg)	Zinc (mg)	Vit A (RAE)	Vit C (mg)	Thia (mg)	Ribo (mg)	Niac (mg)	Vit B6 (mg)	Vit B12 (µg)	Vit E (mg)	Fol (µg)	Alc (g)
71.4	9.35	1.989	17	148.75	255.85	53.55	4.548	0	0	0.06	0.145	2.899	0.196	2.159		5.95	0
25.6	250.88	0.64	25.6	204.8	335.36	117.76	0.947	69.12	0	0.108	0.445	0.353	0.102	1.075		12.8	0
23.94	252.7	0.798	47.88	234.08	457.52	154.28	1.277	69.16	0.266	0.114	0.479	0.378	0.09	1.064	0.16	13.3	0
26.5	259.7	0.557	39.75	241.15	455.8	159	1.087	68.9	0.265	0.143	0.488	0.686	0.122	1.113	0.159	23.85	0
31.8	310.05	0.239	45.05	280.9	484.95	209.35	1.14	87.45	0.53	0.215	0.641	1.375	0.175	1.219	0.329	21.2	0
31.92	292.6	0.213	31.92	228.76	369.74	127.68	0.931	69.16	2.394	0.093	0.42	0.221	0.104	0.878		13.3	0
0	17.7	0.142	17.7	42.48	63.72	10.62	0.106	0	0	0.032	0.106	1.388	0.12	0.035	0	14.16	11.328
0	17.8	0.071	21.36	46.28	89	14.24	0.036	0	0	0.021	0.093	1.613	0.178	0.071	0	21.36	12.816
0	0.52	0.031	1.56	3.12	15.6	4.16	0.016	0	0	0.002	0.006	0.075	0	0		0	13.52
27.26	7.52	0.061	0.94	23.5	15.04	43.24	0.075	81.31	0.094	0.005	0.027	0.037	0.005	0.038	0.211	0.94	6.486
0	0	0.035	0	0	0	2.5	0.02	0	0	0	0	0.002	0	0	0	0	14.9
0	1.8	0.054	1.2	3	12.6	3	0.024	0	0.96	0.008	0.003	0.031	0.005	0	0.018	1.2	13.86
0	0	0	0	0	0	0.84	0	0	0	0	0	0	0	0			15.918
0	0	0.05	0	2.1	0.84	0.42	0.029	0	0	0.003	0	0	0	0			14.028
0	0	0.004	0	2.1	0.42	0.42	0	0	0	0.002	0.003	0	0	0			14.028
0	0	0.008	0	1.26	0.42	0	0.008	0	0	0.003	0	0.021	0	0		0	15.12
0	0.6	0.024	1.2	1.2	9.6	1.8	0.006	0	0	0.002	0.002	0.022	0	0	0	0	20.34
0	11.28	0.296	11.28	9.87	100.11	8.46	0.183	0	6.909	0.041	0.024	0.166	0.063	0	0.028	16.92	13.959
0	1.417	0.028	1.7	1.7	7.085	0.567	0.006	0	0	0	0	0	0	0	0	0	4.563
0	8.24	0.36	9.27	13.39	86.52	6.18	0.062	0	0	0.004	0.016	0.076	0.025	0.01	0	1.03	9.579
0	16.74	0.744	18.6	27.9	163.68	1164.36	0.149	0	0	0	0.019	0.186	0.037	0	0	1.86	6.138
0	8.24	0.247	9.27	9.27	94.76	9.27	0.072	0	0	0.019	0.019	0.219	0	0	0	0	15.759
0	8.24	0.443	13.39	14.42	115.36	5.15	0.093	0	0	0.005	0.029	0.083	0.035	0.01		2.06	9.579
0	8.24	0.391	10.3	15.45	101.97	5.15	0.062	0	0	0.004	0.016	0.076	0.025	0.01		1.03	9.579
0	8.24	0.247	9.27	9.27	94.76	9.27	0.072	0	0	0.019	0.019	0.219	0	0	0	0	15.759
0	9.27	0.33	10.3	14.42	82.4	5.15	0.072	0	0	0.004	0.005	0.069	0.014	0		0	9.579
25.38	250.98	0.902	50.76	253.8	408.9	132.54	1.213	70.5	0	0.11	0.465	0.386	0.09	1.072	0.141	14.1	0
0	90.24	0.749	32.64	134.4	405.12	170.88	0.518	26.88	0.192	0.04	0.209	0.163	0.048	0.25	0.058	1.92	0
2.06	45.32	0.35	24.72	88.58	201.88	146.26	0.433	0	0.412	0.027	0.161	0.167	0.033	0.371	0.144	0	0
1.68	41.16	0.238	16.24	57.96	141.96	96.04	0.204	0	0	0.028	0.118	0.104	0.031	0.118	0.043	1.12	0
0	7.68	0.154	9.6	26.88	119.04	103.68	0.077		0	0.015	0.006	0.323	0	0		0	0
0	7.56	0.019	1.89	41.58	136.08	30.24	0.038		0	0	0.002	0.675	0	0		0	0
0	7.52	0.244	9.4	28.2	118.44	35.72	0.15		0	0.004	0.004	0.259	0	0		0	0
0	4.34	0.057		16.1	71.75	65.03			0								
0	2.37	0.024	4.74	7.11	113.76	2.37	0.024	0	0	0	0.118	0	0.002	0	0.047	4.74	0

EvaluEat Code	Food Name	Amt	Wt (g)	Energy (kcal)	Prot (g)	Carb (g)	Fiber (g)	Fat (g)	Mono (g)	Poly (g)	Sat (g)
14201	Beverage, coffee, brewed, prepared with tap water, decaffeinated	1 cup (8 fl. oz.)	237	9.48	0.332	0	0	1.801	0	0	0
14219	Beverage, coffee, instant powder, decaffeinated, prep	6 fl. oz.	179	3.58	0.215	0.77	0	0	0	0.002	0.002
14215	Beverage, coffee, instant	6 fl. oz.	179	3.58	0.179	0.609	0	0	0	0.004	0.004
14400	Beverage, cola w/caffeine	1 can (12 fl. oz.)	370	155.4	0.185	39.775	0	0	0	0	0
1057	Beverage, eggnog	1 cup	254	342.9	9.677	34.392	0	18.999	5.672	0.861	11.285
14119	Beverage, mixed vegetable and fruit juice drink	1 oz	28.34	32.024	0.071	7.935	0.17	0.014	0.001	0.006	0.002
14137	Beverage, Nestea Ice Tea, lemon flavor	1 cup (8 fl. oz.)	240	88.8	0	20.4	0	0.72			0.058
14121	Beverage, soft drink, club soda	1 can or bottle (16 fl. oz.)	474	0	0	0	0	0	0	0	0
14146	Beverage, soft drink, cola, low calorie, with aspartame, caffeine free	1 can or bottle (16 fl. oz.)	474	4.74	0.474	0.474	0	0	0	0	0
14416	Beverage, soft drink, cola, w/aspartame, low calorie	1 bottle 16 fl. oz.	474	4.74	0.474	0.474	0	0	0	0	0
14148	Beverage, soft drink, cola, with higher caffeine	1 can or bottle (16 fl. oz.)	492	206.64	0.246	52.89	0	0	0	0	0
14130	Beverage, soft drink, cream soda	1 can or bottle (16 fl. oz.)	494	251.94	0	65.702	0	0	0	0	0
14136	Beverage, soft drink, ginger ale	1 can or bottle (16 fl. oz.)	488	165.92	0	42.798	0	0	0	0	0
14142	Beverage, soft drink, grape	1 can or bottle (12 fl. oz.)	372	159.96	0	41.664	0	0	0	0	0
14145	Beverage, soft drink, lemon-lime	1 can or bottle (16 fl. oz.)	491	196.4	0	51.064	0	0	0	0	0
14150	Beverage, soft drink, orange	1 can or bottle (16 fl. oz.)	496	238.08	0	61.008	0	0	0	0	0
14153	Beverage, soft drink, pepper type	1 can or bottle (16 fl. oz.)	491	201.31	0	51.064	0	0.491	0	0	0.344
14157	Beverage, soft drink, root beer	1 can or bottle (16 fl. oz.)	493	202.13	0	52.258	0	0	0	0	0
14376	Beverage, tea mix, instant w/lemon flavor, w/saccharin, dry	1 cup (8 fl. oz.)	237	4.74	0.047	1.043	0	0	0	0.002	0
14369	Beverage, tea mix, Instant w/lemon, unsweetened, dry	1 cup (8 fl. oz.)	238	4.76	0	0.952	0	0	0	0.002	0
14355	Beverage, tea, brewed	1 cup (8 fl. oz.)	237	2.37	0	0.711	0	0	0.002	0.009	0.005
14352	Beverage, tea, brewed, prepared with tap water, decaffeinated	1 cup (8 fl. oz.)	237	2.37	0	0.711	0	0	0.002	0.009	0.005
14545	Beverage, tea, chamomile, brewed	1 cup (8 fl. oz.)	237	2.37	0	0.474	0	0	0.002	0.012	0.005
14381	Beverage, tea, herbal (not chamomile) brewed	1 cup (8 fl. oz.)	237	2.37	0	0.474	0	0	0.002	0.012	0.005
14429	Beverage, water	1 cup (8 fl. oz.)	237	0	0	0	0	0	0	0	0
14155	Beverage, water, carbonated, tonic (quinine)	1 fl. oz.	30.5	10.37	0	2.684	0	0	0	0	0
14553	Beverage, wine, non-alcoholic	1 fl. oz.	29	1.74	0.145	0.319	0	0	0	0	0
18629	Biscuit, buttermilk, refrigerated dough/Pillsbury	1 serving	64	154.24	4.992	30.4		1.408	0.605	0.312	0.285
18017	Biscuit, mixed grain, refrigerated dough	1 biscuit (2-1/2" dia)	44	115.72	2.684	20.856		2.464	1.29	0.387	0.601
18013	Biscuit, plain or buttermilk, refrigerated dough, baked, reduced fat	1 biscuit (2-1/4" dia)	21	62.79	1.638	11.634	0.399	1.092	0.587	0.164	0.272

Chol (g)	Calc (mg)	Iron (mg)	Mag (mg)	Phos (mg)	Pota (mg)	Sodi (mg)	Zinc (mg)	Vit A (RAE)	Vit C (mg)	Thia (mg)	Ribo (mg)	Niac (mg)	Vit B6 (mg)	Vit B12 (µg)	Vit E (mg)	Fol (µg)	Alc (g)
0	2.37	0.024	4.74	7.11	113.76	2.37	0.024	0	0	0	0.118	0	0.002	0	0.047	4.74	0
0	5.37	0.107	8.95	7.16	82.34	3.58	0	0	0	0	0.025	0.505	0	0	0	0	0
0	7.16	0.072	5.37	5.37	53.7	3.58	0.018	0	0	0	0.002	0.422	0	0	0	0	0
0	11.1	0.074	3.7	48.1	3.7	14.8	0.037	0	0	0	0	0	0	0	0	0	0
149.86	330.2	0.508	48.26	276.86	419.1	137.16	1.168	114.3	3.81	0.086	0.483	0.267	0.127	1.143	0.508	2.54	0
0	2.834	0.065	1.417	1.984	51.012	5.668	0.026	29.47	7.085	0.003	0.004	0.044	0.01	0	0.045	1.134	0
						0											0
0	23.7	0.047	4.74	0	9.48	99.54	0.474	0	0	0	0	0	0	0	0	0	0
0	18.96	0.142	4.74	42.66	0	28.44	0.379	0	0	0.024	0.109	0	0	0	0	0	0
0	14.22	0.142	4.74	52.14	28.44	23.7	0	0	0	0.024	0.109	0	0	0	0	0	0
0	14.76	0.098	4.92	63.96	4.92	19.68	0.049	0	0	0	0	0	0	0	0	0	0
0	24.7	0.247	4.94	0	4.94	59.28	0.346	0	0	0	0	0	0	0	0	0	0
0	14.64	0.878	4.88	0	4.88	34.16	0.244	0	0	0	0	0	0	0	0	0	0
0	11.16	0.298	3.72	0	3.72	55.8	0.26	0	0	0	0	0	0	0	0	0	0
0	9.82	0.344	4.91	0	4.91	54.01	0.245	0	0	0	0	0.074	0	0	0	0	0
0	24.8	0.298	4.96	4.96	9.92	59.52	0.496	0	0	0	0	0	0	0	0	0	0
0	14.73	0.196	0	54.01	4.91	49.1	0.196	0	0	0	0	0	0			0	0
0	24.65	0.247	4.93	0	4.93	64.09	0.345	0	0	0	0	0	0	0	0	0	0
0	7.11	0.118	2.37	2.37	30.81	23.7	0.024	0	0	0	0.002	0.047	0.002	0	0	0	0
0	4.76	0.024	4.76	2.38	49.98	14.28	0.071	0	0	0	0.019	0.09	0.005	0	0	0	0
0	0	0.047	7.11	2.37	87.69	7.11	0.047	0	0	0	0.033	0	0	0	0	11.85	0
0	0	0.047	7.11	2.37	87.69	7.11	0.047	0	0	0	0.033	0	0	0	0	11.85	0
0	4.74	0.19	2.37	0	21.33	2.37	0.095	2.37	0	0.024	0.009	0	0	0	0	2.37	0
0	4.74	0.19	2.37	0	21.33	2.37	0.095	0	0	0.024	0.009	0	0	0	0	2.37	0
0	4.74	0	2.37	0	0	4.74	0	0	0	0	0	0	0	0	0	0	0
0	0.305	0.003	0	0	0	1.22	0.031	0	0	0	0	0	0	0	0	0	0
0	2.61	0.116	2.9	4.35	25.52	2.03	0.023	0	0	0	0.003	0.029	0.006	0	0	0.29	0
		1.549				547.2											0
0	7.48	1.21	13.2	103.84	200.64	294.8	0.264	0	0	0.172	0.092	1.496	0.029	0		36.52	0
0	3.99	0.649	3.57	97.65	38.85	304.71	0.097	0	0	0.088	0.049	0.724	0.006	0	0.015	17.43	0

EvaluEat Code	Food Name	Amt	Wt (g)	Energy (kcal)	Prot (g)	Carb (g)	Fiber (g)	Fat (g)	Mono (g)	Poly (g)	Sat (g)
9043	Blackberry juice, canned	1 cup	144	54.72	0.432	11.232	0.144	0.864	0.084	0.495	0.026
42129	Bologna, beef and pork, low-fat	1 oz	28.34	65.182	3.259	0.737	0	5.47	2.592	0.464	2.071
42161	Bologna, beef, low-fat	1 oz	28.34	65.182	3.599	0.879	0	5.356	2.594	0.205	2.269
20034	Bran, oat, cooked	1 cup	219	87.6	7.03	25.054	5.694	1.883	0.637	0.742	0.357
7924	Bratwurst, pork, beef and turkey, lite, smoked	1 serving (2.33 oz)	66	122.76	9.537	1.069	0	8.93	4.729	0.558	3.16
18376	Bread crumbs, dry, grated, seasoned	1 oz	28.35	104.05	4.026	19.958	1.191	0.737	0.274	0.187	0.206
18079	Bread crumbs, plain, grated, dry	1 oz	28.35	111.98	3.785	20.406	1.276	1.503	0.29	0.584	0.341
18080	Bread sticks, plain	1 stick, small (approx 4-1/4" long)	5	20.6	0.6	3.42	0.15	0.475	0.178	0.181	0.071
18085	Bread stuffing, corn, dry mix, prep	.5 cup	100	179	2.9	21.9	2.9	8.8	3.856	2.706	1.755
18082	Bread stuffing, plain, dry mix, prep	.5 cup	100	178	3.2	21.7	2.9	8.6	3.808	2.604	1.734
18019	Bread, banana, Elfin Loaves/Keebler	1 slice	60	195.6	2.58	32.76	0.66	6.3	2.688	1.878	1.342
18023	Bread, corn, dry mix, prepared	1 piece	60	188.4	4.32	28.86	1.44	6	3.084	0.734	1.643
18270	Bread, corn, hushpuppies, homemade	1 cup	152	512.24	11.704	69.92	4.256	20.52	4.96	10.973	3.204
18627	Bread, crusty Italian Bread w/garlic/PepFarm	1 serving	50	186	4.15	20.8		9.6	3.918	1.832	2.411
18027	Bread, egg	1 slice (5" x 3" x 1/2")	40	114.8	3.8	19.12	0.92	2.4	0.921	0.442	0.637
18029	Bread, french/vienna/sourdough	1 slice, medium (4" x 2-1/2" x 1-3/4")	64	175.36	5.632	33.216	1.92	1.92	0.778	0.444	0.41
18604	Bread, garlic, frozen/Campione	1 serving	28	101.36	2.38	12.404	1.316	4.704			0.756
18641	Bread, hamburger rolls/Wonder	1 serving	43	117.39	3.47	21.861	1.118	1.785	0.365	0.936	0.436
18031	Bread, indian (Navajo) Fry	1 piece (10-1/2" dia)	160	526.4	11.36	85.28	2.88	15.2	6.381	4.141	3.701
18032	Bread, Irish soda, homemade, prepared from recipe	1 oz	28.35	82.215	1.871	15.876	0.737	1.418	0.567	0.419	0.315
18033	Bread, Italian	1 slice, medium	20	54.2	1.76	10	0.54	0.7	0.162	0.278	0.171
18035	Bread, mixed grain/7-grain/whole grain	1 slice, large	32	80	3.2	14.848	2.048	1.216	0.488	0.295	0.258
18037	Bread, oatbran	1 slice	30	70.8	3.12	11.94	1.35	1.32	0.477	0.508	0.209
18049	Bread, oatbran, reduced kcal	1 slice	23	46.23	1.84	9.499	2.76	0.736	0.157	0.384	0.102
18039	Bread, oatmeal	1 slice	27	72.63	2.268	13.095	1.08	1.188	0.426	0.46	0.19
18041	Bread, pita, white, enriched	1 pita, large (6-1/2" dia)	60	165	5.46	33.42	1.32	0.72	0.063	0.321	0.1
18042	Bread, pita, whole wheat	1 pita, large (6-1/2" dia)	64	170.24	6.272	35.2	4.736	1.664	0.223	0.675	0.262
18044	Bread, pumpernickel	1 slice, regular	26	65	2.262	12.35	1.69	0.806	0.242	0.322	0.114
18047	Bread, raisin, enriched	1 slice	26	71.24	2.054	13.598	1.118	1.144	0.596	0.177	0.281
18060	Bread, rye	1 slice	32	82.88	2.72	15.456	1.856	1.056	0.42	0.256	0.2
18064	Bread, wheat (includes wheat berry)	1 slice	25	65	2.275	11.8	1.075	1.025	0.43	0.227	0.223
18066	Bread, wheat bran	1 slice	36	89.28	3.168	17.208	1.44	1.224	0.582	0.234	0.28
18068	Bread, wheat germ	1 slice	28	73.08	2.688	13.524	0.588	0.812	0.357	0.187	0.184
18055	Bread, wheat, reduced kcal	1 slice	23	45.54	2.093	10.028	2.76	0.529	0.058	0.223	0.079
18069	Bread, white, commercially prep, crumbs/cubes/slices	1 slice	25	66.5	1.91	12.653	0.6	0.822	0.17	0.339	0.179
18057	Bread, white, reduced kcal	1 slice	23	47.61	2.001	10.189	2.231	0.575	0.248	0.129	0.126
18075	Bread, whole wheat, commercially prep	1 slice	28	68.88	2.716	12.908	1.932	1.176	0.47	0.281	0.257
43100	Breakfast bars, oats, sugar, raisins, coconut (include granola bar)	1 cup	186	863.04	18.228	124.062	5.766	32.736	3.595	3.039	23.603

Chol (g)	Calc (mg)	Iron (mg)	Mag (mg)	Phos (mg)	Pota (mg)	Sodi (mg)	Zinc (mg)	Vit A (RAE)	Vit C (mg)	Thia (mg)	Ribo (mg)	Niac (mg)	Vit B$_6$ (mg)	Vit B$_{12}$ (µg)	Vit E (mg)	Fol (µg)	Alc (g)
0	17.28	0.691	30.24	17.28	194.4	1.44	0.59	11.52	16.27	0.017	0.026	0.642	0.03	0	1.296	14.4	0
11.053	3.117	0.187	3.401	51.295	44.21	314.007	0.425	0	0	0.048	0.037	0.72	0.051	0.371	0.062	1.417	0
10.486	2.551	0.283	3.401	50.445	41.66	319.675	0.519	0	0.283	0.014	0.028	0.709	0.043	0.397	0.054	1.417	0
0	21.9	1.927	87.6	260.61	201.48	2.19	1.161	0	0	0.35	0.074	0.315	0.055	0		13.14	0
36.96	9.24	0.62	9.24	87.12	162.36	648.12	1.769	0	0	0.059	0.11	1.219	0.141	1.056	0.03	3.3	0
0.284	28.067	0.902	10.773	37.706	76.545	751.275	0.258	1.134	0.113	0.045	0.048	0.774	0.042	0.011		30.9	0
0	51.881	1.369	12.191	46.778	55.566	207.522	0.411	0	0	0.274	0.114	1.881	0.034	0.099	0.023	30.34	0
0	1.1	0.214	1.6	6.05	6.2	32.85	0.044	0	0	0.029	0.028	0.264	0.004	0	0.051	8.1	0
0	26	0.94	13	34	62	455	0.23	78	0.8	0.117	0.092	1.247	0.038	0.01	0.85	97	0
0	32	1.09	12	42	74	543	0.28	118	0	0.136	0.107	1.475	0.04	0.01	1.4	39	0
25.8	12.6	0.84	8.4	34.8	80.4	181.2	0.21	63.6	1.02	0.103	0.12	0.868	0.09	0.06	1.071	19.8	0
36.6	43.8	1.14	12	225.6	76.8	466.8	0.378	26.4	0.06	0.146	0.162	1.234	0.062	0.096		33	0
68.4	422.56	4.621	36.48	287.28	218.88	1015.36	1.003	62.32	0.304	0.535	0.505	4.229	0.155	0.289	1.915	135.3	0
5.5		1.185				200											
20.4	37.2	1.216	7.6	42.4	46	196.8	0.316	25.2	0	0.175	0.174	1.939	0.026	0.04	0.104	42	0
0	48	1.619	17.28	67.2	72.32	389.76	0.557	0	0	0.333	0.211	3.039	0.028	0	0.192	94.72	0
		0.302				154											
	37.41	0.955				256.28											
0	372.8	5.76	25.6	251.2	118.4	1112	0.8	0	0	0.688	0.486	5.818	0.043	0	1.235	118.4	0
5.103	22.964	0.763	6.521	32.319	75.411	112.833	0.162	13.61	0.227	0.084	0.076	0.682	0.024	0.014	0.3	13.33	0
0	15.6	0.588	5.4	20.6	22	116.8	0.172	0	0	0.095	0.058	0.876	0.01	0	0.058	38.2	0
0	29.12	1.11	16.96	56.32	65.28	155.84	0.406	0	0.096	0.13	0.109	1.397	0.107	0.022	0.109	37.76	0
0	19.5	0.936	10.5	42.3	44.1	122.1	0.267	0.6	0	0.151	0.104	1.449	0.022	0	0.132	24.3	0
0	13.11	0.725	12.65	31.97	23.46	80.73	0.241	0	0	0.081	0.047	0.865	0.024	0	0.064	18.63	0
0	17.82	0.729	9.99	34.02	38.34	161.73	0.275	1.35	0	0.108	0.065	0.847	0.018	0.008	0.13	16.74	0
0	51.6	1.572	15.6	58.2	72	321.6	0.504	0	0	0.359	0.196	2.779	0.02	0	0.18	64.2	0
0	9.6	1.958	44.16	115.2	108.8	340.48	0.973	0	0	0.217	0.051	1.818	0.17	0	0.39	22.4	0
0	17.68	0.746	14.04	46.28	54.08	174.46	0.385	0	0	0.085	0.079	0.804	0.033	0	0.109	24.18	0
0	17.16	0.754	6.76	28.34	59.02	101.4	0.187	0	0.026	0.088	0.103	0.901	0.018	0	0.073	27.56	0
0	23.36	0.906	12.8	40	53.12	211.2	0.365	0	0.128	0.139	0.107	1.218	0.024	0	0.106	35.2	0
0	26.25	0.827	11.5	37.5	50.25	132.5	0.26	0	0	0.105	0.07	1.031	0.024	0	0.072	22.75	0
0	26.64	1.105	29.16	66.6	81.72	174.96	0.486	0	0	0.143	0.103	1.585	0.063	0	0.115	37.8	0
0	24.92	0.966	7.84	33.88	71.12	154.84	0.274	0	0.056	0.103	0.105	1.259	0.022	0.02	0.143	33.04	0
0	18.4	0.681	8.97	23.46	28.06	117.53	0.258	0	0.023	0.097	0.068	0.894	0.029	0	0.055	20.93	0
0	37.75	0.935	5.75	24.75	25	170.25	0.185	0	0	0.114	0.083	1.096	0.021	0	0.055	27.75	0
0	21.62	0.734	5.29	27.83	17.48	104.19	0.308	0	0.115	0.094	0.066	0.837	0.01	0.064	0.044	21.85	0
0	20.16	0.924	24.08	64.12	70.56	147.56	0.543	0	0	0.098	0.057	1.074	0.05	0.003	0.087	14	0
0	111.6	5.915	187.86	515.22	606.36	517.08	2.976	14.88	1.86	0.521	0.205	3.255	0.651	0	4.352	150.7	0

EvaluEat Code	Food Name	Amt	Wt (g)	Energy (kcal)	Prot (g)	Carb (g)	Fiber (g)	Fat (g)	Mono (g)	Poly (g)	Sat (g)
11097	Broccoli raab, cooked	.5 cup	92	30.36	3.524	2.87	2.576	0.478			
11096	Broccoli raab, raw	.5 cup	92	20.24	2.916	2.622	2.484	0.451	0.024	0.12	0.046
4601	Butter, light, stick, with salt	1 tbsp	12.8	63.872	0.422	0	0	7.053	2.039	0.262	4.393
4602	Butter, light, stick, without salt	1 tbsp	12.8	63.872	0.422	0	0	7.053	2.039	0.262	4.393
1001	Butter, regular (with salt)	1 tbsp	14.2	101.81	0.121	0.009	0	11.518	4.735	0.407	5.799
1145	Butter, unsalted	1 tbsp	14.2	101.81	0.121	0.009	0	11.518	2.985	0.432	7.294
1002	Butter, whipped (with salt)	1 tbsp	9.4	67.398	0.08	0.006	0	7.624	2.202	0.283	4.746
43143	Cabbage, japanese style, fresh, pickled	1 cup	186	55.8	2.976	10.546	5.766	0.186	0.015	0.089	0.024
43144	Cabbage, mustard, salted	1 cup	186	52.08	2.046	10.472	5.766	0.186	0.013	0.089	0.024
18086	Cake, angelfood, commercially prep	1 piece (1/12 of 12 oz cake)	28	72.24	1.652	16.184	0.42	0.224	0.02	0.103	0.034
18090	Cake, boston cream pie, commercially prep	1 piece (1/6 of pie)	92	231.84	2.208	39.468	1.288	7.82	4.18	0.928	2.249
18096	Cake, chocolate w/chocolate icing, commercially prep	1 piece (1/8 of 18 oz cake)	64	234.88	2.624	34.944	1.792	10.496	5.606	1.181	3.053
18101	Cake, chocolate, homemade, w/o icing	1 piece (1/12 of 9"dia)	95	340.1	5.035	50.73	1.52	14.345	5.737	2.623	5.158
18116	Cake, gingerbread, homemade	1 piece (1/9 of 8"square)	74	263.44	2.886	36.408		12.136	5.272	3.12	3.05
18120	Cake, pound, commercially prep w/butter	1 piece (1/12 of 12 oz cake)	28	108.64	1.54	13.664	0.14	5.572	1.652	0.299	3.237
18452	Cake, snack/cupcakes, chocolate w/frosting, low-fat	1 cupcake	43	131.15	1.849	28.896	1.849	1.591	0.795	0.209	0.466
18127	Cake, snack-type cream filled, chocolate w/icing	1 cupcake	50	188	1.7	30.15	0.4	7.25	2.845	2.618	1.429
18133	Cake, sponge, commercially prep	1 piece (1/12 of 16 oz cake)	38	109.82	2.052	23.218	0.19	1.026	0.361	0.17	0.305
18102	Cake, white w/coconut icing, homemade	1 piece (1/12 of 9"dia)	112	398.72	4.928	70.784	1.12	11.536	4.135	2.421	4.365
18139	Cake, white, homemade, w/o icing	1 piece (1/12 of 9"dia)	74	264.18	3.996	42.328	0.592	9.176	3.929	2.33	2.419
18140	Cake, yellow w/chocolate icing, commercially prep	1 piece (1/8 of 18 oz cake)	64	242.56	2.432	35.456	1.152	11.136	6.14	1.352	2.98
18146	Cake, yellow, homemade, w/o icing	1 piece (1/12 of 8"dia)	68	245.48	3.604	36.04	0.476	9.928	4.236	2.428	2.668
9426	Candied fruit	1 oz	28.34	90.971	0.099	23.449	0.453	0.02	0.002	0.006	0.003
43031	Candies, chocolate covered, caramel with nuts	1 cup	186	874.2	17.67	112.8	7.998	39.06	17.566	10.851	8.662
43058	Candies, hard, dietetic or low calorie (sorbitol)	1 cup	186	697.5	0	173.72	0	0	0	0	0
19236	Candies, Hershey's milk chocolate with almond bites	17 pieces	39	214.5	3.806	19.89	1.404	13.935	5.608	0.944	6.782
19279	Candies, milk chocolate coated coffee beans	1 NLEA serving	6	30.78	0.445	3.745	0.342	1.565	0.35	0.051	0.749
19068	Candies, Nestle, Bit-O'-Honey candy chews	18 pieces	40	160	0.84	32.4	0	3	0.781	0.25	2
43046	Candies, nougat	1 cup	186	740.28	6.194	171.85	6.138	3.106	0	0	3.101
19159	Candy bar, 3 Musketeers/M&M Mars	1 bar (.8 oz)	23	95.68	0.736	17.664	0.414	2.967	0.987	0.104	1.495
19065	Candy bar, Almond Joy/Hershey	1 package (1.76 oz)	49	234.71	2.024	29.16	2.45	13.196	2.577	0.578	8.619
19111	Candy bar, Baby Ruth/Nestle	1 bar (0.75 oz)	21	97.44	1.491	12.978	0.504	5.25	1.356	0.694	2.583
19069	Candy bar, Butterfinger Bar and Dessert Topping	1 bar fun size	21	99.96	1.218	15.223	0.357	3.99	1.025	0.517	2.151
19075	Candy bar, Caramello/Hershey	1 bar (1.25 oz)	35	161.7	2.167	22.333	0.42	7.417	1.851	0.22	4.452
19109	Candy bar, Kit Kat Wafer/Hershey	1 bar (1.5 oz)	42	217.14	2.692	26.951	0.798	11.386	2.012	0.214	7.346

Chol (g)	Calc (mg)	Iron (mg)	Mag (mg)	Phos (mg)	Pota (mg)	Sodi (mg)	Zinc (mg)	Vit A (RAE)	Vit C (mg)	Thia (mg)	Ribo (mg)	Niac (mg)	Vit B6 (mg)	Vit B12 (µg)	Vit E (mg)	Fol (µg)	Alc (g)
	108.56	1.168	24.84	75.44	315.56	51.52	0.497	208.8	34.04	0.155	0.129	1.854	0.202		2.328	65.32	
	99.36	1.969	20.24	67.16	180.32	30.36	0.708	120.5	18.58	0.149	0.119	1.123	0.157		1.49	76.36	
13.568	6.144	0.14	0.64	4.352	9.088	57.6	0.033	59.52	0	0.001	0.009	0.003	0.001	0.017	0.202	0.128	0
13.568	6.144	0.14	0.64	4.352	9.088	4.608	0.033	59.52	0	0.001	0.009	0.003	0.001	0.017	0.202	0.128	0
30.53	3.408	0.003	0.284	3.408	3.408	81.792	0.013	97.13	0	0.001	0.005	0.006	0	0.024	0.329	0.426	0
30.53	3.408	0.003	0.284	3.408	3.408	1.562	0.013	97.13	0	0.001	0.005	0.006	0	0.024	0.329	0.426	0
20.586	2.256	0.015	0.188	2.162	2.444	77.738	0.005	64.3	0	0	0.003	0.004	0	0.012	0.218	0.282	0
0	89.28	0.911	22.32	79.98	1586.58	515.22	0.372	16.74	1.302	0	0.074	0.335	0.186	0	0.223	78.12	0
0	124.62	1.302	27.9	50.22	457.56	1333.62	0.558	91.14	0	0.074	0.167	1.339	0.558	0	0.037	133.9	0
0	39.2	0.146	3.36	8.96	26.04	209.72	0.02	0	0	0.029	0.137	0.247	0.009	0.017		9.8	0
34.04	21.16	0.35	5.52	45.08	35.88	132.48	0.147	22.08	0.184	0.375	0.248	0.176	0.024	0.147	0.138	12.88	0
26.88	27.52	1.408	21.76	78.08	128	213.76	0.442	16.64	0.064	0.017	0.085	0.369	0.026	0.09		10.88	0
55.1	57	1.53	30.4	100.7	133	299.25	0.655	38	0.19	0.134	0.202	1.08	0.039	0.152	1.512	25.65	0
23.68	52.54	2.131	51.8	39.96	324.86	241.98	0.289	10.36	0.074	0.141	0.12	1.286	0.141	0.044		24.42	0
61.88	9.8	0.386	3.08	38.36	33.32	111.44	0.129	41.72	0	0.038	0.064	0.367	0.012	0.07		11.48	0
0	15.48	0.662	10.75	78.69	96.32	177.59	0.237	0	0	0.015	0.057	0.307	0.003	0		6.45	0
8.5	36.5	1.68	20.5	46.5	61	212.5	0.255	2.5	0	0.111	0.147	1.214	0.012	0.03	1.09	20	0
38.76	26.6	1.034	4.18	52.06	37.62	92.72	0.194	16.72	0	0.092	0.102	0.734	0.02	0.091	0.091	17.86	0
1.12	100.8	1.299	13.44	78.4	110.88	318.08	0.37	13.44	0.112	0.143	0.212	1.191	0.032	0.067	0.134	34.72	0
1.48	96.2	1.125	8.88	68.82	70.3	241.98	0.237	11.1	0.148	0.138	0.179	1.134	0.016	0.059	0.089	28.12	0
35.2	23.68	1.331	19.2	103.04	113.92	215.68	0.397	21.12	0	0.077	0.1	0.798	0.021	0.109	1.455	14.08	0
36.72	99.28	1.115	8.16	79.56	61.88	233.24	0.306	27.2	0.136	0.124	0.158	0.99	0.024	0.109	0.819	23.12	0
0	5.101	0.048	1.134	1.417	16.154	27.773	0.014	0.283	0	0	0	0	0	0	0.011	0	0
0	145.08	3.162	150.66	308.76	827.7	44.64	3.478	78.12	2.604	0.074	0.298	8.854	0.298	0	2.046	171.1	0
0	0	0	0	0	0	0	0	0	0	0	0	0	0	0	0	0	0
7.41	85.8	0.585	23.01	88.53	183.69	28.86	0.523		0.702	0.027	0.148	0.242	0.027		0.152	6.24	0
1.2	10.14	0.137	3.84	11.28	24.78	4.26	0.106	2.52	0	0.006	0.019	0.02	0.002	0.032	0.104	0.6	0
0	20	0.116	2.8	18	50.4	120	0.084	0	0		0.1	0.024	0.007	0.068	0.396	1.6	0
0	59.52	1.097	59.52	102.3	195.3	61.38	0.781	0	0.558	0.024	0.275	0.889	0.037	0.019	5.152	9.3	0
2.53	19.32	0.168	6.67	20.93	30.59	44.62	0.127	3.45	0.092	0.008	0.032	0.053	0.003	0.044	0.214		0
1.96	31.36	0.622		54.88	124.46	69.58			0.343						0.01		0
0.42	9.45	0.147	15.33	28.98	74.76	44.94	0.25	0	0.021	0.02	0.016	0.583	0.013	0.008	0.393	6.51	0
0	7.35	0.16	17.43	28.35	82.95	44.94	0.25	0	0	0.023	0.016	0.647	0.021	0.004	0.363	6.93	0
9.45	74.55	0.382		52.5	119.35	42.7			0.595						0.077		0
3.78	56.7	0.357	1.26	47.46	121.8	27.3	0.038	10.5	0.546	0.021	0.071	0.088	0.004	0.088	0.147	1.26	0

EvaluEat Code	Food Name	Amt	Wt (g)	Energy (kcal)	Prot (g)	Carb (g)	Fiber (g)	Fat (g)	Mono (g)	Poly (g)	Sat (g)
19110	Candy bar, Krackel/Hershey	1 bar (1.45 oz)	41	209.92	2.714	26.224	0.902	10.898	2.563	0.234	6.527
19115	Candy bar, Mars Almond/M&M Mars	1 bar (1.76 oz)	50	233.5	4.05	31.35	1	11.5	5.346	1.99	3.634
19135	Candy bar, Mars Milky Way/M&M Mars	1 bar (.8 oz)	23	97.29	1.035	16.491	0.391	3.703	1.385	0.138	1.792
19143	Candy bar, Mr. Goodbar/Hershey	1 bar (1.75 oz)	49	263.62	5.008	26.627	1.862	16.273	4.019	2.139	6.924
19118	Candy bar, Oh Henry!/Nestle	1 bar	26	120.12	2.002	17.004	0.546	6.006	1.734	0.707	1.747
19136	Candy bar, Skor Toffee Candy/Hershey	1 bar (1.4 oz)	39	208.65	1.221	24.071	0.507	12.55	3.623	0.499	7.324
19155	Candy bar, Snickers/M&M Mars	1 bar (2 oz)	57	273.03	4.56	33.75	1.425	14.011	5.958	2.803	5.127
19164	Candy bar, Special Dark Sweet Chocolate/Hershey	1 bar (1.45 oz)	41	217.71	2.271	24.358	2.665	13.284	2.107	0.18	7.868
19160	Candy bar, Twix Caramel Cookie/M&M Mars	1 package (2 oz)	57	284.43	2.622	37.381	0.627	13.902	7.638	0.485	5.072
19070	Candy, butterscotch	3 pieces	16	62.56	0.005	14.464	0	0.528	0.136	0.02	0.332
19074	Candy, caramel	1 piece	10.1	38.582	0.465	7.777	0.121	0.818	0.085	0.018	0.665
19071	Candy, carob	1 bar (3 oz)	87	469.8	7.09	48.972	3.306	27.283	0.42	0.257	25.246
19080	Candy, chocolate chips, semisweet	1 cup chips (6 oz package)	168	804.72	7.056	106.01	9.912	50.4	16.75	1.63	29.82
19078	Candy, chocolate, baking, unsweetened, square	1 square	29	145.29	3.741	8.654	4.814	15.17	4.671	0.451	9.382
19081	Candy, chocolate, sweet	1 bar (1.45 oz)	41	207.05	1.599	24.436	2.255	14.022	4.6	0.406	8.233
19011	Candy, fruit leather bar	1 bar	23	80.73	0.414	18.055	0.805	1.219	0.145	0.041	0.925
19013	Candy, fruit leather, pieces	1 package	27	94.77	0.27	22.815	0	0.27	0.141	0.052	0.062
19014	Candy, fruit leather, roll	1 large	21	77.91	0.021	17.997	0.693	0.63	0.311	0.113	0.136
19301	Candy, fudge, chocolate marshmallow nut, homemade	1 oz	28.34	133.77	0.915	19.022	0.595	5.966	1.585	1.152	2.829
19101	Candy, fudge, chocolate w/nuts, homemade	1 oz	28.34	130.65	1.241	19.26	0.709	5.365	1.052	2.099	1.71
19100	Candy, fudge, chocolate, homemade	1 piece	17	69.87	0.406	13.002	0.289	1.77	0.463	0.039	1.006
19106	Candy, gumdrops/gummy bears/fish/worm/dinosaur	10 gumdrops	36	142.56	0	35.604	0.036	0	0	0	0
19107	Candy, hard candy	1 piece	6	23.64	0	5.88	0	0.012	0	0	0
19108	Candy, jellybeans	10 large (1 oz)	28	105	0	26.194	0.056	0.014	0	0	0
19140	Candy, M&M's Peanut chocolate	1 package (1.67 oz)	47	242.52	4.451	28.416	1.598	12.333	5.17	1.974	4.856
19141	Candy, M&M's Plain chocolate	1 box (1.48 oz)	42	206.64	1.819	29.908	1.05	8.875	1.485	0.162	5.494
19116	Candy, marshmallow	1 regular	7.2	22.896	0.13	5.854	0.007	0.014	0.006	0.003	0.004
19120	Candy, milk chocolate	1 bar (1.55 oz)	44	235.4	3.366	26.136	1.496	13.05	5.819	0.358	6.271
19132	Candy, milk chocolate w/almonds	1 bar (1.45 oz)	41	215.66	3.69	21.812	2.542	14.104	5.531	0.935	6.962
19134	Candy, milk chocolate w/rice cereal	1 bar (1.4 oz)	40	198.4	2.52	25.36	1.32	10.6	3.456	0.312	6.356
19148	Candy, peanut brittle, homemade	1 oz	28.34	137.17	2.145	20.025	0.709	5.379	2.285	1.292	1.174
19151	Candy, peanut butter candy/Reese's Pieces/Hershey	10 pieces	8	39.76	0.997	4.789	0.24	1.982	0.357	0.15	1.314
19150	Candy, peanut butter cups, Reese's/Hershey	1 package (0.6 oz, 1 cup)	17	87.55	1.741	9.411	0.612	5.19	2.227	0.952	1.824
19126	Candy, peanuts, milk chocolate coated	10 pieces	40	207.6	5.24	19.76	1.88	13.4	5.168	1.732	5.84
19127	Candy, raisins, milk chocolate coated	10 pieces	10	39	0.41	6.83	0.42	1.48	0.474	0.051	0.88
19152	Candy, Rolo Caramel, milk chocolate/Hershey	1 package (1.91 oz)	54	255.96	2.743	36.693	0.486	11.302	2.03	0.211	7.787
19154	Candy, sesame crunch	1 piece	1.8	9.306	0.209	0.905	0.142	0.599	0.226	0.262	0.08
19370	Candy, Skittles, original bite size candy/M&M Mars	1 package	9979	40415	18.96	9045	0	436.08	295.38	11.975	86.618
19156	Candy, Starburst Fruit Chews/M&M Mars	1 package (2.07 oz)	59	233.64	0.236	49.855	0	4.897	2.106	1.841	0.73
19112	Candy, Twizzlers Strawberry/Hershey	4 pieces from 5 oz package	38	133	0.973	30.301	0	0.882			0
19091	Candy, York Peppermint Patty	1 patty (1.5 oz)	43	165.12	0.942	34.826	0.86	3.083	0.176	0.047	1.866
11683	Carrot, dehydrated	1 tbsp chopped	10	34.1	0.81	7.957	2.36	0.149	0.008	0.073	0.026

Chol (g)	Calc (mg)	Iron (mg)	Mag (mg)	Phos (mg)	Pota (mg)	Sodi (mg)	Zinc (mg)	Vit A (RAE)	Vit C (mg)	Thia (mg)	Ribo (mg)	Niac (mg)	Vit B6 (mg)	Vit B12 (µg)	Vit E (mg)	Fol (µg)	Alc (g)
4.51	64.78	0.435	5.33	50.43	133.25	80.36	0.201		0.328	0.021	0.078	0.107	0.016		0.033	2.46	0
8.5	84	0.55	36	117	162.5	85	0.555	7.5	0.35	0.021	0.156	0.472	0.03	0.18	3.875	4.5	0
3.22	29.9	0.175	7.82	33.12	55.43	55.2	0.163	4.14	0.23	0.008	0.051	0.08	0.012	0.074	0.287	1.38	0
4.9	53.9	0.681	23.03	79.87	193.06	20.09	0.456	17.15	0.441	0.069	0.069	1.686	0.034	0.162	1.553	18.62	0
2.34	21.06	0.161	13.26	36.4	84.24	60.06	0.299	2.6	0.052	0.006	0.042	0.728	0.022	0.052	0.536	11.44	0
20.67	50.7	0.222	3.9	23.79	59.67	123.63	0.066		0.195	0.008	0.039	0.051			0.016	1.17	0
7.41	53.58	0.433	32.49	97.47	169.86	151.62	0.889	23.94	0.342	0.072	0.111	0.901	0.034	0.188	0.627	17.1	0
2.05	12.3	0.873	12.71	20.91	205.82	2.46	0.004		0	0	0.004	0	0	0	0.078	0	0
2.85	51.3	0.462	18.24	62.13	107.73	110.01	0.57	12.54	0.228	0.068	0.109	0.429	0.013	0.165	1.106	10.83	0
1.44	0.32	0.003	0.16	0.16	0.64	62.56	0.002	4.48	0	0	0.003	0.001	0	0	0.014	0	0
0.707	13.938	0.014	1.717	11.514	21.614	24.745	0.044	0.101	0.051	0.001	0.034	0.025	0.004	0	0.28	0.505	0
2.61	263.61	1.122	31.32	109.62	550.71	93.09	3.071	0	0.435	0.087	0.155	0.905	0.113	0.87	1.027	18.27	0
0	53.76	5.258	193.2	221.76	613.2	18.48	2.722	0	0	0.092	0.151	0.717	0.059	0	0.386	5.04	0
0	29.29	5.046	94.83	116	240.7	6.96	2.793	0	0	0.043	0.029	0.393	0.008	0	0.116	8.12	0
0	9.84	1.132	46.33	60.27	118.9	6.56	0.615	0	0	0.008	0.098	0.275	0.018	0	0.107	1.23	0
0	6.67	0.184	5.06	12.65	31.74	17.71	0.044	1.38	16.1	0.01	0.007	0.023	0.069	0		0.92	0
0	4.86	0.203	3.78	6.48	44.28	108.81	0.051	1.62	15.12	0.012	0.027	0.027	0.081	0	0.151	1.08	0
0	6.72	0.212	4.2	6.51	61.74	66.57	0.04	1.26	25.2	0.015	0.004	0.021	0.063	0	0.118	0.84	0.021
6.518	13.887	0.323	13.036	24.939	47.895	27.49	0.218	21.82	0.085	0.012	0.023	0.083	0.015	0.009	0.197	2.267	0
3.401	15.304	0.558	15.587	31.741	51.012	11.619	0.402	10.77	0.057	0.019	0.027	0.09	0.025	0.02	0.185	4.534	0
2.38	7.65	0.301	6.12	11.73	22.27	7.99	0.187	7.48	0	0.004	0.014	0.03	0.002	0.015	0.031	0.68	0
0	1.08	0.144	0.36	0.36	1.8	15.84	0	0	0	0.002	0.005	0.004	0.002	0	0	0	0
0	0.18	0.018	0.18	0.18	0.3	2.28	0.001	0	0	0	0	0	0	0	0	0	0
0	0.84	0.036	0.56	1.12	10.36	14	0.014	0	0	0.001	0.003	0.002	0.001	0	0	0	0
4.23	47.47	0.54	35.72	109.51	163.09	22.56	1.133	12.22	0.235	0.048	0.074	1.922	0.041	0.075	1.203	17.86	0
5.88	44.1	0.466	14.28	47.88	85.26	25.62	0.462	11.34	0.21	0.026	0.071	0.088	0.008	0.143	0.462	2.52	0
0	0.216	0.017	0.144	0.576	0.36	5.76	0.003	0	0	0	0.006	0	0	0	0	0.072	0
10.12	83.16	1.034	27.72	91.52	163.68	34.76	0.884	21.56	0	0.049	0.131	0.17	0.016	0.273	0.889	5.28	0
7.79	91.84	0.668	36.9	108.24	182.04	30.34	0.549	18.04	0.082	0.025	0.178	0.304	0.021	0.135	1.841	5.74	0
7.6	68.4	0.3	19.6	77.2	137.2	58	0.448	24.8	0.12	0.023	0.116	0.185	0.023	0.248	0.8	6	0
3.401	7.652	0.346	11.903	30.04	47.611	126.113	0.247	11.05	0	0.038	0.012	0.75	0.022	0.003	0.726	13.04	0
0	5.52	0.039	7.04	16.56	28.72	15.52	0.092	0	0	0.014	0.018	0.485	0.009	0.01	0.087	4.4	0
1.02	13.26	0.206	10.54	27.37	58.31	53.38	0.218	2.89	0.051	0.027	0.019	0.763	0.017	0.095	0.026	8.5	0
3.6	41.6	0.524	38.4	84.8	200.8	16.4	0.956	13.6	0	0.046	0.07	1.7	0.084	0.176	1.384	3.2	0
0.3	8.6	0.171	4.5	14.3	51.4	3.6	0.081	2.4	0.02	0.008	0.016	0.04	0.008	0.018	0.102	0.7	0
6.48	78.3	0.227	0	38.34	101.52	101.52	0	18.36	0.486	0.011	0.065	0.022	0	0.146	0.481	0	0
0	11.79	0.077	4.518	7.614	5.796	3.006	0.068	0	0.002	0.01	0.003	0.067	0.01	0	0.003	0.936	0
0	0	0.998	99.79	199.58	898.11	1596.64	0.998	0	6676	0.2	2.295	1.497	0.299	0	43.908	0	0
0	2.36	0.077	0.59	4.13	1.18	33.04	0	0	31.21	0.001	0.001	0.003	0	0	0.413	0	0
0	0	0.194				109.06			0								0
0.43	4.73	0.396		0	47.73	12.04			0						0.004		0
0	21.2	0.393	11.8	34.6	254	27.5	0.157	541.6	1.46	0.053	0.042	0.657	0.104	0	0.697	5.5	0

EvaluEat Code	Food Name	Amt	Wt (g)	Energy (kcal)	Prot (g)	Carb (g)	Fiber (g)	Fat (g)	Mono (g)	Poly (g)	Sat (g)
44055	Celery flakes, dried	1 cubic inch	10.2	32.538	1.153	6.497	2.836	0.214	0.041	0.106	0.057
8053	Cereal, 100% bran (wheat bran & barley)	.333 cup									
		(1 NLEA serving)	29	83.23	3.683	22.678	8.294	0.609	0.092	0.319	0.087
8153	Cereal, 40% bran flakes/Ralston Purina	1 cup	49	158.76	5.635	39.102	6.909	0.686			
8001	Cereal, All-Bran/Kellogg	.5 cup									
		(1 NLEA serving)	30	78	3.75	22.2	9.6	0.996	0.222	0.612	0.162
8263	Cereal, Apple Cinnamon Cheerios/General Mills	.75 cup									
		(1 NLEA serving)	30	117.6	1.8	25.2	1.29	1.53	0.713	0.384	0.297
8254	Cereal, Apple Cinnamon Squares Mini-Wheats/Kellogg	.75 cup									
		(1 NLEA serving)	55	182.05	3.96	44.055	4.73	0.99	0.275	0.495	0.22
8003	Cereal, Apple Jacks/Kellogg	1 cup									
		(1 NLEA serving)	30	117	0.9	27.3	0.96	0.6	0.18	0.3	0.12
8262	Cereal, Basic 4/General Mills	1 cup									
		(1 NLEA serving)	55	201.85	4.4	42.35	3.19	2.805	0.99	1.1	0.44
8006	Cereal, Bran Chex (wheat & corn)	1 cup	49	156.31	5.047	39.053	7.938	1.372	0.254	0.671	0.198
8322	Cereal, Bran Flakes/Kraft, Post	.75 cup									
		(1 NLEA serving)	30	96	2.82	24.12	5.28	0.66			0.12
8010	Cereal, Cap'n Crunch/Quaker	.75 cup	27	108.27	1.174	22.901	0.675	1.569	0.289	0.2	0.405
8013	Cereal, Cheerios/General Mills	1 cup									
		(1 NLEA serving)	30	110.7	3.3	22.2	2.7	1.8	0.642	0.216	0.36
8139	Cereal, Cinnamon Grahams/General Mills	.75 cup	30	113.4	1.5	25.8	0.96	0.84	0.304	0.312	0.15
8215	Cereal, Cinnamon Oatmeal Squares/Quaker	1 cup									
		(1 NLEA serving)	60	226.8	6.066	47.898	4.56	2.568	0.864	1.044	0.504
8272	Cereal, Cinnamon Toast Crunch/General Mills	.75 cup									
		(1 NLEA serving)	30	126.6	1.5	23.7	1.2	3.3	1.539	1.015	0.54
8014	Cereal, Cocoa Krispies/Kellogg	.75 cup									
		(1 NLEA serving)	31	118.11	1.054	27.001	0.992	0.992	0.124	0.071	0.617
8271	Cereal, Cocoa Puffs/General Mills	1 cup									
		(1 NLEA serving)	30	117	1.2	26.4	0.69	0.96	0.501	0.184	0.21
8028	Cereal, Complete Wheat Bran Flakes/Kellogg	.75 cup									
		(1 NLEA serving)	29	92.22	2.9	22.91	5.075	0.58	0.145	0.319	0.116
8295	Cereal, Corn Blasts/Quaker	1 cup	33	132.66	1.416	28.034	0.726	1.904	1.033	0.343	0.508
8019	Cereal, Corn Chex	1 cup									
		(1 NLEA serving)	30	111.9	2.1	25.8	0.6	0.27	0.059	0.101	0.06
8020	Cereal, Corn Flakes/Kellogg	1 cup									
		(1 NLEA serving)	28	101.08	1.96	24.08	0.98	0.224	0.031	0.09	0.053
8093	Cereal, corn grits, instant, plain, prep/Quaker	1 cup	245	166.6	3.945	36.897	2.205	0.465	0.066	0.14	0.047
8161	Cereal, corn grits, white, regular/quick, enriched, prep w/salt	1 cup	242	142.78	3.436	31.145	0.726	0.46	0.116	0.201	0.061
8068	Cereal, Corn Pops/Kellogg	1 cup									
		(1 NLEA serving)	31	117.8	1.147	27.9	0.248	0.226	0.084	0.071	0.071
8023	Cereal, Cracklin' Oat Bran/Kellogg	.75 cup									
		(1 NLEA serving)	55	224.95	4.565	39.27	6.435	8.03	4.565	1.155	2.31
8168	Cereal, Cream of Rice, prep w/salt	1 cup	244	126.88	2.196	28.06	0.244	0.244	0.076	0.066	0.049
8171	Cereal, Cream of Wheat, instant, prep w/salt	1 cup	241	149.42	4.434	31.523	1.446	0.578	0.08	0.323	0.092
8169	Cereal, Cream of Wheat, regular, prep w/salt	1 cup	251	125.5	3.665	26.932	1.004	0.477	0.063	0.259	0.075

Chol (g)	Calc (mg)	Iron (mg)	Mag (mg)	Phos (mg)	Pota (mg)	Sodi (mg)	Zinc (mg)	Vit A (RAE)	Vit C (mg)	Thia (mg)	Ribo (mg)	Niac (mg)	Vit B$_6$ (mg)	Vit B$_{12}$ (µg)	Vit E (mg)	Fol (µg)	Alc (g)
0	59.874	0.799	19.992	41.004	447.576	146.37	0.283	9.996	8.823	0.045	0.051	0.473	0.047	0	0.566	10.91	0
0	22.04	8.1	80.62	235.77	274.63	120.93	3.75	225	0	0.374	0.426	5	0.502	0	0.673	100.1	0
0	22.54	7.791	117.6	272.93	286.16	456.19	2.038		25.97	0.637	0.735	8.624	0.882	2.597		173	0
0	99	4.8	114	339	339	77.4	1.8	157.5	6	0.36	0.42	4.8	1.8	6	0.369	393	0
0	99.9	4.5	20.1	65.1	57.6	120.3	3.75	150.3	6	0.375	0.426	5.01	0.501	1.5	0.15	200.1	0
0	20.9	16.225	48.4	154	166.1	19.8	1.485	0	0	0.385	0.44	5.005	0.495	1.485	0.303	110	0
0	7.5	4.17	16.5	37.5	36	142.5	1.5	46.8	13.8	0.51	0.39	4.62	0.45	1.38	0.048	93	0
0	196.35	3.52	40.15	231.55	154.55	315.7	2.97	117.7	0	0.297	0.336	3.905	0.391	1.155	0.594	78.65	0
0	29.4	13.994	69.09	172.97	216.09	345.45	6.483		25.97	0.637	0.265	8.624	0.882	2.597	0.563	173	0
0	16.8	8.1	64.2	152.4	184.8	219.6	1.5		0	0.375	0.426	5.001	0.501	1.5		99.9	
0	4.05	5.16	15.12	45.09	54	202.23	4.285	1.89	0	0.427	0.481	5.711	0.57	0	0.248	420.1	0
0	99.9	8.1	39.9	99.9	96.3	273	3.75	150.3	6	0.375	0.426	5.01	0.501	1.5	0.105	200.1	0
0	99.9	4.5	8.1	20.1	44.1	236.7	3.75	150.3	6	0.375	0.426	5.01	0.501	1.5	0.093	99.9	0
0	116.4	16.86	64.8	201.6	250.2	263.4	4.128	165	6.6	0.408	0.462	5.502	0.546	0	2.214	420	0
0	99.9	4.5	8.1	80.1	42.6	206.1	3.75	150.3	6	0.375	0.426	5.01	0.501	1.5	0.342	99.9	0
0	39.99	4.65	11.78	30.38	49.91	190.03	1.488	152.5	15	0.372	0.434	4.96	0.496	1.519	0.192	102	0
0	99.9	4.5	8.1	20.1	50.4	171.3	3.75	0	6	0.375	0.426	5.01	0.501	1.5	0.063	99.9	0
0	15.37	17.98	40.6	156.6	171.1	207.35	15.23	228.5	60.03	1.566	1.711	20.01	2.03	6.003	26.874	403.1	0
0	10.89	4.95	17.49	60.06	63.69	239.91	4.125		13.2	0.413	0.465	5.498	0.548	0	0.304	109.9	0
0	99.9	9	8.4	21.6	24.9	287.7	3.75	150.6	6	0.375	0.426	5.01	0.501	1.5	0.054	200.1	0
0	1.96	8.4	3.08	14	25.2	203	0.076	150.4	6.16	0.364	0.428	5.012	0.504	1.512	0.039	102.2	0
0	14.7	14.234	17.15	51.45	68.6	514.5	0.318	0	0	0.279	0.333	3.959	0.098	0	0.049	83.3	0
0	7.26	1.452	12.1	26.62	50.82	539.66	0.169	0	0	0.201	0.133	1.747	0.051	0	0.048	79.86	0
0	5.27	1.922	2.17	9.61	26.35	119.66	1.519	151	6.014	0.372	0.434	4.991	0.496	1.519	0.034	102	0
0	22.55	2.035	67.65	178.75	247.5	157.3	1.705	252.5	17.6	0.424	0.479	5.665	0.561	1.705	0.77	112.8	0
0	7.32	0.488	7.32	41.48	48.8	422.12	0.39	0	0	0	0	0.976	0.066	0	0.049	7.32	0
0	154.24	11.954	14.46	43.38	48.2	363.91	0.41	559.1	0	0.559	0.506	7.454	0.745	0	0.048	149.4	0
0	112.95	9.764	12.55	95.38	45.18	336.34	0.351	0	0	0.143	0.065	1.358	0.03	0	0.05	30.12	0

EvaluEat Code	Food Name	Amt	Wt (g)	Energy (kcal)	Prot (g)	Carb (g)	Fiber (g)	Fat (g)	Mono (g)	Poly (g)	Sat (g)
8259	Cereal, Crispix/Kellogg	1 cup									
		(1 NLEA serving)	29	109.33	1.972	24.94	0.145	0.232	0.058	0.116	0.058
8173	Cereal, Farina, enriched, prep w/salt	1 cup	233	111.84	3.309	24.395	0.699	0.163	0.023	0.07	0.023
8244	Cereal, Fiber One/General Mills	.5 cup									
		(1 NLEA serving)	30	59.1	2.4	24.3	14.4	0.81	0.132	0.41	0.12
8030	Cereal, Froot Loops/Kellogg	1 cup									
		(1 NLEA serving)	30	117.9	1.02	26.25	0.93	1.23	0.129	0.204	0.456
8069	Cereal, Frosted Flakes/Kellogg	.75 cup									
		(1 NLEA serving)	31	113.77	1.023	27.993	0.992	0.161	0.028	0.081	0.053
8319	Cereal, Frosted Mini-Wheats, bite size/Kellogg	1 cup, bite size	55	189.2	5.555	44.55	5.5	0.88	0.132	0.55	0.198
8327	Cereal, Fruit & Fiber Dates, Raisins & Walnuts/Kraft, Post	1 cup									
		(1 NLEA serving)	55	211.75	3.905	41.91	5.335	3.08			0.44
8037	Cereal, granola (oats & wheat germ) homemade	1 cup	122	597.8	18.141	64.599	10.492	29.719	9.324	13.066	5.535
8329	Cereal, Grape-Nuts/Kraft, Post	.5 cup									
		(1 NLEA serving)	58	208.22	6.264	47.154	5.046	1.102			0.232
8333	Cereal, Honey Bunches of Oats Honey Roasted/Kraft, Post	.75 cup									
		(1 NLEA serving)	30	118.2	2.13	24.57	1.47	1.65			0.24
8242	Cereal, Just Right w/crunchy nuggets/Kellogg	1 cup									
		(1 NLEA serving)	55	204.05	4.235	46.035	2.805	1.485	0.275	1.045	0.11
8048	Cereal, Kix/General Mills	1.333 cup									
		(1 NLEA serving)	30	113.1	1.8	25.8	0.9	0.6	0.159	0.2	0.15
8049	Cereal, Life, plain/Quaker	.75 cup									
		(1 NLEA serving)	32	120	3.174	24.992	2.112	1.402	0.477	0.451	0.259
8284	Cereal, Low-Fat Granola with Raisins/Kellogg	.667 cup									
		(1 NLEA serving)	55	201.3	4.4	44	2.75	2.75	1.375	0.55	0.825
8050	Cereal, Lucky Charms/General Mills	1 cup									
		(1 NLEA serving)	30	114	2.1	24.9	1.5	1.14	0.252	0.288	0.24
8176	Cereal, Maltex, prep w/salt	1 cup	249	189.24	5.702	39.367	2.241	1.071	0.115	0.386	0.152
8178	Cereal, Malt-O-Meal, plain & chocolate, prep w/salt	1 cup	240	122.4	3.6	25.92	0.96	0.24			0.048
8285	Cereal, Mueslix Apple & Almond Crunch/Kellogg	3/4 cup	55	210.65	5.39	40.865	4.675	4.95	2.585	1.045	1.045
8345	Cereal, Multi-Bran Chex/General Mills	1 cup	49	165.62	3.43	41.16	6.37	1.225	0.299	0.537	0.245
8265	Cereal, Multigrain Cheerios/General Mills	1 cup	30	111.9	2.556	24.45	1.92	1.089	0.297	0.15	0.249
8207	Cereal, Multi-Grain Flakes/Healthy Choice, Kellogg	1 cup	30	103.8	2.55	25.23	2.82	0.36	0.15	0.18	0.03
8291	Cereal, Nutri-Grain Almond and Raisin/Kellogg	1 oz	28.35	104.045	2.268	22	2.268	1.616	0.737	0.822	0.057
8152	Cereal, Nutri-Grain, Wheat	1 oz	28.34	102.02	2.466	23.976	1.785	0.283	0.032	0.119	0.052
8216	Cereal, Oat Bran Cereal/Quaker	1.25 cup	57	212.04	7.057	42.687	5.643	2.913	0.895	1.163	0.519
8214	Cereal, Oatmeal Squares/Quaker	1 cup									
		(1 NLEA serving)	56	211.68	6.182	43.87	3.976	2.419	0.812	0.986	0.504
8125	Cereal, oatmeal, instant, w/apple & cinnamon, prep/Quaker	1 packet, prepared	149	129.63	2.712	26.477	2.682	1.49	0.513	0.428	0.249
8123	Cereal, oats, instant, plain, fortified, prep	1 cup, cooked	234	128.7	5.429	22.441	3.744	2.129	0.672	0.782	0.349
8180	Cereal, oats, regular/quick/instant, cooked w/salt	1 cup	234	145.08	6.084	25.272	3.978	2.34	0.749	0.866	0.421
8196	Cereal, Pop-Tarts Crunch, frosted strawberry/Kellogg	3/4 cup	30	117.9	1.35	26.76	0	0.81	0.24	0.27	0.33
8066	Cereal, Puffed Rice/Quaker	1 cup									
		(1 NLEA serving)	14	53.62	0.98	12.288	0.196	0.126	0.025	0.048	0.045

Chol (g)	Calc (mg)	Iron (mg)	Mag (mg)	Phos (mg)	Pota (mg)	Sodi (mg)	Zinc (mg)	Vit A (RAE)	Vit C (mg)	Thia (mg)	Ribo (mg)	Niac (mg)	Vit B$_6$ (mg)	Vit B$_{12}$ (µg)	Vit E (mg)	Fol (µg)	Alc (g)
0	6.09	8.12	7.25	26.39	37.7	209.96	1.45	150.2	5.8	0.551	0.609	6.989	0.696	2.088	0.058	279.9	0
0	9.32	1.165	4.66	27.96	30.29	766.57	0.186	0	0	0.142	0.1	1.139	0.016	0	0.023	79.22	0
0	99.9	4.5	60	150	232.2	128.7	3.75	0	6	0.375	0.426	5.01	0.501	1.5	0.213	99.9	0
0	23.4	4.23	8.7	19.2	32.7	141.3	1.41	144.9	14.1	0.36	0.39	4.68	0.48	1.41	0.144	93.9	0
0	1.55	4.495	2.48	10.54	22.63	148.49	0.056	160.3	6.2	0.372	0.465	5.022	0.496	1.55	0.016	101.4	0
0	17.6	15.4	64.9	161.7	189.75	4.4	1.76	0	0	0.407	0.456	5.39	0.539	1.617	0	107.8	0
0	23.65	5.401	66	161.7	243.65	279.95	1.502		0	0.374	0.424	5	0.501	1.502		100.1	
0	95.16	5.185	213.5	557.54	655.14	26.84	5.014	1.22	1.464	0.898	0.356	2.58	0.379	0	7.174	101.3	0
0	19.72	16.199	58	138.62	178.06	353.8	1.201		0	0.377	0.423	5	0.499	1.502		99.76	
0	6.3	8.1	16.5	48.3	51.6	192.6	0.3		0	0.375	0.426	5.001	0.501	1.5		99.9	
0	14.3	16.225	34.1	106.15	121	337.7	0.88	375.7	0	0.385	0.44	5.005	0.495	1.485	2.2	102.3	0
0	150	8.1	8.1	39.9	35.1	267.3	3.75	159.6	6.3	0.375	0.426	5.01	0.501	1.5	0.066	200.1	0
0	112	8.954	30.72	132.8	91.2	164.16	4.128	0.64	0	0.403	0.467	5.504	0.55	0	0.176	416	0
0	23.1	1.65	41.25	128.7	165	135.3	3.465	206.3	3.3	0.347	0.385	4.565	1.815	5.5	4.615	369.6	0
0	99.9	4.5	15.9	60	57.3	203.4	3.75	150.3	6	0.375	0.426	5.01	0.501	1.5	0.093	200.1	0
0	22.41	1.793	57.27	176.79	266.43	189.24	1.868	0	0	0.264	0.102	2.373	0.077	0	1.12	29.88	0
0	4.8	9.6	4.8	24	31.2	324	0.168	0	0	0.48	0.24	5.76	0.019	0		4.8	0
0	33.55	4.675	62.7	175.45	209	270.05	3.135		0	0.385	0.44	5.17	0.495	1.265	5.775	110	0
0	89.18	14.455	53.41	178.36	189.63	321.93	3.332	133.8	5.39	0.333	0.377	4.459	0.446	1.323	0.152	356.2	0
0	57	8.1	29.7	114.3	97.2	254.1	3.75		15	0.375	0.426	5.001	0.501	0	0.191	99.9	0
0	8.7	6.3	29.1	86.4	100.2	174	1.5		0	0.54	0.6	6.99	0.69	2.1	3	90	0
0	86.468	0.709	6.521	96.674	101.21	100.643	1.928		0	0.198	0.227	2.58	0.255	0.765	2.835	56.7	0
0	7.935	0.799	22.105	105.992	77.085	192.712	3.741		15.02	0.368	0.425	4.988	0.51	1.502	7.482	100	0
0	108.87	17.072	95.76	295.26	249.66	207.48	3.961	165.3	6.612	0.41	0.467	5.495	0.547	0	2.103	420.1	0
0	112.56	17.069	65.52	205.52	204.96	268.8	4.239	166.9	6.384	0.386	0.476	5.628	0.549	0	1.49	439.6	0
0	110.26	3.844	28.31	93.87	108.77	165.39	0.641	321.8	0.298	0.288	0.346	4.066	0.428	0	0.134	84.93	0
0	131.04	10.156	53.82	126.36	124.02	105.3	1.076	376.7	0	0.339	0.405	4.76	0.501	0	0.234	100.6	0
0	18.72	1.591	56.16	177.84	131.04	374.4	1.147	0	0	0.257	0.047	0.304	0.047	0		9.36	0
0	2.4	4.08	9.6	17.4	27.3	113.7	3.42		13.8	0.33	0.39	4.56	0.45	0	0.083	90	0
0	1.26	0.4	4.2	16.52	16.24	0.7	0.154	0	0	0.062	0.036	0.493	0	0	0.017	21.56	0

EvaluEat Code	Food Name	Amt	Wt (g)	Energy (kcal)	Prot (g)	Carb (g)	Fiber (g)	Fat (g)	Mono (g)	Poly (g)	Sat (g)
8060	Cereal, Raisin Bran/Kellogg	1 cup									
		(1 NLEA serving)	61	194.59	5.185	46.543	7.259	1.525	0.305	0.885	0.336
8287	Cereal, Raisin Squares Mini-Wheats/Kellogg	.75 cup									
		(1 NLEA serving)	55	184.8	5.17	43.56	5.17	0.88	0.192	0.495	0.192
8194	Cereal, Reese's Peanut Butter Puffs/General Mills	.75 cup									
		(1 NLEA serving)	30	127.5	1.8	23.4	0	2.91	1.243	0.903	0.57
8064	Cereal, Rice Chex	1.25 cup									
		(1 NLEA serving)	31	116.87	1.86	26.66	0.31	0.31	0.067	0.069	0.124
8065	Cereal, Rice Krispies/Kellogg	1.25 cup									
		(1 NLEA serving)	33	118.8	2.046	29.04	0.132	0.429	0.132	0.175	0.122
8318	Cereal, Smart Start/Kellogg	1 cup	50	182	3.1	43	2.3	0.6	0.15	0.25	0.2
8264	Cereal, S'mores Grahams/General Mills	3/4 cup	30	117	1.677	25.59	0.84	1.2	0.393	0.15	0.177
8067	Cereal, Special K/Kellogg	1 cup									
		(1 NLEA serving)	31	117.49	6.975	22.01	0.744	0.48	0.124	0.248	0.108
8203	Cereal, Sun Crunchers/General Mills	1 cup	55	215.6	4.857	43.742	2.2	3.157	2.046	0.33	0.341
8059	Cereal, Sweet Crunch/Quisp	1 cup	27	109.35	1.199	22.95	0.702	1.644	0.302	0.205	0.427
8088	Cereal, Team Cheerios/General Mills	1 cup									
		(1 NLEA serving)	30	113.1	2.151	25.068	1.65	1.131	0.329	0.462	0.182
8341	Cereal, The Original Shredded Wheat 'n Bran/Kraft, Post	1.25 cup									
		(1 NLEA serving)	59	197.06	7.375	47.141	7.906	0.826			0.118
8219	Cereal, Toasted Oatmeal Cereal, Honey Nut/Quaker	1 cup									
		(1 NLEA serving)	49	192.08	4.484	37.926	3.479	3.655	1.71	1.005	0.534
8350	Cereal, Toasty O's/Malt-o-Meal	1 cup									
		(1 NLEA serving)	30	111.6	3.321	22.401	2.7	1.809	0.669	0.609	0.369
8247	Cereal, Total Raisin Bran/General Mills	1 cup									
		(1 NLEA serving)	55	171.05	3.85	41.25	4.95	1.1	0.149	0.524	0.22
8077	Cereal, Total/General Mills	.75 cup									
		(1 NLEA serving)	30	97.2	2.4	22.5	2.4	0.75	0.123	0.273	0.159
8078	Cereal, Trix/General Mills	1 cup									
		(1 NLEA serving)	30	117.3	0.9	26.7	0.9	1.14	0.596	0.274	0.18
8305	Cereal, Waffle Crisp/Post	1 cup									
		(1 NLEA serving)	30	129	1.8	23.97	0.54	2.94	1.291	1.225	0.42
8082	Cereal, Wheat Chex	1 cup									
		(1 NLEA serving)	30	103.5	3	24.3	3.3	0.6	0.079	0.242	0.12
8157	Cereal, wheat, puffed, fortified	1 cup	12	43.68	1.764	9.552	0.528	0.144			0.024
8147	Cereal, wheat, shredded, large biscuit	2 biscuits									
		(1 NLEA serving)	46	156.4	5.235	36.138	5.336	1.104	0.161	0.58	0.207
8089	Cereal, Wheaties/General Mills	1 cup									
		(1 NLEA serving)	30	106.5	3	24.3	3	0.96	0.286	0.35	0.18
1163	Cheese fondue	1 cup	215	492.35	30.594	8.106	0	28.961	7.66	1.041	18.75
44048	Cheese food, imitation	1 cubic inch	10.2	14.382	2.285	0.898	0	0.133	0.039	0.005	0.083
19434	Cheese puffs and twists, corn based, low-fat	1 oz	28.35	122.47	2.41	20.511	3.033	3.43	0.992	1.627	0.595
43276	Cheese spread, cream cheese base	1 cup	186	548.7	13.206	6.51	0	53.196	15.012	1.921	33.517
1004	Cheese, blue	1 oz	28.35	100.08	6.067	0.663	0	8.148	2.205	0.227	5.293
1006	Cheese, brie	1 cubic inch	17	56.78	3.528	0.076	0	4.706	1.362	0.14	2.96

Chol (g)	Calc (mg)	Iron (mg)	Mag (mg)	Phos (mg)	Pota (mg)	Sodi (mg)	Zinc (mg)	Vit A (RAE)	Vit C (mg)	Thia (mg)	Ribo (mg)	Niac (mg)	Vit B$_6$ (mg)	Vit B$_{12}$ (µg)	Vit E (mg)	Fol (µg)	Alc (g)
0	29.28	4.636	82.96	258.64	372.1	361.73	1.549	154.9	0.427	0.39	0.439	5.185	0.519	1.549	0.476	103.7	0
0	21.45	15.4	43.45	155.65	264.55	3.3	1.54	0	0	0.391	0.44	5.17	0.517	1.595	0.286	104	0
0	99.9	4.5	15.9	20.1	41.7	166.5	3.75	150.3	6	0.375	0.426	5.01	0.501	1.5	0.36	99.9	0
0	103.23	9.3	9.3	35.34	30.38	291.71	3.875	155.3	6.2	0.387	0.44	5.177	0.518	1.55	0.016	206.8	0
0	5.28	1.815	13.2	45.87	43.89	318.78	0.462	153.1	6.369	0.376	0.462	5.049	0.495	1.485	0.036	104	0
0	17	18	32	101	102	280.5	15.1	231	15.5	1.55	1.7	20	2	6	20.135	402.5	0
0	14.4	4.5	10.8	40.5	48	212.4	3.75		15	0.375	0.426	5.001	0.501	0	0.218	99.9	0
0	9.3	8.37	19.22	67.89	60.76	223.51	0.899	230.3	20.99	0.527	0.589	7.13	1.984	6.045	7.074	399.9	0
0	85.25	4.499	43.45	171.6	129.8	380.05	0.798		15.02	0.374	0.424	5	0.501	0	0.056	99.55	0
0	2.97	4.96	14.85	45.36	51.03	200.07	4.134	10.8	2.916	0.413	0.467	5.511	0.551	0	0.184	420.1	0
	105.9	4.5	21.6	78.3	69.6	223.5	3.75		6	0.375	0.426	5.001	0.501	1.5	0.159	202.5	
0	26.55	2.466	80.83	234.82	247.8	2.95	1.929		0	0.153	0.071	3.723	0.195	0		27.14	
0	133.28	6.806	60.27	166.11	180.81	215.6	5.39	215.6	1.47	0.588	0.666	7.183	0.715	0	2.68	436.6	0
0	39.9	8.1	32.1	99.9	93.9	284.1	3.75	375.3	15	0.375	0.426	5.001	0.501	0	0.189	99.9	0
0	999.9	17.985	40.15	100.1	354.2	239.25	15.02	150.2	0	1.502	1.699	20.02	2.002	5.995	20.301	399.9	0
0	999.9	18	24	80.1	89.4	191.7	15	150.3	60	1.5	1.701	20.01	2.001	6	20.133	399.9	0
0	99.9	4.5	3.6	20.1	17.4	194.1	3.75	150.3	6	0.375	0.426	5.01	0.501	1.5	0.597	99.9	0
0	6	1.8	11.7	33.9	33.6	129.6	0.408	221.1	0	0.375	0.426	5.001	0.501	0	0.225	99.9	0
0	60	8.7	24	90	112.5	267.3	2.4	90	3.6	0.225	0.255	3	0.3	0.9	0.216	240	0
0	3.36	3.804	17.4	42.6	41.76	0.48	0.283	0	0	0.312	0.216	4.236	0.02	0		3.84	0
0	20.24	1.509	62.56	164.68	170.66	5.52	1.426	0	9.246	0.142	0.115	2.636	1.467	0	0.304	27.14	0
0	0	8.1	32.1	99.9	111	217.5	7.5	150.3	6	0.75	0.849	9.99	0.999	3	0.186	200.1	0
96.75	1023.4	0.839	49.45	657.9	225.75	283.8	4.214	234.4	0	0.058	0.421	0.409	0.118	1.785		17.2	0.645
0.612	56.304	0.093	3.57	50.898	34.272	126.378	0.336	1.02	0	0.003	0.049	0.015	0.013	0.125	0.001	0.816	0
0.284	101.21	0.363	11.624	101.21	81.081	364.298	0.607	12.47	6.067	0.153	0.173	2.024	0.201	0.607	1.205	27.5	0
167.4	132.06	2.102	11.16	169.26	208.32	1251.78	0.949	634.3	0	0.037	0.353	1.767	0.074	0.744	1.432	22.32	0
21.263	149.688	0.088	6.521	109.715	72.576	395.483	0.754	56.13	0	0.008	0.108	0.288	0.047	0.346	0.071	10.21	0
17	31.28	0.085	3.4	31.96	25.84	106.93	0.405	29.58	0	0.012	0.088	0.065	0.04	0.28	0.041	11.05	0

EvaluEat Code	Food Name	Amt	Wt (g)	Energy (kcal)	Prot (g)	Carb (g)	Fiber (g)	Fat (g)	Mono (g)	Poly (g)	Sat (g)
1007	Cheese, camembert	1 oz	28.35	85.05	5.613	0.13	0	6.878	1.991	0.205	4.326
1009	Cheese, cheddar	1 cup, shredded	113	455.39	28.137	1.446	0	37.448	10.612	1.064	23.834
1168	Cheese, cheddar or colby, low-fat	1 cup, shredded	113	195.49	27.516	2.158	0	7.91	2.353	0.251	4.906
1012	Cheese, cottage, creamed, large or small curd	4 oz	113	116.39	14.114	3.028	0	5.096	1.452	0.157	3.224
1015	Cheese, cottage, lowfat, 2% fat	4 oz	113	101.7	15.526	4.102	0	2.181	0.622	0.067	1.38
1014	Cheese, cottage, nonfat, uncreamed, dry, large or small curd	4 oz	113	96.05	19.515	2.091	0	0.475	0.124	0.017	0.308
1017	Cheese, cream	1 tbsp	14.5	50.605	1.095	0.386	0	5.056	1.427	0.183	3.185
1186	Cheese, cream, fat-free	1 oz	28.34	27.206	4.084	1.644	0	0.385	0.094	0.017	0.255
1018	Cheese, edam	1 oz	28.35	101.21	7.085	0.405	0	7.881	2.303	0.189	4.982
1019	Cheese, feta	1 oz	28.35	74.844	4.029	1.16	0	6.033	1.311	0.168	4.237
1020	Cheese, fontina	1 cup, shredded	108	420.12	27.648	1.674	0	33.631	9.382	1.786	20.732
1022	Cheese, gouda	1 oz	28.35	100.93	7.07	0.629	0	7.779	2.196	0.186	4.994
1188	Cheese, Kraft Cheez Whiz pasteurized process cheese sauce	2 tbsp	33	91.08	3.96	3.036	0.099	6.93			4.323
1190	Cheese, Kraft Free Singles American nonfat pasteurized process cheese product	1 slice	21	31.08	4.767	2.457	0.042	0.21			0.147
1165	Cheese, Mexican, queso anejo	1 oz	28.35	105.75	6.078	1.313	0	8.499	2.418	0.255	5.396
1025	Cheese, monterey	1 cup, shredded	113	421.49	27.662	0.768	0	34.216	9.889	1.016	21.545
1028	Cheese, mozzarella, part skim milk	1 oz	28.35	72.009	6.878	0.785	0	4.513	1.279	0.134	2.867
1026	Cheese, mozzarella, whole milk	1 oz	28.35	85.05	6.285	0.621	0	6.336	1.863	0.217	3.729
1030	Cheese, muenster	1 cup, shredded	113	415.84	26.453	1.266	0	33.945	9.843	0.747	21.598
1032	Cheese, parmesan, grated	1 tbsp	5	21.55	1.923	0.203	0	1.431	0.419	0.059	0.865
42205	Cheese, pasteurized process, cheddar or American, fat-free	1 cup	186	275.28	41.85	24.924	0	1.488	0.426	0.047	0.937
1035	Cheese, provolone	1 oz	28.35	99.509	7.252	0.607	0	7.547	2.096	0.218	4.842
1037	Cheese, ricotta, part skim milk	1 cup	246	339.48	28.019	12.644	0	19.459	5.692	0.64	12.12
1036	Cheese, ricotta, whole milk	1 cup	246	428.04	27.7	7.478	0	31.931	8.922	0.947	20.406
1038	Cheese, romano	1 oz	28.35	109.72	9.015	1.029	0	7.637	2.222	0.168	4.852
1039	Cheese, roquefort	1 oz	28.35	104.61	6.107	0.567	0	8.686	2.402	0.374	5.461
1040	Cheese, Swiss	1 oz	28.35	107.73	7.635	1.525	0	7.881	2.062	0.276	5.04
18147	Cheesecake, commercially prep	1 piece (1/6 of 17 oz cake)	80	256.8	4.4	20.4	0.32	18	6.907	1.282	7.937
18148	Cheesecake, no bake mix, prep	1 piece (1/12 of 9" dia)	99	271.26	5.445	35.145	1.881	12.573	4.474	0.8	6.624
9367	Cherries, sweet, canned, heavy syrup, drained	1 fruit (2-1/4" high x 2-1/2" dia)	122	101.26	0.891	25.705	3.05	0.256	0.06	0.067	0.049
5028	Chicken liver, simmered	1 container, cooked, yield from 400 g raw liver	256	427.52	62.618	2.227	0	16.666	3.625	3.249	5.274
22703	Chicken & dumplings, canned/Sweet Sue	1 serving	240	218.4	15.12	22.8	2.64	7.44	2.952	1.625	1.795
7932	Chicken breast, fat-free, mesquite flavor, sliced	1 serving 2 slices	42	33.6	7.056	0.945	0	0.164	0.067	0.025	0.055
7933	Chicken breast, oven-roasted, fat-free, sliced	1 serving 2 slices	42	33.18	7.052	0.911	0	0.164	0.051	0.031	0.055
5026	Chicken heart, simmered	1 cup, chopped or diced	145	268.25	38.295	0.145	0	11.484	2.914	3.335	3.277
22527	Chicken pie, frozen/Stouffers	1 package yields	283	571.66	23.206	36.507	3.113	37.073	12.367	10.443	10.726
5058	Chicken, broiler or fryer, breast w/skin, batter fried	1/2 breast, bone removed	140	364	34.776	12.586	0.42	18.48	7.644	4.312	4.928

Chol (g)	Calc (mg)	Iron (mg)	Mag (mg)	Phos (mg)	Pota (mg)	Sodi (mg)	Zinc (mg)	Vit A (RAE)	Vit C (mg)	Thia (mg)	Ribo (mg)	Niac (mg)	Vit B$_6$ (mg)	Vit B$_{12}$ (µg)	Vit E (mg)	Fol (µg)	Alc (g)
20.412	109.998	0.094	5.67	98.375	53.015	238.707	0.675	68.32	0	0.008	0.138	0.179	0.064	0.369	0.06	17.58	0
118.65	814.73	0.768	31.64	578.56	110.74	701.73	3.514	299.5	0	0.031	0.424	0.09	0.084	0.938	0.328	20.34	0
23.73	468.95	0.475	18.08	546.92	74.58	691.56	2.057	67.8	0	0.014	0.25	0.058	0.051	0.554	0.068	12.43	0
16.95	67.8	0.158	5.65	149.16	94.92	457.65	0.418	49.72	0	0.024	0.184	0.142	0.076	0.701	0.045	13.56	0
9.04	77.97	0.181	6.78	170.63	108.48	458.78	0.475	23.73	0	0.027	0.209	0.163	0.086	0.802	0.023	14.69	0
7.91	36.16	0.26	4.52	117.52	36.16	14.69	0.531	10.17	0	0.028	0.16	0.175	0.093	0.938	0	16.95	0
15.95	11.6	0.174	0.87	15.08	17.255	42.92	0.078	53.07	0	0.002	0.029	0.015	0.007	0.061	0.043	1.885	0
2.267	52.429	0.051	3.968	122.996	46.194	154.453	0.249	79.07	0	0.014	0.049	0.045	0.014	0.156	0.003	10.49	0
25.232	207.239	0.125	8.505	151.956	53.298	273.578	1.063	68.89	0	0.01	0.11	0.023	0.022	0.437	0.068	4.536	0
25.232	139.766	0.184	5.387	95.54	17.577	316.386	0.816	35.44	0	0.044	0.239	0.281	0.12	0.479	0.051	9.072	0
125.28	594	0.248	15.12	373.68	69.12	864	3.78	281.9	0	0.023	0.22	0.162	0.09	1.814	0.292	6.48	0
32.319	198.45	0.068	8.222	154.791	34.304	232.187	1.106	46.78	0	0.009	0.095	0.018	0.023	0.437	0.068	5.954	0
24.75	118.47	0.063		265.98	79.2	540.54	0.541		0.132		0.079						
3.36	149.52	0.01		193.83	49.56	272.58	0.525		0.042		0.059						
29.768	192.78	0.133	7.938	125.874	24.665	320.639	0.833	15.31	0	0.006	0.059	0.009	0.013	0.391	0.074	0.284	0
100.57	842.98	0.814	30.51	501.72	91.53	605.68	3.39	223.74	0	0.017	0.441	0.105	0.089	0.938	0.294	20.34	0
18.144	221.697	0.062	6.521	131.261	23.814	175.487	0.782	36.01	0	0.005	0.086	0.03	0.02	0.232	0.04	2.552	0
22.397	143.168	0.125	5.67	100.359	21.546	177.755	0.828	50.75	0	0.009	0.08	0.029	0.01	0.646	0.054	1.985	0
108.48	810.21	0.463	30.51	528.84	151.42	709.64	3.175	336.7	0	0.015	0.362	0.116	0.063	1.661	0.294	13.56	0
4.4	55.45	0.045	1.9	36.45	6.25	76.45	0.193	6	0	0.001	0.024	0.006	0.002	0.113	0.013	0.5	0
20.46	1281.54	0.521	66.96	1740.96	535.68	2842.08	6.361	818.4	0	0.112	0.893	0.391	0.167	2.083	0.502	50.22	0
19.562	214.326	0.147	7.938	140.616	39.123	248.346	0.916	66.91	0	0.005	0.091	0.044	0.021	0.414	0.065	2.835	0
76.26	669.12	1.082	36.9	450.18	307.5	307.5	3.296	263.22	0	0.052	0.455	0.192	0.049	0.713	0.172	31.98	0
125.46	509.22	0.935	27.06	388.68	258.3	206.64	2.854	295.2	0	0.032	0.48	0.256	0.106	0.836	0.271	29.52	0
29.484	301.644	0.218	11.624	215.46	24.381	340.2	0.731	27.22	0	0.01	0.105	0.022	0.024	0.318	0.065	1.985	0
25.515	187.677	0.159	8.505	111.132	25.799	512.852	0.59	83.35	0	0.011	0.166	0.208	0.035	0.181		13.892	0
26.082	224.249	0.057	10.773	160.745	21.83	54.432	1.236	62.37	0	0.018	0.084	0.026	0.024	0.947	0.108	1.701	0
44	40.8	0.504	8.8	74.4	72	165.6	0.408	113.6	0.32	0.022	0.154	0.156	0.042	0.136	1.265	14.4	
28.71	170.28	0.465	18.81	231.66	208.89	376.2	0.455	95.04	0.495	0.12	0.26	0.488	0.051	0.307		29.7	0
0	12.2	0.427	10.98	24.4	180.56	3.66	0.122	14.64	4.392	0.027	0.052	0.483	0.038	0	0.281	6.1	0
1441.28	28.16	29.773	64	1036.8	673.28	194.56	10.19	10191	71.424	0.745	5.102	28.275	1.933	43.136	2.099	1480	0
36		2.568				945.6											0
15.12	1.68	0.126	15.12	107.52	132.72	436.8	0.252	0	0	0.006	0.01	1.152	0.05	0.029	0.022	0.42	0
15.12	2.52	0.134	3.78	25.2	28.14	456.54	0.126	0	0	0.008	0.012	1.44	0.063	0.038	0.028	0.42	0
350.9	27.55	13.094	29	288.55	191.4	69.6	10.59	11.6	2.61	0.102	1.074	4.064	0.464	10.571		116	0
76.41	101.88	3				942.39											0
119	28	1.75	33.6	259	281.4	385	1.33	28	0	0.161	0.204	14.732	0.602	0.42	1.484	21	0

EvaluEat Code	Food Name	Amt	Wt (g)	Energy (kcal)	Prot (g)	Carb (g)	Fiber (g)	Fat (g)	Mono (g)	Poly (g)	Sat (g)
5060	Chicken, broiler or fryer, breast w/skin, roasted	1 cup, chopped or diced	140	275.8	41.72	0	0	10.892	4.242	2.324	3.066
5063	Chicken, broiler or fryer, breast, no skin, fried	1/2 breast, bone and skin removed	86	160.82	28.758	0.439	0	4.051	1.479	0.92	1.109
5064	Chicken, broiler or fryer, breast, no skin, roasted	1 cup, chopped or diced	140	231	43.428	0	0	4.998	1.736	1.078	1.414
5035	Chicken, broiler or fryer, dark meat w/skin, batter fried	yield from 1 lb ready-to-cook chicken	167	497.66	36.489	15.665		31.129	12.659	7.398	8.266
5037	Chicken, broiler or fryer, dark meat w/skin, roasted	yield from 1 lb ready-to-cook chicken	101	255.53	26.23	0	0	15.938	6.252	3.525	4.414
5044	Chicken, broiler or fryer, dark meat, no skin, fried	1 cup	140	334.6	40.586	3.626	0	16.268	6.048	3.878	4.368
5045	Chicken, broiler or fryer, dark meat, no skin, roasted	1 cup, chopped or diced	140	287	38.318	0	0	13.622	4.984	3.164	3.724
5067	Chicken, broiler or fryer, drumstick w/skin, batter fried	1 drumstick, bone removed	72	192.96	15.804	5.962	0.216	11.34	4.63	2.729	2.981
5069	Chicken, broiler or fryer, drumstick w/skin, roasted	1 drumstick, bone removed	52	112.32	14.056	0	0	5.798	2.21	1.3	1.586
5072	Chicken, broiler or fryer, drumstick, no skin, fried	yield from 1 lb ready-to-cook chicken	25	48.75	7.155	0	0	2.02	0.735	0.493	0.533
5073	Chicken, broiler or fryer, drumstick, no skin, roasted	1 drumstick, bone and skin removed	44	75.68	12.448	0	0	2.49	0.823	0.603	0.651
5021	Chicken, broiler or fryer, giblets, floured, fried	1 cup, chopped or diced	145	401.65	47.183	6.307	0	19.517	6.409	4.901	5.51
5022	Chicken, broiler or fryer, giblets, simmered	1 cup, chopped or diced	145	229.1	39.368	0.624	0	6.525	1.395	1.177	1.917
5024	Chicken, broiler or fryer, gizzard, simmered	1 cup, chopped or diced	145	211.7	44.066	0	0	3.886	0.766	0.512	0.972
5076	Chicken, broiler or fryer, leg w/skin, batter fried	1 leg, bone removed	158	431.34	34.397	13.778	0.474	25.549	10.396	6.083	6.762
5078	Chicken, broiler or fryer, leg w/skin, roasted	1 leg, bone removed	114	264.48	29.594	0	0	15.344	5.974	3.42	4.241
5081	Chicken, broiler or fryer, leg, no skin, fried	1 leg, bone and skin removed	94	195.52	26.677	0.611	0	8.761	3.224	2.087	2.341
5082	Chicken, broiler or fryer, leg, no skin, roasted	1 leg, bone and skin removed	95	181.45	25.679	0	0	8.009	2.897	1.872	2.175
5030	Chicken, broiler or fryer, light meat w/skin, batter fried	1/2 chicken, bone removed	188	520.76	44.274	17.86		29.027	11.976	6.768	7.746
5032	Chicken, broiler or fryer, light meat w/skin, roasted	1/2 chicken, bone removed	132	293.04	38.306	0	0	14.322	5.623	3.049	4.026
5040	Chicken, broiler or fryer, light meat, no skin, fried	1 cup	140	268.8	45.948	0.588	0	7.756	2.758	1.764	2.128
5041	Chicken, broiler or fryer, light meat, no skin, roasted	1 cup, chopped or diced	140	242.2	43.274	0	0	6.314	2.156	1.372	1.778

Chol (g)	Calc (mg)	Iron (mg)	Mag (mg)	Phos (mg)	Pota (mg)	Sodi (mg)	Zinc (mg)	Vit A (RAE)	Vit C (mg)	Thia (mg)	Ribo (mg)	Niac (mg)	Vit B_6 (mg)	Vit B_{12} (µg)	Vit E (mg)	Fol (µg)	Alc (g)
117.6	19.6	1.498	37.8	299.6	343	99.4	1.428	37.8	0	0.092	0.167	17.794	0.784	0.448	0.378	5.6	0
78.26	13.76	0.98	26.66	211.56	237.36	67.94	0.929	6.02	0	0.068	0.108	12.713	0.55	0.318	0.361	3.44	0
119	21	1.456	40.6	319.2	358.4	103.6	1.4	8.4	0	0.098	0.16	19.197	0.84	0.476	0.378	5.6	0
148.63	35.07	2.405	33.4	242.15	308.95	492.65	3.474	51.77	0	0.195	0.364	9.364	0.417	0.451		30.06	0
91.91	15.15	1.374	22.22	169.68	222.2	87.87	2.515	60.6	0	0.067	0.209	6.423	0.313	0.293		7.07	0
134.4	25.2	2.086	35	261.8	354.2	135.8	4.074	33.6	0	0.13	0.349	9.898	0.518	0.462		12.6	0
130.2	21	1.862	32.2	250.6	336	130.2	3.92	30.8	0	0.102	0.318	9.167	0.504	0.448	0.378	11.2	0
61.92	12.24	0.972	14.4	105.84	133.92	193.68	1.678	18.72	0	0.081	0.155	3.669	0.194	0.202		12.96	0
47.32	6.24	0.692	11.96	91	119.08	46.8	1.492	15.6	0	0.036	0.112	3.117	0.177	0.166	0.14	4.16	0
23.5	3	0.33	6	46.5	62.25	24	0.805	4.5	0	0.019	0.059	1.536	0.097	0.087	0.123	2.25	0
40.92	5.28	0.572	10.56	80.96	108.24	41.8	1.399	7.92	0	0.033	0.103	2.673	0.172	0.15	0.119	3.96	0
646.7	26.1	14.964	36.25	414.7	478.5	163.85	9.092	5194	12.62	0.141	2.21	15.931	0.885	19.3		549.6	0
640.9	20.3	10.208	20.3	419.05	324.8	97.15	6.134	2542	18.13	0.207	1.525	9.606	0.576	13.688	0.667	372.7	0
536.5	24.65	4.626	4.35	274.05	259.55	81.2	6.409	0	0	0.038	0.305	4.524	0.103	1.508	0.29	7.25	0
142.2	28.44	2.212	31.6	240.16	298.62	440.82	3.429	42.66	0	0.183	0.349	8.584	0.427	0.442		28.44	0
104.88	13.68	1.516	26.22	198.36	256.5	99.18	2.964	44.46	0	0.078	0.243	7.063	0.376	0.342	0.308	7.98	0
93.06	12.22	1.316	23.5	181.42	238.76	90.24	2.801	18.8	0	0.078	0.232	6.287	0.367	0.32		8.46	0
89.3	11.4	1.244	22.8	173.85	229.9	86.45	2.717	18.05	0	0.071	0.22	6.003	0.352	0.304	0.257	7.6	0
157.92	37.6	2.369	41.36	315.84	347.8	539.56	1.993	45.12	0	0.212	0.276	17.213	0.733	0.526		30.08	0
110.88	19.8	1.505	33	264	299.64	99	1.624	43.56	0	0.079	0.156	14.697	0.686	0.422		3.96	0
126	22.4	1.596	40.6	323.4	368.2	113.4	1.778	12.6	0	0.102	0.176	18.711	0.882	0.504		5.6	0
119	21	1.484	37.8	302.4	345.8	107.8	1.722	12.6	0	0.091	0.162	17.389	0.84	0.476	0.378	5.6	0

EvaluEat Code	Food Name	Amt	Wt (g)	Energy (kcal)	Prot (g)	Carb (g)	Fiber (g)	Fat (g)	Mono (g)	Poly (g)	Sat (g)
5007	Chicken, broiler or fryer, meat & skin, batter fried	yield from 1 lb ready-to-cook chicken	280	809.2	63.112	26.376	0.84	48.58	19.852	11.48	12.908
5009	Chicken, broiler or fryer, meat & skin, roasted	1 cup, chopped or diced	140	334.6	38.22	0	0	19.04	7.476	4.158	5.306
5012	Chicken, broiler or fryer, meat only, no skin, fried	1 cup, chopped or diced	140	306.6	42.798	2.366	0.14	12.768	4.69	3.01	3.444
5013	Chicken, broiler or fryer, meat only, no skin, roasted	1 cup, chopped or diced	140	266	40.502	0	0	10.374	3.724	2.366	2.856
5092	Chicken, broiler or fryer, thigh w/skin, batter fried	1 thigh, bone removed	86	238.22	18.585	7.809	0.258	14.216	5.762	3.354	3.793
5094	Chicken, broiler or fryer, thigh w/skin, roasted	1 thigh, bone removed	62	153.14	15.537	0	0	9.604	3.813	2.12	2.685
5097	Chicken, broiler or fryer, thigh, no skin, fried	1 thigh, bone and skin removed	52	113.36	14.654	0.614	0	5.356	1.986	1.264	1.446
5098	Chicken, broiler or fryer, thigh, no skin, roasted	1 thigh, bone and skin removed	52	108.68	13.489	0	0	5.658	2.158	1.29	1.576
5002	Chicken, broiler or fryer, whole, batter fried	1 chicken	1028	2991.5	234.8	92.828		180.21	73.296	42.662	48.008
5001	Chicken, broiler or fryer, whole, raw	1 chicken	1046	2228	191.73	1.36	0	155.12	63.597	33.367	44.35
5004	Chicken, broiler or fryer, whole, roasted	1 chicken	682	1595.9	182.64	0.409	0	90.501	35.259	19.778	25.234
5101	Chicken, broiler or fryer, wing w/skin, batter fried	1 wing, bone removed	49	158.76	9.736	5.361	0.147	10.687	4.39	2.484	2.857
5103	Chicken, broiler or fryer, wing w/skin, roasted	1 wing, bone removed	34	98.6	9.132	0	0	6.616	2.598	1.408	1.853
5106	Chicken, broiler or fryer, wing, no skin, fried	1 wing, bone and skin removed	20	42.2	6.03	0	0	1.83	0.616	0.414	0.5
5107	Chicken, broiler or fryer, wing, no skin, roasted	1 wing, bone and skin removed	21	42.63	6.397	0	0	1.707	0.548	0.374	0.475
22697	Chicken, chicken salad ready to serve sandwich salad/Libby Spreadable	1 serving	118	171.1	5.782	11.918		11.092	3.457	4.224	2.301
5335	Chicken, feet, boiled	1 cup chopped or diced, cooked	174	374.1	33.756	0.348	0	25.404	9.57	5.185	6.821
5277	Chicken, meat only w/broth, canned	1 can (5 oz)	142	234.3	30.913	0	0	11.289	4.473	2.485	3.124
43128	Chicken, meatless	1 cup	186	416.64	43.97	6.77	6.696	23.678	5.072	13.528	3.385
51608	Chicken, nugget, breaded/Pierre product #1879	1 piece	14.2	46.718	2.378	1.889	0.156	3.321	0.977	1.478	0.653
22904	Chili con carne w/beans, canned entree	1 serving	222	255.3	20.18	24.487	8.214	8.147	2.153	1.443	2.109
16059	Chili w/beans, canned	1 cup	256	286.72	14.618	30.49	11.264	14.054	5.97	0.927	6.021
22705	Chili w/o beans, canned entree/Hormel	1 cup	236	193.52	16.992	17.912	3.068	6.561	2.242	0.85	2.195
22720	Chili, vegetarian chili w/beans, canned entree/Hormel	1 cup	247	205.01	11.93	38.013	9.88	0.692	0.074	0.395	0.124
18606	Chocolate cake, snack cake, chocolate creme filling, Ding Dongs/Hostess	1 serving	80	368	3.12	45.36	1.84	19.36	3.992	1.198	11.036
19124	Chocolate, baking, Mexican, squares	1 tablet	20	85.2	0.728	15.482	0.8	3.118	1.009	0.232	1.721
14198	Cocoa mix, No Sugar Added Hot Cocoa Mix/Carnation	1 serving	15	54.75	4.304	8.433	0.75	0.426	0.136	0.014	0.203
14197	Cocoa mix, Rich Chocolate Hot Cocoa Mix/Carnation	1 serving	28	112	1.296	24.237	0.672	1.109	0.348	0.265	0.291
1105	Cocoa, hot, homemade w/whole milk	1 cup	250	192.5	8.8	26.575	2.5	5.825	1.692	0.085	3.577
18103	Coffee cake, cheese	1 piece (1/6 of 16 oz cake)	76	257.64	5.32	33.668	0.76	11.552	5.418	1.25	4.097

Chol (g)	Calc (mg)	Iron (mg)	Mag (mg)	Phos (mg)	Pota (mg)	Sodi (mg)	Zinc (mg)	Vit A (RAE)	Vit C (mg)	Thia (mg)	Ribo (mg)	Niac (mg)	Vit B$_6$ (mg)	Vit B$_{12}$ (µg)	Vit E (mg)	Fol (µg)	Alc (g)
243.6	58.8	3.836	58.8	434	518	817.6	4.676	78.4	0	0.322	0.529	19.72	0.868	0.784	3.472	50.4	0
123.2	21	1.764	32.2	254.8	312.2	114.8	2.716	65.8	0	0.088	0.235	11.882	0.56	0.42	0.378	7	0
131.6	23.8	1.89	37.8	287	359.8	127.4	3.136	25.2	0	0.119	0.277	13.528	0.672	0.476	0.644	9.8	0
124.6	21	1.694	35	273	340.2	120.4	2.94	22.4	0	0.097	0.249	12.842	0.658	0.462	0.378	8.4	0
79.98	15.48	1.247	18.06	133.3	165.12	247.68	1.754	24.94	0	0.102	0.195	4.915	0.224	0.241		16.34	0
57.66	7.44	0.831	13.64	107.88	137.64	52.08	1.463	29.76	0	0.042	0.131	3.946	0.192	0.18	0.167	4.34	0
53.04	6.76	0.759	13.52	103.48	134.68	49.4	1.451	10.92	0	0.046	0.133	3.702	0.198	0.172		4.68	0
49.4	6.24	0.681	12.48	95.16	123.76	45.76	1.336	10.4	0	0.038	0.12	3.393	0.182	0.161	0.14	4.16	0
1058.84	215.88	18.401	215.88	1624.24	1953.2	2919.52	19.64	1861	4.112	1.162	2.549	72.813	3.29	8.532		329	0
941.4	115.06	13.703	209.2	1558.54	1976.94	732.2	15.48	2427	27.2	0.638	1.946	69.444	3.556	11.611	3.849	313.8	0
729.74	102.3	11.321	156.86	1241.24	1445.84	538.78	14.73	1303	3.41	0.43	1.528	53.933	2.592	6.411	2.251	197.8	0
38.71	9.8	0.632	7.84	59.29	67.62	156.8	0.676	16.66	0	0.052	0.074	2.58	0.147	0.123		8.82	0
28.56	5.1	0.432	6.46	51.34	62.56	27.88	0.619	15.98	0	0.014	0.044	2.26	0.143	0.099	0.092	1.02	0
16.8	3	0.228	4.2	32.8	41.6	18.2	0.424	3.6	0	0.009	0.026	1.448	0.118	0.068		0.8	0
17.85	3.36	0.244	4.41	34.86	44.1	19.32	0.449	3.78	0	0.01	0.027	1.536	0.124	0.071	0.057	0.84	0
30.68						552.24											0
146.16	153.12	1.583	8.7	144.42	53.94	116.58	1.201	52.2	0	0.104	0.348	0.696	0.017	0.818	0.47	149.6	0
88.04	19.88	2.244	17.04	157.62	195.96	714.26	2.002	48.28	2.84	0.021	0.183	8.987	0.497	0.412	0.369	5.68	0
0	65.1	6.082	31.62	623.1	100.44	1318.74	1.302	0	0	1.269	0.459	2.704	1.302	4.055	4.985	141.4	0
5.538	5.112	0.315	3.408	31.95	29.962	98.974	0.349		0	0.043	0.035	0.888	0.038	0.099	0.386	4.118	0
24.42	66.6	3.308	55.5	193.14	608.28	1032.3	2.42	44.4	0.888	0.153	0.149	2.073	0.186	0.577	0.284	57.72	
43.52	120.32	8.781	115.2	394.24	934.4	1336.32	5.12	43.52	4.352	0.123	0.269	0.916	0.338	0	1.459	58.88	0
35.4	49.56	2.596	37.76		349.28	969.96	2.596		0								0
0	96.33	3.458	81.51		802.75	778.05	1.729		1.235								0
13.6	3.2	1.84				240.8											0
0	6.8	0.436	19	28.4	79.4	0.6	0.252	0	0.02	0.011	0.021	0.366	0.007	0	0.072	1	0
2.85	123.45	0.39	27	135	288.15	142.05	0.599	0	0.405	0.056	0.218	0.183	0.053	0.447	0.013	5.85	0
1.68	40.04	0.28	27.44	70.84	194.32	101.64	0.358	0	0	0.027	0.116	0.155	0.03	0.104	0.042	1.96	0
20	262.5	1.2	57.5	262.5	492.5	110	1.575	127.5	0.5	0.098	0.455	0.333	0.1	1.05	0.075	12.5	0
64.6	44.84	0.486	11.4	76.76	219.64	257.64	0.448	65.36	0.076	0.08	0.095	0.518	0.044	0.258	1.186	29.64	0

EvaluEat Code	Food Name	Amt	Wt (g)	Energy (kcal)	Prot (g)	Carb (g)	Fiber (g)	Fat (g)	Mono (g)	Poly (g)	Sat (g)
18105	Coffee cake, creme w/chocolate icing	1 piece (1/6 of 19 oz cake)	90	297.9	4.5	48.42	1.8	9.72	5.098	1.319	2.55
14210	Coffee, brewed, espresso, restaurant-prep	1 oz	28.34	2.551	0.003	0.434	0	0.051	0	0.026	0.026
14202	Coffee, brewed, espresso, restaurant-prepared, decaffeinated	1 cup (8 fl. oz.)	237	21.33	0.024	3.626	0	0.427	0	0.218	0.218
2055	Condiment, horseradish, prep	1 tbsp	15	7.2	0.177	1.694	0.495	0.104	0.02	0.051	0.014
2046	Condiment, mustard, prepared, yellow	1 tsp or 1 packet	5	3.3	0.198	0.389	0.16	0.155	0.107	0.029	0.008
11945	Condiment, pickle relish, sweet	1 tbsp	15	19.5	0.056	5.258	0.165	0.071	0.031	0.018	0.008
11935	Condiment, tomato catsup	1 tbsp	15	14.25	0.271	3.582	0.195	0.089	0.014	0.036	0.012
18150	Cookie, animal crackers/Arrowroot/Tea Biscuits	1 oz	28.35	126.44	1.956	21.007	0.312	3.912	2.173	0.531	0.982
18151	Cookie, brownies, commercially prep/Little Debbie	1 square, large (2-3/4" sq x 7/8")	56	226.8	2.688	35.784	1.176	9.128	5.02	1.265	2.372
18154	Cookie, brownies, homemade	1 brownie (2" square)	24	111.84	1.488	12.048		6.984	2.601	2.259	1.757
18159	Cookie, chocolate chip, enriched, commercially prep	1 cookie	12	57.72	0.648	8.016	0.3	2.712	1.401	0.284	0.897
18378	Cookie, chocolate chip, homemade w/butter	1 cookie, medium (2-1/4" dia)	16	78.08	0.912	9.312		4.544	1.319	0.727	2.251
18158	Cookie, chocolate chip, lower fat, commercially prep	1 cookie	10	45.3	0.58	7.33	0.36	1.54	0.609	0.465	0.381
18160	Cookie, chocolate chip, soft, commercially prep	1 cookie	15	68.7	0.525	8.865	0.48	3.645	1.955	0.525	1.112
18608	Cookie, Chocolate Graham Selects/Keebler	1 serving	31	144.15	2.201	22.258		5.146			0.958
18169	Cookie, coconut macaroons, homemade	1 cookie, medium (2" dia)	24	96.96	0.864	17.328	0.432	3.048	0.132	0.034	2.697
18170	Cookie, fig bar	1 individual package (2 oz package containing 2 3"bars)	57	198.36	2.109	40.413	2.622	4.161	1.712	1.58	0.64
18171	Cookie, fortune	1 cookie	8	30.24	0.336	6.72	0.128	0.216	0.108	0.037	0.054
18172	Cookie, ginger snaps	1 cookie	7	29.12	0.392	5.383	0.154	0.686	0.376	0.096	0.172
18609	Cookie, Golden Vanilla Wafers/Keebler	1 serving	31	147.25	1.612	21.607		6.045			1.11
18174	Cookie, graham crackers, chocolate coated	1 cracker (2-1/2" square)	14	67.76	0.812	9.31	0.434	3.248	1.076	0.145	1.873
18173	Cookie, graham crackers, plain/honey/cinnamon	1 large rectangular piece or 2 squares or 4 small rectangular pieces	14	59.22	0.966	10.752	0.392	1.414	0.572	0.536	0.213
18175	Cookie, Ladyfingers/Egg Jumbo w/lemon juice & rind	1 cookie	11	40.15	1.166	6.567	0.11	1.001	0.468	0.177	0.382
18612	Cookie, Little Debbie Nutty Bars, Chocolate Covered Wafers w/Peanut Butter	1 serving	57	312.36	4.56	31.464		18.696			3.585
18177	Cookie, molasses	1 large (3-1/2" to 4" dia)	32	137.6	1.792	23.616	0.32	4.096	2.282	0.553	1.028
18178	Cookie, oatmeal, commercially prep	1 cookie, big (3-1/2" to 4" dia)	25	112.5	1.55	17.175	0.7	4.525	2.506	0.636	1.13
18184	Cookie, oatmeal, homemade w/raisins	1 cookie (2-5/8" dia)	15	65.25	0.975	10.26		2.43	1.033	0.755	0.485
18185	Cookie, peanut butter, commercially prep	1 cookie	15	71.55	1.44	8.835	0.27	3.54	1.855	0.828	0.673
18189	Cookie, peanut butter, homemade	1 cookie (3" dia)	20	95	1.8	11.78		4.76	2.166	1.445	0.888
18186	Cookie, peanut butter, soft, commercially prep	1 cookie	15	68.55	0.795	8.655	0.255	3.66	2.077	0.477	0.922

Chol (g)	Calc (mg)	Iron (mg)	Mag (mg)	Phos (mg)	Pota (mg)	Sodi (mg)	Zinc (mg)	Vit A (RAE)	Vit C (mg)	Thia (mg)	Ribo (mg)	Niac (mg)	Vit B$_6$ (mg)	Vit B$_{12}$ (µg)	Vit E (mg)	Fol (µg)	Alc (g)
62.1	34.2	0.459	13.5	67.5	70.2	290.7	0.396	33.3	0.09	0.072	0.067	0.756	0.037	0.18		36.9	0
0	0.567	0.037	22.672	1.984	32.591	3.968	0.014	0	0.057	0	0.05	1.476	0.001	0	0.006	0.283	0
0	4.74	0.308	189.6	16.59	272.55	33.18	0.118	0	0.474	0.002	0.419	12.341	0.005	0	0.047	2.37	0
0	8.4	0.063	4.05	4.65	36.9	47.1	0.124	0	3.735	0.001	0.004	0.058	0.011	0	0.002	8.55	0
0	4	0.093	1.9	4.4	7.55	56	0.03	0.35	0.145	0.003	0.001	0.023	0.004	0	0.015	0.4	0
0	0.45	0.131	0.75	2.1	3.75	121.65	0.021	1.35	0.15	0	0.005	0.035	0.002	0	0.014	0.15	0
0	2.7	0.076	2.85	4.95	57.3	166.95	0.039	7.05	2.265	0.002	0.07	0.225	0.022	0	0.219	2.25	0
0	12.191	0.78	5.103	32.319	28.35	111.416	0.181	0	0	0.099	0.092	0.984	0.006	0.014	0.034	29.2	0
9.52	16.24	1.26	17.36	56.56	83.44	174.72	0.403	11.2	0	0.143	0.118	0.964	0.02	0.039	0.084	26.32	0
17.52	13.68	0.442	12.72	31.68	42.24	82.32	0.233	42.24	0.072	0.034	0.046	0.236	0.023	0.038		6.96	0
0	3	0.337	3.72	12.96	16.2	37.8	0.077	0	0	0.027	0.034	0.326	0.007	0.001	0.017	6.96	0
11.2	6.08	0.397	8.8	16	35.36	54.56	0.15	22.24	0.032	0.029	0.028	0.218	0.013	0.013		5.28	0
0	1.9	0.307	2.8	8.4	12.3	37.7	0.07	0	0	0.029	0.027	0.277	0.026	0		7	0
0	2.25	0.362	5.25	7.5	13.95	48.9	0.069	0	0	0.016	0.03	0.243	0.024	0		5.85	0
						110.67											0
0	1.68	0.18	5.04	10.32	37.44	59.28	0.17	0	0	0.003	0.026	0.031	0.024	0.007	0.036	0.96	0
0	36.48	1.653	15.39	35.34	117.99	199.5	0.222	5.13	0.171	0.09	0.124	1.068	0.043	0.051	0.37	19.95	0
0.16	0.96	0.115	0.56	2.8	3.28	21.92	0.014	0.08	0	0.015	0.01	0.147	0.001	0.001	0.002	5.28	0
0	5.39	0.448	3.43	5.81	24.22	45.78	0.038	0	0	0.014	0.021	0.226	0.007	0	0.068	6.09	0
						119.66											0
0	8.12	0.501	8.12	18.76	29.26	40.74	0.136	0.7	0	0.02	0.03	0.305	0.01	0	0.038	2.8	0
0	3.36	0.522	4.2	14.56	18.9	84.7	0.113	0	0	0.031	0.044	0.577	0.009	0	0.046	6.44	0
40.15	5.17	0.394	1.32	19.03	12.43	16.17	0.125	0.33	0.407	0.031	0.047	0.231	0.013	0.082	0.069	6.6	0
						127.11				1.14							0
0	23.68	2.058	16.64	30.4	110.72	146.88	0.144	0	0	0.114	0.084	0.97	0.033	0	0.035	28.48	0
0	9.25	0.645	8.25	34.5	35.5	95.75	0.198	1.25	0.125	0.067	0.058	0.557	0.016	0	0.065	14.75	0
4.95	15	0.398	6.3	24.15	35.85	80.7	0.129	21.45	0.075	0.037	0.025	0.189	0.011	0.012		4.5	0
0.15	5.25	0.377	6.75	12.9	25.05	62.25	0.079	0.45	0	0.026	0.027	0.641	0.013	0.006	0.33	10.8	0
6.2	7.8	0.446	7.8	23.2	46.2	103.6	0.164	27.4	0.02	0.044	0.042	0.703	0.017	0.018		11	0
0	1.8	0.134	4.8	13.05	16.05	50.4	0.083	0	0	0.037	0.025	0.324	0.004	0		10.05	0

EvaluEat Code	Food Name	Amt	Wt (g)	Energy (kcal)	Prot (g)	Carb (g)	Fiber (g)	Fat (g)	Mono (g)	Poly (g)	Sat (g)
18166	Cookie, sandwich, chocolate, cream filled	1 cookie	10	47.2	0.47	7.03	0.32	2.06	0.856	0.725	0.366
18190	Cookie, sandwich, peanut butter, regular	1 cookie	14	66.92	1.232	9.184	0.266	2.954	1.567	0.531	0.699
18210	Cookie, sandwich, vanilla, cream filled	1 cookie, oval (3-1/8" x 1-1/4" x 3/8")	15	72.45	0.675	10.815	0.225	3	1.266	1.133	0.447
18193	Cookie, shortbread, pecan, commercially prep	1 cookie (2" dia)	14	75.88	0.686	8.162	0.252	4.55	2.608	0.577	1.149
18192	Cookie, shortbread, plain, commercially prep	1 cookie (1-5/8" square)	8	40.16	0.488	5.16	0.144	1.928	1.074	0.259	0.488
18209	Cookie, sugar wafer, cream filled	1 wafer, large (3-1/2" x 1" x 1/2")	9	45.99	0.369	6.309	0.054	2.187	0.93	0.824	0.326
18206	Cookie, sugar, refrig dough, baked	1 cookie 1 pre-sliced cookie dough	23	111.32	1.081	15.088	0.184	5.313	2.992	0.665	1.358
18213	Cookie, vanilla wafer	1 wafer	6	28.38	0.258	4.266	0.12	1.164	0.665	0.146	0.296
18524	Cookies, Archway Home Style, Coconut Macaroon	1 serving	22	106.04	0.854	12.353	0.506	6.142	0.418	0.077	5.436
18555	Cookies, Archway Home Style, fat-free Oatmeal Raisin	1 serving	31	106.33	1.435	24.363	0.93	0.493	0.174	0.211	0.105
18557	Cookies, Archway Home Style, fat-free Sugar Cookies	1 serving	20	70.8	0.88	16.58	0.24	0.158	0.042	0.066	0.052
18535	Cookies, Archway Home Style, Molasses	1 serving	26	103.48	1.178	18.184	0.312	2.98	1.118	0.208	0.733
18541	Cookies, Archway Home Style, Peanut Butter	1 serving	21	100.8	1.89	12.281	0.588	5.099	2.144	0.888	1.132
18548	Cookies, Archway Home Style, Sugar	1 serving	24	98.4	1.231	16.555	0.264	3.084	1.145	0.202	0.761
13348	Corned beef brisket, canned	1 oz	28.35	70.875	7.683	0	0	4.233	1.69	0.179	1.752
20027	Cornstarch	1 cup	128	487.68	0.333	116.83	1.152	0.064	0.02	0.032	0.012
18214	Cracker, cheese	1 cup, bite size	62	311.86	6.262	36.084	1.488	15.686	7.505	1.533	5.81
18216	Cracker, crispbread, rye	1 cracker	10	36.6	0.79	8.22	1.65	0.13	0.017	0.056	0.014
18217	Cracker, Matzo, plain	1 matzo	28	110.6	2.8	23.436	0.84	0.392	0.036	0.169	0.063
18219	Cracker, Matzo, whole wheat	1 matzo	28	98.28	3.668	22.092	3.304	0.42	0.054	0.183	0.068
18220	Cracker, melba toast rounds, plain	1 cracker	3	11.7	0.363	2.298	0.189	0.096	0.023	0.038	0.013
18221	Cracker, melba toast, rye or pumpernickel	1 toast	5	19.45	0.58	3.865	0.4	0.17	0.045	0.067	0.023
18620	Cracker, Original Premium Saltine Crackers/Nabisco	1 serving	14	58.8	1.526	9.954	0.364	1.428	0.819	0.241	0.259
18228	Cracker, oyster/soda/soup	1 cup	45	195.3	4.14	32.175	1.35	5.31	2.89	0.756	1.319
18621	Cracker, Ritz/Nabisco	1 serving	16	78.72	1.152	10.272	0.304	3.664	2.872	0.283	0.627
18224	Cracker, rusk toast	1 rusk	10	40.7	1.35	7.23		0.72	0.276	0.231	0.138
18425	Cracker, saltine/oyster/soda/soup, low salt	1 cup	45	195.3	4.14	32.175	1.35	5.31	2.89	0.756	1.319
18230	Cracker, sandwich, cheese filled	1 cracker	7	33.39	0.651	4.319	0.133	1.477	0.788	0.18	0.429
18215	Cracker, sandwich, cheese w/peanut butter filling	1 sandwich	6.5	32.24	0.807	3.688	0.221	1.633	0.845	0.331	0.286
18231	Cracker, sandwich, peanut butter filled	1 sandwich	6.5	32.11	0.746	3.795	0.149	1.595	0.895	0.303	0.319
18652	Cracker, Snackwell Wheat Cracker/Nabisco	1 serving	15	62.25	1.191	11.55	0.585	1.5			
18624	Cracker, Wheat Thins, baked/Nabisco	1 serving	29	136.3	2.407	20.039	0.87	5.8	2.03	0.36	0.925
18235	Cracker, whole wheat	10 Triscuit Bits	10	44.3	0.88	6.86	1.05	1.72	0.588	0.66	0.339
18429	Cracker, whole wheat, low sodium	10 Triscuit Bits	10	44.3	0.88	6.86	1.05	1.72	0.588	0.66	0.339
18434	Crackers, cheese, Cheez-its/Goldfish, low sodium	1 gold fish	0.6	3.018	0.061	0.349	0.014	0.152	0.071	0.015	0.058
18457	Crackers, saltines, fat-free, low-sodium	6 saltines	30	117.9	3.15	24.69	0.81	0.48	0.043	0.206	0.073
9079	Cranberries, dried, sweetened	1 cup, whole	95	292.6	0.067	78.242	5.415	1.301	0.188	0.625	0.098
42136	Cream substitute, powdered, light	1 oz	28.34	122.15	0.538	20.802	0	4.449	3.259	0.056	1.077
1058	Cream, filled cream, nonbutterfat sour dressing, cultured	1 tbsp	12	21.36	0.39	0.562	0	1.988	0.235	0.056	1.593
1049	Cream, half and half	1 tbsp	15	19.5	0.444	0.645	0	1.725	0.498	0.064	1.074

Chol (g)	Calc (mg)	Iron (mg)	Mag (mg)	Phos (mg)	Pota (mg)	Sodi (mg)	Zinc (mg)	Vit A (RAE)	Vit C (mg)	Thia (mg)	Ribo (mg)	Niac (mg)	Vit B$_6$ (mg)	Vit B$_{12}$ (µg)	Vit E (mg)	Fol (µg)	Alc (g)
0	2.6	0.388	4.5	9.8	17.5	60.4	0.081	0	0	0.008	0.018	0.207	0.002	0.003	0.158	5.1	0
0	7.42	0.364	6.86	26.32	26.88	51.52	0.148	0.14	0.014	0.045	0.037	0.523	0.019	0.032	0.262	8.54	0
0	4.05	0.332	2.1	11.25	13.65	52.35	0.06	0	0	0.039	0.036	0.404	0.003	0	0.24	7.5	0
4.62	4.2	0.34	2.52	11.9	10.22	39.34	0.081	0.14	0	0.041	0.031	0.347	0.003	0.001		8.82	0
1.6	2.8	0.219	1.36	8.64	8	36.4	0.042	1.44	0	0.026	0.026	0.267	0.006	0.007	0.026	5.6	0
0	1.62	0.176	0.99	5.04	5.31	13.23	0.032	0	0	0.009	0.018	0.219	0.001	0	0.176	4.68	0
7.36	20.7	0.423	1.84	43.01	37.49	107.64	0.062	2.76	0	0.042	0.028	0.555	0.005	0.016	0.048	16.1	0
0	1.5	0.133	0.72	3.84	6.42	18.36	0.02	0	0	0.022	0.013	0.179	0.001	0.002		2.58	0
0	3.3	0.354			57.42	38.28			0	0.007	0.013	0.067				1.1	
0	11.47	0.983			86.8	164.92			0	0.081	0.043	0.505				14.57	
0	2.6	0.436			11.6	80.4			0	0.062	0.04	0.504				15.2	
8.06	8.58	1.136			29.12	143.78			0	0.073	0.06	0.658					
7.77	7.35	0.571			43.89	84.84			0	0.05	0.042	0.918					
5.04	7.2	0.528			19.92	162.24			0	0.074	0.055	0.588					
24.381	3.402	0.59	3.969	31.469	38.556	285.201	1.012	0	0	0.006	0.042	0.689	0.037	0.459	0.043	2.552	0
0	2.56	0.602	3.84	16.64	3.84	11.52	0.077	0	0	0	0	0	0	0	0	0	0
8.06	93.62	2.957	22.32	135.16	89.9	616.9	0.701	17.98	0	0.353	0.265	2.896	0.343	0.285	0.037	94.24	0
0	3.1	0.243	7.8	26.9	31.9	26.4	0.239	0	0	0.024	0.014	0.104	0.021	0	0.081	4.7	0
0	3.64	0.885	7	24.92	31.36	0.56	0.19	0	0	0.108	0.081	1.09	0.032	0	0.017	4.76	0
0	6.44	1.302	37.52	85.4	88.48	0.56	0.731	0	0	0.102	0.076	1.515	0.045	0	0.374	9.8	0
0	2.79	0.111	1.77	5.88	6.06	24.87	0.06	0	0	0.012	0.008	0.123	0.003	0	0.013	3.72	0
0	3.9	0.184	1.95	9.15	9.65	44.95	0.068	0	0	0.024	0.014	0.236	0.004	0	0.032	4.25	0
0	27.02	0.727	2.94	13.86	13.86	177.8			0	0.046	0.062	0.612	0.007			11.76	
0	53.55	2.43	12.15	47.25	57.6	585.9	0.346	0	0	0.254	0.208	2.362	0.017	0	0.054	55.8	
0	23.52	0.648	3.2	48	14.88	124.16	0.232		0	0.04	0.049	0.61	0.006	0		9.6	
7.8	2.7	0.272	3.6	15.3	24.5	25.3	0.11	1.2	0	0.04	0.04	0.463	0.005	0.018		8.7	0
0	53.55	2.43	12.15	47.25	325.8	286.2	0.346	0	0	0.254	0.208	2.362	0.017	0	0.054	55.8	0
0.14	17.99	0.167	2.52	28.42	30.03	98.07	0.043	1.19	0.007	0.031	0.048	0.264	0.003	0.007	0.015	7	0
0	3.25	0.177	3.64	17.42	14.17	46.15	0.068	0	0	0.036	0.019	0.379	0.01	0.018	0.154	6.11	0
0	5.265	0.18	3.575	17.81	13.975	46.67	0.073	0	0	0.032	0.018	0.397	0.01	0.001	0.134	5.59	0
	22.35	0.585	6.9	49.5	28.5	150	0.323			0	0.042	0.055		0			
0	23.2	1.073	15.08	60.32	56.26	167.62				0	0.087	0.087	1.16	0.025		12.18	0
0	5	0.308	9.9	29.5	29.7	65.9	0.215	0	0	0.02	0.01	0.452	0.018	0	0.086	2.8	0
0	5	0.308	9.9	29.5	29.7	24.7	0.215	0	0	0.02	0.01	0.452	0.018	0	0.086	2.8	0
0.078	0.906	0.029	0.216	1.308	0.636	2.748	0.007	0.102	0	0.003	0.003	0.028	0.003	0.003	0.002	0.534	0
0	6.6	2.316	7.8	33.9	34.5	190.8	0.282	0	0	0.155	0.177	1.714	0.026	0	0.036	37.2	0
0	9.5	0.503	4.75	7.6	38	2.85	0.104	0	0.19	0.007	0.015	0.941	0.036	0	1.016	0	0
0	0.283	0.009	0	38.542	255.627	64.899	0.006	0.283	0	0	0	0	0	0	0.074	0.283	0
0.6	13.56	0.004	1.2	10.44	19.44	5.76	0.044	0.36	0.108	0.005	0.02	0.009	0.002	0.04	0.161	1.44	0
5.55	15.75	0.011	1.5	14.25	19.5	6.15	0.076	14.55	0.135	0.005	0.022	0.012	0.006	0.05	0.05	0.45	0

EvaluEat Code	Food Name	Amt	Wt (g)	Energy (kcal)	Prot (g)	Carb (g)	Fiber (g)	Fat (g)	Mono (g)	Poly (g)	Sat (g)
1053	Cream, heavy whipping	1 cup, whipped	120	414	2.46	3.348	0	44.4	12.823	1.649	27.638
1052	Cream, light whipping	1 cup, whipped	120	350.4	2.604	3.552	0	37.092	10.912	1.061	23.204
1056	Cream, sour, cultured	1 tbsp	12	25.68	0.379	0.512	0	2.515	0.726	0.093	1.566
1074	Cream, sour, imitation, cultured	1 oz	28.35	58.968	0.68	1.88	0	5.534	0.167	0.016	5.044
1055	Cream, sour, reduced fat (half and half) cultured	1 tbsp	15	20.25	0.441	0.639	0	1.8	0.52	0.067	1.12
1054	Cream, whipped cream topping, pressurized	1 tbsp	3	7.71	0.096	0.375	0	0.667	0.193	0.025	0.415
18242	Croutons, plain	.5 oz	14.2	57.794	1.69	10.437	0.724	0.937	0.434	0.181	0.214
18243	Croutons, seasoned	1 package, fast food	10	46.5	1.08	6.35	0.5	1.83	0.95	0.237	0.525
19205	Custard, egg, dry mix prep w/reduced fat (2%) milk	100 grams	100	111	4.08	17.42	0	2.74	0.852	0.197	1.357
19170	Custard, egg, dry mix prep w/whole milk	100 grams	100	121	4.04	17.29	0	4.01	1.201	0.244	2.122
9421	Dates, medjool	1 cup, drained	178	493.06	3.222	133.45	11.926	0.267			
18251	Donut, cake, chocolate w/sugar or glaze	1 doughnut (3-3/4" dia)	60	250.2	2.7	34.44	1.32	11.94	6.767	1.486	3.079
18249	Donut, cake, plain w/chocolate icing	1 doughnut, large (approx 3-1/2" dia)	57	270.18	2.85	27.36	1.14	17.67	9.976	2.158	4.621
18250	Donut, cake, plain w/sugar or glaze	1 doughnut, medium (approx 3" dia)	45	191.7	2.34	22.86	0.675	10.305	5.714	1.309	2.667
18248	Donut, cake, plain/old-fashioned	1 doughnut, medium (3-1/4" dia)	47	197.87	2.35	23.359	0.705	10.763	4.37	3.704	1.704
18253	Donut, French cruller, glazed	1 cruller (3" dia)	41	168.92	1.271	24.395	0.492	7.503	4.283	0.937	1.913
18254	Donut, yeast leavened, cream filled	1 doughnut oval (3-1/2" x 2-1/2")	85	306.85	5.44	25.5	0.68	20.825	10.268	2.62	4.615
18255	Donut/Honey Bun, yeast leavened, glazed	1 doughnut, large (approx 4-1/4" dia)	75	302.25	4.8	33.225	0.9	17.1	9.649	2.176	4.36
43287	Dove, cooked (includes squab)	1 cup	186	407.34	44.454	0	0	24.18	10.159	5.083	6.955
5143	Duck liver, domestic, raw	1 liver	44	59.84	8.246	1.553	0	2.042	0.312	0.277	0.634
5140	Duck, domestic, meat & skin, roasted	1 cup, chopped or diced	140	471.8	26.586	0	0	39.69	18.06	5.11	13.538
5142	Duck, domestic, meat, no skin, roasted	1 cup, chopped or diced	140	281.4	32.872	0	0	15.68	5.18	2.002	5.838
1142	Egg substitute, frozen	.25 cup	60	96	6.774	1.92	0	6.666	1.461	3.745	1.158
1143	Egg substitute, liquid	1 cup	251	210.84	30.12	1.606	0	8.308	2.249	4.024	1.654
1144	Egg substitute, powdered	.7 oz	20	88.8	11.1	4.36	0	2.6	1.068	0.337	0.753
1124	Egg, white, raw	1 large	33	17.16	3.597	0.241	0	0.056	0	0	0
1128	Egg, whole, fried	1 large	46	92.5	6.27	0.405	0		2.919	1.224	1.975
1129	Egg, whole, hard-cooked	1 large	50	77.5	6.29	0.56	0	5.305	2.039	0.707	1.633
1131	Egg, whole, poached	1 large	50	73.5	6.265	0.38	0	4.95	1.898	0.679	1.543
1132	Egg, whole, scrambled	1 large	61	101.26	6.765	1.342	0	7.448	2.908	1.31	2.244
1125	Egg, yolk, raw, fresh	1 large	17	54.74	2.696	0.61	0	4.512	1.995	0.715	1.624
43146	Eggplant, pickled	1 cup	186	91.14	1.674	18.172	4.65	1.302	0.117	0.547	0.26
18260	English muffin, mixed grain/granola	1 muffin	66	155.1	6.006	30.558	1.848	1.188	0.546	0.369	0.152
18258	English muffin, plain/sourdough, enriched	1 muffin	57	133.95	4.389	26.22	1.539	1.026	0.172	0.506	0.148
18264	English muffin, wheat	1 muffin	57	127.11	4.959	25.536	2.622	1.14	0.16	0.475	0.164

Chol (g)	Calc (mg)	Iron (mg)	Mag (mg)	Phos (mg)	Pota (mg)	Sodi (mg)	Zinc (mg)	Vit A (RAE)	Vit C (mg)	Thia (mg)	Ribo (mg)	Niac (mg)	Vit B_6 (mg)	Vit B_{12} (µg)	Vit E (mg)	Fol (µg)	Alc (g)
164.4	78	0.036	8.4	74.4	90	45.6	0.276	493.2	0.72	0.026	0.132	0.047	0.031	0.216	1.272	4.8	0
133.2	82.8	0.036	8.4	73.2	116.4	40.8	0.3	334.8	0.72	0.029	0.15	0.05	0.034	0.24	1.056	4.8	0
5.28	13.92	0.007	1.32	10.2	17.28	6.36	0.032	21.24	0.108	0.004	0.018	0.008	0.002	0.036	0.072	1.32	0
0	0.851	0.111	1.701	12.758	45.644	28.917	0.335	0	0	0	0	0	0	0	0.21	0	0
5.85	15.6	0.011	1.5	14.25	19.35	6.15	0.075	15.3	0.135	0.005	0.022	0.01	0.002	0.045	0.051	1.65	0
2.28	3.03	0.002	0.33	2.67	4.41	3.9	0.011	5.64	0	0.001	0.002	0.002	0.001	0.009	0.019	0.09	0
0	10.792	0.579	4.402	16.33	17.608	99.116	0.126	0	0	0.088	0.039	0.772	0.004	0		18.74	0
0.7	9.6	0.282	4.2	14	18.1	123.8	0.094	0.7	0	0.051	0.042	0.465	0.008	0.014	0.04	10.5	0
48	145	0.35	19	138	224	89	0.52	61	0.8	0.054	0.213	0.128	0.069	0.45		9	0
53	143	0.35	19	136	221	88	0.51	37	0.8	0.054	0.211	0.126	0.068	0.44		9	0
	113.92	1.602	96.12	110.36	1238.88	1.78	0.783	12.46	0	0.089	0.107	2.866	0.443			26.7	
34.2	127.8	1.362	20.4	97.2	63.6	204	0.342	7.2	0.06	0.027	0.042	0.282	0.016	0.06	0.126	27	0
34.77	19.95	1.402	22.8	115.14	111.72	244.53	0.348	3.99	0.114	0.072	0.06	0.741	0.029	0.137	0.211	26.79	0
14.4	27	0.477	7.65	52.65	45.9	180.9	0.198	1.35	0.045	0.105	0.089	0.68	0.012	0.108		20.7	0
17.39	20.68	0.917	9.4	126.43	59.69	256.62	0.259	17.86	0.094	0.104	0.113	0.871	0.026	0.127	0.907	24.44	0
4.51	10.66	0.992	4.92	50.43	31.98	141.45	0.107	0.82	0	0.074	0.094	0.873	0.008	0.021	0.066	17.22	0
20.4	21.25	1.556	17	64.6	68	262.65	0.68	9.35	0	0.287	0.126	1.906	0.058	0.119	0.247	59.5	0
4.5	32.25	1.53	16.5	69.75	81	256.5	0.577	3	0.075	0.273	0.161	2.139	0.043	0.068	0.262	36.75	0
215.76	31.62	10.993	48.36	617.52	476.16	106.02	7.124	52.08	5.394	0.521	0.651	14.136	1.06	0.763	0.112	11.16	0
226.6	4.84	13.433	10.56	118.36	101.2	61.6	1.351	5273	1.98	0.247	0.392	2.86	0.334	23.76		324.7	0
117.6	15.4	3.78	22.4	218.4	285.6	82.6	2.604	88.2	0	0.244	0.377	6.755	0.252	0.42	0.98	8.4	0
124.6	16.8	3.78	28	284.2	352.8	91	3.64	32.2	0	0.364	0.658	7.14	0.35	0.56	0.98	14	0
1.2	43.8	1.188	9	43.2	127.8	119.4	0.588	6.6	0.3	0.072	0.232	0.084	0.08	0.204	0.954	9.6	0
2.51	133.03	5.271	22.59	303.71	828.3	444.27	3.263	45.18	0	0.276	0.753	0.276	0.008	0.753	0.678	37.65	0
114.4	65.2	0.632	13	95.6	148.8	160	0.364	73.8	0.16	0.045	0.352	0.115	0.029	0.704	0.252	25	0
0	2.31	0.026	3.63	4.95	53.79	54.78	0.01	0	0	0.001	0.145	0.035	0.002	0.03	0	1.32	0
210.2	27.1	0.911	5.98	95.7	67.6	93.8	0.552	91.1	0	0.035	0.238	0.035	0.071	0.639	0.561	23.5	0
212	25	0.595	5	86	63	62	0.525	84.5	0	0.033	0.257	0.032	0.06	0.555	0.515	22	0
211	26.5	0.915	6	95	66.5	147	0.55	69.5	0	0.034	0.238	0.035	0.071	0.64	0.48	23.5	0
214.72	43.31	0.732	7.32	103.7	84.18	170.8	0.61	87.23	0.122	0.032	0.267	0.048	0.072	0.47	0.519	18.3	0
209.78	21.93	0.464	0.85	66.3	18.53	8.16	0.391	64.77	0	0.03	0.09	0.004	0.06	0.332	0.439	24.82	0
0	46.5	1.432	11.16	16.74	22.32	3113.64	0.428	5.58	0	0.093	0.13	1.228	0.26	0	0.056	37.2	0
0	129.36	1.993	27.06	53.46	102.96	274.56	0.917	0	0	0.284	0.207	2.365	0.025	0	0	52.8	0
0	99.18	1.425	11.97	75.81	74.67	264.48	0.399	0	0	0.252	0.16	2.214	0.025	0.023	0.177	54.15	0
0	101.46	1.636	21.09	60.99	106.02	217.74	0.61	0	0	0.246	0.166	1.913	0.05	0	0.256	36.48	0

EvaluEat Code	Food Name	Amt	Wt (g)	Energy (kcal)	Prot (g)	Carb (g)	Fiber (g)	Fat (g)	Mono (g)	Poly (g)	Sat (g)
21069	Fast food, burrito w/apples or cherries	1 burrito, small	74	230.88	2.501	34.98		9.524	3.42	1.055	4.569
21060	Fast food, burrito w/beans	2 pieces	217	447.02	14.062	71.436		13.497	4.739	1.196	6.888
21061	Fast food, burrito w/beans & cheese	2 pieces	186	377.58	15.066	54.963		11.699	2.483	1.784	6.849
21064	Fast food, burrito w/beans, cheese & beef	2 pieces	203	330.89	14.575	39.686		13.297	4.458	1.019	7.15
21066	Fast food, burrito w/beef	2 pieces	220	523.6	26.598	58.52		20.812	7.41	0.854	10.459
21035	Fast food, chicken, breaded, fried, dark meat (drumstick or thigh)	2 pieces	148	430.68	30.074	15.703		26.699	10.93	6.323	7.049
21036	Fast food, chicken, breaded, fried, light meat (breast or wing)	2 pieces	163	493.89	35.713	19.576		29.519	12.228	6.786	7.844
21037	Fast food, chicken, breaded, fried, no bone, plain	1 piece	18	54.18	3.06	2.594	0	3.499	1.78	0.78	0.79
21038	Fast food, chicken, breaded, fried, no bone, w/BBQ sauce	6 pieces	130	330.2	17.147	25.025		17.966	8.765	2.389	5.57
21042	Fast food, chili con carne	1 cup (8 fl. oz.)	253	255.53	24.617	21.935		8.273	3.408	0.529	3.431
21071	Fast food, chimichanga w/beef & cheese	1 chimichanga	183	442.86	20.057	39.327		23.442	9.434	0.728	11.178
21043	Fast food, clams (shellfish) breaded, fried	.75 cup	115	450.8	12.822	38.813		26.404	11.44	6.773	6.603
21128	Fast food, corn on the cob w/butter	1 ear	146	154.76	4.468	31.945		3.431	1.004	0.612	1.643
21046	Fast food, crab cake (shellfish)	1 cake	60	159.6	11.25	5.112	0.24	10.35	4.308	3.078	2.244
21015	Fast food, Danish pastry, cheese	1 pastry	91	353.08	5.833	28.692		24.625	15.601	2.423	5.123
21016	Fast food, Danish pastry, cinnamon	1 pastry	88	349.36	4.805	46.851		16.72	10.593	1.646	3.479
21017	Fast food, Danish pastry, fruit	1 pastry	94	334.64	4.756	45.064		15.933	10.096	1.568	3.315
21074	Fast food, enchilada w/cheese	1 enchilada	163	319.48	9.633	28.541		18.843	6.311	0.817	10.588
21075	Fast food, enchilada w/cheese & beef	1 enchilada	192	322.56	11.923	30.47		17.645	6.146	1.388	9.047
21076	Fast food, enchirito w/cheese, beef & beans	1 enchirito	193	343.54	17.891	33.794		16.077	6.518	0.328	7.948
21019	Fast food, English muffin w/butter	1 muffin	63	189	4.87	30.36		5.758	1.532	1.348	2.43
21024	Fast food, French toast sticks	5 pieces	141	513.24	8.277	57.852	2.679	29.046	12.648	9.941	4.709
21023	Fast food, French toast w/butter	2 slices	135	356.4	10.341	36.045		18.765	7.074	2.444	7.749
21077	Fast food, frijoles (beans) w/cheese	1 cup	167	225.45	11.373	28.707		7.782	2.617	0.696	4.075
21116	Fast food, ham & cheese sandwich	1 sandwich	146	351.86	20.688	33.346		15.476	6.738	1.375	6.437
21117	Fast food, ham, egg & cheese sandwich	1 sandwich	143	347.49	19.248	30.945		16.302	5.744	1.69	7.4
21202	Fast food, hamburger, large, one meat patty w/condiments	1 sandwich	172	426.56	23.1	36.825	2.064	21.001	9.307	1.594	7.926
21119	Fast food, hot dog w/chili, plain	1 sandwich	114	296.4	13.509	31.293		13.441	6.595	1.188	4.854
21120	Fast food, hot dog w/corn flour coating, corn dog	1 sandwich	175	460.25	16.8	55.79		18.9	9.109	3.497	5.161
21118	Fast food, hot dog, plain	1 sandwich	98	242.06	10.388	18.032		14.543	6.853	1.706	5.109
21129	Fast food, hush puppies	5 pieces	78	256.62	4.875	34.897		11.591	7.819	0.388	2.686
21033	Fast food, ice cream sundae, hot fudge	1 sundae	158	284.4	5.641	47.669	0	8.627	2.331	0.807	5.023
14346	Fast food, milk beverage, chocolate shake/McDonald's	1 medium shake (16 fl. oz.)	333	422.91	11.322	68.265	6.327	12.321	3.58	0.466	7.702
21078	Fast food, nachos w/cheese	1 portion (6–8 nachos)	113	345.78	9.097	36.33		18.95	7.994	2.233	7.78
21080	Fast food, nachos w/cheese, beans, ground beef & peppers	1 portion (6–8 nachos)	255	568.65	19.788	55.819		30.702	10.98	5.689	12.487
21130	Fast food, onion rings, breaded, fried	1 portion (8–9 onion rings)	83	275.56	3.702	31.324		15.513	6.651	0.665	6.953
21048	Fast food, oysters (shellfish) battered/breaded, fried	6 pieces	139	368.35	12.538	39.879		17.931	6.921	4.638	4.579
21025	Fast food, pancakes w/butter & syrup	2 cakes	232	519.68	8.259	90.898		13.99	5.269	1.958	5.851
21049	Fast food, pizza w/cheese	1 slice	63	140.49	7.68	20.5		3.213	0.99	0.491	1.54
21050	Fast food, pizza w/cheese, meat & vegetables	1 slice	79	184.07	13.011	21.291		5.364	2.543	0.915	1.535

Chol (g)	Calc (mg)	Iron (mg)	Mag (mg)	Phos (mg)	Pota (mg)	Sodi (mg)	Zinc (mg)	Vit A (RAE)	Vit C (mg)	Thia (mg)	Ribo (mg)	Niac (mg)	Vit B$_6$ (mg)	Vit B$_{12}$ (µg)	Vit E (mg)	Fol (µg)	Alc (g)
3.7	15.54	1.073	7.4	14.8	104.34	211.64	0.4	20.72	0.74	0.17	0.178	1.857	0.074	0.511		24.42	0
4.34	112.84	4.514	86.8	97.65	653.17	985.18	1.519	17.36	1.953	0.629	0.608	4.058	0.304	1.085		86.8	0
27.9	213.9	2.269	79.98	180.42	496.62	1166.22	1.637	98.58	1.674	0.223	0.707	3.571	0.242	0.893		74.4	0
123.83	129.92	3.735	50.75	140.07	410.06	990.64	2.355	150.2	5.075	0.305	0.711	3.857	0.223	1.096		75.11	0
63.8	83.6	6.094	81.4	173.8	739.2	1491.6	4.73	13.2	1.1	0.242	0.924	6.446	0.308	1.958		129.8	0
165.76	35.52	1.598	37	239.76	445.48	754.8	3.241	66.6	0	0.133	0.429	7.208	0.326	0.829		25.16	0
148.33	60.31	1.483	37.49	306.44	565.61	974.74	1.548	57.05	0	0.147	0.293	11.981	0.571	0.668		29.34	0
10.44	2.34	0.16	4.14	49.14	51.84	87.12	0.169	0.9	0	0.02	0.027	1.269	0.052	0.052	0.221	5.22	0
61.1	20.8	1.456	24.7	214.5	318.5	829.4	1.118	16.9	0.78	0.104	0.156	7.02	0.338	0.299		29.9	0
134.09	68.31	5.186	45.54	197.34	690.69	1006.94	3.567	83.49	1.518	0.126	1.138	2.479	0.329	1.138		45.54	0
51.24	237.9	3.843	60.39	186.66	203.13	957.09	3.367	131.8	2.745	0.384	0.86	4.667	0.22	1.299		91.5	0
87.4	20.7	3.048	31.05	238.05	265.65	833.75	1.633	36.8	0	0.207	0.264	2.863	0.034	1.104		42.55	0
5.84	4.38	0.876	40.88	108.04	359.16	29.2	0.905	33.58	6.862	0.248	0.102	2.175	0.321	0		43.8	0
82.2	202.2	1.116	25.2	226.8	162	491.4	2.124	93	0.18	0.055	0.075	1.166	0.149	4.398		24.6	0
20.02	70.07	1.847	15.47	80.08	116.48	319.41	0.628	44.59	2.639	0.264	0.209	2.548	0.055	0.228		54.6	0
27.28	36.96	1.795	14.08	73.92	95.92	326.48	0.484	5.28	2.552	0.255	0.194	2.2	0.053	0.22		54.56	0
18.8	21.62	1.401	14.1	68.62	109.98	332.76	0.479	25.38	1.598	0.291	0.207	1.795	0.056	0.235		31.02	0
44.01	324.37	1.32	50.53	133.66	239.61	784.03	2.51	99.43	0.978	0.082	0.424	1.907	0.391	0.75		65.2	0
40.32	228.48	3.072	82.56	167.04	574.08	1319.04	2.688	97.92	1.344	0.096	0.403	2.515	0.269	1.018		67.2	0
50.18	218.09	2.393	71.41	223.88	559.7	1250.64	2.76	88.78	4.632	0.174	0.695	2.991	0.212	1.621		94.57	0
12.6	102.69	1.588	13.23	85.05	69.3	386.19	0.422	31.5	0.756	0.252	0.315	2.615	0.038	0.019	0.126	56.7	0
74.73	77.55	2.961	26.79	122.67	126.9	499.14	0.931	0	0	0.226	0.254	2.961	0.254	0.071	2.326	255.2	0
116.1	72.9	1.89	16.2	145.8	176.85	513	0.594	136.4	0.135	0.581	0.5	3.915	0.054	0.365		72.9	0
36.74	188.71	2.238	85.17	175.35	604.54	881.76	1.737	35.07	1.503	0.134	0.334	1.486	0.2	0.685		111.9	0
58.4	129.94	3.241	16.06	151.84	290.54	770.88	1.372	96.36	2.774	0.307	0.482	2.686	0.204	0.54	0.292	75.92	0
245.96	211.64	3.103	25.74	346.06	210.21	1005.29	1.988	165.9	2.717	0.429	0.558	4.204	0.157	1.23	0.586	75.79	0
70.52	134.16	4.145	34.4	213.28	395.6	731	4.764	5.16	2.58	0.342	0.284	6.562	0.246	2.58	0.034	61.92	0
51.3	19.38	3.283	10.26	191.52	166.44	479.94	0.775	3.42	2.736	0.217	0.399	3.739	0.046	0.296		72.96	0
78.75	101.5	6.177	17.5	166.25	262.5	973	1.313	59.5	0	0.28	0.7	4.165	0.087	0.438		103.25	0
44.1	23.52	2.313	12.74	97.02	143.08	670.32	1.98	0	0.098	0.235	0.274	3.646	0.049	0.51		48.02	0
134.94	68.64	1.427	16.38	190.32	187.98	964.86	0.429	8.58	0	0	0.023	2.028	0.101	0.172		57.72	0
20.54	206.98	0.585	33.18	227.52	395	181.7	0.948	58.46	2.37	0.063	0.3	1.074	0.126	0.648	0.664	9.48	0
43.29	376.29	1.032	56.61	339.66	666	323.01	1.365	86.58	1.332	0.193	0.816	0.536	0.167	1.132	0.366	16.65	0
18.08	272.33	1.277	55.37	275.72	171.76	815.86	1.785	149.2	1.243	0.192	0.373	1.537	0.203	0.825		10.17	0
20.4	385.05	2.78	96.9	387.6	451.35	1800.3	3.646	436.1	4.845	0.23	0.688	3.34	0.408	1.02		38.25	0
14.11	73.04	0.847	15.77	86.32	129.48	429.94	0.349	0.83	0.581	0.083	0.1	0.921	0.058	0.124	0.332	54.78	0
108.42	27.8	4.462	23.63	195.99	182.09	676.93	15.64	108.4	4.17	0.306	0.347	4.42	0.028	1.015		30.58	0
58	127.6	2.622	48.72	475.6	250.56	1104.32	1.021	81.2	3.48	0.394	0.557	3.387	0.116	0.232	1.392	51.04	0
9.45	116.55	0.58	15.75	112.77	109.62	335.79	0.813	73.71	1.26	0.183	0.164	2.482	0.044	0.334		34.65	0
20.54	101.12	1.533	18.17	131.14	178.54	382.36	1.114	58.46	1.58	0.213	0.174	1.959	0.095	0.363		32.39	0

EvaluEat Code	Food Name	Amt	Wt (g)	Energy (kcal)	Prot (g)	Carb (g)	Fiber (g)	Fat (g)	Mono (g)	Poly (g)	Sat (g)
21051	Fast food, pizza w/pepperoni	1 slice	71	181.05	10.125	19.866		6.958	3.14	1.165	2.236
21132	Fast food, potato, baked, topped w/cheese & bacon	1 piece	299	451.49	18.418	44.431		25.893	9.715	4.751	10.133
21131	Fast food, potato, baked, topped w/cheese sauce	1 piece	296	473.6	14.622	46.502		28.742	10.7	6.044	10.558
21135	Fast food, potato, baked, topped w/sour cream & chives	1 piece	302	392.6	6.674	50.011		22.318	7.873	3.316	10.011
21138	Fast food, potato, French fried w/vegetable oil	1 large	169	577.98	7.267	67.279	5.915	31.147	17.99	5.288	6.507
21139	Fast food, potato, mashed	.333 cup	80	66.4	1.848	12.896		0.968	0.281	0.234	0.383
21026	Fast food, potatoes, hash brown	.5 cup	72	151.2	1.944	16.15		9.216	3.858	0.47	4.324
21122	Fast food, roast beef sandwich w/cheese	1 sandwich	176	473.44	32.226	45.373		18.005	3.661	3.502	9.029
21121	Fast food, roast beef sandwich, plain	1 sandwich	139	346.11	21.503	33.443		13.761	6.804	1.706	3.606
4021	Fast food, salad dressing, Italian, w/salt, diet (2 kcal/tsp)	1 tbsp	15	11.25	0.071	0.686	0	0.957	0.329	0.256	0.068
4025	Fast food, salad dressing, mayonnaise, soybean oil, w/salt	1 tbsp	13.8	98.946	0.152	0.538	0	10.792	2.705	5.889	1.64
21127	Fast food, salad, cole slaw	.75 cup	99	146.52	1.455	12.751		10.969	2.42	6.394	1.606
21140	Fast food, salad, potato	.333 cup	95	108.3	1.453	12.853		5.728	1.605	2.869	0.978
21083	Fast food, salad, taco	1.5 cup	198	279.18	13.226	23.582		14.771	5.16	1.748	6.823
21084	Fast food, salad, taco w/chili con carne	1.5 cup	261	289.71	17.409	26.57		13.128	4.539	1.537	6
21002	Fast food, sandwich, biscuit w/egg	1 biscuit	136	372.64	11.601	31.906	0.816	22.073	9.073	6.4	4.729
21003	Fast food, sandwich, biscuit w/egg & bacon	1 biscuit	150	457.5	16.995	28.59	0.75	31.095	13.44	7.47	7.95
21004	Fast food, sandwich, biscuit w/egg & ham	1 biscuit	192	441.6	20.429	30.317	0.768	27.034	10.963	7.699	5.914
21005	Fast food, sandwich, biscuit w/egg & sausage	1 biscuit	180	581.4	19.152	41.148	0.9	38.7	16.398	4.446	14.976
21007	Fast food, sandwich, biscuit w/egg, cheese & bacon	1 biscuit	144	476.64	16.258	33.422		31.392	14.226	3.495	11.398
21008	Fast food, sandwich, biscuit w/ham	1 biscuit	113	386.46	13.391	43.787	0.791	18.419	4.833	1.037	11.408
21009	Fast food, sandwich, biscuit w/sausage	1 biscuit	124	484.84	12.115	40.04	1.364	31.781	12.82	3.026	14.22
21093	Fast food, sandwich, cheeseburger (2 patty) condiments & vegetables	1 sandwich	166	416.66	21.248	35.192		21.082	7.809	2.658	8.717
21092	Fast food, sandwich, cheeseburger (2 patty) plain	1 sandwich	155	457.25	27.667	22.056		28.474	11.008	1.914	12.997
21097	Fast food, sandwich, cheeseburger, large, one meat patty w/bacon & condiments	1 sandwich	195	608.4	32	37.128		36.758	14.488	2.711	16.243
21098	Fast food, sandwich, cheeseburger, large, one meat patty w/condiments & vegetables	1 sandwich	219	562.83	28.185	38.391		32.938	12.61	2.026	15.039
21103	Fast food, sandwich, chicken filet w/cheese	1 sandwich	228	631.56	29.412	41.587		38.76	13.65	9.948	12.449
21102	Fast food, sandwich, chicken filet, plain	1 sandwich	182	515.06	24.115	38.693		29.448	10.41	8.383	8.527
21011	Fast food, sandwich, croissant w/egg & cheese	1 croissant	127	368.3	12.789	24.308		24.701	7.541	1.367	14.065
21012	Fast food, sandwich, croissant w/egg, cheese & bacon	1 croissant	129	412.8	16.228	23.646		28.354	9.176	1.758	15.432
21013	Fast food, sandwich, croissant w/egg, cheese & ham	1 croissant	152	474.24	18.924	24.198		33.577	11.392	2.359	17.475
21020	Fast food, sandwich, English muffin w/cheese & sausage	1 muffin	115	393.3	15.341	29.164	1.495	24.265	10.081	2.694	9.851
21021	Fast food, sandwich, English muffin w/egg, cheese & Canadian bacon	1 sandwich	137	289.07	16.687	26.742	1.507	12.59	4.67	1.558	4.665
21105	Fast food, sandwich, fish w/tartar sauce	1 sandwich	158	431.34	16.938	41.017		22.768	7.693	8.248	5.235
21106	Fast food, sandwich, fish w/tartar sauce & cheese	1 sandwich	183	523.38	20.606	47.635		28.603	8.919	9.432	8.14
21114	Fast food, sandwich, hamburger, large (2 patty) w/condiments & vegetables	1 sandwich	226	540.14	34.284	40.273		26.555	10.328	2.796	10.518
21113	Fast food, sandwich, hamburger, large, one meat patty w/condiments & vegetables	1 sandwich	218	512.3	25.833	40.003		27.359	11.423	2.202	10.42
21109	Fast food, sandwich, hamburger, one patty w/condiments & vegetables	1 sandwich	110	279.4	12.914	27.291		13.475	5.29	2.577	4.131

Chol (g)	Calc (mg)	Iron (mg)	Mag (mg)	Phos (mg)	Pota (mg)	Sodi (mg)	Zinc (mg)	Vit A (RAE)	Vit C (mg)	Thia (mg)	Ribo (mg)	Niac (mg)	Vit B6 (mg)	Vit B12 (µg)	Vit E (mg)	Fol (µg)	Alc (g)
14.2	64.61	0.937	8.52	75.26	152.65	266.96	0.518	52.54	1.633	0.135	0.234	3.046	0.057	0.185		36.92	0
29.9	307.97	3.139	68.77	346.84	1178.06	971.75	2.153	188.4	28.7	0.269	0.239	3.977	0.748	0.329		29.9	0
17.76	310.8	3.019	65.12	319.68	1166.24	381.84	1.894	251.6	26.05	0.237	0.207	3.345	0.71	0.178		26.64	0
24.16	105.7	3.111	69.46	184.22	1383.16	181.2	0.906	265.8	33.82	0.272	0.181	3.715	0.785	0.211		33.22	0
0	23.66	1.318	65.91	218.01	1164.41	334.62	0.794	0	19.6	0.135	0.068	4.817	0.605	0	2.569	11.83	0
1.6	16.8	0.376	14.4	44	235.2	181.6	0.256	8.8	0.32	0.072	0.04	0.96	0.184	0.04		6.4	0
9.36	7.2	0.482	15.84	69.12	267.12	290.16	0.216	1.44	5.472	0.079	0.014	1.073	0.166	0.014	0.122	7.92	0
77.44	183.04	5.051	40.48	401.28	344.96	1633.28	5.368	58.08	0	0.387	0.458	5.896	0.334	2.059		63.36	0
51.43	54.21	4.226	30.58	239.08	315.53	792.3	3.392	11.12	2.085	0.375	0.306	5.866	0.264	1.223		56.99	0
0.9	1.35	0.098	0.6	1.65	12.75	204.9	0.029	0.15	0	0	0.002	0	0.011	0	0.03	0	0
5.244	2.484	0.069	0.138	3.864	4.692	78.384	0.022	11.59	0	0	0	0.001	0.08	0.036	0.72	1.104	0
4.95	33.66	0.723	8.91	35.64	177.21	267.3	0.198	35.64	8.316	0.04	0.03	0.079	0.109	0.178		38.61	0
57	13.3	0.693	7.6	53.2	256.5	311.6	0.19	28.5	1.045	0.067	0.104	0.257	0.142	0.114		23.75	0
43.56	192.06	2.277	51.48	142.56	415.8	762.3	2.693	71.28	3.564	0.099	0.356	2.455	0.218	0.634		83.16	0
5.22	245.34	2.662	52.2	153.99	391.5	884.79	3.289	258.4	3.393	0.157	0.496	2.532	0.522	0.731		91.35	0
244.8	81.6	2.897	19.04	387.6	238	890.8	0.993	179.5	0.136	0.303	0.487	2.153	0.112	0.626	3.264	57.12	0
352.5	189	3.735	24	238.5	250.5	999	1.635	106.5	2.7	0.135	0.225	2.4	0.135	1.035	1.965	60	0
299.52	220.8	4.55	30.72	316.8	318.72	1382.4	2.227	236.2	0	0.672	0.595	1.997	0.269	1.19	2.285	65.28	0
302.4	154.8	3.96	25.2	489.6	320.4	1141.2	2.16	160.2	0	0.504	0.45	3.6	0.198	1.368	2.844	64.8	0
260.64	164.16	2.549	20.16	459.36	230.4	1260	1.541	190.1	1.584	0.302	0.432	2.304	0.101	1.051		53.28	0
24.86	160.46	2.723	22.6	553.7	196.62	1432.84	1.65	30.51	0.113	0.508	0.316	3.48	0.136	0.034	1.661	38.42	0
34.72	127.72	2.579	19.84	446.4	198.4	1071.36	1.55	12.4	0.124	0.397	0.285	3.274	0.112	0.508	1.364	45.88	0
59.76	170.98	3.42	29.88	242.36	335.32	1050.78	3.486	71.38	1.66	0.349	0.282	8.051	0.183	1.926		61.42	0
110.05	232.5	3.41	32.55	373.55	308.45	635.5	4.96	99.2	0	0.248	0.372	6.014	0.248	2.309	1.193	68.2	0
111.15	161.85	4.739	44.85	399.75	331.5	1043.25	6.825	81.9	2.145	0.312	0.41	6.63	0.312	2.34		85.8	0
87.6	205.86	4.665	43.8	310.98	444.57	1108.14	4.599	140.2	7.884	0.394	0.46	7.38	0.285	2.562	1.183	81.03	0
77.52	257.64	3.625	43.32	405.84	332.88	1238.04	2.896	164.2	2.964	0.41	0.456	9.074	0.41	0.456		109.4	0
60.06	60.06	4.677	34.58	232.96	353.08	957.32	1.875	30.94	8.918	0.328	0.237	6.807	0.2	0.382		100.1	0
215.9	243.84	2.197	21.59	347.98	173.99	551.18	1.753	276.9	0.127	0.191	0.381	1.511	0.102	0.775		46.99	0
215.43	150.93	2.193	23.22	276.06	201.24	888.81	1.896	141.9	2.193	0.348	0.335	2.193	0.116	0.864		45.15	0
212.8	144.4	2.128	25.84	335.92	272.08	1080.72	2.174	130.7	11.4	0.517	0.304	3.192	0.228	1.003		45.6	0
58.65	167.9	2.254	24.15	186.3	215.05	1036.15	1.679	101.2	1.265	0.701	0.253	4.14	0.149	0.678	1.265	66.7	0
234.27	150.7	2.439	23.29	269.89	198.65	728.84	1.562	176.7	1.781	0.495	0.448	3.335	0.147	0.671	0.562	68.5	0
55.3	83.74	2.607	33.18	211.72	339.7	614.62	0.995	33.18	2.844	0.332	0.221	3.397	0.111	1.074	0.869	85.32	0
67.71	184.83	3.495	36.6	311.1	353.19	938.79	1.171	129.93	2.745	0.458	0.421	4.227	0.11	1.08	1.83	91.5	0
122.04	101.7	5.853	49.72	314.14	569.52	791	5.673	4.52	1.13	0.362	0.384	7.571	0.542	4.068		76.84	0
87.2	95.92	4.927	43.6	233.26	479.6	824.04	4.883	23.98	2.616	0.414	0.371	7.281	0.327	2.376		82.84	0
26.4	62.7	2.629	22	124.3	226.6	503.8	2.057	4.4	1.65	0.231	0.198	3.685	0.121	0.88		51.7	0

EvaluEat Code	Food Name	Amt	Wt (g)	Energy (kcal)	Prot (g)	Carb (g)	Fiber (g)	Fat (g)	Mono (g)	Poly (g)	Sat (g)
21107	Fast food, sandwich, hamburger, plain	1 sandwich	90	274.5	12.321	30.51		11.817	5.456	0.918	4.141
14347	Fast food, shake, vanilla/McDonald's	1 medium shake (16 fl. oz.)	333	369.63	11.655	59.607	0.333	9.99	2.87	0.37	6.187
21059	Fast food, shrimp (shellfish) breaded, fried	6–8 shrimp	164	454.28	18.876	40		24.895	17.379	0.645	5.379
21123	Fast food, steak sandwich	1 sandwich	204	459	30.335	51.959		14.076	5.345	3.346	3.815
21124	Fast food, submarine sandwich, cold cuts	1 sandwich	228	456	21.842	51.049		18.628	8.226	2.282	6.808
21126	Fast food, submarine sandwich, tuna salad	1 sandwich	256	583.68	29.696	55.373		27.981	13.402	7.296	5.33
21082	Fast food, taco	1 large	263	568.08	31.77	41.107		31.613	10.115	1.475	17.484
21085	Fast food, tostada w/beans & cheese	1 piece	144	223.2	9.605	26.525		9.864	3.054	0.749	5.367
21087	Fast food, tostada w/beef & cheese	1 piece	163	314.59	18.99	22.771		16.349	3.345	0.975	10.395
4002	Fat, animal, lard, pork	1 tbsp	12.8	115.46	0	0	0	12.8	5.773	1.434	5.018
6963	Fish broth	.5 cup	125	20	2.5	0.5	0	0.75	0.151	0.203	0.178
43129	Fish sticks, meatless	1 cup	186	539.4	42.78	16.74	11.346	33.48	8.139	17.358	5.299
15187	Fish, bass, freshwater, cooked w/dry heat	3 oz	85	124.1	20.553	0	0	4.021	1.56	1.156	0.851
15188	Fish, bass, striped, cooked w/dry heat	3 oz	85	105.4	19.32	0	0	2.542	0.719	0.854	0.553
15008	Fish, carp, raw	3 oz	85	107.95	15.156	0	0	4.76	1.979	1.216	0.921
15011	Fish, catfish, channel, breaded & fried	3 oz	85	194.65	15.377	6.834	0.595	11.331	4.769	2.826	2.795
15235	Fish, catfish, channel, farmed, cooked w/dry heat	3 oz	85	129.2	15.912	0	0	6.817	3.532	1.183	1.521
15012	Fish, caviar, black/red, granular	1 tbsp	16	40.32	3.936	0.64	0	2.864	0.741	1.185	0.65
15016	Fish, cod, Atlantic, baked/broiled (dry heat)	3 oz	85	89.25	19.406	0	0	0.731	0.105	0.248	0.143
15192	Fish, cod, Pacific, cooked w/dry heat	3 oz	85	89.25	19.508	0	0	0.689	0.089	0.266	0.088
15026	Fish, eel, baked or broiled (dry heat)	3 oz	85	200.6	20.103	0	0	12.708	7.835	1.032	2.57
15034	Fish, haddock, baked or broiled (dry heat)	3 oz	85	95.2	20.604	0	0	0.791	0.128	0.263	0.142
15035	Fish, haddock, smoked	3 oz	85	98.6	21.445	0	0	0.816	0.133	0.273	0.147
15037	Fish, halibut, Atlantic & Pacific, baked or broiled (dry heat)	3 oz	85	119	22.687	0	0	2.499	0.822	0.799	0.354
15196	Fish, halibut, Greenland, cooked w/dry heat	3 oz	85	203.15	15.657	0	0	15.079	9.131	1.49	2.637
15040	Fish, herring, Atlantic, baked or broiled (dry heat)	3 oz	85	172.55	19.576	0	0	9.852	4.072	2.325	2.223
15197	Fish, herring, Pacific, cooked w/dry heat	3 oz	85	212.5	17.859	0	0	15.122	7.486	2.64	3.548
15121	Fish, light tuna, canned in H2O, drained	3 oz	85	98.6	21.684	0	0	0.697	0.135	0.286	0.199
15119	Fish, light tuna, canned in oil, drained	3 oz	85	168.3	24.76	0	0	6.979	2.507	2.452	1.304
15047	Fish, mackerel, Atlantic, baked or broiled (dry heat)	3 oz	85	222.7	20.273	0	0	15.139	5.955	3.655	3.55
15200	Fish, mackerel, king, cooked w/dry heat	3 oz	85	113.9	22.1	0	0	2.176	0.832	0.501	0.395
15058	Fish, ocean perch, Atlantic, baked or broiled (dry heat)	3 oz	85	102.85	20.298	0	0	1.776	0.681	0.465	0.266
15230	Fish, octopus, common, cooked w/moist heat	3 oz	85	139.4	25.347	3.74	0	1.768	0.275	0.405	0.385
15061	Fish, perch, baked or broiled (dry heat)	3 oz	85	99.45	21.131	0	0	1.003	0.166	0.401	0.201
15063	Fish, pike, northern, baked or broiled (dry heat)	3 oz	85	96.05	20.987	0	0	0.748	0.171	0.22	0.128
15204	Fish, pike, walleye, cooked w/dry heat	3 oz	85	101.15	20.859	0	0	1.326	0.32	0.487	0.271
15205	Fish, pollock, Atlantic, cooked w/dry heat	3 oz	85	100.3	21.182	0	0	1.071	0.122	0.529	0.145
15067	Fish, pollock, walleye, baked or broiled	3 oz	85	96.05	19.984	0	0	0.952	0.148	0.445	0.196
15069	Fish, pompano, Florida, baked or broiled (dry heat)	3 oz	85	179.35	20.137	0	0	10.319	2.818	1.239	3.824
15071	Fish, rockfish, Pacific, baked or broiled (dry heat)	3 oz	85	102.85	20.434	0	0	1.709	0.38	0.505	0.403
15207	Fish, roe, cooked w/dry heat	3 oz	85	173.4	24.327	1.632	0	6.995	1.81	2.893	1.586
15232	Fish, roughy, orange, cooked w/dry heat	3 oz	85	75.65	16.023	0	0	0.765	0.523	0.014	0.02

Chol (g)	Calc (mg)	Iron (mg)	Mag (mg)	Phos (mg)	Pota (mg)	Sodi (mg)	Zinc (mg)	Vit A (RAE)	Vit C (mg)	Thia (mg)	Ribo (mg)	Niac (mg)	Vit B_6 (mg)	Vit B_{12} (µg)	Vit E (mg)	Fol (µg)	Alc (g)
35.1	63	2.403	18.9	102.6	144.9	387	1.998	0	0	0.333	0.27	3.717	0.063	0.891	0.495	53.1	0
36.63	406.26	0.3	39.96	339.66	579.42	273.06	1.199	123.2	2.664	0.15	0.606	0.616	0.173	1.199	0.2	16.65	0
200.08	83.64	2.952	39.36	344.4	183.68	1446.48	1.214	36.08	0	0.213	0.902	0	0.066	0.148		100	0
73.44	91.8	5.161	48.96	297.84	524.28	797.64	4.529	20.4	5.508	0.408	0.367	7.303	0.367	1.571		89.76	0
36.48	189.24	2.508	68.4	287.28	394.44	1650.72	2.576	70.68	12.31	1.003	0.798	5.495	0.137	1.094		86.64	0
48.64	74.24	2.637	79.36	220.16	335.36	1292.8	1.869	46.08	3.584	0.461	0.333	11.341	0.23	1.613		102.4	0
86.79	339.27	3.708	107.83	312.97	728.51	1233.47	6.049	165.7	3.419	0.237	0.684	4.944	0.368	1.604		105.2	0
30.24	210.24	1.886	59.04	116.64	403.2	542.88	1.901	44.64	1.296	0.101	0.331	1.325	0.158	0.691		43.2	0
40.75	216.79	2.869	63.57	179.3	572.13	896.5	3.684	50.53	2.608	0.098	0.554	3.146	0.228	1.174		74.98	0
12.16	0	0	0	0	0	0	0.014	0	0	0	0	0	0	0	0.077	0	0
0	37.5	0.262	1.25	37.5	107.5	397.5	0.125	1.25	0	0	0.037	1.712	0.012	0.125	0.188	5	0
0	176.7	3.72	42.78	837	1116	911.4	2.604	0	0	2.046	1.674	22.32	2.79	7.812	7.347	189.7	0
73.95	87.55	1.623	32.3	217.6	387.6	76.5	0.706	29.75	1.785	0.074	0.077	1.294	0.117	1.964		14.45	0
87.55	16.15	0.918	43.35	215.9	278.8	74.8	0.433	26.35	0	0.098	0.031	2.174	0.294	3.748		8.5	0
56.1	34.85	1.054	24.65	352.75	283.05	41.65	1.258	7.65	1.36	0.098	0.047	1.394	0.162	1.301	0.535	12.75	0
68.85	37.4	1.215	22.95	183.6	289	238	0.731	6.8	0	0.062	0.113	1.94	0.162	1.615		25.5	0
54.4	7.65	0.697	22.1	208.25	272.85	68	0.892	12.75	0.68	0.357	0.062	2.136	0.139	2.38		5.95	0
94.08	44	1.901	48	56.96	28.96	240	0.152	89.76	0	0.03	0.099	0.019	0.051	3.2	1.12	8	0
46.75	11.9	0.417	35.7	117.3	207.4	66.3	0.493	11.9	0.85	0.075	0.067	2.136	0.241	0.892	0.689	6.8	0
39.95	7.65	0.281	26.35	189.55	439.45	77.35	0.433	8.5	2.55	0.021	0.043	2.112	0.393	0.884		6.8	0
136.85	22.1	0.544	22.1	235.45	296.65	55.25	1.768	966.5	1.53	0.156	0.043	3.814	0.065	2.457	4.335	14.45	0
62.9	35.7	1.148	42.5	204.85	339.15	73.95	0.408	16.15	0	0.034	0.038	3.937	0.294	1.182		11.05	0
65.45	41.65	1.19	45.9	213.35	352.75	648.55	0.425	18.7	0	0.04	0.042	4.312	0.34	1.36	0.468	12.75	0
34.85	51	0.91	90.95	242.25	489.6	58.65	0.45	45.9	0	0.059	0.077	6.055	0.337	1.164	0.927	11.9	0
50.15	3.4	0.723	28.05	178.5	292.4	87.55	0.433	15.3	0	0.062	0.088	1.635	0.412	0.816		0.85	0
65.45	62.9	1.199	34.85	257.55	356.15	97.75	1.079	30.6	0.595	0.095	0.254	3.505	0.296	11.169	1.164	10.2	0
84.15	90.1	1.224	34.85	248.2	460.7	80.75	0.578	29.75	0	0.062	0.218	2.398	0.441	8.177		5.1	0
25.5	9.35	1.301	22.95	138.55	201.45	287.3	0.655	14.45	0	0.027	0.063	11.288	0.298	2.542	0.281	3.4	0
15.3	11.05	1.182	26.35	264.35	175.95	300.9	0.765	19.55	0	0.032	0.102	10.54	0.094	1.87	0.74	4.25	0
63.75	12.75	1.335	82.45	236.3	340.85	70.55	0.799	45.9	0.34	0.135	0.35	5.823	0.391	16.15		1.7	0
57.8	34	1.938	34.85	270.3	474.3	172.55	0.612	214.2	1.36	0.098	0.493	8.893	0.433	15.3		7.65	0
45.9	116.45	1.003	33.15	235.45	297.5	81.6	0.519	11.9	0.68	0.111	0.114	2.071	0.23	0.978		8.5	0
81.6	90.1	8.109	51	237.15	535.5	391	2.856	76.5	6.8	0.048	0.065	3.213	0.551	30.6	1.02	20.4	0
97.75	86.7	0.986	32.3	218.45	292.4	67.15	1.215	8.5	1.445	0.068	0.102	1.615	0.119	1.87		5.1	0
42.5	62.05	0.604	34	239.7	281.35	41.65	0.731	20.4	3.23	0.057	0.065	2.38	0.115	1.955		14.45	0
93.5	119.85	1.419	32.3	228.65	424.15	55.25	0.672	20.4	0	0.265	0.166	2.381	0.117	1.964		14.45	0
77.35	65.45	0.502	73.1	240.55	387.6	93.5	0.51	10.2	0	0.046	0.191	3.386	0.281	3.128		2.55	0
81.6	5.1	0.238	62.05	409.7	328.95	98.6	0.51	21.25	0	0.063	0.065	1.403	0.059	3.57	0.672	3.4	0
54.4	36.55	0.57	26.35	289.85	540.6	64.6	0.586	30.6	0	0.578	0.128	3.23	0.196	1.02		14.45	0
37.4	10.2	0.45	28.9	193.8	442	65.45	0.45	60.35	0	0.037	0.071	3.331	0.23	1.02	1.326	8.5	0
407.15	23.8	0.655	22.1	437.75	240.55	99.45	1.088	77.35	13.94	0.235	0.807	1.863	0.157	9.809		78.2	0
22.1	32.3	0.196	32.3	217.6	327.25	68.85	0.816	20.4	0	0.098	0.156	3.106	0.294	1.964		6.8	0

EvaluEat Code	Food Name	Amt	Wt (g)	Energy (kcal)	Prot (g)	Carb (g)	Fiber (g)	Fat (g)	Mono (g)	Poly (g)	Sat (g)
15237	Fish, salmon, Atlantic, farmed, cooked w/dry heat	3 oz	85	175.1	18.785	0	0	10.498	3.767	3.762	2.128
15209	Fish, salmon, Atlantic, wild, cooked w/dry heat	3 oz	85	154.7	21.624	0	0	6.911	2.292	2.768	1.068
15087	Fish, salmon, sockeye w/bone, canned, drained	3 oz	85	130.05	17.399	0	0	6.214	2.688	1.605	1.397
15086	Fish, salmon, sockeye, baked or broiled (dry heat)	3 oz	85	183.6	23.214	0	0	9.325	4.497	2.048	1.629
15092	Fish, sea bass, baked or broiled (dry heat)	3 oz	85	105.4	20.086	0	0	2.176	0.462	0.81	0.557
15214	Fish, sea trout, cooked w/dry heat	3 oz	85	113.05	18.241	0	0	3.936	0.963	0.79	1.099
15096	Fish, shark, battered, fried	3 oz	85	193.8	15.8	5.431	0	11.7	5.045	3.146	2.724
15100	Fish, smelt, rainbow, baked or broiled (dry heat)	3 oz	85	105.4	19.21	0	0	2.635	0.699	0.965	0.492
15102	Fish, snapper, baked or broiled (dry heat)	3 oz	85	108.8	22.355	0	0	1.462	0.274	0.5	0.31
15176	Fish, squid, fried	3 oz	85	148.75	15.249	6.622	0	6.358	2.337	1.816	1.596
15105	Fish, sturgeon, baked or broiled	3 oz	85	114.75	17.595	0	0	4.403	2.113	0.752	0.997
15106	Fish, sturgeon, smoked	3 oz	85	147.05	26.52	0	0	3.74	2.003	0.371	0.881
15111	Fish, swordfish, baked or broiled (dry heat)	3 oz	85	131.75	21.582	0	0	4.369	1.684	1.005	1.195
15241	Fish, trout, rainbow, farmed, cooked w/dry heat	3 oz	85	143.65	20.63	0	0	6.12	1.782	1.98	1.789
15116	Fish, trout, rainbow, wild, cooked w/dry heat	3 oz	85	127.5	19.482	0	0	4.947	1.484	1.556	1.376
15128	Fish, tuna salad	1 cup	205	383.35	32.882	19.29	0	18.983	5.918	8.45	3.165
15118	Fish, tuna, bluefin, baked or broiled (dry heat)	3 oz	85	156.4	25.424	0	0	5.338	1.745	1.567	1.37
15221	Fish, tuna, yellowfin, fresh, cooked w/dry heat	3 oz	85	118.2	25.5	0	0	1.037	0.167	0.309	0.256
15222	Fish, turbot, European, cooked w/dry heat	3 oz	85	103.7	17.493	0	0	3.213			
15126	Fish, white tuna, canned in H₂0, drained	3 oz	85	108.8	20.077	0	0	2.525	0.666	0.943	0.673
15124	Fish, white tuna, canned in oil, drained	3 oz	85	158.1	22.551	0	0	6.868	2.773	2.526	1.088
15223	Fish, whitefish, cooked w/dry heat	3 oz	85	146.2	20.799	0	0	6.384	2.175	2.342	0.988
15133	Fish, whiting, baked or broiled (dry heat)	3 oz	85	98.6	19.958	0	0	1.437	0.378	0.499	0.34
15225	Fish, yellowtail, cooked w/dry heat	3 oz	85	158.95	25.22	0	0	5.712			
2050	Flavoring, vanilla extract	1 tsp	4.2	12.096	0.003	0.531	0	0.003	0	0	0
20003	Flour, arrowroot	1 cup	128	456.96	0.384	112.83	4.352	0.128	0.003	0.058	0.024
20130	Flour, barley flour or meal	1 cup	148	510.6	15.54	110.29	14.948	2.368	0.303	1.141	0.496
20011	Flour, buckwheat, whole groat	1 cup	120	402	15.144	84.708	12	3.72	1.139	1.139	0.812
20017	Flour, corn, masa, enriched	1 cup	114	416.1	10.648	86.948	10.944	4.309	1.137	1.965	0.606
20070	Flour, triticale, whole grain	1 cup	130	439.4	17.134	95.082	18.98	2.353	0.238	1.032	0.413
20081	Flour, wheat, white, all purpose, bleached, enriched	1 cup	125	455	12.913	95.387	3.375	1.225	0.109	0.516	0.194
20082	Flour, wheat, white, all purpose, self-rise, enriched	1 cup	125	442.5	12.363	92.775	3.375	1.213	0.108	0.512	0.192
20083	Flour, wheat, white, bread, enriched	1 cup	137	494.57	16.413	99.366	3.288	2.274	0.192	0.996	0.334
20084	Flour, wheat, white, cake, enriched	1 cup unsifted, dipped	137	495.94	11.234	106.9	2.329	1.178	0.1	0.519	0.174
20080	Flour, whole wheat, whole grain	1 cup	120	406.8	16.44	87.084	14.64	2.244	0.278	0.935	0.386
7945	Frankfurter, beef, heated	1 serving	52	169.52	6.001	1.96	0	15.319	7.447	0.553	5.947
18268	French toast, frozen	1 piece	59	125.67	4.366	18.939	0.649	3.599	1.204	0.724	0.904
18269	French toast, homemade w/reduced fat (2%) milk	1 slice	65	148.85	5.005	16.25		7.02	2.941	1.686	1.77
22606	Frozen dinner, cacciatore chicken, pasta w/chicken breast pieces & vegetables in cacci	1 serving	354	265.5	21.983	35.86	4.956	3.965	2.372	0.637	0.991
22602	Frozen dinner, creamed spinach/Stouffer	1 cup	250	337.5	7	18	4.5	26.25	5.67	8.98	7.4
22603	Frozen dinner, spinach au gratin/The Budget Gourmet	1 serving	155	221.65	6.665	11.47	2.325	16.585			7.595
22601	Frozen dinner, Stir Fry 2, white rice & vegetables w/Oriental soy sauce/Hanover	1 serving	137	130.15	4.521	26.989	2.466	0.411			

Chol (g)	Calc (mg)	Iron (mg)	Mag (mg)	Phos (mg)	Pota (mg)	Sodi (mg)	Zinc (mg)	Vit A (RAE)	Vit C (mg)	Thia (mg)	Ribo (mg)	Niac (mg)	Vit B$_6$ (mg)	Vit B$_{12}$ (µg)	Vit E (mg)	Fol (µg)	Alc (g)
53.55	12.75	0.289	25.5	214.2	326.4	51.85	0.366	12.75	3.145	0.289	0.115	6.838	0.55	2.38		28.9	0
60.35	12.75	0.876	31.45	217.6	533.8	47.6	0.697	11.05	0	0.234	0.414	8.565	0.802	2.592		24.65	0
37.4	203.15	0.901	24.65	277.1	320.45	457.3	0.867	45.05	0	0.014	0.164	4.658	0.255	0.255	1.36	8.5	0
73.95	5.95	0.468	26.35	234.6	318.75	56.1	0.433	53.55	0	0.183	0.145	5.67	0.186	4.93		4.25	0
45.05	11.05	0.315	45.05	210.8	278.8	73.95	0.442	54.4	0	0.111	0.128	1.615	0.391	0.255		5.1	0
90.1	18.7	0.298	34	272.85	371.45	62.9	0.493	29.75	0	0.059	0.176	2.485	0.393	2.941		5.1	0
50.2	42.5	0.944	36.5	164.9	131.8	103.7	0.408	45.9	0	0.061	0.082	2.366	0.255	1.029	0	12.8	0
76.5	65.45	0.978	32.3	250.75	316.2	65.45	1.802	14.45	0	0.009	0.124	1.501	0.145	3.375		4.25	0
39.95	34	0.204	31.45	170.85	443.7	48.45	0.374	29.75	1.36	0.045	0.003	0.294	0.391	2.975		5.1	0
221	33.15	0.859	32.3	213.35	237.15	260.1	1.479	9.35	3.57	0.048	0.389	2.212	0.049	1.046		11.9	0
65.45	14.45	0.765	38.25	230.35	309.4	58.65	0.459	223.55	0	0.068	0.077	8.585	0.196	2.125	0.535	14.45	0
68	14.45	0.791	39.95	238.85	322.15	628.15	0.476	238	0	0.077	0.077	9.435	0.23	2.465	0.425	17	0
42.5	5.1	0.884	28.9	286.45	313.65	97.75	1.25	34.85	0.935	0.037	0.099	10.022	0.324	1.717		1.7	0
57.8	73.1	0.281	27.2	226.1	374.85	35.7	0.417	73.1	2.805	0.201	0.068	7.472	0.337	4.224		20.4	0
58.65	73.1	0.323	26.35	228.65	380.8	47.6	0.433	12.75	1.7	0.129	0.082	4.905	0.294	5.355		16.15	0
26.65	34.85	2.05	38.95	364.9	364.9	824.1	1.148	49.2	4.51	0.064	0.144	13.735	0.166	2.46		16.4	0
41.65	8.5	1.113	54.4	277.1	274.55	42.5	0.655	643.5	0	0.236	0.26	8.959	0.446	9.248		1.7	0
49.3	17.9	0.799	54.4	208.2	483.7	40	0.57	17	0.85	0.426	0.048	10.1	0.882	0.51	0	1.7	0
52.7	19.55	0.391	55.25	140.25	259.25	163.2	0.238	10.2	1.445	0.065	0.082	2.277	0.206	2.159		7.65	0
35.7	11.9	0.825	28.05	184.45	201.45	320.45	0.408	5.1	0	0.007	0.037	4.929	0.184	0.994	0.723	1.7	0
26.35	3.4	0.553	28.9	226.95	283.05	336.6	0.4	4.25	0	0.014	0.067	9.943	0.366	1.87	1.955	4.25	0
65.45	28.05	0.4	35.7	294.1	345.1	55.25	1.079	33.15	0	0.145	0.131	3.269	0.294	0.816		14.45	0
71.4	52.7	0.357	22.95	242.25	368.9	112.2	0.45	28.9	0	0.058	0.051	1.419	0.153	2.21	0.255	12.75	0
60.35	24.65	0.535	32.3	170.85	457.3	42.5	0.57	26.35	2.465	0.149	0.043	7.41	0.157	1.063		3.4	0
0	0.462	0.005	0.504	0.252	6.216	0.378	0.005	0	0	0	0.004	0.018	0.001	0	0	0	1.445
0	51.2	0.422	3.84	6.4	14.08	2.56	0.09	0	0	0.001	0	0	0.006	0		8.96	0
0	47.36	3.966	142.08	438.08	457.32	5.92	2.96	0	0	0.548	0.169	9.278	0.586	0	0.844	11.84	0
0	49.2	4.872	301.2	404.4	692.4	13.2	3.744	0	0	0.5	0.228	7.38	0.698	0	0.384	64.8	0
0	160.74	8.219	125.4	254.22	339.72	5.7	2.029	0	0	1.629	0.858	11.221	0.422	0	0.171	265.6	0
0	45.5	3.367	198.9	417.3	605.8	2.6	3.458	0	0	0.491	0.172	3.718	0.524	0	1.17	96.2	0
0	18.75	5.8	27.5	135	133.75	2.5	0.875	0	0	0.981	0.618	7.38	0.055	0	0.075	228.8	0
0	422.5	5.838	23.75	743.75	155	1587.5	0.775	0	0	0.843	0.517	7.29	0.063	0	0.063	245	0
0	20.55	6.042	34.25	132.89	137	2.74	1.164	0	0	1.112	0.701	10.349	0.051	0	0.548	250.71	0
0	19.18	10.028	21.92	116.45	143.85	2.74	0.849	0	0	1.222	0.589	9.302	0.045	0	0.027	254.8	0
0	40.8	4.656	165.6	415.2	486	6	3.516	0	0	0.536	0.258	7.638	0.409	0	0.984	52.8	0
29.12	6.24	0.811	7.28	88.92	76.44	600.08	1.222	0		0.02	0.075	1.224	0.048	0.858	0.104	3.64	0
48.38	63.13	1.304	10.03	82.01	79.06	292.05	0.454	31.86	0.177	0.163	0.225	1.606	0.293	0.991	0.395	30.68	0
75.4	65	1.085	11.05	76.05	87.1	311.35	0.435	80.6	0.195	0.133	0.209	1.058	0.048	0.201		27.95	0
31.86	53.1	2.23		254.88	750.48	552.24											0
32.5	282.5					670											0
41.85	243.35	1.953				654.1								27.13			0
						635.68								16.3			0

EvaluEat Code	Food Name	Amt	Wt (g)	Energy (kcal)	Prot (g)	Carb (g)	Fiber (g)	Fat (g)	Mono (g)	Poly (g)	Sat (g)
22618	Frozen meal, barbecue glazed chicken & sauce w/mixed vegetables/WW Ultimate 200	1 package	209	217.36	18.81	25.916		4.389	1.559	1.099	0.995
22613	Frozen meal, beef & bean burrito/Las Campanas	1 serving	114	296.4	8.664	38.19	0.798	12.084	5.518	0.787	4.184
22682	Frozen meal, beef & bean chimichanga/Fiesta Cafe	1 package	227	422.22	24.062	55.615	6.129	11.577	3.882	3.473	2.156
22402	Frozen meal, beef macaroni/Healthy Choice	1 serving	240	211.2	14.136	33.456	4.56	2.232	1.2	0.336	0.672
22578	Frozen meal, beef pot roast w/whipped potatoes/Stouffer Lean Cuisine Homestyle	1 package	255	206.55	17.34	22.44	3.57	5.355	2.285	0.808	1.306
22616	Frozen meal, beef sirloin salisbury steak w/red skinned potatoes & vegetables/Budget Gourmet	1 package	311	261.24	18.349	33.899	7.153	5.909	1.754	0.936	2.018
22686	Frozen meal, beef stir fry kit: white rice, oriental vegetables, beef strips, Oriental	1 package	810	866.7	51.597	141.59		9.963			
22677	Frozen meal, beef stroganoff and noodles w/carrots & peas/Marie Callender	1 package	368	599.84	30.397	58.696	4.416	27.011	11.96	3.974	11.077
22577	Frozen meal, chicken & vegetables w/vermicelli/Stouffer's Lean Cuisine	1 package	297	252.45	18.711	32.076	5.049	5.643	2.132	1.384	1.028
22581	Frozen meal, chicken a l'orange in sauce w/broccoli & rice/Stouffer's Lean Cuisine	1 package	255	267.75	24.48	38.505		1.785	0.502	0.413	0.418
22610	Frozen meal, chicken alfredo w/fettucini & vegetables/Stouffer's Lunch Express	1 package	272	372.64	19.04	32.64	3.808	18.496	6.256	2.394	6.99
22575	Frozen meal, chicken cordon bleu, filled w/cheese & ham/Barber Food	1 package	340	697	51.68	29.58		41.48	16.694	6.562	11.526
22615	Frozen meal, chicken enchilada & mexican rice w/monterey jack cheese sauce/Stouffer's	1 package	283	376.39	12.452	48.393	4.528	14.716	4.415	3.707	3.368
22687	Frozen meal, chicken fajita kit/Tyson	1 package	756	914.76	56.624	122.77		23.209	9.148	4.158	5.897
22688	Frozen meal, chicken mesquite w/BBQ sauce, corn medley & potatoes au gratin/Tyson	1 package	255	321.3	17.773	44.956	4.335	7.752	2.729	0.484	2.601
22906	Frozen meal, chicken pot pie, frozen entree	1 serving	217	483.91	13.042	42.706	1.736	29.1	12.478	4.488	9.667
22587	Frozen meal, chicken teriyaki w/rice, mixed vegetables w/butter sauce & apple cherry compote	1 package	312	268.32	17.066	37.097	2.808	5.616	2.153	0.468	2.995
22690	Frozen meal, cosmic chicken nuggets w/macaroni & cheese, corn, chocolate pudding	1 package	257	524.28	17.733	52.942	3.084	26.728	10.717	5.962	6.605
22619	Frozen meal, country roast turkey w/mushrooms in brown gravy & rice pilaf/Healthy Choice	1 package	240	223.2	18.984	27.84	3.12	3.936	1.8	0.888	1.248
22579	Frozen meal, creamed chipped beef/Stouffer's	1 package	311	435.4	24.569	17.727		29.545	8.739	2.923	12.533
22614	Frozen meal, escalloped chicken & noodles/Stouffer's	1 package	283	418.84	16.98	31.413		25.187	7.669	13.556	6.566
22617	Frozen meal, French recipe chicken breast, vegetables & potatoes in red wine sauce/Budget Gourmet	1 package	255	178.5	22.95	9.18	6.12	5.61	2.703	0.482	1.446
22710	Frozen meal, gravy & sliced beef, mashed potatoes & carrots/Freezer Queen	1 package	255	206.55	15.3	25.5	3.57	4.845	1.25	1.709	1.3
22585	Frozen meal, homestyle stuffed cabbage w/meat in tomato sauce & whipped pots/Stouffer's	1 package	269	199.06	11.567	25.824	6.456	5.649	2.375	0.748	1.681
22673	Frozen meal, Italian sausage lasagna/Budget Gourmet	1 package	298	455.94	20.562	39.932	2.98	23.84	9.774	1.997	8.165
22570	Frozen meal, lasagna w/meat & sauce/Stouffer's	1 package	595	767.55	51.765	73.185	8.925	29.75	9.639	1.547	13.03
22576	Frozen meal, macaroni & beef in tomato sauce/Stouffer's Lean Cuisine	1 package	283	249.04	13.867	36.507	3.396	5.377	2.057	0.702	1.636

Chol (g)	Calc (mg)	Iron (mg)	Mag (mg)	Phos (mg)	Pota (mg)	Sodi (mg)	Zinc (mg)	Vit A (RAE)	Vit C (mg)	Thia (mg)	Ribo (mg)	Niac (mg)	Vit B$_6$ (mg)	Vit B$_{12}$ (µg)	Vit E (mg)	Fol (µg)	Alc (g)
48.07		1.087				405.46			21.53								0
12.54		3.112				579.12											0
36.32		6.81				803.58			5.902								0
14.4	45.6	2.712	36	134.4	364.8	444	1.224	55.2	58.08	0.276	0.156	3.108	0.194	0.12	1.68	105.6	0
38.25						494.7											0
43.54		3.048				494.49			51								0
						3167.1			50.22								0
69.92	69.92	1.803				1140.8			0								0
23.76	103.95	1.336				582.12			14.55								0
45.9						359.55			18.11								
57.12	146.88					587.52			24.21								0
163.2	292.4					1526.6											0
25.47	254.7					1001.82			15.28								0
90.72						2472.12			73.33								0
25.5						793.05			0								0
41.23	32.55	2.062	23.87	119.35	256.06	857.15	1.02	256.7	1.519	0.254	0.356	4.13	0.202	0.152	3.847	41.23	0
43.68	37.44	1.092		224.64	424.32	602.16			12.17								0
48.83	205.6	2.853				974.03											0
26.4	21.6	1.032				436.8											0
108.85	472.72	2.27				1545.67											0
76.41	116.03	1.132				1211.24											0
25.5						864.45											
30.6						647.7		530.4									0
24.21	104.91					411.57			52.99								0
47.68	315.88	2.682				902.94											0
113.05	636.65					2034.9											0
22.64		2.179				563.17			157.3								0

EvaluEat Code	Food Name	Amt	Wt (g)	Energy (kcal)	Prot (g)	Carb (g)	Fiber (g)	Fat (g)	Mono (g)	Poly (g)	Sat (g)
22675	Frozen meal, meat loaf w/tomato sauce, mashed potatoes & carrots in seasoned sauce/Budget Gourmet	1 package	453	611.55	29.083	33.567	6.342	40.045	17.305	7.248	15.493
22586	Frozen meal, Mexican w/tamales, beef enchiladas & chili sauce, beans & rice	1 package	376	507.6	13.912	68.432	8.272	19.928	7.708	2.707	6.768
22571	Frozen meal, original fried chicken meal w/mashed potatoes & corn in seasoned sauce	1 package	228	469.68	21.455	35.089	2.052	27.041	15.367	2.44	9.257
22569	Frozen meal, pepper, stuffed w/beef in tomato sauce/Stouffer's	1 package	439	377.54	15.804	41.705	10.536	16.243	7.507	1.058	5.444
22672	Frozen meal, roast turkey medallions & mushrooms in sauce w/rice & vegetables/WW Smart	1 package	240	213.6	15.12	34.56	3.12	1.68	0.43	0.451	0.446
22712	Frozen meal, roasted chicken w/garlic sauce, pasta & vegetable medley/Tyson	1 package	255	214.2	16.932	21.522	3.57	6.707	2.346	2.142	1.3
22595	Frozen meal, scrambled eggs & sausage w/hashed brown potatoes	1 package	177	361.08	12.567	17.169	1.416	26.904	12.673	3.628	7.345
22580	Frozen meal, spaghetti w/meat sauce/Stouffer's Lean Cuisine	1 package	326	312.96	14.344	50.53	5.542	5.868	2.282	1.324	1.353
22608	Frozen meal, spaghetti w/meatballs & pomodoro sauce, low-fat/Michelina's	1 package	284	312.4	13.632	48.564	6.248	7.1	2.627	1.051	2.212
22573	Frozen meal, Swedish meatballs w/pasta/Stouffer's Lean Cuisine	1 package	258	276.06	21.672	31.218	2.58	7.224	2.34	1.04	2.423
22599	Frozen meal, turkey w/gravy & dressing w/broccoli/Marie Callender	1 package	397	504.19	31.045	51.848		19.016	8.178	1.747	9.091
42185	Frozen yogurts, chocolate, nonfat milk, with low calorie sweetener	1 cup	186	199.02	8.184	36.642	3.72	1.488	0.398	0.056	0.939
42187	Frozen yogurts, flavors other than chocolate	1 cup	186	236.22	5.58	40.176	0	6.696	1.834	0.186	4.326
14127	Fruit beverage mix, Kool-Aid, sugar free w/aspartame & vit C, dry mix, cherry flavor	.125 envelope	1.2	3.48	0.073	1.019		0.004			
14275	Fruit beverage mix, Kraft Kool-Aid Sugar Sweetened Tropical Punch, powder	1 NLEA serving	17	63.75	0	16.252	0	0			0
14297	Fruit beverage mix, Lemonade Flavor Drink, dry, prep w/H₂O	8 fl. oz.	266	111.72	0	28.728	0	0	0.005	0.011	0.045
14290	Fruit beverage mix, Lemonade w/aspartame, low kcal, dry, prep	8 fl. oz.	237	4.74	0.047	1.232	0	0	0	0.002	0
14408	Fruit beverage mix, orange flavor drink, dry, prep w/H₂O	8 fl. oz.	271	132.79	0	34.281	0.271	0	0	0	0
14403	Fruit beverage mix, orange flavor, Tang, dry mix	8 fl. oz.	25	91.5	0	24.6	0.075	0	0	0	0
14263	Fruit beverage, citrus drink, frozen concentrate, prep w/H₂O	8 fl. oz.	248	124	0.446	30.231	0.248	0.124	0	0	0
14242	Fruit beverage, cranberry cocktail, bottled	8 fl. oz.	253	144.21	0	36.432	0.253	0.253	0.035	0.111	0.023
14431	Fruit beverage, cranberry juice cocktail, frozen concentrate, prep w/H₂O	8 fl. oz.	250	137.5	0	35	0.25	0	0	0	0
14241	Fruit beverage, cranberry-grape drink, bottled	8 fl. oz.	245	137.2	0.49	34.3	0.245	0.245	0.01	0.056	0.081
14267	Fruit beverage, fruit punch, canned	8 fl. oz.	248	116.56	0	29.686	0.496	0	0.005	0.007	0
14269	Fruit beverage, fruit punch, frozen concentrate, prep w/H₂O	8 fl. oz.	247	113.62	0.148	28.8	0.247	0	0.002	0.005	0.002
14277	Fruit beverage, grape drink, canned	8 fl. oz.	250	112.5	0.025	28.875	0	0	0	0.003	0.003
14406	Fruit beverage, juice drink, frozen concentrate, prep	8 fl. oz.	248	124	0.248	30.256	0.248	0.496	0.06	0.122	0.062
14543	Fruit beverage, lemonade, pink, frozen conc, prep w/H₂O	8 fl. oz.	247	98.8	0.247	25.935	0	0	0.005	0.032	0.015
14293	Fruit beverage, lemonade, white, frozen, prep w/H₂O	8 fl. oz.	248	131.44	0.223	34.05	0.248	0.149	0.005	0.042	0.02
14303	Fruit beverage, limeade, frozen concentrate, prep w/H₂O	8 fl. oz.	247	103.74	0.099	26.108	0	0.025	0	0	0

Chol (g)	Calc (mg)	Iron (mg)	Mag (mg)	Phos (mg)	Pota (mg)	Sodi (mg)	Zinc (mg)	Vit A (RAE)	Vit C (mg)	Thia (mg)	Ribo (mg)	Niac (mg)	Vit B$_6$ (mg)	Vit B$_{12}$ (μg)	Vit E (mg)	Fol (μg)	Alc (g)
113.25	77.01	3.941				1943.37			7.701								0
26.32	240.64	2.858				1812.32			4.888								0
88.92	38.76	1.368				1500.24			1.368								0
43.9						1154.57			173								0
24		1.416				504											0
28.05		1.556				466.65											0
283.2		1.664				771.72											0
13.04		2.119				609.62			34.88								0
14.2		2.925				1011.04			8.804								0
46.44		2.064				562.44											0
79.4	131.01	4.367				2036.61			23.82								0
7.44	295.74	0.074	74.4	239.94	630.54	150.66	0.911	3.72	1.302	0.074	0.335	0.372	0.074	0.911	0.149	22.32	0
24.18	186	0.856	18.6	165.54	290.16	117.18	0.521	91.14	1.302	0.074	0.335	0.13	0.074	0.13	0.167	7.44	0
						5.064			6.72								0
0	27.88	0.012		12.75	0.34	1.53			6.001								
0	29.26	0.053	2.66	2.66	2.66	18.62	0.08	0	34.05	0	0.003	0	0	0		0	0
0	52.14	0.095	2.37	23.7	0	4.74	0.024	0	5.925	0	0	0	0	0	0	0	0
0	138.21	0.027	2.71	51.49	65.04	10.84	0.027	208.7	79.95	0	0.236	2.772	0.276	0	0	0	0
0	92.25	0.018	0	42.25	47.5	2	0.01	0	60	0	0.17	2	0.2	0	2.013	0	0
0	12.4	0.124	9.92	9.92	121.52	4.96	0.05	2.48	36.21	0.04	0.02	0.151	0.04	0	0.05	7.44	0
0	7.59	0.38	5.06	5.06	45.54	5.06	0.177	0	89.56	0.023	0.023	0.089	0.048	0	0	0	0
0	12.5	0.225	5	2.5	35	7.5	0.1	2.5	24.75	0.018	0.022	0.03	0.035	0		0	0
0	19.6	0.024	7.35	9.8	58.8	7.35	0.098	0	78.4	0.024	0.044	0.294	0.069	0		2.45	0
0	19.84	0.223	7.44	7.44	62	94.24	0.025	4.96	73.41	0.055	0.057	0.052	0.027	0	0.05	9.92	0
0	9.88	0.222	4.94	2.47	32.11	9.88	0.049	0	108.2	0.025	0.032	0.052	0.015	0		2.47	0
0	5	0.45	2.5	0	30	15	0.3	0	85.25	0.003	0.01	0.025	0.005	0	0	0	0
0	17.36	0.57	9.92	0	190.96	12.4	0.546	0	13.89	0.002	0.161	0.146	0.032	0		0	0
0	7.41	0.395	4.94	4.94	37.05	7.41	0.099	0	9.633	0.015	0.052	0.04	0.015	0		4.94	0
0	9.92	0.521	4.96	7.44	49.6	7.44	0.074	0	12.9	0.02	0.069	0.055	0.017	0	0.025	2.48	0
0	7.41	0.025	2.47	2.47	22.23	4.94	0.025	0	5.928	0.005	0.007	0.02	0.01	0	0	2.47	0

EvaluEat Code	Food Name	Amt	Wt (g)	Energy (kcal)	Prot (g)	Carb (g)	Fiber (g)	Fat (g)	Mono (g)	Poly (g)	Sat (g)
14323	Fruit beverage, orange drink, canned	8 fl. oz.	248	126.48	0	31.992	0	0	0.005	0.007	0.005
14334	Fruit beverage, pineapple & grapefruit juice drink, canned	8 fl. oz.	250	117.5	0.5	29	0.25	0.25	0.025	0.07	0.015
14341	Fruit beverage, pineapple & orange juice drink, canned	8 fl. oz.	250	125	3.25	29.5	0.25	0	0	0	0
9100	Fruit cocktail (peach, pineapple, pear, grape & cherry)canned in heavy syrup	1 cup	248	181.04	0.967	46.897	2.48	0.174	0.032	0.077	0.025
9097	Fruit cocktail (peach, pineapple, pear, grape & cherry)canned in juice	1 cup	237	109.02	1.09	28.108	2.37	0.024	0.005	0.009	0.002
9016	Fruit juice, apple, canned or bottled, unsweetened w/o added vit C	1 cup	248	116.56	0.149	28.966	0.248	0.273	0.012	0.082	0.047
9018	Fruit juice, apple, frozen concentrate, unsweetened w/o added vit C, prep	1 cup	239	112.33	0.335	27.581	0.239	0.239	0.005	0.074	0.043
9036	Fruit juice, apricot nectar, canned w/o added vit C	1 cup	251	140.56	0.929	36.119	1.506	0.226	0.095	0.043	0.015
9124	Fruit juice, grapefruit, canned, sweetened	1 cup	250	115	1.45	27.825	0.25	0.225	0.03	0.052	0.03
9123	Fruit juice, grapefruit, canned, unsweetened	1 cup	247	93.86	1.284	22.131	0.247	0.247	0.032	0.057	0.032
9126	Fruit juice, grapefruit, frozen concentrate, unsweetened, prep	1 cup	247	101.27	1.359	24.033	0.247	0.321	0.044	0.079	0.047
9152	Fruit juice, lemon, fresh	1 fl. oz.	30.5	7.625	0.116	2.632	0.122	0	0	0	0
9160	Fruit juice, lime, fresh	1 fl. oz.	30.8	8.316	0.136	2.775	0.123	0.031	0.003	0.008	0.003
9207	Fruit juice, orange, canned, unsweetened	1 cup	249	104.58	1.469	24.527	0.498	0.349	0.062	0.085	0.045
9206	Fruit juice, orange, fresh	1 cup	248	111.6	1.736	25.792	0.496	0.496	0.089	0.099	0.06
9215	Fruit juice, orange, frozen concentrate, unsweetened, prep	1 cup	249	112.05	1.693	26.842	0.498	0.149	0.025	0.03	0.017
9217	Fruit juice, orange-grapefruit, canned, unsweetened	1 cup	247	106.21	1.482	25.392	0.247	0.247	0.042	0.047	0.027
9229	Fruit juice, papaya nectar, canned	1 cup	250	142.5	0.425	36.275	1.5	0.375	0.103	0.087	0.117
9232	Fruit juice, passion fruit, purple, fresh	1 cup	247	125.97	0.963	33.592	0.494	0.124	0.015	0.072	0.01
9251	Fruit juice, peach nectar, canned w/o added vit C	1 cup	249	134.46	0.672	34.661	1.494	0.05	0.02	0.027	0.005
9273	Fruit juice, pineapple, canned, unsweetened w/o added vit C	1 cup	250	140	0.8	34.45	0.5	0.2	0.022	0.07	0.012
9294	Fruit juice, prune, canned	1 cup	256	181.76	1.562	44.672	2.56	0.077	0.054	0.018	0.008
9223	Fruit juice, tangerine, canned, sweetened	1 cup	249	124.5	1.245	29.88	0.498	0.498	0.045	0.062	0.032
9105	Fruit salad (peach, pineapple, pear, apricot & cherry)canned in heavy syrup	1 cup	255	186.15	0.867	48.73	2.55	0.178	0.036	0.079	0.025
9103	Fruit salad (peach, pineapple, pear, apricot & cherry)canned in juice	1 cup	249	124.5	1.27	32.494	2.49	0.075	0.012	0.027	0.01
9003	Fruit, apple w/skin, raw	1 large (3-1/4" dia) (approx 2 per lb)	212	110.24	0.551	29.277	5.088	0.36	0.015	0.108	0.059
9004	Fruit, apple, peeled, raw, medium	1 medium (2-3/4" dia) (approx 3 per lb)	128	61.44	0.346	16.333	1.664	0.166	0.006	0.047	0.027
9007	Fruit, apple, slices, sweetened, canned, drained	1 cup slices	204	136.68	0.367	34.068	3.468	1	0.041	0.294	0.163
9402	Fruit, applesauce, canned, sweetened w/added vit C	1 cup	255	193.8	0.459	50.771	3.06	0.459	0.018	0.138	0.076
9401	Fruit, applesauce, canned, unsweetened w/added vit C	1 cup	244	104.92	0.415	27.548	2.928	0.122	0.005	0.034	0.02
9027	Fruit, apricot w/skin, canned in heavy syrup	1 cup, halves	258	214.14	1.367	55.393	4.128	0.206	0.085	0.039	0.013
9024	Fruit, apricot w/skin, canned in juice	1 cup, halves	244	117.12	1.537	30.11	3.904	0.098	0.041	0.017	0.007
9035	Fruit, apricot, frozen, sweetened	1 cup	242	237.16	1.694	60.742	5.324	0.242	0.106	0.048	0.017
9023	Fruit, apricot, peeled, canned in H₂O	1 cup, whole, without pits	227	49.94	1.566	12.44	2.497	0.068	0.03	0.014	0.005

Chol (g)	Calc (mg)	Iron (mg)	Mag (mg)	Phos (mg)	Pota (mg)	Sodi (mg)	Zinc (mg)	Vit A (RAE)	Vit C (mg)	Thia (mg)	Ribo (mg)	Niac (mg)	Vit B$_6$ (mg)	Vit B$_{12}$ (µg)	Vit E (mg)	Fol (µg)	Alc (g)
0	14.88	0.694	4.96	2.48	44.64	39.68	0.223	2.48	84.57	0.015	0.007	0.077	0.022	0	0.05	9.92	0
0	17.5	0.775	15	15	152.5	35	0.15	0	115	0.075	0.04	0.667	0.105	0	0.025	22.5	0
0	12.5	0.675	15	10	115	7.5	0.15	2.5	56.25	0.075	0.047	0.517	0.117	0	0.075	22.5	0
0	14.88	0.719	12.4	27.28	218.24	14.88	0.198	24.8	4.712	0.045	0.047	0.928	0.124	0	0.992	7.44	0
0	18.96	0.498	16.59	33.18	225.15	9.48	0.213	35.55	6.399	0.028	0.038	0.955	0.121	0	0.948	7.11	0
0	17.36	0.918	7.44	17.36	295.12	7.44	0.074	0	2.232	0.052	0.042	0.248	0.074	0	0.025	0	0
0	14.34	0.621	11.95	16.73	301.14	16.73	0.096	0	1.434	0.007	0.036	0.091	0.079	0	0.024	0	0
0	17.57	0.954	12.55	22.59	286.14	7.53	0.226	165.7	1.506	0.023	0.035	0.653	0.055	0	0.778	2.51	0
0	20	0.9	25	27.5	405	5	0.15	0	67.25	0.1	0.058	0.798	0.05	0	0.1	25	0
0	17.29	0.494	24.7	27.17	377.91	2.47	0.222	0	72.12	0.104	0.049	0.571	0.049	0	0.099	24.7	0
0	19.76	0.346	27.17	34.58	335.92	2.47	0.124	0	83.24	0.101	0.054	0.536	0.109	0	0.099	9.88	0
0	2.135	0.009	1.83	1.83	37.82	0.305	0.015	0.305	14.03	0.009	0.003	0.031	0.016	0	0.046	3.965	0
0	2.772	0.009	1.848	2.156	33.572	0.308	0.018	0.616	9.024	0.006	0.003	0.031	0.013	0	0.046	2.464	0
0	19.92	1.096	27.39	34.86	435.75	4.98	0.174	22.41	85.66	0.149	0.07	0.782	0.219	0	0.498	44.82	0
0	27.28	0.496	27.28	42.16	496	2.48	0.124	24.8	124	0.223	0.074	0.992	0.099	0	0.099	74.4	0
0	22.41	0.249	24.9	39.84	473.1	2.49	0.124	12.45	96.86	0.197	0.045	0.503	0.11	0	0.498	109.6	0
0	19.76	1.136	24.7	34.58	390.26	7.41	0.173	14.82	71.88	0.138	0.074	0.83	0.057	0	0.346	34.58	0
0	25	0.85	7.5	0	77.5	12.5	0.375	45	7.5	0.015	0.01	0.375	0.022	0	0.6	5	0
0	9.88	0.593	41.99	32.11	686.66	14.82	0.124	88.92	73.61	0	0.324	3.606	0.124	0	0.025	17.29	0
0	12.45	0.473	9.96	14.94	99.6	17.43	0.199	32.37	13.2	0.007	0.035	0.717	0.017	0	0.722	2.49	0
0	42.5	0.65	32.5	20	335	2.5	0.275	0	26.75	0.138	0.055	0.642	0.24	0	0.05	57.5	0
0	30.72	3.021	35.84	64	706.56	10.24	0.538	0	10.5	0.041	0.179	2.01	0.558	0	0.307	0	0
0	44.82	0.498	19.92	34.86	443.22	2.49	0.075	32.37	54.78	0.149	0.05	0.249	0.08	0	0.374	12.45	0
0	15.3	0.714	12.75	22.95	204	15.3	0.178	63.75	6.12	0.038	0.054	0.885	0.082	0	1.02	7.65	0
0	27.39	0.623	19.92	34.86	288.84	12.45	0.349	74.7	8.217	0.027	0.035	0.886	0.067	0		7.47	0
0	12.72	0.254	10.6	23.32	226.84	2.12	0.085	6.36	9.752	0.036	0.055	0.193	0.087	0	0.382	6.36	0
0	6.4	0.09	5.12	14.08	115.2	0	0.064	2.56	5.12	0.024	0.036	0.116	0.047	0	0.064	0	0
0	8.16	0.469	4.08	10.2	138.72	6.12	0.061	6.12	0.816	0.018	0.02	0.149	0.09	0	0.428	0	0
0	10.2	0.892	7.65	17.85	155.55	71.4	0.102	2.55	4.335	0.033	0.071	0.479	0.066	0		2.55	0
0	7.32	0.293	7.32	17.08	183	4.88	0.073	2.44	51.73	0.032	0.061	0.459	0.063	0		2.44	0
0	23.22	0.774	18.06	30.96	361.2	10.32	0.284	160	7.998	0.052	0.057	0.97	0.139	0	1.548	5.16	0
0	29.28	0.732	24.4	48.8	402.6	9.76	0.268	207.4	11.96	0.044	0.046	0.839	0.132	0	1.464	4.88	0
0	24.2	2.178	21.78	45.98	554.18	9.68	0.242	203.3	21.78	0.048	0.097	1.936	0.145	0	2.154	4.84	0
0	18.16	1.226	20.43	36.32	349.58	24.97	0.25	206.6	4.086	0.045	0.054	0.992	0.123	0		4.54	0

EvaluEat Code	Food Name	Amt	Wt (g)	Energy (kcal)	Prot (g)	Carb (g)	Fiber (g)	Fat (g)	Mono (g)	Poly (g)	Sat (g)
9028	Fruit, apricot, peeled, canned in heavy syrup	1 cup, whole, without pits	258	214.14	1.316	55.341	4.128	0.232	0.095	0.044	0.015
9021	Fruit, apricot, raw	1 apricot	35	16.8	0.49	3.892	0.7	0.136	0.06	0.027	0.009
9038	Fruit, avocado, California, peeled, raw	1 fruit without skin and seed	173	288.91	3.391	14.947	11.764	26.659	16.952	3.484	3.678
9040	Fruit, banana, peeled, raw, mashed/sliced	1 medium (7" to 7-7/8" long)	118	105.02	1.286	26.951	3.068	0.389	0.038	0.086	0.132
9048	Fruit, blackberries, frozen, unsweetened	1 cup, unthawed	151	96.64	1.782	23.662	7.55	0.649	0.062	0.37	0.023
9042	Fruit, blackberries, raw	1 cup	144	61.92	2.002	13.838	7.632	0.706	0.068	0.403	0.02
9054	Fruit, blueberries, frozen, unsweetened	1 cup, unthawed	155	79.05	0.651	18.863	4.185	0.992	0.141	0.432	0.082
9050	Fruit, blueberries, raw	1 cup	145	82.65	1.073	21.01	3.48	0.479	0.068	0.212	0.041
9056	Fruit, boysenberries, canned in heavy syrup	1 cup	256	225.28	2.534	57.114	6.656	0.307	0.031	0.174	0.01
9057	Fruit, boysenberries, frozen, unsweetened	1 cup, unthawed	132	66	1.452	16.091	6.996	0.343	0.033	0.195	0.012
9059	Fruit, breadfruit, peeled, raw	1 cup	220	226.6	2.354	59.664	10.78	0.506	0.075	0.145	0.106
9060	Fruit, carambola (starfruit) raw	1 cup, cubes	137	45.21	0.74	10.727	3.699	0.479	0.042	0.262	0.032
9066	Fruit, cherries, sour, red, canned in heavy syrup	1 cup	256	232.96	1.869	59.571	2.816	0.256	0.067	0.074	0.054
9068	Fruit, cherries, sour, red, frozen, unsweetened	1 cup, unthawed	155	71.3	1.426	17.081	2.48	0.682	0.186	0.205	0.155
9064	Fruit, cherries, sour/tart, red, canned in H$_2$O	1 cup	244	87.84	1.879	21.814	2.684	0.244	0.066	0.073	0.056
9074	Fruit, cherries, sweet, canned in heavy syrup	1 cup, pitted	253	209.99	1.518	53.813	3.795	0.38	0.104	0.114	0.086
9072	Fruit, cherries, sweet, canned in juice	1 cup, pitted	250	135	2.275	34.525	3.75	0.05	0.012	0.015	0.01
9070	Fruit, cherries, sweet, raw	1 cup, with pits	117	73.71	1.24	18.732	2.457	0.234	0.055	0.061	0.044
9078	Fruit, cranberries, raw	1 cup, chopped	110	50.6	0.429	13.42	5.06	0.143	0.02	0.06	0.012
9081	Fruit, cranberry sauce, canned, sweetened	1 slice (1/2" thick, approx 8 slices per can)	57	86.07	0.114	22.173	0.57	0.086	0.012	0.038	0.007
9082	Fruit, cranberry-orange relish, canned	1 cup	275	489.5	0.825	127.05	0	0.275			0.033
9084	Fruit, currant, red or white, raw	1 cup	112	62.72	1.568	15.456	4.816	0.224	0.031	0.099	0.019
9085	Fruit, currants, zante, dried	1 cup	144	407.52	5.875	106.68	9.792	0.389	0.068	0.259	0.04
9087	Fruit, dates, domestic, natural, dried	1 cup, pitted, chopped	178	501.96	4.361	133.55	14.24	0.694	0.064	0.034	0.057
9092	Fruit, figs, canned in heavy syrup	1 cup	259	227.92	0.984	59.311	5.698	0.259	0.057	0.124	0.052
9094	Fruit, figs, dried, raw	1 cup	149	371.01	4.917	95.166	14.602	1.386	0.237	0.514	0.215
9089	Fruit, figs, raw	1 large (2-1/2" dia)	64	47.36	0.48	12.275	1.856	0.192	0.042	0.092	0.038
9107	Fruit, gooseberries, raw	1 cup	150	66	1.32	15.27	6.45	0.87	0.076	0.475	0.057
9120	Fruit, grapefruit, canned in juice	1 cup	249	92.13	1.743	22.933	0.996	0.224	0.03	0.052	0.03
9111	Fruit, grapefruit, red, white or pink, peeled, raw	1/2 medium (approx 4" dia)	128	40.96	0.806	10.342	1.408	0.128	0.017	0.031	0.018
9131	Fruit, grapes, American type (slip skin) raw	1 cup	92	61.64	0.58	15.778	0.828	0.322	0.013	0.094	0.105
9139	Fruit, guava, common, raw	1 fruit	90	45.9	0.738	10.692	4.86	0.54	0.049	0.228	0.155
9148	Fruit, kiwifruit (Chinese gooseberry) peeled, raw	1 fruit without skin, medium	76	46.36	0.866	11.142	2.28	0.395	0.036	0.218	0.022
9149	Fruit, kumquat, raw	1 fruit without refuse	19	13.49	0.357	3.021	1.235	0.163	0.029	0.032	0.02
9165	Fruit, lychee (litchi) shelled, dried	1 fruit	2.5	6.925	0.095	1.767	0.115	0.03	0.008	0.009	0.007

Chol (g)	Calc (mg)	Iron (mg)	Mag (mg)	Phos (mg)	Pota (mg)	Sodi (mg)	Zinc (mg)	Vit A (RAE)	Vit C (mg)	Thia (mg)	Ribo (mg)	Niac (mg)	Vit B₆ (mg)	Vit B₁₂ (µg)	Vit E (mg)	Fol (µg)	Alc (g)
0	23.22	1.109	20.64	33.54	345.72	28.38	0.258	160	7.224	0.049	0.059	1.073	0.139	0		5.16	0
0	4.55	0.136	3.5	8.05	90.65	0.35	0.07	33.6	3.5	0.01	0.014	0.21	0.019	0	0.311	3.15	0
0	22.49	1.055	50.17	93.42	877.11	13.84	1.176	12.11	15.22	0.13	0.247	3.308	0.497	0	3.408	107.3	0
0	5.9	0.307	31.86	25.96	422.44	1.18	0.177	3.54	10.27	0.037	0.086	0.785	0.433	0	0.118	23.6	0
0	43.79	1.208	33.22	45.3	211.4	1.51	0.377	9.06	4.681	0.044	0.069	1.823	0.092	0	1.767	51.34	0
0	41.76	0.893	28.8	31.68	233.28	1.44	0.763	15.84	30.24	0.029	0.037	0.93	0.043	0	1.685	36	0
0	12.4	0.279	7.75	17.05	83.7	1.55	0.108	3.1	3.875	0.05	0.057	0.806	0.091	0	0.744	10.85	0
0	8.7	0.406	8.7	17.4	111.65	1.45	0.232	4.35	14.07	0.054	0.059	0.606	0.075	0	0.826	8.7	0
0	46.08	1.101	28.16	25.6	230.4	7.68	0.486	5.12	15.87	0.067	0.074	0.589	0.097	0	1.818	87.04	0
0	35.64	1.122	21.12	35.64	183.48	1.32	0.29	3.96	4.092	0.07	0.049	1.012	0.074	0	1.148	83.16	0
0	37.4	1.188	55	66	1078	4.4	0.264	0	63.8	0.242	0.066	1.98	0.22	0	0.22	30.8	0
0	5.48	0.356	12.33	21.92	223.31	2.74	0.151	4.11	29.04	0.038	0.037	0.563	0.137	0	0.206	19.18	0
0	25.6	3.328	15.36	25.6	238.08	17.92	0.154	92.16	5.12	0.041	0.1	0.43	0.113	0	0.589	20.48	0
0	20.15	0.821	13.95	24.8	192.2	1.55	0.155	68.2	2.635	0.068	0.053	0.212	0.104	0	0.078	7.75	0
0	26.84	3.343	14.64	24.4	239.12	17.08	0.171	92.72	5.124	0.041	0.1	0.432	0.107	0	0.561	19.52	0
0	22.77	0.885	22.77	45.54	366.85	7.59	0.253	20.24	9.108	0.053	0.101	1.002	0.076	0	0.582	10.12	0
0	35	1.45	30	55	327.5	7.5	0.25	15	6.25	0.045	0.06	1.015	0.075	0	0.575	10	0
0	15.21	0.421	12.87	24.57	259.74	0	0.082	3.51	8.19	0.032	0.039	0.18	0.057	0	0.082	4.68	0
0	8.8	0.275	6.6	14.3	93.5	2.2	0.11	3.3	14.63	0.013	0.022	0.111	0.063	0	1.32	1.1	0
0	2.28	0.125	1.71	3.42	14.82	16.53	0.029	1.14	1.14	0.009	0.012	0.057	0.008	0	0.473	0.57	0
0	30.25	0.55	11	22	104.5	88		11	49.5	0.082	0.055	0.275		0			0
0	36.96	1.12	14.56	49.28	308	1.12	0.258	2.24	45.92	0.045	0.056	0.112	0.078	0	0.112	8.96	0
0	123.84	4.694	59.04	180	1284.48	11.52	0.95	5.76	6.768	0.23	0.204	2.326	0.426	0	0.158	14.4	0
0	69.42	1.816	76.54	110.36	1167.68	3.56	0.516	0	0.712	0.093	0.117	2.268	0.294	0	0.089	33.82	0
0	69.93	0.725	25.9	25.9	256.41	2.59	0.285	5.18	2.59	0.057	0.096	1.109	0.181	0	0.311	5.18	0
0	241.38	3.025	101.32	99.83	1013.2	14.9	0.82	0	1.788	0.127	0.122	0.922	0.158	0	0.521	13.41	0
0	22.4	0.237	10.88	8.96	148.48	0.64	0.096	4.48	1.28	0.038	0.032	0.256	0.072	0	0.07	3.84	0
0	37.5	0.465	15	40.5	297	1.5	0.18	22.5	41.55	0.06	0.045	0.45	0.12	0	0.555	9	0
0	37.35	0.523	27.39	29.88	420.81	17.43	0.199	0	84.41	0.072	0.045	0.62	0.05	0	0.224	22.41	0
0	15.36	0.115	10.24	10.24	177.92	0	0.09	58.88	44.03	0.046	0.026	0.32	0.054	0	0.166	12.8	0
0	12.88	0.267	4.6	9.2	175.72	1.84	0.037	4.6	3.68	0.085	0.052	0.276	0.101	0	0.175	3.68	0
0	18	0.279	9	22.5	255.6	2.7	0.207	27.9	165	0.045	0.045	1.08	0.129	0	0.657	12.6	0
0	25.84	0.236	12.92	25.84	237.12	2.28	0.106	3.04	70.45	0.021	0.019	0.259	0.048	0	1.11	19	0
0	11.78	0.163	3.8	3.61	35.34	1.9	0.032	2.85	8.341	0.007	0.017	0.082	0.007	0	0.029	3.23	0
0	0.825	0.043	1.05	4.525	27.75	0.075	0.007	0	4.575	0	0.014	0.078	0.002	0	0.008	0.3	0

EvaluEat Code	Food Name	Amt	Wt (g)	Energy (kcal)	Prot (g)	Carb (g)	Fiber (g)	Fat (g)	Mono (g)	Poly (g)	Sat (g)
9164	Fruit, lychee (litchi) shelled, raw	1 fruit	9.6	6.336	0.08	1.587	0.125	0.042	0.012	0.013	0.01
9176	Fruit, mango, peeled, raw	1 cup, sliced	165	107.25	0.841	28.05	2.97	0.446	0.167	0.084	0.109
9185	Fruit, melon balls (cantaloupe & honeydew) frozen	1 cup, unthawed	173	57.09	1.453	13.736	1.211	0.433	0.01	0.17	0.111
9181	Fruit, melon, cantaloupe (musk) peeled, pieces/balls, raw	1 wedge, large (1/8 of large melon)	102	34.68	0.857	8.323	0.918	0.194	0.003	0.083	0.052
9183	Fruit, melon, casaba, peeled, raw	1 cup, cubes	170	47.6	1.887	11.186	1.53	0.17	0.003	0.066	0.043
9184	Fruit, melon, honeydew, peeled, wedges, raw	1 wedge (1/8 of 6" to 7" dia melon)	160	57.6	0.864	14.544	1.28	0.224	0.005	0.094	0.061
9188	Fruit, mixed (prune, apricot & pear) dried	1 package (11 oz)	293	711.99	7.208	187.7	22.854	1.436	0.68	0.322	0.117
9191	Fruit, nectarine, raw	1 fruit (2-1/2" dia)	136	59.84	1.442	14.348	2.312	0.435	0.12	0.154	0.034
9193	Fruit, olives, ripe, pitted, canned	1 tbsp	8.4	9.66	0.071	0.526	0.269	0.897	0.663	0.077	0.119
9200	Fruit, orange, all varieties, peeled, raw	1 fruit (2-5/8" dia)	131	61.57	1.231	15.392	3.144	0.157	0.03	0.033	0.02
9226	Fruit, papayas, peeled, cubed/mashed, raw	1 medium (5-1/8" long x 3" dia)	304	118.56	1.854	29.822	5.472	0.426	0.116	0.094	0.131
9231	Fruit, passion fruit/granadilla, purple, peeled, raw	1 fruit	18	17.46	0.396	4.208	1.872	0.126	0.015	0.074	0.011
9241	Fruit, peach, canned in heavy syrup	1 cup	262	193.88	1.179	52.243	3.406	0.262	0.092	0.123	0.026
9238	Fruit, peach, canned in juice	1 cup	250	110	1.575	28.925	3.25	0.075	0.03	0.04	0.01
9250	Fruit, peach, frozen, sweetened	1 cup, thawed	250	235	1.575	59.95	4.5	0.325	0.12	0.16	0.035
9236	Fruit, peach, peeled, raw	1 medium (2-1/2" dia) (approx 4 per lb)	98	38.22	0.892	9.349	1.47	0.245	0.066	0.084	0.019
9257	Fruit, pear, canned in heavy syrup	1 cup	266	196.84	0.532	50.992	4.256	0.346	0.072	0.08	0.019
9254	Fruit, pear, canned in juice	1 cup, halves	248	124	0.843	32.091	3.968	0.174	0.035	0.037	0.01
9252	Fruit, pear, raw	1 pear, medium (approx 2-1/2 per lb)	166	96.28	0.631	25.664	5.146	0.199	0.043	0.048	0.01
9265	Fruit, persimmon, native, raw	1 fruit	25	31.75	0.2	8.375		0.1			
9270	Fruit, pineapple, canned in heavy syrup	1 cup, crushed, sliced, or chunks	254	198.12	0.889	51.308	2.032	0.279	0.033	0.102	0.023
9268	Fruit, pineapple, canned in juice	1 cup, crushed, sliced, or chunks	249	149.4	1.046	39.093	1.992	0.199	0.025	0.072	0.015
9278	Fruit, plantain, peeled, cooked	1 cup, mashed	200	232	1.58	62.3	4.6	0.36	0.03	0.066	0.138
9284	Fruit, plum, purple, canned in heavy syrup	1 cup, pitted	258	229.62	0.929	59.959	2.322	0.258	0.17	0.057	0.021
9282	Fruit, plum, purple, canned in juice	1 cup, pitted	252	146.16	1.285	38.178	2.268	0.05	0.035	0.013	0.005
9279	Fruit, plum, raw	1 fruit (2-1/8" dia)	66	30.36	0.462	7.537	0.924	0.185	0.088	0.029	0.011
9286	Fruit, pomegranates, peeled, raw	1 fruit (3-3/8" dia)	154	104.72	1.463	26.442	0.924	0.462	0.071	0.097	0.059
9287	Fruit, prickly pear, peeled, raw	1 cup	149	61.09	1.088	14.259	5.364	0.76	0.112	0.317	0.1
9288	Fruit, prunes, canned in heavy syrup	5 fruits with liquid	86	90.3	0.748	23.908	3.268	0.172	0.112	0.037	0.014
9291	Fruit, prunes, dried	1 prune	8.4	20.16	0.183	5.366	0.596	0.032	0.004	0.005	0.007
9295	Fruit, pummelo, peeled, raw	1 fruit	609	231.42	4.628	58.586	6.09	0.244			
9296	Fruit, quinces, peeled, raw	1 fruit	92	52.44	0.368	14.076	1.748	0.092	0.033	0.046	0.009
9298	Fruit, raisins, seedless	1 cup (not packed)	145	433.55	4.451	114.81	5.365	0.667	0.074	0.054	0.084
9302	Fruit, raspberries, raw	1 cup	123	63.96	1.476	14.686	7.995	0.799	0.079	0.461	0.023
9306	Fruit, raspberries, red, frozen, sweetened	1 cup, unthawed	250	257.5	1.75	65.4	11	0.4	0.037	0.222	0.012

Chol (g)	Calc (mg)	Iron (mg)	Mag (mg)	Phos (mg)	Pota (mg)	Sodi (mg)	Zinc (mg)	Vit A (RAE)	Vit C (mg)	Thia (mg)	Ribo (mg)	Niac (mg)	Vit B6 (mg)	Vit B12 (µg)	Vit E (mg)	Fol (µg)	Alc (g)
0	0.48	0.03	0.96	2.976	16.416	0.096	0.007	0	6.864	0.001	0.006	0.058	0.01	0	0.007	1.344	0
0	16.5	0.214	14.85	18.15	257.4	3.3	0.066	62.7	45.71	0.096	0.094	0.964	0.221	0	1.848	23.1	0
0	17.3	0.502	24.22	20.76	484.4	53.63	0.294	154	10.73	0.287	0.038	1.107	0.183	0	0.26	44.98	0
0	9.18	0.214	12.24	15.3	272.34	16.32	0.184	172.4	37.43	0.042	0.019	0.749	0.073	0	0.051	21.42	0
0	18.7	0.578	18.7	8.5	309.4	15.3	0.119	0	37.06	0.025	0.053	0.394	0.277	0	0.085	13.6	0
0	9.6	0.272	16	17.6	364.8	28.8	0.144	4.8	28.8	0.061	0.019	0.669	0.141	0	0.032	30.4	0
0	111.34	7.94	114.27	225.61	2332.28	52.74	1.465	357.5	11.13	0.129	0.46	5.646	0.466	0		11.72	0
0	8.16	0.381	12.24	35.36	273.36	0	0.231	23.12	7.344	0.046	0.037	1.53	0.034	0	1.047	6.8	0
0	7.392	0.277	0.336	0.252	0.672	73.248	0.018	1.68	0.076	0	0	0.003	0.001	0	0.139	0	0
0	52.4	0.131	13.1	18.34	237.11	0	0.092	14.41	69.69	0.114	0.052	0.369	0.079	0	0.236	39.3	0
0	72.96	0.304	30.4	15.2	781.28	9.12	0.213	167.2	187.9	0.082	0.097	1.028	0.058	0	2.219	115.5	0
0	2.16	0.288	5.22	12.24	62.64	5.04	0.018	11.52	5.4	0	0.023	0.27	0.018	0	0.004	2.52	0
0	7.86	0.707	13.1	28.82	241.04	15.72	0.236	44.54	7.336	0.029	0.063	1.609	0.05	0	1.284	7.86	0
0	15	0.675	17.5	42.5	320	10	0.275	47.5	9	0.02	0.043	1.455	0.047	0	1.225	7.5	0
0	7.5	0.925	12.5	27.5	325	15	0.125	35	235.5	0.032	0.087	1.632	0.045	0	1.55	7.5	0
0	5.88	0.245	8.82	19.6	186.2	0	0.167	15.68	6.468	0.024	0.03	0.79	0.025	0	0.715	3.92	0
0	13.3	0.585	10.64	18.62	172.9	13.3	0.213	0	2.926	0.027	0.059	0.644	0.037	0	0.213	2.66	0
0	22.32	0.719	17.36	29.76	238.08	9.92	0.223	0	3.968	0.027	0.027	0.496	0.035	0	0.198	2.48	0
0	14.94	0.282	11.62	18.26	197.54	1.66	0.166	1.66	6.972	0.02	0.041	0.261	0.046	0	0.199	11.62	0
0	6.75	0.625		6.5	77.5	0.25			16.5					0			0
0	35.56	0.965	40.64	17.78	264.16	2.54	0.305	2.54	18.8	0.229	0.064	0.729	0.188	0	0.025	12.7	0
0	34.86	0.697	34.86	14.94	303.78	2.49	0.249	4.98	23.66	0.237	0.047	0.707	0.184	0	0.025	12.45	0
0	4	1.16	64	56	930	10	0.26	90	21.8	0.092	0.104	1.512	0.48	0	0.26	52	0
0	23.22	2.167	12.9	33.54	234.78	49.02	0.181	33.54	1.032	0.041	0.098	0.751	0.07	0	0.464	7.74	0
0	25.2	0.857	20.16	37.8	388.08	2.52	0.277	126	7.056	0.058	0.149	1.192	0.068	0	0.454	7.56	0
0	3.96	0.112	4.62	10.56	103.62	0	0.066	11.22	6.27	0.018	0.017	0.275	0.019	0	0.172	3.3	0
0	4.62	0.462	4.62	12.32	398.86	4.62	0.185	7.7	9.394	0.046	0.046	0.462	0.162	0	0.924	9.24	0
0	83.44	0.447	126.65	35.76	327.8	7.45	0.179	2.98	20.86	0.021	0.089	0.685	0.089	0	0.015	8.94	0
0	14.62	0.353	12.9	22.36	194.36	2.58	0.163	34.4	2.408	0.029	0.105	0.745	0.175	0		0	0
0	3.612	0.078	3.444	5.796	61.488	0.168	0.037	3.276	0.05	0.004	0.016	0.158	0.017	0	0.036	0.336	0
0	24.36	0.67	36.54	103.53	1315.44	6.09	0.487	0	371.5	0.207	0.164	1.34	0.219	0			0
0	10.12	0.644	7.36	15.64	181.24	3.68	0.037	1.84	13.8	0.018	0.028	0.184	0.037	0	0.506	2.76	0
0	72.5	2.726	46.4	146.45	1086.05	15.95	0.319	0	3.335	0.154	0.181	1.111	0.252	0	0.174	7.25	0
0	30.75	0.849	27.06	35.67	185.73	1.23	0.517	2.46	32.23	0.039	0.047	0.736	0.068	0	1.07	25.83	0
0	37.5	1.625	32.5	42.5	285	2.5	0.45	7.5	41.25	0.047	0.113	0.575	0.085	0	1.8	65	0

EvaluEat Code	Food Name	Amt	Wt (g)	Energy (kcal)	Prot (g)	Carb (g)	Fiber (g)	Fat (g)	Mono (g)	Poly (g)	Sat (g)
9310	Fruit, rhubarb, frozen, cooked w/sugar	1 cup	240	278.4	0.936	74.88	4.8	0.12	0.024	0.06	0.034
9307	Fruit, rhubarb, raw	1 cup, diced	122	25.62	1.098	5.539	2.196	0.244	0.048	0.121	0.065
9319	Fruit, strawberries, frozen, whole, sweetened	1 cup, thawed	255	198.9	1.326	53.55	4.845	0.357	0.048	0.173	0.018
9316	Fruit, strawberries, halves/slices, raw	1 cup, halves	152	48.64	1.018	11.674	3.04	0.456	0.065	0.236	0.023
9322	Fruit, tamarind, raw	1 fruit (3"x 1")	2	4.78	0.056	1.25	0.102	0.012	0.004	0.001	0.005
9326	Fruit, watermelon, balls, raw	1 cup, balls	154	46.2	0.939	11.627	0.616	0.231	0.057	0.077	0.025
17345	Game meat, deer, loin, separable lean only, 1" steak, cooked, broiled	1 serving (3 oz)	85	127.5	25.67	0	0	2.023	0.298	0.088	0.746
17157	Game, bison, roasted	3 oz	85	121.55	24.174	0	0	2.057	0.808	0.204	0.774
5308	Game, cornish game hen w/skin, roasted	1/2 bird	129	335.4	28.728	0	0	23.491	10.32	4.644	6.515
5310	Game, cornish game hens, no skin, roasted	1/2 bird	110	147.4	25.63	0	0	4.257	1.364	1.034	1.089
5145	Game, duck, wild, breast, no skin, raw	1/2 breast, bone and skin removed	83	102.09	16.476	0	0	3.527	1.004	0.481	1.096
5144	Game, duck, wild, meat & skin, raw	1/2 duck	270	569.7	47.034	0	0	41.04	18.36	5.454	13.608
5157	Game, quail, meat & skin, raw	1 quail	109	209.28	21.397	0	0	13.135	4.556	3.248	3.684
17178	Game, rabbit, domestic, composite, roasted	3 oz	85	167.45	24.701	0	0	6.843	1.845	1.326	2.04
5160	Game, squab/pigeon, meat & skin, raw	1 squab	199	585.06	36.755	0	0	47.362	19.343	6.109	16.776
5282	Goose liver pate/pate de fois gras, smoked, canned	1 oz	28.35	130.98	3.232	1.324	0	12.429	7.26	0.238	4.097
5147	Goose, domestic, meat & skin, roasted	1 cup, chopped or diced	140	427	35.224	0	0	30.688	14.35	3.528	9.618
5149	Goose, domestic, meat only, no skin, roasted	yield from 1 lb ready-to-cook goose	143	340.34	41.427	0	0	18.118	6.206	2.202	6.521
20006	Grain, barley, pearled, cooked	1 cup	157	193.11	3.548	44.305	5.966	0.691	0.089	0.336	0.146
20013	Grain, bulgar, cooked	1 cup	182	151.06	5.606	33.816	8.19	0.437	0.056	0.178	0.076
20314	Grain, corn, white	1 cup	166	605.9	15.637	123.27		7.868	2.077	3.591	1.107
20014	Grain, corn, yellow	1 cup	166	605.9	15.637	123.27	12.118	7.868	2.077	3.591	1.107
20038	Grain, oats	1 cup	156	606.84	26.348	103.38	16.536	10.764	3.398	3.955	1.899
20037	Grain, rice, brown, long grain, cooked	1 cup	195	216.45	5.031	44.772	3.51	1.755	0.638	0.63	0.351
20041	Grain, rice, brown, medium grain, cooked	1 cup	195	218.4	4.524	45.845	3.51	1.618	0.585	0.577	0.322
20055	Grain, rice, white, glutinous, cooked	1 cup	174	168.78	3.515	36.697	1.74	0.331	0.122	0.12	0.068
20345	Grain, rice, white, long grain, enriched, cooked w/salt	1 cup	158	205.4	4.25	44.509	0.632	0.442	0.139	0.12	0.122
20049	Grain, rice, white, long grain, precooked/instant, enriched, cooked	1 cup	165	161.7	3.399	35.096	0.99	0.264	0.084	0.073	0.073
20051	Grain, rice, white, medium grain, cooked	1 cup	186	241.8	4.427	53.177	0.558	0.391	0.121	0.104	0.106
20066	Grain, semolina, enriched	1 cup	167	601.2	21.176	121.63	6.513	1.753	0.207	0.718	0.25
20067	Grain, sorghum	1 cup	192	650.88	21.696	143.29		6.336	1.907	2.63	0.877
20068	Grain, tapioca, pearl, dry	1 cup	152	544.16	0.289	134.81	1.368	0.03	0.008	0.005	0.008
20078	Grain, wheat germ, crude	1 cup	115	414	26.622	59.57	15.18	11.178	1.57	6.911	1.915
20087	Grain, wheat, sprouted	1 cup	108	213.84	8.089	45.932	1.188	1.372	0.163	0.602	0.222
6114	Gravy, au jus, canned	1 cup	238	38.08	2.856	5.95	0	0.476	0.19	0.024	0.238
6116	Gravy, beef, canned	1 cup	233	123.49	8.737	11.207	0.932	5.499	2.241	0.186	2.686
6119	Gravy, chicken, canned	1 cup	238	188.02	4.593	12.9	0.952	13.59	6.069	3.57	3.356
6579	Gravy, Home Style Savory Brown Gravy, canned/Heinz	.25 cup	60	24.6	0.9	3.414		0.78	0.276	0.037	0.324
6121	Gravy, mushroom, canned	1 cup	238	119	2.999	13.019	0.952	6.45	2.785	2.428	0.952
6125	Gravy, turkey, canned	1 cup	238	121.38	6.188	12.138	0.952	4.998	2.142	1.166	1.476

Chol (g)	Calc (mg)	Iron (mg)	Mag (mg)	Phos (mg)	Pota (mg)	Sodi (mg)	Zinc (mg)	Vit A (RAE)	Vit C (mg)	Thia (mg)	Ribo (mg)	Niac (mg)	Vit B_6 (mg)	Vit B_{12} (µg)	Vit E (mg)	Fol (µg)	Alc (g)
0	348	0.504	28.8	19.2	230.4	2.4	0.192	9.6	7.92	0.043	0.055	0.48	0.048	0	0.648	12	0
0	104.92	0.268	14.64	17.08	351.36	4.88	0.122	6.1	9.76	0.024	0.037	0.366	0.029	0	0.464	8.54	0
0	28.05	1.198	15.3	30.6	249.9	2.55	0.127	2.55	100.7	0.038	0.196	0.747	0.071	0	0.612	10.2	0
0	24.32	0.638	19.76	36.48	232.56	1.52	0.213	1.52	89.38	0.036	0.033	0.587	0.071	0	0.441	36.48	0
0	1.48	0.056	1.84	2.26	12.56	0.56	0.002	0.04	0.07	0.009	0.003	0.039	0.001	0	0.002	0.28	0
0	10.78	0.37	15.4	16.94	172.48	1.54	0.154	43.12	12.47	0.051	0.032	0.274	0.069	0	0.077	4.62	0
67.15	5.1	3.477	25.5	235.45	338.3	48.45	3.086	0	0	0.238	0.436	9.143	0.643	1.556	0.527	7.65	0
69.7	6.8	2.907	22.1	177.65	306.85	48.45	3.128	0	0	0.085	0.23	3.154	0.34	2.431	0.306	6.8	0
168.99	16.77	1.174	23.22	188.34	316.05	82.56	1.922	41.28	0.645	0.086	0.257	7.607	0.396	0.361	0.464	2.58	0
116.6	14.3	0.847	20.9	163.9	275	69.3	1.683	22	0.66	0.083	0.25	6.9	0.394	0.33	0.264	2.2	0
63.91	2.49	3.743	18.26	154.38	222.44	47.31	0.614	13.28	5.146	0.345	0.257	2.859	0.523	0.631		20.75	0
216	13.5	11.232	54	453.6	672.3	151.2	2.079	70.2	14.04	0.948	0.726	8.956	1.431	1.755	1.893	56.7	0
82.84	14.17	4.327	25.07	299.75	235.44	57.77	2.638	79.57	6.649	0.266	0.283	8.216	0.654	0.469	0.764	8.72	0
69.7	16.15	1.929	17.85	223.55	325.55	39.95	1.929	0	0	0.077	0.178	7.166	0.4	7.055		9.35	0
189.05	23.88	7.045	43.78	493.52	396.01	107.46	4.378	145.3	10.35	0.422	0.446	12.032	0.816	0.796		11.94	0
42.525	19.845	1.559	3.686	56.7	39.123	197.6	0.261	283.8	0.567	0.025	0.085	0.712	0.017	2.665		17.01	0
127.4	18.2	3.962	30.8	378	460.6	98	3.668	29.4	0	0.108	0.452	5.835	0.518	0.574	2.436	2.8	0
137.28	20.02	4.104	35.75	441.87	554.84	108.68	4.533	17.16	0	0.132	0.558	5.836	0.672	0.701		17.16	0
0	17.27	2.088	34.54	84.78	146.01	4.71	1.287	0	0	0.13	0.097	3.239	0.181	0	0.016	25.12	0
0	18.2	1.747	58.24	72.8	123.76	9.1	1.037	0	0	0.104	0.051	1.82	0.151	0	0.018	32.76	0
0	11.62	4.499	210.82	348.6	476.42	58.1	3.669	0	0	0.639	0.334	6.021	1.033	0			0
0	11.62	4.499	210.82	348.6	476.42	58.1	3.669	18.26	0	0.639	0.334	6.021	1.033	0	0.813	31.54	0
0	84.24	7.363	276.12	815.88	669.24	3.12	6.193	0	0	1.19	0.217	1.499	0.186	0	1.092	87.36	0
0	19.5	0.819	83.85	161.85	83.85	9.75	1.229	0	0	0.187	0.049	2.98	0.283	0	0.058	7.8	0
0	19.5	1.033	85.8	150.15	154.05	1.95	1.209	0	0	0.199	0.023	2.594	0.291	0		7.8	0
0	3.48	0.244	8.7	13.92	17.4	8.7	0.713	0	0	0.035	0.023	0.505	0.045	0	0.07	1.74	0
0	15.8	1.896	18.96	67.94	55.3	603.56	0.774	0	0	0.258	0.021	2.332	0.147	0	0.063	91.64	0
0	13.2	1.039	8.25	23.1	6.6	4.95	0.396	0	0	0.124	0.076	1.452	0.016	0	0.016	115.5	0
0	5.58	2.771	24.18	68.82	53.94	0	0.781	0	0	0.311	0.03	3.413	0.093	0		107.9	0
0	28.39	7.281	78.49	227.12	310.62	1.67	1.753	0	0	1.354	0.954	10.003	0.172	0	0.434	305.6	0
0	53.76	8.448		551.04	672	11.52		0	0	0.455	0.273	5.62		0			0
0	30.4	2.402	1.52	10.64	16.72	1.52	0.182	0	0	0.006	0	0	0.012	0	0	6.08	0
0	44.85	7.199	274.85	968.3	1025.8	13.8	14.13	0	0	2.164	0.574	7.835	1.495	0		323.2	0
0	30.24	2.311	88.56	216	182.52	17.28	1.782	0	2.808	0.243	0.167	3.334	0.286	0	0.054	41.04	0
0	9.52	1.428	4.76	71.4	192.78	119	2.38	0	2.38	0.048	0.143	2.142	0.024	0.238		4.76	0
6.99	13.98	1.631	4.66	69.9	188.73	1304.8	2.33	2.33	0	0.075	0.084	1.538	0.023	0.233	0.047	4.66	0
4.76	47.6	1.119	4.76	69.02	259.42	1373.26	1.904	2.38	0	0.04	0.102	1.054	0.024	0.238	0.309	4.76	0
2.4						351.6											0
0	16.66	1.571	4.76	35.7	252.28	1356.6	1.666	0	0	0.079	0.15	1.597	0.048	0		28.56	0
4.76	9.52	1.666	4.76	69.02	259.42	1373.26	1.904	0	0	0.048	0.19	3.094	0.024	0.238	0.119	4.76	0

EvaluEat Code	Food Name	Amt	Wt (g)	Energy (kcal)	Prot (g)	Carb (g)	Fiber (g)	Fat (g)	Mono (g)	Poly (g)	Sat (g)
22700	Hamburger Helper, cheeseburger macaroni, dry mix/Betty Crocker	1 serving	45	177.75	4.95	28.935		4.68			1.269
2003	Herb, basil, ground	1 tsp, leaves	0.7	1.757	0.101	0.427	0.283	0.028	0.003	0.015	0.002
2004	Herb, bay leaf, crumbled	1 tsp, crumbled	0.6	1.878	0.046	0.45	0.158	0.05	0.01	0.014	0.014
11215	Herb, garlic, raw	1 tsp	2.8	4.172	0.178	0.926	0.059	0.014	0	0.007	0.002
11216	Herb, ginger root, peeled, sliced, raw	5 slices (1"dia)	11	8.8	0.2	1.955	0.22	0.082	0.017	0.017	0.022
2029	Herb, parsley, dried	1 tsp	0.3	0.828	0.067	0.155	0.091	0.013	0.01	0.001	0
2036	Herb, rosemary, dried	1 tsp	1.2	3.972	0.059	0.769	0.511	0.183	0.036	0.028	0.088
2042	Herb, thyme, ground	1 tbsp, leaves	2.7	7.452	0.246	1.726	0.999	0.201	0.013	0.032	0.074
18271	Ice cream cone, cake or wafer	1 cone	4	16.68	0.324	3.16	0.12	0.276	0.074	0.131	0.049
18272	Ice cream cone, sugar, rolled	1 cone	10	40.2	0.79	8.41	0.17	0.38	0.147	0.145	0.057
19270	Ice cream, chocolate	.5 cup (4 fl. oz.)	66	142.56	2.508	18.612	0.792	7.26	2.119	0.271	4.488
19264	Ice cream, Eskimo Pie Vanilla Ice Cream Bar w/dark chocolate coating	1 bar	50	165.5	2.05	12.25		12.05			7.25
19262	Ice cream, Klondike Vanilla Ice Cream Bar w/chocolate coating	1 bar (5 fl. oz.)	148	488.4	6.216	35.668		35.668			19.388
19096	Ice cream, light, vanilla, soft serve	.5 cup (4 fl. oz.)	88	110.88	4.312	19.184	0	2.288	0.669	0.088	1.434
19271	Ice cream, strawberry	.5 cup (4 fl. oz.)	66	126.72	2.112	18.216	0.594	5.544			3.425
19095	Ice cream, vanilla	.5 cup	72	144.7	2.52	17	0.504	7.92	2.138	0.325	4.889
7934	Kielbasa, polish, turkey and beef, smoked	2 oz	56	126.56	7.336	2.184	0	9.856	4.631	1.305	3.489
17004	Lamb, domestic, choice, composite, lean (1/4"trim) cooked	3 oz	85	175.1	23.987	0	0	8.092	3.545	0.527	2.89
17002	Lamb, domestic, choice, composite, lean & fat (1/4"trim) cooked	3 oz	85	249.9	20.842	0	0	17.799	7.497	1.284	7.506
18369	Leavening agent, baking powder, double acting, Na Al sulfate	1 tsp	4.6	2.438	0	1.274	0.009	0	0	0	0
18372	Leavening agent, baking soda	1 tsp	4.6	0	0	0	0	0	0	0	0
18373	Leavening agent, cream of tartar	1 tsp	3	7.74	0	1.845	0.006	0	0	0	0
18375	Leavening agent, yeast, Baker's, active	1 tsp	4	11.8	1.532	1.528	0.84	0.184	0.102	0	0.024
11257	Lettuce, red leaf, raw	.5 cup	60	9.6	0.798	1.356	0.54	0.132			
7274	Lunch meat, beef pastrami, cooked, smoked, chopped, pressed/Carl Budding	2 oz	57	80.37	11.172	0.57	0	3.705		0.171	1.71
7272	Lunch meat, beef, smoked, sliced/Carl Budding	2 oz	57	79.23	11.001	0.342	0	3.705		0.171	1.482
7043	Lunch meat, beef, thin slices	1 oz	28.35	50.18	7.969	1.619	0	1.089	0.476	0.057	0.468
7202	Lunch meat, bologna (beef light)/Oscar Mayer	1 slice	28	56	3.29	1.568	0	4.06	2.005	0.132	1.63
7007	Lunch meat, bologna (beef)	1 slice	28	87.08	2.876	1.114	0	7.893	3.421	0.217	3.118
7207	Lunch meat, braunschweiger liver sausage, sliced/Oscar Mayer	1 slice	28	92.68	3.99	0.728	0.056	8.218	4.334	1.044	3.063
7250	Lunch meat, chicken breast, oven roasted deluxe/Louis Rich	1 serving	28	28.28	5.124	0.7	0	0.56	0.23	0.089	0.151
7270	Lunch meat, corned beef, cooked, chopped, pressed/Carl Budding	2 oz	57	80.94	11.001	0.57	0	3.876		0.171	1.596
7253	Lunch meat, franks (turkey & chicken)/Louis Rich	1 serving	45	84.6	5.04	2.385	0	6.075	2.499	1.423	1.728
7029	Lunch meat, ham, slices, regular (11% fat)	1 serving	56	91.28	9.296	2.145	0.728	4.816	2.438	0.442	1.644
7041	Lunch meat, liver sausage (liverwurst)	1 slice (2-1/2" dia x 1/4" thick)	18	58.68	2.538	0.396	0	5.13	2.401	0.468	1.908
7222	Lunch meat, old fashioned loaf/Oscar Mayer	1 serving	28	64.68	3.668	2.24	0	4.564	2.201	0.739	1.568
7051	Lunch meat, olive loaf (pork)	2 slices	57	133.95	6.726	5.244	0	9.405	4.486	1.1	3.334

Chol (g)	Calc (mg)	Iron (mg)	Mag (mg)	Phos (mg)	Pota (mg)	Sodi (mg)	Zinc (mg)	Vit A (RAE)	Vit C (mg)	Thia (mg)	Ribo (mg)	Niac (mg)	Vit B₆ (mg)	Vit B₁₂ (µg)	Vit E (mg)	Fol (µg)	Alc (g)
4.05						913.5											0
0	14.791	0.294	2.954	3.43	24.031	0.238	0.041	3.283	0.428	0.001	0.002	0.049	0.016	0	0.052	1.918	0
0	5.004	0.258	0.72	0.678	3.174	0.138	0.022	1.854	0.279	0	0.003	0.012	0.01	0	0.011	1.08	0
0	5.068	0.048	0.7	4.284	11.228	0.476	0.032	0	0.874	0.006	0.003	0.02	0.035	0	0	0.084	0
0	1.76	0.066	4.73	3.74	45.65	1.43	0.037	0	0.55	0.003	0.004	0.082	0.018	0	0.029	1.21	0
0	4.404	0.294	0.747	1.053	11.415	1.356	0.014	1.527	0.366	0.001	0.004	0.024	0.003	0	0.021	0.54	0
0	15.36	0.351	2.64	0.84	11.46	0.6	0.039	1.872	0.734	0.006	0.005	0.012	0.021	0	0.024	3.684	0
0	51.03	3.337	5.94	5.427	21.978	1.485	0.167	5.13	1.35	0.014	0.011	0.133	0.015	0	0.202	7.398	0
0	1	0.144	1.04	3.88	4.48	5.72	0.027	0	0	0.01	0.014	0.177	0.001	0	0.031	6.92	0
0	4.4	0.443	3.1	10.3	14.5	32	0.075	0	0	0.051	0.041	0.507	0.005	0	0.007	14	0
22.44	71.94	0.614	19.14	70.62	164.34	50.16	0.383	77.88	0.462	0.028	0.128	0.149	0.036	0.191	0.198	10.56	0
14	59.5					34											0
39.96	211.64					108.04											0
10.56	138.16	0.053	12.32	106.48	194.48	61.6	0.466	25.52	0.792	0.046	0.174	0.104	0.04	0.44	0.053	5.28	0
19.14	79.2	0.139	9.24	66	124.08	39.6	0.224	63.36	5.082	0.03	0.168	0.112	0.033	0.198		7.92	0
31.7	92.2	0.065	10.1	75.6	143.3	57.6	0.497	85	0.432	0.03	0.173	0.084	0.035	0.281	0.216	3.6	0.144
39.2		0.694				672		0	8.288								0
78.2	12.75	1.743	22.1	178.5	292.4	64.6	4.48	0	0	0.085	0.238	5.372	0.136	2.218	0.162	19.55	0
82.45	14.45	1.598	19.55	159.8	263.5	61.2	3.791	0	0	0.085	0.213	5.661	0.111	2.168	0.119	15.3	0
0	270.296	0.507	1.242	100.786	0.92	487.6	0	0	0	0	0	0	0	0	0	0	0
0	0	0	0	0	0	1258.56	0	0	0	0	0	0	0	0	0	0	0
0	0.24	0.112	0.06	0.15	495	1.56	0.013	0	0	0	0	0	0	0	0	0	0
0	2.56	0.664	3.92	51.6	80	2	0.256	0	0.012	0.094	0.219	1.59	0.062	0.001	0	93.6	0
	19.8	0.72	7.2	16.8	112.2	15	0.12	225	2.22	0.038	0.046	0.193	0.06		0.09	21.6	
37.05	9.69	1.396			208.05	601.92					0.051	0.131	2.337				0
38.19	7.98	1.288			191.52	815.67					0.051	0.137	2.2				0
11.624	3.119	0.765	5.387	47.628	121.622	407.957	1.128	0	0	0.023	0.054	1.494	0.096	0.729	0.054	3.119	0
12.32	3.64	0.342	3.92	49.84	43.68	322.28	0.535	0	0							3.64	0
15.68	8.68	0.308	3.92	48.16	48.16	302.4	2.548	3.64	4.256	0.007	0.028	0.704	0.048	0.356	0.098	2.52	0
49.84	2.52	2.943	3.92	55.72	56.56	324.52	0.952	1322	2.52	0.064	0.448	2.573	0.092	5.258		13.16	0
13.72	1.96	0.322	6.72	74.48	74.2	332.64	0.204		0								0
37.05	9.69	1.368			200.64	764.94					0.051	0.137	2.394				0
41.4	58.95	0.981	10.35	66.15	72	511.2	0.837		0								0
31.92	13.44	0.571	12.32	85.68	160.72	730.24	0.756	0	2.24	0.351	0.1	1.626	0.184	0.235	0.045	3.92	0
28.44	4.68	1.152	2.16	41.4	30.6	154.8	0.414	1495	0	0.049	0.185	0.774	0.034	2.423		5.4	0
17.08	31.64	0.37	6.44	58.24	82.32	331.52	0.524		0								0
21.66	62.13	0.308	10.83	72.39	169.29	845.88	0.787	34.2	0	0.168	0.148	1.046	0.131	0.718	0.142	1.14	0

EvaluEat Code	Food Name	Amt	Wt (g)	Energy (kcal)	Prot (g)	Carb (g)	Fiber (g)	Fat (g)	Mono (g)	Poly (g)	Sat (g)
13355	Lunch meat, pastrami (beef)	1 slice (1 oz)	28	97.72	4.827	0.854	0	8.17	4.052	0.277	2.918
7052	Lunch meat, pastrami (turkey)	2 slices	57	80.37	10.465	0.946	0	3.54	1.168	0.906	1.032
7225	Lunch meat, pork sausage links, cooked/Oscar Mayer	1 serving, 2 links	48	164.64	7.824	0.48	0	14.64	7.104	1.766	5.131
7226	Lunch meat, salami beef cotto/Oscar Mayer	1 serving, 2 slices	46	94.76	6.532	0.874	0	7.222	3.179	0.359	3.1
7232	Lunch meat, smokie links sausage/Oscar Mayer	1 serving	43	129.86	5.332	0.731	0	11.739	5.663	1.195	4.033
7276	Lunch meat, Spam, pork with ham, minced, canned/Hormel	1 serving, 2 oz	56	173.6	7.414	1.697	0	15.254	7.717	1.652	5.533
7238	Lunch meat, summer sausage thuringer cervalat/Oscar Mayer	1 serving, 2 slices	46	139.84	6.854	0.414	0	12.282	5.585	1.025	4.934
7254	Lunch meat, turkey bacon/Louis Rich	1 serving	14	35	2.114	0.231	0	2.842	1.051	0.658	0.738
7255	Lunch meat, turkey bologna/Louis Rich	1 serving	28	51.52	3.164	1.358	0	3.696	1.487	1.005	1.061
7079	Lunch meat, turkey breast meat	1 slice	28	26.88	2.044	3.822	0.56	0.378	0.151	0.092	0.118
7080	Lunch meat, turkey ham, cured	1 serving, .99 oz	28	35.28	4.9	0.571	0.056	1.355	0.533	0.369	0.427
7266	Lunch meat, turkey salami/Louis Rich	1 serving	28	41.16	4.284	0.112	0	2.632	0.881	0.656	0.779
7242	Lunch meat, wieners (beef franks) bun length/Oscar Mayer	1 serving, 1 link	57	184.68	6.327	1.511	0	17.157	8.333	0.547	7.142
7243	Lunch meat, wieners (beef franks) fat-free/Oscar Mayer	1 serving	50	39	6.6	2.55	0	0.25	0.095	0.024	0.112
7241	Lunch meat, wieners (beef franks)/Oscar Mayer	1 serving	45	147.15	5.108	1.057	0	13.617	6.633	0.612	5.607
22005	Macaroni and Cheese Dinner, Kraft Original Flavor, unprepared	1 NLEA serving (makes about 1 cup prepared)	70	259	11.34	47.53	1.47	2.59			1.26
20100	Macaroni, enriched, cooked	1 cup elbow shaped	140	197.4	6.678	39.676	1.82	0.938	0.111	0.382	0.133
9328	Maraschino cherries, canned, drained	1 cup, balls	154	254.1	0.339	64.634	4.928	0.323	0.075	0.085	0.06
4067	Margarine, hard, corn, soybean-hydrogenated & cottonseed-hydrogenated w/salt	1 tsp	4.7	33.793	0.042	0.042	0	3.783	1.73	1.18	0.705
4611	Margarine, regular, tub, composite, 80% fat, with salt	1 tbsp	12.8	91.648	0.102	0.077	0	10.291	4.616	3.565	1.66
20322	Meal, corn, white, degermed, enriched	1 cup	138	505.08	11.702	107.2	10.212	2.277	0.569	0.98	0.31
20022	Meal, corn, yellow, degermed, enriched	1 cup	138	505.08	11.702	107.2	10.212	2.277	0.569	0.98	0.31
1110	Milk shake, thick, chocolate	1 container (10.6 oz)	300	357	9.15	63.45	0.9	8.1	2.34	0.3	5.043
1111	Milk shake, thick, vanilla	1 container (11 oz)	313	350.56	12.082	55.558	0	9.484	2.739	0.354	5.903
1088	Milk, buttermilk, lowfat, cultured	1 cup	245	98	8.109	11.736	0	2.156	0.622	0.081	1.343
1107	Milk, human, mature breast	1 cup	246	172.2	2.534	16.949	0	10.775	4.079	1.223	4.942
1082	Milk, lowfat, 1% fat w/added vitamin A	1 cup	244	102.48	8.223	12.176	0	2.367	0.676	0.085	1.545
1104	Milk, lowfat, 1% fat, chocolate	1 cup	250	157.5	8.1	26.1	1.25	2.5	0.75	0.087	1.54
1154	Milk, nonfat, dry w/added vit A	.25 cup	30	108.6	10.848	15.594	0	0.231	0.06	0.009	0.15
1097	Milk, nonfat, skim, evaporated, canned	1 cup	256	199.68	19.328	29.056	0	0.512	0.159	0.015	0.31
1085	Milk, nonfat/fat-free, skim w/added vit A	1 cup	245	83.3	8.257	12.152	0	0.196	0.115	0.017	0.287
1079	Milk, reduced fat, 2% fat w/added vitamin A	1 cup	244	122	8.052	11.419	0	4.807	2.042	0.166	2.35
16120	Milk, soy, fluid	1 cup	245	120.05	9.188	11.368	3.185	5.096	0.799	2.041	0.524
1095	Milk, sweetened condensed, canned	1 cup	306	982.26	24.205	166.46	0	26.622	7.427	1.031	16.787
1077	Milk, whole, 3.25% fat	1 cup	244	146.4	7.857	11.029	0	7.93	1.981	0.476	4.551
1102	Milk, whole, chocolate	1 cup	250	207.5	7.925	25.85	2	8.475	2.475	0.31	5.26
1153	Milk, whole, evaporated, canned, w/added vit A	.5 cup	126	168.84	8.581	12.65	0	9.526	2.942	0.309	5.785
1106	Milk, whole, goat	1 cup	244	168.36	8.686	10.858	0	10.102	2.706	0.364	6.507
15250	Mollusks, conch, baked or broiled	3 oz	85	110.5	22.355	1.445	0	1.02	0.284	0.233	0.315
18274	Muffin, blueberry, commercially prep	1 medium	113	313.01	6.215	54.24	2.938	7.345	2.228	2.819	1.579

Chol (g)	Calc (mg)	Iron (mg)	Mag (mg)	Phos (mg)	Pota (mg)	Sodi (mg)	Zinc (mg)	Vit A (RAE)	Vit C (mg)	Thia (mg)	Ribo (mg)	Niac (mg)	Vit B_6 (mg)	Vit B_{12} (µg)	Vit E (mg)	Fol (µg)	Alc (g)
26.04	2.52	0.529	5.04	42	63.84	343.56	1.193	0	0	0.027	0.048	1.418	0.05	0.493	0.07	1.96	0
30.78	5.13	0.946	7.98	114	148.2	595.65	1.231	0	0	0.031	0.142	2.01	0.154	0.137	0.125	2.85	0
36.96	7.68	0.826	8.64	75.84	114.24	401.28	1.248	0									0
38.18	3.22	1.247	7.82	103.04	95.22	602.14	0.961	0									0
27.09	4.3	0.503	7.31	103.2	77.4	433.01	0.899	0									0
39.2	7.84	0.504	7.84		128.24	766.64	1.008	0	0.504							1.68	0
38.64	4.14	1.03	6.9	59.8	104.88	657.8	0.98		0	0.106	0.133	2.019	0.138	1.73		2.3	0
12.6	5.6	0.203	2.66	27.86	29.12	169.82	0.353	0	0							1.12	0
18.76	34.72	0.459	6.16	54.88	42.56	301.56	0.518	0	0							1.68	0
3.36	3.08	0.33	5.88	45.36	58.52	47.04	0.372	0	0	0.003	0.01	0.489	0.036	0.025	0.025	1.12	0
20.16	2.24	0.655	6.16	82.32	80.36	311.92	0.725	1.96	0	0.008	0.042	0.593	0.059	0.064	0.179	1.96	0
21.28	11.2	0.35	6.16	74.48	60.48	281.12	0.65		0								0
33.63	7.41	0.889	8.55	59.85	90.06	584.25	1.283	0	0							6.27	0
15	10	0.975	9.5	64.5	233.5	463.5	1.205	0	0								0
25.2	4.5	0.603	5.85	63	58.5	461.25	0.985	0	0	0.015	0.045	1.031	0.032	0.734		2.7	0
9.8	92.4	2.562		264.6	296.1	561.4	0.35			0.672	0.413	4.536				65.1	
0	9.8	1.96	25.2	75.6	43.4	1.4	0.742	0	0	0.286	0.137	2.341	0.049	0	0.084	107.8	0
0	83.16	0.662	6.16	4.62	32.34	6.16	0.4	3.08	0	0	0	0.006	0.008	0	0.077	0	0
0	1.41	0	0.141	1.081	1.974	44.321	0		38.49	0.009	0	0.002	0.001	0	0.005	0.517	0.047
0	3.328	0	0.256	2.56	4.864	138.112	0		104.8	0.013	0.001	0.004	0.003	0.001	0.01	0.64	0.128
0	6.9	5.699	55.2	115.92	223.56	4.14	0.994	0	0	0.987	0.562	6.947	0.355	0	0.207	321.5	0
0	6.9	5.699	55.2	115.92	223.56	4.14	0.994	15.18	0	0.987	0.562	6.947	0.355	0	0.207	321.5	0
33	396	0.93	48	378	672	333	1.44	54	0	0.141	0.666	0.372	0.075	0.96	0.15	15	0
37.56	456.98	0.313	37.56	359.95	572.79	297.35	1.221	78.25	0	0.094	0.61	0.457	0.131	1.628	0.157	21.91	0
9.8	284.2	0.123	26.95	218.05	369.95	257.25	1.029	17.15	2.45	0.083	0.377	0.142	0.083	0.539	0.123	12.25	0
34.44	78.72	0.074	7.38	34.44	125.46	41.82	0.418	150.1	12.3	0.034	0.089	0.435	0.027	0.123	0.197	12.3	0
12.2	263.52	0.854	26.84	217.16	290.36	122	2.123	141.5	0	0.049	0.451	0.227	0.09	1.074	0.024	12.2	0
7.5	287.5	0.6	32.5	257.5	425	152.5	1.025	145	2.25	0.095	0.415	0.317	0.103	0.85	0.05	12.5	0
6	377.1	0.096	33	290.4	538.2	160.5	1.224	195.9	2.04	0.124	0.465	0.285	0.108	1.209	0	15	0
10.24	742.4	0.742	69.12	499.2	849.92	294.4	2.304	302.1	3.072	0.115	0.791	0.445	0.141	0.614	0	23.04	0
4.9	222.95	1.225	22.05	181.3	237.65	107.8	2.082	149.5	0	0.11	0.446	0.23	0.091	1.298	0.024	12.25	0
19.52	270.84	0.244	26.84	224.48	341.6	114.68	1.171	134.2	0.488	0.095	0.451	0.224	0.093	1.122	0.073	12.2	0
0	9.8	1.421	46.55	120.05	345.45	29.4	0.564	4.9	0	0.394	0.171	0.36	0.1	0	0.024	4.9	0
104.04	869.04	0.581	79.56	774.18	1135.26	388.62	2.876	226.4	7.956	0.275	1.273	0.643	0.156	1.346	0.49	33.66	0
24.4	246.44	0.073	24.4	204.96	324.52	104.92	0.927	68.32	0	0.107	0.447	0.261	0.088	1.074	0.146	12.2	0
30	280	0.6	32.5	252.5	417.5	150	1.025	65	2.25	0.093	0.405	0.313	0.1	0.825	0.15	12.5	0
36.54	328.86	0.239	30.24	255.78	381.78	133.56	0.97	141.1	2.394	0.059	0.398	0.244	0.063	0.202		10.08	0
26.84	326.96	0.122	34.16	270.84	497.76	122	0.732	139.1	3.172	0.117	0.337	0.676	0.112	0.171	0.171	2.44	0
55.25	83.3	1.199	202.3	184.45	138.55	130.05	1.454	5.95	0	0.051	0.068	0.884	0.051	4.463	5.381	152.2	0
33.9	64.41	1.819	18.08	222.61	138.99	505.11	0.554	25.99	1.243	0.158	0.136	1.243	0.025	0.655	0.938	83.62	0

EvaluEat Code	Food Name	Amt	Wt (g)	Energy (kcal)	Prot (g)	Carb (g)	Fiber (g)	Fat (g)	Mono (g)	Poly (g)	Sat (g)
18279	Muffin, corn, commercially prep	1 medium	113	344.65	6.667	57.517	3.842	9.492	2.378	3.633	1.53
18283	Muffin, oatbran	1 medium	113	305.1	7.91	54.579	5.198	8.362	1.915	4.666	1.228
18639	Muffin, Thomas' English Muffins, plain/Best Foods	1 serving	57	131.67	4.959	25.992		0.855	1.052	1.86	0.697
20134	Noodles, rice, cooked	1 cup	176	191.84	1.602	43.824	1.76	0.352	0.046	0.04	0.04
22702	Noodles, alfredo egg noodles in a creamy sauce, dry mix/Lipton	1 cup	93	388.74	14.415	58.032		10.974	3.586	1.157	4.25
20113	Noodles, Chinese, chow mein	1 cup	45	237.15	3.771	25.893	1.755	13.842	3.46	7.799	1.973
20110	Noodles, egg, enriched, cooked w/salt	1 cup	160	212.8	7.6	39.744	1.76	2.352	0.688	0.653	0.496
20115	Noodles, Japanese, soba, cooked	1 cup	114	112.86	5.768	24.442		0.114	0.03	0.035	0.022
12062	Nuts, almonds, dried, blanched	1 tbsp	9.1	52.871	1.997	1.815	0.946	4.606	2.938	1.097	0.354
12566	Nuts, almonds, oil roast, blanched w/salt	1 oz (24 whole kernels)	28.35	173.79	5.398	5.109	3.175	16.026	10.406	3.363	1.519
12077	Nuts, beechnuts, dried	1 oz	28.35	163.3	1.758	9.497		14.175	6.206	5.695	1.621
12078	Nuts, brazilnuts, dried, unblanched	1 oz (6–8 kernels)	28.35	185.98	4.06	3.479	2.126	18.833	6.959	5.834	4.291
12084	Nuts, butternuts, dried	1 oz	28.35	173.5	7.059	3.416	1.332	16.154	2.955	12.117	0.37
12087	Nuts, cashew nuts, raw	1 oz	28.35	160.46	5.165	7.691	0.936	13.302	7.218	2.379	2.361
12585	Nuts, cashews, dry roasted w/salt	1 oz	28.35	162.73	4.34	9.268	0.851	13.14	7.744	2.222	2.596
12094	Nuts, chestnuts, Chinese, dried	1 oz	28.35	102.91	1.933	22.612		0.513	0.268	0.133	0.075
12116	Nuts, coconut cream, canned (liquid expressed from grated meat)	1 cup	296	568.32	7.962	24.716	6.512	52.451	2.232	0.574	46.51
12119	Nuts, coconut water (liquid from coconuts)	1 cup	240	45.6	1.728	8.904	2.64	0.48	0.019	0.005	0.422
12109	Nuts, coconut, sweetened, flakes, dried	1 cup	74	350.76	2.427	35.217	3.182	23.791	1.012	0.26	21.097
12108	Nuts, coconut, unsweetened, dried	1 oz	28.35	187.11	1.95	6.705	4.621	18.294	0.778	0.2	16.221
12122	Nuts, filberts/hazelnuts, dry roasted, unblanched, w/o salt	1 oz	28.35	183.14	4.261	4.99	2.665	17.69	13.213	2.399	1.279
12132	Nuts, macadamia nuts, dry roasted, without salt added	1 oz (10–12 kernels)	28.35	203.55	2.208	3.793	2.268	21.569	16.804	0.425	3.387
12635	Nuts, mixed w/peanuts, dry roasted w/salt	1 oz	28.35	168.4	4.905	7.187	2.552	14.586	8.9	3.053	1.956
12142	Nuts, pecans, dried	1 oz (20 halves)	28.35	195.9	2.6	3.929	2.722	20.403	11.567	6.128	1.752
12147	Nuts, pine nut, pignolias, dried	1 oz (167 kernels)	28.35	190.8	3.881	3.708	1.049	19.383	5.32	9.674	1.389
12652	Nuts, pistachios, dry roasted w/salt	1 oz (49 kernels)	28.35	161.03	6.053	7.592	2.92	13.032	6.865	3.94	1.575
12154	Nuts, walnut, black, dried	1 oz	28.35	175.2	6.821	2.809	1.928	16.727	4.254	9.944	0.955
4589	Oil, fish, cod liver	1 tbsp	13.6	122.67	0	0	0	13.6	6.353	3.066	3.075
4582	Oil, vegetable, canola	1 tbsp	14	123.76	0	0	0	14	8.246	4.144	0.994
4047	Oil, vegetable, coconut	1 tbsp	13.6	117.23	0	0	0	13.6	0.789	0.245	11.764
4518	Oil, vegetable/salad/cooking, corn	1 tbsp	13.6	120.22	0	0	0	13.6	3.291	7.983	1.727
4053	Oil, vegetable/salad/cooking, olive	1 tbsp	13.5	119.34	0	0	0	13.5	9.977	1.35	1.816
4042	Oil, vegetable/salad/cooking, peanut	1 tbsp	13.5	119.34	0	0	0	13.5	6.237	4.32	2.282
4510	Oil, vegetable/salad/cooking, safflower, linoleic >70%	1 tbsp	13.6	120.22	0	0	0	13.6	1.952	10.149	0.844
4511	Oil, vegetable/salad/cooking, safflower, oleic >70%	1 tbsp	13.6	120.22	0	0	0	13.6	10.152	1.952	0.844
4058	Oil, vegetable/salad/cooking, sesame	1 tbsp	13.6	120.22	0	0	0	13.6	5.399	5.671	1.931
4044	Oil, vegetable/salad/cooking, soybean	1 tbsp	13.6	120.22	0	0	0	13.6	3.169	7.874	1.958
11294	Onions, sweet, raw	1 oz	28.34	9.636	0.227	2.14	0.255	0.023			
11292	Onions, young green, tops only	1 tbsp chopped	6	1.86	0.108	0.339	0.21	0.006	0.001	0.002	0.001
18499	Pancake/waffle, buttermilk, Eggo/Kellogg	1 oz	28.34	66.032	1.7	10.798	0.312	1.896	0.833	0.604	0.408

Chol (g)	Calc (mg)	Iron (mg)	Mag (mg)	Phos (mg)	Pota (mg)	Sodi (mg)	Zinc (mg)	Vit A (RAE)	Vit C (mg)	Thia (mg)	Ribo (mg)	Niac (mg)	Vit B$_6$ (mg)	Vit B$_{12}$ (µg)	Vit E (mg)	Fol (µg)	Alc (g)
29.38	83.62	3.175	36.16	320.92	77.97	588.73	0.61	58.76	0	0.308	0.368	2.302	0.095	0.102	0.904	90.4	0
0	71.19	4.746	177.41	424.88	572.91	444.09	2.079	0	0	0.296	0.107	0.475	0.182	0.011	0.746	100.6	0
	76.38	1.704				210.33		0	0.057					0.205	0.994	82.65	0
0	7.04	0.246	5.28	35.2	7.04	33.44	0.44	0	0	0.032	0.007	0.127	0.011	0		5.28	0
104.16	118.11	2.809				1646.1											0
0	9	2.128	23.4	72.45	54	197.55	0.63	0	0	0.26	0.189	2.677	0.049	0	1.566	40.5	0
52.8	19.2	2.544	30.4	110.4	44.8	11.2	0.992	9.6	0	0.298	0.133	2.379	0.058	0.144	0.256	102.4	0
0	4.56	0.547	10.26	28.5	39.9	68.4	0.137	0	0	0.107	0.03	0.581	0.046	0		7.98	0
0	19.656	0.339	25.025	43.68	62.517	2.548	0.284	0	0	0.018	0.051	0.333	0.011	0	2.249	2.73	0
0	54.999	1.503	82.215	163.58	196.466	219.996	0.403		0.284	0.022	0.079	1.106	0.026	0	1.573	18	0
0	0.284	0.697	0	0	288.32	10.773	0.102	0	4.394	0.086	0.105	0.249	0.194	0		32.04	0
0	45.36	0.689	106.596	205.538	186.827	0.851	1.151	0	0.198	0.175	0.01	0.084	0.029	0	1.624	6.237	0
0	15.026	1.14	67.19	126.441	119.354	0.284	0.887	1.701	0.907	0.109	0.042	0.296	0.159	0	0.992	18.71	0
0	10.49	1.894	82.782	168.116	187.11	3.402	1.639	0	0.142	0.12	0.016	0.301	0.118	0	0.255	7.088	0
0	12.758	1.701	73.71	138.915	160.178	181.44	1.588	0	0	0.057	0.057	0.397	0.073	0	0.261	19.56	0
0	8.222	0.649	38.84	43.943	205.821	1.418	0.4	4.536	16.59	0.074	0.083	0.369	0.189	0		31.19	0
0	2.96	1.51	50.32	65.12	298.96	148	1.776	0	5.328	0.065	0.118	0.112	0.086	0	0.385	41.44	0
0	57.6	0.696	60	48	600	252	0.24	0	5.76	0.072	0.137	0.192	0.077	0	0	7.2	0
0	10.36	1.332	35.52	74	233.84	189.44	1.295	0	0	0.022	0.015	0.222	0.193	0	0.281	5.92	0
0	7.371	0.941	25.515	58.401	153.941	10.49	0.57	0	0.425	0.017	0.028	0.171	0.085	0	0.125	2.552	0
0	34.871	1.242	49.046	87.885	214.043	0	0.709	0.851	1.077	0.096	0.035	0.581	0.176	0	4.332	24.95	0
0	19.845	0.751	33.453	56.133	102.911	1.134	0.366	0	0.198	0.201	0.025	0.645	0.102	0	0.162	2.835	
0	19.845	1.049	63.788	123.323	169.25	189.662	1.077	0	0.113	0.057	0.057	1.332	0.084	0	3.101	14.18	0
0	19.845	0.717	34.304	78.53	116.235	0	1.284	0.851	0.312	0.187	0.037	0.331	0.06	0	0.397	6.237	0
0	4.536	1.568	71.159	163.013	169.25	0.567	1.829	0.284	0.227	0.103	0.064	1.244	0.027	0	2.645	19	0
0	31.185	1.191	34.02	137.498	295.407	114.818	0.652	3.686	0.652	0.238	0.045	0.404	0.361	0	0.547	14.18	0
0	17.294	0.885	56.984	145.436	148.271	0.567	0.955	0.567	0.482	0.016	0.037	0.133	0.165	0	0.51	8.789	0
77.52	0	0	0	0	0	0	0	4080	0		0	0	0	0	0	0	0
0	0	0	0	0	0	0	0	0	0	0	0	0	0	0	2.394	0	0
0	0	0.005	0	0	0	0	0	0	0	0	0	0	0	0	0.012	0	0
0	0	0	0	0	0	0	0	0	0	0	0	0	0	0	1.945	0	0
0	0.135	0.089	0	0	0.135	0.405	0	0	0	0	0	0	0	0	1.937	0	0
0	0	0.004	0	0	0	0	0.001	0	0	0	0	0	0	0	2.118	0	0
0	0	0	0	0	0	0	0	0	0	0	0	0	0	0	4.638	0	0
0	0	0	0	0	0	0	0	0	0	0	0	0	0	0	4.638	0	0
0	0	0	0	0	0	0	0	0	0	0	0	0	0	0	0.19	0	0
0	0	0.003	0	0	0	0	0	0	0	0	0	0	0	0	1.253	0	0
	5.668	0.074	2.551	7.652	33.725	2.267	0.037	0	1.36	0.012	0.006	0.038	0.037			6.518	
0	3.66	0.115	1.2	1.98	15.6	0.24	0.027	12	2.736	0.004	0.008	0.012	0.004	0	0.013	0.84	0
3.117	9.919	0.879	5.101	96.639	29.19	150.202	0.17		0.397	0.074	0.082	0.978	0.099	0.292	0	14.74	0

EvaluEat Code	Food Name	Amt	Wt (g)	Energy (kcal)	Prot (g)	Carb (g)	Fiber (g)	Fat (g)	Mono (g)	Poly (g)	Sat (g)
18294	Pancakes, blueberry, homemade	1 pancake (4"dia)	38	84.36	2.318	11.02		3.496	0.88	1.582	0.755
18390	Pancakes, buttermilk, homemade	1 pancake (4"dia)	38	86.26	2.584	10.906		3.534	0.897	1.705	0.696
18293	Pancakes, plain, homemade	1 pancake (4"dia)	38	86.26	2.432	10.754		3.686	0.94	1.69	0.806
18288	Pancakes, plain/buttermilk, frozen	1 pancake (6"dia)	73	167.17	3.796	31.828	1.314	2.409	0.881	0.703	0.56
22515	Pasta, beef ravioli in tomato & meat sauce, canned entree/Chef Boyardee	1 serving	244	229.36	8.369	36.893	3.66	5.392	2.001	0.22	2.489
22516	Pasta, beefaroni, macaroni w/beef in tomato sauce, canned entree/Chef Boyardee	1 serving	212	184.44	8.247	31.143	2.968	2.947	1.272	0.254	1.187
22517	Pasta, mini beef ravioli in tomato & meat sauce, canned entree/Chef Boyardee	1 package	425	403.75	14.833	68.51	5.525	7.99	3.4	0.298	2.975
22518	Pasta, spaghetti & meatballs in tomato sauce, canned entree/Chef Boyardee	1 package	425	442	16.065	60.307	3.825	15.3	6.503	0.68	6.843
20121	Pasta, spaghetti, enriched, cooked w/o salt	1 cup	140	197.4	6.678	39.676	2.38	0.938	0.111	0.382	0.133
20125	Pasta, spaghetti, whole wheat, cooked	1 cup	140	173.6	7.462	37.156	6.3	0.756	0.105	0.298	0.139
22701	Pasta, whole wheat macaroni and cheese dinner, dry mix/Hodgson Mill	1 package	206	774.56	29.046	142.55	15.656	9.682			2.822
18635	Pastry, cinnamon rolls w/icing, refrigerated dough/Pillsbury	1 serving	44	150.04	2.376	23.892		5.016			1.25
18237	Pastry, cream puff/eclair shell, homemade	1 eclair (5"x 2" x 1-3/4")	48	173.76	4.32	10.944	0.384	12.432	5.341	3.542	2.688
18239	Pastry, croissant, butter	1 croissant, mini	28	113.68	2.296	12.824	0.728	5.88	1.547	0.306	3.265
18241	Pastry, croissant, cheese	1 croissant, small	42	173.88	3.864	19.74	1.092	8.778	2.734	1.001	4.464
18245	Pastry, Danish, cheese	1 pastry	71	265.54	5.68	26.412	0.71	15.549	8.032	1.828	4.824
18246	Pastry, Danish, fruit (apple/cinnamon/raisin/lemon/raspberry/strawberry) enriched	1 toaster strudel	53	196.63	2.862	25.334	1.007	9.805	5.314	1.253	2.576
18247	Pastry, Danish, nut (almond/raisin nut/cinnamon nut)	1 pastry (4-1/4"dia)	65	279.5	4.615	29.705	1.3	16.38	8.895	2.783	3.784
18257	Pastry, eclair/cream puff, homemade, custard filled w/chocolate icing	1 cream puff (3-1/2"x 2")	112	293.44	7.168	27.104	0.672	17.584	7.262	4.422	4.613
18338	Pastry, phyllo dough	1 sheet dough	19	56.81	1.349	9.994	0.361	1.14	0.598	0.175	0.279
18354	Pastry, strudel, apple	1 piece	71	194.54	2.343	29.181	1.562	7.952	2.32	3.774	1.451
16097	Peanut butter, chunky w/salt	2 tbsp	32	188.48	8.022	6.749	2.112	15.904	7.539	4.532	3.066
16098	Peanut butter, smooth w/salt	2 tbsp	32	191.68	7.99	5.894	1.888	16.73	7.919	4.764	3.209
16390	Peanuts, all types, dry roasted w/o salt	1 oz	28.35	165.85	6.713	6.098	2.268	14.079	6.985	4.449	1.954
16090	Peanuts, all types, dry roasted w/salt	1 oz	28.35	165.85	6.713	6.098	2.268	14.079	6.985	4.449	1.954
16087	Peanuts, all types, raw	1 oz	28.35	160.75	7.314	4.573	2.41	13.96	6.926	4.411	1.937
16138	Peas, chickpea/garbanzo, falafel, homemade	1 patty (approx 2-1/4"dia)	17	56.61	2.263	5.413		3.026	1.729	0.707	0.405
16158	Peas, chickpea/garbanzo, hummus, commercial	1 tbsp	14	23.24	1.106	2.001	0.84	1.344	0.565	0.506	0.201
16363	Peas, cowpea, common (blackeyed, crowder, southern) mature seed, boiled w/salt	1 cup	171	198.36	13.218	35.5	11.115	0.906	0.075	0.385	0.236
16065	Peas, cowpeas, common (blackeyed, crowder, southern) mature seed, canned w/pork	1 cup	240	199.2	6.576	39.672	7.92	3.84	1.574	0.55	1.452

Chol (g)	Calc (mg)	Iron (mg)	Mag (mg)	Phos (mg)	Pota (mg)	Sodi (mg)	Zinc (mg)	Vit A (RAE)	Vit C (mg)	Thia (mg)	Ribo (mg)	Niac (mg)	Vit B$_6$ (mg)	Vit B$_{12}$ (µg)	Vit E (mg)	Fol (µg)	Alc (g)
21.28	78.28	0.654	6.08	57.38	52.44	156.56	0.205	19	0.836	0.074	0.103	0.579	0.019	0.076		13.68	0
22.04	59.66	0.646	5.7	52.82	55.1	198.36	0.236	11.4	0.152	0.078	0.111	0.599	0.017	0.068		14.44	0
22.42	83.22	0.684	6.08	60.42	50.16	166.82	0.213	20.52	0.114	0.076	0.107	0.595	0.017	0.084		14.44	0
6.57	45.26	2.54	10.22	271.56	53.29	371.57	0.482	21.17	0.219	0.277	0.342	2.927	0.058	0.131	0.204	32.85	0
14.64	19.52	2.416			353.8	1173.64			0.244								0
16.96	16.96	1.505				799.24			0.424								0
29.75	38.25	4.08				2018.75			0.425								0
38.25	29.75	3.145				1666			1.7								0
0	9.8	1.96	25.2	75.6	43.4	1.4	0.742	0	0	0.286	0.137	2.341	0.049	0	0.084	107.8	0
0	21	1.484	42	124.6	61.6	4.2	1.134	0	0	0.151	0.063	0.99	0.111	0	0.42	7	0
16.48	234.84	5.397				1258.66											0
						334.4											0
94.08	17.28	0.97	5.76	57.12	46.56	267.36	0.35	133.4	0	0.099	0.173	0.752	0.036	0.187	1.349	25.44	0
18.76	10.36	0.568	4.48	29.4	33.04	208.32	0.21	57.68	0.056	0.109	0.067	0.613	0.016	0.045	0.235	24.64	0
23.94	22.26	0.903	10.08	54.6	55.44	233.1	0.395	85.68	0.084	0.22	0.136	0.907	0.031	0.134	0.605	31.08	0
11.36	24.85	1.136	10.65	76.68	69.58	319.5	0.497	24.85	0.071	0.135	0.185	1.42	0.028	0.121	0.241	42.6	0
60.42	24.38	0.938	7.95	47.17	43.99	187.62	0.286	7.95	2.067	0.139	0.117	1.056	0.023	0.048	0.18	24.91	0
29.9	61.1	1.17	20.8	71.5	61.75	235.95	0.565	5.85	1.105	0.143	0.156	1.495	0.068	0.136	0.533	53.95	0
142.24	70.56	1.322	16.8	119.84	131.04	377.44	0.683	222.9	0.336	0.129	0.298	0.895	0.066	0.381	2.251	48.16	0
0	2.09	0.61	2.85	14.25	14.06	91.77	0.093	0	0	0.103	0.065	0.774	0.006	0	0.015	16.72	0
4.26	10.65	0.298	6.39	23.43	105.79	190.99	0.135	4.26	1.207	0.028	0.018	0.234	0.033	0.156	1.008	19.88	0
0	16.96	0.653	62.08	125.44	201.92	150.4	1.04	0	0	0.04	0.036	4.38	0.144	0	2.454	29.44	0
0	15.04	0.602	56	105.92	176.64	160	0.938	0	0	0.027	0.034	4.289	0.145	0	2.454	23.68	0
0	15.309	0.641	49.896	101.493	186.543	1.701	0.938	0	0	0.124	0.028	3.834	0.073	0	1.965	41.11	0
0	15.309	0.641	49.896	101.493	186.543	230.486	0.938	0	0	0.124	0.028	3.834	0.073	0	2.211	41.11	0
0	26.082	1.298	47.628	106.596	199.868	5.103	0.927	0	0	0.181	0.038	3.421	0.099	0	2.362	68.04	0
0	9.18	0.581	13.94	32.64	99.45	49.98	0.255	0.17	0.272	0.025	0.028	0.177	0.021	0		15.81	0
0	5.32	0.342	9.94	24.64	31.92	53.06	0.256	0.28	0	0.025	0.009	0.081	0.028	0		11.62	0
0	41.04	4.292	90.63	266.76	475.38	410.4	2.206	1.71	0.684	0.345	0.094	0.846	0.171	0	0.479	355.7	0
16.8	40.8	3.408	103.2	230.4	427.2	840	2.496	0	0.48	0.151	0.12	1.034	0.108	0		122.4	0

EvaluEat Code	Food Name	Amt	Wt (g)	Energy (kcal)	Prot (g)	Carb (g)	Fiber (g)	Fat (g)	Mono (g)	Poly (g)	Sat (g)
16386	Peas, split, mature seed, boiled w/salt	1 cup	196	231.28	16.346	41.356	16.268	0.764	0.159	0.323	0.106
6962	Peppers, hot, chili, immature green, canned, chili sauce	.5 cup	125	25	0.875	6.25	2.375	0.125	0.085	0.015	0.016
6961	Peppers, hot, chili, mature red, canned, chili sauce	.5 cup	125	26.25	1.125	4.875	0.875	0.75	0.514	0.093	0.1
11339	Peppers, sweet, green, sauteed	1 oz	28.34	35.992	0.221	1.196	0.51	3.358	0.662	1.672	0.451
11921	Peppers, sweet, red, sauteed	1 oz	28.34	41.093	0.295	1.862	0.51	3.613	0.735	1.839	0.501
11942	Pickles, cucumber, fresh, (bread and butter pickles)	1 slice	7	5.39	0.063	1.253	0.105	0.014	0	0.006	0.004
18398	Pie crust, chocolate wafer cookie type, chilled	1 piece (1/8 of 9" crust)	28	141.68	1.428	15.232	0.42	8.708	4.124	2.16	1.885
18618	Pie crust, cookie type Nilla Wafer, ready to use/Nabisco	1 serving	28	143.64	0.98	17.668	0.252	7.588	5.236	0.378	1.442
18335	Pie crust, frozen, baked	1 piece (1/8 of 9" crust)	16	82.24	0.704	7.936	0.16	5.248	2.514	0.645	1.693
18399	Pie crust, graham cracker cookie type, chilled	1 piece (1/8 of 9" crust)	30	145.2	1.23	19.17	0.45	7.32	3.343	2.031	1.528
18336	Pie crust, homemade, baked	1 piece (1/8 of 9" crust)	23	121.21	1.472	10.925	0.391	7.958	3.489	2.098	1.983
18628	Pie, apple turnover, frozen, ready to bake/Pepperidge Farm	1 serving	89	283.91	3.738	31.239	1.602	16.02			4.032
18301	Pie, apple, enriched, commercially prep	1 piece (1/8 of 9" dia)	125	296.25	2.375	42.5	2	13.75	5.485	2.747	4.746
18304	Pie, banana cream, homemade	1 piece (1/8 of 9" dia)	144	387.36	6.336	47.376	1.008	19.584	8.235	4.74	5.412
18305	Pie, blueberry, commercially prep	1 piece (1/8 of 9" dia)	125	290	2.25	43.625	1.25	12.5	5.305	4.405	2.099
18308	Pie, cherry, commercially prep	1 piece (1/8 of 9" dia)	125	325	2.5	49.75	1	13.75	7.296	2.569	3.203
18310	Pie, chocolate creme, commercially prep	1 piece (1/4 of 6" pie)	99	300.96	2.574	33.264	1.98	19.206	11.006	2.374	4.918
18312	Pie, chocolate mousse, no bake mix	1 piece (1/8 of 9" dia)	95	247	3.325	28.12		14.63	4.83	0.773	7.785
18313	Pie, coconut creme, commercially prep	1 piece (1/6 of 7" pie)	64	190.72	1.344	23.808	0.832	10.624	4.646	0.988	4.465
18317	Pie, egg custard, commercially prep	1 piece (1/6 of 8" pie)	105	220.5	5.775	21.84	1.68	12.18	5.037	3.909	2.466
18320	Pie, lemon meringue, commercially prep	1 piece (1/6 of 8" pie)	113	302.84	1.695	53.336	1.356	9.831	3.034	4.122	1.996
18322	Pie, mince, homemade	1 piece (1/8 of 9" dia)	165	476.85	4.29	79.2	4.29	17.82	7.679	4.689	4.425
18323	Pie, peach	1 piece (1/6 of 8" pie)	117	260.91	2.223	38.493	0.936	11.7	4.962	4.386	1.764
18324	Pie, pecan, commercially prep	1 piece (1/6 of 8" pie)	113	452	4.52	64.636	3.955	20.905	12.137	3.596	4.006
18326	Pie, pumpkin, commercially prep	1 piece (1/6 of 8" pie)	109	228.9	4.251	29.757	2.943	10.355	4.395	3.434	1.946
18328	Pie, vanilla creme, homemade	1 piece (1/8 of 9" dia)	126	350.28	6.048	41.076	0.756	18.144	7.614	4.332	5.078
22531	Pizza Rolls Pizza Snacks, hamburger, frozen/Totinos	1 serving	85	231.2	9.35	26.435		9.775			

Chol (g)	Calc (mg)	Iron (mg)	Mag (mg)	Phos (mg)	Pota (mg)	Sodi (mg)	Zinc (mg)	Vit A (RAE)	Vit C (mg)	Thia (mg)	Ribo (mg)	Niac (mg)	Vit B$_6$ (mg)	Vit B$_{12}$ (µg)	Vit E (mg)	Fol (µg)	Alc (g)
0	27.44	2.528	70.56	194.04	709.52	466.48	1.96	0	0.784	0.372	0.11	1.744	0.094	0	0.059	127.4	0
0	6.25	0.5	15	17.5	705	31.25	0.188	36.25	85	0.037	0.037	0.875	0.175	0	0.425	15	0
0	11.25	0.625	15	20	705	31.25	0.188	28.75	37.5	0.012	0.113	0.75	0.175	0	0.45	13.75	0
0	2.267	0.085	2.267	4.251	37.976	4.818	0.017	3.968	50.16	0.012	0.014	0.165	0.056	0	0.397	0.567	
	1.984	0.133	3.401	6.518	54.696	5.951	0.043	39.11	46.14	0.016	0.031	0.27	0.103	0	0.876	0.567	0
0	2.24	0.028	0.14	1.89	14	47.11	0.003	0.49	0.63	0	0.002	0	0.001	0	0.011	0.28	0
0.28	8.4	0.84	11.2	29.4	47.04	188.16	0.23	59.08	0	0.043	0.058	0.599	0.001	0.006	0.792	14.84	0
2.8	11.48	0.496	2.24	23.24	19.32	62.72	0.078			0.046	0.054	0.696	0.006	0.031		8.4	0
0	3.36	0.362	2.88	9.44	17.6	103.52	0.054	0	0	0.045	0.061	0.39	0.011	0.003	0.421	8.8	0
0	6	0.636	5.4	19.2	25.8	168	0.138	57.3	0	0.031	0.052	0.627	0.011	0.006	0.684	10.2	0
0	2.3	0.665	3.22	15.41	15.41	124.66	0.101	0	0	0.09	0.064	0.761	0.006	0	0.071	15.41	0
		1.219				176.22											0
0	13.75	0.563	8.75	30	81.25	332.5	0.2	40	4	0.035	0.034	0.329	0.047	0.012	1.9	33.75	0
73.44	108	1.498	23.04	132.48	237.6	345.6	0.691	87.84	2.304	0.2	0.298	1.518	0.192	0.36	0.576	38.88	0
0	10	0.375	6.25	28.75	62.5	406.25	0.2	55	3.375	0.012	0.037	0.375	0.046	0.012	1.3	33.75	0
0	15	0.6	10	36.25	101.25	307.5	0.225	65	1.125	0.029	0.036	0.25	0.051	0.012	0.95	33.75	0
4.95	35.64	1.059	20.79	67.32	125.73	134.64	0.228	0	0	0.036	0.106	0.671	0.02	0.01	2.707	12.87	0
33.25	73.15	1.026	30.4	219.45	270.75	437	0.57	117.8	0.475	0.048	0.14	0.565	0.028	0.199		24.7	0
0	18.56	0.512	12.8	54.4	41.6	163.2	0.301	17.28	0	0.032	0.051	0.128	0.044	0.077	0.096	4.48	0
34.65	84	0.609	11.55	117.6	111.3	252	0.546	59.85	0.63	0.041	0.218	0.307	0.05	0.451	0.987	21	0
50.85	63.28	0.689	16.95	118.65	100.57	164.98	0.554	57.63	3.616	0.07	0.236	0.733	0.034	0.192	1.198	27.12	0
0	36.3	2.458	23.1	69.3	334.95	419.1	0.363	1.65	9.735	0.248	0.173	1.962	0.107	0	0.248	37.95	0
0	9.36	0.585	7.02	25.74	146.25	315.9	0.105	11.7	1.053	0.071	0.039	0.234	0.027	0	1.1	33.93	0
36.16	19.21	1.175	20.34	87.01	83.62	479.12	0.644	57.63	1.243	0.103	0.138	0.281	0.024	0.113	0.362	38.42	0
21.8	65.4	0.861	16.35	77.39	167.86	307.38	0.491	488.3	1.09	0.06	0.167	0.204	0.062	0.283	1.123	26.16	0
78.12	113.4	1.285	16.38	131.04	158.76	327.6	0.668	104.6	0.63	0.175	0.272	1.24	0.062	0.378	0.567	32.76	0
						417.35											0

EvaluEat Code	Food Name	Amt	Wt (g)	Energy (kcal)	Prot (g)	Carb (g)	Fiber (g)	Fat (g)	Mono (g)	Poly (g)	Sat (g)
22533	Pizza Rolls Pizza Snacks, pepperoni, frozen/Totinos	1 serving	141	384.93	14.382	39.48	2.256	18.894	9.236	2.214	4.991
22554	Pizza, deluxe French bread w/sausage, pepperoni & mushroom, frozen/Stouffer's	1 serving	175	428.75	16.1	44.45	3.5	20.65	8.715	2.52	6.37
22542	Pizza, deluxe w/sausage, green & red pepper & mushrooms, frozen/Celeste	1 serving	167	385.77	16.7	33.233		20.708	7.615	2.421	8.116
22556	Pizza, original pepperoni, frozen, 12"/Tombstone	1 serving	113	311.88	14.464	28.25		15.707	5.311	2.045	6
22557	Pizza, original sausage & mushroom, frozen/Tombstone	1 serving	132	306.24	14.388	31.152		13.728	4.435	2.086	5.069
22903	Pizza, pepperoni, frozen	1 serving	146	400.04	16.191	36.208	2.336	21.112	8.439	2.438	7.066
22902	Pizza, sausage & pepperoni, frozen	1 serving	146	385.44	15.768	36.179	2.336	19.695	7.796	2.599	6.336
22598	Pizza, supreme, sausage, mushrooms, pepperoni, frozen/Red Baron	1 serving	136	344.08	13.6	31.824		18.088	7.167	2.475	6.093
43572	Popcorn, microwave, low-fat and sodium	1 cup	148	634.92	18.648	108.62	21.016	14.06	6.046	5.287	2.094
19436	Popcorn, sugar syrup/caramel, fat-free	1 bag (6 oz)	170	647.7	3.4	153.1	4.25	2.38	0.442	1.078	0.34
10193	Pork back rib, fresh, lean & fat, roasted	1 piece, cooked (yield from 1 lb raw meat)	219	810.3	53.129	0	0	64.78	29.477	5.081	24.068
10857	Pork bacon, Canadian style / Hormel	1 serving	56	68.32	9.453	1.047		2.766	1.394	0.347	1.025
10124	Pork bacon, cured, broiled, pan-fried, or roasted	1 slice, cooked	8	43.28	2.963	0.114	0	3.342	1.482	0.364	1.099
10188	Pork composite (leg/loin/shoulder/sparerib) fresh, lean & fat, cooked	3 oz	85	232.05	23.434	0	0	14.603	6.494	1.233	5.287
10227	Pork composite (loin & shoulder blade) fresh, lean & fat, cooked	3 oz	85	214.2	23.613	0	0	12.546	5.568	1.003	4.505
10134	Pork ham, cured, boneless, extra lean (5% fat) roasted	3 oz	85	123.25	17.791	1.275	0	4.701	2.227	0.459	1.538
10136	Pork ham, cured, boneless, regular fat (11% fat) roasted	3 oz	85	151.3	19.227	0	0	7.667	3.774	1.199	2.652
7953	Pork sausage, pre-cooked	1 serving (1 hot dog)	52	196.56	7.535	0	0	18.221	7.888	2.532	6.064
10863	Pork, fresh, variety meats and by-products, stomach, cooked, simmered	1 serving	56	84.56	11.984	0.05	0	4.066	1.191	0.413	1.674
10220	Pork, ground, fresh, cooked	3 oz	85	252.45	21.837	0	0	17.655	7.863	1.59	6.562
10173	Pork, pig's feet, fresh, simmered	3 oz	85	197.2	18.649	0	0	13.642	6.804	1.309	3.692
19823	Potato chips, without salt, reduced fat	1 cup	146	711.02	10.366	98.988	8.906	30.368	7.008	15.972	6.074
11358	Potatoes, red, flesh and skin, baked	1 potato, large (3" to 4-1/4" dia)	299	266.11	6.877	58.574	5.382	0.449	0.006	0.129	0.078
11356	Potatoes, russet, flesh and skin, baked	1 potato, large	299	290.03	7.864	64.106	6.877	0.389	0.006	0.129	
43109	Pretzels, soft	1 cup	186	628.68	15.252	129.07	3.162	5.766	1.992	1.763	1.293
19311	Pudding, banana, ready-to-eat	1 can (5 oz)	142	180.34	3.408	30.104	0.142	5.112	2.173	1.889	0.795
19183	Pudding, chocolate, ready-to-eat	1 can (5 oz)	142	197.38	3.834	32.66	1.42	5.68	2.414	2.031	1.008
19187	Pudding, flan (caramel custard) dry mix	1 portion, amount to make 1/2 cup	21	73.08	0	19.236	0	0	0	0	0
19289	Pudding, Kraft, JELL-O fat-free Pudding Snacks, vanilla, ready-to-eat	1 NLEA serving	113	103.96	2.373	23.165	0.113	0.226			0.226
19276	Pudding, Kraft, JELL-O fat-free Sugar Free Instant, vanilla, asp & ace, powder	1 NLEA serving	8	26.48	0.064	6.232	0.104	0.072			0.008
19277	Pudding, Kraft, JELL-O Sugar Free Cook & Serve, chocolate, asp & ace, powder	1 NLEA serving	10	31	0.61	7.45	0.93	0.3			0.16
19193	Pudding, rice, ready-to-eat	1 can (5 oz)	142	231.46	2.84	31.24	0.142	10.65	4.558	3.962	1.661

Chol (g)	Calc (mg)	Iron (mg)	Mag (mg)	Phos (mg)	Pota (mg)	Sodi (mg)	Zinc (mg)	Vit A (RAE)	Vit C (mg)	Thia (mg)	Ribo (mg)	Niac (mg)	Vit B6 (mg)	Vit B12 (µg)	Vit E (mg)	Fol (µg)	Alc (g)
31.02	102.93					865.74											0
33.25	231	2.712				840			29.93								0
36.74	280.56					764.86											0
31.64	202.27					551.44											0
26.4	200.64					718.08											0
33.58	0	2.613	24.82	221.92	221.92	878.92	1.781	45.26	1.752	0.371	0.352	3.616	0.105	0.058	1.644	54.02	0
30.66	191.26	2.774	26.28	207.32	255.5	854.1	1.606	64.24	3.212	0.372	0.329	3.631	0.098	0.35	1.407	51.1	0
23.12	223.04	2.285				738.48											0
0	16.28	3.374	223.48	390.72	356.68	725.2	5.668	10.36	0	0.518	0.163	3.064	0.252	0	7.415	25.16	0
0	30.6	1.36	45.9	93.5	187	486.2	1.054	3.4	0	0.065	0.099	0.581	0.08	0	0.221	6.8	0
258.42	98.55	3.022	45.99	427.05	689.85	221.19	7.38	6.57	0.657	0.935	0.438	7.774	0.672	1.402		6.57	0
27.44	3.36	0.504	10.64		156.24	568.96	1.008		0.784								0
8.8	0.88	0.115	2.64	42.64	45.2	184.8	0.28	0.88	0	0.032	0.021	0.888	0.028	0.098	0.025	0.16	0
77.35	21.25	0.935	20.4	197.2	300.9	52.7	2.465	1.7	0.255	0.655	0.279	4.187	0.335	0.655	0.17	5.1	0
73.1	20.4	0.842	20.4	192.95	307.7	48.45	2.227	1.7	0.255	0.722	0.275	4.216	0.343	0.629	0.204	5.1	0
45.05	6.8	1.258	11.9	166.6	243.95	1022.55	2.448	0	0	0.641	0.172	3.42	0.34	0.553	0.213	2.55	0
50.15	6.8	1.139	18.7	238.85	347.65	1275	2.1	0	0	0.621	0.281	5.228	0.264	0.595	0.264	2.55	0
38.48	71.24	0.478	6.76	143	159.64	391.04	0.78	9.88	0.364	0.108	0.081	2.106	0.077	0.369	0.276	0.52	0
176.96	8.4	0.689	8.4	72.24	47.6	22.4	1.635	0	0	0.022	0.105	0.773	0.012	0.269	0.05	1.68	0
79.9	18.7	1.097	20.4	192.1	307.7	62.05	2.729	1.7	0.595	0.6	0.187	3.575	0.332	0.459	0.178	5.1	0
90.95	0	0.833	4.25	69.7	28.05	62.05	0.892	0	0	0.014	0.048	0.497	0.032	0.349	0.077	1.7	0
0	30.66	1.971	129.94	281.78	2546.24	11.68	1.475	0	37.52	0.307	0.394	10.22	0.978	0	7.986	14.6	0
0	26.91	2.093	83.72	215.28	1629.55	23.92	1.196	2.99	37.67	0.215	0.149	4.769	0.634	0	0.12	80.73	0
0	53.82	3.199	89.7	212.29	1644.5	23.92	1.046	2.99	38.57	0.2	0.144	4.031	1.058	0	0.12	32.89	0
5.58	42.78	7.291	39.06	146.94	163.68	2611.44	1.748	0	0	0.763	0.539	7.942	0.037	0	1.004	44.64	0
0	120.7	0.185	11.36	97.98	156.2	278.32	0.398	8.52	0.71	0.028	0.209	0.231	0.03	0.256		2.84	0
4.26	127.8	0.724	29.82	113.6	255.6	183.18	0.596	14.2	2.556	0.037	0.22	0.493	0.04	0	0.412	4.26	0
0	5.04	0.017	0	0.21	32.13	90.72	0.008	0	0	0	0	0	0	0		0	0
2.26	85.88	0.045		115.26	123.17	240.69			0.339								0
0	11.76	0.006		189.44	2.48	332.32			0								0
0	6.9	1.183		21.2	139	108.5			0								0
1.42	73.84	0.426	11.36	96.56	85.2	120.7	0.696	35.5	0.71	0.026	0.102	0.229	0.041	0.298	1.954	4.26	0

EvaluEat Code	Food Name	Amt	Wt (g)	Energy (kcal)	Prot (g)	Carb (g)	Fiber (g)	Fat (g)	Mono (g)	Poly (g)	Sat (g)
19218	Pudding, tapioca, ready-to-eat	1 can (5 oz)	142	168.98	2.84	27.548	0.142	5.254	2.244	1.931	0.852
19201	Pudding, vanilla, ready-to-eat	4 oz	113	145.77	2.599	24.747	0	4.068	1.74	1.514	0.644
43282	Quail, cooked, total edible	1 cup	186	435.24	46.686	0	0	26.226	9.097	6.486	7.356
14342	Rice beverage, Rice Dream, canned/Imagine Foods	1 cup	245	120.05	0.417	24.843	0	1.985	1.345	0.309	0.167
18344	Roll, dinner, egg	1 roll (2-1/2" dia)	35	107.45	3.325	18.2	1.295	2.24	1.026	0.395	0.552
18396	Roll, dinner, plain, homemade w/reduced fat (2%) milk	1 roll (2-1/2" dia)	35	110.6	2.975	18.69	0.665	2.555	1.008	0.702	0.628
18347	Roll, dinner, wheat	1 roll (1 oz)	28	76.44	2.408	12.88	1.064	1.764	0.871	0.31	0.419
18349	Roll, french	1 roll	38	105.26	3.268	19.076	1.216	1.634	0.745	0.317	0.366
18350	Roll, hamburger/hot dog, plain	1 roll	43	119.97	4.085	21.264	0.903	1.862	0.478	0.846	0.47
18348	Roll, hamburger/hot dog, whole wheat	1 medium (2-1/2" dia)	36	95.76	3.132	18.396	2.7	1.692	0.432	0.778	0.301
18353	Roll, hard/kaiser	1 roll (3-1/2" dia)	57	167.01	5.643	30.039	1.311	2.451	0.646	0.98	0.345
4017	Salad dressing, 1000 Island, regular, w/salt	1 tbsp	16	59.2	0.174	2.342	0.128	5.61	1.261	2.915	0.815
4635	Salad dressing, 1000 Island dressing, fat-free	1 tbsp	14.6	19.272	0.08	4.273	0.482	0.212	0.05	0.092	0.029
4539	Salad dressing, blue/roquefort cheese, regular w/salt	1 tbsp	15	75.6	0.72	1.11	0	7.845	1.845	4.17	1.485
4367	Salad dressing, French dressing, fat-free	1 tbsp	14	18.48	0.028	4.5	0.308	0.038	0.02	0.009	0.005
4142	Salad dressing, French, low-fat, no salt, diet (5 kcal/tsp)	1 tbsp	16	37.28	0.093	4.685	0.176	2.154	0.944	0.805	0.176
4120	Salad dressing, French, regular w/salt	1 tbsp	16	73.12	0.123	2.493	0	7.17	1.349	3.365	0.904
4636	Salad dressing, Italian dressing, fat-free	1 tbsp	14.6	6.862	0.142	1.278	0.088	0.127	0.034	0.028	0.043
4114	Salad dressing, Italian, regular w/salt	1 tbsp	14.7	42.777	0.056	1.533	0	4.17	0.928	1.902	0.658
4641	Salad dressing, mayonnaise, light	1 tbsp	14.6	47.304	0.128	1.197	0	4.831	1.178	2.621	0.761
4026	Salad dressing, mayonnaise, regular, safflower/soybean oil, w/salt	1 tbsp	13.8	98.946	0.152	0.373	0	10.957	1.794	7.59	1.187
4012	Salad dressing, Miracle Whip Light Dressing / Kraft	1 tbsp	16	36.96	0.096	2.304	0.016	2.976			0.464
4638	Salad dressing, ranch dressing, fat-free	1 tbsp	14.6	17.374	0.036	3.87	0.015	0.28	0.065	0.117	0.075
4640	Salad dressing, ranch dressing, reduced fat	1 tbsp	14.6	32.85	0.15	2.365	0.131	2.526	0.792	0.633	0.194
4015	Salad dressing, Russian w/salt	1 tbsp	15	74.1	0.24	1.56	0	7.62	1.77	4.41	1.095
4016	Salad dressing, sesame seed	1 tbsp	15	66.45	0.465	1.29	0.15	6.78	1.785	3.765	0.93
4135	Salad dressing, vinegar & oil, homemade	1 tbsp	16	71.84	0	0.4	0	8.016	2.368	3.856	1.456
22534	Sandwich, Hot Pockets, beef & cheddar stuffed, frozen	1 serving	142	403.28	16.33	39.192		20.164	6.658	1.221	8.804
22535	Sandwich, Hot Pockets, Croissant Pocket w/chicken, broccoli, & cheddar, frozen	1 serving	128	300.8	11.392	38.912	1.408	11.008	4.378	1.664	3.354
22538	Sandwich, Lean Pockets, glazed chicken supreme stuffed, frozen	1 serving	128	232.96	9.856	34.176		6.272	2.483	0.952	1.92
22364	Sandwich, Sausage Biscuits, breakfast sandwich, frozen/Jimmy Dean	1	48	192.48	4.752	11.568	0.72	14.112			4.306
6140	Sauce, Bulls Eye Original Barbecue/Ridgs	2 tbsp	36	63	0.432	15.156		0.072			
6930	Sauce, cheese, ready-to-eat	.25 cup	63	109.62	4.227	4.303	0.315	8.373	2.408	1.637	3.786
6139	Sauce, Chunky Chili Dip, Salsa, canned/LaVictoria	2 tbsp	30	9.3	0.237	1.962	0.15	0.048			
6901	Sauce, Deluxe Marinara Sauce/Contadina	1 cup	250	145	3.05	17.375	3	7.05	3.428	2.06	1.1
6275	Sauce, Enchilada Sauce/LaVictoria	.25 cup	60	19.8	0.192	2.772	0.42	0.87			
6179	Sauce, fish, ready-to-eat	1 tbsp	18	6.3	0.911	0.655	0	0.002	0	0.001	0.001
6269	Sauce, Green Chile Salsa, mild/LaVictoria	2 tbsp	30	7.5	0.39	1.29	0.12	0.075			
6273	Sauce, Green Salsa Jalapena/LaVictoria	2 tbsp	30	9.6	0.276	1.41	0.27	0.327			
6260	Sauce, Green Taco Sauce, medium/LaVictoria	1 tbsp	15	4.5	0.119	0.873	0.09	0.054			

Chol (g)	Calc (mg)	Iron (mg)	Mag (mg)	Phos (mg)	Pota (mg)	Sodi (mg)	Zinc (mg)	Vit A (RAE)	Vit C (mg)	Thia (mg)	Ribo (mg)	Niac (mg)	Vit B_6 (mg)	Vit B_{12} (µg)	Vit E (mg)	Fol (µg)	Alc (g)
1.42	119.28	0.327	11.36	112.18	136.32	225.78	0.383	0	0.568	0.031	0.139	0.443	0.027	0.298	0.426	4.26	0
7.91	99.44	0.147	9.04	76.84	127.69	152.55	0.282	6.78	0	0.025	0.157	0.285	0.012	0.113	0	0	0
159.96	27.9	8.24	40.92	518.94	401.76	96.72	5.766	130.2	4.278	0.409	0.558	14.731	1.153	0.67	1.302	11.16	0
0	19.6	0.196	9.8	34.3	68.6	85.75	0.245	0	1.225	0.076	0.012	1.909	0.044	0	1.764	90.65	0
17.5	20.65	1.232	8.75	35.35	36.4	190.75	0.392	1.75	0	0.184	0.181	1.15	0.019	0.084	0.126	64.4	0
12.25	21	1.036	6.65	44.1	53.2	145.25	0.245	30.45	0.07	0.138	0.143	1.207	0.021	0.049	0.339	31.5	0
0	49.28	0.994	10.08	29.12	32.2	95.2	0.252	0	0	0.121	0.076	1.14	0.021	0	0.101	16.8	0
0	34.58	1.03	7.6	31.92	43.32	231.42	0.342	0	0	0.199	0.114	1.654	0.015	0	0.114	42.94	0
0	59.34	1.428	9.03	26.66	40.42	205.97	0.284	0	0	0.172	0.137	1.786	0.031	0.086	0.03	47.73	0
0	38.16	0.871	30.6	80.64	97.92	172.08	0.724	0	0	0.089	0.055	1.324	0.07	0	0.324	10.8	0
0	54.15	1.87	15.39	57	61.56	310.08	0.536	0	0	0.272	0.192	2.416	0.02	0	0.239	54.15	0
4.16	2.72	0.189	1.28	4.32	17.12	138.08	0.042	1.76	0	0.231	0.009	0.067	0	0	0.182	0	0
0.73	1.606	0.041	0.584	0.146	17.812	106.434	0.013	0.146	0	0.034	0.007	0.038	0	0	0.109	1.752	0
2.55	12.15	0.03	0	11.1	5.55	164.1	0.041	10.05	0.3	0.002	0.015	0.015	0.006	0.041	0.9	4.2	0
0	0.7	0.081	0.42	0	11.76	111.86	0.014	0.56	0	0.002	0.004	0.016	0	0	0.003	1.96	0
0	1.76	0.139	1.28	2.56	17.12	4.8	0.032	4.32	0	0.004	0.008	0.075	0.009	0	0.458	0.32	0
0	3.84	0.128	0.8	3.04	10.72	133.76	0.046	3.68	0	0.003	0.008	0.03	0	0.022	0.8	0	0
0.292	4.38	0.058	0.73	15.914	14.892	164.834	0.053	0.584	0.058	0.005	0.008	0.02	0	0.045	0.111	1.752	0
0	1.029	0.093	0.441	1.323	7.056	243.138	0.019	0.294	0	0.002	0.003	0	0.009	0	0.735	0	0
5.11	1.168	0.047	0.292	5.11	5.84	98.258	0.026	3.066	0	0.003	0	0	0	0	0.448	0.584	0
8.142	2.484	0.069	0.138	3.864	4.692	78.384	0.017	11.59	0	0	0	0.001	0.08	0.036	3.036	1.104	0
4.16	0.8	0.027		2.08	3.68	131.36			0						0.14		0
1.022	7.3	0.153	1.168	16.498	16.206	110.23	0.058	0.146	0	0.004	0.004	0.001	0.004	0	0.026	0.876	0
3.066	18.25	0.127	0.876	28.178	19.272	136.072	0.091	2.628	0.102	0.003	0.004	0.001	0.004	0	0.234	0.584	0
2.7	2.85	0.09	0.3	5.55	23.55	130.2	0.065	2.25	0.9	0.008	0.008	0.09	0.005	0.045	0.603	1.5	0
0	2.85	0.09	0	5.55	23.55	150	0.015	0.3	0	0	0	0	0	0	0.75	0	0
0	0	0	0	0	1.28	0.16	0	0	0	0	0	0	0	0	0.738	0	0
52.54	336.54	2.925				905.96											0
37.12		3.802				651.52			6.272								0
23.04	121.6					561.92											0
15.84	37.92	0.792				440.64											0
						301.68											0
18.27	115.92	0.132	5.67	98.91	18.9	521.64	0.617	50.4	0.252	0.004	0.072	0.015	0.011	0.088	0.2	2.52	0
	4.2	0.012				147.9			3.15								0
0	47.5	1.5	30	65	517.5	937.5	0.325		17.5	0.108	0.08	1.43	0.21	0	0	22.5	0
0	7.2	0.072				394.8			2.64								0
0	7.74	0.14	31.5	1.26	51.84	1389.6	0.036	0.72	0.09	0.002	0.01	0.416	0.071	0.086	0	9.18	0
	4.5	0.273				172.2			4.02								0
0	4.8	0.12				180			3.6								0
0	1.2	0.008				95.1			0.72								0

EvaluEat Code	Food Name	Amt	Wt (g)	Energy (kcal)	Prot (g)	Carb (g)	Fiber (g)	Fat (g)	Mono (g)	Poly (g)	Sat (g)
6175	Sauce, hoisin	1 tbsp	16	35.2	0.53	7.053	0.448	0.542	0.154	0.272	0.091
6555	Sauce, hollandaise, with butterfat, dehydrated, prepared with water	1 cup (8 fl. oz.)	244	224.48	4.441	12.956	0.732	18.593	5.588	0.878	10.931
6308	Sauce, Kraft Barbecue Sauce Hickory Smoke	2 tbsp	34	39.44	0.17	8.908	0.306	0.102			0
6307	Sauce, Kraft Barbecue Sauce Original	2 tbsp	34	39.44	0.17	8.874	0.306	0.102			0
6136	Sauce, mole poblano, homemade	1 cup, sauce	242	396.88	8.567	31.315	10.164	26.499			
6278	Sauce, Nacho Cheese Sauce with Jalapeno Pepper, medium/LaVictoria	.25 cup	72	122.4	1.31	7.387	0.216	9.713	4.553	1.788	2.692
6933	Sauce, Old World Style Smooth Pasta Sauce, Traditional, jar/Ragu	.5 cup	125	80	1.875	12.112	2.625	2.625	0.546	1.29	0.362
6176	Sauce, oyster	1 tbsp	18	9.18	0.243	1.966	0.054	0.045	0.013	0.012	0.008
6931	Sauce, pasta, spaghetti/marinara	1 cup	250	142.5	3.55	20.55	4	5.15	2.175	1.805	0.737
6168	Sauce, pepper or hot	1 tsp	4.7	0.517	0.024	0.082	0.014	0.017	0.001	0.009	0.002
6151	Sauce, plum	1 tbsp	19	34.96	0.169	8.134	0.133	0.198	0.046	0.112	0.029
6274	Sauce, Red Salsa Jalapena/LaVictoria	2 tbsp	30	12	0.435	2.172	0.39	0.177			
6257	Sauce, Red Taco Sauce, mild/LaVictoria	1 tbsp	16	6.72	0.214	1.314	0.08	0.067			
6265	Sauce, Salsa Picante, mild/LaVictoria	2 tbsp	30	8.1	0.357	1.446	0.09	0.087			
6164	Sauce, salsa	1 cup	259	72.52	3.289	16.162	4.144	0.622	0.065	0.298	0.078
6132	Sauce, Sweet N' Sour, ready-to-eat/Nestle Chef-Mate	1 serving	33	40.26	0.158	8.181	0.264	0.785	0.229	0.377	0.122
6133	Sauce, Szechuan, ready-to-eat/Nestle Chef-Mate	1 tbsp	16	20.8	0.23	2.922	0.048	0.912	0.264	0.439	0.119
6112	Sauce, teriyaki	1 tbsp	18	15.12	1.067	2.871	0.018	0	0	0	0
6166	Sauce, white, medium, homemade	1 cup	250	367.5	9.6	22.925	0.5	26.575	11.05	7.155	7.135
6971	Sauce, worcestershire	.5 cup	125	83.75	0	24.325	0	0	0	0	0
7002	Sausage, beerwurst, beer salami (beef)	2 oz (1 slice)	56	154.56	7.84	2.106	0.504	12.617	5.659	1.165	4.725
7005	Sausage, blood	1 slice	25	94.5	3.65	0.322	0	8.625	3.975	0.865	3.35
7013	Sausage, bratwurst (pork) cooked	1 link cooked	85	281.35	11.662	2.074	0	24.803	12.495	2.244	8.6
7019	Sausage, chorizo (pork & beef)	1 link (4" long)	60	273	14.46	1.116	0	22.962	11.04	2.076	8.628
7023	Sausage, frankfurter (wiener) (beef & pork)	1 frankfurter (5 in long x 3/4 in dia, 10 per lb)	45	137.25	5.188	0.774	1.08	12.438	6.151	1.229	4.846
7022	Sausage, frankfurter (wiener) (beef)	1 frankfurter	45	148.5	5.058	1.827	0	13.306	6.437	0.532	5.26
7024	Sausage, frankfurter (wiener) (chicken)	1 frankfurter	45	115.65	5.819	3.055	0	8.766	3.816	1.818	2.493
7025	Sausage, frankfurter (wiener) (turkey)	1 frankfurter	45	101.7	6.426	0.67	0	7.965	2.511	2.25	2.65
7089	Sausage, Italian, (pork) cooked	1 link, 4/lb	83	268.09	16.625	1.245	0	21.331	9.918	2.731	7.528
7037	Sausage, kielbasa (kolbassy) (pork, beef & NFD Milk)	1 oz	28.35	87.885	3.759	0.607	0	7.697	3.668	0.873	2.809
7038	Sausage, knockwurst (knackwurst) (pork & beef)	1 link	72	221.04	7.992	2.304	0	19.944	9.223	2.102	7.351
7057	Sausage, pepperoni (pork & beef)	1 serving, 15 slices	29	135.14	5.901	1.172	0.435	11.681	5.523	0.764	4.667
7059	Sausage, Polish (pork)	1 sausage (10" long x 1-1/4" dia)	227	740.02	32.007	3.7	0	65.194	30.69	6.992	23.449
7919	Sausage, turkey, breakfast links, mild	1 serving	56	131.6	8.635	0.874	0	10.13	2.801	1.85	4.002
16107	Sausage, vegetarian, meatless	1 link	25	64.25	4.633	2.46	0.7	4.54	1.125	2.32	0.732
12220	Seeds, flax seed	1 tbsp	12	59.04	2.34	4.11	3.348	4.08	0.824	2.693	0.384
12016	Seeds, pumpkin/squash kernels, roasted w/o salt	1 oz	28.35	147.99	9.347	3.807	1.106	11.944	3.714	5.445	2.259
12166	Seeds, sesame, tahini made w/roasted & toasted kernels	1 tbsp	15	89.25	2.55	3.179	1.395	8.064	3.045	3.535	1.129

Chol (g)	Calc (mg)	Iron (mg)	Mag (mg)	Phos (mg)	Pota (mg)	Sodi (mg)	Zinc (mg)	Vit A (RAE)	Vit C (mg)	Thia (mg)	Ribo (mg)	Niac (mg)	Vit B6 (mg)	Vit B12 (µg)	Vit E (mg)	Fol (µg)	Alc (g)
0.48	5.12	0.162	3.84	6.08	19.04	258.4	0.051	0	0.064	0.001	0.035	0.187	0.01	0	0.045	3.68	0
48.8	117.12	0.854	7.32	119.56	117.12	1473.76	0.732	144	0.244	0.049	0.171	0.054	0.488	0.732	0.683	12.2	0
0	5.1	0.211		3.06	27.54	417.52			0.068								0
0	5.1	0.211		3.06	27.54	424.32			0.068								0
	58.08	4.477	77.44	198.44	788.92	324.28	1.113	363	0	0.053	0	3.969	0.607			67.76	0
3.6	64.08	0.864				550.8			1.152								0
		1.025				756.25											0
0	5.76	0.032	0.72	3.96	9.72	491.94	0.016	0	0.018	0.002	0.022	0.265	0.003	0.074	0	2.7	0
0	55	1.8	42.5	80	737.5	1030	0.425	92.5	20	0.135	0.1	2.655	0.285	0	5.1	27.5	0
0	0.376	0.023	0.235	0.517	6.768	124.221	0.005	0.376	3.516	0.002	0.004	0.012	0.007	0	0.006	0.282	0
0	2.28	0.272	2.28	4.18	49.21	102.22	0.036	0.38	0.095	0.003	0.016	0.193	0.015	0	0.037	1.14	0
0	6.3	0.051				146.1			9.63								0
0	3.36	0.029				104.8			2.864								0
0	4.5	0.033				178.8			1.83								0
0	77.7	2.512	33.67	67.34	551.67	1124.06	0.647	88.06	36	0.104	0.083	2.15	0.311	0	3.056	41.44	0
0	5.94	0.281	2.31	2.97	21.78	116.49	0.026		0	0.009	0.005	0.066	0.015	0	0.066	0.66	0
0	1.76	0.12	1.6	5.92	12.8	218.08	0.019		0.256	0.002	0.005	0.096	0.008	0.118	0.069	0.64	0
0	4.5	0.306	10.98	27.72	40.5	689.94	0.018	0	0	0.005	0.013	0.229	0.018	0	0	3.6	0
17.5	295	0.825	35	245	390	885	1.025	225	2	0.172	0.463	1.005	0.1	0.7	0.7	20	0
0	133.75	6.625	16.25	75	1000	1225	0.237	6.25	16.25	0.087	0.162	0.875	0	0	0.1	10	0
34.72	15.12	0.969	10.64	75.6	136.64	409.92	1.238	0	0.336	0.138	0.097	1.666	0.129	0.65	0.106	2.8	0
30	1.5	1.6	2	5.5	9.5	170	0.325	0	0	0.018	0.032	0.3	0.01	0.25	0.032	1.25	0
62.9	23.8	0.45	17.85	191.25	220.15	719.1	2.117	0	0	0.531	0.221	3.94	0.348	0.68	0.017	2.55	0
52.8	4.8	0.954	10.8	90	238.8	741	2.046	0	0	0.378	0.18	3.079	0.318	1.2	0.132	1.2	0
22.5	4.95	0.517	4.5	38.7	75.15	504	0.828	8.1	0	0.09	0.054	1.185	0.058	0.585	0.112	1.8	0
23.85	6.3	0.679	6.3	72	70.2	513	1.107	0	0	0.018	0.066	1.067	0.04	0.774	0.09	2.25	0
45.45	42.75	0.9	4.5	48.15	37.8	616.5	0.468	17.55	0	0.03	0.052	1.39	0.144	0.108	0.099	1.8	0
48.15	47.7	0.828	6.3	60.3	80.55	641.7	1.399	0	0	0.018	0.081	1.859	0.104	0.126	0.279	3.6	0
64.74	19.92	1.245	14.94	141.1	252.32	765.26	1.984	0	1.66	0.517	0.193	3.457	0.274	1.079	0.207	4.15	0
18.995	12.474	0.411	4.536	41.958	76.829	305.046	0.573	0	0	0.065	0.061	0.816	0.051	0.456	0.062	1.418	0
43.2	7.92	0.475	7.92	70.56	143.28	669.6	1.195	0	0	0.246	0.101	1.968	0.122	0.85	0.41	1.44	0
34.22	6.09	0.418	5.22	51.04	91.35	518.52	0.792	0	0.203	0.154	0.067	1.571	0.113	0.455	0.084	1.74	0
158.9	27.24	3.269	31.78	308.72	537.99	1988.52	4.381	0	2.27	1.14	0.336	7.816	0.431	2.225		4.54	0
33.6	17.92	0.599	14	103.6	110.32	327.6	1.193	0	17.02	0.04	0.097	2.058	0.213	0.241	0.186	4.48	0
0	15.75	0.93	9	56.25	57.75	222	0.365	0	0	0.586	0.101	2.799	0.207	0	0.525	6.5	0
0	23.88	0.746	43.44	59.76	81.72	4.08	0.5	0	0.156	0.02	0.019	0.168	0.111	0	0.038	33.36	0
0	12.191	4.235	151.389	332.262	228.501	5.103	2.109	5.387	0.51	0.06	0.09	0.494	0.026	0	0	16.16	0
0	63.9	1.342	14.25	109.8	62.1	17.25	0.693	0.45	0	0.183	0.071	0.817	0.022	0	0.038	14.7	0

EvaluEat Code	Food Name	Amt	Wt (g)	Energy (kcal)	Prot (g)	Carb (g)	Fiber (g)	Fat (g)	Mono (g)	Poly (g)	Sat (g)
12023	Seeds, sesame, whole, dried	1 tbsp	9	51.57	1.596	2.111	1.062	4.47	1.688	1.96	0.626
12037	Seeds, sunflower kernels, dry roast w/o salt	1 oz	28.35	165	5.48	6.824	3.147	14.118	2.695	9.323	1.48
15156	Shellfish, abalone, fried	3 oz	85	160.65	16.685	9.393	0	5.763	2.33	1.425	1.399
15159	Shellfish, clams, boiled/steamed (moist heat)	20 small	190	281.2	48.545	9.747	0	3.705	0.327	1.049	0.357
15158	Shellfish, clams, breaded & fried	3 oz	85	171.7	12.104	8.781		9.477	3.863	2.439	2.281
15160	Shellfish, clams, canned, drained	3 oz	85	125.8	21.718	4.361	0	1.658	0.146	0.469	0.16
15157	Shellfish, clams, raw	1 cup (with liquid and clams)	227	167.98	28.988	5.834	0	2.202	0.182	0.64	0.213
15137	Shellfish, crab, Alaskan king, boiled/steamed	1 leg	134	129.98	25.929	0	0	2.064	0.248	0.718	0.178
15138	Shellfish, crab, Alaskan king, imitation surimi	3 oz	85	86.7	10.217	8.687	0	1.113	0.17	0.57	0.221
15243	Shellfish, crayfish, farmed, cooked w/moist heat	3 oz	85	73.95	14.892	0	0	1.105	0.213	0.351	0.184
15229	Shellfish, cuttlefish, cooked w/moist heat	3 oz	85	134.3	27.608	1.394	0	1.19	0.138	0.228	0.201
15148	Shellfish, lobster, northern, boiled/steamed (moist heat)	3 oz	85	83.3	17.425	1.088	0	0.502	0.136	0.077	0.091
15165	Shellfish, mussel, blue, boiled/steamed	3 oz	85	146.2	20.23	6.281	0	3.808	0.862	1.03	0.723
15170	Shellfish, oyster, east, canned	1 oyster	8	5.52	0.565	0.313	0	0.198	0.02	0.059	0.05
15168	Shellfish, oyster, eastern, breaded & fried	6 medium	88	173.36	7.718	10.226		11.07	4.138	2.915	2.813
15245	Shellfish, oyster, eastern, farmed, raw	6 medium	84	49.56	4.385	4.645	0	1.302	0.128	0.496	0.372
15171	Shellfish, oyster, Pacific, raw	1 medium	50	40.5	4.725	2.475	0	1.15	0.179	0.447	0.255
15173	Shellfish, scallops, breaded, fried	2 large	31	66.65	5.602	3.14		3.391	1.394	0.885	0.827
15151	Shellfish, shrimp, boiled/steamed (moist heat)	4 large	22	21.78	4.6	0	0	0.238	0.043	0.097	0.064
15150	Shellfish, shrimp, breaded & fried	4 large	30	72.6	6.417	3.441	0.12	3.684	1.144	1.526	0.626
19097	Sherbet, orange	.5 cup (4 fl. oz.)	74	106.56	0.814	22.496	2.442	1.48	0.392	0.059	0.858
4615	Shortening, household, composite	1 tbsp	12.8	113.15	0	0	0	12.8	5.711	3.952	2.568
4031	Shortening, vegetable fat, soy hydrogenated & cottonseed hydrogenated	1 tbsp	12.8	113.15	0	0	0	12.8	5.696	3.341	3.2
19400	Snack, banana chips	1 oz	28.35	147.14	0.652	16.556	2.183	9.526	0.553	0.179	8.213
19002	Snack, beef jerky	1 piece, large	20	82	6.64	2.2	0.36	5.12	2.261	0.202	2.17
18501	Snack, cereal bar, mixed berry/Kellogg	1 oz	28.34	104.86	1.219	20.632	0.538	2.154	1.417	0.312	0.425
19033	Snack, Chex Snack Mix	1 oz (approx 2/3 cup)	28.35	120.49	3.119	18.456	1.588	4.905			1.568
19004	Snack, corn chips, BBQ flavor	1 oz	28.35	148.27	1.985	15.933	1.474	9.27	2.688	4.584	1.264
19003	Snack, corn chips, plain	1 oz	28.35	152.81	1.871	16.131	1.389	9.469	2.739	4.672	1.29
19401	Snack, Corn Nuts, BBQ flavor	1 oz	28.35	123.61	2.552	20.327	2.381	4.054	2.087	0.913	0.731
19009	Snack, Corn Nuts, plain	1 oz	28.35	126.44	2.41	20.372	1.956	4.434	2.682	0.865	0.689
19008	Snack, corn puffs or twists, cheese flavor	1 oz	28.35	157.06	2.155	15.252	0.312	9.752	5.749	1.349	1.868
19420	Snack, granola bar, hard, peanut butter	1 bar	24	115.92	2.352	14.952	0.696	5.712	1.68	2.899	0.768
19015	Snack, granola bar, hard, plain	1 bar (1 oz)	28	131.88	2.828	18.032	1.484	5.544	1.226	3.374	0.664
19017	Snack, granola bar, hard, w/chocolate chips	1 bar	24	105.12	1.752	17.304	1.056	3.912	0.631	0.305	2.738
19024	Snack, granola bar, soft, chocolate chip, milk chocolate cover	1 bar (1.25 oz)	35	163.1	2.03	22.33	1.19	8.715	2.72	0.637	4.977
19406	Snack, granola bar, soft, nut & raisin	1 bar (1 oz)	28	127.12	2.24	17.808	1.568	5.712	1.182	1.546	2.671
19020	Snack, granola bar, soft, plain	1 bar (1 oz)	28	124.04	2.072	18.844	1.288	4.816	1.067	1.49	2.027
19407	Snack, meat-based sticks, smoked	1 stick	20	110	4.3	1.08		9.92	4.094	0.884	4.16
19031	Snack, Oriental mix, rice-based	1 oz	28.35	143.45	4.907	14.634	3.742	7.252	2.795	3.017	1.073

Chol (g)	Calc (mg)	Iron (mg)	Mag (mg)	Phos (mg)	Pota (mg)	Sodi (mg)	Zinc (mg)	Vit A (RAE)	Vit C (mg)	Thia (mg)	Ribo (mg)	Niac (mg)	Vit B₆ (mg)	Vit B₁₂ (µg)	Vit E (mg)	Fol (µg)	Alc (g)
0	87.75	1.31	31.59	56.61	42.12	0.99	0.698	0	0	0.071	0.022	0.406	0.071	0	0.023	8.73	0
0	19.845	1.077	36.572	327.443	240.975	0.851	1.5	0.284	0.397	0.03	0.07	1.996	0.228	0	6.03	67.19	0
79.9	31.45	3.23	47.6	184.45	241.4	502.35	0.808	1.7	1.53	0.187	0.111	1.615	0.128	0.586		11.9	0
127.3	174.8	53.124	34.2	642.2	1193.2	212.8	5.187	324.9	41.99	0.285	0.809	6.373	0.209	187.891		55.1	0
51.85	53.55	11.824	11.9	159.8	277.1	309.4	1.241	77.35	8.5	0.085	0.207	1.754	0.051	34.229		30.6	0
56.95	78.2	23.766	15.3	287.3	533.8	95.2	2.321	153.9	18.79	0.128	0.362	2.851	0.094	84.057	0.527	24.65	0
77.18	104.42	31.735	20.43	383.63	712.78	127.12	3.11	204.3	29.51	0.182	0.484	4.007	0.136	112.229	0.704	36.32	0
71.02	79.06	1.018	84.42	375.2	351.08	1436.48	10.21	12.06	10.18	0.071	0.074	1.796	0.241	15.41		68.34	0
17	11.05	0.331	36.55	239.7	76.5	714.85	0.281	17	0	0.027	0.023	0.153	0.025	1.36	0.085	1.7	0
116.45	43.35	0.944	28.05	204.85	202.3	82.45	1.258	12.75	0.425	0.04	0.068	1.417	0.114	2.635		9.35	0
190.4	153	9.214	51	493	541.45	632.4	2.941	172.6	7.225	0.014	1.47	1.861	0.23	4.59		20.4	0
61.2	51.85	0.331	29.75	157.25	299.2	323	2.482	22.1	0	0.006	0.056	0.91	0.065	2.644	0.85	9.35	0
47.6	28.05	5.712	31.45	242.25	227.8	313.65	2.27	77.35	11.56	0.255	0.357	2.55	0.085	20.4		64.6	0
4.4	3.6	0.536	4.32	11.12	18.32	8.96	7.276	7.2	0.4	0.012	0.013	0.1	0.008	1.53	0.068	0.72	0
71.28	54.56	6.116	51.04	139.92	214.72	366.96	76.67	80.08	3.344	0.132	0.178	1.452	0.056	13.754		27.28	0
21	36.96	4.855	27.72	78.12	104.16	149.52	31.85	6.72	3.948	0.088	0.055	1.064	0.05	13.608		15.12	0
25	4	2.555	11	81	84	53	8.31	40.5	4	0.034	0.116	1.005	0.025	8	0.425	5	0
18.91	13.02	0.254	18.29	73.16	103.23	143.84	0.329	7.13	0.713	0.013	0.034	0.467	0.043	0.409		11.47	0
42.9	8.58	0.68	7.48	30.14	40.04	49.28	0.343	14.96	0.484	0.007	0.007	0.57	0.028	0.328	0.304	0.88	0
53.1	20.1	0.378	12	65.4	67.5	103.2	0.414	17.1	0.45	0.039	0.041	0.921	0.029	0.561		5.4	0
0	39.96	0.104	5.92	29.6	71.04	34.04	0.355	7.4	4.292	0.023	0.066	0.056	0.02	0.089	0.022	5.18	0
0	0	0	0	0	0	0	0	0	0	0	0	0	0	0	0.102	0	0
0	0	0	0	0	0	0	0	0	0	0	0	0	0	0	0.102	0	0
0	5.103	0.354	21.546	15.876	151.956	1.701	0.213	1.134	1.786	0.024	0.005	0.201	0.074	0	0.068	3.969	0
9.6	4	1.084	10.2	81.4	119.4	442.6	1.622	0	0	0.031	0.028	0.346	0.036	0.198	0.098	26.8	0
0	11.053	1.389	7.368	27.773	53.279	84.17	1.162		0	0.283	0.312	3.826	0.397	0	0	30.61	0
0	9.923	7.002	17.861	53.015	76.262	288.32	0.593	1.985	13.47	0.441	0.141	4.774	0.441	3.515		14.18	0
0	37.139	0.437	21.83	58.685	66.906	216.311	0.301	8.789	0.482	0.021	0.06	0.466	0.065	0		11.06	0
0	36.005	0.374	21.546	52.448	40.257	178.605	0.357	1.418	0	0.008	0.041	0.335	0.069	0	0.386	5.67	0
0	4.82	0.482	30.902	80.231	81.081	276.696	0.533	4.82	0.113	0.099	0.04	0.427	0.053	0		0	0
0	2.552	0.473	32.036	77.963	78.813	155.642	0.505	0	0	0.012	0.037	0.48	0.065	0	0.561	0	0
1.134	16.443	0.666	5.103	30.618	47.061	297.675	0.108	1.701	0.057	0.075	0.1	0.916	0.038	0.04	1.205	34.02	0
0	9.84	0.576	13.2	33.36	69.84	67.92	0.3	0.24	0.048	0.05	0.022	0.473	0.023	0		4.32	0
0	17.08	0.826	27.16	77.56	94.08	82.32	0.568	2.24	0.252	0.074	0.033	0.443	0.024	0		6.44	0
0	18.48	0.732	17.28	48.96	60.24	82.56	0.463	0.48	0.024	0.043	0.024	0.133	0.014	0.002		3.12	0
1.75	36.05	0.815	23.1	69.65	109.55	70	0.455	2.45	0	0.032	0.087	0.252	0.035	0.199		9.1	0
0.28	23.52	0.61	25.48	67.48	109.76	71.12	0.448	0.56	0	0.053	0.053	0.731	0.034	0.067		8.4	0
0.28	29.4	0.717	20.72	64.4	91	77.84	0.42	0	0	0.083	0.046	0.144	0.028	0.109		6.72	0
26.6	13.6	0.68	4.2	36	51.4	296	0.484	2.6	1.36	0.028	0.087	0.908	0.041	0.2		0	0
0	15.309	0.692	33.453	74.277	92.988	117.086	0.754	0	0.085	0.088	0.04	0.873	0.02	0	1.588	10.77	0

EvaluEat Code	Food Name	Amt	Wt (g)	Energy (kcal)	Prot (g)	Carb (g)	Fiber (g)	Fat (g)	Mono (g)	Poly (g)	Sat (g)
19036	Snack, popcorn cakes	1 cake	10	38.4	0.97	8.01	0.29	0.31	0.092	0.135	0.048
19034	Snack, popcorn, air-popped	1 cup	8	30.56	0.96	6.232	1.208	0.336	0.088	0.152	0.046
19039	Snack, popcorn, caramel coated, no peanuts	1 oz	28.35	122.19	1.077	22.425	1.474	3.629	0.816	1.27	1.023
19040	Snack, popcorn, cheese flavor	1 cup	11	57.86	1.023	5.676	1.089	3.652	1.067	1.691	0.705
19035	Snack, popcorn, oil-popped, yellow corn	1 cup	11	55	0.99	6.292	1.1	3.091	0.899	1.476	0.538
19041	Snack, pork skins, plain	1 oz	28.35	154.51	17.379	0	0	8.874	4.19	1.032	3.223
19042	Snack, potato chips, BBQ flavor	1 oz	28.35	139.2	2.183	14.969	1.247	9.185	1.854	4.641	2.282
19422	Snack, potato chips, light	1 oz	28.35	133.53	2.013	18.966	1.673	5.897	1.361	3.101	1.179
19811	Snack, potato chips, plain, no salt	1 oz	28.35	151.96	1.985	14.997	1.361	9.809	2.79	3.45	3.107
19411	Snack, potato chips, plain, salted	1 oz	28.35	151.96	1.985	14.997	1.276	9.809	2.79	3.45	3.107
19043	Snack, potato chips, sour cream & onion	1 oz	28.35	150.54	2.296	14.6	1.474	9.611	1.735	4.939	2.52
19814	Snack, pretzel, hard, plain, no salt	10 twists	60	228.6	5.46	47.52	1.68	2.1	0.816	0.732	0.45
19047	Snack, pretzel, hard, plain, salted	10 twists	60	228.6	5.46	47.52	1.92	2.1	0.816	0.732	0.45
19053	Snack, rice cake, brown rice & sesame seed	2 cakes	18	70.56	1.368	14.67	0.972	0.684	0.198	0.207	0.097
19051	Snack, rice cake, brown rice, plain	2 cakes	18	69.66	1.476	14.67	0.756	0.504	0.185	0.178	0.103
19524	Snack, taco chips	1 oz	28.35	141.18	0.652	19.306	2.041	7.059	1.256	3.651	1.823
19057	Snack, tortilla chips, nacho flavor	1 oz	28.35	141.18	2.211	17.69	1.503	7.258	4.278	1.004	1.389
19056	Snack, tortilla chips, plain	1 oz	28.35	142.03	1.985	17.832	1.843	7.428	4.38	1.029	1.423
19058	Snack, tortilla chips, ranch flavor	1 oz	28.35	138.92	2.155	18.314	1.106	6.747	3.983	0.936	1.293
19059	Snack, trail mix, regular	1 cup	150	693	20.7	67.35		44.1	18.795	14.475	8.325
19062	Snack, trail mix, regular, chocolate chip, salted nuts & seeds	1 cup	146	706.64	20.732	65.554		46.574	19.768	16.483	8.906
19269	Snacks, Fruit Roll Ups, berry flavored w/vit C/ General Mills-Betty Crocker	2 rolls	28	104.44	0.028	23.856		0.98	0.483	0.026	0.277
19423	Snacks, potato chips, fat-free, made with olestra	1 oz	28.35	75.128	1.88	16.783	1.106	0.198	0.071	0.081	0.045
19438	Snacks, Rice Krispies Treat Squares/Kellogg	1 oz	28.34	117.33	0.964	22.814	0.17	2.551	0.709	1.445	0.397
6190	Soup, bean & ham, canned, reduced sodium, prepared with water or ready-to-serve	1 cup	128	94.72	5.363	17.485	5.12	1.318	0.531	0.344	0.323
6474	Soup, bean w/bacon, dry, made w/H$_2$O	1 cup	265	106	5.485	16.377	9.01	2.147	0.928	0.159	0.954
6978	Soup, beef and mushroom, low sodium, chunk style	.5 cup	125	86.25	5.375	11.975	0.25	2.875	0.493	0.085	2.026
6199	Soup, beef barley, canned/Progresso Healthy Classics	1 cup	241	142.19	11.327	20.003	3.133	1.928	0.689	0.251	0.747
6008	Soup, beef broth or bouillon, canned	1 cup	240	16.8	2.736	0.096	0	0.528	0.216	0.024	0.264
6547	Soup, beef mushroom, canned, made w/H$_2$O	1 cup	244	73.2	5.783	6.344	0.244	3.001	1.244	0.122	1.488
6070	Soup, beef, chunky, canned	1 cup	240	170.4	11.736	19.56	1.44	5.136	2.136	0.216	2.544
6478	Soup, cauliflower, dry, made w/H$_2$O	1 cup	256	69.12	2.893	10.726		1.715	0.742	0.64	0.256
6411	Soup, cheese, canned, made w/H$_2$O	1 cup	247	155.61	5.409	10.522	0.988	10.473	2.964	0.296	6.669
6413	Soup, chicken broth, canned, made w/H$_2$O	1 cup	240	38.4	4.848	0.912	0	1.368	0.576	0.264	0.384
6417	Soup, chicken gumbo, canned, made w/H$_2$O	1 cup	244	56.12	2.635	8.369	1.952	1.44	0.659	0.342	0.317
6549	Soup, chicken mushroom, canned, made w/H$_2$O	1 cup	244	131.76	4.392	9.272	0.244	9.15	4.026	2.318	2.391
6018	Soup, chicken noodle, chunky, canned	1 cup	240	175.2	12.72	17.04	3.84	6	2.664	1.512	1.392
6022	Soup, chicken rice, chunky, ready-to-eat, canned	1 cup	240	127.2	12.264	12.984	0.96	3.192	1.44	0.672	0.96
6024	Soup, chicken vegetable, chunky, canned	1 cup	240	165.6	12.312	18.888		4.824	2.16	1.008	1.44
6015	Soup, chicken, chunky, canned	1 cup	240	170.4	12.144	16.512	1.44	6.336	2.832	1.32	1.896
6203	Soup, cream of broccoli, canned, ready-to-eat/Progresso Healthy Classics	1 cup	244	87.84	2.367	13.322	2.44	2.806	0.92	0.573	0.659
6410	Soup, cream of celery, canned, made w/H$_2$O	1 cup	244	90.28	1.659	8.833	0.732	5.588	1.293	2.513	1.415

Chol (g)	Calc (mg)	Iron (mg)	Mag (mg)	Phos (mg)	Pota (mg)	Sodi (mg)	Zinc (mg)	Vit A (RAE)	Vit C (mg)	Thia (mg)	Ribo (mg)	Niac (mg)	Vit B₆ (mg)	Vit B₁₂ (µg)	Vit E (mg)	Fol (µg)	Alc (g)
0	0.9	0.187	15.9	27.7	32.7	28.8	0.399	0.4	0	0.008	0.018	0.601	0.018	0	0.029	1.8	0
0	0.8	0.213	10.48	24	24.08	0.32	0.275	0.8	0	0.016	0.023	0.156	0.02	0	0.023	1.84	0
1.418	12.191	0.493	9.923	23.531	30.902	58.401	0.164	0.567	0	0.018	0.02	0.624	0.008	0.003	0.34	1.418	0
1.21	12.43	0.246	10.01	39.71	28.71	97.79	0.221	4.18	0.055	0.014	0.027	0.16	0.026	0.058	0.013	1.21	0
0	1.1	0.306	11.88	27.5	24.75	97.24	0.29	0.88	0.033	0.015	0.015	0.17	0.023	0	0.551	1.87	0
26.933	8.505	0.249	3.119	24.098	36.005	521.073	0.159	3.402	0.142	0.028	0.08	0.439	0.007	0.181	0.15	0	0
0	14.175	0.55	21.263	52.731	357.494	212.625	0.266	3.119	9.611	0.061	0.061	1.33	0.176	0	1.418	23.53	0
0	5.954	0.383	25.232	54.716	494.424	139.482	0.02	0	7.286	0.059	0.076	1.985	0.19	0	1.551	7.655	0
0	6.804	0.462	18.995	46.778	361.463	2.268	0.309	0	8.817	0.047	0.056	1.085	0.187	0	2.583	12.76	0
0	6.804	0.462	18.995	46.778	361.463	168.399	0.309	0	8.817	0.047	0.056	1.085	0.187	0	2.583	12.76	0
1.985	20.412	0.454	20.979	49.896	377.339	177.188	0.278	3.969	10.58	0.054	0.057	1.142	0.189	0.284		17.58	0
0	21.6	2.592	21	67.8	87.6	173.4	0.51	0	0	0.277	0.374	3.151	0.07	0	0.21	102.6	0
0	21.6	2.592	21	67.8	87.6	1029	0.51	0	0	0.277	0.374	3.151	0.07	0	0.21	102.6	0
0	2.16	0.284	24.48	67.5	52.2	40.86	0.54	0	0.54	0.009	0.015	1.297	0.028	0		3.24	0
0	1.98	0.268	23.58	64.8	52.2	58.68	0.54	0	0	0.011	0.03	1.405	0.027	0	0.223	3.78	0
0	17.01	0.34	23.814	37.139	214.043	96.957	0.108	1.985	1.418	0.049	0.008	0.146	0.124	0	3.215	5.67	0
0.851	41.675	0.405	23.247	69.174	61.236	200.718	0.34	6.804	0.51	0.036	0.054	0.406	0.081	0.014		3.969	0
0	43.659	0.431	24.948	58.118	55.85	149.688	0.434	1.134	0	0.021	0.052	0.363	0.081	0	1.001	2.835	0
0.284	39.974	0.414	25.232	67.757	69.174	173.502	0.352	4.253	0.255	0.03	0.067	0.412	0.057	0		4.82	0
0	117	4.575	237	517.5	1027.5	343.5	4.83	1.5	2.1	0.693	0.297	7.068	0.447	0		106.5	0
5.84	159.14	4.949	235.06	565.02	946.08	176.66	4.584	2.92	1.898	0.603	0.327	6.431	0.378	0		94.9	0
						88.76		33.6									0
0	9.639	0.422	23.247	46.778	365.715	184.842	0.272	0	8.363	0.098	0.02	1.304	0.519	0	0	8.505	0
0	0.85	0.36	3.684	11.903	11.053	99.473	0.142	91.82	0	0.359	0.387	4.615	0.255	0	0	30.89	0
2.56	48.64	1.306	24.32	16.64	202.24	239.36	0.678	44.8	1.408	0.072	0.037	0.415	0.059	0.038	0.499	37.12	0
2.65	55.65	1.325	29.15	90.1	325.95	927.5	0.689	2.65	1.06	0.053	0.265	0.398	0.026	0.026	0.557	7.95	0
7.5	16.25	1.213	2.5	62.5	175	31.25	1.375	122.5	3.75	0.05	0.138	1.413	0.075	0.325	0.275	6.25	0
19.28	28.92	1.856	31.33	118.09	366.32	469.95	1.542		3.615	0.128	0.125	2.919	0.186	0.362	0.268	24.1	0
0	14.4	0.408	4.8	31.2	129.6	782.4	0	0	0	0.005	0.05	1.872	0.024	0.168	0	4.8	0
7.32	4.88	0.878	9.76	34.16	153.72	941.84	1.464	0	4.636	0.039	0.056	0.954	0.049	0.195		9.76	0
14.4	31.2	2.328	4.8	120	336	866.4	2.64	129.6	6.96	0.058	0.151	2.705	0.132	0.624	0.672	14.4	0
0	10.24	0.512	2.56	51.2	104.96	842.24	0.256	0	2.56	0.077	0.077	0.512	0.026	0.179		2.56	0
29.64	140.79	0.741	4.94	135.85	153.14	958.36	0.642	296.4	0	0.017	0.136	0.398	0.025	0		4.94	0
0	9.6	0.504	2.4	72	206.4	763.2	0.24	0	0	0.01	0.07	3.293	0.024	0.24	0.048	4.8	0
4.88	24.4	0.903	4.88	24.4	75.64	954.04	0.366	7.32	4.88	0.024	0.049	0.664	0.063	0.024	0.366	4.88	0
9.76	29.28	0.878	9.76	26.84	153.72	941.84	0.976	56.12	0	0.024	0.112	1.63	0.049	0.049		0	0
19.2	24	1.44	9.6	72	108	849.6	0.96	67.2	0	0.072	0.168	4.32	0.048	0.312	0.336	38.4	0
12	33.6	1.872	9.6	72	108	888	0.96	292.8	3.84	0.024	0.098	4.104	0.048	0.312	0.576	4.8	0
16.8	26.4	1.464	9.6	105.6	367.2	1068	2.16	300	5.52	0.041	0.166	3.29	0.096	0.24		12	0
28.8	24	1.656	7.2	108	168	849.6	0.96	64.8	1.2	0.082	0.166	4.224	0.048	0.24	0.312	4.8	0
4.88	41.48	1.22	14.64	39.04	161.04	578.28	0.268		5.856	0.029	0.059	0.317	0.073	0	0.383	29.28	0
14.64	39.04	0.634	7.32	36.6	122	949.16	0.146	56.12	0.244	0.029	0.049	0.332	0.012	0.244	0.903	2.44	0

EvaluEat Code	Food Name	Amt	Wt (g)	Energy (kcal)	Prot (g)	Carb (g)	Fiber (g)	Fat (g)	Mono (g)	Poly (g)	Sat (g)
6443	Soup, cream of mushroom, canned, made w/H$_2$O	1 cup	244	129.32	2.318	9.296	0.488	8.979	1.708	4.221	2.44
6453	Soup, cream of potato, canned, made w/H$_2$O	1 cup	244	73.2	1.757	11.468	0.488	2.367	0.561	0.415	1.22
6582	Soup, Cup Noodles, ramen, chicken flavor, dry/Nissin	1 container, individual	64	296.32	5.568	36.8		14.08			6.253
6036	Soup, gazpacho, canned	1 cup	244	46.36	7.076	4.392	0.488	0.244	0.024	0.073	0.024
6449	Soup, green pea, canned, made w/H$_2$O	1 cup	250	165	8.6	26.5	2.75	2.925	1	0.375	1.4
6490	Soup, leek, dry, made w/H$_2$O	1 cup	254	71.12	2.108	11.43	3.048	2.057	0.864	0.076	1.016
6428	Soup, Manhattan clam chowder, canned, made w/H$_2$O	1 cup	244	78.08	2.196	12.224	1.464	2.22	0.383	1.291	0.383
6440	Soup, minestrone, canned, made w/H$_2$O	1 cup	241	81.94	4.266	11.231	0.964	2.506	0.699	1.109	0.554
6445	Soup, onion, canned, made w/H$_2$O	1 cup	241	57.84	3.76	8.17	0.964	1.735	0.747	0.651	0.265
6583	Soup, ramen noodle, any flavor, dehydrated, dry	1 container, individual	64	289.92	5.952	41.92	1.536	10.944	4.096	1.667	4.883
6180	Soup, shark fin, restaurant-prep	1 cup	216	99.36	6.912	8.208	0	4.32	1.259	0.737	1.082
6451	Soup, split pea w/ham, canned, made w/H$_2$O	1 cup	253	189.75	10.322	27.957	2.277	4.402	1.796	0.632	1.771
6174	Soup, stock, fish, homemade	1 cup	233	39.61	5.266	0	0	1.887	0.55	0.322	0.473
6499	Soup, tomato vegetable, dry, made w/H$_2$O	1 cup	241	53.02	1.904	9.736	0.482	0.819	0.289	0.072	0.362
6559	Soup, tomato, canned, made w/H$_2$O	1 cup	244	85.4	2.05	16.592	0.488	1.928	0.439	0.952	0.366
6466	Soup, turkey vegetable, canned, made w/H$_2$O	1 cup	241	72.3	3.085	8.628	0.482	3.037	1.326	0.675	0.892
6471	Soup, vegetable beef, canned, made w/H$_2$O	1 cup	244	78.08	5.588	10.175	0.488	1.903	0.805	0.122	0.854
6974	Soup, vegetable chicken, low sodium	.5 cup	125	86.25	6.375	10.95	0.5	2.5	1.119	0.523	0.746
6468	Soup, vegetarian vegetable, canned, made w/H$_2$O	1 cup	241	72.3	2.097	11.978	0.482	1.928	0.819	0.723	0.289
1180	Sour cream, fat-free	1 oz	28.34	20.972	0.879	4.421	0	0	0	0	0
1179	Sour cream, light	1 oz	28.34	38.542	0.992	2.012	0	3.004	0.879	0.113	1.87
43133	Soyburger	1 cup	186	332.94	33.313	24.924	8.556	11.104	2.055	4.382	1.337
2001	Spice, allspice, ground	1 tsp	1.9	4.997	0.116	1.37	0.41	0.165	0.013	0.045	0.048
2002	Spice, anise seed	1 tsp	2.1	7.077	0.37	1.05	0.307	0.334	0.205	0.066	0.012
2007	Spice, celery seed	1 tsp	2	7.84	0.361	0.827	0.236	0.505	0.319	0.074	0.044
2009	Spice, chili powder	1 tsp	2.6	8.164	0.319	1.421	0.889	0.436	0.093	0.194	0.077
2010	Spice, cinnamon, ground	1 tsp	2.3	6.003	0.089	1.837	1.249	0.073	0.011	0.012	0.015
2011	Spice, cloves, ground	1 tsp	2.1	6.783	0.126	1.285	0.718	0.421	0.031	0.149	0.114
2013	Spice, coriander seed	1 tsp	1.8	5.364	0.223	0.99	0.754	0.32	0.244	0.031	0.018
2014	Spice, cumin seed	1 tsp	2.1	7.875	0.374	0.929	0.22	0.468	0.295	0.069	0.032
2015	Spice, curry powder	1 tsp	2	6.5	0.253	1.163	0.664	0.276	0.111	0.051	0.045
2016	Spice, dill seed	1 tsp	2.1	6.405	0.336	1.159	0.443	0.305	0.198	0.021	0.015
2018	Spice, fennel seed	1 tsp	2	6.9	0.316	1.046	0.796	0.297	0.198	0.034	0.01
2020	Spice, garlic powder	1 tsp	2.8	9.296	0.47	2.036	0.277	0.021	0	0.011	0.004
2021	Spice, ginger, ground	1 tsp	1.8	6.246	0.164	1.274	0.225	0.107	0.018	0.024	0.035
2024	Spice, mustard seed, yellow	1 tsp	3.3	15.477	0.823	1.153	0.485	0.949	0.654	0.178	0.048
2025	Spice, nutmeg, ground	1 tsp	2.2	11.55	0.128	1.084	0.458	0.799	0.071	0.008	0.571
2026	Spice, onion powder	1 tsp	2.4	8.328	0.243	1.936	0.137	0.025	0.004	0.011	0.004
2028	Spice, paprika	1 tsp	2.1	6.069	0.31	1.171	0.785	0.272	0.026	0.175	0.044
2030	Spice, pepper, black	1 tsp	2.1	5.355	0.23	1.361	0.557	0.068	0.021	0.024	0.021

Chol (g)	Calc (mg)	Iron (mg)	Mag (mg)	Phos (mg)	Pota (mg)	Sodi (mg)	Zinc (mg)	Vit A (RAE)	Vit C (mg)	Thia (mg)	Ribo (mg)	Niac (mg)	Vit B$_6$ (mg)	Vit B$_{12}$ (µg)	Vit E (mg)	Fol (µg)	Alc (g)
2.44	46.36	0.512	4.88	48.8	100.04	880.84	0.586	14.64	0.976	0.046	0.09	0.725	0.015	0.049	0.952	4.88	0
4.88	19.52	0.488	2.44	46.36	136.64	1000.4	0.634	70.76	0	0.034	0.037	0.539	0.037	0.049	0.024	2.44	0
		2.182				1433.6											0
0	24.4	0.976	7.32	36.6	224.48	739.32	0.244	14.64	7.076	0.049	0.024	0.927	0.146	0	0.439	19.52	0
0	27.5	1.95	40	125	190	917.5	1.7	10	1.75	0.108	0.068	1.24	0.052	0	0.375	2.5	0
2.54	30.48	0.508	10.16	30.48	88.9	965.2	0.229	2.54	2.54	0.051	0.025	0.254	0.025	0.025	0.178	7.62	0
2.44	26.84	1.635	12.2	41.48	187.88	578.28	0.976	56.12	3.904	0.029	0.039	0.817	0.1	4.05	0.342	9.76	0
2.41	33.74	0.916	7.23	55.43	313.3	910.98	0.747	118.1	1.205	0.053	0.043	0.942	0.099	0	0.072	36.15	0
0	26.51	0.675	2.41	12.05	67.48	1053.17	0.603	0	1.205	0.034	0.024	0.6	0.048	0	0.193	14.46	0
0	10.24	2.733	15.36	69.12	76.8	742.4	0.403	0.64	0	0.422	0.282	3.456	0.039	0.006	1.299	94.08	0
4.32	21.6	2.03	15.12	45.36	114.48	1082.16	1.771	0	0.216	0.058	0.084	1.065	0.056	0.41	6.86	19.44	0
7.59	22.77	2.277	48.07	212.52	399.74	1006.94	1.316	22.77	1.518	0.147	0.076	1.475	0.068	0.253		2.53	0
2.33	6.99	0.023	16.31	130.48	335.52	363.48	0.14	4.66	0.233	0.077	0.177	2.763	0.086	1.608	0.396	4.66	0
0	7.23	0.603	19.28	28.92	98.81	1091.73	0.169	9.64	5.784	0.055	0.043	0.752	0.048	0	0.337	9.64	0
0	12.2	1.757	7.32	34.16	263.52	695.4	0.244	29.28	66.37	0.088	0.051	1.418	0.112	0	2.318	14.64	0
2.41	16.87	0.771	4.82	40.97	175.93	906.16	0.603	122.9	0	0.029	0.039	1.005	0.048	0.169	0.142	4.82	0
4.88	17.08	1.122	4.88	41.48	173.24	790.56	1.537	95.16	2.44	0.037	0.049	1.032	0.076	0.317	0.366	9.76	0
8.75	13.75	0.763	5	55	191.25	43.75	1.125	172.5	2.875	0.025	0.087	1.712	0.05	0.125	0.375	22.5	0
0	21.69	1.084	7.23	33.74	209.67	821.81	0.458	115.7	1.446	0.053	0.046	0.916	0.055	0	0.41	9.64	0
2.551	35.425	0	2.834	26.923	36.559	39.959	0.142	20.69	0	0.011	0.043	0.02	0.006	0.085	0	3.117	0
9.919	39.959	0.02	2.834	20.121	60.081	20.121	0.142	25.51	0.255	0.011	0.034	0.02	0.006	0.119	0.085	3.117	0
0	53.94	3.906	33.48	639.84	334.8	1023	3.348	0	0	1.674	1.116	18.6	2.232	4.464	3.218	145.1	0
0	12.559	0.134	2.565	2.147	19.836	1.463	0.019	0.513	0.745	0.002	0.001	0.054	0.004	0	0.02	0.684	0
0	13.566	0.776	3.57	9.24	30.261	0.336	0.111	0.336	0.441	0.007	0.006	0.064	0.014	0	0.022	0.21	0
0	35.34	0.898	8.8	10.94	28	3.2	0.139	0.06	0.342	0.007	0.006	0.061	0.018	0	0.021	0.2	0
0	7.228	0.37	4.42	7.878	49.816	26.26	0.07	38.56	1.667	0.009	0.021	0.205	0.095	0	0.755	2.6	0
0	28.244	0.876	1.288	1.403	11.5	0.598	0.045	0.322	0.655	0.002	0.003	0.03	0.007	0	0.022	0.667	0
0	13.566	0.182	5.544	2.205	23.142	5.103	0.023	0.567	1.697	0.002	0.006	0.031	0.012	0	0.179	1.953	0
0	12.762	0.294	5.94	7.362	22.806	0.63	0.085	0	0.378	0.004	0.005	0.038		0		0	0
0	19.551	1.394	7.686	10.479	37.548	3.528	0.101	1.344	0.162	0.013	0.007	0.096	0.009	0	0.07	0.21	0
0	9.56	0.592	5.08	6.98	30.86	1.04	0.081	0.98	0.228	0.005	0.006	0.069	0.023	0	0.44	3.08	0
0	31.836	0.343	5.376	5.817	24.906	0.42	0.109	0.063	0.441	0.009	0.006	0.059	0.005	0	0.022	0.21	0
0	23.92	0.371	7.7	9.74	33.88	1.76	0.074	0.14	0.42	0.008	0.007	0.121	0.009	0			0
0	2.24	0.077	1.624	11.676	30.828	0.728	0.074	0	0.504	0.013	0.004	0.019	0.082	0	0.018	0.056	0
0	2.088	0.207	3.312	2.664	24.174	0.576	0.085	0.126	0.126	0.001	0.003	0.093	0.015	0	0.324	0.702	0
0	17.193	0.329	9.834	27.753	22.506	0.165	0.188	0.099	0.099	0.018	0.013	0.26	0.014	0	0.095	2.508	0
0	4.048	0.067	4.026	4.686	7.7	0.352	0.047	0.11	0.066	0.008	0.001	0.029	0.004	0	0	1.672	0
0	8.712	0.061	2.928	8.16	22.632	1.296	0.056	0	0.353	0.01	0.001	0.016	0.029	0	0.006	3.984	0
0	3.717	0.495	3.885	7.245	49.224	0.714	0.085	55.38	1.493	0.014	0.037	0.322	0.084	0	0.626	2.226	0
0	9.177	0.606	4.074	3.633	26.439	0.924	0.03	0.315	0.441	0.002	0.005	0.024	0.007	0	0.015	0.21	0

EvaluEat Code	Food Name	Amt	Wt (g)	Energy (kcal)	Prot (g)	Carb (g)	Fiber (g)	Fat (g)	Mono (g)	Poly (g)	Sat (g)
2033	Spice, poppy seed	1 tsp	2.8	14.924	0.505	0.663	0.28	1.252	0.178	0.863	0.136
2037	Spice, saffron	1 tsp	0.7	2.17	0.08	0.458	0.027	0.041	0.003	0.014	0.011
2043	Spice, turmeric, ground	1 tsp	2.2	7.788	0.172	1.428	0.464	0.217	0.037	0.048	0.069
22905	Stew, beef stew, canned entree	1 serving	232	218.08	11.461	15.706	3.48	12.482	5.522	0.51	5.15
18355	Sweet roll, cheese	1 roll	66	237.6	4.686	28.842	0.792	12.078	5.978	1.341	3.999
18358	Sweet roll, cinnamon w/icing, refrigerated dough, baked	1 roll	30	108.6	1.62	16.83		3.96	2.226	0.518	1.004
18356	Sweet roll, cinnamon-raisin, commercially prep	1 large	83	308.76	5.146	42.247	1.992	13.612	3.982	6.203	2.556
19163	Sweet, chewing gum	1 stick	3	7.41	0	1.982	0.072	0.009	0.002	0.004	0.001
19711	Sweet, frosting, chocolate creamy	1/12 package	38	150.86	0.418	24.016	0.228	6.688	3.428	0.809	2.101
19228	Sweet, frosting, cream cheese flavor	2 tbsp	33	136.95	0.033	22.216	0	5.709	1.239	2.03	1.5
19715	Sweet, frosting, vanilla, creamy	1/12 package	38	159.22	0.038	26.372	0.038	6.384	3.333	0.866	1.858
19294	Sweet, fruit butter, apple	1 tbsp	17	29.41	0.066	7.271	0.255	0	0	0	0
19173	Sweet, gelatin, dry, prep w/H$_2$O	.5 cup	135	83.7	1.647	19.156	0	0	0	0	0
19290	Sweet, gelatin, Kraft, JELL-O Sugar Free Dessert, strawberry, powder	1 NLEA serving	2.5	8.325	1.42	0.123	0	0.003			0
19296	Sweet, honey, strained/extracted	1 tbsp	21	63.84	0.063	17.304	0.042	0	0	0	0
19283	Sweet, ice popsicle	1 bar (1.75 fl. oz.)	52	37.44	0	9.828	0	0	0	0	0
19297	Sweet, jams & preserves	1 tbsp	20	55.6	0.074	13.772	0.22	0.014	0.008	0	0.002
19300	Sweet, jellies	1 packet (0.5 oz)	14	37.24	0.021	9.793	0.14	0.003	0	0.001	0.001
19303	Sweet, marmalade, orange	1 tbsp	20	49.2	0.06	13.26	0.14	0	0	0	0
19304	Sweet, molasses	1 tbsp	20	58	0	14.946	0	0.02	0.006	0.01	0.004
19334	Sweet, sugar, brown	1 tsp packed	4.6	17.342	0	4.477	0	0	0	0	0
19335	Sweet, sugar, granulated, white	1 tsp	4.2	16.254	0	4.199	0	0	0	0	0
19340	Sweet, sugar, maple	1 tsp	3	10.62	0.003	2.727	0	0.006	0.002	0.003	0.001
19336	Sweet, sugar, powdered/confectioner's, white	1 tsp	2.5	9.725	0	2.49	0	0.003	0.001	0.001	0
19113	Sweet, syrup w/butter, pancake	1 tbsp	20	59.2	0	14.82	0	0.32	0.094	0.012	0.202
19348	Sweet, syrup, chocolate, fudge-type	2 tbsp	38	133	1.748	23.902	1.064	3.382	1.466	0.106	1.512
19351	Sweet, syrup, corn, hi-fructose	1 tbsp	19	53.39	0	14.44	0	0	0	0	0
19350	Sweet, syrup, corn, light	1 tbsp	20	58.6	0	15.926	0	0.02	0	0	0
19353	Sweet, syrup, maple	1 tbsp	20	52.2	0	13.418	0	0.04	0.013	0.02	0.007
19129	Sweet, syrup, pancake	1 tbsp	20	46.8	0	12.294	0.14	0	0	0	0
19128	Sweet, syrup, pancake, reduced-kcal	1 tbsp	15	24.6	0	6.645	0	0	0	0	0
19355	Sweet, syrup, sorghum	1 tbsp	21	60.9	0	15.729	0	0	0	0	0
19364	Sweet, topping, butterscotch or caramel	2 tbsp	41	103.32	0.615	27.019	0.369	0.041	0.008	0	0.045
19137	Sweet, topping, strawberry	2 tbsp	42	106.68	0.084	27.846	0.294	0.042	0.006	0.021	0.002
43026	Syrups, dietetic	1 cup	186	74.4	1.488	91.512	5.58	0	0	0	0
18277	Toaster muffin, blueberry	1 muffin	33	103.29	1.518	17.589	0.594	3.135	0.713	1.766	0.461
18281	Toaster muffin, corn	1 muffin	33	114.18	1.749	19.107	0.528	3.729	0.866	2.087	0.555
18361	Toaster pastry, brown sugar—cinnamon	1 pastry	50	206	2.55	34.05	0.5	7.1	4.016	0.901	1.819
18475	Toaster pastry, Pop Tart, Apple Cinnamon/Kellogg	1 pastry	52	205.4	2.288	37.45	0.572	5.304	3.052	1.352	0.879
18491	Toaster pastry, Pop Tart, Frosted Apple Cinnamon, low-fat/Kellogg	1 pastry	52	191.36	2.184	39.988	0.572	2.86	1.456	0.832	0.572

Chol (g)	Calc (mg)	Iron (mg)	Mag (mg)	Phos (mg)	Pota (mg)	Sodi (mg)	Zinc (mg)	Vit A (RAE)	Vit C (mg)	Thia (mg)	Ribo (mg)	Niac (mg)	Vit B$_6$ (mg)	Vit B$_{12}$ (µg)	Vit E (mg)	Fol (µg)	Alc (g)
0	40.544	0.263	9.268	23.772	19.6	0.588	0.286	0	0.084	0.024	0.005	0.027	0.012	0	0.031	1.624	0
0	0.777	0.078	1.848	1.764	12.068	1.036	0.008	0.189	0.566	0.001	0.002	0.01	0.007	0	0.012	0.651	0
0	4.026	0.911	4.246	5.896	55.55	0.836	0.096	0	0.57	0.003	0.005	0.113	0.04	0	0.068	0.858	0
37.12	27.84	1.647	32.48	127.6	403.68	946.56	1.902	192.6	10.21	0.167	0.142	2.856	0.299	0.858	0.172	25.52	0
50.16	77.88	0.502	12.54	64.68	90.42	235.62	0.416		0.132	0.099	0.086	0.548	0.046	0.198		28.38	0
0	10.2	0.795	3.6	104.4	18.9	249.6	0.102	0	0.06	0.123	0.073	1.087	0.01	0.015		16.5	
54.78	59.76	1.328	14.11	63.08	92.13	317.89	0.49	51.46	1.66	0.269	0.22	1.979	0.089	0.116	1.652	59.76	0
0	0	0	0	0	0.06	0.03	0	0	0	0	0	0	0	0	0	0	0
0	3.04	0.54	7.98	22.42	74.48	69.54	0.11		0	0.005	0.006	0.045	0.002	0		0	0
0	0.99	0.053	0.66	0.99	11.55	63.03	0.007	0	0	0	0.002	0.004	0	0	1.401	0	0
0	1.14	0.042	0.38	1.14	14.06	34.2	0		0	0	0.002	0.004	0	0		0	0
0	2.38	0.053	0.85	1.19	15.47	2.55	0.01	0.17	0.17	0.001	0.004	0.011	0.006	0	0.003	0.17	0
0	4.05	0.027	1.35	29.7	1.35	101.25	0.014	0	0	0	0.008	0.001	0	0	0	1.35	0
0.025	0.525	0.029		34.025	0.45	57.05		0									
0	1.26	0.088	0.42	0.84	10.92	0.84	0.046	0	0.105	0	0.008	0.025	0.005	0	0	0.42	0
0	0	0	0.52	0	2.08	6.24	0.01	0	0	0	0	0	0	0	0	0	0
0	4	0.098	0.8	3.8	15.4	6.4	0.012	0.2	1.76	0.003	0.015	0.007	0.004	0	0.024	2.2	0
0	0.98	0.027	0.84	0.84	7.56	4.2	0.004	0	0.126	0	0.004	0.005	0.003	0	0	0.28	0
0	7.6	0.03	0.4	0.8	7.4	11.2	0.008	0.6	0.96	0.001	0.005	0.01	0.004	0	0.012	1.8	0
0	41	0.944	48.4	6.2	292.8	7.4	0.058	0	0	0.008	0	0.186	0.134	0	0	0	0
0	3.91	0.088	1.334	1.012	15.916	1.794	0.008	0	0	0	0	0.004	0.001	0	0	0.046	0
0	0.042	0	0	0	0.084	0	0	0	0	0	0.001	0	0	0	0	0	0
0	2.7	0.048	0.57	0.09	8.22	0.33	0.182	0	0	0	0	0.001	0	0	0	0	0
0	0.025	0.001	0	0	0.05	0.025	0	0	0	0	0	0	0	0	0	0	0
0.8	0.4	0.018	0.4	2	0.6	19.6	0.008	2.8	0	0.002	0.002	0.004	0	0	0.006		0
0.76	38	0.597	24.32	63.84	171.38	131.48	0.319	1.9	0.038	0.027	0.107	0.139	0.029	0.106	0.946	1.9	0
0	0	0.006	0	0	0	0.38	0.004	0	0	0	0.004	0	0	0	0	0	0
0	0.6	0.01	0.4	0.4	0.8	24.2	0.004	0	0	0.002	0.002	0.004	0.002	0	0	0	0
0	13.4	0.24	2.8	0.4	40.8	1.8	0.832	0	0	0.001	0.002	0.006	0	0	0	0	0
0	0.6	0.006	0.4	1.8	3	16.4	0.016	0	0	0.001	0.002	0.002	0.001	0	0	0	0
0	0.15	0.003	0	6.45	0.45	30	0.003	0	0	0.002	0.001	0.003	0	0	0	0	0
0	31.5	0.798	21	11.76	210	1.68	0.086	0	0	0.021	0.033	0.021	0.141	0	0	0	0
0.41	21.73	0.082	2.87	19.27	34.44	143.09	0.078	11.07	0.123	0.005	0.039	0.016	0.006	0.037		0.82	0
0	2.52	0.118	1.68	2.1	21.42	8.82	0.025	0.42	5.754	0.005	0.01	0.068	0.005	0	0.042	2.52	0
0	0	0	0	0	0	39.06	0	0	0	0	0	0	0	0	0	0	0
1.98	4.29	0.168	3.96	19.47	27.39	157.74	0.129	31.02	0	0.079	0.096	0.667	0.009	0.007	0.3	21.45	0
4.29	6.27	0.485	4.62	49.83	30.36	141.9	0.129	5.94	0	0.102	0.122	0.762	0.016	0.01		18.81	0
0	17	2.015	12	66.5	57	212	0.315	148	0.05	0.186	0.288	2.287	0.213	0.11		14.5	0
0	11.96	1.82	5.72	27.56	47.32	173.68	0.338		0	0.151	0.172	1.976	0.198	0	0	41.6	0
0	5.72	1.82	4.68	21.32	28.08	205.92	0.156		0	0.156	0.156	1.976	0.208	0	0	52	0

EvaluEat Code	Food Name	Amt	Wt (g)	Energy (kcal)	Prot (g)	Carb (g)	Fiber (g)	Fat (g)	Mono (g)	Poly (g)	Sat (g)
18495	Toaster pastry, Pop Tart, Frosted Chocolate Fudge, low fat/Kellogg	1 pastry	52	190.32	2.652	39.52	0.572	3.016	1.248	0.884	0.52
18482	Toaster pastry, Pop Tart, Frosted Chocolate Fudge/Kellogg	1 pastry	52	201.24	2.652	37.336	0.572	4.836	2.704	1.144	0.988
3930	Toddler formula, Mead Johnson Next Step Soy, prepared from powder	1 fl. oz.	30.5	20.13	0.641	2.159	0	0.885	0.339	0.169	0.381
43476	Tofu yogurt	1 oz	28.34	26.64	0.992	4.523	0.057	0.51	0.113	0.288	0.073
19125	Topping, chocolate-flavored hazelnut spread	1 oz	28.34	153.32	1.533	17.616	1.53	8.425	4.614	1.919	1.528
22901	Tortellini, pasta with cheese filling	1 cup	236	724.52	31.86	110.92	4.484	17.063	4.876	1.088	8.496
18449	Tortilla, corn, w/o salt, ready to cook	1 tortilla, medium (approx 6" dia)	26	57.72	1.482	12.116	1.352	0.65	0.169	0.292	0.087
18364	Tortilla, flour, ready-to-cook	1 tortilla, medium (approx 6" dia)	46	149.5	4.002	25.576	1.518	3.266	1.733	0.489	0.803
18360	Tortilla, taco shell, baked	1 large (6-1/2" dia)	21	98.28	1.512	13.104	1.575	4.746	1.876	1.784	0.681
42130	Turkey bacon, cooked	1 oz	28.34	108.26	8.389	0.879	0	7.907	3.089	1.929	2.351
22706	Turkey chili w/beans, canned entree/Hormel	1 cup	247	202.54	18.723	25.565	6.422	2.766	0.42	1.21	0.667
5172	Turkey giblets, simmered	1 cup, chopped or diced	145	288.55	30.291	1.16	0	17.197	7.183	1.827	5.688
5174	Turkey gizzard, simmered	1	84	103.32	18.245	0.319	0	3.251	1.016	0.423	0.977
42128	Turkey ham, sliced, extra lean, prepackaged or deli-sliced	1 oz	28.34	33.441	5.555	0.425	0	1.077	0.245	0.322	0.361
5176	Turkey heart, simmered	1 heart	21	27.3	4.509	0.143	0	0.974	0.239	0.25	0.271
5178	Turkey liver, simmered	1 liver	83	226.59	16.617	1.004	0	17.048	7.56	1.678	5.766
5292	Turkey patty, breaded, fried	1 medium slice (approx 3" x 2" x 1/4")	28	79.24	3.92	4.396	0.14	5.04	2.092	1.319	1.313
22528	Turkey pot pie, frozen	1 serving	397	698.72	25.805	70.269	4.367	34.936	13.736	5.479	11.434
5296	Turkey roast, light & dark meat, no bone, frozen, seasoned, cooked	1 cup, chopped or diced	135	209.25	28.782	4.144	0	7.803	1.62	2.241	2.565
5286	Turkey w/gravy, frozen	1 cup	240	160.8	14.112	11.064	0	6.312	2.328	1.128	2.04
5218	Turkey, fryer/roaster, breast w/skin, roasted	1 unit (yield from 1 lb ready-to-cook turkey)	98	149.94	28.489	0	0	3.136	1.176	0.745	0.853
5220	Turkey, fryer/roaster, breast, no skin, roasted	1 unit (yield from 1 lb ready-to-cook turkey)	87	117.45	26.152	0	0	0.644	0.113	0.174	0.209
5208	Turkey, fryer/roaster, dark meat w/skin, roasted	1 unit (yield from 1 lb ready-to-cook turkey)	106	192.92	29.351	0	0	7.484	2.406	1.993	2.247
5206	Turkey, fryer/roaster, light meat w/skin, roasted	1 unit (yield from 1 lb ready-to-cook turkey)	123	201.72	35.387	0	0	5.633	2.091	1.341	1.538
5306	Turkey, ground, cooked	1 patty (4 oz, raw)	82	192.7	22.435	0	0	10.783	4.01	2.649	2.78
7900	Turkey, pork, and beef sausage, low-fat, smoked	1 frankfurter	56	56.56	4.48	6.44	0.336	1.4	0.577	0.185	0.476
17203	Veal liver, braised	1 slice (yield from 116 g raw liver)	80	153.6	22.736	3.016	0	5.008	0.917	0.831	1.589
17204	Veal liver, pan fried	1 slice (yield from 99 g raw liver)	67	129.31	18.338	2.995	0	4.362	0.8	0.745	1.413

Chol (g)	Calc (mg)	Iron (mg)	Mag (mg)	Phos (mg)	Pota (mg)	Sodi (mg)	Zinc (mg)	Vit A (RAE)	Vit C (mg)	Thia (mg)	Ribo (mg)	Niac (mg)	Vit B$_6$ (mg)	Vit B$_{12}$ (µg)	Vit E (mg)	Fol (µg)	Alc (g)
0	13.52	1.82	14.56	39.52	61.88	248.56	0.26		0	0.156	0.156	1.976	0.208	0	0	52	0
0	19.76	1.82	15.08	43.68	82.16	202.8	0.26		0	0.156	0.156	1.976	0.208	0	0	52	0
0	23.18	0.36	1.525	17.995	29.89	8.845	0.241	17.69	2.41	0.016	0.018	0.201	0.018	0.058	0.4	3.05	0
0	33.441	0.3	11.336	10.769	13.32	9.919	0.088	0.567	0.709	0.017	0.006	0.068	0.006	0	0.088	1.7	0
0	30.607	1.241	18.138	43.077	115.344	11.619	0.3	0.283	0	0.034	0.048	0.121	0.024	0.079	1.406	3.968	0
99.12	358.72	3.54	49.56	500.32	210.04	811.84	2.407	89.68	0	0.739	0.732	6.363	0.101	0.378	0.378	174.6	0
0	45.5	0.364	16.9	81.64	40.04	2.86	0.244	0	0	0.029	0.019	0.389	0.057	0	0.04	29.64	0
0	57.5	1.518	11.96	57.04	60.26	219.88	0.327	0	0	0.244	0.135	1.643	0.023	0	0.258	47.84	0
0	33.6	0.525	22.05	52.08	37.59	77.07	0.294	0	0	0.048	0.011	0.283	0.062	0	0.349	27.51	0
27.773	2.551	0.598	8.219	130.364	111.943	647.569	0.859	0	0	0.017	0.068	1	0.091	0.102	0.292	2.551	0
34.58	116.09	3.458	69.16		681.72	1197.95	2.717		1.482								0
419.05	8.7	11.18	26.1	334.95	391.5	92.8	4.524	15569	19.87	0.039	2.179	10.147	0.842	48.213	0.116	485.8	0
170.52	5.88	4.158	14.28	129.36	278.88	56.28	2.831	0	5.292	0.011	0.174	3.587	0.089	6.787	0.042	10.92	0
18.988	1.417	0.383	5.668	86.154	84.737	294.169	0.669	0	0	0.014	0.071	1	0.065	0.074	0.111	1.7	0
38.64	1.47	1.092	5.46	54.39	61.11	18.9	0.934	3.99	0.588	0.007	0.218	0.71	0.089	4.557	0.01	1.68	0
322.04	4.15	8.881	14.11	244.02	175.13	46.48	2.175	18758	18.76	0.032	2.291	8.466	0.863	48.306	0.091	573.5	0
17.36	3.92	0.616	4.2	75.6	77	224	0.403	3.08	0	0.028	0.053	0.644	0.056	0.062	0.353	7.84	0
63.52		3.97				1389.5											0
71.55	6.75	2.201	29.7	329.4	402.3	918	3.429	0	0	0.063	0.22	8.466	0.365	2.052	0.513	6.75	0
43.2	33.6	2.232	19.2	194.4	146.4	1329.6	1.68	31.2	0	0.058	0.305	4.318	0.24	0.576		9.6	0
88.2	14.7	1.539	27.44	211.68	273.42	51.94	1.735	0	0	0.04	0.132	6.823	0.5	0.363		5.88	0
72.21	10.44	1.331	25.23	194.88	254.04	45.24	1.514	0	0	0.037	0.114	6.519	0.487	0.339	0.078	5.22	0
124.02	28.62	2.47	24.38	201.4	251.22	80.56	4.06	0	0	0.051	0.249	3.551	0.35	0.392		9.54	0
116.85	22.14	1.98	31.98	252.15	322.26	70.11	2.558	0	0	0.047	0.171	7.718	0.603	0.443		7.38	0
83.64	20.5	1.583	19.68	160.72	221.4	87.74	2.345	0	0	0.044	0.138	3.952	0.32	0.271	0.279	5.74	0
11.76	5.6	1.232	8.96	41.44	136.08	445.76	0.672	0	1.064	0.073	0.045	0.868	0.056	0.157	0.05	3.36	0
408.8	4.8	4.088	16	368	263.2	62.4	8.984	16916	0.88	0.146	2.288	10.52	0.734	67.68	0.544	264.8	0
324.95	4.69	4.007	15.41	323.61	236.51	56.95	7.973	13450	0.469	0.119	2.05	9.615	0.597	48.575	0.402	234.5	0

EvaluEat Code	Food Name	Amt	Wt (g)	Energy (kcal)	Prot (g)	Carb (g)	Fiber (g)	Fat (g)	Mono (g)	Poly (g)	Sat (g)
17223	Veal tongue, braised	3 oz	85	171.7	21.973	0	0	8.585	3.919	0.323	3.697
17089	Veal, composite, lean & fat, cooked	3 oz	85	196.35	25.585	0	0	9.682	3.74	0.68	3.638
17143	Veal, ground, broiled	3 oz	85	146.2	20.723	0	0	6.426	2.414	0.468	2.584
11655	Vegetable juice, carrot, canned	1 cup	236	94.4	2.242	21.924	1.888	0.354	0.017	0.168	0.064
11886	Vegetable juice, tomato, canned w/o salt	1 cup	243	41.31	1.847	10.303	0.972	0.122	0.022	0.058	0.019
11001	Vege, alfalfa seeds, sprouted, raw	1 tbsp	3	0.87	0.12	0.113	0.075	0.021	0.002	0.012	0.002
11697	Vege, arrowroot, raw	1 cup, sliced	120	78	5.088	16.068	1.56	0.24	0.005	0.11	0.047
11702	Vege, artichokes (globe or French) boiled w/salt, drained	1 artichoke, medium	120	60	4.176	13.416	6.48	0.192	0.006	0.082	0.044
11009	Vege, artichokes (globe or French) frozen	1 package (9 oz)	255	96.9	6.707	19.788	9.945	1.097	0.031	0.456	0.252
11959	Vege, arugula/roquette, raw	1 leaf	2	0.5	0.052	0.073	0.032	0.013	0.001	0.006	0.002
11705	Vege, asparagus, boiled w/salt, drained	4 spears (1/2" base)	60	13.2	1.44	2.466	1.2	0.132	0.006	0.082	0.043
11015	Vege, asparagus, canned, drained	1 spear (about 5" long)	18	3.42	0.385	0.443	0.288	0.117	0.004	0.051	0.026
11011	Vege, asparagus, raw	1 spear, large (7-1/4" to 8-1/2")	20	4	0.44	0.776	0.42	0.024	0.001	0.018	0.009
11712	Vege, bamboo shoots, boiled w/salt, drained	1 cup (1/2" slices)	120	14.4	1.836	2.304	1.2	0.264	0.006	0.118	0.061
11028	Vege, bamboo shoots, canned, drained	1 cup (1/8" slices)	131	24.89	2.253	4.218	1.834	0.524	0.012	0.233	0.121
11026	Vege, bamboo shoots, raw	1 cup (1/2" slices)	151	40.77	3.926	7.852	3.322	0.453	0.011	0.202	0.104
11626	Vege, bean sprouts, mung, mature seeds, sprouted, canned, drained	1 cup	125	15	1.75	2.675	1	0.075	0.01	0.025	0.02
11973	Vege, beans, fava, in pod, raw	1 cup	126	110.88	9.979	22.214		0.92	0.131	0.431	0.149
11716	Vege, beans, lima, baby, immature seeds, frozen, boiled w/salt, drained	.5 cup	90	94.5	5.985	17.505	5.4	0.27	0.015	0.13	0.061
11033	Vege, beans, lima, immature seeds, canned, solids & liquid	.5 cup	124	88.04	5.047	16.529	4.464	0.36	0.02	0.172	0.082
11720	Vege, beans, pinto, immature seeds, boiled w/salt, drained	1 package (10 oz)	284	460.08	26.44	87.699	24.424	1.363	0.099	0.784	0.165
11723	Vege, beans, snap, green, boiled w/salt, drained	1 cup	125	43.75	2.362	9.863	4	0.35	0.014	0.181	0.08
11056	Vege, beans, snap, green, canned, drained	1 cup	135	27	1.553	6.075	2.565	0.135	0.005	0.069	0.03
11052	Vege, beans, snap, green, raw	1 cup	110	34.1	2.002	7.854	3.74	0.132	0.005	0.065	0.029
11725	Vege, beans, snap, yellow, boiled w/salt, drained	1 cup	125	43.75	2.362	9.85	4.125	0.35	0.014	0.181	0.08
11932	Vege, beans, snap, yellow, canned, regular pack, drained	1 cup	135	27	1.553	6.075	1.755	0.135	0.005	0.069	0.03
11722	Vege, beans, snap, yellow, raw	1 cup	110	34.1	2.002	7.854	3.74	0.132	0.005	0.065	0.029
11736	Vege, beet greens, boiled w/salt, drained	1 cup (1" pieces)	144	38.88	3.701	7.862	4.176	0.288	0.055	0.101	0.045
11086	Vege, beet greens, raw	1 cup	38	8.36	0.836	1.645	1.406	0.049	0.01	0.017	0.008
11734	Vege, beets, boiled w/salt, drained	.5 cup slices	85	37.4	1.428	8.466	1.7	0.153	0.03	0.054	0.024
11084	Vege, beets, canned, drained	1 cup, diced	157	48.67	1.429	11.32	2.669	0.22	0.044	0.08	0.036
11080	Vege, beets, peeled, raw	1 cup	136	58.48	2.19	13.002	3.808	0.231	0.045	0.083	0.037
11609	Vege, beets, pickled, canned, solids & liquid	1 cup slices	227	147.55	1.816	36.956	5.902	0.182	0.036	0.066	0.03
11088	Vege, broadbeans, immature seeds, raw	1 cup	109	78.48	6.104	12.753	4.578	0.654	0.019	0.338	0.15
22600	Vege, broccoli in cheese flavored sauce, frozen/Green Giant	1 cup	168	112.56	3.864	14.952		4.2	1.695	0.425	0.806
11741	Vege, broccoli stalks, raw	1 stalk	114	31.92	3.397	5.974		0.399	0.027	0.19	0.062
11742	Vege, broccoli, boiled w/salt, chopped, drained	.5 cup, chopped	78	21.84	2.324	3.947	2.574	0.273	0.019	0.13	0.042
11969	Vege, broccoli, Chinese, cooked	1 cup	88	19.36	1.003	3.353	2.2	0.634	0.044	0.29	0.097
11745	Vege, Brussels sprouts, boiled w/salt, drained	.5 cup	78	31.98	1.989	6.763	2.028	0.398	0.03	0.203	0.082
11098	Vege, Brussels sprouts, raw	1 cup	88	37.84	2.974	7.876	3.344	0.264	0.02	0.135	0.055

Chol (g)	Calc (mg)	Iron (mg)	Mag (mg)	Phos (mg)	Pota (mg)	Sodi (mg)	Zinc (mg)	Vit A (RAE)	Vit C (mg)	Thia (mg)	Ribo (mg)	Niac (mg)	Vit B$_6$ (mg)	Vit B$_{12}$ (µg)	Vit E (mg)	Fol (µg)	Alc (g)
202.3	7.65	1.776	15.3	141.1	137.7	54.4	3.834	0	5.1	0.06	0.298	1.25	0.128	4.505		7.65	0
96.9	18.7	0.978	22.1	203.15	276.25	73.95	4.046	0	0	0.051	0.272	6.774	0.264	1.335	0.34	12.75	0
87.55	14.45	0.842	20.4	184.45	286.45	70.55	3.289	0	0	0.06	0.23	6.826	0.331	1.079	0.128	9.35	0
0	56.64	1.086	33.04	99.12	689.12	68.44	0.425	2256	20.06	0.217	0.13	0.911	0.512	0	2.738	9.44	0
0	24.3	1.045	26.73	43.74	556.47	24.3	0.365	55.89	44.47	0.114	0.075	1.635	0.27	0	0.778	48.6	0
0	0.96	0.029	0.81	2.1	2.37	0.18	0.028	0.24	0.246	0.002	0.004	0.014	0.001	0	0.001	1.08	0
0	7.2	2.664	30	117.6	544.8	31.2	0.756	1.2	2.28	0.172	0.071	2.032	0.319	0		405.6	0
0	54	1.548	72	103.2	424.8	397.2	0.588	10.8	12	0.078	0.079	1.201	0.133	0	0.228	61.2	0
0	48.45	1.275	68.85	147.9	632.4	119.85	0.816	20.4	13.52	0.148	0.357	2.193	0.209	0		321.3	0
0	3.2	0.029	0.94	1.04	7.38	0.54	0.009	2.38	0.3	0.001	0.002	0.006	0.001	0	0.009	1.94	0
0	13.8	0.546	8.4	32.4	134.4	144	0.36	30	4.62	0.097	0.083	0.65	0.047	0		89.4	0
0	2.88	0.329	1.8	7.74	30.96	51.66	0.072	7.38	3.312	0.011	0.018	0.172	0.02	0	0.056	17.28	0
0	4.8	0.428	2.8	10.4	40.4	0.4	0.108	7.6	1.12	0.029	0.028	0.196	0.018	0	0.226	10.4	0
0	14.4	0.288	3.6	24	639.6	288	0.564	0	0	0.024	0.06	0.36	0.118	0		2.4	0
0	10.48	0.419	5.24	32.75	104.8	9.17	0.851	1.31	1.441	0.034	0.034	0.183	0.178	0	0.825	3.93	0
0	19.63	0.755	4.53	89.09	804.83	6.04	1.661	1.51	6.04	0.227	0.106	0.906	0.362	0	1.51	10.57	0
0	17.5	0.538	11.25	40	33.75	175	0.35	0	0.375	0.037	0.087	0.275	0.04	0	0.05	12.5	0
0	46.62	1.953	41.58	162.54	418.32	31.5	1.26	21.42	4.662	0.168	0.365	2.834	0.131	0		186.5	0
0	25.2	1.764	50.4	100.8	369.9	238.5	0.495	7.2	5.22	0.063	0.049	0.693	0.104	0	0.576	14.4	0
0	34.72	1.996	42.16	88.04	353.4	312.48	0.794	9.92	9.052	0.036	0.053	0.66	0.077	0	0.36	19.84	0
0	147.68	7.696	153.36	284	1834.64	905.96	1.96	0	1.988	0.778	0.307	1.795	0.551	0		96.56	0
0	57.5	1.6	31.25	48.75	373.75	298.75	0.45	43.75	12.13	0.093	0.121	0.768	0.07	0	0.563	41.25	0
0	35.1	1.215	17.55	25.65	147.15	353.7	0.391	29.7	6.48	0.02	0.076	0.271	0.05	0	0.378	43.2	0
0	40.7	1.144	27.5	41.8	229.9	6.6	0.264	38.5	17.93	0.092	0.115	0.827	0.081	0	0.451	40.7	0
0	57.5	1.6	31.25	48.75	373.75	298.75	0.45	5	12.13	0.093	0.121	0.768	0.07	0	0.563	41.25	0
0	35.1	1.215	17.55	25.65	147.15	338.85	0.391	6.75	6.48	0.02	0.076	0.271	0.05	0	0.391	43.2	0
0	40.7	1.144	27.5	41.8	229.9	6.6	0.264	5.5	17.93	0.092	0.115	0.827	0.081	0		40.7	0
0	164.16	2.736	97.92	59.04	1308.96	686.88	0.72	367.2	35.86	0.168	0.416	0.719	0.19	0		20.16	0
0	44.46	0.977	26.6	15.58	289.56	85.88	0.144	120.1	11.4	0.038	0.084	0.152	0.04	0	0.57	5.7	0
0	13.6	0.672	19.55	32.3	259.25	242.25	0.298	387.6	3.06	0.023	0.034	0.281	0.057	0	1.836	68	0
0	23.55	2.857	26.69	26.69	232.36	304.58	0.33	1.57	6.437	0.016	0.063	0.246	0.089	0	0.047	47.1	0
0	21.76	1.088	31.28	54.4	442	106.08	0.476	2.72	6.664	0.042	0.054	0.454	0.091	0	0.054	148.2	0
0	24.97	0.931	34.05	38.59	335.96	599.28	0.59	2.27	5.221	0.023	0.109	0.57	0.113	0		61.29	0
0	23.98	2.071	41.42	103.55	272.5	54.5	0.632	19.62	35.97	0.185	0.12	1.635	0.041	0		104.6	0
						806.4			59.47								0
0	54.72	1.003	28.5	75.24	370.5	30.78	0.456	22.8	106.2	0.074	0.136	0.727	0.181	0	1.892	80.94	0
0	31.2	0.523	16.38	52.26	228.54	204.36	0.351	76.44	32.76	0.049	0.096	0.431	0.156	0	1.131	84.24	0
0	88	0.493	15.84	36.08	229.68	6.16	0.343	72.16	24.82	0.084	0.128	0.385	0.062	0	0.422	87.12	0
0	28.08	0.936	15.6	43.68	247.26	200.46	0.257	28.08	48.36	0.083	0.062	0.473	0.139	0		46.8	0
0	36.96	1.232	20.24	60.72	342.32	22	0.37	33.44	74.8	0.122	0.079	0.656	0.193	0	0.774	53.68	0

EvaluEat Code	Food Name	Amt	Wt (g)	Energy (kcal)	Prot (g)	Carb (g)	Fiber (g)	Fat (g)	Mono (g)	Poly (g)	Sat (g)
11109	Vege, cabbage heads, raw	1 cup, chopped	89	21.36	1.282	4.966	2.047	0.107	0.008	0.053	0.014
11112	Vege, cabbage heads, red, raw	1 cup, chopped	89	27.59	1.273	6.559	1.869	0.142	0.017	0.111	0.03
11752	Vege, cabbage, red, boiled w/salt, drained	.5 cup, shredded	75	15.75	0.787	3.48	1.5	0.15	0.011	0.071	0.02
11751	Vege, cabbage, boiled w/salt, drained	.5 cup, shredded	75	16.5	0.765	3.345	1.425	0.322	0.022	0.147	0.04
11754	Vege, cabbage, pak-choi (Chinese) boiled w/salt, drained	1 cup, shredded	170	20.4	2.652	3.026	1.7	0.272	0.02	0.131	0.036
11119	Vege, cabbage, pe-tsai (Chinese) raw	1 cup, shredded	76	12.16	0.912	2.455	0.912	0.152	0.017	0.055	0.033
11960	Vege, carrots, baby, raw	1 medium	10	3.5	0.064	0.824	0.18	0.013	0.001	0.006	0.002
11757	Vege, carrots, boiled w/salt, drained	.5 cup slices	78	27.3	0.593	6.412	2.34	0.14	0.005	0.069	0.023
11128	Vege, carrots, canned, drained	1 cup, sliced	146	36.5	0.934	8.088	2.19	0.277	0.013	0.134	0.053
11124	Vege, carrots, chopped/grated, raw	1 cup, chopped	128	52.48	1.19	12.262	3.84	0.307	0.015	0.131	0.041
11134	Vege, cassava (manioc) raw	1 cup	206	329.6	2.802	78.404	3.708	0.577	0.155	0.099	0.152
11135	Vege, cauliflower head, raw	1 cup	100	25	1.98	5.3	2.5	0.1	0.014	0.099	0.032
11761	Vege, cauliflower, boiled w/salt, drained	.5 cup (1" pieces)	62	14.26	1.141	2.548	1.674	0.279	0.02	0.135	0.043
11764	Vege, celery, boiled w/salt, drained	1 cup, diced	150	27	1.245	6.015	2.4	0.24	0.045	0.113	0.06
11143	Vege, celery, raw	1 cup, diced	120	16.8	0.828	3.564	1.92	0.204	0.038	0.097	0.052
11765	Vege, chard, Swiss, boiled w/salt, drained	1 cup, chopped	175	35	3.29	7.227	3.675	0.14			
11151	Vege, chicory, witloof (Belgian endive) raw	1 head	53	9.01	0.477	2.12	1.643	0.053	0.001	0.023	0.013
11768	Vege, collards, boiled w/salt, drained	1 cup, chopped	190	49.4	4.009	9.329	5.32	0.684	0.049	0.329	0.089
11161	Vege, collards, raw	1 cup, chopped	36	10.8	0.882	2.048	1.296	0.151	0.011	0.072	0.02
11167	Vege, corn ears, yellow, sweet, raw	1 ear, medium	90	77.4	2.898	17.118	2.43	1.062	0.312	0.503	0.164
11908	Vege, corn, white, sweet, canned, vacuum/regular pack	.5 cup	105	82.95	2.53	20.412	2.1	0.525	0.154	0.249	0.081
11900	Vege, corn, white, sweet, ears, raw	1 ear, large	143	122.98	4.605	27.199	3.861	1.687	0.496	0.799	0.26
11770	Vege, corn, yellow, sweet, boiled w/salt, drained	1 cup	164	177.12	5.445	41.18	4.592	2.099	0.613	0.989	0.323
11176	Vege, corn, yellow, sweet, canned, vacuum/regular pack	.5 cup	105	82.95	2.53	20.412	2.1	0.525	0.154	0.249	0.081
11174	Vege, corn, yellow, sweet, cream style, regular pack, canned	1 cup	256	184.32	4.454	46.413	3.072	1.075	0.315	0.507	0.166
11777	Vege, cowpeas (blackeyes), immature seeds, boiled w/salt, drained	1 cup	165	160.05	5.231	33.528	8.25	0.627	0.056	0.266	0.158
11203	Vege, cress, garden, raw	1 cup	50	16	1.3	2.75	0.55	0.35	0.119	0.114	0.012
11205	Vege, cucumber, raw	.5 cup slices	52	7.8	0.338	1.888	0.26	0.057	0.002	0.028	0.018
11207	Vege, dandelion greens, raw	1 cup, chopped	55	24.75	1.485	5.06	1.925	0.385	0.008	0.168	0.094
11783	Vege, eggplant (brinjal) boiled w/salt, drained	1 cup (1" cubes)	99	34.65	0.822	8.643	2.475	0.228	0.02	0.092	0.044
11213	Vege, endive (escarole) raw	.5 cup, chopped	25	4.25	0.313	0.837	0.775	0.05	0.001	0.022	0.012
11957	Vege, fennel bulb, raw	1 cup, sliced	87	26.97	1.079	6.342	2.697	0.174			
11987	Vege, fungi, mushroom, oyster, raw	1 large	148	54.76	6.127	9.206	3.552	0.755			
11798	Vege, fungi, mushroom, shiitake, boiled w/salt, drained	4 mushrooms	72	39.6	1.123	10.282	1.512	0.158	0.049	0.022	0.04
11266	Vege, fungi, mushrooms, brown, Italian, or crimini, raw	1 piece	14	3.08	0.35	0.577	0.084	0.014	0	0.006	0.002
11264	Vege, fungi, mushrooms, canned, caps/slices, drained	1 can	132	33	2.468	6.719	3.168	0.383	0.007	0.149	0.05
11265	Vege, fungi, mushrooms, portabella, raw	1 oz	28.34	7.368	0.709	1.437	0.425	0.057	0.001	0.022	0.007
11260	Vege, fungi, mushrooms, slices, raw	1 medium	18	3.96	0.56	0.583	0.216	0.061	0.001	0.025	0.008
11961	Vege, hearts of palm, canned	1 cup	146	40.88	3.679	6.745	3.504	0.905	0.15	0.295	0.19
11790	Vege, kale, boiled w/salt, drained	1 cup, chopped	130	36.4	2.47	7.319	2.6	0.52	0.039	0.251	0.068
11233	Vege, kale, raw	1 cup, chopped	67	33.5	2.211	6.707	1.34	0.469	0.035	0.226	0.061
11793	Vege, kohlrabi, boiled w/salt, drained	1 cup slices	165	47.85	2.97	11.038	1.815	0.182	0.013	0.087	0.023
11241	Vege, kohlrabi, peeled, raw	1 cup	135	36.45	2.295	8.37	4.86	0.135	0.009	0.065	0.018

Chol (g)	Calc (mg)	Iron (mg)	Mag (mg)	Phos (mg)	Pota (mg)	Sodi (mg)	Zinc (mg)	Vit A (RAE)	Vit C (mg)	Thia (mg)	Ribo (mg)	Niac (mg)	Vit B$_6$ (mg)	Vit B$_{12}$ (μg)	Vit E (mg)	Fol (μg)	Alc (g)
0	41.83	0.525	13.35	20.47	218.94	16.02	0.16	8.01	28.66	0.045	0.036	0.267	0.085	0	0.134	38.27	0
0	40.05	0.712	14.24	26.7	216.27	24.03	0.196	49.84	50.73	0.057	0.061	0.372	0.186	0	0.098	16.02	0
0	27.75	0.262	8.25	21.75	105	183	0.113	0.75	25.8	0.026	0.015	0.15	0.105	0		9.75	0
0	23.25	0.127	6	11.25	72.75	191.25	0.068	5.25	15.08	0.043	0.041	0.212	0.085	0	0.09	15	0
0	158.1	1.768	18.7	49.3	630.7	459	0.289	360.4	44.2	0.054	0.107	0.728	0.282	0	0.153	69.7	0
0	58.52	0.236	9.88	22.04	180.88	6.84	0.175	12.16	20.52	0.03	0.038	0.304	0.176	0	0.091	60.04	0
0	3.2	0.089	1	2.8	23.7	7.8	0.017	69	0.84	0.003	0.004	0.056	0.01	0		3.3	0
0	23.4	0.265	7.8	23.4	183.3	235.56	0.156	659.1	2.808	0.051	0.034	0.503	0.119	0	0.803	1.56	0
0	36.5	0.934	11.68	35.04	261.34	353.32	0.38	814.7	3.942	0.026	0.044	0.806	0.164	0	1.08	13.14	0
0	42.24	0.384	15.36	44.8	409.6	88.32	0.307	770.6	7.552	0.084	0.074	1.258	0.177	0	0.845	24.32	0
0	32.96	0.556	43.26	55.62	558.26	28.84	0.7	2.06	42.44	0.179	0.099	1.759	0.181	0	0.391	55.62	0
0	22	0.44	15	44	303	30	0.28	1	46.4	0.057	0.063	0.526	0.222	0	0.08	57	0
0	9.92	0.205	5.58	19.84	88.04	150.04	0.112	0.62	27.47	0.026	0.032	0.254	0.107	0	0.043	27.28	0
0	63	0.63	18	37.5	426	490.5	0.21	43.5	9.15	0.065	0.071	0.479	0.129	0	0.525	33	0
0	48	0.24	13.2	28.8	312	96	0.156	26.4	3.72	0.025	0.068	0.384	0.089	0	0.324	43.2	0
0	101.5	3.955	150.5	57.75	960.75	726.25	0.578	535.5	31.5	0.06	0.15	0.63	0.149	0	3.307	15.75	0
0	10.07	0.127	5.3	13.78	111.83	1.06	0.085	0.53	1.484	0.033	0.014	0.085	0.022	0		19.61	0
0	266	2.204	38	57	220.4	478.8	0.437	771.4	34.58	0.076	0.201	1.092	0.243	0	1.672	176.7	0
0	52.2	0.068	3.24	3.6	60.84	7.2	0.047	119.9	12.71	0.019	0.047	0.267	0.059	0	0.814	59.76	0
0	1.8	0.468	33.3	80.1	243	13.5	0.405	9	6.12	0.18	0.054	1.53	0.049	0	0.063	41.4	0
0	5.25	0.441	24.15	67.2	195.3	285.6	0.483	0	8.505	0.043	0.077	1.225	0.058	0		51.45	0
0	2.86	0.744	52.91	127.27	386.1	21.45	0.643	0	9.724	0.286	0.086	2.431	0.079	0	0.1	65.78	0
0	3.28	1	52.48	168.92	408.36	414.92	0.787	21.32	10.17	0.353	0.118	2.647	0.098	0	0.148	75.44	0
0	5.25	0.441	24.15	67.2	195.3	285.6	0.483	4.2	8.505	0.043	0.077	1.225	0.058	0	0.042	51.45	0
0	7.68	0.973	43.52	130.56	343.04	729.6	1.357	10.24	11.78	0.064	0.136	2.458	0.161	0	0.179	115.2	0
0	211.2	1.848	85.8	84.15	689.7	396	1.699	66	3.63	0.167	0.244	2.315	0.107	0	0.363	209.6	0
0	40.5	0.65	19	38	303	7	0.115	173	34.5	0.04	0.13	0.5	0.123	0	0.35	40	0
0	8.32	0.146	6.76	12.48	76.44	1.04	0.104	2.6	1.456	0.014	0.017	0.051	0.021	0	0.016	3.64	0
0	102.85	1.705	19.8	36.3	218.35	41.8	0.226	135.9	19.25	0.105	0.143	0.443	0.138	0	2.635	14.85	0
0	5.94	0.248	10.89	14.85	121.77	236.61	0.119	1.98	1.287	0.075	0.02	0.594	0.085	0	0.406	13.86	0
0	13	0.207	3.75	7	78.5	5.5	0.198	27	1.625	0.02	0.019	0.1	0.005	0	0.11	35.5	0
0	42.63	0.635	14.79	43.5	360.18	45.24	0.174	6.09	10.44	0.009	0.028	0.557	0.041	0		23.49	0
0	8.88	2.575	29.6	208.68	763.68	45.88	1.154	2.96	0	0.081	0.533	5.297	0.181	0		69.56	0
0	2.16	0.317	10.08	20.88	84.24	172.8	0.958	0	0.216	0.027	0.122	1.08	0.114	0		15.12	0
0	2.52	0.056	1.26	16.8	62.72	0.84	0.154	0	0	0.013	0.069	0.532	0.015	0.014	0.016	1.96	0
0	14.52	1.043	19.8	87.12	170.28	561	0.95	0	0	0.112	0.028	2.103	0.081	0	0.013	15.84	0
0	2.267	0.17	3.117	36.842	137.166	1.7	0.17	0	0	0.022	0.136	1.275	0.028	0.014	0.037	6.235	0
0	0.54	0.094	1.62	15.3	56.52	0.72	0.094	0	0.432	0.016	0.075	0.694	0.021	0.007	0.002	2.88	0
0	84.68	4.57	55.48	94.9	258.42	621.96	1.679	0	11.53	0.016	0.083	0.638	0.032	0		56.94	0
0	93.6	1.17	23.4	36.4	296.4	336.7	0.312	885.3	53.3	0.069	0.091	0.65	0.179	0	1.105	16.9	0
0	90.45	1.139	22.78	37.52	299.49	28.81	0.295	515.2	80.4	0.074	0.087	0.67	0.182	0	0.536	19.43	0
0	41.25	0.66	31.35	74.25	561	424.05	0.512	3.3	89.1	0.066	0.033	0.643	0.254	0	0.858	19.8	0
0	32.4	0.54	25.65	62.1	472.5	27	0.041	2.7	83.7	0.068	0.027	0.54	0.203	0	0.648	21.6	0

EvaluEat Code	Food Name	Amt	Wt (g)	Energy (kcal)	Prot (g)	Carb (g)	Fiber (g)	Fat (g)	Mono (g)	Poly (g)	Sat (g)
11246	Vege, leeks (bulb & lower leaf-portion) raw	1 leek	89	54.29	1.335	12.593	1.602	0.267	0.004	0.148	0.036
11795	Vege, leeks (bulbs & lower leaves) boiled w/salt, drained	1 leek	124	38.44	1.004	9.449	1.24	0.248	0.004	0.138	0.033
11250	Vege, lettuce, butterhead (Boston/bibb) leaves, raw	1 leaf, medium	7.5	0.975	0.101	0.167	0.083	0.016	0.001	0.009	0.002
11251	Vege, lettuce, cos/romaine, raw	1 inner leaf	10	1.7	0.123	0.329	0.21	0.03	0.001	0.016	0.004
11252	Vege, lettuce, iceberg, head, raw	1 head, medium	539	53.9	4.366	11.265	5.39	0.593	0.022	0.296	0.075
11253	Vege, lettuce, looseleaf, raw	1 leaf	10	1.5	0.136	0.279	0.13	0.015	0.001	0.008	0.002
11799	Vege, mustard greens, boiled w/salt, drained	1 cup, chopped	140	21	3.164	2.94	2.8	0.336	0.154	0.064	0.017
11270	Vege, mustard greens, raw	1 cup, chopped	56	14.56	1.512	2.744	1.848	0.112	0.052	0.021	0.006
11803	Vege, okra, boiled w/salt, drained	.5 cup slices	80	17.6	1.496	3.608	2	0.168	0.022	0.037	0.036
11278	Vege, okra, raw	1 cup	100	31	2	7.03	3.2	0.1	0.017	0.027	0.026
11296	Vege, onion rings, breaded, par fried, frozen, oven heated	10 rings, large	71	288.97	3.791	27.094	0.923	18.957	7.715	3.63	6.095
11805	Vege, onions, boiled w/salt, chopped, drained	1 cup	210	92.4	2.856	21.315	2.94	0.399	0.057	0.153	0.065
11282	Vege, onions, chopped, raw	1 cup, chopped	160	67.2	1.472	16.176	2.24	0.128	0.037	0.099	0.042
11291	Vege, onions, spring (tops & bulb) chopped, raw	1 cup, chopped	100	32	1.83	7.34	2.6	0.19	0.027	0.074	0.032
11808	Vege, parsnip, boiled w/salt, drained	.5 cup, sliced	78	63.18	1.03	15.233	3.12	0.234	0.087	0.037	0.039
11298	Vege, parsnip, peeled, raw	1 cup, sliced	133	99.75	1.596	23.927	6.517	0.399	0.149	0.063	0.067
11318	Vege, peas & carrots, canned, regular pack, solids & liquid	1 cup	255	96.9	5.534	21.624	5.1	0.688	0.059	0.329	0.125
11809	Vege, peas w/edible pod-snow/sugar, boiled w/salt, drained	1 cup	160	67.2	5.232	11.28	4.48	0.368	0.037	0.16	0.07
11300	Vege, peas w/edible pod-snow/sugar, raw	1 cup, chopped	98	41.16	2.744	7.399	2.548	0.196	0.021	0.087	0.038
11811	Vege, peas, green, boiled w/salt, drained	1 cup	160	134.4	8.576	25.024	8.8	0.352	0.03	0.163	0.062
11308	Vege, peas, green, canned, regular pack, drained	1 cup	170	117.3	7.514	21.386	6.97	0.595	0.053	0.277	0.105
11304	Vege, peas, green, raw	1 cup	145	117.45	7.859	20.967	7.395	0.58	0.051	0.271	0.103
11980	Vege, pepper, chili, green, canned	1 cup	139	29.19	1.001	6.394	2.363	0.375	0.024	0.213	0.039
11979	Vege, pepper, jalapeno, raw	1 cup, sliced	90	27	1.215	5.319	2.52	0.558	0.03	0.287	0.056
11977	Vege, pepper, serrano, raw	1 pepper	6.1	1.952	0.106	0.409	0.226	0.027	0.001	0.014	0.004
11333	Vege, pepper, sweet, green, chopped/sliced, raw	1 medium	119	23.8	1.023	5.522	2.023	0.202	0.01	0.074	0.069
11821	Vege, pepper, sweet, red, raw	1 medium	119	30.94	1.178	7.176	2.38	0.357	0.008	0.186	0.07
11951	Vege, pepper, sweet, yellow, raw	1 medium	186	50.22	1.86	11.755	1.674	0.391			0.058
11937	Vege, pickles, cucumber, dill	1 medium	65	11.7	0.403	2.678	0.78	0.123	0.002	0.05	0.031
11940	Vege, pickles, cucumber, sweet, gherkins	1 gherkin (2-3/4" long)	25	29.25	0.093	7.952	0.275	0.065	0.001	0.026	0.017
11943	Vege, pimiento, canned	1 tbsp	12	2.76	0.132	0.612	0.228	0.036	0.002	0.019	0.005
11383	Vege, potato mashed, granules w/milk, prep w/water & margarine	1 cup	210	243.6	4.599	33.768	2.73	10.059	4.105	2.824	2.541
11672	Vege, potato pancakes, homemade	1 pancake	76	206.72	4.682	21.766	1.52	11.582	3.526	4.971	2.313
11414	Vege, potato salad, homemade	1 cup	250	357.5	6.7	27.925	3.25	20.5	6.2	9.342	3.572
11373	Vege, potato, au gratin, homemade w/butter	1 cup	245	323.4	12.397	27.612	4.41	18.596	5.265	0.676	11.596
11833	Vege, potato, boiled w/o skin & w/salt	1 medium	167	143.62	2.856	33.417	3.34	0.167	0.003	0.072	0.043
11376	Vege, potato, canned, drained	1 cup	180	108	2.538	24.498	4.14	0.378	0.009	0.16	0.097
11838	Vege, potato, french fries, frozen, oven heated, w/salt	10 strips	50	100	1.585	15.595	1.6	3.78	2.381	0.389	0.631
11391	Vege, potato, hashed brown, plain, frozen, cooked	1 patty, (approx 3" x 1-1/2" x 1/2")	29	63.22	0.916	8.149	0.58	3.335	1.49	0.384	1.303
11387	Vege, potato, scalloped, mix, prep w/H₂O, whole milk & butter	1 cup (unprepared)	245	227.85	5.194	31.287	2.695	10.535	2.972	0.475	6.451

Chol (g)	Calc (mg)	Iron (mg)	Mag (mg)	Phos (mg)	Pota (mg)	Sodi (mg)	Zinc (mg)	Vit A (RAE)	Vit C (mg)	Thia (mg)	Ribo (mg)	Niac (mg)	Vit B$_6$ (mg)	Vit B$_{12}$ (µg)	Vit E (mg)	Fol (µg)	Alc (g)
0	52.51	1.869	24.92	31.15	160.2	17.8	0.107	73.87	10.68	0.053	0.027	0.356	0.207	0	0.819	56.96	0
0	37.2	1.364	17.36	21.08	107.88	305.04	0.074	2.48	5.208	0.032	0.025	0.248	0.14	0		29.76	0
0	2.625	0.093	0.975	2.475	17.85	0.375	0.015	12.45	0.278	0.004	0.005	0.027	0.006	0	0.014	5.475	0
0	3.3	0.097	1.4	3	24.7	0.8	0.023	29	2.4	0.007	0.007	0.031	0.007	0	0.013	13.6	0
0	107.8	1.886	43.12	118.58	819.28	48.51	0.862	86.24	21.02	0.199	0.113	0.668	0.248	0	0.162	301.8	0
0	3.6	0.086	1.3	2.9	19.4	2.8	0.018	37	1.8	0.007	0.008	0.038	0.009	0	0.029	3.8	0
0	103.6	0.98	21	57.4	282.8	352.8	0.154	442.4	35.42	0.057	0.088	0.606	0.137	0	1.694	102.2	0
0	57.68	0.818	17.92	24.08	198.24	14	0.112	294	39.2	0.045	0.062	0.448	0.101	0	1.126	104.7	0
0	61.6	0.224	28.8	25.6	108	4.8	0.344	11.2	13.04	0.106	0.044	0.697	0.15	0	0.216	36.8	0
0	81	0.8	57	63	303	8	0.6	19	21.1	0.2	0.06	1	0.215	0	0.36	88	0
0	22.01	1.2	13.49	57.51	91.59	266.25	0.298	7.81	0.994	0.199	0.099	2.563	0.055	0		46.86	0
0	46.2	0.504	23.1	73.5	348.6	501.9	0.441	0	10.92	0.088	0.048	0.347	0.271	0	0.042	31.5	0
0	35.2	0.304	16	43.2	230.4	4.8	0.256	0	10.24	0.077	0.04	0.133	0.235	0	0.032	30.4	0
0	72	1.48	20	37	276	16	0.39	50	18.8	0.055	0.08	0.525	0.061	0	0.55	64	0
0	28.86	0.452	22.62	53.82	286.26	191.88	0.203	0	10.14	0.065	0.04	0.565	0.073	0		45.24	0
0	47.88	0.785	38.57	94.43	498.75	13.3	0.785	0	22.61	0.12	0.067	0.931	0.12	0	1.982	89.11	0
0	58.65	1.912	35.7	117.3	255	663	1.479	737	16.83	0.189	0.135	1.482	0.224	0		45.9	0
0	67.2	3.152	41.6	88	384	384	0.592	86.4	76.64	0.205	0.122	0.862	0.23	0	0.624	46.4	0
0	42.14	2.038	23.52	51.94	196	3.92	0.265	52.92	58.8	0.147	0.078	0.588	0.157	0	0.382	41.16	0
0	43.2	2.464	62.4	187.2	433.6	382.4	1.904	64	22.72	0.414	0.238	3.234	0.346	0	0.224	100.8	0
0	34	1.615	28.9	113.9	294.1	428.4	1.207	45.9	16.32	0.206	0.133	1.244	0.109	0	0.051	74.8	0
0	36.25	2.132	47.85	156.6	353.8	7.25	1.798	55.1	58	0.386	0.191	3.03	0.245	0	0.189	94.25	0
0	50.04	1.849	5.56	15.29	157.07	551.83	0.125	8.34	47.54	0.014	0.042	0.872	0.167	0		75.06	0
0	9	0.63	17.1	27.9	193.5	0.9	0.207	36	39.87	0.13	0.051	1.005	0.457	0	0.423	42.3	0
0	0.671	0.052	1.342	2.44	18.605	0.61	0.016	2.867	2.739	0.003	0.005	0.094	0.031	0	0.042	1.403	0
0	11.9	0.405	11.9	23.8	208.25	3.57	0.155	21.42	95.68	0.068	0.033	0.571	0.267	0	0.44	13.09	0
0	8.33	0.512	14.28	30.94	251.09	2.38	0.298	186.8	226.1	0.064	0.101	1.165	0.346	0	1.88	21.42	0
0	20.46	0.856	22.32	44.64	394.32	3.72	0.316	18.6	341.3	0.052	0.047	1.655	0.312	0		48.36	0
0	5.85	0.344	7.15	13.65	75.4	833.3	0.091	5.85	1.235	0.009	0.019	0.039	0.008	0	0.058	0.65	0
0	1	0.147	1	3	8	234.75	0.02	2.25	0.3	0.002	0.008	0.043	0.004	0	0.023	0.25	0
0	0.72	0.202	0.72	2.04	18.96	1.68	0.023	15.96	10.19	0.002	0.007	0.074	0.026	0	0.083	0.72	0
4.2	67.2	0.441	42	130.2	325.5	361.2	0.504	98.7	13.65	0.189	0.181	1.814	0.336	0.21	1.071	16.8	0
72.96	18.24	1.186	25.08	84.36	597.36	386.08	0.631	5.32	16.72	0.103	0.131	1.629	0.288	0.144		17.48	0
170	47.5	1.625	37.5	130	635	1322.5	0.775	80	25	0.192	0.15	2.225	0.353	0		17.5	0
56.35	291.55	1.568	49	276.85	970.2	1060.85	1.691	156.8	24.26	0.157	0.284	2.433	0.426	0		26.95	0
0	13.36	0.518	33.4	66.8	547.76	402.47	0.451	0	12.36	0.164	0.032	2.191	0.449	0	0.017	15.03	0
0	9	2.268	25.2	50.4	412.2	394.2	0.504	0	9.18	0.122	0.023	1.647	0.338	0	0.09	10.8	0
0	4	0.62	11	41	209	133	0.2	0	5.05	0.056	0.014	1.044	0.154	0		6	0
0	4.35	0.438	4.93	20.88	126.44	9.86	0.093	0	1.827	0.032	0.006	0.702	0.037	0	0.055	2.03	0
26.95	88.2	0.931	34.3	137.2	497.35	835.45	0.613	85.75	8.085	0.047	0.137	2.521	0.103	0	0.368	24.5	0

EvaluEat Code	Food Name	Amt	Wt (g)	Energy (kcal)	Prot (g)	Carb (g)	Fiber (g)	Fat (g)	Mono (g)	Poly (g)	Sat (g)
11830	Vege, potato, skin only, baked w/salt	1 skin	58	114.84	2.488	26.715	4.582	0.058	0.001	0.025	0.015
11426	Vege, pumpkin pie mix, canned	1 cup	270	280.8	2.943	71.253	22.41	0.351	0.043	0.019	0.175
11846	Vege, pumpkin, canned w/salt	1 cup	245	83.3	2.695	19.796	7.105	0.686	0.091	0.037	0.358
11952	Vege, radicchio, raw	1 cup, shredded	40	9.2	0.572	1.792	0.36	0.1	0.004	0.044	0.024
11430	Vege, radish, oriental (daikon) raw	1 radish (7" long)	338	60.84	2.028	13.858	5.408	0.338	0.057	0.152	0.101
11429	Vege, radish, slices, raw	1 large (1" to 1-1/4" dia)	9	1.44	0.061	0.306	0.144	0.009	0.002	0.004	0.003
11851	Vege, rutabaga, boiled w/salt, drained	.5 cup, mashed	120	46.8	1.548	10.488		0.264	0.032	0.114	0.035
11439	Vege, sauerkraut, canned, solids & liquid	1 cup	142	26.98	1.292	6.078	3.55	0.199	0.018	0.087	0.05
11445	Vege, seaweed, kelp, raw	2 tbsp (1/8 cup)	10	4.3	0.168	0.957	0.13	0.056	0.01	0.005	0.025
11667	Vege, seaweed, spirulina, dried	1 cup	15	43.5	8.621	3.585	0.54	1.158	0.101	0.312	0.398
11677	Vege, shallots, peeled, raw	1 tbsp, chopped	10	7.2	0.25	1.68		0.01	0.001	0.004	0.002
11658	Vege, spinach egg souffle, homemade	1 cup	136	218.96	10.989	2.829		18.36	6.835	3.082	7.148
11854	Vege, spinach, boiled w/salt, drained	1 cup	180	41.4	5.346	6.75	4.32	0.468	0.013	0.194	0.076
11461	Vege, spinach, canned, drained	1 cup	214	49.22	6.013	7.276	5.136	1.07	0.03	0.447	0.173
11457	Vege, spinach, raw	1 cup	30	6.9	0.858	1.089	0.66	0.117	0.003	0.05	0.019
11864	Vege, squash, acorn, peeled, baked w/salt	1 cup, cubes	205	114.8	2.296	29.889	9.02	0.287	0.02	0.121	0.059
11866	Vege, squash, butternut, baked w/salt	1 cup, cubes	205	82	1.845	21.504		0.185	0.014	0.078	0.039
11870	Vege, squash, spaghetti, baked or boiled w/salt, drained	1 cup	155	41.85	1.023	10.013	2.17	0.403	0.034	0.195	0.096
11857	Vege, squash, summer, all varieties, boiled w/salt, drained	1 cup, sliced	180	36	1.638	7.758	2.52	0.558	0.041	0.236	0.115
11863	Vege, squash, winter, all varieties, baked w/salt	1 cup, cubes	205	79.95	1.824	17.938	5.74	1.291	0.096	0.543	0.266
11477	Vege, squash, zucchini w/skin, slices, raw	1 cup, chopped	124	19.84	1.5	4.154	1.364	0.223	0.017	0.094	0.046
11861	Vege, squash, zucchini w/skin, boiled w/salt, drained	.5 cup, sliced	90	14.4	0.576	3.537	1.26	0.045	0.004	0.019	0.009
11871	Vege, succotash (corn & lima beans) boiled w/salt, drained	1 cup	192	220.8	9.734	46.81		1.536	0.298	0.732	0.284
11875	Vege, sweet potato, baked in skin w/salt	1 medium (2" dia, 5" long, raw)	114	102.6	2.291	23.609	3.762	0.171	0.001	0.073	0.039
11647	Vege, sweet potato, canned w/syrup, drained	1 cup	196	211.68	2.509	49.706	5.88	0.627	0.024	0.276	0.135
11878	Vege, taro, cooked w/salt	1 cup, sliced	132	187.44	0.686	45.672	6.732	0.145	0.012	0.061	0.03
11954	Vege, tomatillos, raw	1 medium	34	10.88	0.326	1.986	0.646	0.347	0.053	0.142	0.047
11887	Vege, tomato paste, canned w/salt	1 can (6 oz)	170	139.4	7.344	32.147	7.65	0.799	0.141	0.381	0.182
11888	Vege, tomato puree, canned w/salt	1 cup	250	95	4.125	22.45	4.75	0.525	0.078	0.215	0.072
11549	Vege, tomato sauce, canned	1 cup	245	78.4	3.234	18.056	3.675	0.588	0.091	0.24	0.083
11533	Vege, tomato, red, canned, stewed	1 cup	255	66.3	2.321	15.785	2.55	0.484	0.074	0.196	0.066
11531	Vege, tomato, red, canned, whole	1 cup	240	40.8	1.92	9.384	2.16	0.312	0.05	0.13	0.043
11883	Vege, tomato, red, cherry, ripe, raw, June–October	1 cup	149	31.29	1.266	6.914	1.639	0.492	0.075	0.201	0.067
11529	Vege, tomato, red, ripe, whole, raw	1 cup, chopped or sliced	180	32.4	1.584	7.056	2.16	0.36	0.09	0.243	0.081
11955	Vege, tomato, sun-dried	1 cup	54	139.32	7.619	30.11	6.642	1.604	0.263	0.602	0.23
11696	Vege, tomato, yellow, raw	1 tomato	212	31.8	2.078	6.318	1.484	0.551	0.085	0.229	0.076
11891	Vege, turnip greens, boiled w/salt, drained	1 cup, chopped	144	28.8	1.642	6.278	5.04	0.331	0.022	0.131	0.076
11889	Vege, turnip, boiled w/salt, drained	1 cup, cubes	156	32.76	1.108	7.644	3.12	0.125	0.008	0.066	0.012
11990	Vege, wasabi, root, raw	1 cup, sliced	130	141.7	6.24	30.602	10.14	0.819			
11590	Vege, waterchestnut, Chinese, canned, solids & liquid	.5 cup, sliced	70	35	0.616	8.61	1.75	0.042	0.001	0.018	0.011
11591	Vege, watercress, raw	1 cup, chopped	34	3.74	0.782	0.439	0.17	0.034	0.003	0.012	0.009
11897	Vege, yam, boiled or baked w/salt	1 cup, cubes	136	157.76	2.026	37.509	5.304	0.19	0.007	0.082	0.039

Chol (g)	Calc (mg)	Iron (mg)	Mag (mg)	Phos (mg)	Pota (mg)	Sodi (mg)	Zinc (mg)	Vit A (RAE)	Vit C (mg)	Thia (mg)	Ribo (mg)	Niac (mg)	Vit B₆ (mg)	Vit B₁₂ (µg)	Vit E (mg)	Fol (µg)	Alc (g)
0	19.72	4.083	24.94	58.58	332.34	149.06	0.284	0.58	7.83	0.071	0.061	1.778	0.356	0	0.023	12.76	0
0	99.9	2.862	43.2	121.5	372.6	561.6	0.729	1121	9.45	0.043	0.319	1.01	0.429	0		94.5	0
0	63.7	3.405	56.35	85.75	504.7	590.45	0.417	2702	10.29	0.059	0.132	0.899	0.137	0		29.4	0
0	7.6	0.228	5.2	16	120.8	8.8	0.248	0.4	3.2	0.006	0.011	0.102	0.023	0	0.904	24	0
0	91.26	1.352	54.08	77.74	767.26	70.98	0.507	0	74.36	0.068	0.068	0.676	0.155	0	0	94.64	0
0	2.25	0.031	0.9	1.8	20.97	3.51	0.025	0	1.332	0.001	0.004	0.023	0.006	0	0	2.25	0
0	57.6	0.636	27.6	67.2	391.2	304.8	0.42	0	22.56	0.098	0.049	0.858	0.122	0	0.384	18	0
0	42.6	2.087	18.46	28.4	241.4	938.62	0.27	1.42	20.87	0.03	0.031	0.203	0.185	0	0.142	34.08	0
0	16.8	0.285	12.1	4.2	8.9	23.3	0.123	0.6	0.3	0.005	0.015	0.047	0	0	0.087	18	0
0	18	4.275	29.25	17.7	204.45	157.2	0.3	4.35	1.515	0.357	0.551	1.923	0.055	0	0.75	14.1	0
0	3.7	0.12	2.1	6	33.4	1.2	0.04	6	0.8	0.006	0.002	0.02	0.034	0		3.4	0
183.6	229.84	1.346	38.08	231.2	201.28	762.96	1.292	266.6	2.992	0.091	0.305	0.477	0.12	1.36		80.24	0
0	244.8	6.426	156.6	100.8	838.8	550.8	1.368	943.2	17.64	0.171	0.425	0.882	0.436	0	3.744	262.8	0
0	271.78	4.922	162.64	94.16	740.44	57.78	0.984	1049	30.6	0.034	0.295	0.83	0.214	0	4.152	209.7	0
0	29.7	0.813	23.7	14.7	167.4	23.7	0.159	140.7	8.43	0.023	0.057	0.217	0.058	0	0.609	58.2	0
0	90.2	1.906	88.15	92.25	895.85	492	0.348	43.05	22.14	0.342	0.027	1.806	0.398	0		38.95	0
0	84.05	1.23	59.45	55.35	582.2	492	0.266	717.5	30.96	0.148	0.035	1.986	0.254	0		38.95	0
0	32.55	0.527	17.05		181.35	393.7	0.31	9.3	5.425	0.059	0.034	1.255	0.153	0		12.4	0
0	48.6	0.648	43.2	70.2	345.6	426.6	0.702	246.6	9.9	0.079	0.074	0.923	0.117	0	0.126	36	0
0	28.7	0.677	16.4	41	895.85	485.85	0.533	364.9	19.68	0.174	0.049	1.437	0.148	0		57.4	0
0	18.6	0.434	21.08	47.12	324.88	12.4	0.36	12.4	21.08	0.06	0.176	0.604	0.27	0	0.149	35.96	0
0	11.7	0.315	19.8	36	227.7	215.1	0.162	50.4	4.14	0.037	0.037	0.385	0.07	0	0.108	15.3	0
0	32.64	2.918	101.76	224.64	787.2	485.76	1.21	28.8	15.74	0.323	0.184	2.548	0.223	0		63.36	0
0	43.32	0.787	30.78	61.56	541.5	280.44	0.365	1096	22.34	1.65	0.121	1.695	0.326	0	0.809	6.84	0
0	33.32	1.862	23.52	49	378.28	76.44	0.314	701.7	21.17	0.049	0.074	0.666	0.122	0	0.549	15.68	0
0	23.76	0.95	39.6	100.32	638.88	331.32	0.356	0	6.6	0.141	0.037	0.673	0.437	0		25.08	0
0	2.38	0.211	6.8	13.26	91.12	0.34	0.075	2.04	3.978	0.015	0.012	0.629	0.019	0	0.129	2.38	0
0	61.2	5.066	71.4	141.1	1723.8	1343	1.071	129.2	37.23	0.102	0.26	5.229	0.367	0	7.31	20.4	0
0	45	4.45	57.5	100	1097.5	997.5	0.9	65	26.5	0.063	0.2	3.665	0.315	0	4.925	27.5	0
0	31.85	2.499	39.2	63.7	810.95	1283.8	0.49	41.65	17.15	0.059	0.162	2.389	0.238	0	5.096	22.05	0
0	86.7	3.391	30.6	51	527.85	563.55	0.433	22.95	20.15	0.117	0.089	1.821	0.043	0	2.116	12.75	0
0	74.4	2.328	26.4	45.6	451.2	307.2	0.336	14.4	21.6	0.108	0.113	1.764	0.216	0	1.704	19.2	0
0	7.45	0.67	16.39	35.76	330.78	13.41	0.134	46.19	38.74	0.088	0.072	0.936	0.119	0	0.507	22.35	0
0	18	0.486	19.8	43.2	426.6	9	0.306	75.6	22.86	0.067	0.034	1.069	0.144	0	0.972	27	0
0	59.4	4.909	104.76	192.24	1850.58	1131.3	1.075	23.76	21.17	0.285	0.264	4.887	0.179	0	0.005	36.72	0
0	23.32	1.039	25.44	76.32	546.96	48.76	0.594	0	19.08	0.087	0.1	2.499	0.119	0		63.6	0
0	197.28	1.152	31.68	41.76	292.32	381.6	0.202	548.6	39.46	0.065	0.104	0.592	0.259	0	2.707	169.9	0
0	34.32	0.343	12.48	29.64	210.6	446.16	0.312	0	18.1	0.042	0.036	0.466	0.105	0		14.04	0
0	166.4	1.339	89.7	104	738.4	22.1	2.106	2.6	54.47	0.17	0.148	0.966	0.356	0		23.4	0
0	2.8	0.609	3.5	13.3	82.6	5.6	0.266	0	0.91	0.008	0.017	0.252	0.111	0	0.35	4.2	0
0	40.8	0.068	7.14	20.4	112.2	13.94	0.037	79.9	14.62	0.031	0.041	0.068	0.044	0	0.34	3.06	0
0	19.04	0.707	24.48	66.64	911.2	331.84	0.272	8.16	16.46	0.129	0.038	0.751	0.31	0	0.517	21.76	

EvaluEat Code	Food Name	Amt	Wt (g)	Energy (kcal)	Prot (g)	Carb (g)	Fiber (g)	Fat (g)	Mono (g)	Poly (g)	Sat (g)
11601	Vege, yam, peeled, raw	1 cup, cubes	150	177	2.295	41.82	6.15	0.255	0.009	0.114	0.056
11603	Vege, yambean (jicama) peeled, slices, raw	1 cup, sliced	120	45.6	0.864	10.584	5.88	0.108	0.006	0.052	0.025
14187	Vegetable beverage, clam & tomato juice, canned	1 can (5.5 oz)	166	79.68	0.996	18.177	0.332	0.332	0.013	0.033	0.08
11578	Vegetable juice cocktail, canned	1 cup	242	45.98	1.525	11.011	1.936	0.218	0.034	0.092	0.031
11159	Vegetable salad, coleslaw, homemade	.5 cup	60	41.4	0.774	7.446	0.9	1.566	0.425	0.811	0.231
11894	Vegetables, mixed, frozen, boiled w/salt, drained	.5 cup	91	53.69	2.603	11.912	4.004	0.137	0.009	0.066	0.028
43134	Vegetarian fillets	1 cup	186	539.4	42.78	16.74	11.346	33.48	8.139	17.358	5.299
43137	Vegetarian meatloaf or patties	1 cup	186	366.42	39.06	14.88	8.556	16.74	4.07	8.679	2.65
43136	Vegetarian stew	1 cup	186	228.78	31.62	13.02	2.046	5.58	1.356	2.892	0.883
22121	Vegetarian, Better'n Burgers/vegan burgers, frozen/Worthington, Morningstar	1 patty	85	90.95	13.906	7.531	4.25	0.535	0.318	0.173	0.107
22122	Vegetarian, breakfast patties/Worthington, Morningstar	1 patty	38	79.42	9.918	3.716	1.976	2.77	0.688	1.319	0.509
22120	Vegetarian, burger crumbles/Worthington, Morningstar	1 cup	110	231	22.154	6.622	5.06	12.925	4.628	4.925	3.257
22215	Vegetarian, chili w/beans, canned entree/Nestle Chef-Mate	1 cup	253	412.39	17.735	29.044	11.132	25.022	10.747	1.397	10.93
22119	Vegetarian, deli franks/Worthington, Morningstar	1 serving	45	111.6	10.386	3.699	2.745	6.16	1.953	3.314	0.893
22118	Vegetarian, garden patties, frozen/Worthington, Morningstar	1 patty	67	119.26	11.209	10.204	4.02	3.765	1.065	2.161	0.539
22125	Vegetarian, Harvest Burger, original flavor, vegetable protein patty	1 patty	90	137.7	18	7.02	5.67	4.14	2.135	0.265	1.017
22223	Vegetarian, macaroni and cheese, canned entree/Nestle Chef-Mate	1 cup	253	283.36	10.803	35.42	3.289	11.005	3.026	0.524	6.199
22128	Vegetarian, Natural Touch Vegan Burgers, frozen/Worthington	1 patty	85	90.95	13.906	7.531	4.25	0.535	0.318	0.173	0.107
22123	Vegetarian, Spicy Black Bean Burger/Worthington, Morningstar	1 patty	78	114.66	11.786	15.202	4.758	0.78	0.25	0.351	0.179
2048	Vinegar, cider	1 tbsp	15	2.1	0	0.885	0	0	0	0	0
2053	Vinegar, distilled	1 tbsp	13	1.56	0	0.65	0	0	0	0	0
48052	Vital wheat gluten	1 cup	148	547.6	111.24	20.409	0.888	2.738	0.231	1.199	0.403
18505	Waffle, Eggo Lowfat Homestyle/Kellogg	1 waffle, round (4" dia)	35	82.6	2.471	15.453	0.35	1.246	0.35	0.375	0.315
18367	Waffle, plain, homemade	1 waffle, round (7" dia)	75	218.25	5.925	24.675		10.575	2.641	5.089	2.149
18365	Waffle, plain/buttermilk, frozen, ready-to-heat	1 waffle square	39	97.89	2.301	15.054	0.858	3.042	1.23	1.081	0.505
1072	Whipped dessert topping, nondairy, pressurized can	1 tbsp	4	10.56	0.039	0.643	0	0.892	0.077	0.01	0.756
1073	Whipped dessert topping, nondairy, semi-solid, frozen	1 tbsp	4	12.72	0.05	0.922	0	1.012	0.065	0.021	0.871
42135	Whipped topping, frozen, low-fat	1 oz	28.34	62.348	0.85	6.688	0	3.713	0.237	0.076	3.195
43406	Yeast extract spread	1 fl. oz.	29.8	47.084	8.284	3.516	0.894	0	0	0	0
19393	Yogurt, frozen, chocolate, soft serve	.5 cup (4 fl. oz.)	72	115.2	2.88	17.928	1.584	4.32	1.26	0.158	2.614
43261	Yogurt, fruit variety, nonfat	1 cup	186	174.84	8.184	35.34	0	0.372	0.093	0.03	0.221
1121	Yogurt, lowfat w/fruit, 10 g protein/8 oz	1 cup (8 fl. oz.)	245	249.9	10.707	46.673	0	2.646	0.728	0.076	1.708
1117	Yogurt, lowfat, plain, 12 g protein/8 oz	1 cup (8 fl. oz.)	245	154.35	12.863	17.248	0	3.797	1.044	0.108	2.45
1116	Yogurt, whole milk, plain, 8 g protein/8 oz	1 cup (8 fl. oz.)	245	149.45	8.502	11.417	0	7.963	2.188	0.225	5.135

Chol (g)	Calc (mg)	Iron (mg)	Mag (mg)	Phos (mg)	Pota (mg)	Sodi (mg)	Zinc (mg)	Vit A (RAE)	Vit C (mg)	Thia (mg)	Ribo (mg)	Niac (mg)	Vit B₆ (mg)	Vit B₁₂ (µg)	Vit E (mg)	Fol (µg)	Alc (g)
0	25.5	0.81	31.5	82.5	1224	13.5	0.36	10.5	25.65	0.168	0.048	0.828	0.44	0	0.585	34.5	0
0	14.4	0.72	14.4	21.6	180	4.8	0.192	1.2	24.24	0.024	0.035	0.24	0.05	0	0.552	14.4	0
0	19.92	0.996	36.52	129.48	149.4	600.92	1.793	18.26	6.806	0.066	0.05	0.315	0.139	50.796		26.56	0
0	26.62	1.016	26.62	41.14	467.06	653.4	0.484	188.8	67.03	0.104	0.068	1.757	0.339	0	12.1	50.82	0
4.8	27	0.354	6	19.2	108.6	13.8	0.12	31.8	19.62	0.04	0.037	0.163	0.076	0		16.2	0
0	22.75	0.746	20.02	46.41	153.79	246.61	0.446	194.7	2.912	0.065	0.109	0.774	0.067	0		17.29	0
0	176.7	3.72	42.78	837	1116	911.4	2.604	0	0	2.046	1.674	22.32	2.79	7.812	6.417	189.7	0
0	53.94	3.906	33.48	639.84	334.8	1023	3.348	0	0	1.674	1.116	18.6	2.232	4.464	3.218	145.1	0
0	57.66	2.418	236.22	409.2	223.2	744	2.046	87.42	0	1.302	1.116	22.32	2.046	4.092	0.911	191.6	0
0	86.7	2.899	16.15	181.05	433.5	382.5	0.748			0	0.256	0.553	4.113	0.198	0	0.009	245.7	0
0.76	18.24	1.919	1.14	106.4	101.84	259.16	0.369		0	5.385	0.133	1.835	0.19	1.497	0.298		0
0	79.2	6.402	2.2	173.8	178.2	476.3	1.639		0	9.922	0.352	2.981	0.539	4.367	0.689		0
55.66	88.55	4.832	45.54	166.98	511.06	1171.39	3.871		0.759	0.106	0.202	3.476	0.228	1.442	1.209		0
0.45	17.1	0.608	3.6	42.3	49.95	430.65	0.378		0	0.144	0.022	0	0.012	0.009	1.256		0
0.67	48.24	1.213	29.48	123.95	179.56	381.9	0.576	134	0	6.465	0.101	0	0	0	0.549	58.96	0
0	101.7	3.852	70.2	225	432	411.3	8.073		0	0.315	0.198	6.3	0.387	0	1.557	21.6	0
27.83	202.4	1.923	32.89	250.47	151.8	1343.43	1.569		0	0.319	0.331	2.505	0.071	0.202	0.159		0
0	86.7	2.899	16.15	181.05	433.5	382.5	0.748		0	0.256	0.553	4.113	0.198	0	0.009	245.7	0
0.78	56.16	1.841	43.68	149.76	269.1	499.2	0.928		0	8.057	0.14	0	0.211	0.07	0.359		0
0	0.9	0.09	3.3	1.35	15	0.15	0	0	0	0	0	0	0	0	0	0	0
0	0	0	2.86	0	1.95	0.13	0	0	0	0	0	0	0	0	0	0	0
0	210.16	7.696	37	384.8	148	42.92	1.258	0	0	0	0	0	0	0	0	0	0
8.75	20.3	1.946	23.8	28.35	50.05	154.7			0	0.308	0.259	2.593	0.164	0.549		26.95	
51.75	191.25	1.732	14.25	142.5	119.25	383.25	0.51	48.75	0.3	0.197	0.26	1.555	0.042	0.188		34.5	0
12.48	86.19	1.657	8.19	155.61	47.58	291.72	0.214	149	0	0.178	0.196	1.826	0.369	0.928	0.246	23.79	0
0	0.2	0.001	0.04	0.72	0.76	2.48	0	0.16	0	0	0	0	0	0	0.034	0	0
0	0.24	0.005	0.08	0.32	0.72	1	0.001	0.28	0	0	0	0	0	0	0.038	0	0
0.567	20.121	0.028	1.984	20.972	28.623	20.405	0.028	1.134	0	0.006	0.026	0.028	0.006	0.057	0.142	0.85	0
0	25.628	1.103	53.64	30.992	774.8	1072.8	0.626	0	0	2.891	4.261	28.906	0.387	0.149	0	301	0
3.6	105.84	0.9	19.44	100.08	187.92	70.56	0.353	31.68	0.216	0.026	0.152	0.22	0.053	0.209	0.097	7.92	0
3.72	282.72	0.13	27.9	221.34	360.84	107.88	1.376	3.72	1.302	0.074	0.335	0.186	0.074	0.874	0.112	16.74	0
9.8	372.4	0.171	36.75	291.55	477.75	142.1	1.813	24.5	1.715	0.091	0.436	0.233	0.098	1.151	0.049	22.05	0
14.7	448.35	0.196	41.65	352.8	573.3	171.5	2.181	34.3	1.96	0.108	0.524	0.279	0.12	1.372	0.073	26.95	0
31.85	296.45	0.123	29.4	232.75	379.75	112.7	1.446	66.15	1.225	0.071	0.348	0.184	0.078	0.907	0.147	17.15	0

Appendix B *Calculations and Conversions*

Calculation and Conversion Aids

Commonly Used Metric Units

millimeter (mm): one-thousandth of a meter (0.001)
centimeter (cm): one-hundredth of a meter (0.01)
kilometer (km): one-thousand times a meter (1000)
kilogram (kg): one-thousand times a gram (1000)
milligram (mg): one-thousandth of a gram (0.001)
microgram (μg): one-millionth of a gram (0.000001)
milliliter (ml): one-thousandth of a liter (0.001)

International Units

Some vitamin supplements may report vitamin content as International Units (IU).

To convert IU to:

- Micrograms of vitamin D (cholecalciferol), divide the IU value by 40 or multiply by 0.025.
- Milligrams of vitamin E (alpha-tocopherol), divide the IU value by 1.5 if vitamin E is from natural sources. Divide the IU value by 2.22 if vitamin E is from synthetic sources.
- Vitamin A: 1 IU = 0.3 μg retinol or 3.6 μg beta-carotene

Retinol Activity Equivalents

Retinol Activity Equivalents (RAE) are a standardized unit of measure for vitamin A. RAE account for the various differences in bioavailability from sources of vitamin A. Many supplements will report vitamin A content in IU, as shown above, or Retinol Equivalents (RE).

1 RAE = 1 μg retinol
12 μg beta-carotene
24 μg other vitamin A carotenoids

To calculate RAE from the RE value of vitamin carotenoids in foods, divide RE by 2.
For vitamin A supplements and foods fortified with vitamin A, 1 RE = 1 RAE.

Folate

Folate is measured as Dietary Folate Equivalents (DFE). DFE account for the different factors affecting bioavailability of folate sources.

1 DFE = 1 μg food folate
0.6 μg folate from fortified foods
0.5 μg folate supplement taken on an empty stomach
0.6 μg folate as a supplement consumed with a meal

To convert micrograms of synthetic folate, such as that found in supplements or fortified foods, to DFE:

$$\mu g \text{ synthetic folate} \times 1.7 = \mu g \text{ DFE}$$

For naturally occurring food folate, such as spinach, each microgram of folate equals 1 microgram DFE:

$$\mu g \text{ folate} = \mu g \text{ DFE}$$

Conversion Factors

Use the following table to convert U.S. measurements to metric equivalents:

Original Unit	Multiply by	To Get
ounces avdp	28.3495	grams
ounces	0.0625	pounds
pounds	0.4536	kilograms
pounds	16	ounces
grams	0.0353	ounces
grams	0.002205	pounds
kilograms	2.2046	pounds
liters	1.8162	pints (dry)
liters	2.1134	pints (liquid)
liters	0.9081	quarts (dry)
liters	1.0567	quarts (liquid)
liters	0.2642	gallons (U.S.)
pints (dry)	0.5506	liters
pints (liquid)	0.4732	liters
quarts (dry)	1.1012	liters
quarts liquid	0.9463	liters
gallons (U.S.)	3.7853	liters
millimeters	0.0394	inches
centimeters	0.3937	inches
centimeters	0.03281	feet
inches	25.4000	millimeters
inches	2.5400	centimeters
inches	0.0254	meters
feet	0.3048	meters
meters	3.2808	feet
meters	1.0936	yards
cubic feet	0.0283	cubic meters
cubic meters	35.3145	cubic feet
cubic meters	1.3079	cubic yards
cubic yards	0.7646	cubic meters

Length: U.S. and Metric Equivalents

¼ inch = 0.6 centimeters
1 inch = 2.5 centimeters
1 foot = 0.3048 meter
    30.48 centimeters
1 yard = 0.91144 meter
1 millimeter = 0.03937 inch
1 centimeter = 0.3937 inch
1 decimeter = 3.937 inches
1 meter = 39.37 inches
    1.094 yards
1 micron = 0.00003937 inch

Weights and Measures

Food Measurement Equivalencies from U.S. to Metric

Capacity

⅕ teaspoon = 1 milliliter
¼ teaspoon = 1.25 milliliters
½ teaspoon = 2.5 milliliters
1 teaspoon = 5 milliliters
1 tablespoon = 15 milliliters
1 fluid ounce = 28.4 milliliters
¼ cup = 60 milliliters
⅓ cup = 80 milliliters
½ cup = 120 milliliters
1 cup = 225 milliliters
1 pint (2 cups) = 473 milliliters
1 quart (4 cups) = 0.95 liter
1 liter (1.06 quarts) = 1,000 milliliters
1 gallon (4 quarts) = 3.84 liters

Weight

0.035 ounce = 1 gram
1 ounce = 28 grams
¼ pound (4 ounces) = 114 grams
1 pound (16 ounces) = 454 grams
2.2 pounds (35 ounces) = 1 kilogram

U.S. Food Measurement Equivalents

3 teaspoons = 1 tablespoon
½ tablespoon = 1-½ teaspoons
2 tablespoons = ⅛ cup
4 tablespoons = ¼ cup
5 tablespoons + 1 teaspoon = ⅓ cup
8 tablespoons = ½ cup
10 tablespoons + 2 teaspoons = ⅔ cup
12 tablespoons = ¾ cup
16 tablespoons = 1 cup
2 cups = 1 pint
4 cups = 1 quart
2 pints = 1 quart
4 quarts = 1 gallon

Volumes and Capacities

1 cup = 8 fluid ounces
½ liquid pint
1 milliliter = 0.061 cubic inches
1 liter = 1.057 liquid quarts
0.908 dry quart
61.024 cubic inches
1 U.S. gallon = 231 cubic inches
3.785 liters
0.833 British gallon
128 U.S fluid ounces
1 British Imperial gallon = 277.42 cubic inches
1.201 U.S gallons
4.546 liters
160 British fluid ounces
1 U.S. ounce, liquid or fluid = 1.805 cubic inches
29.574 milliliters
1.041 British fluid ounces
1 pint, dry = 33.600 cubic inches
0.551 liter
1 pint, liquid = 28.875 cubic inches
0.473 liter
1 U.S. quart, dry = 67.201 cubic inches
1.101 liters
1 U.S. quart, liquid = 57.75 cubic inches
0.946 liter
1 British quart = 69.354 cubic inches
1.032 U.S. quarts, dry
1.201 U.S. quarts, liquid

Energy Units

1 kilocalorie (kcal) = 4.2 kilojoules
1 millijoule (MJ) = 240 kilocalories
1 kilojoule (kJ) = 0.24 kcal
1 gram (g) carbohydrate = 4 kcal
1 g fat = 9 kcal
1 g protein = 4 kcal

Temperature Standards

	°Fahrenheit	°Celsius
Body temperature	98.6°	37°
Comfortable room temperature	65–75°	18–24°
Boiling point of water	212°	100°
Freezing point of water	32°	0°

Temperature Scales

To Convert Fahrenheit to Celsius:

[(°F − 32) × 5]/9

1. subtract 32 from °F
2. multiply (°F − 32) by 5, then divide by 9

To Convert Celsius to Fahrenheit:

[(°C × 9)/5] + 32

1. multiply °C by 9, then divide by 5
2. add 32 to (°C × 9/5)

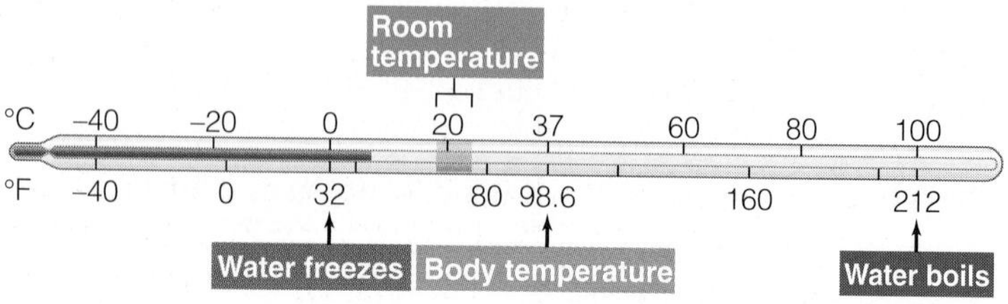

Contents

Introduction

In the last decade, nutrition scientists have been working to make the dietary advice given to Americans and Canadians more consistent. The new Dietary Reference Intakes (DRIs), used in the United States and Canada, are an example of harmonized recommendations between the two countries.

However, there are still some differences in the nutrition advice given to consumers in Canada from that given in the United States. This appendix highlights the key elements in food guides, labels, and government regulations provided by the Canadian government. It also provides a guide for physical activity and some useful web-based resources for readers who want additional information.

Nutrition Advice for Canadians

The Canadian government first issued nutrition advice to Canadians in 1942. The world was at war and some foods, such as milk, were rationed or hard to get, and many people didn't have enough money to buy the food they needed. The government felt it should provide guidance on how to eat to stay healthy despite food shortages. *Canada's Official Food Rules* (1942) listed the amounts of "health protective foods" to be eaten every day.

Over the years, as the Canadian food supply changed, Canadians changed their eating habits, and as new scientific information became available, nutrition advice given by the government also changed. *Canada's Official Food Rules* became *Canada's Food Rules* (1944, revised in 1949), then *Canada's Food Guide* (1961, with two subsequent revisions in 1977 and 1982), and finally, the present *Canada's Food Guide to Healthy Eating*, released in 1992 and 1997.

Although the original purpose of nutrition advice was to prevent nutrition deficiencies, few people in Canada today suffer from malnutrition due to lack of food. In fact, many Canadians are overweight or obese and are at risk for diseases that are linked to consumption of too many calories or too much fat in their diets. Today's nutrition advice for Canadians is designed to: (1) help people get all the nutrients they need for good health, and (2) reduce the risk of chronic diseases such as heart disease, diabetes, and stroke.

Nutrition Recommendations for Canadians

In 1990, an expert committee of scientists developed and released a set of *Nutrition Recommendations for Canadians*. Based on the best nutrition research available at the time, these recommendations were intended for healthy Canadians over the age of two, and were written for health professionals to use. Currently, the information for carbohydrates and fats given by the *Nutrition Recommendations* differ from the DRI values, which have been created using more current research. The *Nutrition Recommendations* are now under review and are slated to be revised. For reference, the *Nutrition Recommendations* are listed as follows:

- The Canadian diet should provide energy consistent with the maintenance of body weight within the recommended range.
- The Canadian diet should include essential nutrients in amounts specified in the Recommended Nutrient Intakes.
- The Canadian diet should include no more than 30% of energy as fat (33 g/1000 kcal or 39 g/5000 kJ) and no more than 10% as saturated fat (11 g/1000 kcal or 13 g/5000 kJ).
- The Canadian diet should provide 55% of energy as carbohydrates (138 g/1000 kcal or 165 g/5000 kJ) from a variety of sources.
- The sodium content of the Canadian diet should be reduced.
- The Canadian diet should include no more than 5% of total energy as alcohol, or two drinks daily, whichever is less.

- The Canadian diet should contain no more caffeine than the equivalent of four cups of regular coffee per day.
- Community water supplies containing less than 1 mg/liter should be fluoridated to that level.

Canada's Guidelines for Healthy Eating

From the *Nutrition Recommendations* came a set of five short, positive, and action-oriented messages called *Canada's Guidelines to Healthy Eating* (Health & Welfare Canada, 1990). These guidelines tell Canadians how to practice healthy eating.

1. Enjoy a VARIETY of foods.
2. Emphasize cereals, breads, other grain products, vegetables, and fruit.
3. Choose lower-fat dairy products, leaner meats, and food prepared with little or no fat.
4. Achieve and maintain a healthy body weight by enjoying regular physical activity and healthy eating.
5. Limit salt, alcohol, and caffeine.

These five guidelines were then used along with the *Nutrition Recommendations for Canadians* to develop *Canada's Food Guide to Healthy Eating.*

Canada's Food Guide to Healthy Eating

The most important tool available to teach Canadians about healthy eating is the *Food Guide to Healthy Eating* (Figure C.1). The *Food Guide* is intended to be used to plan meals that enable people to meet their daily energy and nutrient needs while reducing their risk of chronic diseases. The scientific basis for the current version of the *Food Guide* comes from the *1990 Nutrition Recommendations for Canadians* and *Canada's Guidelines for Healthy Eating* (Health & Welfare Canada, 1990).

Earlier versions of food guides in Canada provided advice on what was called a "foundation diet," the minimum number of servings from each food group needed each day to prevent undernutrition. The current version of *Canada's Food Guide to Healthy Eating* is significantly different from earlier versions, and from the U.S. Food Guide Pyramid, because it takes a total diet approach. That is, it gives a range of servings in each food group to acknowledge that "different people need different amounts of food" (Health & Welfare Canada, 1992). The recommendations are written for healthy Canadians aged four years and over.

What Does the Food Guide to Healthy Eating Tell You?

The rainbow side of the *Food Guide* tells people how to choose healthy foods. There are two general messages:

Enjoy a variety of foods from each group every day.
Choose lower-fat foods more often.

Four messages accompany each of the food groups:

Choose whole grain and enriched products more often.
Choose dark green and orange vegetables and orange fruit more often.
Choose lower-fat milk products more often.
Choose leaner meats, poultry and fish, as well as dried peas, beans and lentils more often.

The bar side of the *Food Guide* shows the amounts of various foods that are equal to one serving and the number of servings recommended each day. The recommended number of servings depends on your age, body size, activity level, whether you are male or female, and if female, whether you are pregnant or breastfeeding. The lower number in the range of servings per day is probably appropriate for older people who are not very active. Most people will need to have more than the lower number of servings; male teenagers and very active people should aim for the higher number of servings each day.

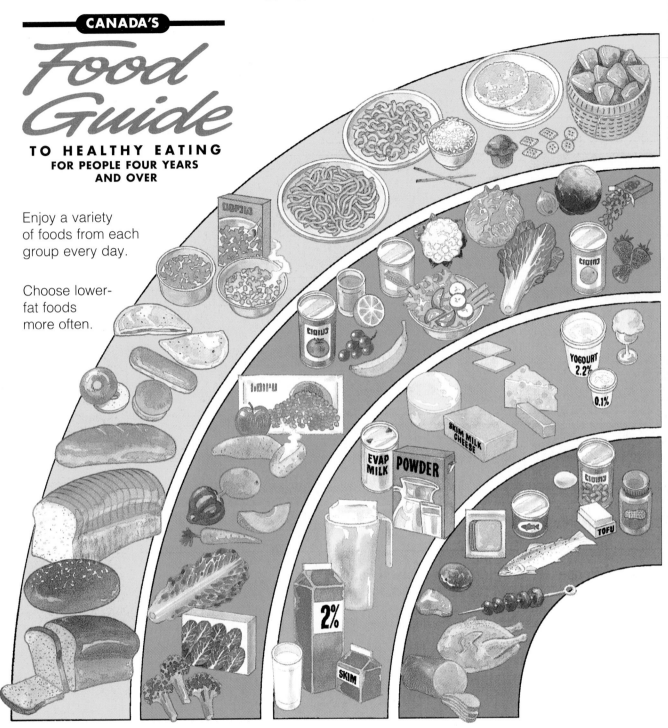

CANADA'S
Food Guide

TO HEALTHY EATING
FOR PEOPLE FOUR YEARS AND OVER

Enjoy a variety of foods from each group every day.

Choose lower-fat foods more often.

Grain Products
Choose whole grain and enriched products more often.

Vegetables and Fruit
Choose dark green and orange vegetables and orange fruit more often.

Milk Products
Choose lower-fat milk products more often.

Meat and Alternatives
Choose leaner meats, poultry and fish, as well as dried peas, beans and lentils more often.

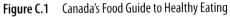

Canada

Figure C.1   Canada's Food Guide to Healthy Eating

(*Source:* © Minister of Public Works and Government Services Canada, 1997. Cat. No. H39-252/1992. No changes permitted.)

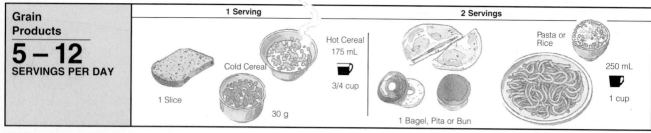

Grain Products

5 – 12 SERVINGS PER DAY

1 Serving

1 Slice

Cold Cereal
30 g

Hot Cereal
175 mL
3/4 cup

2 Servings

1 Bagel, Pita or Bun

Pasta or Rice
250 mL
1 cup

Vegetables and Fruit

5 – 10 SERVINGS PER DAY

1 Serving

1 Medium Size Vegetable or Fruit

Fresh, Frozen or Canned Vegetables or Fruit
125 mL
1/2 cup

Salad
250 mL
1 cup

Juice
125 mL
1/2 cup

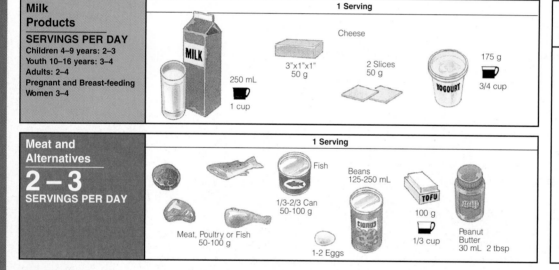

Milk Products

SERVINGS PER DAY
Children 4–9 years: 2–3
Youth 10–16 years: 3–4
Adults: 2–4
Pregnant and Breast-feeding Women 3–4

1 Serving

MILK
250 mL
1 cup

Cheese
3"x1"x1"
50 g

2 Slices
50 g

YOGOURT
175 g
3/4 cup

Other Foods

Taste and enjoyment can also come from other foods and beverages that are not part of the 4 food groups. Some of these foods are higher in fat or Calories, so use these foods in moderation.

Meat and Alternatives

2 – 3 SERVINGS PER DAY

1 Serving

Meat, Poultry or Fish
50-100 g

Fish
1/3-2/3 Can
50-100 g

1-2 Eggs

Beans
125-250 mL

TOFU
100 g
1/3 cup

Peanut Butter
30 mL 2 tbsp

Different People Need Different Amounts of Food

The amount of food you need every day from the 4 food groups and other foods depends on your age, body size, activity level, whether you are male or female and if you are pregnant or breast-feeding. That's why the Food Guide gives a lower and higher number of servings for each food group. For example, young children can choose the lower number of servings, while male teenagers can go to the higher number. Most other people can choose servings somewhere in between.

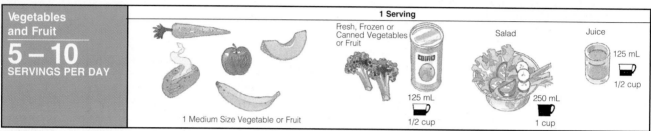

Consult *Canada's Physical Activity Guide to Healthy Active Living* to help you build physical activity into your daily life

Enjoy eating well, being active and feeling good about yourself. That's VITALIT

© Minister of Public Works and Government Services Canada, 1997
Cat. No. H39-252/1992E   ISBN 0-662-19648-1
No changes permitted. Reprint permission not required.

Figure C.1   Continued

"Other Foods" are foods and beverages that are not part of any food group. They include:

- foods that are mostly fats and oils such as butter, margarine, and cooking oils
- foods that are mostly sugar such as jam, honey, syrup, and candies
- high-fat and/or high-salt snack foods such as potato chips
- all beverages except juice (e.g., water, tea, coffee, alcohol, and soft drinks)
- herbs, spices, and condiments such as pickles, mustard, and ketchup

In the U.S. Food Guide Pyramid, the Other Foods are found on the top of the pyramid. In *Canada's Food Guide to Healthy Eating*, they are not shown on the rainbow design.

Canada's Food Guide to Healthy Eating is currently under review by Health Canada, and an updated version is expected to be ready by March 2006.

Dietary Reference Intakes

Until recently, Canada used the 1990 Recommended Nutrient Intakes (RNIs) to determine whether Canadians were getting sufficient amounts of energy and nutrients in their diets and for deciding if public health programs, such as food fortification, were needed. The RNIs have now been replaced by the Dietary Reference Intakes (DRIs), used by the United States and Canada. The DRIs were issued in a series of 11 reports by the National Academy of Sciences from 1997 through 2004. You can see the latest DRI values on the inside back cover of your book.

Understanding Canadian Food Labels

While ingredient lists have been required on packaged foods in Canada for a long time, nutrition information was provided on a voluntary basis. When nutrition information was given, sometimes only a few nutrients were listed. Also, manufacturers often used different formats for different types of foods and this confused consumers.

In January 2003, Health Canada announced its new nutrition labeling policy that requires nutrition labeling on most pre-packaged foods. For the first time, five specific claims that link health and diet are allowed on food packaging. Nutrient content claims, such as, "low in saturated fat," can also appear on packaging, and the new policy revised and added the list of nutrient content claims approved for use. The ingredient list, which lists all ingredients in order from largest to smallest by weight, remains the same.

The Nutrition Facts Table

A food's nutrient information must be listed in a table called *Nutrition Facts* (Figure C.2). The amount of calories (energy) and 13 "core" nutrients (fat, saturated fat, *trans* fat, cholesterol, sodium, carbohydrate, fiber, sugar, protein, vitamin A, vitamin C, calcium, and iron) in one serving of the food must be provided. This is the first time that information has been given about the *trans* fat content of packaged foods.

Manufacturers may also state the amounts of other nutrients if they wish: potassium, soluble and insoluble fiber, sugar alcohol, starch, and the following vitamins and minerals: vitamin D, vitamin E, vitamin K, thiamine, riboflavin, niacin, vitamin B_6, folate, vitamin B_{12}, biotin, pantothenic acid, phosphorus, iodine, magnesium, zinc, selenium, copper, manganese, chromium, molybdenum, and chloride.

The amounts of fat, saturated fat and *trans* fat, sodium, carbohydrate, and fiber in one serving are stated in grams or milligrams, as well as a percent Daily Value (%DV). The remaining nutrients are listed as a %DV only. The %DV is based on recommendations for a healthy 2000-calorie diet and is an easy way of determining the relative amount (i.e., a little or a lot) of a nutrient in one serving. For example, using a 2000-calorie diet with 30% of its calories (energy) as fat, the %DV for fat

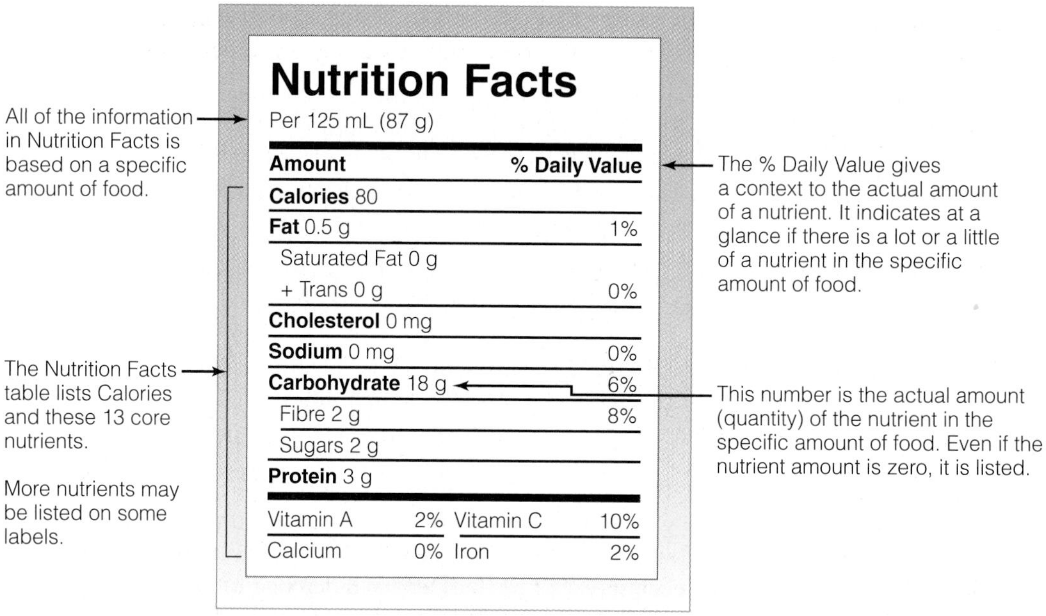

All of the information in Nutrition Facts is based on a specific amount of food.

The Nutrition Facts table lists Calories and these 13 core nutrients.

More nutrients may be listed on some labels.

Nutrition Facts
Per 125 mL (87 g)

Amount	% Daily Value
Calories 80	
Fat 0.5 g	1%
Saturated Fat 0 g	
+ Trans 0 g	0%
Cholesterol 0 mg	
Sodium 0 mg	0%
Carbohydrate 18 g	6%
Fibre 2 g	8%
Sugars 2 g	
Protein 3 g	

Vitamin A	2%	Vitamin C	10%
Calcium	0%	Iron	2%

The % Daily Value gives a context to the actual amount of a nutrient. It indicates at a glance if there is a lot or a little of a nutrient in the specific amount of food.

This number is the actual amount (quantity) of the nutrient in the specific amount of food. Even if the nutrient amount is zero, it is listed.

Figure C.2   Canadian Nutrition Facts Table
(*Source:* From Nutrition Recommendations, Health Canada, 2002. Reproduced with the permission of the Minister of Public Works and Government Services Canada, 2004.)

would be 65 grams. A product with 13 grams of fat in one serving, has a %DV of $13/65 \times 100 = 20\%$. In other words, one serving of this food would provide 20% of the %DV for fat.

Consumers need to understand that the amount listed as "one serving" on a package label may not be the same as a serving according to *Canada's Food Guide to Healthy Eating*.

For foods that are made specifically for children under the age of two years, a simplified version of the Nutrition Facts panel is used. The amount of calories and 10 nutrients are listed; saturated and *trans* fats and cholesterol are not required.

Health Claims

Five statements or "health claims" about some specific diet/health relationships are now allowed on food products:

- A healthy diet low in sodium and high in potassium may reduce the risk of high blood pressure, a risk factor for stroke and heart disease;
- A healthy diet adequate in calcium and vitamin D, and regular physical activity, help to achieve strong bones and may reduce the risk of osteoporosis;
- A healthy diet low in saturated fat and *trans* fats may reduce the risk of heart disease;
- A healthy diet rich in a variety of vegetables and fruit may help reduce the risk of some types of cancer.
- Foods very low in starch and fermentable sugars can make the following health claims:
  will not cause cavities;
  does not promote tooth decay;
  does not promote dental caries; and are
  non-carcinogenic.

Nutrient Content Claims

The Canadian government has strict rules for terms such as "reduced in fat," "very high source of fiber," and "low fat." Before these terms can be used on a label or advertisement, the exact amount of a nutrient in one serving has to be determined and has to meet set criteria (e.g., "low fat" means no more than 3 grams of fat in one serving).

These nutrient content claims are usually on the front of food packages where they can be easily seen by consumers. Any of the following words may indicate a nutrient content claim:

free	very high
low	light/lite
less	source of
more	high source of
reduced	good source of
lower	excellent source of

Manufacturers can decide whether they want to have nutrient content claims on their products.

Some of the more important recent changes to nutrient content claims include:

- "Free" claims mean that the number of calories or the amount of a nutrient is nutritionally insignificant in a specified amount of food.
- Claims for saturated fatty acids now include a restriction on levels of both saturated and *trans* fatty acids.
- The claim "(naming the percent) fat-free" is allowed only if accompanied by the statement "low fat" or "low in fat."
- The nutrient content claim "light" is allowed only on foods that meet the criteria for either "reduced in fat" or "reduced in calories."
- The use of "light" must be accompanied by a statement that explains what makes the food "light;" this is also true if "light" refers to a sensory characteristic such as "light in color."

The only nutrient content claims that are permitted for foods for children under two years of age are "source of protein," "excellent source of protein," "more protein," "no added salt," and "no added sugar."

Physical Activity Advice for Canadians

Canada's Physical Activity Guide

While Canada's *Food Guide* has been in existence, in one form or another, for more than 60 years, it is only recently that the Canadian government developed a guide to help people include physical activity in their daily routines. In 1997, Health Canada and the Canadian Society for Exercise Physiology partnered to produce *Canada's Physical Activity Guide to Healthy Active Living* (Figure C.3). The current version was published in 1998, and is accompanied by a handbook for people who want more detailed information. *The Physical Activity Guide* uses the familiar rainbow format of the *Food Guide*, and shows people a range of activities to build endurance and strength.

Two other similar guides have been developed. *Canada's Physical Activity Guide to Healthy Active Living for Older Adults* was developed in 1999 by Health Canada, the Canadian Society for Exercise Physiology and the Active Living Coalition of Older Adults. Copies of this guide are available from: http://www.hc-sc.gc.ca/hbbp/fitness/pdf/guide_older.pdf.

In 2002, Health Canada, the Canadian Society for Exercise Physiology, the College of Family Physicians of Canada, and the Canadian Pediatric Society published *Canada's Physical Activity Guide for Children* (2002). It can be downloaded from: http://www.hc-sc.gc.ca/hppb/paguide/child_youth/pdf/guide_k_en.pdf.

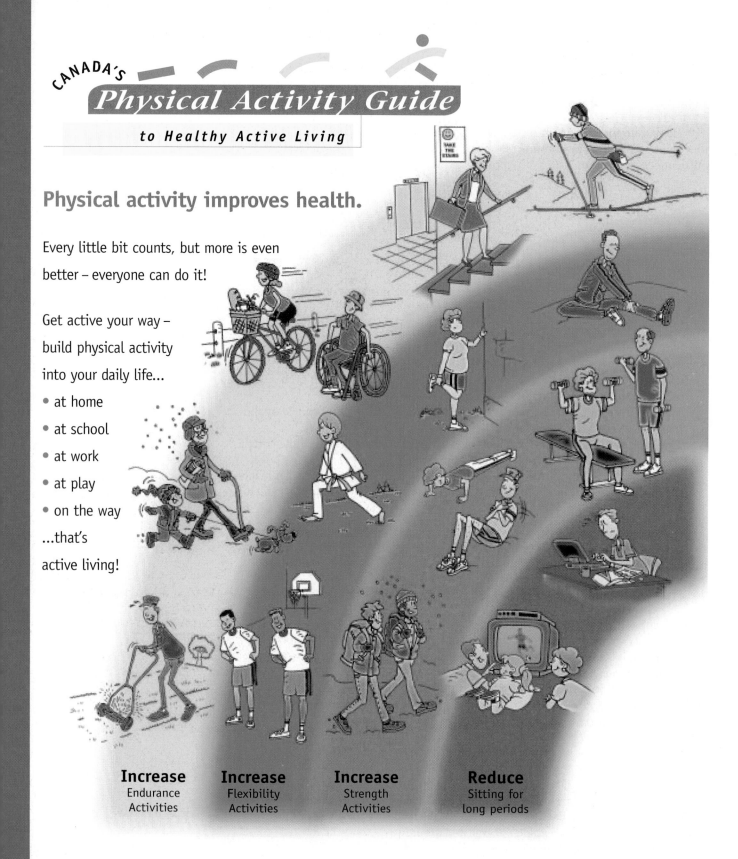

Physical activity improves health.

Every little bit counts, but more is even better – everyone can do it!

Get active your way – build physical activity into your daily life...

- at home
- at school
- at work
- at play
- on the way

...that's active living!

Increase Endurance Activities

Increase Flexibility Activities

Increase Strength Activities

Reduce Sitting for long periods

 Health Canada Santé Canada

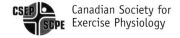 CSEP SCPE Canadian Society for Exercise Physiology

Figure C.3 Canada's Physical Activity Guide to Healthy Active Living

(Source: From Canada's Physical Activity Guide, Health Canada, 1998. Reproduced with the permission of the Minister of Public Works and Government Services Canada, 2004.)

Choose a variety of activities from these three groups:

Endurance

4-7 days a week
Continuous activities for your heart, lungs and circulatory system.

Flexibility

4-7 days a week
Gentle reaching, bending and stretching activities to keep your muscles relaxed and joints mobile.

Strength

2-4 days a week
Activities against resistance to strengthen muscles and bones and improve posture.

Starting slowly is very safe for most people. Not sure? Consult your health professional.

For a copy of the *Guide Handbook* and more information: **1-888-334-9769**, or **www.paguide.com**

Eating well is also important. Follow *Canada's Food Guide to Healthy Eating* to make wise food choices.

Get Active Your Way, Every Day – For Life!

Scientists say accumulate 60 minutes of physical activity every day to stay healthy or improve your health. As you progress to moderate activities you can cut down to 30 minutes, 4 days a week. Add-up your activities in periods of at least 10 minutes each. Start slowly… and build up.

Time needed depends on effort

Very Light Effort	Light Effort *60 minutes*	Moderate Effort *30-60 minutes*	Vigorous Effort *20-30 minutes*	Maximum Effort
• Strolling • Dusting	• Light walking • Volleyball • Easy gardening • Stretching	• Brisk walking • Biking • Raking leaves • Swimming • Dancing • Water aerobics	• Aerobics • Jogging • Hockey • Basketball • Fast swimming • Fast dancing	• Sprinting • Racing

Range needed to stay healthy

You Can Do It – Getting started is easier than you think

Physical activity doesn't have to be very hard. Build physical activities into your daily routine.

- Walk whenever you can – get off the bus early, use the stairs instead of the elevator.
- Reduce inactivity for long periods, like watching TV.
- Get up from the couch and stretch and bend for a few minutes every hour.
- Play actively with your kids.
- Choose to walk, wheel or cycle for short trips.

- Start with a 10 minute walk – gradually increase the time.
- Find out about walking and cycling paths nearby and use them.
- Observe a physical activity class to see if you want to try it.
- Try one class to start – you don't have to make a long-term commitment.
- Do the activities you are doing now, more often.

Benefits of regular activity:	Health risks of inactivity:
• better health • improved fitness • better posture and balance • better self-esteem • weight control • stronger muscles and bones • feeling more energetic • relaxation and reduced stress • continued independent living in later life	• premature death • heart disease • obesity • high blood pressure • adult-onset diabetes • osteoporosis • stroke • depression • colon cancer

No changes permitted. Permission to photocopy this document in its entir ety not required.
Cat. No. H39-429/1998-1E ISBN 0-662-86627-7

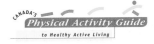

Figure C.3   Continued

Useful Web sites

http://www.hc-sc.gc.ca/hpfb-dgpsa/onpp-bppn/index_e.html

Health Canada, Office of Nutrition Policy and Promotion

This Web site provides all of Canada's nutrition policies and government documents, including *Canada's Food Guide to Healthy Eating, Nutrition Recommendations for Canadians,* Healthy Weights, Nutrition Labeling, Infant Feeding Guidelines, and more.

http://www.dietitians.ca/

Dietitians of Canada

This is the Web site for Canada's national association of dietitians, but it is also an excellent source of nutrition information for consumers. There are FAQs and factsheets, a Meal Planner, Healthy Body Quiz, Virtual Kitchen, and Virtual Grocery Store to teach consumers how to assess their food choices and to read product labels.

http://www.diabetes.ca/

Canadian Diabetes Association

Consumers can find up-to-date information about diabetes in English, French, and Chinese on this Web site. Health Professionals can access the 2003 Clinical Practice Guidelines.

http://www.cpha.ca/

Canadian Public Health Association

The latest "hot topics" in public health (such as mad cow disease), national public health programs, and Public Policy Statements on a wide range of public health topics, are available at this site.

http://www.canadian-health-network.ca

Canadian Health Network

This national, non-profit collaboration of hundreds of health organizations, provincial and territorial governments, universities, hospitals, libraries, community organizations, and Health Canada is a valuable source of e-health information for consumers.

http://www.cihr-irsc.gc.ca

Canadian Institutes of Health Research

CIHR is comprised of 13 Institutes, including *Nutrition, Metabolism and Diabetes.* This is Canada's main federal funding agency for health research.

http://ww2.heartandstroke.ca/

Heart and Stroke Foundation of Canada

Consumers can find the latest information on heart disease, stroke, and healthy living, as well as an e-newsletter, recipes, activities designed to help them assess their risks of heart disease and stroke on this Web site. Health professionals can search for research funding opportunities.

http://www.healthcheck.org/

Health Check

"Health Check™ . . . tells you it's a healthy choice" is a product logo program created by the Heart and Stroke Foundation of Canada. This Web site lists the participating food companies and product brands that meet the Heart and Stroke Foundation's criteria for healthy food choices.

www.healthyeatingisinstore.ca/

Healthy Eating Is In Store for You

"Healthy Eating Is In Store for You™" is an online program created by the Canadian Diabetes Association and Dietitians of Canada to teach consumers how to read product labels.

www.missionnutrition.ca

Mission Nutrition

"Mission Nutrition™" is an educational program developed by the Registered Dietitians at Kellogg Canada Inc. and Dietitians of Canada. Teachers can download lesson plans and activities for grades K–8. Students in grades 6–8 can enjoy fun and challenging games online.

Appendix D *Traditional Organization of Nutrients*

Nutrient Classification	Nutrient	Primary Functions	Recommended Intake	Toxicity Symptoms/ Side Effects	Deficiency Symptoms/ Side Effects	Chapter Reference
Water-soluble vitamin	Thiamin vitamin B$_1$	Part of the coenzyme thiamin pyrophosphate (TPP) involved in carbohydrate metabolism Coenzyme involved in branched-chain amino acid metabolism	RDA: Men = 1.2 mg/day Women = 1.1 mg/day	None known at this time	Beriberi Anorexia and weight loss Apathy Decreased short-term memory Confusion and irritability Muscle weakness Enlarged heart	10
Water-soluble vitamin	Riboflavin vitamin B$_2$	Coenzymes involved in oxidation-reduction reactions, including flavin mononucleotide (FMN) and flavin adenine dinucleotide (FAD).	RDA: Men = 1.3 mg/day Women = 1.1 mg/day	None known at this time	Ariboflavinosis Sore throat Swelling of mouth and throat Cheilosis Angular stomatitis Glossitis (magenta tongue) Seborrheic dermatitis Anemia	10
Water-soluble vitamin	Niacin (nicotinamide and nicotinic acid)	Coenzymes in carbohydrate and fatty acid metabolism, including nicotinamide adenine dinucleotide (NAD$^+$ and NADH) and nicotinamide adenine dinucleotide phosphate (NADP$^+$) Plays role in DNA replication and repair and cell differentiation	RDA: Men = 16 mg/day Women = 14 mg/day	Flushing Liver dysfunction and damage Glucose intolerance Blurred vision and edema of eyes	Pellagra Pigmented rash Vomiting Constipation or diarrhea Bright red tongue Depression Apathy Headache Fatigue Loss of memory	10
Water-soluble vitamin	Vitamin B$_6$ (pyridoxine)	Part of coenzyme (pyridoxal phosphate, or PLP) involved in amino acid metabolism, synthesis of blood cells, and carbohydrate metabolism	RDA: Men aged 19 to 50 = 1.3 mg/day Men aged > 50 = 1.7 mg/day Women aged 19 to 50 = 1.3 mg/day Women aged > 50 = 1.5 mg/day	Sensory neuropathy Lesions of the skin	Seborrheic dermatitis Microcytic anemia Convulsions Depression and confusion	10
Water-soluble vitamin	Folate (folic acid)	Coenzyme tetrahydrofolate (THF) (or tetrahydrofolic acid, THFA) involved in DNA synthesis and amino acid metabolism Involved in the metabolism of homocysteine	RDA: Men = 400 μg/day Women = 400 μg/day	Masks symptoms of vitamin B$_{12}$ deficiency Neurological damage	Macrocytic anemia Weakness and fatigue Difficulty concentrating Irritability Headache Palpitations Shortness of breath Elevated levels of homocysteine in the blood Neural tube defects in the developing fetus	10

continued

Nutrient Classification	Nutrient	Primary Functions	Recommended Intake	Toxicity Symptoms/ Side Effects	Deficiency Symptoms/ Side Effects	Chapter Reference
Water-soluble vitamin	Vitamin B$_{12}$ (cobalamin)	Part of coenzymes that assist with formation of blood, nervous system function, and homocysteine metabolism	RDA: Men = 2.4 µg/day Women = 2.4 µg/day	None known at this time	Pernicious anemia Pale skin Diminished energy and low exercise tolerance Fatigue Shortness of breath Palpitations Tingling and numbness in extremities Abnormal gait Memory loss Poor concentration Disorientation Dementia	10
Water-soluble vitamin	Pantothenic Acid	Component of coenzymes (coenzyme A) that assist with fatty acid metabolism	AI: Men = 5 mg/day Women = 5 mg/day	None known at this time	Rare; only seen in people fed diets with virtually no pantothenic acid	10
Water-soluble vitamin	Biotin	Component of coenzymes involved in carbohydrate, fat, and protein metabolism	AI: Men = 30 µg/day Women = 30 µg/day	None known at this time	Red, scaly skin rash Depression Lethargy Hallucinations Paresthesia of the extremities	10
Water-soluble vitamin	Vitamin C	Antioxidant in extracellular fluid and lungs Regenerates oxidized vitamin E Reduces formation of nitrosamines in stomach Assists with collagen synthesis Enhances immune function Assists in the synthesis of hormones, neurotransmitters, and DNA Enhances absorption of iron	RDA: Men = 90 mg Women = 75 mg Smokers = 35 mg more per day than RDA	Nausea and diarrhea Nosebleeds Abdominal cramps Increased oxidative damage Increased formation of kidney stones in those with kidney disease	Scurvy Bleeding gums and joints Loose teeth Weakness Hemorrhaging of hair follicles Poor wound healing Swollen ankles and wrists Diarrhea Bone pain and fractures Depression Anemia	8
Fat-soluble vitamin	Vitamin A	Necessary for our ability to adjust to changes in light Protects color vision Cell differentiation Necessary for sperm production in men and fertilization in women Contributes to healthy bone growth	RDA: Men = 900 µg Women = 700 µg	Spontaneous abortions and birth defects of fetus in pregnant women Loss of appetite Blurred vision Hair loss Abdominal pain, nausea, diarrhea Liver and nervous system damage	Night blindness Xerophthalmia, which leads to permanent blindness Impaired immunity and increased risk of illness and infection Inability to reproduce Failure of normal growth	8
Fat-soluble vitamin	Vitamin D	Regulates blood calcium levels Maintains bone health Cell differentiation	AI (based on the assumption that a person does not get adequate sun exposure): Men aged 19 to 50 = 5 µg/day	Hypercalcemia, including weakness, loss of appetite, diarrhea, mental confusion, vomiting, excessive urine output, extreme thirst, and formation of calcium deposits in kidney, heart, and liver	Rickets (in children), leading to bone weakness and deformities Osteomalcia (in adults), leading to bone weakness and increased rate of fractures	9

continued

Nutrient Classification	Nutrient	Primary Functions	Recommended Intake	Toxicity Symptoms/ Side Effects	Deficiency Symptoms/ Side Effects	Chapter Reference
			Men aged 50 to 70 = 10 µg/day Men aged > 70 = 15 µg/day Women aged 19 to 50 = 5 µg/day Women aged 50 to 70 = 10 µg/day Women aged > 70 = 15 µg/day	Increased bone loss	Osteoporosis, leading to increased rate of fractures	
Fat-soluble vitamin	Vitamin E	Protects cell membranes from oxidation Protects polyunsaturated fatty acids (PUFAs) from oxidation Protects vitamin A from oxidation Protects white blood cells and enhances immune function Improves absorption of vitamin A	RDA: Men = 15 mg alpha-tocopherol Women = 15 mg alpha-tocopherol	Inhibition of blood clotting Increased risk of hemorrhagic stroke Intestinal discomfort	Red blood cell hemolysis Anemia Impairment of nerve transmission Muscle weakness and degeneration Leg cramps Difficulty walking Fibrocytic breast disease	8
Fat-soluble vitamin	Vitamin K	Serves as a coenzyme during production of specific proteins that assist in blood coagulation and bone metabolism	AI: Men = 120 µg/day Women = 90 µg/day	No known side effects or toxicity symptoms from consuming excess vitamin K	Reduced ability to form blood clots, leading to excessive bleeding and easy bruising Effect on bone health is controversial	9 and 10
Major mineral	Sodium	Major positively charged electrolyte in extracellular fluid Maintains proper acid-base balance Assists with transmission of nerve signals Aids muscle contraction Assists in the absorption of glucose and other nutrients	AI: Men = 1.5 g/day (1,500 mg/day) Women = 1.5 g/day (1,500 mg/day)	Water retention High blood pressure May increase loss of calcium in urine	Muscle cramps Loss of appetite Dizziness Fatigue Nausea Vomiting Mental confusion	7
Major mineral	Potassium	Major positively charged electrolyte in intracellular fluid Regulates contraction of muscles Regulates transmission of nerve impulses Assists in maintaining healthy blood pressure levels	AI: Men = 4.7 g/day (4,700 mg/day) Women = 4.7 g/day (4,700 mg/day)	Muscle weakness Vomiting Irregular heartbeat	Muscle weakness Muscle paralysis Mental confusion	7
Major mineral	Phosphorus	Major negatively charged electrolyte in intracellular fluid Maintains proper fluid balance Plays critical role in bone formation as a major component of hydroxyapatite crystals Component of ATP, which provides energy for our bodies Helps regulate biochemical reactions by activating and inactivating enzymes	RDA: Men = 700 mg/day Women = 700 mg/day	High blood phosphorus levels Muscle spasms Convulsions Low blood calcium levels	Low blood phosphorus levels Muscle weakness Muscle damage Bone pain Dizziness	7 and 9

continued

Nutrient Classification	Nutrient	Primary Functions	Recommended Intake	Toxicity Symptoms/ Side Effects	Deficiency Symptoms/ Side Effects	Chapter Reference
		Major part of genetic materials (DNA, RNA)				
		A component in cell membranes, LDL, and HDL				
Major mineral	Calcium	Primary component of bone and teeth structure	AI:	Potential mineral imbalances; calcium can interfere with absorption of iron, zinc, and magnesium	Osteoporosis	9
		Helps maintain optimal acid-base balance	Men aged 19 to 50 = 1,000 mg/day		Bone fractures	
		Maintains normal nerve transmission	Men aged > 50 = 1,200 mg/day	Shock	Convulsions and muscle spasms	
		Supports muscle contraction and relaxation	Women aged 19 to 50 = 1,000 mg/day	Kidney failure	Heart failure	
		Regulates blood pressure, blood clotting, and various hormones and enzymes	Women aged > 50 = 1,200 mg/day	Fatigue	Bleeder's disease	
				Mental confusion		
Major mineral	Magnesium	An essential component of bone tissue	RDA:	No known toxicity symptoms of consuming excess in diet	Hypomagnesemia, resulting in low blood calcium levels, muscle cramps, spasms or seizures, nausea, weakness, irritability, and confusion	9
		Influences formation of hydroxyapatite crystals and bone growth	Men aged 19 to 30 = 400 mg/day	Toxicity from pharmacological use includes diarrhea, nausea, abdominal cramps; in severe cases, massive dehydration, cardiac arrest, and death can result		
		Cofactor for more than 300 enzyme systems, including ATP, DNA and protein synthesis and vitamin D metabolism and action	Men aged > 30 = 420 mg/day		Chronic diseases such as heart disease, high blood pressure, osteoporosis, and type 2 diabetes	
			Women aged 19 to 30 = 310 mg/day			
		Supports muscle contraction and blood clotting	Women aged > 30 = 320 mg/day			
Major mineral	Sulfur	Component of B vitamins thiamin and biotin	No DRI	No known symptoms	No known symptoms	10
		As part of the amino acids methionine and cysteine, helps stabilize the three-dimensional shapes of proteins in our bodies				
		Assists liver in the detoxification of alcohol and various drugs				
		Assists in maintaining acid-base balance				
Trace mineral	Chloride	Assists with maintaining fluid balance	AI:	Vomiting	Dangerous changes in pH	7
		Aids in preparing food for digestion (as HCl)	Men = 2.3 g/day (2,300 mg/day)		Irregular heartbeat	
		Helps kill bacteria				
		Assists in the transmission of nerve impulses	Women = 2.3 g/day (2,300 mg/day)			
Trace mineral	Selenium	Part of glutathione peroxidase, an antioxidant enzyme	RDA:	Brittle hair and nails	Keshan disease: a specific form of heart disease	8
		Indirectly spares vitamin E from oxidation	Men = 55 µg/day	Skin rashes	Kashin-Beck disease: deforming arthritis	
		Assists in production of thyroid hormone	Women = 55 µg/day	Vomiting, nausea	Impaired immune function	
		Assists in maintaining immune function		Weakness	Increased risk of viral infections	
				Cirrhosis of liver	Infertility	
					Depression, hostility	
					Muscle pain and wasting	

continued

Nutrient Classification	Nutrient	Primary Functions	Recommended Intake	Toxicity Symptoms/ Side Effects	Deficiency Symptoms/ Side Effects	Chapter Reference
Trace mineral	Fluoride	Maintains health of teeth and bones Protects teeth against dental caries Stimulates new bone growth	AI: Men = 4 mg/day Women = 3 mg/day	Teeth fluorosis, which causes staining and pitting of teeth Skeletal fluorosis, which ranges from mild to severe; causes joint pain and stiffness, and in extreme cases can cause crippling, wasting of muscles, and osteoporosis of the extremities	High occurrence of dental caries and tooth decay Low fluoride intakes may also be associated with lower bone density	9
Trace mineral	Iodine	Critical for synthesis of thyroid hormones Assists in temperature regulation, maintenance of resting metabolic rate, and supports reproduction and growth	RDA: Men = 150 µg/day Women = 150 µg/day	Goiter, or enlargement of thyroid gland	Goiter, or enlargement of thyroid gland Hypothyroidism, which includes decreased body temperature, inability to tolerate cold temperatures, weight gain, fatigue, and sluggishness Iodine deficiency during pregnancy causes a form of mental retardation in the infant called cretinism	10
Trace mineral	Chromium	Enhances the ability of insulin to transport glucose from the bloodstream into the cells Plays an important role in the metabolism of RNA and DNA Important for healthy immune function and growth	AI: Men aged 19 to 50 = 35 µg/day Men aged > 50 = 30 µg/day Women aged 19 to 50 = 25 µg/day Women aged > 50 = 20 µg/day	No known symptoms	Inhibition of uptake of glucose by the cells, leading to rise in blood glucose and insulin Elevated blood lipid levels Damage to brain and nervous system	10
Trace minerals	Manganese	Coenzyme involved in energy metabolism and in the formation of urea Assists in the synthesis of the protein matrix found in bone tissue and in building cartilage An integral component of superoxide dismutase, an antioxidant enzyme	AI: Men = 2.3 mg/day Women = 1.8 mg/day	Impairment of the neuromuscular system, causing muscle spasms and tremors	Impaired growth and reproductive function Reduced bone density and impaired skeletal growth Impaired glucose and lipid metabolism Skin rash	10
Trace mineral	Iron	As a component of hemoglobin, assists with oxygen transport in our blood As a component of myoglobin, assists in the transport of oxygen into muscle cells Coenzyme for enzymes involved in energy metabolism Part of the antioxidant enzyme system that combats free radicals	RDA: Men aged 19 to 50 years = 8 mg/day Med aged > 50 = 8 mg/day Women aged 19 to 50 = 18 mg/day Women aged > 50 = 8 mg/day	Nausea Vomiting Diarrhea Dizziness, confusion Rapid heart beat Damage to heart, central nervous system, liver, kidneys Death	First stage of iron deficiency: decrease in iron stores with no physical symptoms Second stage of iron deficiency: decrease in iron transport, causing reduced work capacity Third stage of iron deficiency: anemia, causing impaired work performance, general fatigue, pale skin, depressed immune function, impaired cognitive and nerve function, and impaired memory	10

continued

Nutrient Classification	Nutrient	Primary Functions	Recommended Intake	Toxicity Symptoms/ Side Effects	Deficiency Symptoms/ Side Effects	Chapter Reference
Trace mineral	Zinc	Coenzyme that assists with hemoglobin production Part of superoxide dismutase antioxidant enzyme system that combats free radicals Facilitates folding of proteins, which assists in gene regulation Plays role in cell replication and normal growth and sexual maturation Plays a role in proper development and function of immune system	RDA: Men = 11 mg/day Women = 8 mg/day	Intestinal pain and cramps Nausea Vomiting Loss of appetite Diarrhea Headaches Depressed immune function Reduced absorption of copper	Growth retardation Diarrhea Delayed sexual maturation and impotence Eye and skin lesions Hair loss Impaired appetite Increased incidence of illness and infections	10
Trace mineral	Copper	Coenzyme in metabolic pathways that produce energy Coenzyme that assists in production of collagen and elastin Part of superoxide dismutase antioxidant enzyme system that combats free radicals Component of ceruloplasmin, which allows for the proper transport of iron	RDA: Men = 900 µg/day Women = 900 µg/day	Abdominal pain and cramps Nausea Diarrhea Vomiting Liver damage occurs in extreme cases that result from Wilson's disease and other rare disorders	Anemia Reduced levels of white blood cells Osteoporosis in infants and growing children	10

Appendix E *Foods Containing Caffeine*

Source: Values are obtained from the USDA Nutrient Database for Standard Reference, Release 16.

Beverages

Food Name	Serving	Caffeine/serving (mg)
Beverage Mix, chocolate flavor, dry mix, prep w/milk	1 cup (8 fl. oz.)	7.98
Beverage Mix, chocolate malt powder, fortified, prepared w/milk	1 cup (8 fl. oz.)	5.3
Beverage Mix, chocolate malted milk powder, no added nutrients, prepared w/milk	1 cup (8 fl. oz.)	7.95
Beverage, chocolate syrup w/o added nutrients, prepared w/milk	1 cup (8 fl. oz.)	5.64
Beverage, chocolate syrup, fortified, mixed w/milk	1 cup milk and 1 tbsp syrup	2.63
Cocoa Mix w/aspartame and calcium and phosphorus, no sodium or vitamin A, low kcal, dry, prepared	6 fl. oz. water and 0.53 oz packet	15.36
Cocoa Mix w/aspartame, dry, low kcal, prepared w/water	1 packet dry mix with 6 fl. oz. water	1.92
Cocoa Mix, dry mix	1 serving (3 heaping tsp or 1 envelope)	5.04
Cocoa Mix, dry, w/o added nutrients, prepared w/water	1 oz packet with 6 fl. oz. water	4.12
Cocoa Mix, fortified, dry, prepared w/water	6 fl. oz. H_2O and 1 packet	6.27
Cocoa, dry powder, hi-fat or breakfast, plain	1 piece	6.895
Cocoa, hot, homemade w/whole milk	1 cup	5
Coffee Liqueur 53 proof	1 fl. oz.	9.048
Coffee Liqueur 63 proof	1 fl. oz.	9.048
Coffee w/Cream Liqueur, 34 proof	1 fl. oz.	2.488
Coffee Mix w/sugar (cappuccino) dry, prepared w/water	6 fl. oz. H_2O and 2 rounded tsp mix	74.88
Coffee Mix w/sugar (French) dry, prepared w/water	6 fl. oz. H_2O and 2 rounded tsp mix	51.03
Coffee Mix w/sugar (mocha) dry, prepared w/water	6 fl. oz. and 2 round tsp mix	33.84
Coffee, brewed	1 cup (8 fl. oz.)	85.32
Coffee, brewed, prepared with tap water, decaffeinated	1 cup (8 fl. oz.)	2.37
Coffee, instant, prepared	1 fl. oz.	7.748
Coffee, instant, regular, powder, half the caffeine	1 cup (8 fl. oz.)	3723.27
Coffee, instant powder, decaffeinated, prepared	6 fl. oz.	1.79
Coffee and cocoa (mocha) powder, with whitener and low calorie sweetener	1 cup	405.48
Coffee, brewed, espresso, restaurant-prepared	1 ounce	60.081
Coffee, brewed, espresso, restaurant-prepared, decaffeinated	1 cup (8 fl. oz.)	2.37
Energy drink, with caffeine, niacin, pantothenic acid, vitamin B_6	1 fl. oz.	9.517
Milk Beverage Mix, dairy drink w/aspartame, low kcal, dry, prep	6 fl. oz.	4.08
Milk, lowfat, 1% fat, chocolate	1 cup	5
Milk, whole, chocolate	1 cup	5
Soft Drink, cola w/caffeine	1 fl. oz.	3.1
Soft Drink, cola, w/higher caffeine	1 fl. oz.	8.37
Soft Drink, cola or Pepper type, low kcal w/saccharin and caffeine	1 fl. oz.	3.256
Soft Drink, cola, low kcal w/saccharin and aspartame, w/caffeine	1 fl. oz.	4.144
Soft Drink, lemon-lime soda, w/caffeine	1 fl. oz.	4.605
Soft Drink, low kcal, not cola or Pepper, with aspartame and caffeine	1 fl. oz.	4.44
Soft Drink, Pepper type	1 fl. oz.	3.07
Tea Mix, instant w/lemon flavor, w/saccharin, dry, prepared	1 cup (8 fl. oz.)	16.59
Tea Mix, instant w/lemon, unsweetened, dry, prepared	1 cup (8 fl. oz.)	26.18
Tea Mix, instant w/sugar and lemon, dry, no added vitamin C, prepared	1 cup (8 fl. oz.)	28.49
Tea Mix, instant, unsweetened, dry, prepared	1 cup (8 fl. oz.)	30.81
Tea, brewed	1 cup (8 fl. oz.)	47.4
Tea, brewed, prepared with tap water, decaffeinated	1 cup (8 fl. oz.)	2.37
Tea, instant, unsweetened, powder, decaffeinated	1 tsp	1.183
Tea, instant, w/sugar, lemon-flavored, w/added vitamin C, dry prepared	1 cup (8 fl. oz.)	28.49
Tea, instant, with sugar, lemon-flavored, decaf, no added vitamin	1 cup	9.1

Cake, Cookies, and Desserts

Food Name	Serving	Caffeine/serving (mg)
Brownies, commercially prepared, Little Debbie	1 oz	0.567
Cake, chocolate pudding, dry mix	1 oz	1.701
Cake, chocolate, dry mix, regular	1 oz	3.118
Cake, German chocolate pudding, dry mix	1 oz	1.985
Cake, marble pudding, dry mix	1 oz	1.985
Candies, chocolate covered, caramel with nuts	1 cup	35.34
Candies, chocolate covered, dietetic or low calorie	1 cup	16.74
Candy, milk chocolate w/almonds	1 bar (1.45 oz)	9.02
Candy, milk chocolate w/rice cereal	1 bar (1.4 oz)	9.2
Candy, raisins, milk chocolate coated	1 cup	45
Chocolate Chips, semisweet	1 cup chips (6 oz package)	104.16
Chocolate, baking, unsweetened, square	1 cup, grated	105.6
Chocolate, baking, Mexican, squares	1 tablet	2.8
Chocolate, sweet	1 oz	18.711
Cookie Cake, Snackwell Fat Free Devil's Food, Nabisco	1 serving	1.28
Cookie, Snackwell Caramel Delights, Nabisco	1 serving	1.44
Cookie, chocolate chip, enriched, commercially prepared	1 oz	3.118
Cookie, chocolate chip, homemade w/margarine	1 oz	4.536
Cookie, chocolate chip, lower fat, commercially prepared	1 oz	1.985
Cookie, chocolate chip, refrigerated dough	1 portion, dough spoon from roll	2.61
Cookie, chocolate chip, soft, commercially prepared	1 oz	1.985
Cookie, chocolate wafers	1 cup, crumbs	7.84
Cookie, graham crackers, chocolate coated	1 oz	13.041
Cookie, sandwich, chocolate, cream filled	1 oz	3.686
Cookie, sandwich, chocolate, cream filled, special dietary	1 oz	0.85
Cupcakes, chocolate w/frosting, low-fat	1 oz	0.567
Donut, cake, chocolate w/sugar or glaze	1 oz	0.284
Donut, cake, plain w/chocolate icing	1 oz	0.567
Fast Food, ice cream sundae, hot fudge	1 sundae	1.58
Fast Food, milk beverage, chocolate shake	1 cup (8 fl. oz.)	1.66
Frosting, chocolate, creamy, ready to eat	2 tbsp creamy	0.82
Frozen Yogurts, chocolate	1 cup	5.58
Fudge, chocolate w/nuts, homemade	1 ounce	1.984
Granola Bar, soft, milk chocolate coated, peanut butter	1 ounce	0.85
Granola Bar, with coconut, chocolate coated	1 cup	5.58
Ice Cream, chocolate	1 individual (3.5 fl. oz.)	1.74
Ice Cream, chocolate, light	1 ounce	0.85
Ice Cream, chocolate, rich	1 cup	5.92
M&M's Peanut Chocolate	1 cup	18.7
M&M's Plain Chocolate	1 cup	22.88
Milk chocolate	1 cup chips	33.6
Milk chocolate coated coffee beans	1 NLEA serving	48
Milk Dessert, frozen, fat-free milk, chocolate	1 ounce	0.85
Milk Shake, thick, chocolate	1 fl. oz.	0.568
Pastry, eclair/cream puff, homemade, custard filled w/chocolate	1 oz	0.567
Pie Crust, chocolate wafer cookie type, chilled	1 crust, single 9″	11.15
Pie, chocolate mousse, no bake mix	1 oz	0.284
Pudding, chocolate, instant dry mix prep w/reduced fat (2%) milk	1 ounce	0.283
Pudding, chocolate, regular dry mix prep w/reduced fat (2%) milk	1 ounce	0.567
Pudding, chocolate, ready-to-eat, fat free	1 ounce	0.567
Syrups, chocolate, genuine chocolate flavor, lite, Hershey	2 tbsp	1.05
Topping, chocolate-flavored hazelnut spread	1 ounce	1.984
Yogurt, chocolate, nonfat milk	1 ounce	0.567
Yogurt, frozen, chocolate, soft serve	.5 cup (4 fl. oz.)	2.16

Source: © 2003, American Diabetes Association/American Dietetic Association. Used with permission.

Starch List

1 starch exchange = 15 g carbohydrate, 3 g protein, 0–1 g fat, and 80 cal

Food	Serving Size
Bread	
Bagel, 4 oz	¼ (1 oz)
Bread, reduced-calorie	2 slices (1½ oz)
Bread, white, whole-wheat, pumpernickel, rye	1 slice (1 oz)
Bread sticks, crisp, 4″ × ½″	4 (⅔ oz)
English muffin	½
Hot dog bun or hamburger bun	½ (1 oz)
Naan, 8″ × 2″	¼
Pancake, 4″ across, ¼″ thick	1
Pita, 6″ across	½
Roll, plain small	1 (1 oz)
Raisin bread, unfrosted	1 slice (1 oz)
Tortilla, corn, 6″ across	1
Tortilla, flour, 6″ across	1
Tortilla, flour, 10″ across	⅓
Waffle, 4″ square or across, reduced-fat	1
Cereals and Grains	
Bran cereals	½ c
Bulgur	½ c
Cereals, cooked	½ c
Cereals, unsweetened, ready-to-eat	¾ c
Cornmeal (dry)	3 tbs
Couscous	⅓ c
Flour (dry)	3 tbs
Granola, low-fat	¼ c
Grape-Nuts®	¼ c
Grits	½ c
Kasha	½ c
Millet	⅓ c
Muesli	¼ c
Oats	½ c
Pasta	⅓ c
Puffed cereal	1½ c
Rice, white or brown	⅓ c
Shredded Wheat®	½ c
Sugar-frosted cereal	½ c
Wheat germ	3 tbs

Food	Serving Size
Starchy Vegetables	
Baked beans	⅓ c
Corn	½ c
Corn on cob, large	½ cob (5 oz)
Mixed vegetables with corn, peas, or pasta	1 c
Peas, green	½ c
Plantain	½ c
Potato, boiled	½ c or ½ medium (3 oz)
Potato, mashed	½ c
Squash, winter (acorn, butternut, pumpkin)	1 c
Yam, sweet potato, plain	½ c
Crackers and Snacks	
Animal crackers	8
Graham crackers, 2½″ square	3
Matzoh	¾ oz
Melba toast	4 slices
Oyster crackers	24
Popcorn (popped, no fat added or low-fat microwave)	3 c
Pretzels	¾ oz
Rice cakes, 4″ across	2
Saltine-type crackers	6
Snack chips, fat-free or baked (tortilla, potato)	15–20 (¾ oz)
Whole-wheat crackers, no fat added	2–5 (¾ oz)
Beans, Peas, and Lentils	
(Count as 1 starch exchange, plus 1 very lean meat exchange)	
Beans and peas (garbanzo, pinto, kidney, white, split, black-eyed)	½ c
Lima beans	⅔ c
Miso*	3 tbs
Starchy Foods Prepared with Fat	
(Count as 1 starch exchange plus 1 fat exchange)	
Biscuit, 2½″ across	1
Chow mein noodles	½ c
Corn bread, 2″ cube	1 (2 oz)
Crackers, round butter type	6
Croutons	1 c
French-fried potatoes (oven-baked) (see also the fast foods list)	1 c (2 oz)
Granola	¼ c
Muffin, 5 oz	⅕ (1 oz)
Popcorn, microwaved	3 c
Sandwich crackers, cheese or peanut butter filling	3
Stuffing, bread (prepared)	⅓ c
Taco shell, 6″ across	2
Waffle, 4″ square or across	1
Whole-wheat crackers, fat added	4–7 (1 oz)

* = 400 mg or more sodium per exchange.

Fruit List

1 fruit exchange = 15 g carbohydrate and 60 cal
Weight includes skin, core, seeds, and rind.

Food	Serving Size	Food	Serving Size
Apples, unpeeled, small	1 (4 oz)	Orange, small	1 (6½ oz)
Applesauce, unsweetened	½ c	Papaya	½ (8 oz) or 1 c cubes
Apples, dried	4 rings	Peach, medium, fresh	1 (4 oz)
Apricots, fresh	4 whole (5½ oz)	Peaches, canned	½ c
Apricots, dried	8 halves	Pear, large, fresh	½ (4 oz)
Apricots, canned	½ c	Pears, canned	½ c
Banana, small	1 (4 oz)	Pineapple, fresh	¾ c
Blackberries	⅓ c	Pineapple, canned	½ c
Blueberries	⅓ c	Plums, small	2 (5 oz)
Cantaloupe, small	⅓ melon (11 oz)	Plums, canned	½ c
	or 1 c cubes	Plums, dried (prunes)	3
Cherries, sweet, fresh	12 (3 oz)	Raisins	2 tbs
Cherries, sweet, canned	½ c	Raspberries	1 c
Dates	3	Strawberries	1¼ c whole berries
Figs, fresh	1½ large or 2 medium	Tangerines, small	2 (8 oz)
	(3½ oz)	Watermelon	1 slice (13½ oz)
Figs, dried	1½		or 1¼ c cubes
Fruit cocktail	½ c		
Grapefruit, large	½ (11 oz)	**Fruit Juice, Unsweetened**	
Grapefruit sections, canned	¾ c	Apple juice/cider	½ c
Grapes, small	17 (3 oz)	Cranberrry juice cocktail	⅓ c
Honeydew melon	1 slice (10 oz)	Cranberry juice cocktail, reduced-calorie	1 c
	or 1 c cubes	Fruit juice blends, 100% juice	⅓ c
Kiwi	1 (3½ oz)	Grape juice	⅓ c
Mandarin oranges, canned	¾ c	Grapefruit juice	½ c
Mango, small	½ (5½ oz) or ½ c	Orange juice	½ c
Nectarine, small	1 (5 oz)	Pineapple juice	½ c
		Prune juice	⅓ c

Milk List

1 milk exchange = 12 g carbohydrate and 8 g protein

Food	Serving Size	Food	Serving Size
Fat-Free and Low-Fat Milk		**Reduced-Fat Milk**	
(0–3 g fat per serving)		*(5 g fat per serving)*	
Fat-free milk	1 c	2% milk	1 c
½% milk	1 c	Soy milk	1 c
1% milk	1 c	Sweet acidophilus milk	1 c
Buttermilk, low-fat or fat-free	1 c	Yogurt, plain, low-fat	6 oz
Evaporated fat-free milk	½ c	**Whole Milk**	
Fat-free dry milk	⅓ c dry	*(8 g fat per serving)*	
Soy milk, low-fat or fat-free	1 c	Whole milk	1 c
Yogurt, plain, fat-free	6 oz	Evaporated whole milk	½ c
Yogurt, fat-free, flavored, sweetened with		Goat's milk	1 c
nonnutritive sweetener and fructose	1 c	Kefir	1 c
		Yogurt, plain (made from whole milk)	8 oz

Other Carbohydrates List

1 other carbohydrate exchange = 15 g carbohydrate, or 1 starch, or 1 fruit, or 1 milk

Food	Serving Size	Exchanges per Serving
Angel food cake, unfrosted	¹⁄₁₂ cake (about 2 oz)	2 carbohydrates
Brownies, small, unfrosted	2" square (about 1 oz)	1 carbohydrate, 1 fat
Cake, unfrosted	2" square (about 1 oz)	1 carbohydrate, 1 fat
Cake, frosted	2" square (about 2 oz)	2 carbohydrates, 1 fat
Cookie, sugar-free	3 small or 1 large (¾ oz–1oz)	1 carbohydrate
Cookie or sandwich cookie with creme filling	2 small (about ⅔ oz)	1 carbohydrate, 1 fat
Cupcakes, frosted	1 small (about 2 oz)	2 carbohydrates, 1 fat
Cranberry sauce, jellied	¼ c	1½ carbohydrates
Doughnut, plain cake	1 medium, (1½ oz)	1½ carbohydrates, 2 fats
Doughnut, glazed	3¾" across (2 oz)	2 carbohydrates, 2 fats
Energy, sport, or breakfast bar	1 bar (1⅓ oz)	1½ carbohydrates, 0–1 fat
Energy, sport, or breakfast bar	1 bar (2 oz)	2 carbohydrates, 1 fat
Fruit juice bars, frozen, 100% juice	1 bar (3 oz)	1 carbohydrate
Fruit snacks, chewy (pureed fruit concentrate)	1 roll (¾ oz)	1 carbohydrate
Fruit spreads, 100% fruit	1½ tbs	1 carbohydrate
Gelatin, regular	½ c	1 carbohydrate
Gingersnaps	3	1 carbohydrate
Granola or snack bar regular or low-fat	1 bar (1 oz)	1½ carbohydrates
Honey	1 tbs	1 carbohydrate
Ice cream	½ c	1 carbohydrate, 2 fats
Ice cream, light	½ c	1 carbohydrate, 1 fat
Ice cream, fat-free, no sugar added	½ c	1 carbohydrate
Jam or jelly, regular	1 tbs	1 carbohydrate
Milk, chocolate, whole	1 c	2 carbohydrates, 1 fat
Pie, fruit, 2 crusts	⅙ of 8-inch commercially prepared pie	3 carbohydrates, 2 fats
Pie, pumpkin or custard	⅛ of 8-inch commercially prepared pie	2 carbohydrates, 2 fats
Pudding, regular (made with reduced-fat milk)	½ c	2 carbohydrates
Pudding, sugar-free, or sugar-free and fat-free (made with fat-free milk)	½ c	1 carbohydrate
Reduced-calorie meal replacement (shake)	1 can (10–11 oz)	1½ carbohydrates, 0–1 fat
Rice milk, low-fat or fat-free, plain	1 c	1 carbohydrate
Rice milk, low-fat, flavored	1 c	1½ carbohydrates
Salad dressing, fat-free*	¼ c	1 carbohydrate
Sherbet, sorbet	½ c	2 carbohydrates
Spaghetti or pasta sauce, canned*	½ c	1 carbohydrate, 1 fat
Sports drinks	8 oz (1 c)	1 carbohydrate
Sugar	1 tbs	1 carbohydrate
Sweet roll or Danish	1 (2½ oz)	2½ carbohydrates, 2 fats
Syrup, light	2 tbs	1 carbohydrate
Syrup, regular	1 tbs	1 carbohydrate
Syrup, regular	¼ c	4 carbohydrates
Vanilla wafers	5	1 carbohydrate, 1 fat
Yogurt, frozen, fat-free	⅓ c	1 carbohydrate
Yogurt, frozen, fat-free, no sugar added	½ c	1 carbohydrate, 0–1 fat
Yogurt, low-fat with fruit	1 c	3 carbohydrates, 0–1 fat

* = 400 mg or more sodium per exchange.

Vegetable List

1 vegetable exchange = 5 g carbohydrate, 2 g protein, 0 g fat, 25 cal

Artichoke
Artichoke hearts
Asparagus
Beans (green, wax, Italian)
Bean sprouts
Beets
Broccoli
Brussels sprouts
Cabbage
Carrots
Cauliflower
Celery
Cucumber
Eggplant
Green onions or scallions
Greens (collard, kale, mustard, turnip)
Kohlrabi
Leeks
Mixed vegetables (without corn, peas, or pasta)
Mushrooms
Okra
Onions
Pea pods
Peppers (all varieties)
Radishes
Salad greens (endive, escarole, lettuce, romaine, spinach)
Sauerkraut*
Spinach
Summer squash
Tomato
Tomatoes, canned
Tomato sauce*
Tomato /vegetable juice*
Turnips
Water chestnuts
Watercress
Zucchini

* = 400 mg or more sodium per exchange.

Meat and Meat Substitutes List

Food	Serving Size

Very Lean Meat and Substitutes

1 very lean meat exchange = 7 g protein, 0–1 g fat, 35 cal, 0 g carbohydrate

Poultry: Chicken or turkey (white meat, no skin),

Cornish hen (no skin) . . . . .1 oz

Fish: Fresh or frozen cod, flounder, haddock, halibut,

trout, lox (smoked salmon)*; tuna, fresh or canned in water   1 oz

Shellfish: Clams, crab, lobster, scallops, shrimp,

imitation shellfish . . . . .1 oz

Game: Duck or pheasant (no skin), venison, buffalo,

ostrich . . . . .1 oz

Cheese with ≤ *1 g fat/oz:*

Fat-free or low-fat cottage cheese . . . . .¼ c

Fat-free cheese . . . . .1 oz

Other:

Processed sandwich meats with ≤ 1 g fat/oz

(such as deli thin, shaved meats, chipped beef*,

turkey ham) . . . . .1 oz

Egg whites 2

Egg substitutes, plain . . . . .¼ c

Hot dogs with ≤1 g fat/oz* . . . . .1 oz

Kidney (high in cholesterol) . . . . .1 oz

Sausage with ≤ 1 g fat/oz . . . . .1 oz

Count as one very lean meat and one starch exchange:

Beans, peas, lentils (cooked) . . . . .½ c

Lean Meat and Substitutes

1 lean meat exchange = 7g protein, 3 g fat, 55 cal, 0 g carbohydrate

Beef: USDA Select or Choice grades of lean beef

trimmed of fat (round, sirloin, and flank steak);

tenderloin; roast (rib, chuck, rump); steak (T-bone,

porterhouse, cubed); ground round . . . . .1 oz

Pork: Lean pork (fresh ham); canned, cured, or boiled

ham; Canadian bacon*; tenderloin, center loin chop . . . . .1 oz

Lamb: Roast, chop, leg . . . . .1 oz

Veal: Lean chop, roast . . . . .1 oz

Poultry: Chicken, turkey (dark meat, no skin), chicken

white meat (with skin), domestic duck or goose (well

drained of fat, no skin) . . . . .1 oz

Fish:

Herring (uncreamed or smoked) . . . . .1 oz

Oysters . . . . .6 medium

Salmon (fresh or canned), catfish . . . . .1 oz

Sardines (canned) . . . . .2 medium

Tuna (canned in oil, drained) . . . . .1 oz

Game: Goose (no skin), rabbit . . . . .1 oz

Food	Serving Size

Cheese:

4.5% fat cottage cheese . . . . .¼ c

Grated Parmesan . . . . .2 tbs

Cheeses with ≤ 3 g fat/oz . . . . .1 oz

Other:

Hot dogs with ≤ 3 g fat/oz* . . . . .1½ oz

Processed sandwich meat with ≤ 3 g fat/oz (turkey

pastrami or kielbasa) . . . . .1 oz

Liver, heart (high in cholesterol) . . . . .1 oz

Medium-Fat Meat and Substitutes

1 medium-fat meat exchange = 7 g protein, 5 g fat, and 75 cal, 0 g carbohydrate

Beef: Most beef products (ground beef, meatloaf,

corned beef, short ribs, Prime grades of meat trimmed

of fat, such as prime rib) . . . . .1 oz

Pork: Top loin, chop, Boston butt, cutlet . . . . .1 oz

Lamb: Rib roast, ground . . . . .1 oz

Veal: Cutlet (ground or cubed, unbreaded) . . . . .1 oz

Poultry: Chicken dark meat (with skin), ground turkey

or ground chicken, fried chicken (with skin) . . . . .1 oz

Fish: Any fried fish product . . . . .1 oz

Cheese with ≤ *5 g fat/oz:*

Feta . . . . .1 oz

Mozzarella . . . . .1 oz

Ricotta . . . . .¼ c (2 oz)

Other:

Egg (high in cholesterol, limit to 3/week) 1

Sausage with ≤ 5 g fat/oz . . . . .1 oz

Tempeh . . . . .¼ c

Tofu . . . . .4 oz or ½ c

High-Fat Meat and Substitutes

1 high-fat meat exchange = 7 g protein, 8 g fat, 100 cal, 0 g carbohydrate

Pork: Spareribs, ground pork, pork sausage . . . . .1 oz

Cheese: All regular cheeses (American* cheddar,

Monterey Jack, Swiss) . . . . .1 oz

Other:

Proceesed sandwich meats with ≤ 8 g fat/oz

(bologna, pimento loaf, salami) . . . . .1 oz

Sausage (bratwurst, Italian, knockwurst, Polish,

smoked) . . . . .1 oz

Hot dog (turkey or chicken)* 1 (10/lb)

Bacon . . . . .3 slices (20 slices/lb)

Peanut butter (contains unsaturated fat) . . . . .1 tbs

Count as one high-fat meat plus one fat exchange:

Hot dog (beef, pork, or combination)* 1 (10/lb)

* = 400 m or more of sodium per serving.

Fat List
1 fat exchange = 5 g fat, 45 cal

Food	Serving Size

Monounsaturated Fats

Avocado, medium	2 tbs (1 oz)
Oil (canola, olive, peanut)	1 tsp
Olives, ripe (black)	8 large
Olives, green, stuffed*	10 large
Almonds, cashews	6 nuts
Mixed nuts (50% peanuts)	6 nuts
Peanuts	10 nuts
Pecans	4 halves
Peanut butter, smooth or crunchy	½ tbs
Sesame seeds	1 tbs
Tahini paste	2 tsp

Polyunsaturated Fats

Margarine, stick, tub, or squeeze	1 tsp
Margarine, lower-fat (30% to 50% vegetable oil)	1 tbs
Mayonnaise, regular	1 tsp
Mayonnaise, reduced-fat	1 tbs
Nuts, walnuts, English	4 halves
Oil (corn, safflower, soybean)	1 tsp
Salad dressing, regular*	1 tbs
Salad dressing, reduced-fat	2 tbs
Miracle Whip Salad Dressing®, regular	2 tsp
Miracle Whip Salad Dressing®, reduced-fat	1 tbs
Seeds: pumpkin, sunflower	1 tbs

Saturated Fats

Bacon, cooked	1 slice (20 slices/lb)
Bacon, grease	1 tsp
Butter, stick	1 tsp
Butter, whipped	2 tsp
Butter, reduced-fat	1 tbs
Chitterlings, boiled	2 tbs (½ oz)
Coconut, sweetened, shredded	2 tbs
Coconut milk	1 tbs
Cream, half and half	2 tbs
Cream, cheese, regular	1 tbs (½ oz)
Cream cheese, reduced-fat	1½ tbs (¾ oz)
Fatback or salt pork*a	
Shortening or lard	1 tsp
Sour cream, regular	2 tbs
Sour cream, reduced-fat	3 tbs

* = 400 mg or more sodium per exchange.
aUse a piece 1″ × 1″ × ¼″ if you plan to eat the fatback cooked with vegetables.
Use a piece 2″ × 1″ × ½″ when eating only the vegetables with the fatback removed.

Free Foods List
A *free food* is any food or drink that contains less than 20 calories or less than 5 grams of carbohydrate per serving. Foods with a serving size listed should be limited to three servings per day. Be sure to spread them out throughout the day. If you eat all three servings at one time, it could affect you blood glucose level. Foods listed without a serving size can be eaten as often as you like.

Fat-Free or Reduced-Fat Foods

Cream cheese, fat-free	1 tbs (½ oz)
Creamers, nondairy, liquid	1 tbs
Creamers, nondairy, powdered	2 tsp
Mayonnaise, fat-free	1 tbs
Mayonnaise, reduced-fat	1 tsp
Margarine, spread fat-free	4 tbs
Margarine, spread reduced-fat	1 tsp
Miracle Whip®, fat-free	1 tbs
Miracle Whip®, reduced-fat	1 tsp
Nonstick cooking spray	
Salad dressing, fat-free or low-fat	1 tbs
Salad dressing, fat-free, Italian	2 tbs
Sour cream, fat-free, reduced-fat	1 tbs
Whipped topping, regular	1 tbs
Whipped topping, light or fat-free	2 tbs

Sugar-Free Foods

Candy, hard, sugar-free	1 candy
Gelatin dessert, sugar-free	
Gelatin, unflavored	
Gum, sugar-free	
Jam or jelly, light	2 tsp
Sugar substitutesa	
Syrup, sugar-free	2 tbs

Drinks

Bouillon, broth, consommé*	
Bouillon or broth, low-sodium	
Carbonated or mineral water	
Club soda	
Cocoa powder, unsweetened	1 tbs
Coffee	
Diet soft drinks, sugar-free	
Drink mixes, sugar-free	
Tea	
Tonic water, sugar-free	

Condiments

Catsup	1 tbs
Horseradish	
Lemon juice	
Lime juice	
Mustard	
Pickles, dill*	1½ medium
Salsa	¼ c

aSugar substitutes, alternatives, or replacements that are approved by the Food and Drug Administration (FDA) are safe to use. Common brand names include:
Equal® (aspartame), Splenda® (sucralose), Sprinkle Sweet® (saccharin), Sweet One® (acesulfame K), Sweet-10® (saccharin), Sugar Twin® (saccharin), Sweet 'n Low® (saccharin).

Soy sauce, regular or light* ....1 tbs
Taco sauce ....1 tbs
Vinegar
Yogurt ....2 tbs

Seasonings

Be careful with seasonings that contain sodium or are salts, such as garlic or celery salt, and lemon pepper.

Flavoring extracts

Garlic

Herbs, fresh or dried

Pimento

Spices

Tabasco® or hot pepper sauce

Wine, used in cooking

Worcestershire sauce

* = 400 mg or more of sodium per choice.

Combination Foods List

Food	Serving Size	Exchanges per Serving
Entrées		
Tuna noodle casserole, lasagna, spaghetti with meatballs, Chili with beans, macaroni and cheese*	1 c (8 oz)	2 carbohydrates, 2 medium-fat meats
Chow mein (without noodles or rice)	2 c (16 oz)	1 carbohydrate, 2 lean meats
Frozen Entrées		
Dinner-type meal*	generally 14–17 oz	3 carbohydrates, 3 medium-fat meats, 3 fats
Meatless burger, soy based	3 oz	½ carbohydrate, 2 lean meats
Meatless burger, vegetable and starch based	3 oz	1 carbohydrate, 1 lean meat
Pizza, cheese, thin crust* (5 oz)	¼ of 12″ (6 oz)	2 carbohydrates, 2 medium-fat meats
Pizza, meat topping, thin crust* (5 oz)	¼ of 12″ (6 oz)	2 carbohydrates, 2 medium-fat meats, 1½ fats
Potpie*	1 (7 oz)	2½ carbohydrates, 1 medium-fat meat, 3 fats
Entrée with less than 340 calories*	about 8–11 oz	2–3 carbohydrates, 1–2 lean meats
Soups		
Bean*	1 c	1 carbohydrate, 1 very lean meat
Cream (made with water)*	1 c (8 oz)	1 carbohydrate, 1 fat
Split pea (made with water)*	½ c (4 oz)	1 carbohydrate
Tomato (made with water)*	1 c (8 oz)	1 carbohydrate
Vegetable beef, chicken noodle, or other broth-type*	1 c (8 oz)	1 carbohydrate

* = 400 mg or more sodium per exchange.

Fast Foods List[a]

Food	Serving Size	Exchanges per Serving
Burrito with beef*	1 (5–7 oz)	3 carbohydrates, 1 medium-fat meat, 1 fat
Chicken nuggets*	6	1 carbohydrate, 2 medium-fat meats, 1 fat
Chicken breast and wing, breaded and fried*	1 each	1 carbohydrate, 4 medium-fat meats, 2 fats
Chicken sandwich, grilled*	1	2 carbohydrates, 3 very lean meats
Chicken wings, hot*	6 (5 oz)	1 carbohydrate, 3 medium-fat meats, 4 fats
Fish sandwich/tartar sauce*	1	3 carbohydrates, 1 medium-fat meat, 3 fats
French fries, thin	20–25	2 carbohydrates, 2 fats
Hamburger, regular	1	2 carbohydrates, 2 medium-fat meats
Hamburger, large*	1	2 carbohydrates, 3 medium-fat meats, 1 fat
Hot dog with bun*	1	1 carbohydrate, 1 high-fat meat, 1 fat
Individual pan pizza*	1	5 carbohydrates, 3 medium-fat, meats, 3 fats
Pizza, cheese, thin crust*	¼ of 12″ (about 6 oz)	2½ carbohydrates, 2 medium-fat meats, 1½ fats
Pizza, meat, thin crust*	¼ of 12″ (about 6 oz)	2½ carbohydrates, 2 medium-fat meats, 2 fats
Soft serve cone	1 medium	2 carbohydrates, 1 fat
Submarine sandwich*	1 (6 ″)	3 carbohydrates, 1 vegetable, 2 medium-fat meats, 1 fat
Taco, hard shell*	1 (6 oz)	2 carbohydrates, 2 medium-fat meats, 2 fats
Taco, soft shell*	1 (3 oz)	1 carbohydrate, 1 medium-fat meat, 1 fat

* = 400 mg or more sodium per exchange.

[a]Ask at your fast-food restaurant for nutrition information about your favorite fast foods or check websites.

CDC Growth Charts: United States
Stature-for-age percentiles: Boys, 2 to 20 years

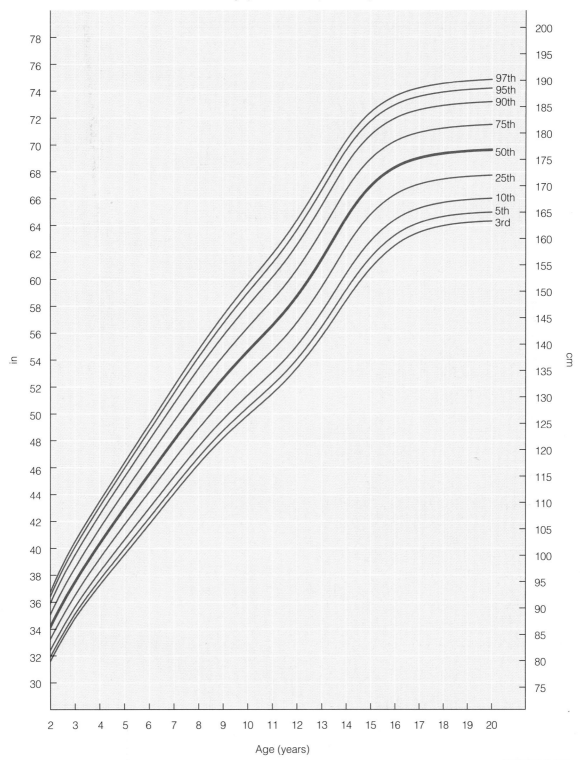

Published May 30, 2000.
SOURCE: Developed by the National Center for Health Statistics
in collaboration with the National Center for Chronic
Disease Prevention and Health Promotion (2000).

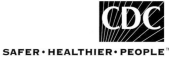

SAFER·HEALTHIER·PEOPLE™

http://www.cdc.gov/nchs/data/nhanes/growthcharts/set1/chart07.pdf

CDC Growth Charts: United States
Stature-for-age percentiles: Girls, 2 to 20 years

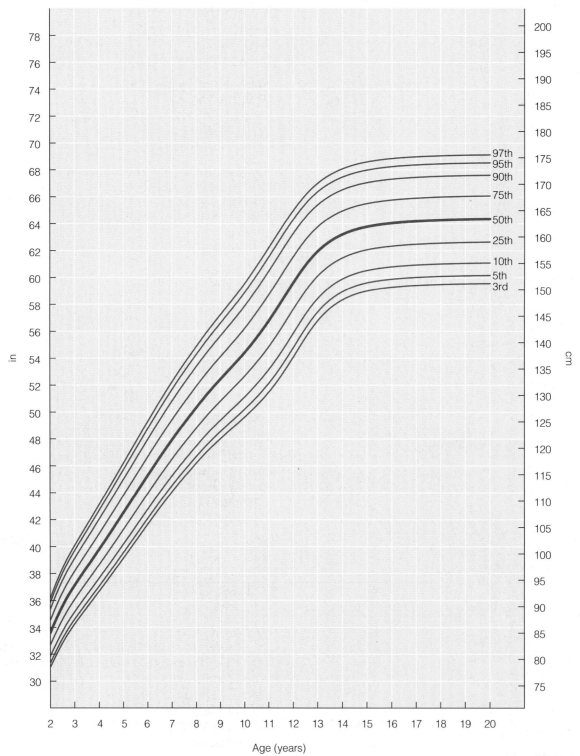

Age (years)

Published May 30, 2000.
SOURCE: Developed by the National Center for Health Statistics
in collaboration with the National Center for Chronic
Disease Prevention and Health Promotion (2000).

http://www.cdc.gov/nchs/data/nhanes/growthcharts/set1/char14.pdf

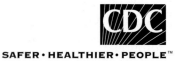

SAFER · HEALTHIER · PEOPLE™

Academic Journals

International Journal of Sport Nutrition and Exercise Metabolism
Human Kinetics
P.O. Box 5076
Champaign, IL 61825-5076
(800) 747-4457
http://www.humankinetics.com/IJSNEM

Journal of Nutrition
A. Catharine Ross, Editor
Department of Nutrition
Pennsylvania State University
126-S Henderson Building
University Park, PA 16802-6504
(814) 865-4721
http://www.nutrition.org/

Nutrition Research
Elsevier: Journals Customer Service
6277 Sea Harbor Drive
Orlando, FL 32887
(877) 839-7126
http://www.journals.elsevierhealth.com/periodicals/NTR

Nutrition
Elsevier: Journals Customer Service
6277 Sea Harbor Drive
Orlando, FL 32887
(877) 839-7126
http://www.journals.elsevierhealth.com/periodicals/NUT

Nutrition Reviews
International Life Sciences Institute
Subscription Office
P.O. Box 830430
Birmingham, AL 35283
(800) 633-4931
http://www.ilsi.org/publications/

Obesity Research
North American Association for the Study of Obesity (NAASO)
8630 Fenton Street, Suite 918
Silver Spring, MD 20910
(301) 563-6526
http://www.obesityresearch.org/

International Journal of Obesity
Journal of the International Association for the Study of Obesity
Nature Publishing Group
The Macmillan Building
4 Crinan Street
London N1 9XW
United Kingdom
http://www.nature.com/ijo/

Journal of the American Medical Association
American Medical Association
P.O. Box 10946
Chicago, IL 60610-0946
(800) 262-2350
http://jama.ama-assn.org/

New England Journal of Medicine
10 Shattuck Street
Boston, MA 02115-6094
(617) 734-9800
http://content.nejm.org/

American Journal of Clinical Nutrition
The American Journal of Clinical Nutrition
9650 Rockville Pike
Bethesda, MD 20814-3998
(301) 634-7038
http://www.ajcn.org/

Journal of the American Dietetic Association
Elsevier, Health Sciences Division
Subscription Customer Service
6277 Sea Harbor Drive
Orlando, FL 32887
(800) 654-2452
http://www.adajournal.org/

Aging

Administration on Aging
U.S. Health & Human Services
200 Independence Avenue, SW
Washington, DC 20201
(877) 696-6775
www.aoa.gov

American Association of Retired Persons (AARP)
601 E. Street, NW
Washington, DC 20049
(888) 687-2277
www.aarp.org

Health and Age
Sponsored by the Novartis Foundation for Gerontology & The Web-Based Health Education Foundation
Robert Griffith MD
Executive Director
573 Vista de la Ciudad
Santa Fe, NM 87501
www.healthandage.com

National Council on the Aging
300 D Street, SW, Suite 801
Washington, DC 20024
(202) 479-1200
www.ncoa.org

International Osteoporosis Foundation
5 Rue Perdtemps
1260 Nyon
Switzerland
41 22 994 01 00
www.osteofound.org

Osteogenesis Imperfecta Foundation
804 W. Diamond Avenue, Suite 210
Gaithersburg, MD 20878
(800) 981-2663
www.oif.org

National Institute on Aging
Building 31, Room 5C27
31 Center Drive, MSC 2292
Bethesda, MD 20892
(301) 496-1752
www.nia.nih.gov

Osteoporosis and Related Bone Diseases National Resource Center
2 AMS Circle
Bethesda, MD 20892-3676
(800) 624-BONE
www.osteo.org

American Geriatrics Society
The Empire State Building
350 Fifth Avenue, Suite 801
New York, NY 10118
(212) 308-1414
http://www.americangeriatrics.org/

National Osteoporosis Foundation
1232 22nd Street, NW
Washington, DC 20037-1292
(202) 223-2226
http://www.nof.org/

Alcohol and Drug Abuse

National Institute on Drug Abuse
6001 Executive Boulevard, Room 5213
Bethesda, MD 20892-9561
(301) 443-1124
www.nida.nih.gov

National Institute on Alcohol Abuse and Alcoholism
5635 Fishers Lane, MSC 9304
Bethesda, MD 20892-9304
http://www.niaaa.nih.gov

Alcoholics Anonymous
Grand Central Station
P.O. Box 459
New York, NY 10163
www.alcoholics-anonymous.org

Narcotics Anonymous
P.O. Box 9999
Van Nuys, California 91409
(818) 773-9999
http://www.na.org/

National Council on Alcoholism and Drug Dependence
20 Exchange Place, Suite 2902
New York, NY 10005
(212) 269-7797
http://www.ncadd.org/

National Clearinghouse for Alcohol and Drug Information
11420 Rockville Pike
Rockville, MD 20852
(800) 729-6686
http://www.health.org/

Canadian Government

Health Canada
A.L. 0900C2
Ottawa, ON
K1A 0K9
(613) 957-2991
http://www.hc-sc.gc.ca/english/

National Institute of Nutrition
408 Queen Street, 3rd Floor
Ottawa, ON K1R 5A7
(613) 235-3355
http://www.nin.ca/public_html/index.html

Agricultural and Agri-Food Canada
Public Information Request Service
Sir John Carling Building
930 Carling Avenue
Ottawa, ON K1A 0C5
(613) 759-1000
http://www.agr.gc.ca/

Bureau of Nutritional Sciences
Sir Frederick G. Banting Research Centre
Tunney's Pasture (2203A)
Ottawa, ON K1A 0L2
(613) 957-0352
http://www.hc-sc.gc.ca/food-aliment/ns-sc/e_nutrition.html

Canadian Food Inspection Agency
59 Camelot Drive
Ottawa, ON K1A 0Y9
(613) 225-2342
http://www.inspection.gc.ca/english/toce.shtml

Canadian Institute for Health Information
CIHI Ottawa
377 Dalhousie Street, Suite 200
Ottawa, ON K1N 9N8
(613) 241-7860
www.cihi.ca/

Canadian Public Health Association
1565 Carling Avenue, Suite 400
Ottawa, ON K1Z 8R1
(613) 725-3769
http://www.cpha.ca/

Canadian Nutrition and Professional Organizations

Dietitians of Canada
480 University Avenue, Suite 604
Toronto, ON M5G 1V2
(416) 596-0857
http://www.dietitians.ca/

Canadian Diabetes Association
National Life Building
1400-522 University Avenue
Toronto, ON M5G 2R5
(800) 226-8464
http://www.diabetes.ca/

National Eating Disorder Information Centre
CW 1-211, 200 Elizabeth Street
Toronto, ON M5G 2C4
(866) NEDIC-20
http://www.nedic.ca/

Canadian Pediatric Society
100-2204 Walkley Road
Ottawa, ON K1G 4G8
(613) 526-9397
http://www.cps.ca/

Canadian Dietetic Association
480 University Avenue, Suite 604
Toronto, ON M5G 1V2
(416) 596-0857
http://www.dietitians.ca/

Disordered Eating/Eating Disorders

American Psychiatric Association
1000 Wilson Boulevard, Suite 1825
Arlington, VA 22209
(703) 907-7300
http://www.psych.org/

Harvard Eating Disorders Center
WACC 725
15 Parkman Street
Boston, MA 02114
(617) 236-7766
www.hedc.org

National Institute of Mental Health
Office of Communications
6001 Executive Boulevard, Room 8184, MSC 9663
Bethesda, MD 20892
(866) 615-6464
www.nimh.nih.gov

National Association of Anorexia Nervosa and Associated Disorders (ANAD)
Box 7
Highland Park, IL 60035
(847) 831-3438
www.anad.org

National Eating Disorders Association
603 Stewart Street, Suite 803
Seattle, WA 98101
(206) 382-3587
www.nationaleatingdisorders.org

Eating Disorder Referral and Information Center
2923 Sandy Pointe, Suite 6
Del Mar, CA 92014
(858) 792-7463
www.edreferral.com

Anorexia Nervosa and Related Eating Disorders, Inc. (ANRED)
Email: jarinor@rio.com
www.anred.com

Overeaters Anonymous
P.O. Box 44020
Rio Rancho, NM 87174
(505) 891-2664
http://www.oa.org/

Exercise, Physical Activity, and Sports

American College of Sports Medicine (ACSM)
P.O. Box 1440
Indianapolis, IN 46206-1440
(317) 637-9200
http://www.acsm.org/

American Physical Therapy Association (ASNA)
1111 North Fairfax Street
Alexandria, VA 22314
(800) 999-APTA
www.apta.org

Gatorade Sports Science Institute (GSSI)
617 West Main Street
Barrington, IL 60010
(800) 616-GSSI
http://www.gssiweb.com/

National Coalition for Promoting Physical Activity (NCPPA)
1010 Massachusetts Avenue, Suite 350
Washington, DC 20001
(202) 454-7518
http://www.ncppa.org/

Sports, Wellness, Eating Disorder and Cardiovascular Nutritionists (SCAN)
P.O. Box 60820
Colorado Springs, CO 80960
(719) 635-6005
http://www.scandpg.org/

President's Council on Physical Fitness and Sports
Department W
200 Independence Avenue, SW
Room 738-H
Washington, DC 20201-0004
(202) 690-9000
http://www.fitness.gov/

American Council on Exercise
4851 Paramount Drive
San Diego, CA 92123
(858) 279-8227
http://www.acefitness.org/

The International Association for Fitness Professionals (IDEA)
10455 Pacific Center Court
San Diego, CA 92121
(800) 999-4332, ext. 7
www.ideafit.com

International Society of Sports Nutrition
Executive Director, Maelu Fleck
600 Pembrook Drive
Woodland Park, CO 80863
(866) 472-4650
http://www.sportsnutritionsociety.org/

Food Safety

Food Marketing Institute
655 15th Street, NW
Washington, DC 20005
(202) 452-8444
http://www.fmi.org/

Agency for Toxic Substances and Disease Registry (ATSDR)
ORO Washington Office
Ariel Rios Building
1200 Pennsylvania Avenue, NW
M/C 5204G
Washington, DC 20460
(888) 422-8737
http://www.atsdr.cdc.gov/

Food Allergy and Anaphylaxis Network
11781 Lee Jackson Highway, Suite 160
Fairfax, VA 22033-3309
(800) 929-4040
http://www.foodallergy.org/

Foodsafety.gov
www.foodsafety.gov

The USDA Food Safety and Inspection Service
Food Safety and Inspection Service
United States Department of Agriculture
Washington, DC 20250
www.fsis.usda.gov

Consumer Reports
Web Site Customer Relations Department
101 Truman Avenue
Yonkers, NY 10703
www.consumerreports.org

Center for Science in the Public Interest: Food Safety
1875 Connecticut Avenue, NW
Washington, DC 20009
(202) 332-9110
http://www.cspinet.org/foodsafety/index.html

Center for Food Safety and Applied Nutrition
5100 Paint Branch Parkway
College Park, MD 20740
(888) SAFEFOOD
http://www.cfsan.fda.gov

Food Safety Project
Dan Henroid, MS, RD, CFSP
HRIM Extension Specialist and Website Coordinator
Hotel, Restaurant and Institution Management
9e MacKay Hall
Iowa State University
Ames, IA 50011
(515) 294-3527
http://www.extension.iastate.edu/foodsafety/

Organic Consumers Association
6101 Cliff Estate Road
Little Marais, MN 55614
(218) 226-4164
www.organicconsumers.org

Infancy and Childhood

Administration for Children and Families
370 L'Enfant Promenade, SW
Washington, DC 20447
http://www.acf.dhhs.gov/

The American Academy of Pediatrics
141 Northwest Point Boulevard
Elk Grove Village, IL 60007
(847) 434-4000
http://www.aap.org/

Kidnetic.com
Email: contactus@kidnetic.com
http://www.kidnetic.com

Kidshealth: The Nemours Foundation
12735 West Gran Bay Parkway
Jacksonville, FL 32258
(866) 390-3610
www.kidshealth.org

National Center for Education in Maternal Health & Child Health
Georgetown University
Box 571272
Washington, DC 20057
(202) 784-9770
www.ncemch.org

Birth Defects Research for Children, Inc.
930 Woodcock Road, Suite 225
Orlando, FL 32803
(407) 895-0802
www.birthdefects.org

USDA/ARS Children's Nutrition Research Center at Baylor College of Medicine
1100 Bates Street
Houston, TX 77030
http://www.kidsnutrition.org

Keep Kids Healthy.com
www.keepkidshealthy.com

International Agencies

UNICEF
3 United Nations Plaza
New York, NY 10017
(212) 326-7000
www.unicef.org/

World Health Organization
Avenue Appia 20
1211 Geneva 27
Switzerland
41 22 791 21 11
http://www.who.int/en/

The Stockholm Convention on Persistent Organic Pollutants
11-13 Chemin des Anémones
1219 Châtelaine
Geneva, Switzerland
41 22 917 8191
http://www.pops.int/

Food and Agricultural Organization of the United Nations
Viale delle Terme di Caracalla
00100 Rome, Italy
39 06 57051
http://www.fao.org/

International Food Information Council Foundation
1100 Connecticut Avenue, NW
Suite 430
Washington, DC 20036
(202) 296-6540

Pregnancy and Lactation

San Diego County Breastfeeding Coalition
c/o Children's Hospital and Health Center
3020 Children's Way, MC 5073
San Diego, CA 92123
(800) 371-MILK
www.breastfeeding.org

National Alliance for Breastfeeding Advocacy
Barbara Heiser, Executive Director
9684 Oak Hill Drive
Ellicott City, MD 21042-6321
OR
Marsha Walker, Executive Director
254 Conant Road
Weston, MA 02493-1756
http://www.naba-breastfeeding.org/

American College of Obstetricians and Gynecologists
409 12th Street, SW, P.O. Box 96920
Washington, DC 20090
http://www.acog.org/

La Leche League
1400 N. Meacham Road
Schaumburg, IL 60173
(847) 519-7730
www.lalecheleague.org

National Organization on Fetal Alcohol Syndrome
900 17th Street, NW
Suite 910
Washington, DC 20006
(800) 66 NOFAS
www.nofas.org

March of Dimes Birth Defects Foundation
1275 Mamaroneck Avenue
White Plains, NY 10605
(888) 663-4637
http://modimes.org

Professional Nutrition Organizations

Association of Departments and Programs of Nutrition (ANDP)
Dr. Carolyn M. Bednar, ANDP Chair
Dept. of Nutrition and Food Sciences
Texas Woman's University
P.O. Box 425888
Denton, TX 76204-5888
(940) 898-2658
http://andpnet.org/

North American Association for the Study of Obesity (NAASO)
8630 Fenton Street, Suite 918
Silver Spring, MD 20910
(301) 563-6526
www.naaso.org/

American Dental Association
211 East Chicago Avenue
Chicago, IL 60611-2678
(312) 440-2500
http://www.ada.org/

American Heart Association
National Center
7272 Greenville Avenue
Dallas, TX 75231
(800) 242-8721
http://www.americanheart.org/

American Dietetic Association (ADA)
120 South Riverside Plaza, Suite 2000
Chicago, IL 60606-6995
(800) 877-1600
www.eatright.org

The American Society for Clinical Nutrition (ASCN)
9650 Rockville Pike
Bethesda, MD 20814-3998
(301) 634-7110
http://www.ascn.org/

The Society for Nutrition Education
7150 Winton Drive, Suite 300
Indianapolis, IN 46268
(800) 235-6690
http://www.sne.org/

American College of Nutrition
300 S. Duncan Avenue, Suite 225
Clearwater, FL 33755
(727) 446-6086
http://www.amcollnutr.org/

American Obesity Association
1250 24th Street, NW, Suite 300
Washington, DC 20037
(800) 98-OBESE

American Council on Health and Science
1995 Broadway
Second Floor
New York, NY 10023
(212) 362-7044
http://www.acsh.org/

The American Society for Nutritional Sciences (ASNS)
9650 Rockville Pike, Suite 4500
Bethesda, MD 20814
(301) 634-7050
http://www.asns.org/

American Diabetes Association
ATTN: National Call Center
1701 North Beauregard Street
Alexandria, VA 22311
(800) 342-2383
http://www.diabetes.org/

Institute of Food Technologies
525 W. Van Buren, Suite 1000
Chicago, IL 60607
(312) 782-8424
www.ift.org

ILSI Human Nutrition Institute
One Thomas Circle, Ninth Floor
Washington, DC 20005
(202) 659-0524
http://hni.ilsi.org

Trade Organizations

American Meat Institute
1700 North Moore Street
Suite 1600
Arlington, VA 22209
(703) 841-2400
http://www.meatami.com/

National Dairy Council
10255 W. Higgins Road, Suite 900
Rosemont, IL 60018
(312) 240-2880
http://www.nationaldairycouncil.org/

United Fresh Fruit and Vegetable Association
1901 Pennsylvania Ave. NW, Suite 1100
Washington, DC 20006
(202) 303-3400
http://www.uffva.org/

U.S.A. Rice Federation
Washington, DC
4301 North Fairfax Drive, Suite 425
Arlington, VA 22203
(703) 236-2300
http://www.usarice.com

U.S. Government

The USDA National Organic Program
Agricultural Marketing Service
USDA-AMS-TMP-NOP
Room 4008-South Building
1400 Independence Avenue, SW
Washington, DC 20250-0020
(202) 720-3252
www.ams.usda.gov

U.S. Department of Health and Human Services
200 Independence Avenue, SW
Washington, DC 20201
(877) 696-6775
http://www.os.dhhs.gov/

Food and Drug Administration (FDA)
5600 Fishers Lane
Rockville, MD 20857
(888) 463-6332
http://www.fda.gov/

Environmental Protection Agency
Ariel Rios Building
1200 Pennsylvania Avenue, NW
Washington, DC 20460
(202) 272-0167
http://www.epa.gov/

Federal Trade Commission
600 Pennsylvania Avenue, NW
Washington, DC 20580
(202) 326-2222
www.ftc.gov

Partnership for Healthy Weight Managment
www.consumer.gov/weightloss

Office of Dietary Supplements
National Institutes of Health
6100 Executive Boulevard, Room 3B01, MSC 7517
Bethesda, MD 20892
(301) 435-2920
http://dietary-supplements.info.nih.gov

Nutrient Data Laboratory Homepage
Beltsville Human Nutrition Center
10300 Baltimore Avenue
Building 307-C Room 117
BARC-East

Beltsville, MD 20705
(301) 504-8157
www.nal.usda.gov/fnic/foodcomp

National Digestive Disease Clearinghouse
2 Information Way
Bethesda, MD 20892-3570
(800) 891-5389
http://digestive.niddk.nih.gov

The National Cancer Institute
NCI Public Inquiries Office
Suite 3036A
6116 Executive Boulevard, MSC 8322
Bethesda, MD 20892-8322
(800) 4-CANCER
http://www.cancer.gov/

The National Eye Institute
31 Center Drive MSC 2510
Bethesda, MD 20892-2510
(301) 496-5248
http://www.nei.nih.gov/

The National Heart, Lung, and Blood Institute
Building 31, Room 5A52
31 Center Drive MSC 2486
Bethesda, MD 20892
(301) 592-8573
http://www.nhlbi.nih.gov/index.htm

Institute of Diabetes and Digestive and Kidney Diseases
Office of Communications and Public Liaison
NIDDK, NIH, Building 31, Room 9A04
Center Drive, MSC 2560
Bethesda, MD 20892
(301) 496-4000
http://www.niddk.nih.gov/

National Center for Complementary and Alternative Medicine
NCCAM Clearinghouse
P.O. Box 7923
Gaithersburg, MD 20898
(888) 644-6226
http://nccam.nih.gov/

U.S. Department of Agriculture (USDA)
14th Street, SW
Washington, DC 20250
(202) 720-2791
http://www.usda.gov/

Centers for Disease Control and Prevention (CDC)
1600 Clifton Rd
Atlanta, GA 30333
(404) 639-3311 / Public Inquiries: (800) 311-3435
http://www.cdc.gov/

National Institutes of Health (NIH)
9000 Rockville Pike
Bethesda, MD 20892
(301) 496-4000
http://www.nih.gov/

Food and Nutrition Information Center
Agricultural Research Service, USDA
National Agricultural Library, Room 105
10301 Baltimore Avenue
Beltsville, MD 20705-2351
(301) 504-5719
http://www.nal.usda.gov/fnic/

National Institute of Allergy and Infectious Diseases
NIAID Office of Communications and Public Liaison
6610 Rockledge Drive, MSC 6612
Bethesda, MD 20892
(301) 496-5717
www.niaid.nih.gov

Weight and Health Management

The Vegetarian Resource Group
P.O. Box 1463, Dept. IN
Baltimore, MD 21203
(410) 366-VEGE
http://www.vrg.org

American Obesity Association
1250 24th Street, NW
Suite 300
Washington, DC 20037
(202) 776-7711
http://www.obesity.org/

Anemia Lifeline
(888) 722-4407
www.anemia.com

The Arc
(301) 565-3842
Email: info@thearc.org
www.thearc.org

Bottled Water Web
P.O. Box 5658
Santa Barbara, CA 93150
(805) 879-1564
http://www.bottledwaterweb.com/

The Food and Nutrition Board
Institute of Medicine
500 Fifth Street, NW
Washington, DC 20001
(202) 334-2352
http://www.iom.edu/board.asp?id-3788

The Calorie Control Council
http://www.caloriecontrol.org/

TOPS (Take Off Pounds Sensibly)
4575 South Fifth Street
P.O. Box 07360
Milwaukee, WI 53207
(800) 932-8677
www.tops.org

Shape Up America!
15009 Native Dancer Road
N. Potomac, MD 20878
(240) 631-6533
www.shapeup.org

World Hunger

Center on Hunger, Poverty, and Nutrition Policy
Tufts University
Medford, MA 02155
(617) 627-3020
www.tufts.edu/nutrition/

Freedom from Hunger
1644 DaVinci Court
Davis, CA 95616
(800) 708-2555
http://www.freefromhunger.org/

Oxfam International
1112 16th Street, NW, Suite 600
Washington, DC 20036
(202) 496-1170
http://www.oxfam.org/

WorldWatch Institute
1776 Massachusetts Avenue, NW
Washington, DC 20036
(202) 452-1999
www.worldwatch.org

Food First
398 60th Street
Oakland, CA 94618
(510) 654-4400
www.foodfirst.org

The Hunger Project
15 East 26th Street
New York, NY 10010
(212) 251-9100
http://www.thp.org/

U.S. Agency for International Development
Information Center
Ronald Reagan Building
Washington, DC 20523
(202) 712-0000
http://www.usaid.gov/

Answers to Review Questions

Please find answers to Review Questions 11–15 of each chapter on the Companion Website, www.aw-bc.com/thompson.

Chapter 1

1. **d.** micronutrients.
2. **a.** a set of health-related goals and objectives for the United States.
3. **c.** contain 90 kilocalories of energy.
4. **d.** "A high-protein diet increases the risk for porous bones," is an example of a hypothesis.
5. **d.** all of the above
6. False. Vitamins do not provide any energy, although many vitamins are critical to the metabolic processes that assist us in generating energy from carbohydrates, fats, and proteins.
7. True.
8. True.
9. True.
10. True.

Chapter 2

1. **d.** The % Daily Values of select nutrients in a serving of the packaged food.
2. **b.** provides enough of the energy, nutrients, and fiber to maintain a person's health.
3. **a.** 6 to 11 servings of whole grains, cereals, and breads each day.
4. **c.** Being physically active each day.
5. **b.** Foods with a lot of nutrients per calorie, such as fish, are more nutritious choices than foods with fewer nutrients per calorie, such as candy.
6. False. There is no standardized definition for a serving size for foods.
7. True. General categories are listed, but no clear distinction is made for low-fat and low-calorie food choices.
8. False. The six exchange lists are starch/bread, meat and meat substitutes, fruits, vegetables, milk, and fats.
9. True. Pasta is listed at the top of the Healthy Eating Pyramid as a food that should be eaten sparingly.
10. False. This program was instituted by the National Cancer Institute.

Chapter 3

1. **c.** atoms, molecules, cells, tissues, organs, systems
2. **d.** emulsifies fats.
3. **c.** hypothalamus.
4. **a.** seepage of gastric acid into the esophagus.
5. **a.** a bean and cheese burrito
6. True.
7. True.

8. False. Vitamins and minerals are not really "digested" the same way that macronutrients are. These compounds do not have to be broken down because they are small enough to be readily absorbed by the small intestine. For example, fat-soluble vitamins, such as vitamins A, D, E, and K, are soluble in lipids and are absorbed into the intestinal cells along with the fats in our foods. Water-soluble vitamins, such as the B vitamins and vitamin C, typically undergo some type of active transport process that helps assure the vitamin is absorbed by the small intestine. Minerals are absorbed all along the small intestine, and in some cases in the large intestine as well, by a wide variety of mechanisms.
9. False. A person with celiac disease cannot tolerate products with gluten, a protein found in wheat, rye, and barley.
10. False. Cells are the smallest units of life. Atoms are the smallest units of matter in nature.

Chapter 4

1. **b.** the potential of foods to raise blood glucose and insulin levels.
2. **d.** carbon, hydrogen, and oxygen.
3. **d.** sweetened soft drinks.
4. **a.** monosaccharides.
5. **a.** phenylketonuria.
6. False. Sugar alcohols are considered nutritive sweeteners because they contain 2 to 4 kcal of energy per gram.
7. True.
8. False. A person with lactose intolerance has a difficult time tolerating milk and other dairy products. This person does not have an allergy to milk, as he or she does not exhibit an immune response indicative of an allergy. Instead, this person does not digest lactose completely, which causes intestinal distress and symptoms such as gas, bloating, diarrhea, and nausea.
9. False. Plants store glucose as starch.
10. False. Salivary amylase breaks starches into maltose and shorter polysaccharides.

Chapter 5

1. **d.** found in leafy green vegetables, flax seeds, soy milk, and fish.
2. **b.** exercise regularly.
3. **a.** lipoprotein lipase.
4. **d.** high-density lipoproteins.
5. **a.** monounsaturated fats.
6. True.
7. False. Fat is an important source of energy during rest and during exercise, and adipose tissue is our primary storage site for fat. We rely significantly on

the fat stored in our adipose tissue to provide energy during rest and exercise.

8. False. A triglyceride is a lipid comprised of a glycerol molecule and three fatty acids. Thus, fatty acids are a component of triglycerides.

9. False. While most *trans* fatty acids result from the hydrogenation of vegetable oils by food manufacturers, a small amount of *trans* fatty acids are found in cow's milk.

10. False. A serving of food labeled *reduced fat* has at least 25% less fat than a standard serving, but may not have fewer calories than a full-fat version of the same food.

Chapter 6

1. **d.** mutual supplementation.
2. **a.** Rice, pinto beans, acorn squash, soy butter, and almond milk.
3. **c.** protease.
4. **b.** amine group.
5. **c.** carbon, oxygen, hydrogen, and nitrogen.
6. True.
7. False. Both shape and function are lost when a protein is denatured.
8. False. Some hormones are made from lipids.
9. False. Buffers help the body maintain acid-base balance.
10. False. Depending upon the type of sport, athletes may require the same or up to two times as much protein as nonactive people.

Chapter 7

1. **b.** It can be found in fresh fruits and vegetables.
2. **d.** A healthy infant of average weight.
3. **a.** extracellular fluid.
4. **d.** It is freely permeable to water, but impermeable to solutes.
5. **b.** Losing weight.
6. False. In addition to water, the body needs electrolytes, such as sodium and potassium, to prevent fluid imbalances during long-distance events such as a marathon. As purified water contains no electrolytes, this would not be the ideal beverage to prevent fluid imbalances during a marathon.
7. False. Our thirst mechanism is triggered by an increase in the concentration of electrolytes in our blood.
8. False. Hypernatremia is commonly caused by a rapid intake of high amounts of sodium.
9. False. Quenching our thirst does not guarantee adequate hydration. Urine that is clear or light yellow in color is one indicator of adequate hydration.
10. False. These conditions are associated with decreased fluid loss or an increase in body fluid. Diarrhea,

blood loss, and low humidity are conditions that increase fluid loss.

Chapter 8

1. **d.** It is destroyed by exposure to high heat.
2. **b.** an atom loses an electron.
3. **a.** cardiovascular disease.
4. **d.** nitrates.
5. **a.** vitamin A.
6. True.
7. True.
8. False. Vitamin C helps regenerate vitamin E.
9. True.
10. False. Pregnant women should not consume beef liver very often, as it can lead to vitamin A toxicity and potentially serious birth defects.

Chapter 9

1. **a.** calcium and phosphorus.
2. **c.** has normal bone density as compared to an average, healthy 30-year old.
3. **d.** It provides the scaffolding for cortical bone.
4. **c.** a fair-skinned retired teacher living in a nursing home in Ohio
5. **d.** structure of bone, nerve transmission, and muscle contraction.
6. True.
7. True.
8. False. The fractures that result from osteoporosis cause an increased risk of infection and other related illnesses that can lead to premature death.
9. True.
10. False. Our body makes vitamin D by converting a cholesterol compound in our skin to the active form of vitamin D that we need to function. We do not absorb vitamin D from sunlight, but when the ultraviolet rays of the sun hit our skin, they react to eventually form calcitriol, which is considered the primary active form of vitamin D in our bodies

Chapter 10

1. **d.** thiamin, pantothenic acid, and biotin.
2. **b.** vitamin K.
3. **b.** Iron is a component of hemoglobin, myoglobin, and certain enzymes.
4. **c.** an amino acid.
5. **d.** Choline is necessary for the synthesis of phospholipids and other components of cell membranes.
6. True.
7. True.
8. False. Iron deficiency causes iron deficiency anemia; pernicious anemia occurs at the end stage of an

autoimmune disorder that causes the loss of various cells in the stomach, which leads to a deficiency of vitamin B_{12}.

9. False. Neural tube defects occur during the first four weeks of pregnancy; this is often before a woman even knows she is pregnant. Thus, the best way for a woman to protect her fetus against neural tube defects is to make sure she is consuming adequate folate before she is pregnant.

10. False. Wilson's disease is a rare disorder that causes copper toxicity.

Chapter 11

1. **d.** body mass index.
2. **a.** basal metabolic rate, thermal effect of food, and effect of physical activity.
3. **b.** take in more energy than they expend.
4. **c.** all people have a genetic set-point for their body weight.
5. **a.** hunger.
6. False. It is the apple-shaped fat patterning, or excess fat in the trunk region, that is known to increase a person's risk for many chronic diseases.
7. True
8. False. Weight-loss medications are typically prescribed for people with a body mass index greater than or equal to 30 kg/m^2, or for people with a body mass index greater than or equal to 27 kg/m^2 who also have other significant health risk factors such as heart disease, high blood pressure, and type 2 diabetes.
9. False. Healthful weight gain includes eating more energy than you expend and also exercising to maintain both aerobic fitness and to build muscle mass.
10. True.

Chapter 12

1. **c.** 50 to 80% of your estimated maximal heart rate.
2. **a.** 1 to 3 seconds.
3. **b.** fat
4. **c.** seems to increase strength gained in resistance exercise.
5. **a.** An intensity of 12 to 15, or somewhat hard to hard, is recommended to achieve physical fitness.
6. True.
7. False. A dietary fat intake of 15 to 25% of total energy intake is generally recommended for athletes.
8. False. Carbohydrate loading involves altering duration and intensity of exercise and intake of carbohydrate such that the storage of carbohydrate is maximized.
9. False. Sports anemia is not true anemia, but a transient decrease in iron stores that occurs at the start of an

exercise program. This is a result of an initial increase in plasma volume (or water in our blood) that is not matched by an increase in hemoglobin.

10. True.

Chapter 13

1. **b.** bulimia nervosa
2. **a.** increases your risk of developing a psychiatric eating disorder.
3. **d.** disordered eating, menstrual dysfunction, and osteoporosis.
4. **a.** exercise regularly.
5. **b.** I wish I could change the way I look in the mirror.
6. False. People with binge-eating disorder typically do not purge to compensate for the binge; thus, these individuals are usually overweight or obese.
7. False. Although it is suspected that media images of idealized female bodies may contribute to an increase in eating disorder in adolescent girls, there is no scientific evidence to support this suspicion.
8. True.
9. False. People with anorexia typically deny they are hungry and may lie about eating.
10. False. People who suffer from binge-eating disorder may also suffer from chronic overeating behaviors. However, chronic overeating is defined as regularly overeating without losing control, whereas binge-eating involves the loss of control during a binge episode that prevents a person from stopping him- or herself from overeating.

Chapter 14

1. **a.** oxygen, heat, and light.
2. **c.** a type of fungus used to ferment foods.
3. **b.** a flavor enhancer used in a variety of foods.
4. **a.** contain only organically produced ingredients, excluding water and salt.
5. **d.** cooling, canning, pasteurization, irradiation
6. False. The appropriate temperatures for cooking foods varies according to the food.
7. True.
8. True.
9. True.
10. True.

Chapter 15

1. **b.** neural tube defects
2. **c.** oxytocin
3. **a.** fiber
4. **b.** women who begin thei
5. **d.** iron-fortified rice cerea
6. False. These issues are mo trimester of pregnancy.

7. True.
8. True.
9. True.
10. True.

Chapter 16

1. **b.** vitamin D
2. **c.** 45 to 60%
3. **d.** dental caries
4. **a.** ½ cup of iron-fortified cooked oat cereal, two tablespoons of mashed pineapple, and one cup of whole milk
5. **a.** Cigarette smoking can interfere with the absorption of nutrients.
6. False. Preschool children are able to understand the basic information about which foods are more nutritious and those that should be eaten in moderation. Also, parents are important role models for preschool children.
7. True.
8. False. Although eating disorders frequently begin during adolescence, the rates of obesity are significantly higher than those for eating disorders in this age group.
9. False. There is no DRI for fat for toddlers; however, it is recommended that toddlers consume 30 to 40% of their total daily energy intake as fat.
10. True.

Glossary

24-hour recall   A data collection that assesses everything a person has consumed over the past 24 hours.

5-A-Day for Better Health Program   A major public health initiative developed by the National Cancer Institute to promote nutrition and prevent cancer; recommends that Americans consume at least five servings of fruits and vegetables daily.

A

absorption   The physiologic process by which molecules of food are taken from the gastrointestinal tract into the body.

acceptable daily intake (ADI)   An estimate made by the Food and Drug Administration of the amount of a non-nutritive sweetener that someone can consume each day over a lifetime without adverse effects.

Acceptable Macronutrient Distribution Range (AMDR)   A range of intakes for a particular energy source that is associated with reduced risk of chronic disease while providing adequate intakes of essential nutrients.

acidosis   A disorder in which the blood becomes acidic; that is, the level of hydrogen in the blood is excessive. It can be caused by respiratory or metabolic problems.

added sugars   Sugars and syrups that are added to food during processing or preparation.

adenosine triphosphate (ATP)   The common currency of energy for virtually all cells of the body.

adequate diet   A diet that provides enough of the energy, nutrients, and fiber to maintain a person's health.

Adequate Intake (AI)   A recommended average daily nutrient intake level based on observed or experimentally determined estimates of nutrient intake by a group of healthy people.

alkalosis   A disorder in which the blood becomes basic; that is, the level of hydrogen in the blood is deficient. It can be caused by respiratory or metabolic problems.

alpha-linolenic acid   An essential fatty acid found in leafy green vegetables, flax seed oil, soy oil, fish oil and fish products; an omega-3 fatty acid.

amenorrhea   Lack of menstruation for at least three consecutive months in the absence of pregnancy.

amino acids   Nitrogen-containing molecules that combine to form proteins.

amniotic fluid   The watery fluid contained within the innermost membrane of the sac containing the fetus. It cushions and protects the growing fetus.

anabolic   Refers to a substance that builds muscle and increases strength.

anaerobic   Means "without oxygen." Term used to refer to metabolic reactions that occur in the absence of oxygen.

anencephaly   A fatal neural tube defect in which there is partial absence of brain tissue most likely caused by failure of the neural tube to close.

anorexia nervosa   A serious, potentially life-threatening eating disorder that is characterized by self-starvation, which eventually leads to a deficiency in energy and essential nutrients that are required by the body to function normally. For an individual to be considered to have anorexia nervosa, he/she must be medically diagnosed by a physician and meet specific diagnostic criteria.

antibodies   Defensive proteins of the immune system. Their production is prompted by the presence of bacteria, viruses, toxins, allergens, and so on.

antioxidant   A compound that has the ability to prevent or repair the damage caused by oxidation.

anti-resorptive   Characterized by an ability to slow or stop bone resorption without affecting bone formation. Anti-resorptive medications are used to reduce the rate of bone loss in people with osteoporosis.

appetite   A psychological desire to consume specific foods.

atom   A discrete, irreducible unit of matter. It is the smallest unit of an element and is identical to all other atoms of that element.

B

balanced diet   A diet that contains the combinations of foods that provide the proper proportions of nutrients.

basic metabolic rate (BMR)   The energy the body expends to maintain its fundamental physiologic functions.

Behavioral Risk Factor Surveillance Systems (BRFSS)   The world's largest telephone survey that tracks lifestyle behaviors that increase our risks for chronic diseases.

bile   Fluid produced by the liver and stored in the gallbladder; it emulsifies fats in the small intestine.

binge eating   Consumption of a large amount of food in a short period of time, usually accompanied by a feeling of loss of self-control.

binge-eating disorder   A disorder characterized by binge eating an average of twice a week or more.

bioavailability   The degree to which our bodies can absorb and utilize any given nutrient.

blood volume   The amount of fluid in blood.

body composition   The amount of bone, muscle, and fat tissue in the body. Also, the ratio of a person's body fat to lean body mass.

body image   A person's perception of his or her body's appearance and functioning.

body mass index (BMI)   A measurement representing the ratio of a person's body weight to his or her height.

bone density   The degree of compactness of bone tissue, reflecting the strength of the bones. *Peak bone density* is the point at which a bone is strongest.

brush border   Term that describes the microvilli of the small intestine's lining. These microvilli tremendously increase the small intestine's absorptive capacity.

buffers   Proteins that help maintain proper acid-base balance by attaching to, or releasing, hydrogen ions as conditions change in the body.

bulimia nervosa   A serious eating disorder characterized by recurrent episodes of binge eating and recurrent inappropriate compensatory behaviors (such as self-induced vomiting; misuse of laxatives, diuretics, enemas, or other medications; fasting or excessive exercise) in order to prevent weight gain.

C

calcitriol   The primary active form of vitamin D in the body.

cancer   A group of diseases characterized by cells that reproduce spontaneously and independently and may invade other tissues and organs.

carbohydrate loading   Also known as glycogen loading. A process that involves altering training and carbohydrate intake so that muscle glycogen storage is maximized.

carbohydrate   One of the three macronutrients; a compound made up of carbon, hydrogen, and oxygen that is derived from plants and provides energy. Also, the primary fuel source for our bodies, particularly for our brain and for physical exercise.

carcinogen   Any substance capable of causing the cellular mutations that lead to cancer.

carcinogens   Cancer-causing agents, such as certain pesticides, industrial chemicals, and pollutants.

cardiorespiratory fitness   Fitness of the heart and lungs; achieved through regular participation in aerobic-type activities.

cardiovascular disease   A general term that refers to abnormal conditions involving dysfunction of the heart and blood vessels; cardiovascular disease can result in heart attack or stroke.

carotenoids   Fat-soluble plant pigments that the body stores in the liver and adipose tissues. The body is able to convert certain carotenoids to vitamin A.

cataract   A damaged portion of the eye's lens, which causes cloudiness that impairs vision.

celiac disease   Genetic disorder characterized by a total intolerance for gluten that causes an immune reaction that damages the lining of the small intestine.

cell differentiation   The process by which immature, undifferentiated stem cells develop into highly specialized functional cells of discrete organs and tissues.

cell membrane   The boundary of an animal cell, composed of a phospholipid bilayer that separates its internal cytoplasm and organelles from the external environment.

cell   The smallest unit of matter that exhibits the properties of living things, such as growth, reproduction, and metabolism.

Centers for Disease Control and Prevention (CDC)   The leading federal agency in the United States that protects the health and safety of people. It's mission is to promote health and quality of life by preventing and controlling disease, injury, and disability.

cephalic phase   Earliest phase of digestion in which the brain thinks about and prepares the digestive organs for the consumption of food.

childhood overweight   Having a body mass index (BMI) at or above the 85th percentile.

cholecalciferol   Vitamin D_3, a form of vitamin D found in animal foods and the form we synthesize from the sun.

chronic dieting   Consistently and successfully restricting energy intake to maintain an average or below average body weight.

chylomicron   A lipoprotein produced in the mucosal cell of the intestine; transports dietary fat out of the intestinal tract.

chyme   Semifluid mass consisting of partially digested food, water, and gastric juices.

coenzyme   An organic compound that combines with an inactive enzyme to form an active enzyme.

cofactor   A compound that is needed to allow enzymes to function properly.

colic   Unconsolable infant crying that lasts for hours at a time.

collagen   A protein found in all connective tissues in our body.

colostrum   The first fluid made and secreted by the breasts from late in pregnancy to about a week after birth. It is rich in immune factors and protein.

complementary proteins   Two or more foods that together contain all nine essential amino acids necessary for a complete protein. It is not necessary to eat complementary proteins at the same meal.

complete proteins   Foods that contain all nine essential amino acids.

complex carbohydrate   A nutrient compound consisting of long chains of glucose molecules, such as starch, glycogen, and fiber.

conception   (also called *fertilization*) The uniting of an ovum (egg) and sperm to create a fertilized egg, or zygote.

constipation   Condition characterized by the absence of bowel movements for a period of time that is significantly longer than normal for the individual. When a bowel movement does occur, stools are usually small, hard, and difficult to pass.

cool-down   Activities done after an exercise session is completed. Should be gradual and allow your body to slowly recover from exercise.

cortical bone (compact bone)   A dense bone tissue that makes up the outer surface of all bones as well as the entirety of most small bones of the body.

creatine phosphate (CP)   A high-energy compound that can be broken down for energy and used to regenerate ATP.

cystic fibrosis   A genetic disorder that causes an alteration in chloride transport, leading to the production of thick, sticky mucus that causes life-threatening respiratory and digestive problems.

cytoplasm   The liquid within an animal cell.

D

Daily Reference Values (DRV)   Standardized food label values for food components that do not have an RDA, such as fiber, cholesterol, and saturated fats.

DASH diet   The diet developed in response to research into hypertension funded by the National Institutes of Health (NIH); stands for "Dietary Approaches to Stop Hypertension."

deamination   The process by which an amine group is removed from an amino acid. The nitrogen is then transported to the kidneys for excretion in the urine, while the carbon and other components are metabolized for energy or used to make other compounds.

dehydration   Depletion of body fluid that results when fluid excretion exceeds fluid intake.

denature   Term used to describe the action of unfolding proteins. Proteins must be denatured before they can be digested.

dental caries   Dental erosion and decay caused by acid-secreting bacteria in the mouth and on the teeth. The acid produced is a by-product of bacterial metabolism of carbohydrates deposited on the teeth.

diabetes   A chronic disease in which the body can no longer regulate glucose.

diarrhea   Condition characterized by the frequent passage of loose, watery stools.

dietary fiber   The nondigestible carbohydrate part of plants that form the support structures of leaves, stems, and seeds.

Dietary Guidelines for Americans   A set of principles developed by the U.S. Department of Agriculture and the U.S.

Department of Health and Human Services to assist Americans in designing a healthful diet and lifestyle. These guidelines are updated every five years.

Dietary Reference Intakes (DRI) A set of nutritional reference values for the United States and Canada that apply to healthy people.

digestion The process by which foods are broken down into their component molecules, either mechanically or chemically.

disaccharide A carbohydrate compound consisting of two sugar molecules joined together.

disordered eating Disordered eating is a general term used to describe a variety of abnormal or atypical eating behaviors that are used to keep or maintain a lower body weight. Individuals with disordered eating behaviors do not have severe enough eating disturbances to be medically diagnosed with an eating disorder such as anorexia nervosa or bulimia nervosa. The designation of "Eating Disorders Not Otherwise Specified" is the medical term used to describe these individuals.

diuretic A substance that increases fluid loss via the urine. Common diuretics include coffee, tea, cola, and other caffeine-containing beverages, as well as prescription medications for high blood pressure and other disorders.

docosahexaenoic acid (DHA) Metabolic derivative of alpha-linolenic acid; together with EPA, it appears to reduce our risk of a heart attack.

dual energy x-ray absorptiometry (DXA or DEXA) Currently the most accurate tool for measuring bone density.

E

eating disorder An eating disorder is a psychiatric disorder that must be clinically diagnosed by a physician and is characterized by severe disturbances in body image and eating behaviors. Anorexia nervosa and bulimia nervosa are two examples of eating disorders for which specific diagnostic criteria must be present for diagnosis.

edema A disorder in which fluids build up in the tissue spaces of the body, causing fluid imbalances and a swollen appearance.

eicosapentaenoic acid (EPA) A metabolic derivative of alpha-linolenic acid.

electrolyte A substance that disassociates in solution into positively and negatively charged ions and is thus capable of carrying an electric current.

electron A negatively charged particle orbiting the nucleus of an atom.

elimination The process by which the undigested portions of food and waste products are removed from the body.

embryo Human growth and developmental stage lasting from the third week to the end of the eighth week after fertilization.

energy cost of physical activity The energy that expanded on body movement and muscular work above basal levels.

energy expenditure The energy the body expends to maintain its basic functions and to perform all levels of movement and activity.

energy intake The amount of food a person eats; in other words, it is the number of kilocalories consumed.

enteric nervous system The nerves of the GI tract.

enzymes Small chemicals, usually proteins, that act on other chemicals to speed up body processes but are not apparently changed during those processes.

epiphyseal plates Plates of cartilage located toward the end of long bones that provide for growth in the length of long bones.

ergocalciferol Vitamin D_2, a form of vitamin D found exclusively in plant foods.

ergogenic aids Substances used to improve exercise and athletic performance.

esophagus Muscular tube of the GI tract connecting the back of the mouth to the stomach.

essential amino acids Amino acids not produced by the body that must be obtained from food.

essential fatty acids (EFA) Fatty acids that must be consumed in the diet because they cannot be made by our bodies. The two essential fatty acids are linoleic acid and alpha-linolenic acid.

Estimated Average Requirements (EAR) The average daily nutrient intake level estimated to meet the requirement of half of the healthy individuals in a particular life stage or gender group.

Estimated Energy Requirements (EER) The average dietary energy intake that is predicted to maintain energy balance in a healthy adult. Also, the total amount of energy needed per day for any age group.

evaporative cooling Another term for sweating, which is the primary way in which we dissipate heat.

exchange system Diet planning tool developed by the American Dietetic Association and the American Diabetes Association in which exchanges, or portions, are organized according to the amount of carbohydrate, protein, fat, and calories in each food.

exercise A subcategory of leisure-time physical activity; any activity that is purposeful, planned, and structured.

extracellular fluid The fluid outside of the body's cells, either in the body's tissues, or as the liquid portion of blood, called *plasma*.

F

fats An important energy source for our bodies at rest and during low intensity exercise.

fat-soluble vitamins Vitamins that are not soluble in water, but soluble in fat. These include vitamins A, D, E, and K.

fatty acids Long chains of carbon atoms bound to each other as well as to hydrogen atoms.

female athlete triad A condition characterized by the co-existence of three disorders in some athletic females: an eating disorder, amenorrhea, and osteoporosis.

fetal alcohol effects (FAE) A milder set of alcohol-related birth defects characterized by behavioral problems such as hyperactivity, attention deficit disorder, poor judgment, sleep disorders, and delayed learning.

fetal alcohol syndrome (FAS) A set of serious, irreversible alcohol-related birth defects characterized by certain physical and mental abnormalities.

fetus Human growth and developmental stage lasting from the beginning of the ninth week after conception to birth.

FIT principle The principle used to achieve an appropriate overload for physical training. Stands for frequency, intensity, and time of activity.

flexibility The ability to move a joint through its full range of motion.

fluid   A substance composed of molecules that move past one another freely. Fluids are characterized by their ability to conform to the shape of whatever container holds them.

fluorohydroxyapatite   A mineral compound in human teeth which contains fluoride, calcium, and phosphorous and is more resistant to destruction by acids and bacteria than hydroxyapatite.

fluorosis   A condition marked by the staining and pitting of the teeth; caused by an abnormally high intake of fluoride.

food allergy   An allergic reaction to food, caused by a reaction of the immune system.

Food Guide Pyramid   Illustration developed by the U.S. Department of Agriculture (USDA) to provide Americans with a conceptual framework for the types and amounts of foods we can eat in combination to achieve a healthful diet.

food intolerance   Gastrointestinal discomfort characterized by certain foods that is not a result of an immune system reaction.

free radical   A highly unstable atom with an unpaired electron in its outermost shell.

frequency   Refers to the number of activity sessions per week you perform.

fructose   The sweetest natural sugar; a monosaccharide that occurs in fruits and vegetables. Also called *levulose,* or *fruit sugar.*

functional fiber   The nondigestible forms of carbohydrates that are extracted from plants or manufactured in the laboratory and have known health benefits.

G

galactose   A monosaccharide that joins with glucose to create lactose, one of the three most common disaccharides.

gallbladder   A tissue sac beneath the liver that stores bile and secretes it into the small intestine.

gastric juice   Acidic liquid secreted within the stomach; it contains hydrochloric acid, pepsin, and other compounds.

gastroesophageal reflux disease (GERD)   The painful type of heartburn that occurs more than twice per week.

gastrointestinal (GI) tract   A long, muscular tube consisting of several organs: the mouth, esophagus, stomach, small intestine, and large intestine.

gene expression   The process of using a gene to make a protein.

gestation   The period of intrauterine development from conception to birth.

gestational diabetes   Insufficient insulin production or insulin resistance that results in consistently high blood glucose levels, specifically during pregnancy; condition typically resolves after birth occurs.

glucagon   Hormone secreted by the alpha cells of the pancreas in response to decreased blood levels of glucose. Causes breakdown of liver storage of glycogen into glucose.

gluconeogenesis   The generation of glucose from the breakdown of proteins into amino acids.

glucose   The most abundant sugar molecule; monosaccharide generally found in combination with other sugars. The preferred source of energy for the brain and an important source of energy for all cells.

glycemic index   Rating of the potential of foods to raise blood glucose and insulin levels.

glycerol   An alcohol composed of three carbon atoms; it is the backbone of a triglyceride molecule.

glycogen   A polysaccharide stored in animals; the storage form of glucose in animals.

glycolysis   The breakdown of glucose; yields two ATP molecules and two pyruvic acid molecules for each molecule of glucose.

grazing   Consistently eating small meals throughout the day; done by many athletes to meet their high energy demands.

H

healthful diet   A diet that provides the proper combination of energy and nutrients and is adequate, moderate, balanced, and varied.

Healthy People 2010   An agenda that emphasizes health promotion and disease prevention across the United States by identifying goals and objectives that we hope to reach as a nation by the year 2010.

heartburn   The painful sensation that occurs over the sternum when hydrochloric acid backs up into the lower esophagus.

heat cramps   Muscle spasms that occur several hours after strenuous exercise; most often occur when sweat losses and fluid intakes are high, urine volume is low, and sodium intake is inadequate.

heat exhaustion   A heat illness that is characterized by excessive sweating, weakness, nausea, dizziness, headache, and difficulty concentrating. Unchecked heat exhaustion can lead to heat stroke.

heat stroke   A potentially fatal response to high temperature characterized by failure of the body's heat-regulating mechanisms. Symptoms include rapid pulse, reduced sweating, hot, dry skin, high temperature, headache, weakness, and sudden loss of consciousness. Commonly called *sunstroke.*

heat syncope   Dizziness that occurs when people stand for too long in the heat or when they stop suddenly after a race or stand suddenly from a lying position; results from blood pooling in the lower extremities.

hemorrhoids   Swollen varicose veins in the rectum.

hormone   Chemical messenger that is secreted into the bloodstream by one of the many glands of the body and acts as regulator of the physiological processes at a site remote from the gland which secreted it.

hunger   A physiologic sensation that prompts us to eat.

hydrogenation   The process of adding hydrogen to unsaturated fatty acids, making them more saturated and thereby more solid at room temperature.

hypercalcemia   A condition marked by an abnormally high concentration of calcium in the blood.

hyperkalemia   A condition in which potassium levels are dangerously high.

hypermagnesemia   A condition marked by an abnormally high concentration of magnesium in the blood.

hypernatremia   A condition in which blood sodium levels are dangerously high.

hypertension   A chronic condition characterized by above-average blood pressure readings; specifically, systolic blood pressure over 140 mm Hg or diastolic blood pressure over 90 mm Hg.

hypocalcemia   A condition characterized by an abnormally low concentration of calcium in the blood.

hypoglycemia   A condition marked by blood glucose levels that are below normal fasting levels.

hypokalemia   A condition in which blood potassium levels are dangerously low.

hypomagnesemia   A condition characterized by an abnormally low concentration of magnesium in the blood.

hyponatremia   A condition in which blood sodium levels are dangerously low.

hypothalamus   A region of the forebrain below the thalamus where visceral sensations such as hunger and thirst are regulated.

I

incomplete proteins   Foods that do not contain all of the essential amino acids in sufficient amounts to support growth and health.

inorganic   A substance or nutrient that does not contain the element carbon.

insensible water loss   The loss of water from the skin in the form of sweat and from the lungs during breathing.

insulin   Hormone secreted by the beta cells of the pancreas in response to increased blood levels of glucose. Facilitates uptake of glucose by body cells.

intensity   Refers to the amount of effort expended during the activity, or how difficult the activity is to perform.

intracellular fluid   The fluid held at any given time within the walls of the body's cells.

invisible fats   Fats that are hidden in foods, such as the fats found in baked goods, regular-fat dairy products, marbling in meat, and fried foods.

ion   Any electrically charged particle, either positively or negatively charged.

iron-deficiency anemia   A reduction in the number of red blood cells or hemoglobin or both, resulting in pallor and fatigue. Caused by a lack of the mineral iron, in this case.

irritable bowel syndrome   A bowel disorder that interferes with normal functions of the colon. Symptoms are abdominal cramps, bloating, and constipation or diarrhea.

K

Keshan disease   A heart disorder caused by selenium deficiency. It was first identified in children in the Keshan province of China.

ketoacidosis   A condition in which excessive ketones are present in the blood causing the blood to become very acidic, which alters basic body functions and damages tissues. Untreated ketoacidosis can be fatal. This condition is found in individuals with untreated diabetes mellitus.

ketones   Substances produced during the breakdown of fat when carbohydrate intake is insufficient to meet energy needs. Provide an alternative energy source for the brain when glucose levels are low.

ketosis   The process by which the breakdown of fat during fasting results in the production of ketones.

kwashiorkor   A form of protein-energy malnutrition that is typically seen in developing countries in infants and toddlers who are weaned early because of the birth of a subsequent child. Denied breast milk, they are fed a cereal diet that provides adequate energy but inadequate protein.

L

lactase   A digestive enzyme that breaks lactose into glucose and galactose.

lactation   The production of breast milk.

lacteal   A small lymph vessel located inside of the villi of the small intestine.

lactic acid   A compound that results when pyruvic acid is metabolized in the presence of insufficient oxygen.

lactose intolerance   A disorder in which the body does not produce sufficient lactase enzyme and therefore cannot digest foods that contain lactose, such as cow's milk.

lactose   Also called *milk sugar,* a disaccharide consisting of one glucose molecule and one galactose molecule. Found in milk, including human breast millk.

large intestine   Final organ of the GI tract consisting of cecum, colon, rectum, and anal canal, and in which most water is absorbed and feces are formed.

leisure-time activity   Any activity not related to a person's occupation; includes competitive sports, recreational activities, and planned exercise training.

leptin   A hormone that is produced by body fat that acts to reduce food intake and to decrease body weight and body fat.

limiting amino acid   The essential amino acid that is missing or in the smallest supply in the amino acid pool and is thus responsible for slowing or halting protein synthesis.

linoleic acid   An essential fatty acid found in vegetable and nut oils; also known as omega-6 fatty acid.

lipids   A diverse group of organic substances that are insoluble in water; lipids include triglycerides, phospholipids, and sterols.

lipoprotein   A spherical compound in which fat clusters in the center and phospholipids and proteins form the outside of the sphere.

lipoprotein lipase   An enzyme that sits on the outside of cells and breaks apart triglycerides so that their fatty acids can be removed and taken up by the cell.

liver   The largest auxiliary organ of the GI tract and one of the most important organs of the body. Its functions include production of bile and processing of nutrient-rich blood from the small intestine.

long-chain fatty acids   Fatty acids that are fourteen or more carbon atoms in length.

low intensity activities   Activities that cause very mild increases in breathing, sweating, and heart rate.

low-birth weight   A weight of less than 5.5 pounds at birth.

M

macronutrients   Nutrients that our bodies need in relatively large amounts to support normal function and health. Carbohydrates, fats, and proteins are macronutrients.

macular degeneration   A vision disorder caused by deterioration of the central portion of the retina and marked by loss or distortion of the central field of vision.

mad cow disease   A fatal brain disorder prompted by consumption of food containing *prions,* which are an abnormal form of protein found in the brains and other organs of infected sheep, cows, and other livestock.

major minerals Minerals we need to consume in amounts of at least 100 milligrams per day and of which the total amount in our bodies is at least 5 grams.

maltase A digestive enzyme that breaks maltose into glucose.

maltose A disaccharide consisting of two molecules of glucose. Does not generally occur independently in foods but results as a by-product of digestion. Also called *malt sugar*.

marasmus A form of protein-energy malnutrition that results from grossly inadequate intakes of protein, energy, and other nutrients.

maximal heart rate The rate at which your heart beats during maximal intensity exercise.

medium-chain fatty acids Fatty acids that are six to twelve carbon atoms in length.

megadose A dose of a nutrient that is ten or more times greater than the recommended amount.

menaquinone The form of vitamin K produced by bacteria in the large intestine.

menarche The beginning of menstruation, or the menstrual period.

metabolic water The water formed as a by-product of our body's metabolic reactions.

micronutrients Nutrients needed in relatively small amounts to support normal health and body functions. Vitamins and minerals are micronutrients.

minerals Inorganic substances that are not broken down during digestion and absorption and are not destroyed by heat or light. Minerals assist in the regulation of many body processes and are classified as major minerals or trace minerals.

moderate intensity activities Activities that cause moderate increases in breathing, sweating, and heart rate.

moderation Eating the right amounts of foods to maintain a healthy weight and to optimize our bodies' metabolic processes.

monosaccharide The simplest of carbohydrates. Consists of one sugar molecule, the most common form of which is glucose.

monosaturated fatty acids (MUFA) Fatty acids that have two carbons in the chain bound to each other with one double bond; these types of fatty acids are generally liquid at room temperature.

morbid obesity A condition in which a person's body weight exceeds 100% of normal, putting him or her at very high risk for serious health consequences.

morning sickness Varying degrees of nausea and vomiting associated with pregnancy, most commonly in the first trimester.

multifactorial disease Any disease which may be attributable to one or more of a variety of causes.

muscle cramps Involuntary, spasmodic, and painful muscle contractions that last for many seconds or even minutes; electrolyte imbalances are often the cause of muscle cramps.

muscular endurance A subcomponent of musculoskeletal fitness defined as the ability of a muscle to maintain submaximal force levels for extended periods of time.

muscular strength A subcomponent of musculoskeletal fitness defined as the maximal force or tension level that can be produced by a muscle group.

musculoskeletal fitness Fitness of the muscles and bones.

mutual supplementation The process of combining two or more incomplete protein sources to make a complete protein.

N

National Health and Nutrition Examination Survey (NHANES) A survey conducted by the National Center for Health Statistics and the CDC; this survey tracks the nutrient and food consumption of Americans.

National Institutes of Health (NIH) The world's leading medical center and the focal point for medical research in the United States.

neonatal Term referring to a newborn.

neural tube Embryonic tissue that forms a tube, which eventually becomes the brain and spinal cord.

night blindness A vitamin A–deficiency disorder that results in the loss of the ability to see in dim light.

nonessential amino acids Amino acids that can be manufactured by the body in sufficient quantities and therefore do not need to be consumed regularly in our diet.

non-nutritive sweeteners Also called *alternative sweeteners;* manufactured sweeteners that provide little or no energy.

nucleus The positively charged, central core of an atom. It is made up of two types of particles—protons and neutrons—bound tightly together. The nucleus of an atom contains essentially all of its atomic mass.

nutrient density The relative amount of nutrients per amount of energy (or number of calories).

nutrients Chemicals found in foods that are critical to human growth and function.

Nutrition Facts Panel The label on a food package that contains the nutrition information required by the FDA.

nutrition The science that studies food and how food nourishes our bodies and influences our health.

nutritive sweeteners Sweeteners such as sucrose, fructose, honey, and brown sugar that contribute calories (or energy).

O

obesity Having an excess body fat that adversely affects health, resulting in a person having a weight that is substantially greater than some accepted standard for a given height.

organ A body structure composed of two or more tissues and performing a specific function, for example, the esophagus.

organelle A tiny "organ" within a cell that performs a discrete function necessary to the cell.

organic A substance or nutrient that contains the element carbon.

osteoblasts Cells that prompt the formation of new bone matrix by laying down the collagen-containing component of bone that is then mineralized.

osteoclasts Cells that erode the surface of bones by secreting enzymes and acids that dig grooves into the bone matrix.

osteogenesis imperfecta (OI) A bone disease caused by a genetic defect that affects collagen production, resulting in a significantly increased rate of fractures, often from no apparent cause.

osteomalacia Vitamin D deficiency disease in adults, in which bones become weak and prone to fractures.

osteoporosis A disease characterized by low bone mass and deterioration of bone tissue, leading to increased bone fragility and fracture risk.

overhydration Dilution of body fluid. It results when water intake or retention is excessive.

overload principle   Placing an extra physical demand on your body in order to improve your fitness level.

overweight   Having a moderate amount of excess body fat, resulting in a person having a weight that is greater than some accepted standard for a given height but is not considered obese.

ovulation   The release of an ovum (egg) from a woman's ovary.

oxidation   A chemical reaction in which molecules of a substance are broken down into their component atoms. During oxidation, the atoms involved lose electrons.

P

Paget's disease   A bone disease characterized by excessive breakdown and formation of bone tissue, causing bones to enlarge, weaken, become deformed, and eventually fracture.

pancreas   Gland located behind the stomach; it secretes digestive enzymes.

pancreatic amylase   An enzyme secreted by the pancreas into the small intestine that digests any remaining starch into maltose.

pepsin   An enzyme in the stomach that begins the breakdown of proteins into shorter polypeptide chains and single amino acids.

peptic ulcer   Area of the GI tract that has been eroded by the acidic gastric juice of the stomach. The two main causes of peptic ulcers are an *H. pylori* infection or use of nonsteroidal anti-inflammatory drugs.

peptide bonds   Unique types of chemical bonds in which the amine group of one amino acid binds to the acid group of another in order to manufacture dipeptides and all larger peptide molecules.

percent daily values (% DV)   Information on a Nutrition Facts Panel that identifies how much a serving of food contributes to your overall intake of nutrients listed on the label; based on an energy intake of 2,000 calories per day.

peristalsis   Wave of squeezing and pushing contractions that move food in one direction through the length of the GI tract.

pH   Stands for percentage of hydrogen. It is a measure of the acidity—or level of hydrogen—of any solution, including human blood.

phospholipids   A type of lipid in which a fatty acid is combined with another compound that contains phosphate; unlike other lipids, phospholipids are soluble in water.

photosynthesis   Process by which plants use sunlight to fuel a chemical reaction that combines carbon and water into glucose, which is then stored in their cells.

phylloquinone   The form of vitamin K found in plants.

physical activity   Any movement produced by muscles that increases energy expenditure; includes occupational, household, leisure-time, and transportation activities.

Physical Activity Pyramid   A pyramid similar to the Food Guide Pyramid that makes recommendations for the type and amount of activity that should be done weekly to increase physical activity levels.

physical fitness   The ability to carry out daily tasks with vigor and alertness, without undue fatigue, and with ample energy to enjoy leisure-time pursuits and met unforeseen emergencies.

phytic acid   The form of phosphorus stored in plants.

phytochemicals   Chemicals found in plants (*phyto-* is from the Greek word for plant,) such as pigments and other substances, that may reduce our risk for diseases such as cancer and heart disease.

pica   An abnormal craving to eat something not fit for food, such as clay, paint, etc.

placebo effect   The belief that a product improves performance although it has been proven to have no physiologic benefits.

placenta   A pregnancy-specific organ formed from both maternal and embryonic tissues. It is responsible for oxygen, nutrient, and waste exchange between the mother and fetus.

polysaccharide   A complex carbohydrate consisting of long chains of glucose.

polyunsaturated fatty acids (PUFA)   Fatty acids that have more than one double bond in the chain; these types of fatty acids are generally liquid at room temperature.

preeclampsia   High blood pressure that is pregnancy-specific and accompanied by protein in the urine, edema, and unexpected weight gain.

preterm   Birth of a baby prior to 38 weeks gestation.

prooxidant   A nutrient that promotes oxidation and oxidative cell and tissue damage.

proteases   Enzymes that continue the breakdown of polypeptides in the small intestine.

protein digestibility corrected amino acid score (PDCAAS)   A measurement of protein quality that considers the balance of amino acids as well as the digestibility of the protein in the food.

protein-energy malnutrition   A disorder caused by inadequate consumption of protein. It is characterized by severe wasting.

proteins   The only macronutrient that contains nitrogen; the basic building blocks of proteins are amino acids.

provitamin   An inactive form of a vitamin that the body can convert to an active form. An example is beta-carotene.

puberty   The period in life in which secondary sexual characteristics develop and people are biologically capable of reproducing.

purging   An attempt to rid the body of unwanted food by vomiting or other compensatory means, such as excessive exercise, fasting, or laxative abuse.

pyruvic acid   The primary end product of glycolysis.

R

rating of perceived exertion (RPE)   A scale that defines the difficulty level of any activity; this scale can be used to estimate intensity during exercise.

Recommended Dietary Allowance (RDA)   The average daily nutrient intake level that meets the nutrient requirements of 97 to 98% of healthy individuals in a particular life stage and gender group.

Reference Daily Intakes (RDI)   Standardized food label values for nutrients with RDAs, including protein and vitamins.

remodeling   The two-step process by which bone tissue is recycled; includes the breakdown of existing bone and the formation of new bone.

resistance training   Exercises in which our muscles act against resistance.

resorption   The process by which the surface of bone is broken down by cells called osteoclasts.

retina   The delicate light-sensitive membrane lining the inner eyeball and connected to the optic nerve. It contains retinal.

retinal An active, aldehyde form of vitamin A that plays an important role in healthy vision and immune function.

retinoic acid An active, acid form of vitamin A that plays an important role in cell growth and immune function.

retinol An active, alcohol form of vitamin A that plays an important role in healthy vision and immune function.

rickets Vitamin D deficiency disease in children. Symptoms include deformities of the skeleton such as bowed legs and knocked knees.

S

saliva A mixture of water, mucus, enzymes, and other chemicals that moistens the mouth and food, binds food particles together, and begins the digestion of carbohydrates.

salivary amylase An enzyme in saliva that breaks starch into smaller particles and eventually into the disaccharide maltose.

salivary glands Group of glands found under and behind the tongue and beneath the jaw which release saliva continually as well as in response to the thought, sight, smell, or presence of food.

saturated fatty acids (SFA) Fatty acids that have no carbons joined together with a double bond; these types of fatty acids are generally solid at room temperature.

seizures Uncontrollable muscle spasms caused by increased nervous system excitability that can result from electrolyte imbalances.

set-point theory A theory that suggests that the body raises or lowers energy expenditure in response to increased and decreased food intake and physical activity. This action serves to maintain an individual's body weight within a narrow range.

short-chain fatty acids Fatty acids fewer than six carbon atoms in length.

sickle cell anemia A genetic disorder that causes red blood cells to be sickle-, or crescent-, shaped. These cells cannot travel smoothly through the blood vessels, causing cell breakage and anemia.

simple carbohydrate Commonly called *sugar;* a monosaccharide or disaccharide such as a glucose.

small intestine The longest portion of the GI tract where most digestion and absorption takes place.

solvent A substance that is capable of mixing with and breaking apart a variety of compounds. Water is an excellent solvent.

sphincter A tight ring of muscle separating some of the organs from the GI tract and opening in response to nerve signals indicating that food is ready to pass into the next station.

spontaneous abortion (also called *miscarriage*) Natural termination of a pregnancy and expulsion of pregnancy tissues because of a genetic, developmental, or physiological abnormality that is so severe that the pregnancy cannot be maintained.

starch A polysaccharide stored in plants; the storage form of glucose in plants.

sterols A type of lipid found in foods and the body that has a ring structure; cholesterol is the most common sterol that occurs in our diets.

stomach A J-shaped organ where food is partially digested, churned, and stored until release into the small intestine.

sucrase A digestive enzyme that breaks sucrose into glucose and fructose.

sucrose A disaccharide composed of one glucose molecule and one fructose molecule. Sweeter than lactose or maltose.

sudden infant death syndrome (SIDS) The sudden death of a previously healthy infant; the most common cause of death in infants over one month of age.

system A group of organs that work together to perform a unique function, for example, the gastrointestinal system.

T

teratogen Any substance that can cause a birth defect.

thermic effect of food (TEF) The energy expended as a result of processing food consumed.

thirst mechanism A cluster of nerve cells in the hypothalamus that stimulate our conscious desire to drink fluids in response to an increase in the concentration of salt in our blood or a decrease in blood pressure and blood volume.

thrifty gene theory A theory that suggests that some people possess a gene (or genes) that causes them to be energetically thrifty, resulting in them expending less energy at rest and during physical activity.

time of activity How long each exercise session lasts.

tissue A sheet or other grouping of similar cells that performs a particular set of functions, for example, muscle tissue.

tocopherol The active form of vitamin E in our bodies.

tocotrienol A form of vitamin E that does not play an important biological role in our bodies.

Tolerable Upper Intake Level (UL) The highest average daily nutrient intake level likely to pose no risk of adverse health effects to almost all individuals in a particular life stage and gender group.

total fiber The sum of dietary fiber and functional fiber.

trabecular bone (spongy or cancellous bone) A porous bone tissue that makes up only 20% of our skeleton and is found within the ends of the long bones, inside the spinal vertebrae, inside the flat bones (breastbone, ribs, and most bones of the skull) and inside the bones of the pelvis.

trace minerals Minerals we need to consume in amounts less than 100 milligrams per day and of which the total amount in our bodies is less than 5 grams.

transamination The process of transferring the amine group from one amino acid to another in order to manufacture a new amino acid.

transcription The process through which messenger RNA copies genetic information from DNA in the nucleus.

translation The process that occurs when the genetic information carried by messenger RNA is translated into a chain of amino acids at the ribosome.

transport proteins Protein molecules that help to transport substances throughout the body and across cell membranes.

triglyceride A molecule consisting of three fatty acids attached to a three-carbon glycerol backbone.

trimester Any one of three stages of pregnancy, each lasting 13 to 14 weeks.

T-score A comparison of an individual's bone density to the average peak bone density of a 30-year-old healthy adult.

tumor Any newly formed mass of undifferentiated cells.

type 1 diabetes Disorder in which the body cannot produce enough insulin.

type 2 diabetes Progressive disorder in which body cells become less responsive to insulin.

U

umbilical cord   The cord containing arteries and veins that connect the baby (from the navel) to the mother via the placenta.

underweight   Having too little body fat to maintain health, causing a person to have a weight that is below an acceptably defined standard for a given height.

urinary tract infection   A bacterial infection of the urethra, the tube leading from the bladder to the body exterior.

V

variety   Eating a lot of different foods each day.

vegetarianism   The practice of restricting the diet to food substances of plant origin, including vegetables, fruit, grains, and nuts.

vigorous intensity activities   Activities that produce significant increases in breathing, sweating, and heart rate; talking is difficult when exercising at a vigorous intensity.

visible fats   Fat we can see in our foods or see added to foods, such as butter, margarine, cream, shortening, salad dressings, chicken skin, and untrimmed fat on meat.

vitamins   Organic compounds that assist us in regulating our bodies' processes.

W

warm-up   lso called preliminary exercise; includes activities that prepare you for an exercise bout, including stretching, calisthenics, and movements specific to the exercise bout.

water-soluble vitamins   Vitamins that are soluble in water. These include vitamin C and the B vitamins.

weight cycling   The condition of successfully dieting to lose weight, regaining the weight, and repeating the cycle again.

wellness   A multidimensional, lifelong process that includes physical, emotional, and spiritual health.

Z

zygote   A fertilized egg (ovum) consisting of a single cell.

Index

Credits

Figure and Text Credits